Exercise Testing and Prescription

A HEALTH-RELATED APPROACH

FOURTH EDITION

David C. Nieman, DrPH, FACSM
Appalachian State University

Mayfield Publishing Company
Mountain View, California
London • Toronto

To my wife Cathy,
dietitian, editor, loving companion,
and award-winning quilter

Library of Congress Cataloging-in-Publication Data

Nieman, David C.,
    [Fitness and sports medicine]
    Exercise testing and prescription : a health-related approach /
David C. Nieman.—4th ed.
      p. cm.
    Previously published under the title: Fitness and sports medicine.
    Includes bibliographical references and index.
    ISBN 0-7674-0474-2
    1. Exercise—Physiological aspects.   2. Physical fitness.
3. Sports medicine.   4. Exercise tests.   5. Exercise therapy.
I. Title.
QP301.N53   1998
613.7—dc21   98-10359
                                                  CIP

Manufactured in the United States of America
10   9   8   7   6   5   4

Mayfield Publishing Company
1280 Villa Street
Mountain View, CA 94041

Sponsoring editor, Michele Sordi; *production editor,* Julianna Scott Fein; *manuscript editor,* Shari Hatch; *art director and cover designer,* Jeanne M. Schreiber; *text designer,* Dick Kharibian; *cover art,* Glen Mitsui; *art manager,* Robin Mouat; *illustrators,* Joan Carol, Lotus Art, and Joanne Bales; *manufacturing manager,* Randy Hurst. The text was set in 9/12 Palatino by Thompson Type and printed on acid-free 50# Somerset Matte by R. R. Donnelley & Sons Company.

All photographs are reprinted with permission of Robert O. Parriott.

Preface

More than 12 years have passed since the publication of the first edition of this book in 1986. The first edition was written to assist readers in preparing for the American College of Sports Medicine (ACSM) Health and Fitness Instructor certification. That is still a major purpose of the book, and the book retains the basic structure of past editions to ensure successful preparation for certification.

Since the 1980s, much progress has been made in advancing our understanding of exercise testing and prescription, the health-related benefits of regular physical activity, and fitness-related public policy issues. In this fourth edition, I have attempted to provide the most current information possible on each of these topics. Over 1,100 new references have been integrated into the fourth edition. The title of the book has been changed to *Exercise Testing and Prescription: A Health-Related Approach,* which best represents the content of this edition. Accordingly, the chapters dealing with exercise and fitness testing, exercise prescription, and the relationship between physical activity and health have been expanded and updated to ensure that readers have the most current information.

New chapters have been added on cancer and diabetes, and major new or updated sections have been integrated on the following topics: cardiovascular screening of competitive athletes, American Heart Association risk-stratification criteria, bioelectrical impedance and body density formulas, low-back pain, abdominal testing, gender and life-cycle issues, the U.S. Surgeon General's report on physical activity and health, strategies of physical activity promotion, 1998 ACSM exercise prescription guidelines, medications, basic nutrition, "fat loading," creatine supplementation, antioxidants, fluid replacement, the glycemic index, dietary supplements, NHANES III national health data, lipoproteins, prevention of coronary heart disease and stroke, new hypertension guidelines, cardiac rehabilitation, drug therapy for obesity, strategies for obesity treatment, 1998 NIH obesity detection and treatment guidelines, sleep, stress management, osteoporosis, arthritis, exercise-induced asthma, heat illness, and overtraining. World Wide Web Internet site addresses have been integrated throughout the book to give the reader access to further information. In addition, I have included 2,436 references from the literature (46% of them dated 1994 and later), 430 illustrations and photographs, and over 200 tables and boxes.

Two features in this edition (as in the third) enhance its use as a textbook. These are the Sports Medicine Insight, and the Physical Fitness Activity. The Sports Medicine In-

sight precedes the end-of-chapter summary and highlights interesting topics of special concern in sports medicine. The Physical Fitness Activity outlines practical and useful laboratory activities for students, and new ones have been added in the fourth edition.

The chapters of this fourth edition have been ordered and organized in such a way that there is a natural progression of information. The reader will find it most satisfactory to start with Chapter 1 and continue chapter by chapter to the end of the book. The book is organized into four parts. Part 1 deals with public policy issues in physical activity, trends in physical activity patterns and wellness, and basic definitions. Part 2 describes the various tests for each of the major elements of physical fitness: cardiorespiratory endurance, body composition, and musculoskeletal fitness. Part 3 reviews the basics of exercise physiology, the process of writing exercise prescriptions, and the relationship between nutrition and performance. Part 4 summarizes current understanding regarding the association of physical activity and heart disease, obesity, aging, osteoporosis, arthritis, psychological health, diabetes, cancer, and other concerns. In addition, a complete review of exercise risks is given in Chapter 16. The appendixes have been updated, expanded, and improved. Appendix A contains 39 tables of physical fitness testing norms (which complement those found within the chapters). Addresses of professional organizations and equipment suppliers are listed in Appendix B. A detailed listing of the energy cost of human physical activities is provided in Appendix E. Finally, following the appendixes is a comprehensive glossary.

Ancillaries are available with this book: A test bank with more than 700 questions is available both as a bound hard copy and on a diskette for instructors; and the physical fitness test norms and all formulas used in this book have been organized into a comprehensive computer software package. This software program allows readers to input test data and then print results that are classified according to the normative tables found in this book. (See "The Fitness Publisher" on the following page.)

I am grateful to the reviewers of this edition: Steven Aldana, Brigham Young University; Sue Bloomfield, Texas A&M University; Lorrie Brilla, Western Washington University; Rebecca A. Glass, Ed.D., Austin Peay State University; Ellen Glickman-Weiss, Ph.D., FACSM, Kent State University; Brenda Reeves, Grand Valley State University; and Pamela Swan, Arizona State University.

Health and Fitness Software

BSDI

Advanced Assessment, Training,
and Motivation Systems
PO Box 81
Chester, NJ 07930
Phone: (888) BSDI-FIT
Fax: (908) 879-9344
http://www.BSDIFitness.com

Company Background:

BSDI is now one of the world's leading health and fitness software companies, with more than 1000 systems installed in 17 countries. Founded by Dr. Mark Brittingham in 1991, BSDI has prospered by emphasizing high-quality software and a drive for innovation. From its first few dozen systems sold in 1992 to the nearly 400 systems sold last year, BSDI's strengths in product quality and innovation have placed it in the top tier of health and fitness companies.

Additional Products:

- **Retention Manager™**
Manage all of your client-retention activities: training schedule, incentive programs, fitness testing appointments, and more.

- **Motivation™**
Client Check-In and Attendance Tracking

The Fitness Publisher

BSDI has worked with Dr. Nieman for nearly a decade in the construction of a comprehensive software tool supporting many of the calculations, norms, and questionnaires found in this book. The result of this collaboration is a software system called the *Fitness Publisher™*.

The Fitness Publisher supports a broad range of fitness tests, health risk assessments, and medical screening tools. You can track change over time and progress toward a goal for:

- Fitness tests,
- Aerobic activities (calories, points, heart rate, etc.),
- Body circumferences,
- Blood pressure,
- Total energy expenditure,
- Blood chemistry measurements, and
- Athletic or rehabilitation performance values.

The Fitness Publisher supports exercise programming with a large library of illustrated strength exercises as well as a complete set of aerobic activities. The software is highly customizable—it is built to adapt to the exercises or methods that you prefer.

The Fitness Publisher is the most analytically complete fitness appraisal software available. Now supporting over 100 fitness tests (all documented online), it is a comprehensive guide to the science of fitness appraisal.

The software also provides a complete charting facility, an extensive help system, and a "Publishing Center" where you can select from over 75 customizable reports. The Fitness Publisher even includes a powerful word processor that can be integrated with your client database to help you communicate results and ideas easily and efficiently.

The Fitness Publisher has been subjected to exhaustive "usability testing" to ensure that it is easy to use. The result of this testing is our unique "folder and page" user interface. This interface gives you access to the power of the software even if you have little or no computer software experience.

There are Fitness Publisher editions for all types of users. Whether you are a solo personal trainer or work for a large multi-user site, there is a system tailored to your needs and budget.

Brief Contents

Contents

Chapter 4 Cardiorespiratory Fitness 80

Chapter 5 Body Composition 120

Chapter 9   Nutrition and Performance   262

P A R T

I

Trends and Definitions

CHAPTER

1

Health and Fitness Trends

Despite common knowledge that exercise is healthful, more than 60 percent of American adults are not regularly active, and 25 percent of the adult population are not active at all. Moreover, although many people have enthusiastically embarked on vigorous exercise programs at one time or another, most do not sustain their participation.

—*Physical Activity and Health: A Report of the Surgeon General,* 1996

The focus of public health has changed in recent years. Attention has shifted from mainly trying to minimize sickness and avoid premature death toward chiefly emphasizing health promotion.[1]

America began to get serious about health promotion during the 1970s. *Health promotion* is defined as the science and art of helping people change their lifestyle to move toward a state of optimal health.[2] This modern emphasis on health promotion is inspired in part by the World Health Organization's definition of *health:* "Health is physical, mental, and social well-being, not merely the absence of disease and infirmity" (see Figure 1.1).

As depicted in Figure 1.2, the absence of health is death, but before death comes disease, and before disease, most people go through a sustained period of high-risk behavior. Health represents a dynamic state of positive well-being, involving the practice of habits that promote health, thereby lowering the risk of premature disease and death.

In 1979, the U.S. Surgeon General issued his report on health promotion and disease prevention, *Healthy People.*[3] Noting that the nation's first public health revolution against infectious diseases had been very successful, he issued a challenge to begin a second public health revolution—this time against *chronic diseases,* or lifestyle-related diseases

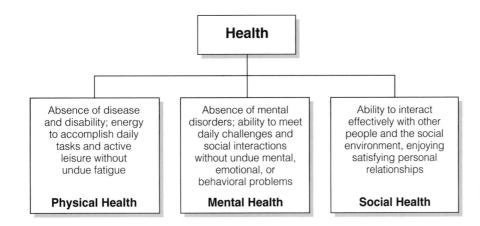

Figure 1.1 According to the World Health Organization, "Health is physical, mental, and social well-being, not merely the absence of disease and infirmity."

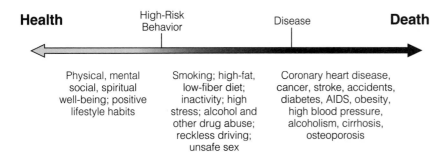

Figure 1.2 The health continuum. The health continuum shows that between optimal health and death lies disease, which is preceded by a prolonged period of negative lifestyle habits.

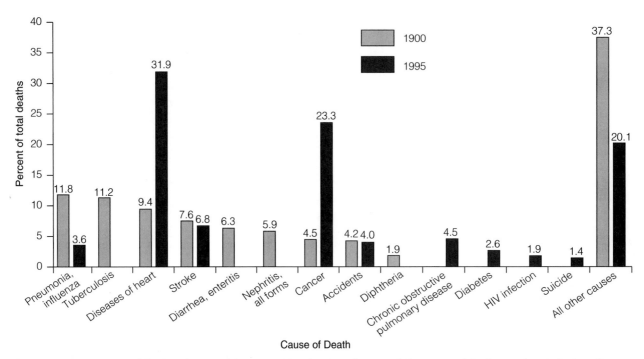

Figure 1.3 Major causes of death in the United States in 1900 and 1995. A dramatic shift in cause of death away from infectious disease toward chronic disease took place between 1900 and 1995. *Sources:* U.S. Department of Health and Human Services. Prevention '86/'87: Federal Programs and Progress. Washington, DC: U.S. Government Printing Office, 1987; Monthly Vital Statistics Report 45 (No. 11, supplement 2): June 12, 1997.

such as heart disease, cancer, stroke, and diabetes, which together account for two thirds of all deaths in America (see Figure 1.3).

With the release of the surgeon general's report, the U.S. Public Health Service launched an unprecedented initiative, calling on professionals and laypeople alike to take steps to reduce preventable death and disease. Following up on the surgeon general's report, *Promoting Health/Preventing Disease: Objectives for the Nation* was published in 1980.[4] It set out 226 health objectives for 1990, emphasizing 15 areas of particular importance. In response to the growing body of evidence that regular physical activity produces significant health benefits, "physical fitness and exercise" was specified as one of those 15 areas.[4]

In 1990, a new document was published, *Healthy People 2000: National Health Promotion and Disease Prevention Objectives,*[5] which provided a strategy for improving the health of the nation. A framework for *Healthy People 2010* goals has

been established (see Figure 1.15 in Physical Fitness Activity 1.2). (*HealthyPeople2000/2010* has its own website on the Internet: http://odphp.osophs.dhhs.gov/pubs/hp2000/. See Physical Fitness Activity 1.2 at the end of this chapter for a full listing of *Healthy People 2000/2010* websites on the Internet and the proposed *Healthy People 2010* framework.) As stated in the initial pages of this landmark document, "Perhaps more than any other age group, adults have the opportunity to assume personal responsibility for their health. Many of the leading causes of death for people between the ages of 25 and 65 are preventable, wholly or in part, through changes in lifestyle."[5] The Public Health Service specified 12 objectives to increase physical activity and fitness of Americans by the year 2000.[5] Table 1.1 summarizes 7 of the 12 objectives.

Reaching the physical fitness and exercise objectives for the year 2000 and beyond will entail a coordinated effort by educational systems; mass media; local, state, and federal

TABLE 1.1   Year 2000 Objectives to Increase Physical Activity and Fitness

Year 2000 Goals (selected)	Best Estimate of Current Status
Risk reduction	
Increase to at least 30% the proportion of people age 6 and older who engage regularly, preferably daily, in light-to-moderate physical activity for at least 30 minutes per day.	22% (5 times/week) 17% (7 times/week)
Increase to at least 20% the proportion of people age 18 and older and to at least 75% the proportion of children and adolescents ages 6–17 who engage in vigorous physical activity that promotes the development and maintenance of cardiorespiratory fitness three or more days per week for 20 or more minutes per occasion.	15% (age ≥ 18 yrs) 54% (ages 12–21) 66% (ages 10–17)
Reduce to no more than 15% the proportion of people age 6 and older who engage in no leisure-time physical activity.	25% (of adults)
Increase to at least 40% the proportion of people age 6 and older who regularly perform physical activities that enhance and maintain muscular strength, muscular endurance, and flexibility.	16% (adults, weight training)
Services and protection	
Increase to at least 50% the proportion of children and adolescents in first through twelfth grades who participate in daily school physical education.	36% (1st–12th grade) 25% (9th–12th grade)
Increase to at least 50% the proportion of school physical education class time that students spend being physically active, preferably engaged in lifetime physical activities.	27% (1st–12th grade) 33% (9th–12th grade)
Increase the proportion of worksites offering employer-sponsored physical activity and fitness programs, as follows:	
• 50–99 employees 20%	33%
• 100–249 employees 35%	47%
• 250–749 employees 50%	66%
• ≥750 employees 80%	83%
Increase community availability and accessibility of physical activity and fitness facilities.	

Source: U.S. Department of Health and Human Services, Public Health Service. Healthy People 2000: National Health Promotion and Disease Prevention Objectives (1991). DHHS Publication No. (PHS) 91-50212. Government Printing Office, Washington, DC 20402-9325. Healthy People 2000 Review, 1997. DHHS Publication No. (PHS) 98-1256. Hyattsville, MD: Public Health Service, 1997.

governments; health-care providers; private industry; volunteer organizations; and the American public.

As Table 1.1 shows, the proportion of American children and adults who are exercising appropriately falls short of year 2000 goals. Worksites, however, have exceeded year 2000 goals in providing fitness programs for their employees. This chapter focuses on progress toward the national health and fitness goals for adults, children, and youths, and at worksites.

THE SURGEON GENERAL'S REPORT ON PHYSICAL ACTIVITY AND HEALTH*

In 1994, the Office of the Surgeon General authorized the Centers for Disease Control and Prevention (CDC) to serve as the lead agency for preparing the first report on physical activity and health by the surgeon general.[6] This landmark review of the research on physical activity and health was

*Additional information on the surgeon general's report can be obtained at this site on the World Wide Web: http://www.cdc.gov/nccdphp/sgr/sgr.htm

published in 1996 and has helped initiate a new awareness of the importance of regular exercise. The main message of the surgeon general's first report on physical activity and health was that "Americans can substantially improve their health and quality of life by including moderate amounts of physical activity in their daily lives."

The report's major conclusions included the following:

• People of all ages, both males and females, benefit from regular physical activity.

• People can obtain significant health benefits by including a moderate amount of physical activity (e.g., 30 minutes of walking briskly or raking leaves, 15 minutes of running, or 45 minutes of playing volleyball) on most, if not all, days of the week. Through a modest increase in daily activity, most Americans can improve their health and quality of life.

• People can gain additional health benefits through greater amounts of physical activity. People who can maintain a regular regimen of activity that is of longer duration or of more vigorous intensity are likely to derive greater benefit.

- Physical activity reduces the risk of premature mortality in general, and of coronary heart disease, hypertension, colon cancer, and diabetes mellitus in particular. Physical activity also improves mental health and is important for the health of muscles, bones, and joints.

- More than 60% of American adults are not regularly physically active. In fact, 25% of all adults are not active at all. Physical inactivity is more prevalent among women than men, among blacks and Hispanics than whites, among older than younger adults, and among the less affluent than the more affluent.

- The most popular leisure-time physical activities among adults are walking and gardening or yard work.

- Nearly half of American youths 12–21 years of age are not vigorously active on a regular basis. Moreover, physical activity declines dramatically during adolescence.

- Daily attendance in physical education classes has declined among high school students from 42% in 1991 to 25% in 1995.

- Research on understanding and promoting physical activity is at an early stage, but some interventions to promote physical activity through schools, worksites, and health-care settings have been evaluated and found to be successful.

- Consistent influences on physical activity patterns among adults and youths include confidence in one's ability to engage in regular physical activity, enjoyment of physical activity, support from others, positive beliefs concerning the benefits of physical activity, and lack of perceived barriers to being physically active.

EXERCISE AND PHYSICAL FITNESS IN AMERICA

Although the modern-day fitness movement falls short in attracting the majority of Americans, it has been a major force in shaping societal norms and standards. In addition, the contemporary movement has roots in various events dating from the previous century.

A Brief Historical Review

During the mid- to late 1800s, as America experienced increasing urbanization and industrialization, the health of Americans became a growing concern of many leaders.[7,8] The new nation grew from 17 million people in 1840 to more than 50 million in 1880, becoming more urban in the

process. Many farmers became factory workers, travel changed from horses to trains, and the invention of the telegraph vastly accelerated communication. Greatly expanded numbers of industrial laborers worked 12 to 16 hours a day, six days a week.

In response to these changing conditions, America's first health and fitness reform movement took shape, led by social reformers such as Oliver Wendell Holmes, Sr., Catharine Beecher, and Dioclesian Lewis, and by health reformers such as Sylvester Graham and William Alcott. The reform movement was directed at the increasingly poor health of the general population, particularly in the cities. Gymnasiums opened, and various organizations such as the YMCA, YWCA, and settlement houses organized exercise programs. The health reformers also urged people to pay attention to improving their diets, while avoiding the abuse of drugs such as alcohol—themes still embraced today.

In the schools, several progressive colleges hired medical doctors—including Edward Hitchcock (Amherst), Dudley Allen Sargent (Harvard), Edward Hartwell (Johns Hopkins), and William Anderson (Yale)—to teach students about health, gymnastic exercises with light dumbbells and other apparatus, weight lifting, European gymnastics, and anthropometric measurements. Most of the programs were based on German and Swedish gymnastic programs, which consisted of marching, free exercises with rings and clubs, and work with apparatus such as the balance board, rings, and vaulting box.[9] These programs emphasized the health-related values of proper physical exercise, with muscular strength and size seen as most important.

Dioclesian Lewis, a medical doctor, gave up his medical practice to become a leading figure in the health and fitness movement from 1850 to 1880. An animated and inspirational speaker (it was said people could "inhale hygiene in his presence"), he developed a system of "New Gymnastics" that swept the country in the early 1860s.[7] His exercise program was structured around several sets of light exercises, including beanbag games; calisthenic movements with 6-inch wooden rings, wooden dumbbells, and wands; and dancing and marching to musical accompaniment (the original aerobic-dance system).

Catharine Beecher warned against the poor health of women and against the societal conventions that limited women's participation in physical activity; her stand was supported strongly by Lewis and other reformers.[8] Her famous brother, the Reverend Henry Ward Beecher of Brooklyn, was an advocate of the "muscular Christianity movement," which aimed at "breadth of shoulders as well as of doctrines." He favored vigorous outdoor recreation and urged that churches and other Christian associations provide opportunities for young adults of the city to exercise in wholesome environments.

In 1845, when Alexander Cartwright and his friends took what was essentially a child's game and turned it into an adult male sport called "baseball," they initiated America's love affair with sports.[8] Other games were organized into sports during the latter half of the 1800s, and a growing public interest in sports spread onto the college campus.

At the same time that Amherst, Harvard, Johns Hopkins, and Yale were hiring medical doctors to maintain and improve students' health, the growing popularity of intercollegiate sport introduced thousands of students to the fun and stimulation of vigorous games and athletics. The students began to organize a series of intercollegiate sporting contests. The relatively dull routine of gymnastic drills paled in comparison to sport participation, and soon after the turn of the century, sports surpassed gymnastics as the students' exercise of choice; the trend was supported by such educational leaders as John Dewey, William Kilpatrick, and Thomas Wood.

Schools gradually shifted from medical doctors to "physical educators" who promoted sports and games as the best way to develop intellectual awareness, character, and improved moral and social behavior, along with physical fitness.[10] John Dewey, for example, believed that to be effective centers of learning, schools must be interesting and must emphasize the role of play in the education of the student. Luther Gulick stressed the role of sports in the "toughening of the individual for the achievements of life." Many educators melded these viewpoints, believing that the objectives of physical education could best be met through a "sports for all" program, therefore shifting the curriculum from the goal of health through gymnastics to the goals of character, sportsmanship, and fitness through sport.

According to some critics, however, the promotion of physical fitness became secondary to the development of game and sport skills (motor fitness), and the attainment of psychosocial goals. This was the beginning of a furious debate that has continued to this day—should physical education emphasize health-related physical activities (exercises that develop the heart, lungs, and musculoskeletal systems), or should it emphasize motor-fitness-related activities (exercises that develop coordination, balance, agility, speed and power)?[11]

Between World War I and World War II, the United States became a nation in which sport was a part of its very being, as entertainment, as an integral part of education, and as an accepted and worthwhile way for all Americans to spend leisure time.

The Contemporary Fitness Movement

In the 1940s and 1950s, several major events prompted Americans to take a closer look at both school physical education programs and adult fitness.

For one thing, statistics on draftees during World War II spurred the media to report that school sports programs were not adequately enhancing students' physical fitness. Out of 9 million registrants examined for the armed services in early 1943, almost 3 million (one third) were rejected for physical and mental reasons.[9] The chief of Athletics and Recreation of the Services Division of the U.S. Army responded by recommending at the 1943 War Fitness Conference that "physical education through play must be discarded and a more rugged program substituted."

Later, in 1953, the shocking results of the Kraus–Weber tests of minimum muscular fitness of schoolchildren were released, arousing massive public and official concern.[12] The tests consisted of six simple movements of key muscle groups. Among U.S. children, 57.9% failed, while only 8.7% of European children failed. When President Eisenhower's attention was called to the report of this study, he immediately called for a special White House Conference on the subject, which was finally held in June, 1956. As a result, the President's Council on Youth Fitness and a President's Citizens Advisory Committee on the Fitness of American Youth were formed.

Among adults in the general population, the stage was being set for the second popular fitness movement. After World War II, heart disease had reached epidemic proportions, obesity had become a major public health problem, and health-care costs had begun to skyrocket. A growing sentiment among some health researchers and administrators was that technological advances in transportation, communication, and industry had created a society in which physical activity was no longer necessary or even likely, so if people were to get adequate exercise, they would have to make an effort to interject it into their normal sedentary routine.

Finally, the late 1960s brought a sudden change in adult fitness awareness. In 1967, Oregon track coach Bill Bowerman toured New Zealand and discovered "jogging." He returned to America and wrote *Jogging*,[13] igniting the first running boom in the United States, with his book selling more than 300,000 copies.

In 1968, Kenneth H. Cooper, a medical doctor for the Air Force, published his book *Aerobics*,[14] followed two years later by *The New Aerobics*.[15] In these books, Cooper challenged Americans to take personal charge of their lifestyles and to counter the epidemics of heart disease, obesity, and rising health-care costs by engaging in regular exercise.

To Cooper, the best form of exercise is "aerobic," a word he coined to represent activities that stimulated the heart, lungs, and blood vessels. Stated Cooper: "The best exercises are running, swimming, cycling, walking, stationary running, handball, basketball, and squash, and in just about that order. . . . Isometrics, weight lifting, and calisthenics, though good as far as they go, don't even make the list, despite the fact that most exercise books are based on one of these three, especially calisthenics."[14]

These two books provided the necessary theoretical fuel for an adult fitness revolution that soon zoomed across the country. Millions took up the aerobic challenge and began jogging, cycling, walking, and swimming programs.[16] Ken Cooper's wife, Mildred Cooper, joined her husband in 1972 in writing *Aerobics for Women*.[17] Within nine years, these three books on aerobics sold more than 6 million copies and were translated into 15 foreign languages and into braille.

In 1972, Frank Shorter won the Olympic marathon gold medal in Munich. The extensive television coverage of this marathon and Shorter's silver-medal effort in 1976 (Montreal) helped to spawn the road-racing movement that has since become so popular.[18]

Running, which quickly became a symbol of the American exercise movement, was promoted by a spate of successful books by Henderson,[19] Ullyot,[20] Sheehan,[21] and others, climaxing in *The Complete Book of Running* by Jim Fixx,[22] which topped the best-seller lists for nearly two years. In the space of one year, 1977 to 1978, the magazine *Runner's World* more than tripled its circulation from 85,000 to 270,000.[18]

Just as the running movement was starting, another popular form of adult exercise, aerobic dance, emerged. By making exercise fun and socially oriented, aerobic dance attracted millions who otherwise might not have joined the fitness movement.[23] Aerobic dance, now one of the most popular, organized fitness activities for women in the United States, traces its origins to Jacki Sorenson, the wife of a naval pilot, who began conducting exercise classes at a U.S. Navy base in Puerto Rico in 1969. The growth of aerobic dance has been stimulated more recently by the production of videotaped dance exercise program (see Figure 1.4).

The original aerobic-dance programs consisted of an eclectic combination of various dance forms, including ballet, modern jazz, disco, and folk, as well as calisthenic-type exercises. More recent innovations include water aerobics (done in a swimming pool), nonimpact or low-impact aer-

obics (one foot on the ground at all times), specific types of dance aerobics, step aerobics (using a low stool), and assisted aerobics (with weights worn on the wrists and/or ankles).

The fitness movement experienced strong growth during the 1970s and 1980s but appears to have plateaued during the 1990s. Nevertheless, some 1990s surveys by the National Sporting Goods Association have shown that despite little growth, millions of Americans continue to participate regularly in aerobic forms of exerise.

The most popular fitness activity continues to be fitness walking, followed by gardening or yard work, stretching exercises, bicycling, strengthening exercises, stair climbing, jogging or running, aerobic dancing, and swimming. According to the Fitness Products Council, core fitness participants (those who report at least 100 days per year in a particular fitness activity) now number over 54 million.

Health clubs (as we know them today) evolved in the mid- to late 1970s when racquetball, tennis, and aerobic dance grew in popularity.[24] Many of the early clubs were not run professionally, and some unscrupulous operators crowded their clubs with too many members while delivering little service (or in some instances, closing shop and leaving town after receiving "lifetime" membership dues).

To combat this problem and ensure quality control over the fitness movement, universities have developed sophisticated graduate-degree programs, and various professional groups provide certification and continuing education programs. In 1988, the International Health, Racquet and Sportsclub Association (IHRSA) and a health-club-industry trade group adopted a code of conduct and, in 1993, established a list of minimum standards.[24] In 1992, the American College of Sports Medicine (ACSM) published an exhaustive standards manual, which listed 353 mandatory policies and procedures and 397 guidelines that were

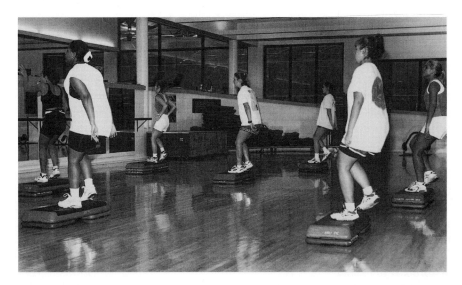

Figure 1.4 Aerobic dance is one of the most popular forms of exercise for women.

strongly recommended for health clubs.[25] In 1997, the ACSM published a revised list of standards and guidelines for health and fitness facilities[26] (see Box 1.1). Memberships at commercial clubs grew by 51% between 1987 and 1996, with huge gains being recorded among members age 65

Box 1.1

American College of Sports Medicine Standards for Health and Fitness Facilities

ACSM has identified six fundamental standards to which all health and fitness facilities should adhere. Collectively, these standards ensure that every physical activity or program offered by a facility is held in a relatively safe environment and is conducted in an appropriate manner.

Standard 1

The staff of a facility must be able to respond in a timely manner to any reasonably foreseeable emergency event that threatens the health and safety of facility users. Toward this end, a facility must have an appropriate emergency plan that can be executed by qualified personnel in a timely manner.

Standard 2

A facility must offer each adult member a preactivity screening that is appropriate to the physical activities to be performed by the member.

Standard 3

Each person who has supervisory responsibilities for a physical activity program or an area at a facility must have demonstrable professional competence in that physical activity program or area.

Standard 4

A facility must post appropriate signage alerting users to the risks involved in their use of those areas of a facility that present potential increased risk.

Standard 5

A facility that offers youth services or programs must provide appropriate supervision.

Standard 6

A facility must conform to all relevant laws, regulations, and published standards.

Source: Reprinted by permission of American College of Sports Medicine. *ACSM's Health/Fitness Facility Standards and Guidelines* (2nd ed.). Champaign, IL: Human Kinetics, 1997.

---

and older. The number of health-club members reached a record high in 1996, rising to 21 million. IHRSA estimates that by the year 2010, club memberships will nearly double, reaching 40 million.

Also joining the fitness movement have been many hospitals and corporations that provide programs for their employees, employees' families, and, in most instances, the community. An estimated 150 fitness centers are owned or operated by hospitals.[24] Also, as described later in this chapter, a 1992 government-sponsored survey of worksites revealed that 81% offer at least one health-promotion activity, with exercise and physical fitness programs second in popularity only to injury-prevention programs.

Current Activity Levels of American Adults

Since the early 1990s, many surveys of the activity levels of American adults have attempted to evaluate the magnitude of the present adult fitness revolution in the United States.[6] Measurement of physical activity is difficult, and no single technique is suitable for all purposes. More than 30 methods for assessment of physical activity have been described, and these can be divided into three broad categories: self-report surveys, mechanical and electronic monitors, and physiological measurement.

Time and cost restraints have led to the predominant use of self-report surveys in national studies investigating the physical activity patterns of American adults.[6] All of the other techniques are simply too burdensome and costly for a general population survey. Self-report survey methods include telephone or mail questionnaires using short- or long-term recall of typical habits, and personal diaries, which are used for varying lengths of time (e.g., activities recorded every 15 minutes for three days in a row).

Three government-sponsored national surveys have provided the most useful data on the physical activity habits of American adults: (1) the National Health Interview Survey of Health Promotion and Disease Prevention (NHIS) from the National Center for Health Statistics (NCHS); (2) the Behavioral Risk Factor Surveillance System (BRFSS), administered in cooperation with the CDC; and (3) the Third National Health and Nutrition Examination Survey (NHANES III) of U.S. adults from 1988 to 1994.[6]

The NHIS was a two-week recall survey conducted in 1985, 1990, and 1991, which assessed the frequency, duration, and intensity of 22 physical activities (see the questionnaire at the end of this chapter, Physical Fitness Activity 1.1). Data were collected on a national representative sample of a large number of American adults, representing one of the best current sources of descriptive information on American physical activity habits.[6,27,28]

The BRFSS consists of annual random-digit-dialed telephone surveys conducted by state health departments in cooperation with the CDC. These surveys routinely collect risk-factor data, including the prevalence of sedentary lifestyles.[29] In addition, physical activity data were collected from 1986 through 1992 and in 1994. In 1994, a total of 105,853 people in 50 states were asked questions on their physical activity habits.[6,29]

In the first phase of NHANES III, 9,488 adults were asked questions about the type and frequency of their physically active hobbies, sports, and exercises.[6]

Based on these surveys, several important conclusions can be drawn:[6]

1. Few Americans engage in appropriate levels of physical activity. Only 15% of American adults report exercising vigorously (at an intensity of at least 50% $\dot{V}O_{2max}$, for 20 or more minutes a session, three or more times per week), the level generally recommended for cardiovascular benefit. As stated earlier, the year 2000 goal has been set at 20%, and most experts feel this goal will not be reached because little change has been measured between surveys of the 1980s and those of the 1990s.

Approximately 22% of Americans report they exercise moderately or vigorously for 30 minutes or more five or more times per week, while 25% report essentially sedentary lifestyles. The rest of Americans (53%) report exercising irregularly (see Figure 1.5). For sake of comparison, data show that 52% of Canadians exercise less than is recommended.[30]

2. Women and the elderly are more sedentary. As Figure 1.6 shows, at any given age, more females than males are physically sedentary. As age increases, both genders tend to report a greater avoidance of physical activity. Similarly, men are somewhat more likely than women to engage in regular, sustained activity, and the rate of this activity tends to decrease as age increases.

3. People with higher incomes and more education tend to exercise more often. People of higher socioeconomic status (SES) (as indicated by income, education, and occupation) are more likely to be physically active (especially when considering total time devoted to physical exercise) than are those of lower SES (see Table 1.2). In general, managers and professionals are more active in their leisure time

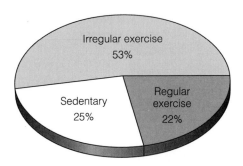

Figure 1.5 Physical activity patterns of U.S. adults. Fewer than one in four Americans exercise on a regular basis (five or more times a week, 30 minutes or more per occasion, light-to-vigorous intensity).

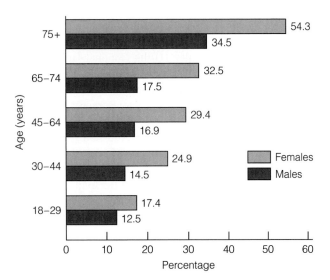

Figure 1.6 Percentage of adults reporting no leisure-time physical activity. Females are more sedentary than males; with increases in age, both sexes report an increasing avoidance of physical activity. *Source:* Data from NHANES III.[6]

TABLE 1.2 Percentage of Adults Who Exercise on a Regular Basis (Five or More Times a Week for 30 or More Minutes Per Session), by Education Level and Income

Characteristic	Percentage of All Adults
Education level	
<12 years	15.6
12 years	17.8
13–15 years	22.7
>15 years	23.5
Income	
<$10,000	17.6
$10,000–$19,999	18.7
$20,000–$34,999	20.3
$35,000–$49,999	20.9
≥$50,000	23.5

Source: Physical Activity and Health: A Report of the Surgeon General, 1996.

than are other white-collar workers, who in turn exercise more frequently than do blue-collar workers. However, about 40% of the U.S. population report that they have jobs requiring at least a moderate amount of physical work, and the proportion tends to be higher among people with lower incomes and education (Figure 1.7). Among men under 45 years of age, for example, about two thirds of those with 12 years of education or less report that they have physically demanding jobs, in contrast with about one fifth of college graduates. The NHIS has also revealed that 16% of employees in the United States report working in jobs requiring four or more hours daily of repeated strenuous physical activity.[31] As a matter of comparison, 49% of Canadians reported at least moderate amounts of physical activity demands at work.[30]

When considering both on-the-job and leisure-time exercise, there probably is little difference between upper- and lower-SES groups. The various races also tend to be equally active in their leisure time, when age and SES are held constant.[6,28,30]

4. **Walking and other convenient activities are most popular.** The most popular physical activity reported by both Americans and Canadians is walking (see Figure 1.8). Other activities that consistently account for large numbers of participants include gardening, calisthenics, bicycling, exercising with indoor equipment (such as stationary bicycles, stair climbers, treadmills, weights, etc.), aerobic dancing, and jogging–running.[6] These activities have several important features in common, including low cost, casual scheduling, and convenience.

5. **A greater proportion of people in the western states exercise.** Regionally, the northeast and the south have the lowest proportion of physically active residents; the midwest and west have the highest proportion who have "regular, sustained activity." In the 1994 BRFSS survey, 49 states reported the proportion of adults who were physically active. As shown in Figure 1.9, the western half of the nation tends to be more active than the eastern half.[6]

6. **The exercise boom appears to have plateaued.** Unfortunately, there is no adequate series of statistics available to gauge trends in activity since the mid-1950s or so in America. One problem is that no satisfactory definition of physical activity has been consistently used in comparable national surveys. Nonetheless, using various national probability samples by Gallup (1961 to 1984), Louis Harris and Associates (1979 to present), the CDC (1982 to present, BRFSS), and the NCHS (1985 and 1990, NHIS), the data suggest that at any given age, the proportion of people who exercise regularly tended to in-

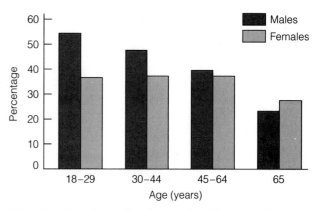

Figure 1.7 Americans whose jobs require at least a moderate amount of physical work. A surprisingly high percentage of American adults report that their jobs require at least a moderate amount of physical work (39.3% overall).[28]

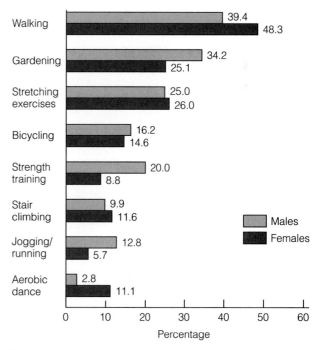

Figure 1.8 Percentage of adults reporting participation in selected activities. Americans tend to engage in physical activities that are low cost, convenient, and easy to schedule.[6]

crease strongly throughout the 1970s and early 1980s, before plateauing during the late 1980s and 1990s.[6]

A series of national biannual surveys conducted from 1983 to the present for *Prevention* magazine by Louis Harris & Associates has not shown any significant change in the percentage of Americans who have answered "yes" to the question, "Do you exercise strenuously (that is, so you breathe heavily and your heart and pulse rate are accelerated for a period lasting at least 20 minutes) three days or more a week?"[32] About one third of Americans have claimed to meet these exercise criteria since 1983.

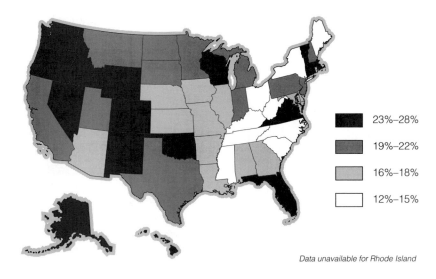

23%–28%

19%–22%

16%–18%

12%–15%

Data unavailable for Rhode Island

Figure 1.9 Regular, sustained activity by American adults. Adults from the western half of the nation tend to be more active than their eastern counterparts.[6] *Source:* Behavioral Risk Factor Surveillance System, 1994.

Future Challenges

Results from these surveys point out some very basic problems with the modern-day fitness movement. In particular, despite all of the media hype, the majority of Americans are *not* exercising. Less than one in four Americans is exercising appropriately (only 15% if intensity is considered). Physical inactivity is even more common among those with less education and income, the elderly, and females.[6]

Perhaps two principles from the national surveys discussed in this chapter stand out as we consider the year 2000 objectives: (1) Americans appear more inclined to exercise if it can be done at moderate- versus high-intensity levels, suggesting that we more strongly emphasize activities such as walking in our public health endeavors rather than activities such as running; (2) A surprising number of Americans claim to exercise on the job, indicating that we should direct more attention to helping people exercise during their regular daily routine instead of seeking time and energy to add exercise to an already crowded schedule.

YOUTH FITNESS STUDIES

There is a perceived fitness crisis among American children and youths. In general, most experts feel that American children and youths are less healthy, active, and physically fit than is recommended.[6] Baseline data on the health-related fitness level of school-age children were made available in 1984 with the release of the First National Children and Youth Fitness Study (NCYFS I);[33] in 1985 with the President's Council on Physical Fitness and Sports School Population Fitness Survey;[34] in 1987 with the Second National Children and Youth Fitness Study (NCYFS II);[35–38] in 1991, 1993, and 1995 from the national school-based

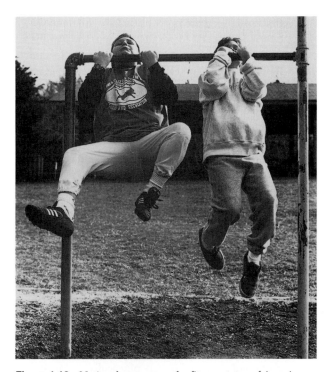

Figure 1.10 National surveys on the fitness status of American children and youths have aroused much public concern.

Youth Risk Behavior Survey of youths in grades 9–12; and in 1992 from the NHIS, Youth Risk Behavior Survey of all young people ages 12–21.[6,39] Results from these five surveys have caused much public concern about the fitness of American youths (see Figure 1.10).

In general, although some experts differ on their interpretation of the test results, the general perception is that American children and youths are less active and physically fit than is recommended for optimal protection against future chronic disease.

Important findings from these four surveys include the following:

- Youths are increasingly overweight. Among children and youths ages 6–17, 22% (about 10 million) are overweight, an increase of 6 percentage points from the late 1970s. This finding is disturbing because a high proportion of overweight youths end up obese as adults (about half of obese school-age children become obese adults, and more than 80% of obese adolescents remain obese into adulthood) (see Chapter 13).

- Only half exercise vigorously. *Healthy People 2000* proposed to increase to at least 75% the proportion of children and adolescents ages 6–17 years who engage regularly in vigorous aerobic physical activity. However, only 54% of U.S. young people (ages 12–21 years) regularly participate in vigorous physical activity, while one fourth get none at all. As Figure 1.11 shows, this proportion falls sharply with increasing age. Only about one in three students in grades 5

through 12 takes physical education daily, with this proportion falling to one in four among high school students (Figure 1.12). Even among students taking physical education, observers have noted that many students do not participate in moderate to vigorous physical activity. Overall, only 19% of all high school students were physically active for at least 20 minutes on a daily basis in physical education classes.

- Girls exercise less than boys. Activity levels of girls are below those of boys and tend to drop sharply as age or grade in school increases (see Figure 1.11).

- Upper body strength is poor for many children and youths. For example, among girls ages 9–17, about half cannot perform more than one pull-up. For boys ages 6–12, 40% cannot do more than one pull-up, while 25% cannot do any. About one half of males and two thirds of females, ages 12–21 years do not participate regularly in strengthening or toning activities (e.g., push-ups, sit-ups, or weight lifting).

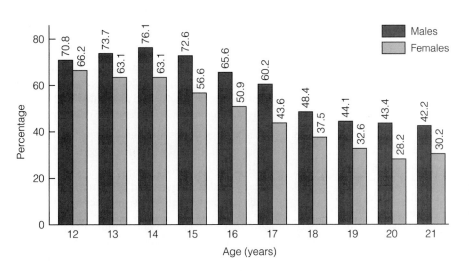

Figure 1.11 Vigorous exercise among young people during three or more of the seven days preceding the survey. Female young people exercise vigorously less often than males, and the percentage for both males and females falls sharply with increasing age.[6]

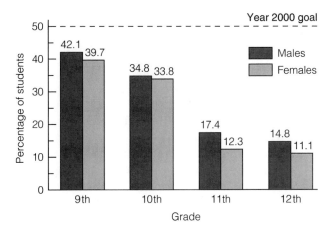

Figure 1.12 Percentage of high school students attending physical education classes daily. A year 2000 goal is that 50% of students have daily P.E. Overall, only 25.4% of high school students have daily P.E., with 40% not enrolled in any P.E. classes.[6]

- Aerobic (heart and lung) fitness is lower than recommended for many young people. About half of girls ages 6–17 and 60% of boys ages 6–12 cannot run a mile in less than 10 minutes, for example.

- Many young people have disease risk factors. About 12% of children and youths ages 12–17 smoke, with the proportion rising to 25% among high school seniors. Close to one in three children and adolescents have serum cholesterol levels that exceed 170 mg/dl, the level deemed "acceptable" by the National Cholesterol Education Program. A national survey by the CDC revealed that 63% of adolescents have two or more of five major risk factors for chronic disease. Risk factors tend to cluster and show tracking from childhood and adolescence to adulthood, meaning that every attempt should be made to bring risk factors under control while people are young.

GUIDELINES FOR PROMOTING LIFELONG PHYSICAL ACTIVITY AMONG YOUNG PEOPLE

Most experts feel that children and youths need daily physical activity to keep fit and healthy.[6] Chapter 8 outlines some specific recommended exercise prescriptions for young people. In general, parents and teachers are urged to provide many opportunities for play and simple sports for children and youths.[40,41] Enjoyment and excitement have been identified as major reasons why children and youths engage in physical activity such as sports. Physically active parents and role models provide support for children to be active. The American Academy of Pediatrics has emphasized that children need active play, good physical education programs, parental involvement, and generally active lifestyles, rather than specific vigorous exercise training.

In 1997,* the CDC released guidelines urging schools and communities to encourage physical activity among young people so that they will continue to engage in physical activity in adulthood and will obtain the health benefits of physical activity throughout life.[42] The CDC guidelines included recommendations about 9 aspects of school and community programs:

1. Establish policies that promote enjoyable, lifelong physical activity among young people (e.g., require comprehensive and daily physical education for students in kindergarten through grade 12).

2. Provide physical and social environments that encourage and facilitate safe and enjoyable physical activity (e.g., increase availability of hiking, biking, and fitness trails; swimming pools; parks; playgrounds; and other open spaces for recreation.)

3. Implement physical education and health curricula and instruction that emphasize enjoyable participation in physical activity and that help students develop the knowledge, attitudes, motor skills, behavioral skills, and confidence needed to adopt and maintain physically active lifestyles (e.g., emphasize skills for lifetime physical activities such as dance, strength training, jogging, swimming, bicycling, cross-country skiing, walking, and hiking, rather than those for competitive sports).

4. Provide extracurricular physical activity programs that meet the needs and interests of all students.

5. Include parents and guardians in physical activity instruction and in extracurricular and community physical activity programs, and encourage them to support their children's participation in enjoyable physical activities.

6. Provide training for education, coaching, recreation, health-care, and other school and community personnel that imparts the knowledge and skills needed to effectively promote enjoyable, lifelong physical activity among young people.

7. Assess physical activity patterns among young people, counsel them about physical activity, refer them to appropriate programs, and advocate for physical-activity instruction and programs for young people.

8. Provide a range of developmentally appropriate community sports and recreation programs that are attractive to all young people.

9. Regularly evaluate school and community physical-activity instruction, programs, and facilities.

According to the CDC, "School and community programs that promote regular physical activity among young people could be among the most effective strategies for reducing the public health burden of chronic diseases associated with sedentary lifestyles. Programs that provide students with the knowledge, attitudes, motor skills, behavioral skills, and confidence to participate in physical activity may establish active lifestyles among young people that continue into and throughout their adult lives."[42]

WORKSITE HEALTH-PROMOTION AND FITNESS ACTIVITIES

Since the mid-1970s, there have been major changes in employer attitudes toward workplace health-promotion programs. Interest in worksite health programs has increased, fueled in part by a supportive science base and a desire to

---

*This report is available on the World Wide Web: http://www.cdc.gov/epo/mmwr/mmwr.html

help contain spiraling health-care costs while improving productivity and morale and reducing employee absenteeism and turnover.[43]

There are several advantages in using the workplace as a setting for health and fitness programs, including convenience, easy accessibility, supportive company policies and incentives, and the opportunity to affect the lives of family members. Also, the worksite is an effective location for offering health screening and educational programs otherwise inaccessible to at-risk persons. By the year 2000, 140 million Americans are projected to be in the civilian labor force.

In 1985 and 1992, the Office of Disease Prevention and Health Promotion, Public Health Service, conducted national surveys to determine the extent of health-promotion activities in the private sector.[43] Overall, the 1992 survey of more than 1,500 worksites revealed an increase in worksite health-promotion activities since 1985 and substantial progress toward achieving many of the worksite-related health objectives for the year 2000. The 1992 survey found that 81% of worksites offer at least one health-promotion activity, compared with 66% in 1985. Figure 1.13 shows the relationship between worksite size and health-promotion activity; Figure 1.14 shows the most popular activities offered. A 1994 survey by a benefits consulting firm showed that 76% of employers nationwide reported using some type of health-promotion initiative to encourage healthy lifestyles among employees, up 12% from a similar study conducted in 1992.[44] Worksite health-promotion programs are expected to continue to grow and expand.

Worksite size is a strong indicator of health-promotion activity, with the larger companies more involved than the smaller ones.[43] Seventy-two percent of worksites allow employees to use official company time to participate in health-promotion activities, and 45% allow the use of flextime. Employers use several types of incentives to encourage healthy practices, including flexible spending accounts and risk-rated health insurance premiums. Some also offer subsidized discounts or reduced fees for participation in community-based health programs.

The eight benefits cited most frequently by worksites offering health-promotion programs in the 1992 survey were[43]

1. Improved employee health—28%
2. Improved employee morale—26%
3. Reduced health insurance cost—19%
4. Reduced absenteeism—19%
5. Increased output / productivity—16%
6. Reduced accidents on the job—9%
7. Improved education on health issues—7%
8. Reduced workers' compensation claims—4%

The three most common barriers to implementing worksite health promotion were cost, lack of management support, and lack of interest by employees.[43]

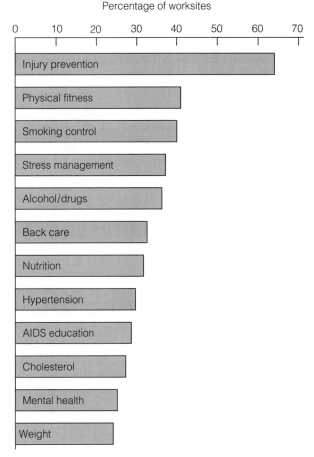

Figure 1.14 Health-promotion programs offered at worksites, 1992. Injury prevention, fitness programs, and smoking programs are most popular at the worksite.[43]

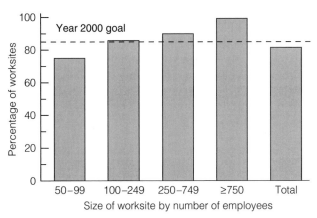

Figure 1.13 Percentage of worksites with at least one health-promotion activity, 1992. The year 2000 goal is for 85% of worksites to have health programs. As the size of the worksite increases, opportunities for employee health-promotion programs increase.[43]

Box 1.2

Wellness Outreach at Work

Wellness Outreach at Work was developed by the Worker Health Program, a research unit of the Institute of Labor and Industrial Relations at the University of Michigan. The program offers comprehensive risk-reduction services to all employees at a workplace. It encompasses screening for cardiovascular risks, referral for medical treatment, follow-up counseling, and health-improvement programs. The program has been implemented in more than 100 worksites and has reached more than 75,000 employees in organizations ranging in size from 5 employees to 6,000 employees, both blue collar and white collar, at an average cost of about $100 per employee each year.

The Wellness Outreach at Work Program consists of three main components: planning, implementation, and evaluation.

1. Planning. This component involves appointing a wellness committee and hiring wellness professionals, setting goals, promoting the program, and establishing procedures to ensure confidentiality. Based on information from 100 worksites and 75,000 employees, employee risk factors typically are as follows:

   a. Exercise fewer than three times a week (65–72%)

   b. Have high or borderline-high cholesterol ($\geq$200 mg/dl) (45–60%)

   c. Smoke cigarettes (18–45%)

   d. Are overweight by 20% or more (26–40%)

   e. Have high blood pressure ($\geq$140/90 mm Hg) (22–38%)

   f. Report high levels of stress (21–35%)

2. Implementation. This component consists of five major tasks:

   a. Screening and referral. Five waves of screening are recommended to identify high-risk employees.

   b. Follow-up and counseling of employees. The keys to a successful wellness program are persistent and long-term one-to-one outreach and follow-up counseling to encourage adherence, promote changes in lifestyle, and prevent relapse. Experts urge contacting employees at least every six months throughout their careers at the worksite. People with several health risks, people in key positions, and those in need of medical evaluation should receive the highest priority.

   c. Follow-up with physicians. Inform the physician or clinic of each employee who has gone through screening, and supply basic results.

   d. Health-improvement programs. Offer three types of programs—classes, minigroups, and guided self-help.

   e. Organizing worksite activities. Organize and support activities and worksite policies that promote a healthy work environment.

3. Evaluation. The final component involves monitoring the programs to find out what is working and how to refine the various programs. Achievable objectives for most worksites for the first year include the following:

   a. At least 70% of the employees participate in initial screening.

   b. At least 80% of the employees with targeted health risks receive follow-up counseling by a wellness counselor.

   c. At least 50% of the employees interviewed by a counselor begin a risk-reduction program.

Following the implementation of the Wellness Outreach at Work Program, typical results include these changes:

- About 50% of workers with high blood pressure bring it under control.

- About 55% of those with high cholesterol reduce it by 20 mg/dl or more.

- About 28% of overweight employees lose at least 10 pounds and keep it off.

- About 25% of smokers quit and do not relapse.

- About 50% of all workers exercise at least three times a week.

- About 30% of all workers make changes in their lives to reduce stress.

Source: Erfurt JC, Foote A, Heirich MA, Brock BM. *The Wellness Outreach at Work Program: A Step-by-Step Guide.* NIH Publication No. 95-3043, August, 1995.

In response to financial pressures, employer-based health-promotion programs are emphasizing activities most likely to save money *and* improve health. Employers are paying increased attention to (a) identifying those employees at greatest risk of health-care utilization and (b) using social marketing strategies to engage them in health-promotion programs. Box 1.2 describes a recommended strategy for improving the health status of employees at worksite settings.[45] Studies show that a comprehensive health-promotion program focused on high-risk individuals can achieve long-term positive health effects.[45–47]

Benefits of Worksite Exercise Programs

A growing number of companies, especially large ones, have worksite physical fitness programs (see Table 1.3). Since 1985, physical fitness programs have showed the most impressive gains of all worksite health-promotion programs.[43] In fact, the year 2000 goals have been exceeded for each worksite size category (see Table 1.3). Government officials in both Canada and the United States view the worksite as an effective place to encourage exercise habits among the general population.[48,49]

What benefits can be expected from worksite exercise programs? A summary of the major research in this area was developed through a cooperative effort by the Office of Disease Prevention and Health Promotion, U.S. Department of Health and Human Services, and a team of researchers from the Institute for Aerobics Research, Dallas.[48]

In general, the research results support the notion that worksite exercise programs improve fitness and help reduce health risks. The findings consistently show improvements in aerobic capacity and exercise habits, as well as in other fitness-related measures. In most cases, health risk factors such as smoking and elevated blood lipids also respond to the worksite programs. The impact of these programs on job performance, including productivity and job-related attitudes, and the effect on health-care costs, are less well established.

A major challenge for worksite fitness directors is employee adherence to on-site programs, with most studies showing that less than 20% of employees became long-term participants.[49] Often these participants have been generally active to begin with, and at lower risk for chronic disease than nonparticipants.

Impact of Exercise on Absenteeism

Employers are very interested in the relationship between worksite exercise programs and "bottom-line" variables, such as absenteeism and health-care costs. The results from the few programs that measured these variables show mostly favorable effects.[48–50]

- Among Canadian Life employees, there were modest differences in absenteeism between those that were and those that were not in the fitness program.[51] However, the average absentee rate of "high adherent" participants dropped almost 50% the first year they participated in the fitness program.

TABLE 1.3 Summary of Progress Toward the Year 2000 Objectives

Year 2000 Worksite Objective	1985	1992	Year 2000 Target
Health promotion activities	66%	81%	85%
High blood pressure and / or cholesterol education	17%	35%	50%
Formal smoking policy	27%	59%	75%
Physical activity and fitness for worksites with:			
50 to 99 employees	14%	33%	20%
100 to 249 employees	23%	47%	35%
250 to 749 employees	32%	66%	50%
750 or more employees	54%	83%	80%
Nutrition education and / or weight control	Joint data point not available	37%	50%
Stress management	27%	37%	40%
Alcohol and drug policies	Not available	87%	60%
Occupant protection systems	Not available	82%	75%
Back injury prevention and rehabilitation	29%	32%	50%

Source: Office of Disease Prevention and Health Promotion National Survey of Worksite Health Promotion Activities, 1992.

- In a large study of more than 14,000 DuPont Company employees, involvement in a comprehensive health-promotion program, which included exercise, reduced illness absenteeism by 12% over a two-year period.[52]

- In the U.S., average absenteeism rates are 3.5% of work hours/year. In one study of 8,300 employees nationwide, absenteeism was significantly lower by one day/year for highly fit than for poorly fit employees.[53]

- At Prudential, there was a 20.1% reduction in average disability days for one group of program participants.[54]

- At Tenneco, there was a trend for exercisers to have fewer sick hours than nonexercisers, although this difference was statistically significant only for female employees.[55]

- During a four-year period in a group of 4,972 Duke University employees, participants in a fitness and wellness program experienced 3.3 to 6.5 fewer absentee hours per year than did nonparticipants.[56]

- At both the Dallas and the H-E-B Independent School Districts, there were reductions in absences of 1.25 days per year and 0.43 days per year, respectively, for program participants relative to those not enrolled. These absenteeism reductions yielded actual savings of $149,578 for the Dallas district and $4,127 for the H-E-B district.[57,58]

Healthy and fit workers tend to be absent less often, and most studies suggest they are more productive (e.g., have less fatigue, make fewer errors).[49] In addition, worksites with on-site fitness programs tend to experience reduced employee turnover.

Impact of Exercise on Medical- and Health-Care Costs

Direct medical- and health-care cost savings also have been documented in several studies of worksite exercise programs.[45,49] Most studies report the short-term (one- to two-year) effects.

- For example, in the Canadian Life program,[59] researchers showed that the total costs for medical care increased by 35% in a company without a program but only by 1% at Canadian Life.

- At Prudential,[54] researchers found a 46% ($262) reduction in average major medical costs for one group of program participants. The higher the level of fitness achieved during the program, the lower the postentry medical-care costs.

- Similarly, there was a 48% ($553) difference between exercisers and nonexercisers at Tenneco.[55]

- An average $253 reduction in medical-care costs was reported for the comprehensive program participants at the H-E-B Independent School District.

Two long-term medical-care studies extend the findings of the short-term programs:

- The Los Angeles County Firefighters showed a 45% reduction in workers' compensation costs during the first 10 years of their program. Compensation costs, especially those for back injuries, were substantially lower for those firefighters who were most flexible, who were strongest, and who had the highest physical work capacity.[60]

- At Blue Cross and Blue Shield of Indiana, there was a long-term (4.75 years) difference of $519 in discounted average medical-care costs between a group of program participants and a matched group of nonparticipants.[61] For every $1.00 in medical-care costs spent on participating employees, $1.75 was spent on nonparticipating employees.

Cost–Benefit Analyses of Worksite Exercise Programs

Although logic suggests that health and fitness programs should reduce health-care costs, a reduction in the *need* for services may not always mean a reduction in the actual *use* of services.[62] Thus, it may be inappropriate to evaluate the worth of worksite health and fitness programs solely in terms of their *direct* financial benefits. However, if all the *indirect* economic benefits are included (e.g., lower employee turnover, gains in productivity, reduced absenteeism, fewer industrial injuries), the financial value of the total benefits usually exceeds that of costs to the corporation (e.g., promotion, facilities, equipment, professional leadership).[49]

Worksite exercise programs are not free, so in an attempt to factor in the costs associated with conducting these programs, several researchers have published cost–benefit analyses. Nearly every study has shown that the financial value of benefits is greater than that of costs, with ratios varying from 1.1 to 5.8.[45,49] Cost per participant per year usually ranges from $150 to $500.

- At Prudential, with a facility-based program that includes physical examinations, laboratory testing, exercise classes and instruction, educational seminars, and periodic rescreening, researchers estimated that for every $1.00 spent on the programs, Prudential realized a $1.91 savings in short-term disability and medical-care costs.[54]

- At the H-E-B Independent School District, in a program that used the existing facilities and resources of the school district, the benefit-to-cost ratio for program participants during the experimental period was $1.41 benefit for every $1.00 of cost.[63]

- In the Blue Cross and Blue Shield of Indiana program, the original evaluation showed the benefit-to-cost ratio for the entire five years of the program to be $1.45 to $1.00.[60]
- After 12 years of implementing a fitness program for the salaried employees of a Toronto Life Assurance Company, benefit estimates average $340 versus a cost of only $70 per worker.[64]

Predicted Future Growth for Worksite Health Programs

Projections for the next decade indicate that worksite health programs will continue to grow in importance.[44,45] Most experts are predicting, however, that construction of on-site fitness facilities will decline as companies attempt to make better use of existing facilities and community resources and encourage self-help programs in the employees' homes, and as other alternative health-promotion programs are offered.[44] Physical activities that can be built into the normal day of the employee (e.g., walking or cycling to and from work) may prove more acceptable and more cost-effective than formal classes at the worksite. (See Box 1.3 for organizations devoted to worksite health promotion.)

STRATEGIES FOR INCREASING PHYSICAL ACTIVITY IN AMERICA

The challenges set forth in *Healthy People 2000* are directed to people throughout the nation—health professionals, com-munity groups, employers, the media, professional organizations, government agencies, and individuals. Meeting these challenges and objectives will require both individual and collective effort. No single person, family, business, organization, or government has the resources to bring about the changes needed to implement the broad and far-reaching physical activity objectives for the year 2000.

As this book shows, regular physical activity is associated with a wide array of health benefits. This association legitimates the development of national directives to promote physical activity across all segments of this society, as an aid to preventing chronic disease and improving the quality of life. As an example, sedentary living is estimated to cause one third of deaths due to coronary heart disease, colon cancer, and diabetes.[65] Therefore, encouraging people to become physically active would do much to reduce mortality and enhance quality of life.

Since the late 1960s, this nation has experienced a health and fitness revolution unparalleled in its history. Despite decades of fitness enthusiasm, programs, and media coverage and promotion, however, nearly one fourth of Americans are sedentary, and only 22% exercise moderately for at least 30 minutes, five or more times per week.[6]

At the worksite, considered one of the most promising places for adults to get regular exercise, less than 20% of eligible workers join exercise programs, and up to 50% of them drop out of the program over the first 6–12 months.[66] In supervised exercise programs, a dropout or noncompliance rate near 50% is typically seen over a 3- to 12-month period. Larger numbers of participants leave exercise programs within the first few weeks. Even in well-structured programs for cardiac patients, 30–70% of them drop out, the majority within the first 3 months.

Exercise participation continues to deteriorate thereafter, leveling off at 50–70% attrition at 12–24 months. This is remarkable, in light of the acknowledged benefits of exercise, especially for patients who stand to benefit the most.

Tremendous challenges lie ahead if the physical activity and fitness objectives for the years 2000 and 2010 are to be met. To meet these objectives, Americans need population-based strategies, which seek to reach all Americans, using tools such as mass media and community organization (e.g., environmental change).

Box 1.3

Organizations Devoted to Worksite Health Promotion

These organizations can supply information on conducting health-promotion programs at the worksite.

Association for Worksite
  Health Promotion
60 Revere Drive, Suite 500
Northbrook, IL 60062
708-480-9574

American Association
  of Occupational Health
  Nurses
50 Lenox Pointe
Atlanta, GA 30324-3176
404-262-1162

Washington Business Group
  on Health
777 North Capitol Street, NE,
  Suite 800
Washington, DC 20002
202-408-9320

Wellness Councils
  of America
Community Health Plaza
7101 Newport Avenue,
  Suite 311
Omaha, NE 66152-2100
402-572-3590

Population-Based Strategies

The goal of population- or community-based interventions is to achieve risk reduction across a broad segment of the population.[67–69] A variety of strategies are utilized to focus on four targets of change: (1) the person; (2) organizations (e.g., worksites); (3) the environment (e.g., development of fitness trails); and (4) public policies (e.g., federal or state reimbursement for preventive services). The key concept here is that multifaceted intervention strategies are needed to reach a wide variety of people.

Specific strategies include the following:

- Enhancement of physical activity throughout the day by encouraging stair climbing and exercise breaks, providing trails and paths for transportation-related activity, and increasing the number of parks and recreation areas for leisure-time activity

- Support of legislative and regulatory policies that promote physical activity at school, at the worksite, and in the community

- Increases in funding for school, worksite, and community health/fitness programs; for research that supports physical activity for all Americans; and for insurance reimbursement of health/fitness activities.

- Use of the electronic and print media to repeatedly transmit relevant information

- Cooperation among community leaders and power structures involving the private sector, organizations of health professionals, the mass media, schools, and other community groups, to promote behavioral change

- Development of community programs tailored to the needs and preferences of specific target groups (especially those at high risk and various minority groups)

Of particular usefulness are community and worksite risk-factor screening programs, with an emphasis on measurement, immediate counseling, and referral of high-risk individuals. Such programs have proven to be an effective way of reaching large numbers of people.[45,46]

To enhance people's long-term participation in regular physical activity, several factors should be considered, especially those that pertain to the person, the exercise regimen itself, and the environment.[67-69]

Personal Factors

Factors such as gender, age, occupational status, health status, education, and prior exercise experience should be considered when helping establish community-based exercise programs.[67-69] In general, women tend to participate in less strenuous activities than men. Older people are less active and appear to enjoy such activities as walking and gardening more than young people. Blue-collar workers are less formally active than white-collar workers, overweight people and smokers are less active, and less-educated people tend to exercise less than those with more education.[6,67-69]

Self-efficacy (an "I can do it" attitude) has consistently been found to predict long-term adherence to regular physical activity regimens.[70-72] Those who perceive important barriers are unlikely to exercise regularly. Interestingly, other personal characteristics such as knowledge have been inconsistently related to physical activity habits.

The Exercise Regimen

The 1996 surgeon general's report on physical activity and health places emphasis on reducing inactivity and increasing light-to-moderate physical activity.[6] Moderate intensity, longer duration activities, such as walking, are being promoted more and more by fitness leaders because these types of activities are more acceptable to the average person, increasing the likelihood of a permanent change in lifestyle.

Also, the musculoskeletal risks are less, and studies show that health benefits are still realized, especially when the total caloric expenditure averages at least 1000 calories per week. It has been demonstrated that people tend to adhere better to moderate-intensity than to vigorous-intensity physical activity programs, and that injuries from high-intensity workouts are a major cause of relapse from exercise.[73,74]

The Environment

In general, more people tend to participate in physical activity when community facilities and conducive environments are nearby and available. A 12-month study of 357 adults showed that adherence to home-based exercise programs (75%) was much greater than to group-based, travel-to-site programs (53%).[75] In a study of more than 2,000 San Diego residents, the density of exercise facilities around people's homes was positively associated with increased adherence to exercise.[76]

Time is a major obstacle to regular physical activity, and greater availability of community exercise facilities, trails, and parks that are close to homes is a major factor in helping people become more involved. Thus, community efforts are more effectively applied when promoting low-cost, home- or near-home-based, physical activity patterns, than when trying to encourage people to join programs that involve substantial travel time.

Programs that emphasize the availability of appropriate exercise facilities can have a substantial impact on the health of the community.[6] This is the essence of effective public health intervention, and officials should consider the potential positive effects of altering policies related to the distribution of exercise facilities and trails in the community.

The family has been shown to be a powerful influence on several health-promoting behaviors, including physical activity.[77] Studies indicate that support from a variety of sources—including family members and spouse, exercise partners and staff, and co-workers and employers—can have a positive impact on long-term adherence to exercise.

Environmental support also includes the use of federal, state, and county public health departments to provide economic support and to establish public policies to facilitate local community efforts.

The DHHS Contribution

In November 1990, then Department of Health and Human Services (DHHS) Secretary Louis W. Sullivan announced a broad multiyear plan to "improve the health and well-being of individuals through improved preventive health care and promotion of personal responsibility." Part of this effort is still being coordinated by the U.S. Public Health Service's Office of Disease Prevention and Health Promotion, through its Healthy Difference Program.[78]

Using the slogan "Healthy People 2000: You CAN make a difference!" the DHHS has provided information about what people can do on behalf of their own health and the health of their families and communities, distributed to 30,000 community-based DHHS agencies and offices. The topics emphasized in 1991 were physical activity, diet, smoking, alcohol, and immunization.

The DHHS is also implementing the Healthy People 2000 initiatives in many other specific and tangible ways, including working through interagency ad hoc committees, establishing hotlines, encouraging progressive new programs by the President's Council on Physical Fitness and Sports, conducting market research regarding communication of health messages, and developing worksite health-promotion programs.[78] In addition, the DHHS is encouraging homes, families, churches, schools, neighborhood groups, communities, cities, worksites, foundations, and hospitals to "join the battle."

National Coalition for Promoting Physical Activity (NCPPA)

The NCPPA was created in May, 1995, and comprises more than 100 member and participating organizations. The NCPPA objective is to unite the strengths of public, private, and industry efforts into a collaborative partnership to inspire Americans to lead physically active lifestyles to enhance their health and quality of life. Five areas of priority for action are education, research, health care and health insurance, community and employer, and target populations. The NCPPA seeks to convey one consistent physical-activity message to clarify for Americans the confusing array of messages that currently exist, to coordinate education efforts between the public and private sectors, and to support public policy as it relates to exercise. More information on the NCPPA can be obtained at their Internet site: http://www.ncppa.org. (Box 1.4 provides a resource list of some organizations that promote safe and enjoyable physical activity.)

Box 1.4

Physical Activity Information Resource List

Several resources for promoting safe and enjoyable physical activity among Americans are available from government agencies, professional organizations, and voluntary organizations. On the state and local levels, these materials might be available from affiliates of voluntary health organizations (e.g., the American Heart Association); state and local health departments; governors' councils on physical fitness and sports; state associations for health, physical education, recreation, and dance; state and local organizations that serve young people (e.g., the Young Women's Christian Association); and state physical activity contact networks. On the national level, materials can be obtained from the following agencies and organizations:

American Alliance for
Health, Physical
Education, Recreation,
and Dance
1900 Association Drive
Reston, VA 20191-1599
703-476-3400
800-213-7193

American Cancer Society
1599 Clifton Road, NE
Atlanta, GA 30329-4251
800-227-2345

American Heart Association
7272 Greenville Avenue
Dallas, TX 75231-4596
800-242-8721

American School Health
Association
PO Box 708
Kent, OH 44240-0708
330-678-1601

National Association for
Sport and Physical
Education
1900 Association Drive
Reston, VA 20191-1599
703-476-3410
800-213-7193, ext. 410

National Association of
Governors' Councils
on Physical Fitness
and Sports
201 South Capitol Avenue,
Suite 560
Indianapolis, IN 46225
317-237-5630

Division of Adolescent
and School Health
Resource Room
National Center for Chronic
Disease Prevention and
Health Promotion
Centers for Disease Control
and Prevention
MS K-32
4770 Buford Highway, NE
Atlanta, GA 30341-3724
888-CDC-4NRG

National Heart, Lung,
and Blood Institute
Information Center
PO Box 30105
Bethesda, MD 20824-0105
301-251-1222

National Recreation and
Park Association
2775 South Quincy Street,
Suite 300
Arlington, VA 22206-2204
703-578-5558
800-649-3042

President's Council
on Physical Fitness
and Sports
HHH Building, Rm 738H
200 Independence Ave., SW
Washington, DC 20201
202-690-9000

The ACSM Commitment

The ACSM has been very active in cooperating with the DHHS and the NCPPA. During 1990 and 1991, ACSM established an organizational structure, introduced ACSM to the governors of each state, developed two lecture/slide presentations ("The Recommended Quantity and Quality of Exercise for Developing and Maintaining Cardiorespiratory and Muscular Fitness" and "The Prevention of Thermal Injuries during Distance Running"), worked with the media to publicize the Healthy People 2000 physical activity objectives, and encouraged each ACSM regional chapter to devote at least one session at its annual meeting to a Healthy People 2000 topic. More information on ACSM can be obtained at their Internet site, http://www.acsm.org.

The Role of Physicians

Although medical education and training have not emphasized health promotion and disease prevention, systematic efforts are now underway to increase physician cooperation in addressing the personal health practices of patients. Research tends to support the view that adults perceive their personal physician as someone who believes that they should exercise.[79] Approximately 80% of American adults have confidence in their physicians and see them at least

SPORTS MEDICINE INSIGHT
The Wellness Revolution

As this chapter indicates, many Americans have joined the fitness movement. The fitness movement, however, is only one part of a much larger "wellness revolution" that is sweeping the United States. Let's consider some facts about this wellness revolution.[5,28] Much of this textbook is devoted to reviewing this information in greater detail.

THE HOPEFUL FACTS ABOUT THE WELLNESS REVOLUTION

1. Life expectancy is increasing. The age-adjusted death rate from all causes in 1995 was the lowest ever recorded in the United States. As a result, life expectancy in 1995 was 75.8 years, the highest in our history.

2. Death rates for heart disease are declining. Between 1950 and 1995, the American death rate for stroke fell 70%, and for heart disease, 55%. Heart disease deaths, however, are still the leading cause of death in America, now closely followed by cancer deaths.

3. Diets are improving. Recent U.S. government surveys of adults find that Americans consume 33% of calories in the form of fat, down from the 1970s. Other surveys show that the percentage of people consuming poultry and fish has increased, while the consumption of beef and pork has declined. Consumption of whole milk and eggs also declined, while intake of low-fat and skim milk products increased.

4. Cigarette consumption is falling. In 1965, 52% of men and 33% of women smoked. Now only 25% of all Americans smoke. This is among our greatest national health success stories of the past half century.

5. Alcohol consumption is falling. Per capita rates of alcohol consumption rose approximately 21% during the 1960s, and 10.3% during the 1970s, peaking in 1980 and 1981. Since then, alcohol consumption has fallen, due in part to the public's increasing awareness of alcohol's associated dangers.

6. Death rates for the elderly are falling. In 1900, only about 4% of the population was elderly; by 1984 the number was approximately 28 million, or roughly 12% of the population. By the year 2030, the percentage will be 18%. Between 1950 and 1995, the age-adjusted death rate for older adults dropped by about one fifth, primarily because of steep decreases in heart disease and stroke death rates.

7. Prevalence of high blood pressure and high cholesterol is falling. Recent national surveys indicate that the proportion of Americans with these two heart disease risk factors is decreasing (although much more progress needs to be made). Between 1960–1962 and 1988–1994, prevalence of hypertension declined from 39% to 24%; high blood cholesterol dropped from 32% to 19%.[82]

HEALTH-PROMOTION CONCERNS

Despite the successes, however, many areas still need much improvement.

1. Stress levels are high. About 60% of adults report that they experience moderate to high levels of stress. People with higher education and income are more likely to experience stress than are people with lower education and income. Four in 10 adults feel that stress has had at least some effect on their health in the past year.

2. Cancer death rates are rising. Although heart disease is our number one killer, cancer is a close second and will soon surpass heart disease as our major cause of death. For various reasons—most of them related to diet, smoking, and other lifestyle habits—we are not winning the war against cancer.

3. Too many Americans are obese. About 35% of the adult population is 20% or more above desirable body weight, a proportion that has been steadily rising during the twentieth century.

4. Too many Americans have high blood pressure. Fifty million have high blood pressure. This is a major risk factor for heart disease.

5. Too many Americans have high blood cholesterol levels. One out of five (19%) Americans has blood cholesterol levels above 240 mg/dl; one out of two are above 200 mg/dl. This is another major risk factor for heart disease.

6. Too many Americans still smoke. One out of four Americans still smoke, especially those with little education or blue-collar workers.

7. Too few Americans exercise regularly. Only 15% of American adults exercise vigorously, and 22% of adults exercise regularly at moderate levels. Inactivity is a major risk factor for heart disease, cancer, diabetes, obesity, osteoporosis, and frailty in old age.

once each year, and a substantial proportion (85%) believe that a physician's recommendation would increase their involvement in sports and exercise. Nonetheless, only a minority of physicians counsel their patients about exercise, and when they do, they typically spend less than three minutes on the subject.

Many physicians are uncomfortable about their ability to properly counsel and advise patients about physical activity and other health-related subjects. There are several reasons for this discomfort, including a lack of time, a perception that patients are not receptive to advice or willing to change, a perceived lack of skills or resources to counsel patients about lifestyle, a lack of reimbursement for preventive services, and a sense of confusion on the best advice to give patients because of disagreement among experts.

Obviously, physicians would benefit from more training on exercise, nutrition, and other health-related topics. Recommendations by the U.S. Preventive Services Task Force should do much to alleviate some of the confusion regarding the strengths and weaknesses of specific preventive services. This task force has observed that:[80]

> Effective interventions that address personal health practices are likely to lead to substantial reductions in the incidence and severity of the leading causes of disease and disability in the U.S. Primary prevention as it relates to such risk factors as smoking, physical inactivity, poor nutrition, alcohol and [other] drug abuse, and inadequate attention to safety precautions holds greater promise for improving overall health than many secondary preventive measures such as routine screening for early disease.... Counseling to promote physical activity is recommended for all children and adults.

Some medical groups have hired health-promotion experts to provide individualized counseling for high-risk patients. The theory is that it may be better for some physicians to refer their patients to health-promotion specialists who have the time and resources to meet the health-behavior change needs of patients.

Regarding reimbursement, the Office of Disease Prevention and Health Promotion, DHHS, is developing strategies for increasing the provision for preventive services within third-party insurance plans, self-funded health benefit plans, managed-care plans, and Medicare. In addition, that office is advising the Office of Personnel Management to facilitate the inclusion of preventive services within the reformed federal employee health-benefits plan.

SUMMARY

1. The year 2000 health objectives for the nation were reviewed, with emphasis on the physical activity and fitness objectives. The objectives were evaluated in relation to adult exercise habits, youth fitness, and worksite exercise programs.

2. The problem of inactivity in this country can be viewed in a historical context, showing how concepts of healthful exercise have changed. A turning point in adult fitness awareness took place in 1968, with the publication of Ken Cooper's first book, *Aerobics.*

3. National surveys have tried to evaluate the magnitude of the present fitness revolution. Only 15% of the American public is exercising at levels generally recommended for basic aerobic fitness. The year 2000 goal of having more than 20% of adults exercising at this level is unlikely to be reached.

4. Those exercising effectively tend to be of upper socioeconomic status, young, male, and from the western region of the nation.

5. Several major surveys of child and youth fitness have been conducted during the 1980s and 1990s. They show that large numbers of American children and youths exercise at less than desirable levels. Of particular concern are test results showing poor upper-body strength and cardiorespiratory fitness. Skinfold measurements show larger fat percentages now than in the mid-1970s.

6. Exercise programs are offered by 41% of worksites with 50 or more employees. Studies show that through worksite exercise programs, fitness status can be improved, and absenteeism and health risks and costs can be lowered.

7. Population strategies to increase physical activity in America should be multifaceted, with an emphasis on four targets of change—the person, organizations, the environment, and public policies.

REFERENCES

1. Breslow L. Setting objectives for public health. *Ann Rev Public Health* 8:289–307, 1987.

2. O'Donnell MP. Definition of health promotion: Part II: Levels of programs. *Am J Health Promotion* 1(2):6–9, 1986.

3. Office of the Assistant Secretary for Health and Surgeon General. *Healthy People: The Surgeon General's Report on Health Promotion and Disease Prevention.* DHEW (PHS) Publication No. 79-55071. Washington, DC: U.S. Government Printing Office, 1979.

4. Department of Health and Human Services. *Promoting Health/Preventing Disease: Objectives for the Nation.* Washington, DC: U.S. Government Printing Office, Fall 1980.

5. Public Health Service, U.S. Department of Health and Human Services. *Healthy People 2000: National Health Promotion and Disease Prevention Objectives.* DHHS Publication No. (PHS) 91-50212. Washington, DC: U.S. Government Printing Office, 1991.

6. U.S. Department of Health and Human Services. *Physical Activity and Health: A Report of the Surgeon General.* Atlanta, GA: U.S. Department of Health and Human Services, Centers for Disease Control and Prevention, National Center for Chronic Disease Prevention and Health Promotion, 1996.

7. Wharton JC. *Crusaders for Fitness: The History of American Health Reformers.* Princeton, NJ: Princeton University Press, 1982.

8. Spears B, Swanson RA. *History of Sports and Physical Activity in the United States.* Dubuque, IA: W.C. Brown Co., 1978.

9. Rice EA, Hutchinson JL, Lee M. *A Brief History of Physical Education.* New York: The Ronald Press Co., 1958.

10. Corbin DH. *Recreation Leadership.* Englewood Cliffs, NJ: Prentice-Hall, Inc., 1970.

11. Pate RR. A new definition of youth fitness. *Physician Sportsmed* 11:77–83, 1983.

12. Kraus H, Hirschland RP. Muscular fitness and health. *JAMA,* 17–19, December, 1953. See also: Kraus H, Hirschland RP. Minimum muscular fitness tests in school children. *Res Q Am Assoc Health Phys Educ* 25:178–188, 1954.

13. Bowerman WJ, Harris WE. *Jogging.* New York: Grosset & Dunlap, 1967, 1977.

14. Cooper KH. *Aerobics.* New York: Bantam Books, Inc., 1968.

15. Cooper KH. *The New Aerobics.* New York: M. Evans and Company, Inc., 1970.

16. Cooper KH. *The Aerobics Way.* New York: M. Evans and Company, Inc., 1977.

17. Cooper M, Cooper KH. *Aerobics for Women.* New York: M. Evans and Co., Inc., 1972.

18. Higdon H. Running after 40. *Runner's World,* August 1978, 36.

19. Henderson J. *Long Slow Distance: The Humane Way to Train.* Mountain View, CA: World Publications, 1969.

20. Ullyot J. *Women's Running.* Mountain View, CA: World Publications, 1976.

21. Sheehan GA. *Dr. Sheehan on Running.* Mountain View, CA: World Publications, 1976.

22. Fixx IF. *The Complete Book of Running.* New York: Random House, 1977.

23. Garrick JG, Requa RK. Aerobic dance: A review. *Sports Med* 6: 169–179, 1988.

24. Amend PC. Health clubs: A new resource for health promotion. *Med Exerc Nutr Health* 2:170–176, 1993.

25. Sol N, Foster C. *ACSM's Health/Fitness Facility Standards and Guidelines.* Champaign, IL: Human Kinetics, 1992.

26. Tharrett SJ, Peterson JA. *ACSM's Health/Fitness Facility Standards and Guidelines* (2nd ed.). Champaign, IL: Human Kinetics, 1997.

27. National Center for Health Statistics, Schoenborn CA. *Health Promotion and Disease Prevention: United States, 1985. Vital and Health Statistics.* Series 10, No. 163, DHHS Pub. No. (PHD) 88-1591, U.S. Public Health Service. Washington, DC: U.S. Government Printing Office, 1988.

28. Piani A, Schoenborn C. Health promotion and disease prevention: United States, 1990. National Center for Health Statistics. *Vital Health Stat* 10(185), 1993.

29. Caspersen CJ, Merritt RK. Physical activity trends among 26 states, 1986–1990. *Med Sci Sports Exerc* 27:713–720, 1995.

30. Stephens T, Craig CL. *The Well-being of Canadians: Highlights of the 1988 Campbell's Survey.* Ottawa: Canadian Fitness and Lifestyle Research Institute, 1990.

31. Wagener PC. *Health Conditions among the Currently Employed: United States, 1988.* National Center for Health Statistics, Series 10 No. 186 (PHS) 93-1412. Washington, DC: U.S. Government Printing Office, 1993.

32. Dybdahl T. *The Prevention Index '97: A Report Card on the Nation's Health.* Emmaus, PA: Rodale Press, Inc., 1997.

33. Office of Disease Prevention and Health Promotion, Public Health Service. Summary of findings from National Children and Youth Fitness Study. *JOPERD,* January 1985.

34. Youth Physical Fitness in 1985. *The President's Council on Physical Fitness and Sports School Population Fitness Survey.* President's Council on Physical Fitness and Sports, 450 Fifth St., NW, Suite 7103, Washington, DC 20001, 1985.

35. Ross, JG, Pate RR, Delpy LA, Gold RS, Svilar M. New health-related fitness norms. *JOPERD,* November/December 1987, 66–77.

36. Pate RR, Ross JG. Factors associated with health-related fitness. *JOPERD,* November/December 1987, 93–96.

37. Ross JG, Pate RR. The National Children and Youth Fitness Study II: A summary of findings. *JOPERD,* November/December 1987, 51–56.

38. Ross JG, Delpy LA, Christenson GM, Gold RS, Damberg CL. The National Children and Youth Fitness Study II: Study procedures and quality control. *JOPERD,* November/December 1987, 57–62.

39. Centers for Disease Control. Participation of high school students in school physical education—United States, 1990. *MMWR* 40:607–615, 1991.

40. Simons-Morton BG, Taylor WC, Snider SA, Huang IW. The physical activity of fifth-grade students during physical education classes. *Am J Public Health* 83:262–264, 1993.

41. Kuntzleman CT, Reiff GG. The decline in American children's fitness levels. *Res Quart Exerc Sport* 63:107–111, 1992.

42. Centers for Disease Control and Prevention. Guidelines for school and community programs to promote lifelong physical activity among young people. *MMWR* 46 (No. RR-6): 1–35, 1997.

43. U.S. Department of Health and Human Services, Public Health Service. *1992 National Survey of Worksite Health Promotion Activities.* Washington, DC: U.S. Government Printing Office, 1993. Published also in: *Am J Health Promotion* 7(6):452–463, 1993.

44. Office of Disease Prevention and Health Promotion. Worksite programs target health and cost benefits. *Prevention Report,* August/September 1994.

45. Erfurt JC, Foote A, Heirich MA, Brock BM. *The Wellness Outreach at Work Program: A Step-by-Step Guide.* NIH Publication No. 95-3043, August 1995.

46. Goetzel RZ, Kahr TY, Aldana SG, Kenny GM. An evaluation of Duke University's Live for Life health promotion program and its impact on employee health. *Am J Health Promotion* 10: 340–342, 1996.

47. Wilson MG. A comprehensive review of the effects of worksite health promotion on health-related outcomes: An update. *Am J Health Promotion* 11:107–108, 1996.

48. Washington Business Group on Health. Physical fitness programs in the workplace, 1987. 220½ Pennsylvania Ave., SE, Washington, DC 20003. Reported in *Employee Health & Fitness* (April):44–46, 1987.

49. Shephard RJ. A critical analysis of worksite fitness programs and their postulated economic benefits. *Med Sci Sports Exerc* 24: 354–370, 1992.

50. Blake SM, Caspersen CJ, Finnegan J, Crow RA, Mittlemark MB, Ringhofer KR. The shape up challenge: A community-based worksite exercise competition. *Am J Health Promotion* 11: 23–34, 1996.

51. Cox MC, Shephard RJ, Corey P. Influence of an employees fitness program upon fitness, productivity, and absenteeism. *Ergonomics* 24:795–806, 1981.

52. Bertera RL. Behavioral risk factor and illness day changes with workplace health promotion: Two-year results. *Am J Health Promotion* 7(5):365–373, 1993.

53. Tucker LA, Aldana SG, Friedman GM. Cardiovascular fitness and absenteeism in 8,301 employed adults. *Am J Health Promotion* 5(2): 140–145, 1990.

54. Bowne DW, Russell ML, Morgan JL, Optenberg SA, Clarke AK. Reduced disability and health care costs in an industrial fitness program. *J Occup Med* 26:809–815, 1984.

55. Baun WB, Bernacki EJ, Tsai SP. A preliminary investigation: Effect of a corporate fitness program on absenteeism and health care cost. *J Occup Med* 28:18–22, 1986.

56. Knight KK, Goetzel RZ, Fielding JE, Eisen M, Jackson GW, Kahr TY, Kenny GM, Wade SW, Duann S. An evaluation of Duke University's Live for Life health promotion program on changes in worker absenteeism. *JOM* 36:533–536, 1994.

57. Blair SN, Smith M, Collingwood TR, Reynolds R, Prentice MC, Sterline CL. Health promotion for educators: Impact on absenteeism. *Prev Med* 15:166–175, 1986.

58. Blair SN, Piserchia PV, Wilbur CS, Crowder JH. A public health intervention model for worksite health promotion: Impact on exercise and physical fitness in a health promotion plan after 24 months. *JAMA* 255:921–926, 1986.

59. Shephard RJ, Corey P, Renzland P, Cox M. The influence of an employee fitness and lifestyle modification program upon medical care costs. *Can J Public Health* 73:259–263, 1982.

60. Cady LD, Thomas PC, Karwasky RJ. Program for increasing health and physical fitness of fire fighters. *J Occup Med* 27: 110–114, 1985.

61. Gibbs JO, Mulvaney D, Henes C, Reed RW. Work-site health promotion: Five-year trend in employee health care costs. *J Occup Med* 27:826–830, 1985.

62. Sciacca J, Seehafer R, Reed R, Mulvaney D. The impact of participation in health promotion on medical costs: A reconsideration of the Blue Cross and Blue Shield of Indiana study. *Am J Health Promotion* 7(5):374–383, 1993.

63. Rogers T, Cole JA, Erwin PG. "Heart at work": Cost–benefit analysis of a new worksite health promotion program. In *Proceedings of the Seventh Annual Meeting of the Society of Behavioral*

Medicine. San Francisco: Society of Behavioral Medicine, 1986, 10–11.

64. Shephard RJ. Twelve years experience of a fitness program for the salaried employees of a Toronto Life Assurance Company. *Am J Health Promotion* 6(4):292–301, 1992.

65. Powell KE, Blair SN. The public health burdens of sedentary living habits: Theoretical but realistic estimates. *Med Sci Sports Exerc* 26:851–856, 1994.

66. Dishman RK. *Exercise Adherence: Its Impact on Public Health.* Champaign, IL: Human Kinetics, 1988.

67. King AC. Community intervention for promotion of physical activity and fitness. *Exerc Sport Sci Rev* 19:211–259, 1991.

68. King AC. Community and public health approaches to the promotion of physical activity. *Med Sci Sports Exerc* 26:1405–1412, 1994.

69. Pate RR, Pratt M, Blair SN, et al. Physical activity and public health: A recommendation from the Centers for Disease Control and Prevention and the American College of Sports Medicine. *JAMA* 273:402–407, 1995.

70. Sallis JF, Hovell MF. Determinants of exercise behavior. *Exerc Sport Sci Rev* 18:307–330, 1990.

71. Hovell MF, Sallis JF, Hofstetter CR, Spry VM, Faucher P, Caspersen CJ. Identifying correlates of walking for exercise: An epidemiological prerequisite for physical activity promotion. *Prev Med* 18:856–866, 1989.

72. Sallis JF, Hovell MF, Hofstetter CR, et al. A multivariate study of determinants of vigorous exercise in a community sample. *Prev Med* 18:20–34, 1989.

73. Sallis JF, Haskell WL, Fortmann SP, Wood PD, Vranizan KM. Moderate-intensity physical activity and cardiovascular risk factors: The Stanford five-city project. *Prev Med* 15:561–568, 1986.

74. Sallis JF, Hovell MF, Hofstetter CR, Elder JP, Faucher P, Spry VM, Barrington E, Hackley M. Lifetime history of relapse from exercise. *Addict Beh* 15:573–579, 1990.

75. King AC, Haskell WL, Taylor CB, Kraemer HC, DeBusk RF. Home-based exercise training in healthy older men and women. *JAMA* 266:1535–1542, 1991.

76. Sallis JF, Hovell MF, Hofstetter CR, Elder JP, Hackley M, Caspersen CJ, Powell KE. Distance between homes and exercise facilities related to frequency of exercise among San Diego residents. *Pub Health Reports* 105:179–185, 1990.

77. Sallis JF, Patterson TL, Buono MJ, Atkins CJ, Nader PR. Aggregation of physical activity habits in Mexican American and Anglo families. *J Beh Med* 11:31–41, 1988.

78. Sullivan LW. Partners in prevention: A mobilization plan for implementing Healthy People 2000. *Am J Health Promotion* 5: 291–297, 1991.

79. Godin G, Shephard RJ. An evaluation of the potential role of the physician in influencing community exercise behavior. *Am J Health Promotion* 4:255–259, 1990.

80. U.S. Preventive Services Task Force. *Guide to Clinical Preventive Services* (2nd ed.). Alexandria, VA: International Medical Publishing, 1996.

81. Anderson RN, Kochanek KD, Murphy SL. Report of final mortality statistics, 1995. *Monthly Vital Statistics Report* 45(11)(suppl 2), June 12, 1997.

82. National Center for Health Statistics. *Health, United States, 1996–97, and Injury Chartbook.* Hyattsville, MD: U.S. Public Health Service, 1997.

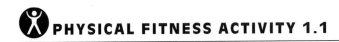

PHYSICAL FITNESS ACTIVITY 1.1

What Is Your Personal Exercise Program?

This chapter fully described the exercise habits of Americans. The 1990 National Health Interview Survey (NHIS) by the National Center for Health Statistics is presently one of the best data sources for this type of information.[28] Data from NHIS have been collected continuously since 1957. In 1985 and 1990, a special section on Health Promotion and Disease Prevention was included.

In this Physical Fitness Activity, you will be answering questions on exercise taken directly from the NHIS section on Health Promotion and Disease Prevention. Fill in the blanks in the table on the next page, and then summarize your exercise program by answering the following questions.

Physical Fitness Activity Questions

1. Summarize your answers to the NHIS questionnaire by filling in the following:

    a. What was your average frequency per week of exercise during the past 2 weeks? *Note:* Count only the sessions where intensity was high or moderate.

    _____ average frequency / week

    Note: Total the number of times in past 2 weeks and divide by 2. For example, if you jogged 2 times in the past 2 weeks, biked 2 times, and played soccer once, your average frequency per week would be 5 divided by 2, or 2.5 times / week.

    b. What was your average *duration per exercise session in minutes* (from "a")?

    _____ average duration per exercise session (in minutes)

    Note: Total the number of minutes spent in exercise during the past 2 weeks, and divide that by the number of exercise sessions. For example, if the jogging sessions lasted 15 minutes each, the biking sessions 30 minutes each, and soccer 40 minutes, the average duration per exercise session in minutes would be 130 min / 5 = 26 minutes per session. *Note:* Only include sessions from part "a."

2. How do you compare with ACSM standards?

    The American College of Sports Medicine recommends that people exercise at least three times per week, for at least 20 to 30 minutes, at moderate-to-high intensity levels (at least 50% maximal oxygen capacity) (see Chapter 8).

    Did you exercise:

    Yes   No

    _____   _____   3 or more times / week?

    _____   _____   20 or more minutes / session?

    _____   _____   At moderate or high heart rate / breathing levels for each session?

National Health Interview Survey, 1990
Health Promotion and Disease Prevention Supplement

A			B	C	D			
In the past 2 weeks, have you done any of the following exercises, sports, or physically active hobbies?			How many times in the past 2 weeks did you [play / go / do] (*activity in A*)?	On average, about how many minutes did you actually spend (*activity in A*) on each occasion?	What usually happened to your heart rate or breathing when you undertook (*activity in A*). Did you have a small, moderate, or large increase, or no increase at all in your heart rate or breathing?			
	Yes	No	Times	Minutes	Small	Moderate	Large	None
1. Walking for exercise	——	——	——	——	——	——	——	——
2. Jogging or running	——	——	——	——	——	——	——	——
3. Hiking	——	——	——	——	——	——	——	——
4. Gardening / yard work	——	——	——	——	——	——	——	——
5. Aerobic dancing	——	——	——	——	——	——	——	——
6. Other dancing	——	——	——	——	——	——	——	——
7. Calisthenics	——	——	——	——	——	——	——	——
8. Golf	——	——	——	——	——	——	——	——
9. Tennis	——	——	——	——	——	——	——	——
10. Bowling	——	——	——	——	——	——	——	——
11. Biking	——	——	——	——	——	——	——	——
12. Swimming	——	——	——	——	——	——	——	——
13. Weight lifting	——	——	——	——	——	——	——	——
14. Basketball	——	——	——	——	——	——	——	——
15. Baseball	——	——	——	——	——	——	——	——
16. Football	——	——	——	——	——	——	——	——
17. Soccer	——	——	——	——	——	——	——	——
18. Volleyball	——	——	——	——	——	——	——	——
19. Handball / racquetball	——	——	——	——	——	——	——	——
20. Skating	——	——	——	——	——	——	——	——
21. Skiing	——	——	——	——	——	——	——	——
22. Any other type of exercise not mentioned here	——	——	——	——	——	——	——	——
List here			——	——	——	——	——	——

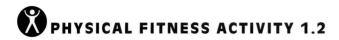

PHYSICAL FITNESS ACTIVITY 1.2

Using the Internet to Explore Health and Fitness

In this Physical Fitness Activity, choose a World Wide Web Internet site that deals with health, physical fitness, or Healthy People 2000/2010 goals; explore the site; and print out a topic that updates information presented in this chapter. Prepare a one- to three-minute oral report to the students of your class.

Health and Fitness Websites

- American Alliance for Health, Physical Education, Recreation, and Dance *www.aahperd.org*
- American College of Sports Medicine *www.acsm.org*
- CDC National Center for Chronic Disease Prevention and Health Promotion *www.cdc.gov/nccdphp/nccdhome.htm*
- Physical Activity and Health Network (PAHnet) *www.pitt.edu/~pahnet*
- President's Council on Physical Fitness and Sports *www.dhhs.gov/progorg/ophs/pcpfs.htm*

Lack of regular physical activity claims about 250,000 lives per year in this country. In this information age, trends show that more people are taking up sedentary lifestyles. Public health, medical, and mental-health professionals recognize the vital importance of physical activity and fitness for the general population.

The lead agency for this high-priority area is the President's Council on Physical Fitness and Sports (PCPFS). The CDC serves as the science advisor. These two agencies posted *Physical Activity and Health: A Report of the Surgeon General* online even before it was published in hard copy. PCPFS also has available an online text version of *How to Celebrate National Physical Fitness and Sports Month.* Within CDC, the National Center for Chronic Disease Prevention and Health Promotion (NCCDPHP) lists online its study of physical inactivity and cardiovascular health and chronic conditions. NCCDPHP and the ACSM collaborated on and helped disseminate online a recommendation that every adult should accumulate 30 minutes or more of daily moderate-intensity physical activity.

Consortium member ACSM provides electronic abstracts of its journal, *Medicine and Science in Sports and Exercise,* for its users. ACSM also features an online version of the NIH Consensus Development Conference Statement on Physical Activity and Cardiovascular Health.

The American Alliance for Health, Physical Education, Recreation, and Dance site features research, information on its national convention, and "Physical Best at a Glance."

The PAHnet home page offers news of current research, activity and health recommendations, reference material, professional organizations, online journals, and listservs. PAHnet also offers a directory of professionals in the field, including their e-mail addresses. Several consortium members are represented on PAHnet.

Healthy People 2000/2010 Websites

The following agencies have assumed responsibility for the Healthy People 2000/2010 priority areas indicated:

Centers for Disease Control and Prevention (**www.cdc.gov**)

- Clinical preventive services
- Diabetes and other chronic disabling conditions

- Educational and community-based programs
- Environmental health
- HIV infection
- Immunizations and infectious diseases
- Occupational safety and health
- Oral health
- Tobacco use and addiction
- Sexually transmitted diseases
- Surveillance and data systems
- Unintentional injuries
- Violent and abusive behavior

Food and Drug Administration (www.fda.gov)

- Food and drug safety
- Nutrition

Health Resources and Services Administration (www.hrsa.dhhs.gov)

- Clinical preventive services
- Educational and community-based programs
- Maternal and infant health

National Institutes of Health (www.nih.gov)

- Cancer
- Diabetes and other chronic disabling conditions
- Environmental health
- Heart disease and stroke
- Mental health and mental disorders
- Nutrition
- Oral health

Office of Population Affairs (www.dhhs.os.gov/progorg/opa/)

- Family planning

President's Council on Physical Fitness and Sports (www.dhhs.gov/progorg/ophs/pcpfs.htm)

- Physical activity and fitness

Substance Abuse and Mental Health Services Administration (www.samhsa.gov)

- Mental health and mental disorders

Figure 1.15 shows the framework within which these agencies operate in addressing the Healthy People 2000/2010 goals.

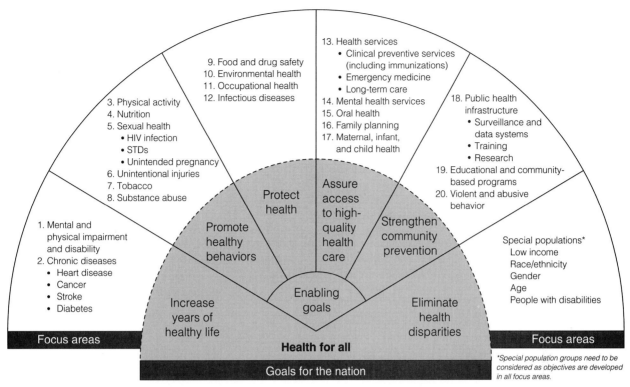

Figure 1.15 Proposed Healthy People 2010 framework: vision of 2010: healthy people in healthy Communities.

2

Physical Fitness Defined

Over the years, I have come to look upon physical fitness as the trunk of a tree that supports the many branches which represent all the activities that make life worth living: intellectual life, spiritual life, occupation, love life and social activities.

—Thomas Kirk Cureton, Jr.

Although many definitions of physical fitness have been proposed, there still is much disagreement among physical educators and exercise scientists as to its real meaning. During the first half of the twentieth century, for example, muscular strength was emphasized by many fitness leaders as the primary goal of an exercise program. During the 1970s and 1980s, the pendulum swung the other way toward a focus on cardiorespiratory fitness through aerobic activity.

Among physical educators, a furious debate has raged since the late 1800s as to whether youth fitness programs should stress the development of skills important for athletic ability (e.g., hand–eye coordination, agility, balance, speed) or attributes that some researchers feel are more important to health (e.g., cardiorespiratory endurance, optimal body composition, flexibility). Since the mid-1980s, several organizations have attempted to redefine physical fitness and exercise in light of modern evidence and understanding. This chapter discusses the contemporary definitions of physical fitness terms important to sport and exercise science. Box 2.1 summarizes the definitions of key terms that are explored in this chapter and other chapters of this book.

PHYSICAL ACTIVITY

Physical activity has been defined as any bodily movement produced by skeletal muscles, which results in energy expenditure.[1,2,3] The energy expenditure can be measured in kilocalories (kcal) or kilojoules (kJ). One kcal is equivalent to 4.184 kJ. In this book, we also use the term *Calories* to denote kcals. One banana, for example, provides about 100 Calories, approximately the amount of energy expended in running a mile.

Everyone performs physical activity in order to sustain life. The amount, however, varies considerably from one individual to another, based on personal lifestyles and other factors. A compendium of physical activities has been developed to provide researchers and practitioners with an estimation of the energy cost for a wide variety of human physical activities. This comprehensive table is available in Appendix E of this book.[4]

Measurement of physical activity is difficult, and researchers have utilized a wide array of methods. Over 50 different measures have been described and can be classified into four general categories:[2]

- *Calorimetry*—direct heat exchange (in an insulated chamber or suit), or indirect measurement through measurement of oxygen consumption and carbon-dioxide production
- *Physiological markers*—heart rate monitoring and use of doubly labeled water (DLW)
- *Mechanical and electronic motion detectors*—pedometers, in-shoe step counters, electronic motion sensors, and accelerometers
- *Occupational and leisure-time survey instruments*—job classification, activity diaries or records, and physical activity recall questionnaires

Box 2.1

Glossary of Terms

Following are key terms related to physical fitness. Review this list, as needed, to investigate terms used in this chapter and throughout the book.

aerobic training: Training that improves the efficiency of the aerobic energy-producing systems and that can improve cardiorespiratory endurance.

agility: A skill-related component of physical fitness that relates to the ability to rapidly change the position of the entire body in space, with speed and accuracy.

anaerobic training: Training that improves the efficiency of the anaerobic energy-producing systems and that can increase muscular strength and tolerance for acid–base imbalances during high-intensity effort.

balance: A skill-related component of physical fitness that relates to the maintenance of equilibrium while either stationary or in motion.

body composition: A health-related component of physical fitness that relates to the relative amounts of muscle, fat, bone, and other vital body tissues.

calorimetry: Methods used to calculate the rate and quantity of energy expenditure when the body is at rest and during physical exertion.

    direct calorimetry: A method that gauges the body's rate and quantity of energy production by direct measurement of the body's heat production; the method uses a *calorimeter,* which is a chamber that measures the heat expended by the body.

    indirect calorimetry: A method of estimating energy expenditure by measuring respiratory gases; given that the amount of O_2 and CO_2 exchanged in the lungs normally equals that used and released by body tissues, caloric expenditure can be measured by CO_2 production and O_2 consumption.

cardiorespiratory endurance (cardiorespiratory fitness): A health-related component of physical fitness that relates to the ability of the circulatory and respiratory systems to supply oxygen during sustained physical activity.

coordination: A skill-related component of physical fitness that relates to the ability to use the senses, such as sight and hearing, together with body parts, in performing motor tasks smoothly and accurately.

detraining: Changes the body undergoes in response to a reduction or cessation of regular physical training.

endurance training and **endurance activities:** Repetitive aerobic use of large muscles (e.g., walking, bicycling, swimming).

exercise (exercise training): Planned, structured, and repetitive bodily movement done to improve or maintain one or more components of physical fitness.

flexibility: A health-related component of physical fitness that relates to the range of motion available at a joint.

kilocalorie (kcal): A measurement of energy: 1 kilocalorie = 1 Calorie = 4,184 joules = 4.184 kilojoules.

kilojoule (kjoule or kJ): A measurement of energy: 4.184 kilojoules = 4,184 joules = 1 Calorie = 1 kilocalorie.

maximal heart rate (HR_{max}): The highest heart rate value attainable during an all-out effort to the point of exhaustion.

maximal heart rate reserve: The difference between maximal heart rate and resting heart rate.

maximal oxygen uptake ($\dot{V}O_{2max}$): The maximal capacity for oxygen consumption by the body during maximal exertion; also known as aerobic power, maximal oxygen consumption, and cardiorespiratory endurance capacity.

metabolic equivalent (MET): A unit used to estimate the metabolic cost (oxygen consumption) of physical activity; 1 MET equals the resting metabolic rate of approximately 3.5 ml O_2 per kilogram of body weight per minute.

muscular endurance: The ability of the muscle to continue to perform without fatigue.

physical activity: Bodily movement that is produced by the contraction of skeletal muscle and that substantially increases energy expenditure.

physical fitness: a set of attributes that people have or achieve, which relates to the ability to perform physical activity.

power: A skill-related component of physical fitness that relates to the rate at which one can perform work.

reaction time: A skill-related component of physical fitness that relates to the time elapsed between a stimulus and the beginning of the reaction to it.

relative perceived exertion (RPE): A person's subjective assessment of how hard he or she is working; the Borg scale is a numerical scale for rating perceived exertion.

resistance training: Training designed to increase strength, power, and muscle endurance.

resting heart rate: The heart rate at rest, averaging 60 to 80 beats per minute.

retraining: Recovery of conditioning after a period of inactivity.

speed: A skill-related component of physical fitness relating to the ability to perform a movement within a short period of time.

strength: The ability of the muscle to exert force.

training heart rate (THR): A heart rate goal established by using the heart rate equivalent to a selected training level (percentage of $\dot{V}O_{2max}$). For example, if a training level of 75% $\dot{V}O_{2max}$ is desired, the $\dot{V}O_{2max}$ at 75% is determined and the heart rate corresponding to this $\dot{V}O_2$ is selected as the THR.

Source: U.S. Department of Health and Human Services. *Physical Activity and Health: A Report of the Surgeon General.* Atlanta, GA: U.S. Department of Health and Human Services, Centers for Disease Control and Prevention, National Center for Chronic Disease Prevention and Health Promotion, 1996.

Questionnaire methods are currently the most popular and practical approaches for large groups of individuals. A collection of physical activity questionnaires for health-related research has been published.[5] Physical Fitness Activity 1.1 from the previous chapter contains the physical activity questionnaire used in the 1991 National Health Interview Survey.

Calorimetry and DLW can provide accurate measurements of average daily energy expenditure under controlled laboratory conditions for small groups of subjects. Measurement of energy expenditure away from the laboratory has been enhanced with the development of light metabolic units that can be worn on the chest. DLW is an effective but expensive method for measuring energy expenditure in free-living humans.[6] Briefly, the DLW method requires that the subject ingest a dose of water containing both the isotope deuterium ($^2H_2$) and the stable oxygen isotope ^{18}O (as $^2H_2{}^{18}O$). The technique is safe because the isotopes employed are naturally occurring rather than radioactive. Subjects provide urine, blood, or saliva samples before and 3 hours after ingestion, as well as each day for several days. Through use of mass spectrometers, energy expenditure is calculated by measuring the difference in the rate of loss between the two isotope labels (which is related to carbon dioxide production and through calculation to oxygen consumption).

Total 24-hour energy expenditure consists of three major categories (as discussed in more detail in Chapter 11):[7]

1. Resting metabolic rate (RMR). *Resting metabolic rate* is generally the largest component of energy expenditure for most people except for some athletes. This is the amount of energy expended to maintain body systems while resting quietly in a comfortable environment several hours following a meal or physical activity.

2. Thermic effect of physical activity. The second largest component of daily energy expenditure for most people is the energy expended for physical activity. The amount of energy expended by muscular work depends on the duration and intensity of the physical activity.

Energy is expended in physical activity during occupational duties, leisure-time activities, and even sleep. Table 2.1 outlines the average energy expenditure of American adults in various types of occupations.[8] The 24-hour Calorie totals represent the contribution of both resting metabolic rate and energy expended during physical activity.

Notice (from Table 2.1) that endurance athletes tend to have energy expenditure patterns quite similar to those of sedentary office workers, except for

TABLE 2.1 Patterns of Average Daily Physical Activity and Energy Expenditure for Athletes and Nonathletes

Males	Sedentary (office)	Light Occupation	Heavy Occupation	Endurance Training	Heavy Sports Training
Rest/Maintenance					
sleep	8 hrs / 530 Calories	8 hrs / 530 Calories	8 hrs / 530 Calories	8 hrs / 600 Calories	8 hrs / 600 Calories
sit / stand	14 hrs / 1700 Calories	6 hrs / 750 Calories	6 hrs / 750 Calories	12 hrs / 1500 Calories	10 hrs / 1250 Calories
Physical activity					
45% $\dot{V}O_{2max}$	2 hrs / 350 Calories	10 hrs / 1500 Calories	6 hrs / 1125 Calories	3 hrs / 525 Calories	2 hrs / 400 Calories
45–70% $\dot{V}O_{2max}$	< ... >	< ... >	4 hrs / 1200 Calories	< ... >	3 hrs / 1500 Calories
70%+ $\dot{V}O_{2max}$	< ... >	< ... >	< ... >	1 hr / 1100 Calories	1 hr / 750 Calories
Total 24 hrs	2580 Calories	2780 Calories	3605 Calories	3725 Calories	4500 Calories

Females	Sedentary (office)	Light Occupation		Endurance Training	Heavy Sports Training
Rest/Maintenance					
sleep	8 hrs / 400 Calories	8 hrs / 420 Calories		8 hrs / 460 Calories	8 hrs / 460 Calories
sit / stand	15 hrs / 1100 Calories	12 hrs / 990 Calories		12 hrs / 1290 Calories	10 hrs / 1170 Calories
Physical activity					
45% $\dot{V}O_{2max}$	1 hr / 130 Calories	4 hrs / 550 Calories		3 hrs / 400 Calories	3 hrs / 430 Calories
45–70% $\dot{V}O_{2max}$	< ... >	< ... >		< ... >	2 hrs / 940 Calories
70%+ $\dot{V}O_{2max}$	< ... >	< ... >		1 hr / 790 Calories	1 hr / 590 Calories
Total 24 hrs	1630 Calories	1960 Calories		2940 Calories	3590 Calories

Source: Adapted from Brotherhood JR. Nutrition and sports performance. *Sports Med* 1:350–389, 1984. With permission from ADIS Press Limited, Auckland 10, New Zealand.

TABLE 2.2   Energy Intake by American Adults and Percent Calories as Fat (% Fat), from National Surveys[9,10]

Population Studied		Name of Study	Calories	(% Fat)
Men	20 and over	NHANES[a]	2492	(34%)
Women	20 and over		1718	(34%)
Men	20 and over	CSFII[b]	2470	(34%)
Women	20 and over		1633	(33%)

[a]National Health and Nutrition Examination Survey (1988–1991)[6]
[b]Continuing Survey of Food Intakes by Individuals (1994–1995)[10]

the large amount of energy expended during short but intense training sessions. When endurance athletes are compared to workers in heavy labor occupations, the total energy expenditure is nearly the same, but once again, the athletes' energy expenditure patterns are characterized by short but intense sessions, whereas heavy laborers expend the majority of their Calories in lower intensity physical activity. The nutritional implications of these different energy-expenditure patterns are discussed in Chapter 9.

Table 2.2 outlines the average energy intakes of Americans.[9,10] Results from the 1994–1995 Continuing Survey of Food Intakes by Individuals[8] show that the average American male is consuming about 2,500 Calories/day, and the average American female about 1,600 Calories/day. These energy intake levels approximate closely the average energy expenditures of sedentary males and females.

3. Thermic effect of food (TEF). The third component of energy expenditure is the *thermic effect of food* or the energy expended above RMR over the several hours (usually 4–6) following a meal.[7] The largest part of the energy expended immediately following meals is due to the metabolic costs of processing the meal, and these include the costs of digestion ("internal exercise" by the muscular gastrointestinal tract), absorption, transport, and storage. The TEF accounts for approximately 10% of daily energy expenditure but can vary, depending on the amount and the composition of the diet (high-carbohydrate diets elevate the TEF more than high-fat diets). (See Chapter 11.)

EXERCISE

Exercise is not synonymous with physical activity.[1,2,3] It is a subcategory of physical activity. Exercise is physical activity that is planned, structured, repetitive, and purposive, in the sense that improvement or maintenance of physical fitness is an objective.[3] Virtually all conditioning and many sports activities are considered exercise because they are generally performed to improve or maintain physical fitness. Household and occupational tasks are usually accomplished with little regard to physical fitness. However, a person can structure work and home tasks in a more active form and thus build up physical fitness at the same time the tasks are accomplished. Many people find this more motivating than "running in circles" for exercise.

A COMPREHENSIVE APPROACH TO PHYSICAL FITNESS

During the boom years of the aerobic movement in the 1970s and 1980s, development of cardiorespiratory fitness was emphasized, often to the detriment of musculoskeletal fitness. Although this was a much needed reform from the undue preoccupation with muscular strength and size, which had dominated since the late 1800s, most fitness experts today believe in a more balanced approach to all the components of fitness.[11,12,13] The focus of the 1990s is on a comprehensive approach to physical fitness in which three major components—cardiorespiratory fitness, body composition, and musculoskeletal fitness (comprising flexibility, muscular strength, and muscular endurance)—are given equal attention.

The Meaning of Physical Fitness

Several organizations have submitted philosophical definitions of physical fitness. The World Health Organization, for example, has defined it simply as "the ability to perform muscular work satisfactorily."[14] The Centers for Disease Control and Prevention sponsored a workshop, bringing together a group of experts who concluded that physical fitness "is a set of attributes that people have or achieve that relates to the ability to perform physical activity."[3] The American College of Sports Medicine has proposed that "fitness is the ability to perform moderate to vigorous levels of physical activity without undue fatigue and the capability of maintaining such ability throughout life."[15]

The President's Council on Physical Fitness and Sports has offered one of the more widely used definitions, describing physical fitness as the "ability to carry out daily tasks with vigor and alertness, without undue fatigue and with ample energy to enjoy leisure-time pursuits and to meet unforeseen emergencies."[16] Finally, as summarized by one physical education textbook author, "physical fitness is the ability to last, to bear up, to withstand stress, and to persevere under difficult circumstances where an unfit person would give up. Physical fitness is the opposite to being fatigued from ordinary efforts, to lacking the energy to enter zestfully into life's activities, and to becoming exhausted from unexpected, demanding physical exertion.... It is a positive quality, extending on a scale from death to 'abundant life.'"[17]

All of these definitions place an emphasis on having vigor and energy to perform work and exercise. Vigor and energy are not easily measured, however, and physical fitness experts have debated for more than a century the important measurable components of physical fitness.[17,18]

The most frequently cited components fall into two groups, one related to health and the other related to athletic skills.[3,11,12,18] Figure 2.1 summarizes the components of health- and skill-related fitness, with examples of the continuum of physical activities that represent each group.

It is felt by some researchers that while the elements of skill-related fitness are important for participation in various dual and team sports, they have little significance for the day-to-day tasks of Americans or for their general health.[3,18] On the other hand, individuals who engage in regular physical activity to develop cardiorespiratory endurance, musculoskeletal fitness, and optimal body fat levels appear to improve their basic energy levels and place themselves at lower risk for the common diseases of our time, including heart disease, cancer, diabetes, osteoporosis, and other chronic disorders.[2]

In accordance with this viewpoint, the American College of Sports Medicine has defined health-related physical fitness as "a state characterized by an ability to perform daily activities with vigor and a demonstration of traits and capacities that are associated with low risk of premature

development of the hypokinetic diseases (i.e., those associated with physical inactivity)."[11] This definition implies that athletes who excel in throwing a ball or swinging a golf club should understand that they may not have optimal levels of body fat or cardiorespiratory fitness, and as a consequence may be at higher risk for chronic disease. Also, even though individuals may possess poor coordination, they can still be physically fit and healthy by engaging regularly in aerobic and musculoskeletal exercise. Of course, there are athletes who by the nature of their sport (e.g., soccer or basketball) would be rated high in both the health- and skill-related elements.

Among the general population, many individuals would rather play sports while getting fit than engage in "pure" fitness activities such as running, swimming, or using indoor exercise equipment. Fitness leaders need to individualize their recommendations to fit the goals and interests of their clients, realizing that many need the socialization and "fun" of sports to participate regularly in exercise.

The definitions of skill-related components of physical fitness have been defined as follows:[1,3]

Agility—the ability to rapidly change the position of the entire body in space, with speed and accuracy

Balance—the maintenance of equilibrium while stationary or in motion

Coordination—the ability to use the senses, such as sight and hearing, together with body parts, in performing motor tasks smoothly and accurately

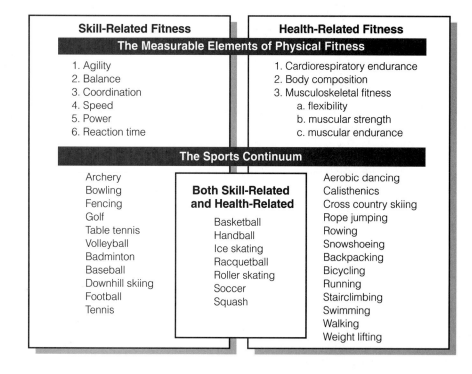

Figure 2.1 Most physical activities exist on a continuum between health- and skill-related fitness. *Source:* Adapted from Caspersen CJ, Powell KE, Christenson GM. Physical activity, exercise, and physical fitness: Definitions and distinctions for health-related research. *Public Health Rep* 100:126–131, 1985.

Speed—the ability to perform a movement within a short period of time

Power—the rate at which a person can perform work (strength over time)

Reaction time—the time elapsed between a stimulus and the beginning of the reaction to it

The trend today in public policy recommendations is to emphasize the development of the health-related fitness elements, and to push for their prominence in school, work-site, and community programs.[1,2,3,13,19] Exercise testing batteries have been developed for children and adults to ensure that each of the health-related fitness elements is measured, followed by appropriate counseling to improve areas that may be deficient.[13,20–25]

The Elements of Health-Related Physical Fitness

Each of the components of health-related physical fitness can be measured separately from the others, and specific exercises may be applied to the development of each component.[11] In other words, the degree to which each of the five health-related components of physical fitness is developed in any one particular individual can vary widely. For example, a person may be strong but lack flexibility or may have good cardiorespiratory endurance but lack muscular strength. To develop "total" physical fitness for health, each of the components (cardiorespiratory endurance, body composition, and musculoskeletal fitness) must be tested separately and then included within the exercise prescription.

Cardiorespiratory Endurance

Cardiorespiratory endurance can be defined as the ability to continue or persist in strenuous tasks involving large-muscle groups for extended periods of time.[1,26–28] It is the ability of the circulatory and respiratory systems to adjust to and recover from the effects of whole-body exercise or work. According to the American College of Sports Medicine, cardiorespiratory endurance is considered health related because low levels have been consistently linked with markedly increased risk of premature death from all causes, especially heart disease.[11]

For many people, being in good shape means having good cardiorespiratory endurance, exemplified by such feats as being able to run, cycle, and swim for prolonged periods of time (Figure 2.2). High levels of cardiorespiratory endurance indicate a high physical work capacity, which is the ability to release relatively high amounts of energy over an extended period of time. To many top fitness leaders, cardiorespiratory endurance is the most important of the health-related physical fitness components.

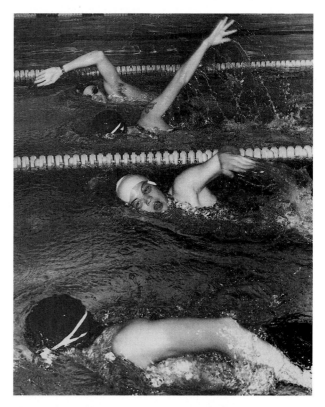

Figure 2.2 *Cardiorespiratory endurance* can be defined as the ability to continue or persist in strenuous tasks involving large muscle groups for extended periods of time. Swimming is one example.

The laboratory test generally regarded as the best measure of cardiorespiratory endurance is the direct measurement of oxygen uptake during maximal, graded exercise. The exercise is usually performed using a bicycle ergometer or treadmill, which allows the progressive increase in workload from light to exhaustive (maximal) exercise. However, laboratory measurement of $\dot{V}O_{2max}$ is expensive, time-consuming, and requires highly trained personnel and therefore is not practical for mass testing situations or the testing of most patients on a day-to-day basis.

Various tests to estimate $\dot{V}O_{2max}$ have been developed as substitutes. These include field tests, stair-climbing tests, submaximal bicycle tests, and maximal treadmill and cycle ergometer tests. These tests are described in detail in Chapter 4.

Based on existing evidence concerning exercise prescription for the enhancement of health and cardiorespiratory fitness, the American College of Sports Medicine has recommended that large-muscle-group activity corresponding to either 40–85% $\dot{V}O_{2max}$ or 55–90% of maximal heart rate be engaged in for 15–60 minutes, 3–5 days a week.[11]

This recommendation has been subjected to a great deal of scrutiny since the late 1980s. In general, there is a growing consensus that when development of fitness is the major concern, higher intensity and longer, continuous duration of aerobic effort is required; when improvement of health is the goal, lower intensity physical activity spread throughout the day appears sufficient. Exercise prescription is discussed in Chapter 8.

Body Composition

Body composition refers to the body's relative amounts of fat, and lean body tissue or fat-free mass (e.g., muscle, bone, water).[1,2] Body weight can be subdivided simply into two components: fat weight (the weight of fat tissue) and fat-free weight (the weight of the remaining lean tissue).[11,21,26] *Percent body fat*, the percentage of total weight represented by fat weight, is the preferred index used to evaluate a person's body composition. Obesity is defined as an excessive accumulation of fat weight. Men have optimal body fat levels when the percent of body fat is 15% or less; they are considered obese when the body fat percentage is 25% and higher. The optimal body fat level for women is 23% or less, and they are considered obese when their body fat percentage is 33% or higher.

Interest in measurement of body composition has grown tremendously since the mid-1970s, largely because of its relationship to both sports performance and health. Elite athletes, individuals seeking to reach or maintain optimal body weight, and patients in hospitals have all benefited from the increased popularity and accuracy of body composition measurement.

Research to establish ways of determining body composition through indirect methods began during the 1940s. Since then, a wide variety of methods have been developed. The most precise measure for assessing body composition using the two-compartment model is hydrostatic (underwater) weighing, although skinfold testing is the method of choice for many physical educators and exercise scientists (Figure 2.3). When conducted appropriately, estimation of percent body fat from skinfold measurements correlates well with hydrostatic weighing ($r > .80$). Chapter 5 deals with these methods, as well as some newer techniques for determining body composition.

Musculoskeletal Fitness

Musculoskeletal fitness has three components: flexibility, muscular strength, and muscular endurance.

1. *Flexibility* is the functional capacity of the joints to move through a full range of movement.[1,3,11,21,26] Flexibility is specific to each joint of the body. Muscles, ligaments, and tendons largely determine the amount of movement possible at each joint (Figure 2.4).

2. *Muscular strength* is the maximal one-effort force that can be exerted against a resistance,[1,3,26] the max-

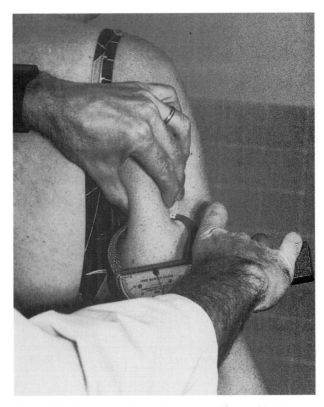

Figure 2.3 *Body composition* is the body's relative amounts of fat and lean body tissue, or fat-free mass (muscle, bone, water). Chapter 5 reviews procedures for measuring body fat through the use of skinfold calipers.

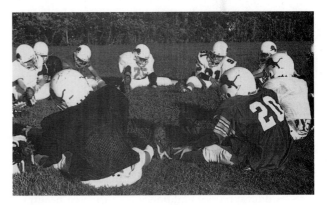

Figure 2.4 *Flexibility* is defined as the functional capacity of the joints to move through a full range of movement.

imum amount of force that one can generate in an isolated movement of a single muscle group. The stronger the individual, the greater the amount of force that can be generated. Lifting heavy weights maximally once or twice, or exerting maximal force when gripping a hand dynamometer, provides measurements of muscular strength (Figure 2.5).

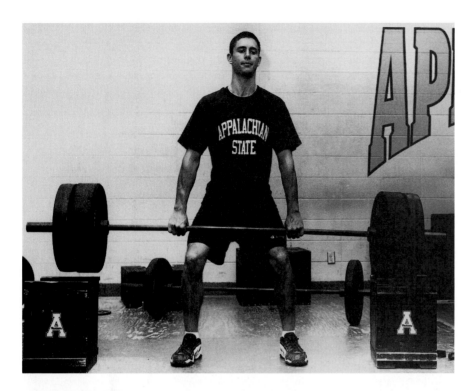

Figure 2.5 *Strength* is the maximal one-effort force that can be exerted against a resistance.

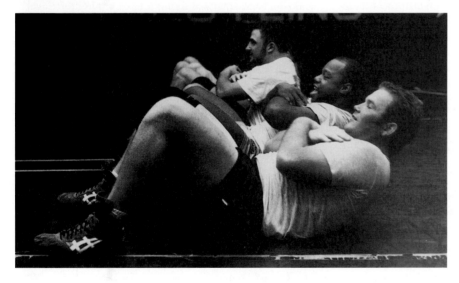

Figure 2.6 *Muscular endurance* is defined as the ability of the muscles to apply a submaximal force repeatedly or to sustain a muscular contraction for a certain period of time.

3. *Muscular endurance* is the ability of the muscles to apply a submaximal force repeatedly or to sustain a submaximal muscular contraction for a certain period of time.[1,3,11,26] Common muscular-endurance exercises are sit-ups, push-ups, chin-ups, or lifting weights 10–15 times in succession (Figure 2.6).

Elaborate and expensive musculoskeletal fitness testing equipment is available, and books have been written describing the sophisticated testing that can be done with it.[28] For most people, however, simple and inexpensive musculoskeletal fitness tests such as the sit-and-reach flexibility test, push-ups, sit-ups, pull-ups, and various weight-lifting measures are available with extensive norms.[20–25] These are described in Chapter 6. Most of the health-related benefits of musculoskeletal fitness have focused on the contribution of abdominal muscle strength and endurance, and lower back–hamstring flexibility for the prevention of low-back pain, a topic also explored in Chapter 6.

Chapter 8 deals with conditioning principles to improve musculoskeletal fitness. The American College of Sports Medicine recommends that static stretching exercises be sustained for 10–30 seconds and then repeated three to five times, at least three times per week, to develop flexibility.[11] It is also recommended that an active aerobic warm-up precede vigorous stretching exercises.

For the development of muscular strength and endurance, the American College of Sports Medicine recommends a minimum of one set of 8–12 repetitions of 8–10 exercises that condition the major muscle groups at least 2 days per week.[15] Optimal gains in strength are provided by three sets of 5–7 repetitions of a weight-resistance exercise.

SPORTS MEDICINE INSIGHT
Physical Fitness of Children and Youths

Chapter 1 reviewed data from national surveys on the status of physical fitness of children and youths. In general, although experts disagree on the interpretation of the results, the studies indicate that many American youths are not exercising enough or are not at a level of physical fitness thought to be conducive to future health and longevity. At the center of the debate on the fitness status of American youths are two testing issues: (1) Should performance- or health-related tests and standards be used? (2) Are criterion-referenced standards or percentile norms the better method for interpeting test results?

Fitness experts are currently divided into two well-entrenched camps on these issues. On the one side is the President's Council on Physical Fitness and Sports (PCPFS), which supports a youth-testing battery incorporating elements related to both health and performance, with test results scored using percentile norms organized by age and sex.[25] For example, the PCPFS testing battery included the following tests: pull-ups / flexed-arm hang, 1-minute bent-knee sit-ups, sit-and-reach test for flexibility, 1-mile run / walk, and the shuttle run. The PCPFS offers the "Presidential Physical Fitness Award" for those who meet the 85th percentile on all test items, the "National Physical Fitness Award" for those who score at or above the 50th percentile on all test items, and the "Participant Award" for those who attempt the tests but fall below the 50th percentile on one or more test items. Appendix A contains the tables and norms for the PCPFS 1985 survey on which the awards are based.

In the other camp is the American Alliance for Health, Physical Education, Recreation, and Dance (AAHPERD) and the Cooper Institute for Aerobics Research (CIAR)[20] both of which have testing batteries (Physical Best and FITNESSGRAM®, respectively) containing only health-related tests, with scores graded according to criterion-referenced health standards. (See Appendix A for a listing of the tests and norms.) In 1993, AAHPERD and CIAR decided to promote just one testing package (the FITNESS-GRAM®), and as a consequence, the Physical Best testing program has been discontinued. See Box 2.2 for further information on the FITNESSGRAM® and Physical Best.

In the FITNESSGRAM®, test results are compared against a basic standard thought to be a minimum level needed to promote health. For example, the criterion-referenced health (CRH) standard (or "healthy fitness zone") for pull-ups is one to two for a 10-year-old boy, and five to eight for 17-year-old boys. A sit-and-reach box with the footline set at 9 inches is used for the flexibility test, and boys and girls of all ages who are able to reach 8 inches on the scale (or to within 1 inch of the footline) meet the CRH standards.

Scoring of test results using percentile norms organized by age and sex allows evaluation in relation to peers but does not address the problem of how fit is fit enough.[29] The CRH standards attempt to address this issue by setting a single cutoff score, meant to represent "desirable health standards" attainable by those who regularly engage in appropriate physical activity. The great difficulty with CRH standards is determining what the cutoff scores should be.

Various studies suggest that about 75% of boys and 50% of girls are able to attain CRH standards on all tests given in the FITNESSGRAM® testing package.[29,30] Yet it appears that many children may be achieving these standards despite not engaging in appropriate levels of physical activity. Thus, the CRH standards may be below the minimum level where physical activity would make a difference and should probably be increased to reflect a higher standard.

Currently, many of the CRH standards correspond to scores below the twentieth percentile, using national norms. Many of the CRH standards for children and youths are based on adult data, with various equations used to adjust the data so that they can be applied to young people. Cardiorespiratory and body composition CRH standards have a stronger scientific foundation than those for muscular strength, endurance, and flexibility. CRH standards are often based on expert opinion from an analysis of normative data provided from national youth fitness-test results. Much more research is needed to provide CRH standards that correctly classify children and youths. Researchers continue to test the reliability and validity of many of the FITNESSGRAM® test items, and revision of the testing battery itself is likely.[20,31–35]

Hoping to bring a resolution to some of these issues, the ACSM published an opinion statement on the physical fitness of children and youths.[26] Although this opinion statement has not stopped the debate, it does reflect the viewpoints of many exercise scientists who have a "concern about the physical fitness of children and youth in the United States."[36] Following are several key statements from this document:

1. "It is the opinion of the ACSM that physical fitness programs for children and youth should be developed with the primary goal of encouraging the adoption of appropriate lifelong exercise behavior in order to develop and maintain sufficient physical fitness for adequate functional capacity and health enhancement."

2. "Until more definitive evidence is available, current recommendations are that children and youth obtain 20–30 minutes of vigorous exercise each day. . . . Recreational and fun aspects of exercise should be emphasized."

3. "The focus of physical fitness testing should be health-related rather than athletic-related. Characteristics such as speed, muscular power, and agility are important for athletic success and are primarily genetically determined . . . Aerobic power, body composition, joint flexibility, and strength and endurance of the skeletal muscular are partly influenced by heredity but can be changed significantly by appropriate exercise patterns."

4. "The ACSM recommends that physical fitness test scores be interepreted in relation to acceptable standards, rather than by normative comparison.

It is illogical to declare that American children and youth are physically unfit as a group and then use group norms to interpret a student's fitness test scores. A standards approach establishes a desirable physical fitness score for each fitness component. Current research is inadequate to establish with scientific precision acceptable standards for all fitness components, but preliminary standards should be developed based on the best available evidence and professional opinion."

CRH standards have recently been developed for adults by the Canadian Society for Exercise Physiology (CSEP), in its "Canadian Physical Activity, Fitness & Lifestyle Appraisal" (CPAFLA) plan.[13] (Call CSEP at 613-234-3755 to obtain the CPAFLA package.) According to the CSEP, "It has become evident in recent years that the health benefits derived from regular physical activity participation may not be related to improvements in physical fitness. For example, many health benefits are gained at exercise intensities below the threshold required to bring about an increase in aerobic fitness. Hence, the results from a fitness assessment (and particularly a follow-up fitness assessment), may not truly reflect the health benefits derived from a client's participation in physical activity." The CPAFLA fitness-appraisal results are now interpreted in terms of associated health benefits instead of percentile distributions of the Canadian population. The CPAFLA in 1996 was adapted as follows:

Earlier	*1996*
Performance related	Health related
Emphasis on fitness	Emphasis on physical activity
Focus on prescribed exercise	Considers broader lifestyle issues

The YMCA and Human Kinetics have produced a software package that gives CRH standards for adults tested at YMCA centers. (Call Human Kinetics at 217-351-5076 for more information on the "YMCA Fitness Analyst.") The *YMCA Youth Fitness Test Manual* also advocates CRH standards for children and youths, using "good," "borderline," and "needs work" labels for the five test items.[22]

Box 2.2

FITNESSGRAM®

FITNESSGRAM® is the fitness assessment of choice for thousands of schools and is used for millions of children and youths annually. The program is much more than an assessment of physical fitness. Youths who participate in the health-related test receive personalized reports on their performance. Here are some key features of FITNESSGRAM®:[20]

1. Each of the test items was selected to assess important aspects of a student's health-related fitness, not skill or agility.

2. Students are compared not to each other, but to health fitness standards, established for each age and gender, which indicate good health.

3. Participants receive objective, personalized feedback and positive reinforcement, which are vital to changing behavior and serve as a communications link between teachers and parents.

FITNESSGRAM® system software is available for PC-DOS, Windows 3.1, and Macintosh. The software, *Test Administration Manual,* and *Computer Reference Guide* are provided free of charge with the initial purchase of blank FITNESSGRAM® report forms. The instructor may also generate group summary reports and a statistical report that provides an overview of group results. FITNESS-GRAM® can be ordered through the Cooper Institute for Aerobics Research (800-635-7050, or through the Internet, http://www.cooperinst.org).

Used in conjunction with its youth fitness partners, Physical Best and *You Stay Active!*, FITNESSGRAM® is part of a complete fitness-education program available for use by schoolteachers and youth fitness leaders. *You Stay Active!* is a new recognition system designed to provide recognition for regular participation in physical activity, rather than an award for a specific fitness performance. The system provides teachers and fitness leaders with 19 different events that can be conducted throughout the year to encourage children and youths to be active almost every day. *You Stay Active!* also provides national recognition to teachers and fitness leaders who conduct program events. The *You Stay Active!* notebook includes master copies to be used in making materials for an entire school. The notebook is available for $37.45. *You Stay Active!* was designed by the Cooper Institute for Aerobics Research and the American Alliance for Health, Physical Education, Recreation, and Dance. You may purchase *You Stay Active!* materials from the Cooper Institute by faxing a purchase order to 972-991-4626 or by purchasing online with a credit card. Physical Best is a companion product to the Prudential FITNESSGRAM®. Developed by AAHPERD, Physical Best is a complete educational program for teaching health-related fitness concepts. Learning activities are included for the areas of health-related fitness: aerobic capacity, body composition, and muscular strength, endurance, and flexibility. To order Physical Best materials, call 800-321-0789.

FITNESSGRAM® Test Items

Aerobic Capacity (select one)

- The Pacer—a 20-meter progressive, multistage shuttle run set to music
- Walk/Run (1 mile)

Body Composition (select one)

- Percent Body Fat—calculated from triceps and calf skinfold measurements
- Body Mass Index—calculated from height and weight

Muscle Strength, Endurance, and Flexibility

- Abdominal Strength Curl-up Test
- Trunk Extensor Strength and Flexibility Trunk Lift
- Upper-Body Strength (select one)—90-degree push-up, pull-up, flexed-arm hang, modified pull-up
- Flexibility (select one)—back-saver sit-and-reach, shoulder stretch

SUMMARY

1. "Physical activity," "exercise," and "physical fitness" are terms that describe different concepts. Physical activity is defined as any bodily movement produced by skeletal muscles, which results in energy expenditure. Total energy expenditure is the sum of the energy expended in basal metabolism, the thermic effect of physical activity, and the thermic effect of food. Physical activity includes sleep and occupational and leisure-time activities.

2. Exercise is a subcategory of physical activity, which is planned, structured, repetitive, and purposive, in the sense that improvement or maintenance of physical fitness is an objective.

3. Several organizations have proposed definitions of physical fitness, most of them emphasizing the ability to perform work and exercise without undue fatigue throughout life.

4. The measurable elements of physical fitness fall into two groups: "skill-related fitness" and "health-related fitness." The former includes agility, balance, coordination, speed, power, and reaction time. The latter includes cardiorespiratory endurance, body composition, and musculoskeletal fitness, which includes flexibility, muscular strength, and muscular endurance.

REFERENCES

1. U.S. Department of Health and Human Services. *Physical Activity and Health: A Report of the Surgeon General.* Atlanta, GA: U.S. Department of Health and Human Services, Centers for Disease Control and Prevention, National Center for Chronic Disease Prevention and Health Promotion, 1996.

2. Bouchard C, Shephard RJ, Stephens T. *Physical Activity, Fitness, and Health: International Proceedings and Consensus Statement.* Champaign, IL: Human Kinetics, 1994.

3. Caspersen CJ, Powell KE, Christenson GM. Physical activity, exercise, and physical fitness: Definitions and distinctions for health-related research. *Public Health Rep* 100:120–131, 1985.

4. Ainsworth BE, Haskell WL, Leon AS, Jacobs DR, Montoye HJ, Sallis JF, Paffenbarger RS. Compendium of physical activities: Classification of energy costs of human physical activities. *Med Sci Sports Exerc* 25:71–80, 1993.

5. Kriska AM, Caspersen CJ. A collection of physical activity questionnaires for health-related research. *Med Sci Sports Exerc* 29(suppl):S1–S205, 1997.

6. Stager JM, Lindemann A, Edwards J. The use of doubly labeled water in quantifying energy expenditure during prolonged activity. *Sports Med* 19:166–173, 1995.

7. Danforth E. Diet and obesity. *Am J Clin Nutr* 41:1132–1145, 1985.

8. Brotherhood JR. Nutrition and sports performance. *Sports Med* 1:350–389, 1984.

9. National Center for Health Statistics. Daily dietary fat and total food-energy intakes—Third National Health and Nutrition Examination Survey, Phase I, 1988–91. *MMWR* 43(7):116–125, 1994.

10. Wilson JW, Enns CW, Goldman JD, Tippett KS, Mickle SJ, Cleveland LE, Chahil PS. *Data Tables: Combined Results from USDA's 1994 and 1995 Continuing Survey of Food Intakes by Individuals and 1994 and 1995 Diet and Health Knowledge Survey* [Online]. ARS Food Surveys Research Group. Available (under "Releases"): http://www.barc.usda.gov/bhnrc/foodsurvey/home.htm [visited 1997, June 2].

11. American College of Sports Medicine. *Guidelines for Exercise Testing and Prescription.* Philadelphia: Lea & Febiger, 1995.

12. Nieman DC. The exercise test as a component of the total fitness evaluation. *Prim Care* 21:569–587, 1994.

13. Canadian Society for Exercise Physiology. *The Canadian Physical Activity, Fitness & Lifestyle Appraisal.* Ottawa, Ontario: Canadian Society for Exercise Physiology, 1996.

14. Anderson KL, Shephard RJ, Denolin H, et al. *Fundamentals of Exercise Testing.* Geneva: World Health Organization, 1971.

15. American College of Sports Medicine. The recommended quantity and quality of exercise for developing and maintaining cardiorespiratory and muscular fitness in healthy adults. *Med Sci Sports Exerc* 22:265–274, 1990.

16. President's Council on Physical Fitness and Sports. *Physical Fitness Research Digest* (Series 1, No. 1). Washington, DC, 1971.

17. Clarke HH. *Application of Measurement to Health and Physical Education.* Englewood Cliffs, NJ: Prentice-Hall, Inc., 1967.

18. Pate RR. A new definition of youth fitness. *Physician Sportsmed* 11:77–83, 1983.

19. Public Health Service, U.S. Department of Health and Human Services. *Healthy People 2000: National Health Promotion and Disease Prevention Objectives* DHHS Publication No. (PHSO) 91-50212. Washington, DC: U.S. Government Printing Office, 1991.

20. Morrow JR, Falls HB, Kohl HW. *The Prudential FITNESSGRAM Technical Reference Manual.* Dallas: Cooper Institute for Aerobics Research, 1994.

21. Golding LA, Myers CR, Sinning WE. *The Y's Way to Physical Fitness* (4th ed.). Champaign, IL: Human Kinetics, 1998.

22. Franks B. *YMCA Youth Fitness Test Manual.* Champaign, IL: Human Kinetics, 1989.

23. Cooper Institute for Aerobics Research. *The Strength Connection.* Dallas: Author, 1990.

24. American College of Sports Medicine. *ACSM Fitness Book.* Champaign, IL: Human Kinetics, 1992.

25. President's Council on Physical Fitness and Sports. *Get Fit: A Handbook for Youth Ages 6–17.* Washington, DC: Author, 1993.

26. American College of Sports Medicine. *Resource Manual for Guidelines for Exercise Testing and Prescription* (2nd ed.). Philadelphia: Lea & Febiger, 1993.

27. Baranowski T, Bouchard C, Bar-Or O, et al. Assessment, prevalence, and cardiovascular benefits of physical activity and fitness in youth. *Med Sci Sports Exerc* 24(suppl 6):S237–S246, 1992.

28. Heyward VH. *Advanced Fitness Assessment and Exercise Prescription* (2nd ed.). Champaign, IL: Human Kinetics, 1991.

29. Looney MA, Plowman SA. Passing rates of American children and youth on the FITNESSGRAM criterion referenced physical fitness standards. *Res Q Exerc Sport* 61:215–223, 1990.

30. Corbin CB, Pangrazi RP. Are American children and youth fit? *Res Q Exerc Sport* 63:96–106, 1992.

31. Jackson AW, Morrow JR, Jensen RL, Jones NA, Schultes SS. Reliability of the Prudential FITNESSGRAM trunk lift test in young adults. *Res Q Exerc Sport* 67:115–117, 1996.

32. Rikli RE, Petray C, Baumgartner TA. The reliability of distance run tests for children in grades K–4. *Res Q Exerc Sport* 63: 270–276, 1992.

33. Cureton KJ, Sloniger MA, Black DM, McCormack WP, Rowe DA. Metabolic determinants of the age-related improvement in one-mile run/walk performance in youth. *Med Sci Sports Exerc* 29:259–267, 1997.

34. Patterson P, Wiksten DL, Ray L, Flanders C, Sanphy D. The validity and reliability of the back saver sit-and-reach test in middle school girls and boys. *Res Q Exerc Sport* 67:448–451, 1996.

35. Cureton KJ, Warren GL. Criterion-reference standards for youth health-related fitness tests: A tutorial. *Res Q Exerc Sport* 61:7–19, 1990.

36. American College of Sports Medicine. Opinion statement on physical fitness in children and youth. *Med Sci Sports Exerc* 20: 422–423, 1988.

⊗ PHYSICAL FITNESS ACTIVITY 2.1

Ranking Activities by Health-Related Value

As discussed in this chapter, there are five measurable elements of health-related fitness:

Cardiorespiratory endurance
Body composition

Musculoskeletal fitness }   **Flexibility**
Muscular endurance
Muscular strength

Sports and other forms of physical activity vary in their capacity to develop each component. In this physical fitness activity, you will be ranking different sports and exercises in terms of their capacity to promote such development, using a 5-point scale for each of the five health-related fitness components. Answer the questions to the best of your ability, and then *compare* your answers in a group session with your teacher or your local fitness expert.

Rate each physical activity or sport in terms of its capacity to develop each of the five health-related components: 1 = not at all; 2 = somewhat or just a little bit; 3 = moderately; 4 = strongly; 5 = very strongly. Then answer the following question.

What five activities received the highest total score (add the five component scores for each activity)?

#1 Overall activity _____

#2 Overall activity _____

#3 Overall activity _____

#4 Overall activity _____

#5 Overall activity _____

Physical Activity—Recreational	Cardiorespiratory Endurance	Body Composition	Flexibility	Muscular Endurance	Muscular Strength	Total
Archery						
Backpacking						
Badminton						
Basketball						
nongame						
game play						
Bicycling						
pleasure						
15 mph						
Bowling						
Calisthenics						
Canoeing, rowing, kayaking						
Dancing						
social and square						
aerobic						
Fencing						
Fishing						
bank, boat, or ice						
stream, wading						
Football (touch)						

Physical Activity—Recreational	Cardiorespiratory Endurance	Body Composition	Flexibility	Muscular Endurance	Muscular Strength	Total
Golf						
power cart						
walking, with bag						
Handball						
Hiking, cross-country						
Horseback riding						
Paddleball, racquetball						
Rope jumping						
Running						
12 min per mile						
6 min per mile						
Sailing						
Scuba diving						
Skating						
ice						
roller						
Skiing, snow						
downhill						
cross-country						
Skiing, water						
Sledding, tobogganing						
Snowshoeing						
Soccer						
Squash						
Stair climbing						
Swimming						
Table Tennis						
Tennis						
Volleyball						
Walking briskly						
Weight training, circuit						
Physical Activity—Nonrecreational						
Bricklaying, plastering						
Digging ditches						
Shoveling light earth						
Splitting wood						

P A R T
II

Screening and Testing

CHAPTER

3

Testing Concepts

Obviously, there is no precise and completely reliable way of gauging a person's physical fitness. The real test is intuitive, and the truly fit person can know that he is truly fit only by sensing that he is deriving the most possible satisfaction from living.

—Thomas K. Cureton, Jr.

As emphasized in Chapter 16, about 75,000 Americans suffer a heart attack during or after exercise each year. These victims tend to be men who were sedentary, already had heart disease or were at high risk for it, and then exercised too hard for their fitness level.[1] Also of concern is congenital cardiovascular disease, now the major cause of athletic death in high school and college. According to the American College of Sports Medicine, "the incidence of cardiovascular problems during physical activity is reduced by nearly 50 percent when individuals are first screened and those identified with risk factors or disease are diverted to other professionally established activity programs."[2] (See Figure 3.1.)

This chapter focuses on some of the steps that individuals can take to help protect themselves when initiating exercise or athletic programs. In addition to health screening through the use of questionnaires, physical fitness testing is useful in identifying adverse signs and symptoms or conditions that might compromise well-being during exercise. Physical fitness testing also provides an opportunity for individuals to be educated and motivated to adopt more healthful lifestyles and to establish goals to progress toward. This chapter emphasizes six issues regarding the screening and testing of individuals prior to participation in an exercise program:

1. The American College of Sports Medicine classification categories

2. Medical/health status questionnaire

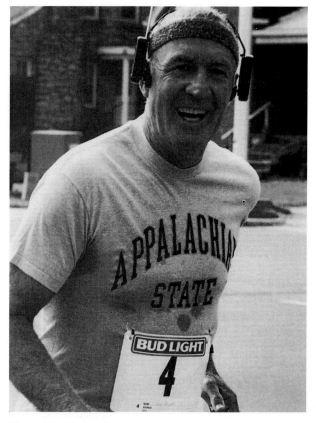

Figure 3.1 The incidence of cardiovascular problems during vigorous exercise can be cut in half by proper screening and testing procedures.

3. Medical evaluation and the graded exercise test
4. Informed consent
5. Physical fitness testing concepts and the purposes of testing
6. Choosing a physical fitness testing battery

THE AMERICAN COLLEGE OF SPORTS MEDICINE CLASSIFICATION CATEGORIES

The American College of Sports Medicine (ACSM) has advised that people wishing to enter an exercise program should be classified first, according to one of the categories described in Table 3.1. Box 3.1 contains a similar classification system from the American Heart Association.[3] This "risk stratification" is important to ensure the safety of exercise testing and participation, to determine the appropri-

ate type of exercise test or program, to identify those in need of more extensive medical evaluation, and to make appropriate recommendations for an exercise program.[1]

Notice from Table 3.1 that there are three risk strata: (1) apparently healthy, (2) increased risk, (3) known disease. Physical Fitness Activity 3.1, at the end of this chapter, contains a questionnaire that simplifies the process of classifying individuals into one of these three categories. Also useful is the medical/health questionnaire in Physical Fitness Activity 3.2. These questionnaires are discussed first before reviewing the ACSM risk categories in more detail.

MEDICAL/HEALTH STATUS QUESTIONNAIRE

To classify an individual according to the ACSM categories and to aid in the exercise prescription process, the medical/health status questionnaire should be given to each potential participant as a first step.

TABLE 3.1 Classification of Individuals by Health Status Prior to Exercise Testing or Exercise Prescription

Category	Description
Apparently healthy	Those who are asymptomatic* and apparently healthy, with no more than one major coronary risk factor**
Increased risk	Those who have signs or symptoms suggestive of possible cardiopulmonary or metabolic disease (see next category) and/or two or more major coronary risk factors
Known disease	Those with known cardiac, pulmonary, or metabolic disease (diabetes, thyroid disorders, renal disease, liver disease)

*Major symptoms or signs suggestive of cardiopulmonary or metabolic disease include (1) pain or discomfort in the chest or surrounding areas that appear to be ischemic (deficiency of blood supply due to obstruction of the circulation) in nature; (2) unaccustomed shortness of breath at rest or with mild exertion; (3) dizziness or fainting; (4) difficulty in breathing when standing or sudden breathing problems during the night; (5) ankle edema; (6) rapid throbbing or fluttering of the heart; (7) severe pain in leg muscles during walking; (8) known heart murmur; (9) unusual fatigue or shortness of breath with usual activities.

**If an individual has two or more of the following coronary risk factors, the classification is "increased risk":

Positive Risk Factors	Defining Criteria
1. Age	Men >45 years; women >55 or premature menopause without estrogen replacement therapy
2. Family history	MI or sudden death before 55 years of age in father or other male first-degree relative, or before 65 years of age in mother or other female first-degree relative
3. Current cigarette smoking	
4. Hypertension	Blood pressure ≥140/90 mm Hg, confirmed by measurements on at least two separate occasions; or on antihypertensive medication
5. Hypercholesterolemia	Total serum cholesterol >200 mg/dl (if lipoprotein profile is unavailable) or HDL < 35mg/dl. (Most other organizations use >240 mg/dl.)
6. Diabetes mellitus	Persons with insulin-dependent diabetes mellitus (type 1) who are >30 years of age, or have had type 1 for >15 years, and persons with non–insulin-dependent diabetes mellitus (type 2) who are >35 years of age should be classified as patients with disease
7. Sedentary lifestyle	Persons composing the least active 25% of the population, as defined by the combination of sedentary jobs involving sitting for a large part of the day and no regular exercise or active recreational pursuits

Negative Risk Factor	Comments
1. High serum HDL cholesterol	>60 mg/dl

Notes: (1) It is common to sum risk factors in making clinical judgments. If HDL is high, subtract one risk factor from the sum of positive risk factors because high HDL decreases CAD risk; (2) obesity is not listed as an independent positive risk factor because its effects are exerted through other risk factors (e.g., hypertension, hyperlipidemia, diabetes). Obesity should be considered as an independent target for intervention, however.

Source: American College of Sports Medicine. *ACSM's Guidelines for Exercise Testing and Prescription* (5th ed.). Baltimore: Williams & Wilkins, 1995. Used with permission.

There are many questionnaires available for preexercise screening (see Physical Fitness Activity 3.2). The medical/health status questionnaire should include the following:[2,4]

- Medical diagnoses
- Previous physical examination findings
- History of symptoms
- Recent illness, hospitalization, or surgical procedures
- Orthopedic problems
- Medication use and drug allergies
- Lifestyle habits
- Exercise history
- Work history
- Family history of disease

The information obtained from the questionnaire will enable each participant to be classified in one of the ACSM categories. In addition, questionnaire data enhance a professional's ability to interpret exercise testing data. In Chapter 8, emphasis is placed on using the medical/health status questionnaire to individualize the exercise prescription. The more background information is obtained, the greater is the ability to meet individual needs.

In some circumstances, particularly when testing large numbers of people in relatively short time periods, a shorter, simpler medical/health questionnaire is preferable. A simple, brief medical questionnaire called the *Physical Activity Readiness Questionnaire* (PAR-Q) has been used very successfully in Canada.[5-9] (See Figure 3.2.)

The PAR-Q was designed in the 1970s as an economical and safe procedure for identifying individuals for whom increased physical activity may be imprudent. Following its development, the PAR-Q was endorsed by the Canadian government and used in conjunction with the Canadian Standard Test of Fitness. Since the 1970s, the PAR-Q has been administered to more than 1 million people, with no

---

Box 3.1

American Heart Association Risk-Stratification Criteria

After the medical clearance stratification is complete, subjects can be classified by risk, based on their characteristics. The following classifications are recommended, and subsequent electrocardiogram (ECG) monitoring is advised, based on this classification.

Class A: Apparently Healthy

There is no evidence of increased cardiovascular risk for exercise. This classification includes (1) individuals under age 40 who have no symptoms or known presence of heart disease or major coronary risk factors, and (2) individuals of any age without known heart disease or major risk factors and who have a normal exercise test.

Activity guidelines: No restrictions other than basic guidelines

ECG and blood pressure monitoring: Not required

Supervision required: None

Class B: Presence of Known, Stable Cardiovascular Disease with Low Risk for Vigorous Exercise but Slightly Greater Than for Apparently Healthy Individuals

Moderate activity is not believed to be associated with increased risk in this group. This classification includes individuals with (1) coronary artery disease (CAD) (myocardial infarction, coronary artery bypass surgery, per-cutaneous transluminal coronary angioplasty, angina pectoris, abnormal exercise test, and abnormal coronary angiograms) whose condition is stable and who have the following clinical characteristics; (2) valvular heart disease; (3) congenital heart disease; (4) cardiomyopathy; and (5) exercise test abnormalities that do not meet the criteria outlined in class C.

Clinical characteristics—(1) New York Heart Association (NYHA) class 1 or 2, (2) exercise capacity over 6 METs, (3) no evidence of heart failure, (4) free of ischemia or angina at rest or on the exercise test at or below 6 METs, (5) appropriate rise in systolic blood pressure during exercise, (6) no sequential ectopic ventricular contractions, and (7) ability to satisfactorily self-monitor intensity of activity

Activity guidelines—individualized activity with exercise prescription by qualified personnel trained in basic CPR or with electronic monitoring at home

ECG and blood pressure monitoring—only during the early prescription phase of training, usually 6–12 sessions

Supervision required—medical supervision during prescription sessions and nonmedical supervision for other exercise sessions until the individual understands how to monitor his or her activity

(continued)

American Heart Association Risk-Stratification Criteria *(continued)*

Class C: Those at Moderate-to-High Risk for Cardiac Complications during Exercise and/or Unable to Self-Regulate Activity or to Understand Recommended Activity Level

This classification includes individuals with (1) CAD with the following clinical characteristics, (2) cardiomyopathy, (3) valvular heart disease, (4) exercise test abnormalities not directly related to ischemia, (5) previous episode of ventricular fibrillation or cardiac arrest that did not occur in the presence of an acute ischemic event or cardiac procedure, (6) complex ventricular arrhythmias that are uncontrolled at mild-to-moderate work intensities with medication, (7) three-vessel disease or left main disease, and (8) low-ejection fractions (less than 30%).

Clinical characteristics—(1) Two or more myocardial infarctions, (2) NYHA class 3 or greater, (3) exercise capacity less than 6 METs, (4) ischemic horizontal or downsloping ST depression of 4 mm or more or angina during exercise, (5) fall in systolic blood pressure with exercise, (6) a medical problem that the physician believes may be life-threatening, (7) previous episode of primary cardiac arrest, and (8) ventricular tachycardia at a workload of less than 6 METs

Activity guidelines—individualized activity with exercise prescription by qualified personnel

ECG and blood pressure monitoring—continuous during exercise sessions until safety is established, usually in 6–12 sessions or more

Supervision—medical supervision during all exercise sessions until safety is established

Class D: Unstable Disease with Activity Restriction

This classification includes individuals with (1) unstable ischemia, (2) heart failure that is not compensated, (3) uncontrolled arrhythmias, (4) severe and symptomatic aortic stenosis, and (5) other conditions that could be aggravated by exercise.

Activity guidelines—no activity recommended for conditioning purposes. Attention should be directed to treating the subject and restoring him or her to class C or higher. Daily activities must be prescribed based on individual assessment by the subject's personal physician.

The foregoing classifications are presented as a means of beginning exercise with the lowest possible risk. They do not consider accompanying morbidities (e.g., insulin-dependent diabetes mellitus, morbid obesity, severe pulmonary disease, or debilitating neurological or orthopedic conditions) that may necessitate closer supervision during training sessions. As the individual gains experience, the decision may be made to place the subject in another category. In most cases, as the safety of exercise and improvement in working capacity are demonstrated, graduation to classes nearer A and B is appropriate.

Source: Fletcher GF, Balady G, Froelicher VF, Hartley LH, Haskell WL, Pollock ML. Exercise standards: A statement for healthcare professionals from the American Heart Association. *Circulation* 91: 580–615, 1995.

---

serious cardiovascular complications reported.[8] ACSM has recommended the PAR-Q as a safe, preparticipatory exercise-screening measure prior to increased low-to-moderate (but not vigorous) exercise training.[1,4] One of the chief criticisms of the PAR-Q has been that it unnecessarily excludes people (especially the elderly) for whom physical activity participation is safe. The revised PAR-Q (see Figure 3.2) was published in 1994 and has been shown to screen out fewer people for whom exercise training is safe.[7,8]

MEDICAL EVALUATION AND THE GRADED EXERCISE TEST

A careful evaluation prior to exercise testing or participation in an exercise program is important to assure safety, to aid in diagnosis of potential cardiovascular disease, to assess heart and lung fitness, to provide a baseline from which to follow progress, and to develop early rapport with the participant.[1,10] The process of exercise prescription is greatly enhanced when physicians and exercise leaders have an adequate background knowledge of the individual seeking to initiate an exercise program.

A physical examination for any potential individual is sometimes recommended, the depth of evaluation depending on the health status of the individual.[1] Laboratory tests such as total cholesterol and high-density lipoprotein (HDL) cholesterol are helpful in determining whether an individual is at higher risk. The most important part of the pretest evaluation, however, is the medical history.[1]

In general, most individuals, except for those with known serious disease, can begin a moderate exercise program such as walking (40–60% $\dot{V}O_{2max}$) without a medical

Physical Activity Readiness
Questionnaire-PAR-Q
(revised 1994)

PAR-Q & YOU

(A Questionnaire for People Aged 15 to 69)

Regular physical activity is fun and healthy, and increasingly more people are starting to become more active every day. Being more active is very safe for most people. However, some people should check with their doctor before they start becoming much more physically active.

If you are planning to become much more physically active than you are now, start by answering the seven questions in the box below. If you are between the ages of 15 and 69, the PAR-Q will tell you if you should check with you doctor before you start. If you are over 69 years of age, and you are not used to being very active, check with your doctor.

Common sense is your best guide when you answer these questions. Please read the questions carefully and answer each one honestly: check YES or NO.

YES	NO	
☐	☐	1. Has your doctor ever said that you have a heart condition *and* that you should only do physical activity recommended by a doctor?
☐	☐	2. Do you feel pain in your chest when you do physical activity?
☐	☐	3. In the past month, have you had chest pain when you were not doing physical activity?
☐	☐	4. Do you lose your balance because of dizziness or do you ever lose consciousness?
☐	☐	5. Do you have a bone or joint problem that could be made worse by a change in your physical activity?
☐	☐	6. Is your doctor currently prescribing drugs (for example, water pills) for your blood pressure or heart condition?
☐	☐	7. Do you know of *any other reason* why you should not do physical activity?

If you answered

YES to one or more questions

Talk with your doctor by phone or in person BEFORE you start becoming much more physically active or BEFORE you have a fitness appraisal. Tell your doctor about the PAR-Q and which questions you answered YES.
- You may be able to do any activity you want—as long as you start slowly and build up gradually. Or, you may need to restrict your activities to those which are safe for you. Talk with your doctor about the kinds of activities you wish to participate in and follow his/her advice.
- Find out which community programs are safe and helpful for you.

NO to all questions

If you answered NO honestly to *all* PAR-Q questions, you can be reasonably sure that you can:

- start becoming much more physically active—begin slowly and build up gradually. This is the safest and easiest way to go.
- take part in the fitness appraisal—this is an excellent way to determine your basic fitness so that you can plan the best way for you to live actively.

DELAY BECOMING MUCH MORE ACTIVE:
- If you are not feeling well because of a temporary illness such as a cold or a fever—wait until you feel better; or
- If you are or may be pregnant—talk to your doctor before you start becoming more active.

Please note: If your health changes so that you then answer YES to any of the above questions, tell your fitness or health professional. Ask whether you should change your physical activity plan.

Informed Use of the PAR-Q: The Canadian Society for Exercise Physiology, Health Canada, and their agents assume no liability for persons who undertake physical activity, and if in doubt after completing this questionnaire, consult your doctor prior to physical activity.

You are encouraged to copy the PAR-Q but only if you use the entire form.

Note: If the PAR-Q is being given to a person before he or she participates in a physical activity program or a fitness appraisal, this section may be used for legal or administrative purposes.

I have read, understood and completed this questionnaire. Any questions I had were answered to my full satisfaction.

NAME _____

SIGNATURE _____ DATE _____

SIGNATURE OF PARENT _____ WITNESS _____
or GUARDIAN (for participants under the age of majority)

Figure 3.2 The Physical Activity Readiness Questionnaire (PAR-Q) offers an easy, brief evaluation prior to starting an exercise program.

TABLE 3.2 Guidelines for Medical Examination, Exercise Testing, and Physician Supervision Prior to Participation

	Apparently Healthy		Increased Risk		Known Disease
	Younger*	Older	No Symptoms	Symptoms	
Medical exam and diagnostic exercise test recommended prior to					
Moderate exercise (40–60% $\dot{V}O_{2max}$)	No**	No	No	Yes	Yes
Vigorous exercise (>60% $\dot{V}O_{2max}$)	No	Yes	Yes	Yes	Yes
Physician supervision recommended* during**					
Submaximal testing	No	No	No	Yes	Yes
Maximal testing	No	Yes	Yes	Yes	Yes

*≤40 years for men, ≤50 years for women.

**The "no" responses in this table mean that an item is "not necessary." The "no" response does not mean that the item should not be done. The "yes" response means that an item is recommended.

***For physician supervision, a "yes" response suggests that a physician is in close proximity and readily available should there be an urgent need.

Source: American College of Sports Medicine. *ACSM's Guidelines for Exercise Testing and Prescription* (5th ed.). Baltimore: Williams & Wilkins, 1995. Used with permission.

evaluation or exercise test.[1] Whenever people are in doubt about their own personal safety while exercising, a medical evaluation is recommended. Exercise testing is not recommended as a routine screening procedure in adults who have no evidence of heart disease.[3,11] Risk of serious medical complications during exercise is low unless an individual is at high risk for cardiovascular disease.

Guidelines for exercise testing and physician supervision vary according to the ACSM "risk stratification" (Table 3.2).[1]

Apparently Healthy Individuals

Apparently healthy individuals can begin moderate (intensities of 40–60% $\dot{V}O_{2max}$) exercise programs such as walking or increasing usual daily activities, without the need for exercise testing or medical examination.[1,3] This is especially true when the moderate exercise program proceeds gradually and the individual is alert to the development of the signs and symptoms listed in Table 3.1.

Prior to starting a vigorous exercise program (>60% $\dot{V}O_{2max}$), apparently healthy men above age 40 or women above age 50 would do well to have a medical examination and a maximal exercise test (with physician supervision). The distinction between moderate and vigorous exercise is an important one. While untrained individuals can usually exercise moderately, safely, and comfortably for about 60 minutes, they cannot sustain vigorous exercise for more than 15 to 20 minutes, and such exercise results in a significant increase in their heart rate and breathing. In most studies of sudden death during exercise, high-intensity ex-

ercise has been found to be a significant risk factor (see Chapter 16).[1,3]

At any age, the information garnered from a maximal exercise test is useful to establish an effective and safe exercise prescription (Figure 3.3). Submaximal testing up to 75% of age-predicted maximal heart rates can be conducted without physician supervision but provides less valuable information for exercise prescription or fitness status determination (see Chapter 4).

Exercise testing is relatively safe, with only one death per 20,000 tests reported in the literature.[1] At the Institute for Aerobics Research, after more than 70,000 maximal exercise tests, no deaths have been reported, and there have been only six major medical complications.[1]

Individuals at Increased Risk

Individuals at increased risk are those with two or more major coronary risk factors and/or symptoms suggestive of heart, lung, or metabolic disease (metabolic diseases include diabetes mellitus, thyroid disorders, kidney disease, liver disease, and other less common forms) (see Table 3.1). A maximal graded exercise test (GXT) prior to a vigorous exercise program is desirable for high-risk individuals of any age, especially those with symptoms.[1] For those without symptoms, an exercise test or medical examination may not be necessary if moderate exercise (such as walking) is undertaken gradually, with appropriate guidance (Figure 3.4). The maximal GXT should be physician supervised. Although submaximal exercise tests are of little diagnostic value for individuals at increased risk, if such a test is given

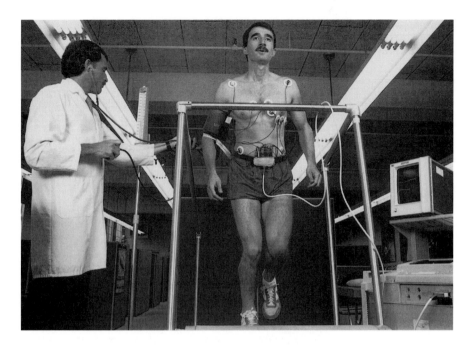

Figure 3.3 For people of all ages, information from the maximal graded exercise test is valuable in establishing an effective and safe exercise prescription.

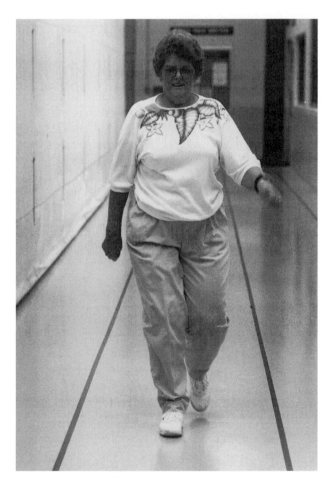

Figure 3.4 For individuals at increased risk without symptoms, an exercise test or medical evaluation may not be necessary if moderate exercise is undertaken gradually, with appropriate guidance.

for fitness assessment purposes, it is not necessary to have a physician present if the patient has no symptoms of disease.

Patients with Known Disease

A complete medical evaluation with a physician-supervised maximal GXT is recommended before starting an exercise program for all individuals with known heart, blood vessel, lung, or metabolic disease. Test results can help the physician make appropriate decisions to ensure the safety of exercise for the patient and also allow progress to be monitored.[1,3]

Astrand, the European exercise physiologist who has done much to mold thought and opinion about exercise since the mid-1970s, summarizes this discussion as follows:[12]

> Anyone who is in doubt about the condition of his health should consult his physician. But as a general rule, moderate activity is less harmful to the health than inactivity. You could also put it this way: A medical examination is more urgent for those who plan to remain inactive than for those who intend to get into good physical shape.

Contraindications for Exercise and Exercise Testing

Although most people in the United States can be safely evaluated and started on an exercise program, there are some who should not exercise. The risks for such people

TABLE 3.3 Contraindications for Exercise and Exercise Testing in Out-of-Hospital Settings

Absolute Contraindications	Relative Contraindications (benefits of evaluation often exceed risk)
A recent significant change in the resting ECG, suggesting infarction or other acute cardiac events	Resting diastolic blood pressure over 115 mm Hg; systolic over 200 mm Hg
Recent complicated myocardial infarction	Moderate valvular heart disease
Unstable angina	Known electrolyte abnormalities (hypokalemia, hypomagnesemia)
Uncontrolled ventricular dysrhythmia	
Uncontrolled atria dysrhythmia that compromises cardiac function	Fixed-rate artificial pacemaker (rarely used)
	Frequent or complex ventricular ectopy
Third degree A–V block without pacemaker	Ventricular aneurysm
Acute congestive heart failure	Uncontrolled metabolic disease (diabetes, thyrotoxicosis, myxedema, etc.)
Severe aortic stenosis	
Suspected or known dissecting aneurysm	Chronic infectious disease (mononucleosis, hepatitis, AIDS, etc.)
Active or suspected myocarditis or pericarditis	Neuromuscular, musculoskeletal, or rheumatoid disorders that are exacerbated by exercise
Thrombophlebitis or intracardiac thrombi	
Recent systemic or pulmonary embolus	Advanced or complicated pregnancy
Acute infections	
Significant emotional distress (psychosis)	

Source: American College of Sports Medicine. *ACSM's Guidelines for Exercise Testing and Prescription* (5th ed.). Baltimore: Williams & Wilkins, 1995. Used with permission.

Note: The American Heart Association has also published absolute and relative contraindications for exercise testing.[3]

outweigh the benefits. The American College of Sports Medicine has established contraindications for exercise and exercise testing in out-of-hospital settings.[1] A *contraindication* means that most experts would agree that it is inadvisable for the individual to be exercise tested or to engage in active exercise. These contraindications should be diagnosed only by medical doctors. The exercise leader should draw the attention of the attending physician to this ACSM contraindication listing (summarized in Table 3.3).

CARDIOVASCULAR SCREENING OF COMPETITIVE ATHLETES

An average of 12–20 athletes, most of them high school students, die suddenly each year from congenital heart defects that are not detected during normal physical examinations.[13–15] About a third of the cases of sudden cardiac death are caused by a congenital heart defect called "hypertrophic cardiomyopathy" (thickened heart muscle), with the next most frequent cause being congenital coronary anomalies.

In the United States, there are nearly 6 million scholastic athletes. Although most states require a regular physical once every 1 or 2 years for these athletes, the cost for the more sensitive tests (e.g., two-dimensional echocardiography) that would detect heart defects ranges from $400

to $2,000 a screening. However, even with echocardiography, some athletes are incorrectly classified (e.g., false-positive or false-negative).[14]

The sudden death of a young athlete is tragic, but the financial, ethical, medical, and legal issues involved in preparticipation screening have created huge barriers. In 1996, the American Heart Association (AHA) published a consensus statement on this issue from a panel of experts.[14] Here are the key recommendations.

1. "The AHA recommends that some form of preparticipation cardiovascular screening for high school and collegiate athletes is justifiable and compelling, based on ethical, legal, and medical grounds."[14] Although such tests as 12-lead electrocardiography, echocardiography, or graded exercise testing improve detection of cardiovascular disease in large populations of young or older athletes, the AHA expert panel concluded that "it is not prudent to recommend routine use" of these tests because of practical and cost-efficiency considerations.

2. "Consequently, we conclude that a complete and careful personal and family history and physical examination designed to identify (or raise suspicion of) those cardiovascular lesions known to cause sudden death or disease progression in young athletes is the best available and most practical approach to screening populations of competitive

sports participants, regardless of age. Such cardio-vascular screening is an obtainable objective and should be mandatory for all athletes. We recommend that both a history and a physical examination be performed before participation in organized high school (grades 9 through 12) and collegiate sports. Screening should then be repeated every 2 years. In intervening years an interim history should be obtained."[14] The AHA panel emphasized that because states vary so much in their screening standards and procedures, "we also recommend developing a national standard for preparticipation medical evaluations."

3. "We strongly recommend that athletic screening be performed by a healthcare worker with the requisite training, medical skills, and background to reliably obtain a detailed cardiovascular history, perform a physical examination, and recognize heart disease."[14] The AHA panel urged that "while it is preferable that such an individual be a licensed physician, this may not always be feasible, and under certain circumstances it may be acceptable for an appropriately trained registered nurse or physician assistant to perform the screening examination."

4. "Athletic screening evaluations should include a complete medical history and physical examination, including brachial artery blood pressure measurement."[14] The cardiovascular history (with input from both the athletes and the parents) should include key questions designed to determine (1) prior occurrence of exertional chest pain/discomfort or syncope/near-syncope, as well as excessive, unexpected, and unexplained shortness of breath or fatigue associated with exercise; (2) past detection of a heart murmur or increased systemic blood pressure; and (3) family history of premature death (sudden or otherwise), or significant disability from cardiovascular disease in close relative(s) younger than 50 years old or specific knowledge of the occurrence of certain conditions (e.g., hypertrophic cardiomyopathy, dilated cardiomyopathy, long QT syndrome, Marfan syndrome, or clinically important arrhythmias).

The cardiovascular physical examination should emphasize (but not necessarily be limited to) (1) precordial auscultation in both the supine and standing positions to identify, in particular, heart murmurs consistent with dynamic left ventricular outflow obstruction; (2) assessment of the femoral artery pulses to exclude coarctation of the aorta; (3) search for and recognition of any of the physical stigmata of Marfan syndrome; and (4) brachial blood pressure measurement in the sitting position. When cardio-vascular abnormalities are identified or suspected, the athlete should be referred to a cardiovascular specialist for further evaluation or confirmation.

INFORMED CONSENT

Like it or not, we live in an increasingly litigious society.[16] Today's exercise program director, recreation administrator, or exercise testing program director is much more likely to be sued than his or her predecessors. In general, legal claims against exercise professionals are based on either alleged violations of contract law or tort principles.[4] A legal contract is a promise or performance bargained for and given in exchange for another. Most tort claims affecting the exercise professional are based on allegations of either negligence or malpractice, and commonly involve the following:[4,16-22]

- Failure to monitor an exercise test properly
- Failure to evaluate physical impairments competently
- Failure to prescribe a safe exercise intensity or program
- Failure to provide appropriate supervision
- Rendition of advice later construed to represent medical diagnosis
- Failure to refer participants to physician
- Failure to respond adequately to an untoward event
- Failure to disclose certain information in the informed-consent process

By law, any subject, patient, or client who is exposed to possible physical, psychological, or social injury must give informed consent prior to participation in a program.[16,23] *Informed consent* can be defined as the knowing consent of an individual or that person's legally authorized representative, with free power of choice and the absence of undue inducement or any element of force, fraud, deceit, duress, or other form of constraint or coercion.

The subject should read the informed-consent form and then sign it in the presence of a witness, indicating that the document has been read and consent given to participation under the described conditions. The consent form should be written so as to be easily understood by each participant, in the language in which the person is fluent.

Separate forms should be used for diagnostic exercise testing and for the exercise program itself. (See Figures 3.5 and 3.6 for sample forms.) No sample form should be adopted unless approved by local legal counsel. The following items should be included in the informed-consent form:[1,4,23,24]

Testing Objectives: I understand that the tests that are about to be administered to me are for the purpose of determining my physical fitness status, including heart, lung, and blood vessel capacities for whole body activity, body composition (ratio of body fat to muscle, bone, and water), muscular endurance and strength, and joint flexibility.

Explanation of Procedures: I understand that the tests that I will undergo will be performed on a treadmill, bicycle, or steps. The tests are designed to increase the demands on the heart, lung, and blood vessel system. This increase in effort will continue until exhaustion or other symptoms prohibit further exercise. During the test, heart rate, blood pressure, and electrocardiographic data will be periodically measured. Body composition will be determined through use of skinfolds or underwater weighing to determine levels of body fat versus fat-free weight. Muscular endurance and strength will be determined through the use of body calisthenics and/or equipment. The sit-and-reach test will be used to determine the flexibility of the hip joint.

Description of Potential Risks: I understand that there exists the possibility that certain abnormal changes may occur during the testing. These changes could include abnormal heart beats, abnormal blood pressure response, various muscle and joint strains or injuries, and in rare instances, heart attack. Professional care throughout the entire testing process should provide appropriate precaution against such problems.

Benefits to Be Expected: I understand that the results of these tests will aid in determining my physical fitness status and in determining potential health hazards. These results will facilitate a better individualized exercise prescription.

I have read the foregoing information and understand it. Questions concerning these procedures have been answered to my satisfaction. I also understand that I am free to deny answering any questions during the evaluation process, or to withdraw consent and discontinue participating in any procedures. I have also been informed that the information derived from these tests is confidential and will not be disclosed to anyone other than my physician or others who are involved in my care or exercise prescription, without my permission. However, I am in agreement that information from these tests not identifiable to me can be used for research purposes.

Participant's Signature _____   Date _____

Witness Signature _____   Date _____

Figure 3.5   Consent to graded exercise testing and other physical fitness tests.

General Statement of Program Objectives and Procedures: I understand that this physical fitness program may include exercises to build the cardiorespiratory system (heart and lungs), the musculoskeletal system (muscle endurance and strength, and flexibility), and to improve body composition (decrease of body fat in individuals needing to lose fat, with an increase in weight of muscle and bone). Exercises may include aerobic activities (treadmill walking/running, bicycle riding, rowing machine exercise, group aerobic activity, swimming, and other such activities), calisthenics, and weight lifting to improve muscular strength and endurance, and flexibility exercises to improve joint range of motion.

Description of Potential Risks: I understand that the reaction of the heart, lung, and blood vessel system to such exercise cannot always be predicted with accuracy. I know there is a risk of certain abnormal changes occurring during or following exercise, which may include abnormalities of blood pressure or heart rate, ineffective functioning of the heart, and in rare instances, heart attacks. Use of the weight-lifting equipment , and engaging in heavy body calesthenics, can lead to musculoskeletal strains, pain, and injury if adequate warm-up, gradual progression, and safety procedures are not followed. Safety procedures are listed on the wall of the fitness facility. In addition, trained staff members will be supervising during all times to help ensure that these risks are minimized. The staff members are trained in CPR and first aid and regularly practice emergency procedures. Equipment is inspected and maintained on a regular basis.

Description of Potential Benefits: I understand that a program of regular exercise for the heart and lungs, muscles, and joints has many associated benefits. These may include a decrease in body fat, improvement in blood fats and blood pressure, improvement in psychological function, and a decrease in risk of heart disease.

I have read the foregoing information and understand it. Any questions that may have occurred to me have been answered to my satisfaction. I understand that I am free to withdraw from this program without prejudice at any time I desire. I am also free to decline answering specific items or questions during interviews or when filling out questionnaires. The information that is obtained will be treated as privileged and confidential and will not be released or revealed to any person other than my physician without my express written consent. The information obtained, however, may be used for a statistical or scientific purpose with my right of privacy retained.

Signature of Participant _____ Date_____

Signature of Witness _____ Date _____

Figure 3.6   Consent for physical fitness programs.

1. A general statement of the background of the program and objectives

2. A fair explanation of the procedures to be followed

3. A description of any and all risks attendant to the procedures

4. A description of the benefits that can reasonably be expected

5. An offer to answer any of the subject's queries

6. An instruction that the subject, client, or patient is free to withdraw consent and to discontinue participation in the program at any time without prejudice to the person

7. An instruction that, in the case of questionnaires and interviews, the participant is free to refuse to answer specific items or questions

8. An explanation of the procedures to be taken to ensure the confidentiality of the information derived from the participant

While it should be understood that execution of an informed-consent form does not protect the exercise or medical director from legal action, if the program is in accordance with established guidelines and run by a qualified staff, and the participant voluntarily assumes risk as outlined in the consent form, the possibility of legal action is minimized.[1,4,16]

HEALTH/FITNESS FACILITY STANDARDS AND GUIDELINES

In 1997, ACSM established six standards and nearly 500 guidelines for health/fitness facilities, which are expected to have a rather dramatic effect on the industry.[24] (See Box 1.1 in Chapter 1.) These standards should be regarded as a benchmark of competency that probably will be used in a court of law to assess performance and service.[24–26] In their 211-page book, the ACSM has provided an extensive list of guidelines for physical plant safety, effective signage, organizational structure and professional staffing, user screening, emergency and safety procedures, external grounds, the control desk, laundry room, locker rooms, fitness testing and wellness areas, exercise classrooms, pool areas, and specialty areas (e.g., the spa, physical therapy area, climbing walls).[24]

Box 3.2 summarizes the "user screening" guidelines given by the ACSM for health/fitness facilities. In regard to staffing, ACSM has recommended that "each person who has supervisory responsibility for a physical activity program or area at a facility must have demonstrable professional competence in that physical activity program or area."[24] ACSM defines demonstrable professional competence as "some combination of education and professional experience that would be recognized by both the industry and the public at large as representing a relatively high level of competence and credibility."[24] Within the health and fitness industry, an indication of professional competence for four different program areas includes the following:

1. Fitness director—4-year college education in a health- or fitness-related field or substantially equivalent work experience; certification from a nationally recognized association or organization in the health and fitness industry; CPR certification and first-aid training; 1 year or more of work experience in the fitness field

2. Aerobics coordinator; physical activity instructor— 2-year college education in a health- or fitness-related field or substantially equivalent work experience; certification from a nationally recognized association or organization in the health and fitness industry; CPR certification and first-aid training

3. Aquatics director—certification in advanced lifesaving; certification in water-safety instruction; at least 1 year of work experience in aquatics; pool-operation training; CPR certification and first-aid training

4. Fitness testing staff—4-year college education in a health- or fitness-related field or related exercise-science field; current professional certification from a nationally recognized association or organization in the health and fitness industry; CPR certification and first-aid training

(See the Sports Medicine Insight and Box 3.3, at the end of this chapter, for more information on professional certification.)

All health/fitness facilities must be prepared to handle situations that arise unexpectedly and must have a comprehensive emergency plan that provides guidelines for the staff. Emergency plan guidelines, according to the ACSM, include the following:[24]

1. Provisions for physical access to all areas of the facility, as well as a plan for the handling and disposition of bystanders

2. Provisions for documenting all events to provide a basis for the orderly evaluation of a situation after it occurs and the subsequent follow-up actions that may be taken

3. Provisions for securing and using specific protocols and emergency supplies, including the development of a written emergency plan, listing specific steps that the staff should perform to satisfy the basic emergency goals

Box 3.2

ACSM's Guidelines for User Screening: Standards for Health/Fitness Facilities

Considerable evidence supports the fact that physically active individuals are less likely to suffer from a wide array of medical conditions, including coronary heart disease. On the other hand, when participating in physical activity, the risk of cardiovascular incident or death is greater than when not participating in physical activity. Because of the increased risk of cardiovascular incident during physical activity, staff members prescribing programmed physical activity for facility users should ensure that users are screened for conditions that might indicate the heightened possibility of cardiovascular incident or death. This recommendation is also applicable in instances where facility users participate without staff guidance.

Research indicates that individuals with coronary risk factors or other medically significant risk factors, as identified through a preactivity screening process, run a greater chance of a cardiovascular incident during physical activity than do individuals with no risk factors. As a result, it is prudent that individuals be screened for coronary and other medical risk factors with a preactivity screening protocol before engaging in any physical activity program. In addition, users should undergo fitness evaluations prior to engaging in a physical activity program. One of the benefits of such an evaluation is that it affords the staff an opportunity to better educate and motivate users to adopt healthier lifestyles. Fitness evaluations also allow staff members to identify adverse signs and symptoms that might otherwise compromise user well-being and that should be promptly evaluated and assessed by qualified medical personnel.

ACSM has published recommended guidelines that should govern the screening of users prior to their participation in a physical activity program. These guidelines are designed to protect users from troublesome medical events or death while engaging in physical activity and to enhance the ability of the facility to meet an appropriate standard of care. Among the issues related to user screening are the following:

- Preactivity screening
- Informed consent
- User screening

Preactivity Screening

A screening procedure given to an individual before that person engages in a physical activity program should incorporate either a general screening device (e.g., PAR-Q and YOU) or a specific screening device (e.g., the Health History Questionnaire). Refer to forms in Figure 3.2, Physical Fitness Activity 3.1, and Physical Fitness Activity 3.2 for samples of preactivity screening devices.

When an individual who has completed a preactivity screening instrument, fitness test, or health-promotion evaluation is identified as having a condition or risk factor that could be adversely aggravated by physical activity, that person should be advised in writing or verbally to see a physician before engaging in physical activity. For a clarification of coronary risk factors, facility staff members should refer to the fifth edition of *ACSM's Guidelines for Graded Exercise Testing and Prescription*[1] and the American Heart Association's *Exercise Standards: A Statement for Health Professionals*.[3] Examples of the forms that can be used to obtain physician approval for individuals with identified coronary risk factors are illustrated in Note 3.

Informed Consent

As part of their efforts to prescreen users, to conduct fitness-evaluation protocols, and to prescribe physical activity, health/fitness facilities should encourage all users to complete an informed-consent form. An informed-consent form is generally designed to advise all users of the benefits and risks of participation, testing, and physical activity and to advise users that their participation is voluntary in nature. Samples of informed-consent sheets are provided in Figures 3.5 and 3.6.

User Screening

Individuals who decide not to participate in preactivity screening prior to engaging in programmed physical activity should be required to complete and sign an assumption of risk or a prospective release or waiver of claims form (or other form legally recognized as such within the jurisdiction of the facility), by the terms of which the individual assumes all risks of participation. Examples of prospective release, assumption of risk, and waiver of claims forms are provided in *ACSM's Health/Fitness Facility Standards and Guidelines*.[24]

Source: Tharrett SJ, Peterson JA. *ACSM's Health/Fitness Facility Standards and Guidelines* (2nd ed.). Champaign, IL: Human Kinetics, 1997. Used with permission.

4. Provisions in an emergency plan for contact and interaction with a predetermined community emergency resource

CONCEPTS AND PURPOSES IN PHYSICAL FITNESS TESTING

Reduced to its simplest terms, the function of measurement is to determine status.[27–29] Ideally, status should be determined before individualized exercise counseling is conducted. The information from the physical fitness testing can be used along with the medical test information to better meet the individual's needs.

When conducting physical fitness tests, several important test criteria should be considered:[27–30]

1. *Validity*—refers to the degree to which the test measures what it was designed to measure; a valid test is one that measures accurately what it is used to measure

2. *Reliability*—deals with how consistently a certain element is measured by the particular test; concerned with the repeatability of the test—if a person is measured two separate times by the same tester or by two different people, the results should be close to the same

3. *Norms*—represent the achievement level of a particular group to which the measured scores can be compared; norms provide a useful basis for interpretation and evaluation of test results

4. *Economy*—refers to ease of administration, the use of inexpensive equipment, the limitation of time needed to administer the test, and the simplicity of the test so that the person taking it can easily understand the purpose and results

So in other words, a good physical fitness test accurately measures what it is supposed to measure, can be consistently used by different people, produces results that can be compared to a data set, and is relatively inexpensive, simple, and easy to administer.

In a complete physical fitness program, testing of participants before, during, and after participation is important for several reasons:[1,4,31]

1. To assess current fitness levels (both strengths and weaknesses)

2. To identify special needs for individualized counseling

3. To evaluate progress

4. To motivate and educate

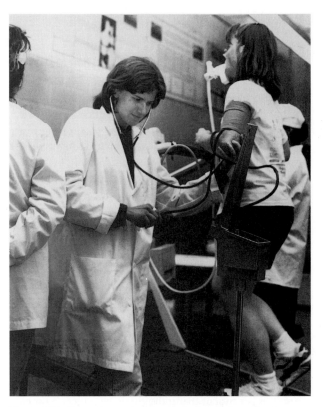

Figure 3.7 Expensive and elaborate testing such as direct measurement of $\dot{V}O_{2max}$ during graded exercise testing is seldom needed for the average fitness participant.

Test results are best viewed as a means to an end, not as an end in themselves. In other words, the testing process should be used to help individuals know more about themselves so that appropriate health and fitness goals can be established. Expensive, elaborate, and lengthy testing is seldom needed (except in research) and can be distractive (Figure 3.7). Scores on the various items of the simple and inexpensive test batteries noted at the end of this chapter are adequate to identify the strengths and weaknesses of participants, so that special attention can be given to individualized goals and objectives. If anything, it is better to undertest than overtest so that more time and attention can be given to counseling and guiding each participant through the exercise program.

PHYSICAL FITNESS TESTING BATTERIES

The very process of administering a fitness test draws attention to what is considered worthy of special attention in a person's lifestyle. The test results can therefore be used to educate, motivate, and stimulate interest in exercise and other health-related topics.

Recommended Order for Fitness-Evaluation Tests

The evaluation procedure has a recommended order for both safety and efficiency. In general, it is best for the participant to fill out the medical/health status questionnaire at home before coming to the testing center. The testing batteries listed at the end of this chapter usually take only about 1 hour.

Precise instructions should be given to the participants before they come to the testing site. In general they should come in exercise attire (and bring a swimsuit if necessary); avoid eating or drinking for 3 hours before the test; avoid alcohol, tobacco, and coffee for at least 3 hours before the test; avoid exercise the day of the test; try to get a good night's sleep; bring the medical/health status questionnaire.

If blood is to be analyzed, alcohol consumption and vigorous exercise should be avoided for 24 hours beforehand, and a 12-hour fast is recommended. Diabetics should be allowed to keep their dietary habits and injections of insulin as regular as possible. According to the ACSM, patients should continue their medication regimen on their usual schedule so that the exercise test responses will be consistent with responses expected during exercise training.[1]

The organization of the testing session is important. It should begin with the quiet, resting tests (heart rate, blood pressure, blood drawing, all after a 5-minute rest). Body composition measures should follow next, then the graded exercise test for cardiorespiratory endurance. Finally, the musculoskeletal tests should be given.

If musculoskeletal tests precede the graded exercise test, the heart rate can be elevated, giving false information on fitness status, especially when submaximal tests are conducted.

Immediate feedback and counseling should follow the testing. Follow-up evaluations should be conducted after 3–6 months, after 1 year of training, and yearly thereafter.[1,4]

Health-Related Fitness Testing Batteries

The YMCA, Canadian Society for Exercise Physiology, Cooper Institute for Aerobics Research, AAHPERD, and President's Council on Physical Fitness and Sports have each developed physical fitness testing batteries that follow the recommended criteria of testing outlined in this chapter. They are valid, reliable, and economical, and they have sound norms. In addition, most follow a comprehensive health-related fitness approach, testing each of the five components.[30,32]

The norms for the various tests within these batteries are found in Appendix A. Descriptions of how to conduct the tests are found in the following chapters of this book. A brief outline of each testing battery is listed in this section.

YMCA

The YMCA physical fitness testing battery for adults is administered in the following order:[31]

- Standing height
- Weight
- Resting heart rate
- Resting blood pressure
- Skinfold tests for men and women (at three or four sites)
- Submaximal cycle test for cardiorespiratory endurance; 3-minute step test for mass testing
- Sit-and-reach test (for flexibility)
- Bench-press test (35 pounds, women; 80 pounds, men) at a rate of 30 times per minute for muscular endurance and strength
- Timed (1 minute) sit-ups for abdominal muscular endurance; or abdominal curl-ups

The YMCA also has a testing manual for youths:[33]

- Skinfolds (triceps and calf)
- Run (1 mile)
- Sit-and-reach test (for flexibility)
- Modified pull-ups
- Curl-ups (40 maximum)

Canadian Physical Activity, Fitness & Lifestyle Appraisal (CPAFLA)

In 1981, the Canada Fitness Survey was initiated and funded by Fitness and Amateur Sport in Canada.[9,34] A major objective of the survey was to provide reliable statistics on physical activity patterns and fitness levels of the Canadian population. The survey sample consisted of 11,884 households that had been identified by Statistics Canada and that were located in urban and rural areas of each province. Members of these households, 15,519 between the ages of 7 and 69, undertook the Canadian Standardized Test of Fitness; this was the largest and most comprehensive study of physical activity and fitness ever undertaken. In 1996, these data were repackaged by the Canadian Society for Exercise Physiology as the "Canadian Physical Activity, Fitness & Lifestyle Appraisal" (CPAFLA).[9] (See Appendix A for norms.) The CPAFLA is administered in the following order (after pretest screening using the PAR-Q and a consent form):[9]

- Resting heart rate
- Resting blood pressure
- Standing height
- Body mass (weight)

- Waist girth
- Skinfolds (triceps, biceps, subscapular, iliac crest, medial calf)
- Canadian aerobic fitness step test
- Grip strength (right and left hands)
- Push-ups
- Trunk-forward flexion
- Partial curl-ups
- Vertical jump

A software program called "The Fitness Analyst" incorporates the CPAFLA tests and norms and has been approved by the Canadian Society for Exercise Physiology. (Call BSDI Inc. at 908-879-4991 for more information.)

Cooper Institute for Aerobics Research: FITCHECK® for Adults

The Cooper Institute for Aerobics Research (CIAR) published their physical fitness test for adults, FITCHECK®, in 1990.[35] The test items are as follows:

- Waist-to-hip ratio (ratio of the circumferences of the waist to the hip)
- Body mass index (height and weight)
- Walking test (1 mile)
- Sit-and-reach test (for flexibility)
- Shoulder flexibility (touching right hand to left hand behind the back)
- Timed (1 minute) bent-knee sit-ups
- Timed (1 minute) push-ups
- Flexed-arm hang
- One-repetition maximum bench-press lift (optional)
- One-repetition maximum leg press (optional)

AAHPERD: Health-Related Fitness Test for College Students

AAHPERD released the results of their testing program for college students in 1985.[36] The study population consisted of 5,158 young adults in colleges from all geographic regions of the United States. The data for the study were collected under the supervision of 24 coinvestigators. The test items in order are as follows (see Appendix A for norms):

- Two-site skinfold test (triceps and subscapular)
- Mile run or 9-minute run for cardiorespiratory endurance
- Sit-and-reach test for flexibility
- Timed (1 minute) sit-ups for abdominal muscular endurance

AAHPERD: Physical Best

The U.S. Public Health Service, in response to the landmark government report, *Promoting Health/Preventing Disease: Objectives for the Nation*, launched the National Children and Youth Fitness Study (NCYFS I) to determine how fit and how active first- through twelfth-grade students actually were.[37] Data on 10- to 18-year-olds were collected from a random sample of 10,275 students from 140 public and private schools in 19 states between February and May, 1984. The NCYFS I was the first nationwide assessment of the physical fitness of American young people in nearly a decade and the most rigorous study of fitness among our youth ever conducted. Test items from the NCYFS I were as follows (see Appendix A for norms):

- Two-site skinfold test (triceps and subscapular)
- Mile run (for cardiorespiratory endurance)
- Sit-and-reach test (for flexibility)
- Chin-ups (for upper-body muscular strength and endurance)
- Timed (1 minute) sit-ups (for abdominal muscular endurance)

As described in Chapter 1, the second National Children and Youth Fitness Study (NCYFS II)[38] was launched to study the physical fitness and physical activity habits of 4,678 children ages 6 to 9. The study was the first to assess the fitness and activity patterns of 6- to 9-year-olds.

Test items of the NCYFS II included

- Triceps, subscapular, and medial calf skinfolds (for body composition)
- Walk/run (for cardiorespiratory endurance): 1 mile (age 8 or 9) or ½ mile (age 6 or 7)
- Sit-and-reach test (for lower back–hamstring flexibility)
- Modified pull-up (for upper-body muscular strength and endurance)
- Timed (1 minute) bent-knee sit-ups (for abdominal strength/endurance)

Physical Best from AAHPERD is a comprehensive, physical fitness education and assessment program that utilizes the testing procedures and norms developed from the NCYFS.[39] Physical Best is the first program to combine assessment of health-related fitness with practical classroom instructional materials that teach why and how to stay fit for a lifetime.

Three components make up the complete Physical Best program:

1. A health-related fitness assessment

2. An educational component, contained in a kit available from AAHPERD

3. A set of awards, to reinforce positive behavior change and recognize personal achievement

In December of 1993, the Cooper Institute for Aerobics Research (CIAR) and AAHPERD announced a partnership agreement. AAHPERD will endorse the FITNESSGRAM® assessment program (with the Physical Best testing phase terminated) while CIAR will endorse Physical Best educational materials. For many years, AAHPERD had problems with their Physical Best testing computer software program and finally decided it would be best to switch to the FITNESSGRAM® assessment program and software.

FITNESSGRAM®

FITNESSGRAM® is a youth fitness testing system developed by the Cooper Institute for Aerobics Research and sponsored by the Prudential Insurance Company of America.[40] It consists of a fitness assessment phase, a computerized reporting program, a behavior-oriented recognition system, and educational materials for teachers to use in assisting students in establishing daily physical fitness as a part of their lifestyles. The test items are health related and, as discussed in the Sports Medicine Insight of Chapter 2, criterion-referenced standards have been established for each age and sex group. These standards are similar to those originally used in the Physical Best program and are thought to represent minimum levels of performance that most often correlate with health. FITNESSGRAM® has also adopted an award system based primarily on exercise behaviors.

Recommended test items of the FITNESSGRAM® include

- Height and weight (to determine body mass index)
- Two-site skinfold test (triceps and calf)
- Run/walk (1 mile, for cardiorespiratory endurance)
- Sit-and-reach test (for flexibility); shoulder stretch optional

- Push-ups (for upper-body muscular strength and endurance); other optional tests include pull-ups and the flexed-arm hang
- Curl-up test (for abdominal muscular endurance)
- Trunk lift test (for trunk extensor strength and flexibility)

The President's Challenge

As described in Chapter 1, the President's Council on Physical Fitness and Sports School Population Fitness Survey was conducted in 1985.[41] Data were collected to assess the physical fitness status of American public school children ages 6 to 17. A four-stage probability sample was designed to select approximately 19,200 boys and girls from 57 school districts and 187 schools.

Data from this survey provide the norms for the current Presidential Physical Fitness Award Program, or "President's Challenge" (about 2 million awards distributed each year).[42] The test battery consists of five required items:

- Run/walk (1 mile, for cardiorespiratory endurance)
- Timed (1 minute) sit-ups (for abdominal muscular endurance)
- V-sit and reach (for flexibility)
- Pull-ups (for upper-body strength and endurance)
- Shuttle run (for body coordination)

Awards for the President's Challenge are based on three different levels of physical fitness exhibited:

1. Presidential (85th percentile or higher on all tests)

2. National (50th percentile or higher on all tests)

3. Participant (below 50th on one or more tests but attempted all of them)

The President's Challenge differs from the Physical Best in that no test for body composition is given, the shuttle run is included, and awards are percentile based instead of criterion based.

SPORTS MEDICINE INSIGHT

Certification for Health and Fitness Professionals

Certification provides health/fitness professionals with public recognition of their knowledge, technical skills, and experience in their particular field. It certifies that the individual is qualified to practice in accordance with the standards deemed to be essential by the certifying body.[43,44] See Box 3.3 for a listing of 10 organizations that provide certifications for the health/fitness industry.

The most prestigious health and fitness certification program is conducted by the American College of Sports Medicine (ACSM). This Sports Medicine Insight provides a description of their certification program. This textbook was written to help individuals prepare for the ACSM Health/Fitness Instructor certification written and practical exams, and the reader is urged to send for the full application packet (ACSM, PO Box 1440, Indianapolis, IN 46206-1440).

ABOUT THE AMERICAN COLLEGE OF SPORTS MEDICINE

The American College of Sports Medicine includes more than 16,000 members in almost 60 countries, who are dedicated to improving the quality of life for people around the world. ACSM's mission statement reflects this goal: "The American College of Sports Medicine promotes and integrates scientific research, education, and practical applications of sports medicine and exercise science to maintain and enhance physical performance, fitness, health, and quality of life."

ACSM was established in 1954 in Madison, Wisconsin. Since that time, ACSM members have applied their knowledge, training, and dedication in sports medicine and exercise science to promote healthier lifestyles for people around the globe. In 1984, the national center was relocated to Indianapolis, Indiana.

Working in a wide range of medical specialties, allied health professions, and scientific disciplines, ACSM members are committed to the diagnosis, treatment, and prevention of sports-related injuries and the advancement of the science of exercise. ACSM members' diversity and expertise makes ACSM the largest, most respected sports-medicine and exercise-science organization in the world. From astronauts to athletes, from people with chronic diseases to those with physical challenges, ACSM continues to look for and find better methods to allow everyone to live longer and more productively. Healthier people make a healthier society.

What started as a group of only 11 physicians, physiologists, and educators back in 1954 has evolved into a diversified professional association, comprising more than 16,000 members in more than 50 different professions today. These many and varied professions are divided into three main categories: basic and applied science, education and allied health, and medicine.

ACSM is also committed to developing students into exceptional professionals. Students are the foundation of the future. The importance of student members is exemplified by their presence on ACSM's Board of Trustees, with a designation for an elected student trustee. A student newsletter is available on ACSM's home page to facilitate the needs of the student members.

ACSM offers five types of new memberships:

- Professional
- Professional-in-Training
- Graduate Student
- Undergraduate Student
- Associate

ACSM also offers the status of "Fellow" to those who meet the required standards. The ACSM member benefits include the following: ACSM members in the "Professional," "Professional-in-Training," "Graduate Student," and "Undergraduate Student" categories receive subscriptions to ACSM's monthly scientific journal, *Medicine and Science in Sports and Exercise* (MSSE); ACSM's quarterly newsmagazine, *Sports Medicine Bulletin* (SMB); the *ACSM Membership Directory;* and the annual review of current research topics in exercise science found in *Exercise and Sport Sciences Reviews* (ESSR). "Associate" members receive SMB and the membership directory. All ACSM members enjoy discounts on rental cars, meeting-registration fees, certification examinations, and other products and services. In addition, they have the opportunity to purchase the best liability insurance policy available today.

ACSM interest groups provide a forum for focused discussion, activity, debate, and networking among members with similar interests. In addition, interest groups allow members to network on a more formal basis. Each recognized interest group works toward fulfilling the mission of the college.

Twelve regional chapters broaden the base of participation and encourage networking at the grassroots level for members, as well as provide valuable professional growth for student members. Local concerns are addressed through annual regional chapter scientific meetings and publications.

ACSM's mailing address: PO Box 1440, Indianapolis, IN 46206-1440

Street address: 401 West Michigan Street, Indianapolis, IN 46202-3233

Telephone, voice: 317-637-9200; fax: 317-634-7817

Internet address: http://www.acsm.org/sportsmed

ACSM CERTIFICATIONS FOR HEALTH AND FITNESS PROFESSIONALS

In the mid-1970s, the American College of Sports Medicine identified a goal of increasing the competency of individuals involved in health and fitness and in cardiovascular rehabilitative exercise programs. With increased public awareness of the benefits of exercise, the college also saw the importance of consumers being able to recognize professional competence.

With the publication of the ACSM's first edition of *ACSM's Guidelines for Graded Exercise Testing and Prescription*, the college was able to set the standards and objectives for its clinical track certifications. Since 1975, more than 6,000 individuals have been certified in one or more of the clinical track's three levels. At the height of the health and fitness awakening in the early 1980s, ACSM introduced its health and fitness track certifications for those working with healthy individuals. In only 15 years, more than 11,000 health/fitness professionals have been certifiedby ACSM.

In 1996, ACSM established the Certification Resource Center (CRC), which can be reached by calling 800-486-5643. In its first year, the CRC fielded more than 30,000 calls from individuals interested in ACSM certifications. The CRC is a one-stop resource for ACSM certification information, workshop dates, and study packets, as well as for a complete line of certification review, reference, and resource materials.

ACSM certification is available to any professional in the preventive and rehabilitative exercise field who meets the established prerequisites. Each of the six progressive levels of ACSM certification requires individuals to pass a written exam that tests knowledge and a practical exam that measures hands-on skills. Many educational workshops, taught by ACSM-member experts, are offered but are not required to earn certification.

Clinical Track Certifications

The particular levels of this track recognize competence of personnel working in clinical exercise programs for individuals with cardiovascular, pulmonary, and metabolic diseases: ACSM Program Director(SM), ACSM Exercise Specialist(SM), and ACSM Exercise Test Technologist(SM). Most individuals with ACSM clinical certifications are found in cardiac rehabilitation programs.

Health and Fitness Track Certifications

The three progressive levels of certification for this track are targeted to professionals who work with those apparently healthy individuals who have no history of disease or who have controlled disease: ACSM Health/Fitness Director(R), ACSM Health/Fitness Instructor(SM), and ACSM Exercise Leader(SM). ACSM health and fitness personnel can be found in corporate fitness centers, fitness clubs, wellness programs, and the like.

Certifications of Enhanced Qualification

ACSM has expanded the education and certification opportunities available to those certified at the Exercise Specialist level and the Health/Fitness Instructor level or above with the Certification of Enhanced Qualification (CEQ). The procedure to qualify for the CEQ involves a 1-day workshop followed by a 1-hour exam. The workshop consists of five or six lectures presented by experts in the topic areas. There is no practicum section. ACSM's first CEQs focused on the "Advanced Personal Trainer" and "Exercise and the Older Adult."

The primary objective of the CEQ workshops is to present selected topics that are relevant to professionals in clinical exercise and applied fitness. These topics focus on a subject and provide the latest research, as well as information about applied skills. Exercise professionals are emerging as key players in the continuum of health care, and it is critical that they be prepared to work with all populations. The CEQ is a vehicle that ACSM has created to advance professional training to meet these expanded roles in health care.

After Certification

Once certification has been earned, individuals are reviewed every 4 years to ensure that competence and the

(continued)

Certification for Health and Fitness Professionals (continued)

ACSM's high level of standards are maintained. Individuals are required to document continuing education credits (CECs) or continuing education units (CEUs) and to maintain a current CPR certification. CEQs are good for 4 years and must be repeated to be maintained. ACSM is developing a new CEQ each year.

For information about workshop and certification dates and sites, recommended study material, and applications for registration, please call ACSM's Certification Resource Center at 800-486-5643.

ACSM HEALTH/FITNESS INSTRUCTOR℠ WORKSHOP/CERTIFICATION

The ACSM Health/Fitness Instructor certification is granted to candidates successfully completing both the written and the practical examinations. The two components are scored separately, and a passing score is required for each component, as indicated in the *ACSM Health/Fitness Instructor Study Packet*.

The ACSM Health/Fitness Instructor certification provides professionals with recognition of their practical experience and demonstrated competence in conducting exercise programs for people who are apparently healthy or who have a controlled disease. These exercise programs apply both scientific principles of conditioning and motivational techniques for establishing an appropriate lifestyle that includes healthy exercise habits. In addition, it is recommended that an ACSM Health/Fitness Instructor meet the following criteria:

1. Work-related experience or any educational degree within the health and fitness field
2. Educational training comparable to an undergraduate degree in a health and fitness or closely related field
3. Adequate knowledge of and skill in risk-factor and health status identification, fitness appraisal, and exercise prescription
4. Demonstrated ability to evaluate the physiological and psychological effects of regular exercise
5. Demonstrated ability to incorporate suitable and innovative activities that will improve an individual's functional capacity
6. Demonstrated ability to effectively educate or counsel individuals regarding lifestyle modification

7. Demonstrated competence in the knowledge and skills required of the ACSM Exercise Leader
8. Knowledge of exercise science, including kinesiology, functional anatomy, exercise physiology, nutrition, risk-factor identification, lifestyle modification techniques, and injury prevention
9. Current CPR certification

The written examination is multiple choice and is based on the expectations as outlined in *ACSM's Guidelines for Graded Exercise Testing and Prescription*, 5th edition. The practical examination consists of evaluating the candidate's performance at a variety of stations that require the candidate to perform tasks routinely performed by ACSM Health/Fitness Instructors. The expectations for the ACSM Health/Fitness Instructor and ACSM Exercise Leaders, outlined in *ACSM's Guidelines for Graded Exercise Testing and Prescription*, are used for constructing the stations for the practical examination.

The candidate will identify and demonstrate proper techniques in estimating body composition using standard anthropometric protocols (including skinfold and circumference assessments). The candidate will also assess flexibility exercises for specific muscle groups. The candidate will demonstrate the ability to assess muscular strength and endurance and to instruct a client on specific muscular strength and endurance exercises. The candidate will discuss the necessary preparation for the testing site and equipment, including emergency procedures, testing environment, and the preparation of equipment. The candidate will also explain the informed consent, including the benefits and risks of the test. The candidate will explain and demonstrate proper procedures before, during, and after the exercise test, including the measurement of heart rate, blood pressure, and the use of perceived exertion. The candidate will administer selected segments of a submaximal graded exercise test. The *ACSM Health/Fitness Instructor Study Packet* includes complete information regarding the protocols to be utilized and references for further study.

A multiday workshop may be conducted in conjunction with the ACSM Health/Fitness Instructor Certification exam. The purposes of the workshops are to provide a forum for the acquisition of new knowledge and the updating of techniques and skills. Workshops are not a prerequisite for certification, nor are they intended to provide the full experience and knowledge necessary for the examination. Workshops are designed to provide a review of the principles for ACSM Health/Fitness Instructor. There are no prerequisites to attend the workshop. However, the program content is based on scientific principles of exercise physiology, nutrition and weight control, exercise programming, emergency procedures, health appraisal and fitness evaluation techniques, exercise psychology, human development and aging, functional anatomy and kinesiology, and risk-factor identification.

Participants should have prior experience and competence in monitoring heart rate and blood pressure, both at rest and during exercise. Blood pressure training sessions are usually available from the local chapter of the American Heart Association if additional training is warranted. Experience in leading an exercise class, providing basic counseling skills, and demonstrating knowledge of functional anatomy and exercise physiology are also expected prior to attendance. Workshop candidates must complete the PAR-Q & YOU form in the application and must send it directly to the workshop site.

The study packet includes information regarding the written and practical components of the examination, reference materials for further study, as well as the specific protocols that will be utilized. However, all candidates are encouraged to purchase *ACSM's Guidelines for Exercise Testing and Prescription,* 5th edition; and ACSM's *Resource Manual for Guidelines for Exercise Testing and Prescription* (3rd edition), 1998. Both are published by Williams & Wilkins, PO Box 64380, Baltimore, MD 21264-4380. The guidelines are available for $23.95 (U.S. funds only). The resource manual is available for $55 (U.S. funds only). To order, call 800-638-0672; outside the continental United States call 410-528-4223 for foreign distributors and rates.

Separate fees have been established for the ACSM Health/Fitness Instructor workshop, certification, written retest, and practical retest. All fees must accompany applications and must be paid by check or money order, made payable to ACSM.

Workshop Fee: $280

Certification Fee: $170 ACSM member;
$220 non–ACSM member

Retest Fee: $30 written; $100 practical

Workshop participants must provide the following:

- Submit a completed written application for the optional workshop of choice. The application must be received by ACSM at least 30 days prior to the scheduled date of the workshop. Mail to the ACSM National Center.

- Submit a PAR-Q & YOU form (enclosed) for each workshop candidate. This form must be mailed to the workshop site director of your first choice.

Certification candidates must provide the following:

- Submit a completed written application. Applications and one photocopy of the application must be postmarked 30 days prior to the start of the certification session. Apply as early as possible to ensure your primary choice.

- Mail the materials to the ACSM National Center: ACSM National Center, Certification Department, PO Box 1440, Indianapolis, IN 46206-1440.

SUMMARY

1. The American College of Sports Medicine takes the position that candidates for an exercise program or testing for physical fitness status be categorized as "apparently healthy," "at increased risk," or "with known disease."

2. A medical/health status questionnaire should be used for such ACSM classification.

3. Depending on the ACSM risk stratification and the type of exercise program planned (moderate versus vigorous), Table 3.2 summarizes ACSM recommendations for preexercise medical exams and diagnostic exercise testing.

4. Various relative and absolute contraindications to exercise have been submitted by ACSM. Physicians are responsible for diagnosing the presence and significance of these factors for those planning to start an exercise program.

5. We live in an increasingly litigious society. Proper informed-consent forms and the adoption of appropriate strategies for reducing liability exposure are needed.

6. The function of measurement is to determine health and fitness status. Tests should be valid, reliable, have sound norms, and be economical in terms of money, time, and testing expertise.

Box 3.3

Ten of the Most Prominent Certifying Organizations in the Health/Fitness Industry

Three criteria are often used to judge whether one is qualified to assist someone on basic health, wellness, and exercise-related issues:[43, 44]

1. Formal academic preparation
2. Professional experience
3. Professional certification

It has been estimated that more than 60 organizations offer some form of certification for health and fitness professionals. A list of 10 of the more prominent certifying organizations is presented here. Certification is recommended to gain a competitive advantage in the hiring process and to stay abreast of issues related to health and fitness.

Aerobics and Fitness Association of America (AFAA). Offers two types of certification: primary certification and emergency-response certification. Contact: 800-446-2322.

American College of Sports Medicine (ACSM). Offers three levels of certification within two specific tracks: a clinical track and a health and fitness track. Contact: 317-637-9200.

American Council on Exercise (ACE). Offers three types of certification: aerobics, personal trainer, and the lifestyle and weight-management consultant. Contact: 800-529-8227.

International Sports Sciences Association (ISSA). Offers certification in six different subject areas: personal training, sports nutrition, sports conditioning, therapeutic and rehabilitation exercise, fitness for physically challenged individuals, and youth fitness. Contact: 800-892-4772.

International Weightlifting Association (IWA). Offers certification in strength training. Contact: 216-655-9644.

National Academy of Sports Medicine (NASM). Offers a professional certification course for personal fitness trainers. Contact: 312-929-5101.

National Dance-Exercise Instructor's Training Association (NDEITA). Offers certification for aerobics instructors. Contact: 800-237-6242.

National Federation of Professional Trainers (NFPT). Offers certification in personal training. Contact: 800-729-6378.

National Strength and Conditioning Association (NSCA). Offers certification for two groups: strength and conditioning professionals and personal trainers. Contact: 402-476-6669, ext. 115.

Young Men's Christian Association (YMCA). Offers 10 levels of health and fitness certification: fitness leader, fitness instructor, strength training instructor, strength training director, youth fitness, healthy back instructor, prenatal and postpartum exercise instructor, fitness walking instructor, and weight-management consultant. Contact: 312-269-0520.

Source: Peterson JA, Bryant CX, Stevenson R. Making professional certification work for your facility. *Fitness Management,* July 1996, 36–38. Copyright © 1996 Leisure Publications, Inc., Los Angeles, CA.

---

7. Physical fitness tests have several purposes, including assessment of status, identification of special needs, evaluation of progress, and motivation.

8. Evaluation procedures should follow a certain order for both safety and efficiency.

9. The YMCA, Canadian Society for Exercise Physiology, AAHPERD, Cooper Institute for Aerobics Research, and President's Council on Physical Fitness and Sports have developed health-related physical fitness testing batteries.

REFERENCES

1. American College of Sports Medicine. *ACSM's Guidelines for Graded Exercise Testing and Prescription* (5th ed.). Baltimore: Williams & Wilkins, 1995.

2. American College of Sports Medicine; Sol N, Foster C (eds). *Health/Fitness Facility Standards and Guidelines.* Champaign, IL: Human Kinetics, 1992.

3. Fletcher GF, Balady G, Froelicher VF, Hartley LH, Haskell WL, Pollock ML. Exercise standards: A statement for healthcare professionals from the American Heart Association. *Circulation* 91:580–615, 1995.

4. American College of Sports Medicine. *ACSM's Resource Manual for Guidelines for Exercise Testing and Prescription* (3rd ed.). Baltimore: Williams & Wilkins, 1998.

5. Shephard RJ, Thomas S, Weller I. The Canadian Home Fitness Test: 1991 update. *Sports Med* 11:358–366, 1991.

6. Shephard RJ. PAR-Q Canadian Home Fitness Test and exercise screening alternatives. *Sports Med* 5:185–195, 1988.

7. Cardinal BJ, Cardinal MK. Screening efficiency of the Revised Physical Activity Readiness Questionnaire in Older Adults. *J Aging Phys Act* 3:299–308, 1995.

8. Cardinal BJ, Esters J, Cardinal MK. Evaluation of the Revised Physical Activity Readiness Questionnaire in Older Adults. *Med Sci Sports Exerc* 28:468–472, 1996.

9. Canadian Society for Exercise Physiology. *The Canadian Physical Activity, Fitness & Lifestyle Appraisal.* Ottawa, Ontario: Canadian Society for Exercise Physiology, 1996.

10. Kohl HW, Gibbons LW, Gordon NF, Blair SN. An empirical evaluation of the ACSM guidelines for exercise testing. *Med Sci Sports Exerc* 22:533–539, 1990.

11. Gibbons RJ, Balady GJ, Beasley JW, et al. ACC/AHA Guidelines for Exercise Testing: Executive Summary. A report of the American College of Cardiology/American Heart Association task force on practice guidelines (Committee on Exercise Testing). *Circulation* 96:345–354, 1997.

12. Sharkey BJ. *Physiology of Fitness.* Champaign, IL: Human Kinetics, 1979, 60.

13. Maron BJ, Shirani J, Poliac LC, Mathenge R, Roberts WC, Mueller FO. Sudden death in young competitive athletes: Clinical, demographic, and pathological profiles. *JAMA* 276: 199–204, 1996.

14. American Heart Association. Cardiovascular preparticipation screening of competitive athletes. *Circulation* 94:850–856, 1996.

15. Thompson PD. The cardiovascular complications of vigorous physical activity. *Arch Intern Med* 156:2297–2302, 1996.

16. Herbert DL. *Legal Aspects of Sports Medicine* (2nd ed.). Canton, OH: PRC Publishing, Inc., 1995.

17. Herbert DL. Practice guidelines take center court. *Physician Sportsmed* 24(3):81–87.

18. Herbert DL. Cardio exercise death results in costly verdict. *Fitness Management*, March 1996, 46.

19. Herbert DL. GXT use raises more litigation. *Fitness Management*, August 1994, 21, 22.

20. Herbert DL. Release form clarification. *Fitness Management*, September 1996, 22.

21. Herbert DL. Failure to enforce policy may lead to suit. *Fitness Management*, February 1997, 42.

22. Herbert DL. Health club release upheld in the state of Washington. *Fitness Management*, May 1997, 36.

23. Sloan J, Resnick GD. The consent form revisited. *Arch Intern Med* 153:1170–1173, 1993.

24. Tharrett SJ, Peterson JA. *ACSM's Health/Fitness Facility Standards and Guidelines* (2nd ed.). Champaign, IL: Human Kinetics, 1997.

25. Peterson JA, Tharrett SJ. How and why the ACSM standards were revised. *Fitness Management*, July 1997, 43–46.

26. Herbert DL. Legal implications of ACSM's new facility standards & guidelines. *Fitness Management*, August 1997, 20.

27. Maud PJ, Foster C. *Physiological Assessment of Human Fitness.* Champaign, IL: Human Kinetics, 1995.

28. Clarke HH. *Application of Measurement to Health and Physical Education.* Englewood Cliffs: Prentice-Hall, Inc., 1967.

29. Johnson BL, Nelson JK. *Practical Measurements for Evaluation in Physical Education.* Minneapolis: Burgess Publishing Co., 1979.

30. Pate RR, Hohn RC. *Health and Fitness through Physical Education.* Champaign IL: Human Kinetics, 1994.

31. Golding LA, Myers CR, Sinning WE. *The Y's Way to Physical Fitness* (4th ed.). Champaign, IL: Human Kinetics, 1998.

32. Nieman DC. The exercise test as a component of the total fitness evaluation. *Prim Care* 21:569–587, 1994.

33. Franks B. *YMCA Youth Fitness Test Manual.* Champaign, IL: Human Kinetics, 1989.

34. *Canadian Standardized Test of Fitness (CSTF) Operations Manual* (3rd ed.) (for 15 to 69 years of age). Ottawa, Ontario: Fitness and Amateur Sport, 1987.

35. Institute for Aerobics Research. *The Strength Connection.* Dallas: Author, 1990.

36. Pate RR. *Norms for College Students: Health Related Physical Fitness Test.* Reston, VA: American Alliance for Health, Physical Education, Recreation, and Dance, 1985.

37. Ross JG. Summary of findings from National Children and Youth Fitness Study. *JOPERD*, January 1985, 4–90.

38. Ross JG, Pate RR. The National Children and Youth Fitness Study II: A summary of findings. *JOPERD*, November/December 1987, 51–56.

39. AAHPERD. *Physical Best: The American Alliance Physical Fitness Education & Assessment Program.* Reston, VA: American Alliance for Health, Physical Education, Recreation, and Dance, 1988.

40. Cooper Institute for Aerobics Research. *The Prudential FITNESSGRAM.* Dallas: Author, 1992.

41. President's Council on Physical Fitness and Sports. *Youth Physical Fitness in 1985: The President's Council on Physical Fitness and Sports School Population Fitness Survey.* Washington, DC: President's Council on Physical Fitness and Sports, 1985.

42. President's Council on Physical Fitness and Sports. *Get Fit: A Handbook for Youth Ages 6–17.* Washington, DC: Author, 1993.

43. Peterson JA, Bryant CX, Stevenson R. Making professional certification work for your facility. *Fitness Management*, July 1996, 36–38.

44. DuBois PC. Certification: How to spot the real thing. *Fitness Management*, August 1995, 46–48.

PHYSICAL FITNESS ACTIVITY 3.1

Are You Ready to Exercise?

NAME _____

Age _____

Sex ____ M ____ F

1. Turn to the questionnaire on the following page (*Pre-exercise Test/Program Health Questionnaire*), and carefully answer all of the questions.

2. Based on your questionnaire responses, in what ACSM category would you put yourself (see Table 3.1)? For example, if you did not check any of the blanks under "suggestive symptoms" or "known diseases," and you checked no more than one of the blanks under "heart disease risk factors," then you are categorized as "apparently healthy." If you did not check any of the blanks under "known diseases" but did check at least one blank under "suggestive symptoms" or two or more blanks under "heart disease risk factors," then you are classified as an "individual at increased risk." If you checked any of the blanks under "known disease," then you are an "individual with disease."

    _____ Apparently healthy

    _____ Individual at increased risk

    _____ Individual with disease

3. Based on your ACSM category, and whether you plan to exercise moderately or vigorously, what guidelines for exercise testing and participation apply to you (from Table 3.2)?

    _____

    _____

    _____

    _____

    _____

    _____

    _____

4. Do you need a medical exam and diagnostic exercise test prior to starting your exercise program?

    _____ Yes

    _____ No

Pre-exercise Test/Program Health Questionnaire

Suggestive Symptoms

Put a check in blank if your answer is "yes."

_____ Have you experienced unusual pain or discomfort in your chest (pain due to blockage in coronary arteries of heart)?

_____ Have you experienced unusual shortness of breath during moderate exercise (such as climbing stairs)?

_____ Have you had any problems with dizziness or fainting?

_____ When you stand up, or sometimes during the night, do you have difficulty breathing?

_____ Do you suffer from swelling of the ankles (ankle edema)?

_____ Have you experienced a rapid throbbing or fluttering of the heart?

_____ Have you experienced severe pain in your leg muscles during walking?

_____ Has a doctor told you that you have a heart murmur?

_____ Have you felt unusual fatigue or shortness of breath with usual activities?

Heart Disease Risk Factors

Check those that apply to you.*

_____ Are you a male over age 45 years, or a female over age 55 years; or a female who has experienced premature menopause and is not on estrogen replacement therapy?

_____ Has your father or brother had a heart attack or died suddenly of heart disease before age 55 years; has your mother or sister experienced these heart problems before age 65 years?

_____ Are you a current cigarette smoker?

_____ Is your blood pressure over 140/90 mm Hg, or are you on medication to control your blood pressure?

_____ Is your total serum cholesterol greater than 240 mg/dL?

_____ Do you have diabetes mellitus?

_____ Are you physically inactive and sedentary (little physical exercise on the job or after work)?

Known Diseases

Check those that apply to you.

_____ Do you have a personal history of heart disease?

_____ Do you have a personal history of kidney, liver, or thyroid disease?

_____ Are you a long-term diabetic (over age 30 with a long history of this disease)?

---

*If your HDL cholesterol is 60 mg/dl, count this as a positive factor. For example, if you are a 60-year-old male with high blood pressure (2 risk factors), but also have an HDL cholesterol of 60 mg/dl, your net count is only 1.

PHYSICAL FITNESS ACTIVITY 3.2

Medical/Health Questionnaire

According to the American College of Sports Medicine, a medical examination and clinical exercise test is recommended prior to (1) moderate exercise training for those at increased risk for disease with symptoms, or those with known disease; (2) vigorous exercise training for older apparently healthy individuals, those at increased risk for disease (with or without symptoms), or (3) patients with known disease.[1] ACSM recommends that the pretest medical history be thorough and include 11 components: medical diagnoses, previous physical examination findings, history of symptoms, recent illness, hospitalization or surgical procedures, orthopedic problems, medication use and drug allergies, lifestyle habits, exercise history, work history, and family history of disease. The following medical and health questionnaire meets these criteria and can be used to gain a useful history on clients at fitness testing facilities located in worksites, hospitals, and universities. In this activity, select a faculty member or member of the community that you feel would benefit from this process. Have the person answer the questions in the medical questionnaire, and then summarize important findings in the following blanks.

1. Symptoms or signs of disease: _____

_____

_____

_____

2. Chronic disease risk factors: _____

_____

_____

_____

3. Personal and family medical history: _____

_____

_____

_____

4. Medications: _____

_____

_____

_____

_____

5. Summary of lifestyle habits: _____

_____

_____

_____

Medical/Health Questionnaire

Personal Information

Today's Date _____   Please print your name _____

How old are you? _____ years   Sex ❑ Male; ❑ Female

Please circle the highest grade in school you have completed:

Elementary school   1   2   3   4   5   6   7   8

High school   9   10   11   12

College/Postgrad   13   14   15   16   17   18   19   20+

What is your marital status? ❑ Single; ❑ Married; ❑ Widowed; ❑ Divorced/Separated

Race or ethnic background:

❑ White, not of Hispanic origin   ❑ American Indian/Alaskan native   ❑ Asian

❑ Black, not of Hispanic origin   ❑ Pacific Islander   ❑ Hispanic

What is your job or occupation? Check the one that applies to the greatest percentage of your time.

❑ Health professional   ❑ Disabled, unable to work   ❑ Service

❑ Manager, educator, professional   ❑ Operator, fabricator, laborer   ❑ Unemployed

❑ Skilled crafts   ❑ Homemaker   ❑ Student

❑ Technical, sales, support   ❑ Retired   ❑ Other

Symptoms or Signs Suggestive of Disease

Place a check in the box if your answer is "yes."

❑ 1. Have you experienced unusual pain or discomfort in your chest, neck, jaw, arms, or other areas that may be due to heart problems?

❑ 2. Have you experienced unusual fatigue or shortness of breath at rest, during usual activities, or during mild-to-moderate exercise (e.g., climbing stairs, carrying groceries, brisk walking, cycling)?

❑ 3. Have you had any problems with dizziness or fainting?

❑ 4. When you stand up, or sometimes during the night while you are sleeping, do you have difficulty breathing?

❑ 5. Do you suffer from swelling of the ankles (ankle edema)?

❑ 6. Have you experienced an unusual and rapid throbbing or fluttering of the heart?

❑ 7. Have you experienced severe pain in your leg muscles during walking?

❑ 8. Has a doctor told you that you have a heart murmur?

Chronic Disease Risk Factors

Place a check in the box if your answer is "yes."

❑ 9. Are you a male over age 45 years, or a female over age 55 years, or a female who has experienced premature menopause and is not on estrogen replacement therapy?

❑ 10. Has your father or brother had a heart attack or died suddenly of heart disease before age 55 years; has your mother or sister experienced these heart problems before age 65 years?

❑ 11. Are you a current cigarette smoker?

❑ 12. Has a doctor told you that you have high blood pressure (more than 140/90 mm Hg), or are you on medication to control your blood pressure?

❑ 13. Is your total serum cholesterol greater than 240 mg/dl, or has a doctor told you that your cholesterol is at a high-risk level?

❑ 14. Do you have diabetes mellitus?

❑ 15. Are you physically inactive and sedentary (little physical activity on the job or during leisure time)?

❑ 16. During the past year, would you say that you experienced enough stress, strain, and pressure to have a significant effect on your health?

❑ 17. Do you eat foods nearly every day that are high in fat and cholesterol such as fatty meats, cheese, fried foods, butter, whole milk, or eggs?

Chronic Disease Risk Factors (continued)

❏ **18.** Do you tend to avoid foods that are high in fiber such as whole-grain breads and cereals, fresh fruits or vegetables?

❏ **19.** Do you weigh 30 or more pounds more than you should?

❏ **20.** Do you average more than two alcoholic drinks each day?

Medical History

21. *Please check which of the following conditions you have had or now have. Also check medical conditions in your family (father, mother, brother(s), or sister(s)). Check as many as apply.*

Personal	Family	Medical Condition
❏	❏	Coronary heart disease, heart attack, coronary artery surgery
❏	❏	Angina
❏	❏	High blood pressure
❏	❏	Peripheral vascular disease
❏	❏	Phlebitis or emboli
❏	❏	Other heart problems (specify: _____)
❏	❏	Lung cancer
❏	❏	Breast cancer
❏	❏	Prostate cancer
❏	❏	Colorectal cancer (bowel cancer)
❏	❏	Skin cancer
❏	❏	Other cancer (specify: _____)
❏	❏	Stroke
❏	❏	Chronic obstructive pulmonary disease (emphysema)
❏	❏	Pneumonia
❏	❏	Asthma
❏	❏	Bronchitis
❏	❏	Diabetes mellitus
❏	❏	Thyroid problems
❏	❏	Kidney disease
❏	❏	Liver disease (cirrhosis of the liver)
❏	❏	Hepatitis
❏	❏	Gallstones / gallbladder disease
❏	❏	Osteoporosis
❏	❏	Arthritis
❏	❏	Gout
❏	❏	Anemia (low iron)
❏	❏	Bone fracture
❏	❏	Major injury to foot, leg, knee, hip, or shoulder
❏	❏	Major injury to back or neck
❏	❏	Stomach / duodenal ulcer
❏	❏	Rectal growth or bleeding
❏	❏	Cataracts
❏	❏	Glaucoma
❏	❏	Hearing loss
❏	❏	Depression
❏	❏	High anxiety, phobias
❏	❏	Substance abuse problems (alcohol, other drugs, etc.)
❏	❏	Eating disorders (anorexia, bulimia)

❏	❏	Problems with menstruation
❏	❏	Hysterectomy
❏	❏	Sleeping problems
❏	❏	Allergies
❏	❏	Any other health problems (please specify, and include information on any recent illnesses, hospitalizations, or surgical procedures):

_____

_____

22. *Please check any of the following medications you currently take regularly. Also give the name of the medication.*

Medication	**Name of Medication**
❏ Heart medicine	_____
❏ Blood pressure medicine	_____
❏ Blood cholesterol medicine	_____
❏ Hormones	_____
❏ Birth control pills	_____
❏ Medicine for breathing / lungs	_____
❏ Insulin	_____
❏ Other medicine for diabetes	_____
❏ Arthritis medicine	_____
❏ Medicine for depression	_____
❏ Medicine for anxiety	_____
❏ Thyroid medicine	_____
❏ Medicine for ulcers	_____
❏ Painkiller medicine	_____
❏ Allergy medicine	_____
❏ Other (please specify)	_____

Physical Fitness, Physical Activity/Exercise

23. In general, compared to other persons your age, rate how physically fit you are:

1 ❏   2 ❏   3 ❏   4 ❏   5 ❏   6 ❏   7 ❏   8 ❏   9 ❏   10 ❏

Not at all   Somewhat   Extremely
physically fit   physically fit   physically fit

24. Outside of your normal work or daily responsibilities, how often do you engage in exercise that at least moderately increases your breathing and heart rate and makes you sweat, for at least 20 minutes (such as brisk walking, cycling, swimming, jogging, aerobic dance, stair climbing, rowing, basketball, racquetball, vigorous yard work).

❏ 5 or more times per week   ❏ 3–4 times per week   ❏ 1–2 times per week

❏ Less than 1 time per week   ❏ Seldom or never

25. How much hard physical work is required on your job?

❏ A great deal   ❏ A moderate amount   ❏ A little   ❏ None

Physical Fitness, Physical Activity Exercise (continued)

26. How long have you exercised or played sports regularly?

❏ I do not exercise regularly   ❏ Less than 1 year   ❏ 1–2 years

❏ 2–5 years   ❏ 5–10 years   ❏ More than 10 years

Diet

27. On average, how many servings of fruit do you eat per day? (One serving = 1 medium apple, banana, orange, etc.; ½ cup of chopped, cooked, or canned fruit; ¾ cup of fruit juice).

❏ None   ❏ 1   ❏ 2   ❏ 3   ❏ 4 or more

28. On average, how many servings of vegetables do you eat per day? (One serving = ½ cup cooked or chopped raw, 1 cup raw leafy, ¾ cup of vegetable juice).

❏ None   ❏ 1–2   ❏ 3   ❏ 4   ❏ 5 or more

29. On average, how many servings of bread, cereal, rice, or pasta do you eat per day? (One serving = 1 slice of bread, 1 ounce of ready-to-eat cereal, ½ cup of cooked cereal, rice, or pasta).

❏ None   ❏ 1–3   ❏ 4–6   ❏ 7–9   ❏ 10 or more

30. When you use grain and cereal products, do you emphasize:

❏ Whole grain, high fiber   ❏ Mixture of whole grain and refined   ❏ Refined, low fiber

31. On average, how many servings of red meat (not lean) do you eat per day? (One serving = 2–3 ounces of steak, roast beef, lamb, pork chops, ham, burgers, etc.).

❏ None   ❏ 1   ❏ 2   ❏ 3   ❏ 4 or more

32. On average, how many servings of fish, poultry, lean meat, cooked dry beans, peanut butter, or nuts do you eat per day? (One serving = 2–3 ounces of meat, ½ cup of cooked dry beans, two tablespoons of peanut butter, or ⅓ cup of nuts).

❏ None   ❏ 1   ❏ 2   ❏ 3   ❏ 4 or more

33. On average, how many servings of dairy products do you eat per day? (One serving = 1 cup of milk or yogurt, 1.5 ounces of natural cheese, 2 ounces of processed cheese).

❏ None   ❏ 1   ❏ 2   ❏ 3   ❏ 4 or more

34. When you use dairy products, do you emphasize

❏ Regular   ❏ Low fat   ❏ Nonfat

35. How would you characterize your intake of fats and oils (e.g., regular salad dressings, butter or margarine, mayonnaise, vegetable oils).

❏ High   ❏ Moderate   ❏ Low

Body Weight

36. How tall are you (without shoes)? _____ feet _____ inches

37. How much do you weigh (minimal clothing and without shoes)? _____ pounds

38. What is the most you have ever weighed? _____ pounds

39. Are you *now* trying to

❏ Lose weight   ❏ Gain weight   ❏ Stay about the same   ❏ Not trying to do anything

Psychological Health

40. How have you been feeling in general during the past month?

❏ In excellent spirits   ❏ In very good spirits

❏ In good spirits mostly   ❏ I've been up and down in spirits a lot

❏ In low spirits mostly   ❏ In very low spirits

41. During the past month, would you say that you experienced _____ stress?

❏ A lot of   ❏ Moderate   ❏ Relatively little   ❏ Almost none

42. In the past year, how much effect has stress had on your health:

❏ A lot   ❏ Some   ❏ Hardly any or none

43. On average, how many hours of sleep do you get in a 24-hour period?

❏ Less than 5   ❏ 5–6.9   ❏ 7–9   ❏ More than 9

Substance Use

44. Have you smoked at least 100 cigarettes in your entire life?

❏ Yes   ❏ No

45. How would you describe your cigarette smoking habits?

❏ Never smoked

❏ Used to smoke
   How many years has it been since you smoked? _____ *years*

❏ Still smoke
   How many cigarettes a day do you smoke on average? _____ *cigarettes/day*

46. How many alcoholic drinks do you consume? (A "drink" is a glass of wine, a wine cooler, a bottle/can of beer, a shot glass of liquor, or a mixed drink).

❏ Never use alcohol   ❏ Less than 1 per week   ❏ 1–6 per week

❏ 1 per day   ❏ 2–3 per day   ❏ More than 3 per day

Occupational Health

47. Please describe your main job duties.

_____

_____

	All of the time	Most of the time	Some of the time	Rarely or never
48. After a day's work, do you often have pain or stiffness that lasts for more than 3 hours?	❏	❏	❏	❏
49. How often does your work entail repetitive pushing and pulling movements or lifting while bending or twisting, leading to back pain?	❏	❏	❏	❏

CHAPTER

4

Cardiorespiratory Fitness

An exercise test is often used to evaluate the safety of an exercise training program and is useful in formulating an exercise prescription. In general, a sedentary individual who at the age of 40 years decides to enter an exercise program of a higher intensity than walking at 50% to 60% of maximum heart rate reserve should undergo an exercise test. Testing should also be recommended for younger individuals with coronary risk factors or a strong family history of coronary artery disease.

—American Heart Association[1]

The laboratory test generally regarded as the best measure of heart and lung endurance is the direct measurement of oxygen uptake during maximal exercise.[1–4] The exercise is usually performed using a bicycle ergometer or treadmill, which allows the progressive increase in workload from light-to-exhaustive (maximal) exercise. The amount of oxygen consumed during the exercise test is measured using various methods (douglas bag collection of expired air, mixing box and gas-flow meter, or computerized metabolic carts).[5] (See Figure 4.1.) New portable metabolic systems that can be strapped to the chest have been developed, which should revolutionize measurement of oxygen consumption outside of laboratory settings.[6] Measurement of $\dot{V}O_{2max}$ should be specific to the sport practiced by the individual being tested because of the very unique muscular, circulatory, and metabolic adaptations that occur.

Maximal oxygen uptake ($\dot{V}O_{2max}$) is defined as the greatest rate at which oxygen can be consumed during exercise or the maximal rate at which oxygen can be taken up, distributed, and used by the body during physical activity.[5] ("$\dot{V}$" is the volume used per minute, "O_2" is oxygen, and "max" represents maximal exercise conditions.)[1–5]

$\dot{V}O_{2max}$ is usually expressed in terms of milliliters of oxygen consumed per kilogram of body weight per minute ($ml \cdot kg^{-1} \cdot min^{-1}$). By factoring in body weight, it becomes possible to compare the $\dot{V}O_{2max}$ of people of varying size in different environments. It should be noted that expressing $\dot{V}O_{2max}$ in $ml \cdot kg^{-1} \cdot min^{-1}$ may unfairly underestimate the aerobic fitness of individuals with large amounts of body fat.[7]

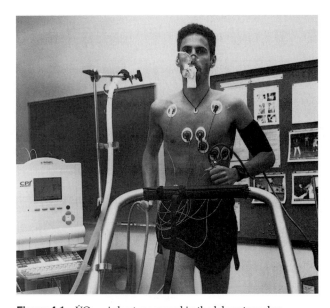

Figure 4.1 $\dot{V}O_{2max}$ is best measured in the laboratory during a maximal exercise test in which the oxygen consumed is measured by a computerized metabolic cart.

A high level of $\dot{V}O_{2max}$ depends on the proper functioning of three important systems in the body:

1. The *respiratory system*, which takes up oxygen from the air in the lungs and transports it into the blood
2. The *cardiovascular system*, which pumps and distributes the oxygen-laden blood throughout the body

3. The *musculoskeletal system,* which uses the oxygen to convert stored carbohydrates and fats into adenosine triphosphate (ATP) for muscle contraction and heat production[5]

In the laboratory, several criteria are used to determine whether an individual's true $\dot{V}O_{2max}$ has been achieved:[8,9]

- Oxygen consumption plateaus during the last minutes of a graded exercise test (defined as a rise of less than 2 ml $\cdot$ kg^{-1} $\cdot$ min^{-1} between the final test stages).

- The *respiratory exchange ratio* (RER) (ratio of the volume of carbon dioxide produced to the volume of oxygen consumed) increases to 1.15 or higher.

- The subject's heart rate increases to within 10 beats of the age-predicted maximum (maximum heart rate is estimated by subtracting the age from 220).

- Blood lactate levels rise above 8 mmol / liter.

Laboratory measurement of $\dot{V}O_{2max}$ is expensive and time-consuming, requires highly trained personnel, and therefore is not practical for most testing situations. Various formulas and tests have been developed as substitutes and are the focus of this chapter:

- Nonexercise test $\dot{V}O_{2max}$ prediction equations
- Field tests of cardiorespiratory endurance
- Submaximal laboratory tests
- Maximal laboratory tests

It is assumed that before these tests are conducted, the preliminary considerations outlined in the previous chapter have been attended to (medical / health status questionnaire, consent form, and for those at high risk, a physical examination by a physician, treadmill test, and possibly a blood lipid analysis). It is also assumed that the order outlined for each testing battery is followed, with subjects following the appropriate pretest preparation routine (abstention from food, tobacco, alcohol, and caffeine for 3 hours, proper hydration, comfortable exercise clothes, adequate sleep, and avoidance of exercise the day of the test).

RESTING AND EXERCISE BLOOD PRESSURE AND HEART RATE DETERMINATION

When conducting a bicycle or treadmill test, the tester should include heart rate, blood pressure, and electrocardiogram (ECG) monitoring on all high-risk individuals. The test can then be used for determination of both cardiorespiratory fitness and potential health problems such as high blood pressure and heart disease (as diagnosed by a physician). Although blood pressure and ECG monitoring is not necessary when testing apparently healthy subjects, some testing facilities do it as an extra precaution.

Resting Blood Pressure

Blood pressure is the force of blood against the walls of the arteries and veins created by the heart as it pumps blood to every part of the body. *Hypertension* is simply a condition in which the blood pressure is chronically elevated above optimal levels. The 1997 Joint National Committee on Detection, Evaluation, and Treatment of High Blood Pressure has established blood pressure classifications.[10] (See Table 4.1.)

Hypertension is diagnosed for adults when *diastolic* measurements (blood pressure when the heart is resting) on at least two separate visits average 90 mm Hg or higher, and / or systolic measurements (while the heart is beating) are 140 mm Hg or higher. There are three stages of hypertension, with stage 3 diagnosed when measurements are equal to or greater than 180 / 100 mm Hg. High normal blood pressure (130–139 / 85–89 mm Hg) is included as a separate category because this is now considered to be a risk factor for future hypertension and cardiovascular disease.[10] Recommended follow-up testing procedures for hypertension are given in Table 4.2.

As many as 50 million people in the United States have hypertension.[10] Prevalence increases with age and is higher among blacks than whites[11] (see Figure 4.2). (See Chapter 10 for more information on hypertension.) Health-care professionals are urged to measure blood pressure at each patient visit.

To take the resting blood pressure, a sphygmomanometer and a stethoscope are needed.[12–14] The *sphygmomanometer* consists of an inflatable compression bag enclosed in an unyielding covering called the cuff, plus an inflating bulb, a manometer from which the pressure is read, and a controlled exhaust valve to deflate the system. The *stethoscope* is made of rubber tubing attached to a device that amplifies the sounds of blood passing through the blood vessels (see Figure 4.3). This equipment can be obtained in most drug stores for about $30, though more expensive blood pressure equipment is available.

Those taking blood pressure should be trained by qualified instructors. For each patient, blood pressure should be measured two or three times until consistency is achieved. A single blood pressure reading does not provide an accurate measure.[12–14] Several blood pressure readings by different observers, or on different occasions by the same observer, are recommended to check the validity of initially high values.

For best results in taking blood pressure:[12–14]

- Measurements should be taken with a mercury-stand sphygmomanometer, a recently calibrated aneroid manometer, or a validated electronic device. Aneroid

TABLE 4.1   Blood Pressure Classifications

Category[a]	Systolic (mm Hg)		Diastolic (mm Hg)
Optimal[b]	<120	and	<80
Normal	<130	and	<85
High normal	130–139	or	85–89
Hypertension[c]			
Stage 1	140–159	or	90–99
Stage 2	160–179	or	100–109
Stage 3	≥180	or	≥110

[a]Not taking antihypertensive drugs and not acutely ill. When systolic and diastolic blood pressures fall into different categories, the higher category should be selected to classify the individual's blood pressure status. For example, 160/92 mm Hg should be classified as stage 2 hypertension, and 174/120 mm Hg should be classified as stage 3 hypertension. Isolated systolic hypertension is defined as SBP of 140 mm Hg or greater and DBP below 90 mm Hg and staged appropriately (e.g., 170/82 mm Hg is defined as stage 2 isolated systolic hypertension). In addition to classifying stages of hypertension on the basis of average blood pressure levels, clinicians should specify presence or absence of target organ disease and additional risk factors. This specificity is important for risk classification and treatment.
[b]Optimal blood pressure with respect to cardiovascular risk is below 120/80 mm Hg. However, unusually low readings should be evaluated for clinical significance.
[c]Based on the average of two or more readings taken at each of two or more visits after an initial screening.

Source: National High Blood Pressure Education Program. *The Sixth Report of the Joint National Committee on Detection, Evaluation, and Treatment of High Blood Pressure.* National Heart, Lung, and Blood Institute, National Institutes of Health, NIH Publication No. 98-4080. Bethesda, MD: National Institutes of Health, 1997.

TABLE 4.2   Recommended Follow-up Testing for Hypertension

Initial Blood Pressure (mm Hg)[a]		Follow-up Recommended[b]
Systolic	Diastolic	
<130	<85	Recheck in 2 years
130–139	85–89	Recheck in 1 year[c]
140–159	90–99	Confirm within 2 months[c]
160–179	100–109	Evaluate or refer to source of care within 1 month
≥180	≥110	Evaluate or refer to source of care immediately or within 1 week, depending on clinical situation

[a]If systolic and diastolic categories are different, follow recommendations for shorter time follow-up (e.g., 160/86 mm Hg should be evaluated or referred to source of care within 1 month).
[b]Modify the scheduling of follow-up according to reliable information about past blood pressure measurements, other cardiovascular risk factors, or target organ disease.
[c]Provide advice about lifestyle modifications.

Source: National High Blood Pressure Education Program. *The Sixth Report of the Joint National Committee on Detection, Evaluation, and Treatment of High Blood Pressure.* National Heart, Lung, and Blood Institute, National Institutes of Health, NIH Publication No. 98-4080. Bethesda, MD: National Institutes of Health, 1997.

and electronic devices should be checked against a mercury manometer at least once a year.

- Two or more readings should be taken 30–60 seconds apart, and averaged. If the first two readings differ by more than 5 mm Hg, additional readings should be obtained.

- Take the measurement in a quiet room with the temperature approximately 70–74° Fahrenheit (21–23° C).

- Having the upper arm bare makes it easier to adjust the cuff.

- With older people, because of potential arterial obstructions, it is best to take readings on both arms. If the pressures differ by more than 10 mm Hg, obtain simultaneous readings in the two arms and thereafter use the arm with the higher pressure.

- Use the proper size cuff. The rubber bladder should encircle at least 80% of the arm. If the person's arm is large, the adult normal size cuff will be too small (making the reading larger than it actually should be) and the "obese" size bladder is strongly recommended.

- Between determinations, allow at least 30 seconds for normal circulation to return to the arm.

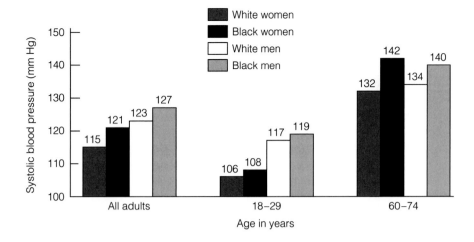

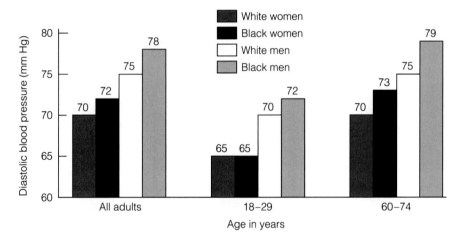

Figure 4.2   Mean systolic (left) and diastolic (right) blood pressure by race, sex, and age. The average blood pressure in the United States varies among subgroups, being higher in blacks versus whites and older versus younger adults.   *Source:* National Health and Nutrition Examination Survey III, 1988–1991.[11]

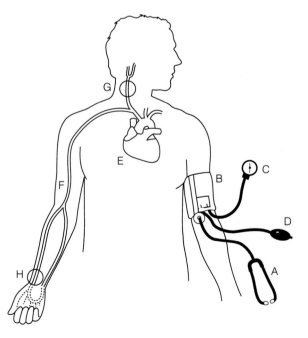

Figure 4.3   Blood pressure is taken with a stethoscope (A) and sphygmomanometer, which consists of an inflatable cuff (B) connected by rubber tubes to a manometer, which measures pressure in millimeters of mercury (C), and a rubber bulb that regulates air during the measurements (D). Blood pressure is the force of blood against the walls of the arteries and veins created by the heart (E) as it pumps. The blood pressure cuff fits over the brachial artery (F). The upper circle (G) represents the common carotid artery, and the lower circle (H) the radial artery, for sensing the heart rate.

- The subject should be comfortably seated, with the arm straight (just slightly flexed), palm up, and the whole forearm supported at heart level on a smooth surface.

- Anxiety, emotional turmoil, food in the stomach, bladder distension, climate variation, exertion, and pain all may influence blood pressure, and when possible, should be controlled or avoided. Heavy exercise or eating should be avoided, and the individual being tested should sit quietly for at least 5 minutes before the test. The tested person should also avoid smoking or ingesting caffeine for at least 30 to 60 minutes prior to measurement. If the individual is on medication for hypertension, the time since the prior dose should be noted (it may be useful to take readings at the end of a dosing interval).

- Place the cuff (deflated) with the lower margin about 1 inch above the inner elbow crease (antecubital space). The rubber bag should be over the brachial artery (in the inner part of the upper arm; see Figure 4.3).

- Place the earpieces of the stethoscope into the ear canals, angled forward to fit snugly. For resting blood pressures, switch the stethoscope head to the bell, or low-frequency, position.

- The stethoscope should be applied lightly just above and medial to the antecubital space (but make sure that the head makes contact with the skin around its entire circumference). Excessive pressure on the stethoscope head can erroneously lower diastolic readings. The stethoscope should not touch clothing, the cuff, or the cuff tubing (to avoid unnecessary rubbing sounds). The tubing should come from the top of the cuff, to avoid interference.

- With the stethoscope in place, the pressure should be raised 20–30 mm Hg above the point at which the pulse sound disappears. (Listen carefully through the stethoscope as the cuff bladder is inflated. The pressure will close off the blood flow in the brachial artery, causing the pulse sound to stop.)

- The pressure should be slowly released at a rate of 2 mm Hg / second or heart beat. Do not go slower than this, however, because it can cause pain and also raise blood pressure.

- As the pressure is released, the blood pressure sounds (the *Korotkoff sounds*) become audible and pass through several phases. Phase 1 (the systolic pressure) is marked by the appearance of faint, clear tapping sounds, which gradually increase in intensity. This represents the blood pressure when the heart is contracting.

- A true systolic blood pressure cannot be obtained unless the Korotkoff sounds are relatively sharp. Korotkoff sounds can be made louder by having the person open and clench the fist five or six times while the arm is raised and then starting over again.

- To obtain the diastolic blood pressure, the following rules should be followed:

    At rest—diastolic blood pressure equals the disappearance of the pulse sound (also called the fifth sound).

    During exercise testing—sometimes the disappearance of sound drops all the way to zero. Therefore, the point at which there is an abrupt muffling sound (fourth phase) should be used for the diastolic blood pressure.

Exercise Blood Pressure

Blood pressure should be taken at least every 3 minutes during exercise testing on the treadmill or bicycle (see Figure 4.4). Several important principles should be followed when taking blood pressure readings during exercise:[15,16]

- If the exercise stages are 3 minutes long (as in the Bruce treadmill protocol, for example), blood pressure readings should be taken at 2 minutes and 15 seconds into each stage. The cuff should be taped onto the person being tested for the entire test, but the inflating bulb should be removed between readings.

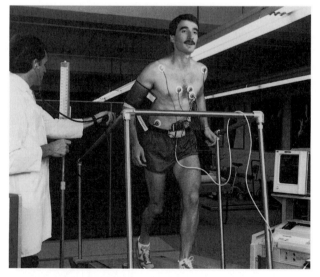

Figure 4.4   Blood pressure determination during exercise is a difficult skill and requires considerable experience. Korotkoff sounds are easier to hear if the tubes are not allowed to rub or bump the subject or the treadmill. The stethoscope head should be attached to the subject's arm. The manometer should be at the level of the subject's heart.

- It is best to stand on a stool and have the person being tested raise their arm to heart level while you support it. The subject's arm should be relaxed and not grasping a treadmill or cycle bar. If you are using a mercury-stand sphygmomanometer, the mercury column should be elevated to the person's heart level.

- Taking blood pressure during exercise is somewhat difficult because of the noise. It is best to raise the cuff pressure quickly until pulse sounds disappear and then, because the heart rate is higher than at rest, let the cuff pressure fall 5–6 mm Hg per second. Try to focus only on the pulse sounds through the stethoscope and keep the various tubes from flapping and rubbing against objects. Keep ambient noise in the testing room to a minimum. If you can't hear the pulse sounds, it may be necessary to stop the test for 15 seconds for a quick blood pressure determination.

- During exertion, the diastolic reading stays basically the same as the resting diastolic, whereas the systolic rises linearly with the increase in workload (see Figure 4.5).

- Peak exercise blood pressures vary according to age and gender[17] (see Figure 4.6).

- If the systolic rises above 260 mm Hg, or the diastolic rises above 115 mm Hg, the test should be terminated.[18] The test should also be stopped if the systolic blood pressure drops with increasing workload.

- During recovery, blood pressure should be taken every 2 to 3 minutes.

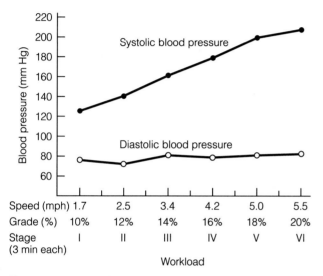

Figure 4.5 Pattern of systolic and diastolic blood pressures during graded exercise testing.

Resting Heart Rate

The resting heart rate can be obtained through *auscultation* (using the bell of the stethoscope), *palpation* (feeling the pulse with your fingers), or ECG recordings. When taking heart rate by auscultation, the bell of the stethoscope is placed to the left of the sternum, just above the level of the nipple. The heart beats (lub-dub) can be counted for 30 seconds and then multiplied by two for beats per minute (bpm).

In using palpation techniques, the pulse is best determined during rest, at the radial artery (lateral aspect of the palm side of the wrist, in line with the base of the thumb) (see Figure 4.3). The tip of the middle and index fingers

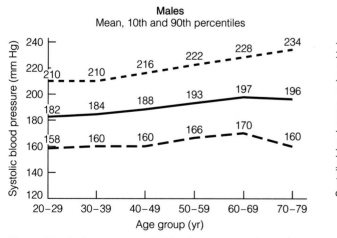

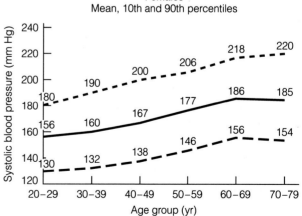

Figure 4.6 Peak exercise systolic blood pressures are higher in men than women, and they increase with advancing age. Data are from 7,863 male and 2,406 female apparently healthy people (Bruce treadmill max test). *Source:* Daida H, et al. *Mayo Clin Proc* 71: 445–452, 1996.

should be used (not the thumb, which has a pulse of its own). Start the stopwatch simultaneously with the pulse beat. Count the first beat as zero. Continue counting for 30 seconds and then multiply by two to get the total heart beats per minute.

During exercise, the carotid artery is easier to palpate because it is bigger than the radial (see Figure 4.3). When palpating the carotid (in the neck just lateral to the larynx), heavy pressure should not be applied, because pressure receptors (baroreceptors) in the carotid arteries can detect the pressure and cause a reflex slowing of the heart rate.

The heart rate is a variable that fluctuates widely and easily, due to the same factors that influence blood pressure. Resting heart rate is best determined upon awakening, and averaged from measurements taken on at least three separate mornings. Lower heart rates are usually (but not always) indicative of a heart conditioned by exercise training —a heart able to push out more blood with each beat (having a larger stroke volume) and therefore needing fewer beats. (See Appendix A, Table 2.) Accordingly, the resting heart rate usually drops with regular exercise, decreasing approximately one beat every 1 or 2 weeks for the first 10 to 20 weeks of the program. Some of the best endurance athletes in the world have resting heart rates as low as 30– 45 bpm. For example, Miguel Indurain, one of the best cyclists in history, had a resting heart rate of 28 bpm. Women have slightly higher resting pulse rates than men, while age appears to have little effect.[19] Resting pulse rates are also slightly higher in the fall and winter than in spring and summer, and higher in smokers versus nonsmokers.

Exercise Heart Rate

Heart rate during exercise is best determined through the use of an *electrocardiogram* (ECG), a record of the electrical activity of the heart. Several methods are used:

- Using a heart rate ruler, count two or three R waves (depending on the ruler) from the reference arrow, and then read the heart rate from the ruler (see Figure 4.7).
- Counting the number of larger squares between R waves and dividing into 300 (for example, if two large blocks are between R waves, then the heart rate is 300/2 or 150 bpm).
- Counting the number of millimeters between four R waves and dividing into 6,000 (for example, if 40 mm separate four R waves, then the heart rate is 6,000/40, or 150 bpm).

Figure 4.8 shows a form for practicing ECG heart rate determination.

Another method involves auscultation with the stethoscope. The blood pressure cuff can be filled, the systolic blood pressure taken, and then midway between the systolic and diastolic blood pressures (usually around 100 to 110 mm Hg), the release of pressure can be stopped and the pulse counted through the stethoscope for 10 seconds. (Often, the pulse sounds are very loud when this method is used.) The pressure can then be released for diastolic blood pressure determination.

Several types of heart rate measuring devices have been developed. Heart rate monitors using chest electrodes are very accurate, stable, and functional. A telemetry device with permanent electrodes is attached to the chest, with the heart rate signal sent to a receiver worn on the wrist. Heart rate and elapsed time are displayed (the heart rate is updated every 5 seconds). These heart rate monitors can now be purchased for as little as $100. Heart rate monitors using photocells to measure the opacity of blood flow (earlobe or fingertip) are not recommended.

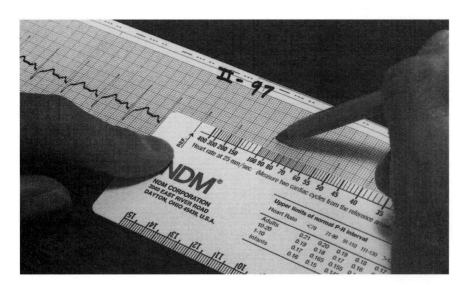

Figure 4.7   The heart rate can be determined from an ECG recording by using a heart rate ruler. With this particular ruler, heart rate is determined by reading the ruler after counting two heart rate cycles to the right of the reference arrow.

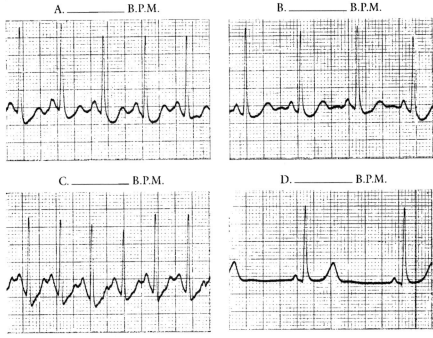

A. _____ B.P.M. B. _____ B.P.M.

C. _____ B.P.M. D. _____ B.P.M.

Figure 4.8 Use this form to practice heart rate determination from ECG recording strips. Practice each of the three methods described in this section (ECG ruler, large-square method, four-R method).

Quick Method—Number of squares between R waves divided into 300 gives the rate per minute.
Use of Ruler—Be sure to count the appropriate number of R waves from the reference point.

NONEXERCISE TEST $\dot{V}O_{2max}$ PREDICTION EQUATIONS

Direct measurement of $\dot{V}O_{2max}$ with computerized metabolic carts is the most valid and reliable marker of cardiorespiratory fitness. However, the time, expense, and technical supervision required have made laboratory measurements of $\dot{V}O_{2max}$ impractical for large populations involved in epidemiological studies of exercise and disease. Several researchers have developed regression equations that predict $\dot{V}O_{2max}$ using nonexercise test variables such as age, gender, body composition, and level of physical activity.[20-25] Although these prediction equations are not as accurate as laboratory testing of $\dot{V}O_{2max}$, they do allow researchers to broadly classify people as having poor, average, or good cardiorespiratory fitness.

One of the most commonly used nonexercise prediction equations for $\dot{V}O_{2max}$ was developed by researchers at the University of Houston, using age, physical activity status, and percent body fat or body mass index (BMI).[20] The percent body fat equation is slightly more accurate than the BMI equation. Physical activity is rated from the subject's exercise habits, using the following code:

1. Does not participate regularly in programmed recreation, sport, or physical activity.

   0 points: Avoids walking or exertion (e.g., always uses elevator, drives whenever possible instead of walking)

   1 point: Walks for pleasure, routinely uses stairs, occasionally exercises sufficiently to cause heavy breathing or perspiration

2. Participates regularly in recreation or work requiring modest physical activity, such as golf, horseback riding, calisthenics, gymnastics, table tennis, bowling, weight lifting, or yard work:

   2 points: 10–60 minutes per week

   3 points: More than 1 hour per week

3. Participates regularly in heavy physical exercise (such as running or jogging, swimming, cycling, rowing, skipping rope, running in place) or engages in vigorous aerobic activity (such as tennis, basketball, or handball).

   4 points: Runs less than 1 mile per week or spends less than 30 minutes per week in comparable physical activity

   5 points: Runs 1–5 miles per week or spends 30–60 minutes per week in comparable physical activity

   6 points: Runs 5–10 miles per week or spends 1–3 hours per week in comparable physical activity

   7 points: Runs more than 10 miles per week or spends more than 3 hours per week in comparable physical activity

The physical activity rating (PA-R) is used in the following equations to estimate $\dot{V}O_{2max}$ in ml · kg^{-1} · min^{-1}:[20]

- % fat model (R = 0.81, SEE = 5.35 ml · kg⁻¹ · min⁻¹)

$$\dot{V}O_{2max}\ ml \cdot kg^{-1} \cdot min^{-1} = 50.513 + 1.589\ (PA\text{-}R)$$
$$- 0.289\ (age) - 0.552\ (\%\ fat)$$
$$+ 5.863\ (F{=}0,\ M{=}1)$$

- BMI model (R = 0.783, SEE = 5.70 ml · kg⁻¹ · min⁻¹)

$$\dot{V}O_{2max}\ ml \cdot kg^{-1} \cdot min^{-1} = 56.363 + 1.921\ (PA\text{-}R)$$
$$- 0.381\ (age)$$
$$- 0.754\ (BMI)$$
$$+ 10.987\ (F{=}0,\ m{=}1)$$

For example, the estimated $\dot{V}O_{2max}$ for a 45-year-old woman with 25% body fat and a physical activity rating of 5 would be

$$\dot{V}O_{2max} = 50.513 + (1.589 \times 5) - (0.289 \times 45)$$
$$- (0.552 \times 25) + (5.863 \times 0)$$
$$= 31.7\ ml \cdot kg^{-1} \cdot min^{-1}$$

FIELD TESTS FOR CARDIORESPIRATORY FITNESS

A number of performance tests such as maximal endurance runs on a track have been devised and validated for testing large groups in field situations.[26–41] These tests are practical, inexpensive, less time-consuming than laboratory tests, easy to administer for large groups, and quite accurate when properly conducted. Although outdoor cycling and pool swimming tests have been developed for estimating $\dot{V}O_{2max}$, they do not appear to be as valid as running tests.[30–32]

Endurance runs should be of 1 mile or greater to test the aerobic system. For ease of administration, the 1-mile and 1.5-mile runs are most commonly used. Various set-timed runs such as the 12-minute run are hard to administer because exact distance determination is difficult. With the 1-mile or 1.5-mile runs, those being tested run the set distance around a track (or exactly measured course) while their time is measured (see Figure 4.9). The objective is to cover the distance in the shortest possible time.[26] The effort should be maximal and only made by those properly motivated and experienced in running.

The 1-mile run is used in several fitness test batteries (see Chapter 3). Norms are found in Appendix A (Tables 9, 10, 17, 19, 20). Researchers from the University of Georgia have developed a generalized equation for prediction of $\dot{V}O_{2max}$ in ml · kg⁻¹ · min⁻¹ for males and females between the ages of 8 and 25.[26] The equation is based on a total sample of 490 males and 263 females and has a standard error of estimate of 4.8 ml · kg⁻¹ · min⁻¹, giving it an accuracy that is as good as or better than that of most other field methods for estimating $\dot{V}O_{2max}$ in children and adults. The regression equation for prediction of $\dot{V}O_{2max}$ from the 1-mile run time (MRT) is

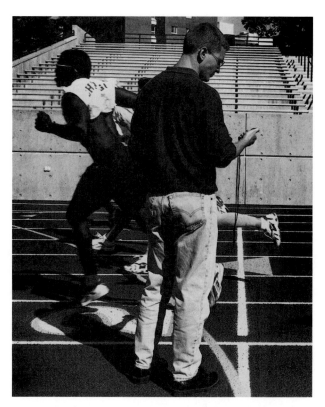

Figure 4.9 $\dot{V}O_{2max}$ can be estimated quite accurately from the time taken to run 1 mile as fast as possible. This test is recommended only for those who are apparently healthy and accustomed to running.

$$\dot{V}O_{2max}\ ml \cdot kg^{-1} \cdot min^{-1}$$
$$= (-8.41 \times MRT) + (0.34 \times MRT^2)$$
$$+ (0.21 \times age \times sex) - (0.84 \times BMI) + 108.94$$

[MRT = mile run time in minutes; sex = 0 for females, 1 for males; BMI = body mass index, kg/m²]

For example, if a 15-year-old can run a mile in 6.5 minutes and has a BMI of 21, the equation would estimate a $\dot{V}O_{2max}$ of 54.2 ml · kg⁻¹ · min⁻¹:

$$(-8.41 \times 6.5) + (0.34 \times 6.5^2)$$
$$+ (0.21 \times 15 \times 1) - (0.84 \times 21) + 108.94$$
$$= 54.2\ ml \cdot kg^{-1} \cdot min^{-1}$$

Normative data for the 1.5-mile run are found in Table 4.3 and Appendix A, Table 23. $\dot{V}O_{2max}$ can be estimated from the 1.5-mile run for college students using the following equation:[28]

$$\dot{V}O_{2max}\ (ml \cdot kg^{-1} \cdot min^{-1})$$
$$= 88.02 + (3.716 \times gender)$$
$$- (0.1656 \times kg) - (2.767 \times time)$$

[gender = 0 for female and 1 for male; kg = body weight; time = total run time in minutes]

TABLE 4.3 Norms for the 1.5-Mile Run Test (for People between the Ages of 17 and 35)

Fitness Category	Time: Ages 17–25	Time: Ages 26–35
Superior		
Males	< 8:30	< 9:30
Females	< 10:30	< 11:30
Excellent		
Males	8:30–9:29	9:30–10:29
Females	10:30–11:49	11:30–12:49
Good		
Males	9:30–10:29	10:30–11:29
Females	11:50–13:09	12:50–14:09
Moderate		
Males	10:30–11:29	11:30–12:29
Females	13:10–14:29	14:10–15:29
Fair		
Males	11:30–12:29	12:30–13:29
Females	14:30–15:49	15:30–16:49
Poor		
Males	> 12:20	> 13:29
Females	> 15:49	> 16:49

Note: Before taking this running test, it is highly recommended that the student or individual be "moderately fit." Sedentary people should first start an exercise program and slowly build up to 20 minutes of running, 3 days per week, before taking this test.

Source: Draper DO, Jones GL. The 1.5 mile run revisited—An update in women's times. *JOPERD*, September 1990:78–80. Reprinted with permission. *JOPERD* is a publication of the American Alliance for Health, Physical Education, Recreation and Dance, 1990 Association Drive, Reston, VA 20191.

For example, if a 70-kg male can run 1.5 miles in 9 minutes, his estimated $\dot{V}O_{2max}$ would be

$$55.2 \text{ ml} \cdot \text{kg}^{-1} \cdot \text{min}^{-1} = \times [88.02 + (3.716 \times 1) - (0.1656 \times 70) - (2.767 \times 9)]$$

Equations have also been developed to predict $\dot{V}O_{2max}$ from ability to run other distances at maximal speed.[35] Table 4.4 summarizes these equations for various racing distances. Notice that the correlations of calculated values of $\dot{V}O_2$ with actual measured $\dot{V}O_2$ are very high (0.88 to 0.98).

These equations assume that the person being tested has run the distance at maximum speed. The average running speed is computed in kilometers per hour (kmh), and the equation is used to calculate the $\dot{V}O_{2max}$ in METs.

One *MET* is equal to the resting oxygen consumption of the reference average human, which equals 3.5 ml · kg^{-1} · min^{-1}. To get $\dot{V}O_{2max}$, the number of METs is multiplied by 3.5 ml · kg^{-1} · min^{-1}. (See example in Table 4.4.)

Table 4.5 summarizes calculations from the equations in Table 4.4. Equivalent relationships between $\dot{V}O_{2max}$ and running performance for races ranging from 1.5 km to 42.195 km (marathon) are given. Notice, for example, that running a mile in 6:01 demands the same $\dot{V}O_{2max}$ (56 ml · kg^{-1} · min^{-1}) as running the 5 km in 21:23, the 10 km in 46:17, or the marathon in 3:49:28.

The maximal endurance run tests are only for the healthy (ACSM "apparently healthy" category). Cooper suggests that the 1.5-mile run test should not be taken unless the subject can already jog nonstop for 15 minutes.[32] In

TABLE 4.4 Estimation of $\dot{V}O_{2max}$ from Average Running Speed during Racing

Racing Distance	Equation to Calculate $\dot{V}O_{2max}$	Correlation
1.5 km	METs = 2.4388 + (0.8343 × kmh)	0.95
1.6093 km (mile)	METs = 2.5043 + (0.8400 × kmh)	0.95
3 km	METs = 2.9226 + (0.8900 × kmh)	0.98
5 km	METs = 3.1747 + (0.9139 × kmh)	0.98
10 km	METs = 4.7226 + (0.8698 × kmh)	0.88
42.195 km = (marathon)	METs = 6.9021 + (0.8246 × kmh)	0.85

Note: kmh = average racing speed in competition in kilometers per hour. 1 MET = 3.5 ml · kg^{-1} · min^{-1}. To calculate total oxygen power, multiply number of METs times 3.5 ml · kg^{-1} · min^{-1}. For example, if you can run a 5-km race in 18:30 (which is 16.2 kmh, calculated by multiplying the number of kilometers in the race by 60, and then dividing by the race time in decimal form (5 × 60) / 18.5 = 16.2 kmh), using the preceding equation, $\dot{V}O_{2max}$ in METs is equal to

$$\text{METs} = 3.1747 + (0.9139 \times 16.2) = 18 \text{ METs}$$

$\dot{V}O_{2max}$ in ml · kg^{-1} · min^{-1} = 18 METs × 3.5 ml · kg^{-1} · min^{-1} = 63 ml · kg^{-1} · min^{-1}.

Source: Tokmakidis SP, Léger L, Mercier D, Péronnet F, Thibault G. New approaches to predict $\dot{V}O_{2max}$ and endurance from running performance. *J Sports Med* 27:401–409, 1987.

TABLE 4.5 Equivalent Performances for Various Distances

$\dot{V}O_{2max}$ (ml · kg^{-1} · min^{-1})	Performance Time for Various Distances (hours:minutes:seconds)				
	1.5 km	1 mile	5 km	10 km	42.2 km
28	13:30	14:46	56:49	2:39:14	31:41:25
31.5	11:27	12:29	47:04	2:02:00	16:35:05
35	9:56	10:49	40:10	1:38:53	11:13:52
38.5	8:46	9:33	35:02	1:23:08	8:29:26
42	7:51	8:33	31:04	1:11:43	6:49:30
45.5	7:07	7:44	27:54	1:03:03	5:42:21
49	6:30	7:03	25:20	0:56:15	4:54:07
52.5	5:59	6:29	23:11	0:50:47	4:17:48
56	5:32	6:01	21:23	0:46:17	3:49:28
59.5	5:09	5:36	19:50	0:42:30	3:26:44
63	4:50	5:14	18:30	0:39:33	3:08:06
66.5	4:32	4:55	17:20	0:36:33	2:52:34
70	4:17	4:38	16:18	0:34:10	2:39:23
73.5	4:03	4:23	15:23	0:32:12	2:28:05
77	3:50	4:09	14:34	0:30:12	2:18:16
80.5	3:39	3:57	13:50	0:28:33	2:09:41
84	3:29	3:46	13:10	0:27:04	2:02:06
87.5	3:20	3:36	12:34	0:25:44	1:55:21

Source: Tokmakidis SP, Léger L, Mercier D, Péronnet F, Thibault G. New approaches to predict $\dot{V}O_{2max}$ and endurance from running performance. *J Sports Med* 27:401–409, 1987.

addition, there always should be proper warm-up of slow jogging and calisthenics. After the test, there should be an adequate "warm-down" or "cool-down," with several minutes of walking, followed by flexibility exercises.

A 1-mile walk test is available for testing a wide variety of people.[37] Walking is safer than running and more easily performed by most Americans. Three hundred and forty-three males and females, 30 to 69 years of age, were tested using a 1-mile walk test. They walked a mile as fast as possible, performing the test a minimum of two times, with heart rates monitored. They then were given a treadmill $\dot{V}O_{2max}$ test, and the 1-mile walk results correlated very highly with actual measured $\dot{V}O_2$ ($r = 0.93$).

The following equation was developed to determine $\dot{V}O_{2max}$ from 1-mile walk test results:[37]

$$\dot{V}O_{2max} \text{ (L · min}^{-1}\text{)}$$
$$= 6.9652 + (0.0091 \times \text{body weight, lb})$$
$$- (0.0257 \times \text{age}) + (0.5955 \times \text{gender})$$
$$- (0.2240 \times \text{mile walk time in minutes})$$
$$- (0.0115 \times \text{ending heart rate})$$

For example, if a male subject weighs 150 pounds, is 30 years old, and can walk 1 mile in 12 minutes with an ending heart rate of 120 beats · min^{-1} (gender, 1 = male, 0 = female):

$$\dot{V}O_{2max} = 6.9652 + (0.0091 \times 150 \text{ lb}) - (0.0257 \times 30)$$
$$+ (0.5955 \times 1) - (0.2240 \times 12 \text{ min})$$
$$- (0.0115 \times 120 \text{ bpm})$$
$$= 4.09 \text{ liters of oxygen per minute (L · min}^{-1}\text{)}$$

To change the $\dot{V}O_{2max}$ units from liters per minute to milliliters per kilogram body weight (in order to use fitness classification tables), first multiply 4.09 · min^{-1} by 1000 to get milliliters (4.09 L · min^{-1} × 1000 = 4090 ml · min^{-1}). Next divide the body weight (lb) by 2.2046 to get kilograms (150 lb/2.2046 lb/kg = 68.04 kg). Next divide the $\dot{V}O_{2max}$ by body weight (4090 ml · min^{-1}/68.04 kg = 60.1 ml · kg^{-1} · min^{-1}). Using the $\dot{V}O_{2max}$ norms in Appendix A (Table 24), this 30-year-old male would be classified as being in "athletic" cardiorespiratory shape.

The 1-mile walk test has been shown to be valid for elderly subjects if they are accustomed to walking.[42] This test can be administered outdoors on a track or indoors on a treadmill and will give similar results.[38]

A 1-mile track jog test has been developed for college students.[28] Although the mile run is commonly used to measure cardiorespiratory fitness in the college setting, there is considerable dissatisfaction with it because students dislike the maximum effort required. In the 1-mile track jog test, students self-select a steady, comfortable pace (recommended total mile times are greater than 8 minutes for males and 9 minutes for females, with an ending heart rate of less than 180 bpm). After jogging the mile at the same pace throughout, the ending time and heart rate are recorded, with $\dot{V}O_{2max}$ estimated using this equation:[28]

$$\dot{V}O_{2max} \ (ml \cdot kg^{-1} \cdot min^{-1})$$
$$= 100.5 + (8.344 \times gender) - (0.1636 \times kg)$$
$$- (1.438 \times time) - (0.1928 \times bpm)$$

[gender = 0 for female, 1 for male; kg = body weight; time = mile jog time; bpm = ending heart rate]

For example, if a female college student weighing 60 kg jogs a mile in 10 minutes with an ending heart rate of 150 bpm, her $\dot{V}O_{2max}$ would be

$$47.4 \ ml \cdot kg^{-1} \cdot min^{-1} = \times [100.5 + (8.344 \times 0)$$
$$- (0.1636 \times 60) - (1.438 \times 10)$$
$$- (0.1928 \times 150)]$$

Using Table 24 in Appendix A, her fitness level would be rated "good." This formula has been shown to correlate highly ($r = .87$) with directly measured $\dot{V}O_{2max}$.

SUBMAXIMAL LABORATORY TESTS

During submaximal testing, physiological responses (usually heart rate) to exercise are measured. The workload is usually fixed—for example, a particular grade and speed on a treadmill, a fixed rate and resistance on a cycle *ergometer* (an apparatus for measuring the amount of work performed), or a fixed rate of stepping and fixed height of bench in a step test. Usually heart rate is measured during and at the end of such exercise.

On the other hand, the physiological response may be fixed and the exercise required to reach the response measured (e.g., work required to reach a heart rate of 170 bpm). The reasoning underlying both types of submaximal tests is that the person with the higher $\dot{V}O_{2max}$ is able to accomplish a given amount of exercise with less effort (or more exercise at a particular heart rate).[43]

The submaximal exercise test makes three assumptions:[3,5,43–45]

1. That a linear relationship exists between heart rate, oxygen uptake, and workload

2. That the maximum heart rate at a given age is uniform

3. That the mechanical efficiency (oxygen uptake at a given workload) is the same for everyone

These assumptions are not entirely accurate, however, and can result in a 10–20% error in estimating $\dot{V}O_{2max}$. Figure

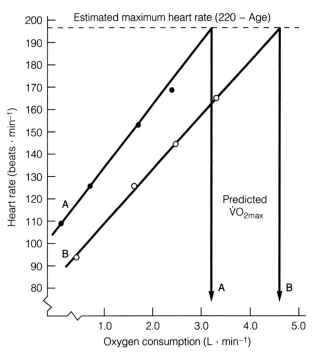

Figure 4.10 In most submaximal tests, heart rates at submaximal workloads are plotted (A or B), then extrapolated to an estimated maximum heart rate level, and then further extrapolated to an estimated workload that has been associated with an average oxygen consumption. These extrapolations can result in substantial error. *Source:* McArdle WO, Katch FI, Katch VL. *Exercise Physiology: Energy, Nutrition, and Human Performance.* Philadelphia: Lea & Febiger, 1991.

4.10 shows that in most submaximal tests, heart rates at submaximal workloads are plotted, then extrapolated to an estimated maximum heart rate level, and then further extrapolated to an average oxygen consumption. These extrapolations can result in substantial error.

The *maximum heart rate* is the fastest heart rate that can be measured when the individual is brought to total exhaustion during a graded exercise test. A formula has been developed to represent the average maximum heart rate in humans:

$$maximum \ heart \ rate = 220 - age$$

The maximum heart rate varies substantially among different people of the same age, however. (One standard deviation is ±12 bpm, which means that two thirds of the population varies an average of plus-or-minus 12 heart beats from the average.) If the line connecting submaximal heart rates is extrapolated to an average maximum heart rate level that is really 12 beats lower than the real maximum heart rate in an individual, the final extrapolation to the workload and estimated oxygen consumption will underestimate the true cardiorespiratory fitness of the individual (see Figure 4.10).

Oxygen uptake at any given workload can vary 15% among different people.[44,45] In other words, people vary in the amount of oxygen they require to perform a certain exercise workload. Some are more efficient than others, and thus the average oxygen consumption associated with a given workload may differ significantly from one person to another.

For these reasons, $\dot{V}O_{2max}$ predicted by submaximal stress tests tends to be overestimated for those who are highly trained (who respond with a low heart rate to a given workload and are mechanically efficient), and underestimated for the untrained (those with a high heart rate for a given workload, who are also inefficient).

Nonetheless, submaximal exercise testing has its place in cardiorespiratory fitness determination.[18,43] Sometimes large populations are required to be tested, and the time, equipment, and skill needed to measure $\dot{V}O_{2max}$ are prohibitive. The measurement of $\dot{V}O_{2max}$ through maximal testing requires an all-out physical effort. For some people, such effort can be hazardous and at the very least often requires medical supervision and evaluation. Also, maximal testing, while definitely the most accurate way to determine fitness status, requires a high level of motivation. Submaximal exercise testing, though not as valid, can still give a somewhat accurate picture of fitness status without the expense, risk, and hard effort.

Step Tests

Prior to the widespread use of treadmills and cycle ergometers for exercise testing, maximal step-testing protocols were recommended by the American Heart Association.[46,47] However, adjustable steps were required, and the extreme up and down stepping action for fit subjects made measurement of heart rate and blood pressure extremely difficult. Maximal step testing constitutes a safety hazard for some subjects and is no longer a recommended protocol for estimation of aerobic fitness. Submaximal step-test protocols, however, have been developed for estimation of aerobic fitness and $\dot{V}O_{2max}$, the two most common ones being the modified Canadian Aerobic Fitness Test (mCAFT) and the YMCA 3-minute step test.

The Modified Canadian Aerobic Fitness Test

The modified Canadian Aerobic Fitness Test (mCAFT) is a practical, fairly accurate, inexpensive, and fun way to determine cardiorespiratory endurance.[48–52]

The original CAFT was developed in the mid-1970s, when the Canadian government suggested that many Canadians would be motivated to increase their habitual exercise if there were a simple exercise test that indicated their current physical condition.[49]

The CAFT was designed using double steps, each 8 inches high and wide, as in a domestic staircase. The double step is climbed to an age- and sex-specific rhythm set by a cassette tape. Fitness is assessed from test duration and the radial or carotid pulse count immediately following exercise.

Since the 1970s, the CAFT has been used by millions worldwide, with the only reported complications being a very small number of minor muscle pulls (caused by stumbling) and very rare episodes of dizziness or transient loss of consciousness (arising from preexisting conditions).[48,49] The test has been well received and has achieved its primary objective of stimulating an interest in endurance exercise.

Using the CAFT with an electrocardiogram or chest heart rate monitor for heart rate determination gives a closer approximation of aerobic fitness than the Astrand-Rhyming bicycle test.[50] A properly administered mCAFT, with postexercise heart rate accurately recorded, offers a convenient submaximum tool for evaluating cardiorespiratory fitness, particularly in such settings as employee fitness programs.[52] With the relatively high correlation with directly measured maximum oxygen uptake, it provides a means of accurately testing large populations without sophisticated equipment.[48]

The Canadian Physical Activity, Fitness & Lifestyle Appraisal (CPAFLA), which includes all the instructions on how to take the mCAFT test, plus the cassette tape and other fitness materials, can be obtained from

The Canadian Society for Exercise Physiology
185 Somerset St., W, Ste. 202
Ottawa, Ontario, Canada K2P 0J2

The mCAFT is a modified step test performed on two 8-inch (20.3-cm) steps (see Figure 4.11). Based on the age of the person being tested, the tape is set at a certain stepping tempo. The person then steps up and down the steps at the given rate for 3 minutes. The cassette gives instructions and time signals as to when to start and stop exercising and how to measure the postexercise heart rate.

Table 4.6a gives the stepping cadence for the modified CAFT.[52] After an initial stepping level is chosen according to the age group (Table 4.6b), subjects step for 3 minutes on the double steps in time to the musical tape or metronome, set at the proper cadence. Subjects step at progressively higher cadences until they reach a ceiling heart rate (85% of age-predicted maximum heart rate) or the end of level 8. Notice from Table 4.6a that a single 16-inch step is used during the highest exercise levels to provide a suitable intensity for the very fit. Some people need a bit of coaching to get used to the rhythm of the beat. The stepping procedure for the double step follows a six-count format:

1—(right foot on the first step); 2—(left foot on top of the second step); 3—(right foot on top of the second step along with the left); 4—(left foot down

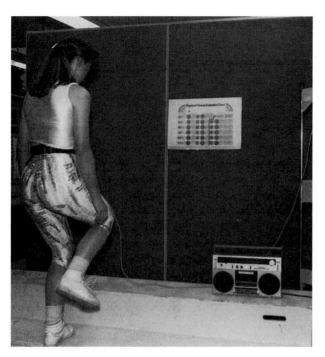

Figure 4.11 The modified Canadian Aerobic Fitness Test is a modified step test performed on two 8-inch (20.3-cm) steps.

to the first step); 5—(right foot down to the floor); 6—(left foot down to the floor along with the right). For the highest exercise levels (7 and 8 for men, 8 for women), a four-step cycle is used on the single 16-inch step.

The pulse is taken immediately after each 3-minute stepping exercise level, while the participant stands motionless. If the pulse is low enough (below 85% of maximum heart rate), another 3-minute stepping exercise is undertaken at a faster rate, with the process continuing until the ceiling heart rate or top exercise level is reached.

The mCAFT should not be taken after a large meal, after performing vigorous exercise, after using alcohol, coffee, or tobacco, or in hot rooms. Once the mCAFT has been completed, an aerobic fitness score should be established, using the following equation:[52]

aerobic fitness score
$$= 400 + (200 \times O_2 \text{ cost}) - (2.125 \times \text{kg}) - (3 \times \text{age})$$

The oxygen cost for the different stages of the mCAFT are given in Table 4.6c. For example, if a male subject 35 years of age and weighing 70 kg (154 pounds) begins stepping stage 4 and completes stages 5, 6, and 7 (oxygen cost of 2.4 liters per minute) before reaching his heart rate ceiling of 157 bpm (85% of maximum heart rate), then the aerobic fitness score would be

aerobic fitness score
$$= 400 + (200 \times 2.4) - (2.125 \times 70) - (3 \times 35)$$
$$= 626$$

TABLE 4.6a   Stepping Cadences for Men and Women Performing the Modified Canadian Aerobic Fitness Test (mCAFT)

Exercise Level	Cadence (steps/minute)	
	Males	Females
1	66	66
2	84	84
3	102	102
4	114	114
5	132	120
6	144	132
7	118*	144
8	132*	118*

*All exercise levels use two 8-inch (20.3-cm) steps except for levels 7 and 8 in men, and 8 in women, which use a single 16-inch step. The double-step exercise levels use a six-step cycle, whereas for single-step levels there are four steps per cycle.

TABLE 4.6b   Starting Levels for Performing the mCAFT in Each Gender and Age Group[30]

Age Group (yr)	Starting Level	
	Males	Females
15–19	5	4
20–29	5	3
30–39	4	3
40–49	3	2
50–59	2	1
60–69	1	1

TABLE 4.6c   Oxygen Cost in Liters of Oxygen per Minute for Stages of the mCAFT

Stage	Males	Females
1	1.00	0.94
2	1.34	1.08
3	1.65	1.30
4	1.86	1.42
5	2.10	1.52
6	2.28	1.72
7	2.40	2.08
8	2.75	2.22

Source (Tables 4.6a, b, and c): Reprinted with permission from the Canadian Society for Exercise Physiology. *The Canadian Physical Activity, Fitness & Lifestyle Appraisal.* Ottawa, Ontario: Canadian Society for Exercise Physiology, 1996.

Table 4.7 summarizes the classification system used by CPAFLA for the mCAFT.[52] An aerobic fitness score of 626 for a 35-year-old male is classified as "very good" (an aerobic fitness level that is generally associated with optimal health benefits). The mCAFT step test should be discontinued if subjects begin to stagger, complain of dizziness, extreme leg pain, nausea, or chest pain, or if they show facial pallor.

TABLE 4.7   Health Zone from Aerobic Fitness Score

	Males	Females
Ages 15–19		
Excellent	750+	646+
Very good	691–750	576–645
Good	656–690	541–575
Fair	626–655	520–540
Needs improvement	<626	<520
Ages 20–29		
Excellent	740+	556+
Very good	671–740	516–555
Good	641–670	491–515
Fair	610–640	470–490
Needs improvement	<610	<470
Ages 30–39		
Excellent	645+	530+
Very good	621–645	491–530
Good	576–620	466–490
Fair	530–575	445–465
Needs improvement	<530	<445
Ages 40–49		
Excellent	590+	466+
Very good	551–590	441–465
Good	511–550	411–440
Fair	461–510	370–410
Needs improvement	<461	<370
Ages 50–59		
Excellent	520+	410+
Very good	476–520	318–410
Good	431–475	341–380
Fair	371–430	310–340
Needs improvement	<371	<310
Ages 60–69		
Excellent	445+	380+
Very good	401–445	356–380
Good	341–400	311–355
Fair	276–340	226–310
Needs improvement	<276	<226

Source: Reprinted with permission from the Canadian Society for Exercise Physiology. *The Canadian Physical Activity, Fitness & Lifestyle Appraisal.* Ottawa, Ontario: Canadian Society for Exercise Physiology, 1996.

The YMCA 3-Minute Step Test

The YMCA uses the 3-minute step test for mass testing of participants. (See norms, Appendix A, Table 22.)[53]

The equipment involved includes a 12-inch-high, sturdy bench; a metronome set at 96 bpm (four clicks of the metronome equals one cycle, up 1,2, down 3,4), which should be properly calibrated with a wrist watch; a timing clock for the 3-minute stepping exercise and 1-minute recovery; and preferably a stethoscope to count the pulse rate.[53]

It is important to first demonstrate the stepping technique to the person to be tested (four counts—right foot up onto the bench on 1, left foot up on 2, right foot down to the floor on 3, and left foot down on 4). The exerciser should have some preliminary practice and should be well rested, with no prior exercise of any kind.

The test involves stepping up and down at the 24-steps-per-minute rate for 3 minutes, then immediately sitting down. Within 5 seconds the tester should be counting the pulse with the stethoscope and should *count for 1 full minute.* The person being tested can take her or his own pulse at the same time by palpating the radial artery, providing a double check of the count. The 1-minute count limit reflects the heart's ability to recover quickly, with a low versus high count reflecting better fitness.

The total 1-minute postexercise heart rate is the score for the test and should be recorded. It can be affected by many factors other than fitness, such as emotion, tiredness, prior exercise, resting and maximum heart rates that differ from population averages, and miscounting.

Other Step Tests

McArdle and colleagues have devised a step test (the Queens College Step Test) for college students to predict $\dot{V}O_{2max}$.[54] Subjects step at a rate of 22 steps per minute (females) or 24 steps per minute (males) for 3 minutes. The bench height is 16.25 inches (about the height of a gymnasium bleacher). After exercise, the subject remains standing, waits 5 seconds, and takes a 15-second heart rate count. The $\dot{V}O_{2max}$ (ml · kg^{-1} · min^{-1}) is predicted using this equation:

Males

predicted $\dot{V}O_{2max} = 111.33 - (0.42 \times \text{heart rate})$

Females

predicted $\dot{V}O_{2max} = 65.81 - (0.1847 \times \text{heart rate})$

The standard error of prediction using the equation is within plus or minus 16% of the actual $\dot{V}O_{2max}$ and is considered suitable for mass testing.[30,54]

There are additional step tests described in the literature. The Harvard Step Test is for young men, who step 30 times per minute for 5 minutes on a 20-inch bench. A description of the test is given by Brouha.[55] There is also the Astrand-Rhyming nomogram, which may be used to predict $\dot{V}O_{2max}$ from postexercise heart rate and body weight during bench stepping. The subject steps at a rate of 22.5 steps per minute for 5 minutes. The bench height is 33 cm for women and 40 cm for men. The postexercise heart rate is obtained by counting the number of beats between 15 and 30 seconds immediately after exercise (then multiplying by 4).[56]

ACSM Bench-Stepping Equation

The American College of Sports Medicine has published an equation for estimating the energy expenditure for stepping in terms of METs.[18] (See Table 4.8 and Box 4.1.) To use this and other ACSM metabolic equations, two units must be understood: METs and kcal $\cdot$ min^{-1}. As explained earlier, 1 MET is equal to 3.5 ml $\cdot$ kg^{-1} $\cdot$ min^{-1} or the oxygen consumption during rest. One MET is also equal to 1 kcal $\cdot$ kg^{-1} $\cdot$ hour^{-1}. Thus the energy expenditure in kcal $\cdot$ min^{-1} can be determined by multiplying the MET value of the exercise by the body weight of the person tested in kilograms, and then dividing by 60 (minutes per hour). (See Box 4.1. See also Physical Fitness Activity 4.1 at the end of this chapter.)

Treadmill Submaximal Laboratory Tests

Submaximal testing is conducted not only on steps but also with the treadmill. Submaximal testing on treadmills can use a cutoff point based on a predetermined heart rate—for example, 85% of the predicted heart rate range.

TABLE 4.8 Energy Expenditure in METs during Stepping at Different Rates on Steps of Different Heights

Step Height		Steps per Minute			
(cm)	(inches)	12	18	24	30
0	0	1.2	1.8	2.4	3.0
4	1.6	1.5	2.3	3.1	3.8
8	3.2	1.9	2.8	3.7	4.6
12	4.7	2.2	3.3	4.4	5.5
16	6.3	2.5	3.8	5.0	6.3
20	7.9	2.8	4.3	5.7	7.1
24	9.4	3.2	4.8	6.3	7.9
28	11.0	3.5	5.2	7.0	8.7
32	12.6	3.8	5.7	7.7	9.6
36	14.2	4.1	6.2	8.3	10.4
40	15.8	4.5	6.7	9.0	11.2

Source: American College of Sports Medicine. *ACSM's Guidelines for Exercise Testing and Prescription* (5th ed.). Baltimore: Williams & Wilkins, 1995. Used with permission.

There are limitations, however, when using the test heart rate as a single measure of fitness. Heart rate does not always correlate closely with $\dot{V}O_2$ and is often affected by emotional state, environmental noise, stress, age, and previous meal and beverage intake. For these reasons, several submaximal treadmill tests have been developed using multiple regression techniques to estimate $\dot{V}O_{2max}$ from measured factors.[57-63] One submaximal treadmill test was developed and cross-validated on males and females spanning a wide range of age and fitness levels.[57] In this test, a brisk walking pace, ranging from 2.0 to 4.5 mph and eliciting a heart rate within 50–70% of age-predicted maximum, should be established during a 4-minute warm-up at 0% grade. This should be followed by a second 4-minute stage in which the speed remains the same, but the treadmill is raised to a 5% grade. The ending heart rate should be measured and used in the following equation to estimate $\dot{V}O_{2max}$:

Box 4.1

MET Value Calculations

Each MET is equal to 3.5 ml of oxygen per kilogram of body weight per minute (3.5 ml $\cdot$ kg^{-1} $\cdot$ min^{-1}). Total oxygen uptake can thus be determined by multiplying the MET value by 3.5 ml $\cdot$ kg^{-1} $\cdot$ min^{-1}. The data in this box are based on submaximal, steady-state exercise; thus, caution should be taken in extrapolating to $\dot{V}O_{2max}$ (data may overpredict $\dot{V}O_{2max}$ by 1 to 2 METs). This table is based on formulas derived from the ACSM as follows:

$$\left(\frac{m}{step} \times \frac{steps}{min} \times 2.4 \, \frac{ml \cdot kg^{-1} \cdot min^{-1}}{m \cdot min^{-1}} \right)$$
$$+ \left(\frac{steps}{min} \times 0.35 \, \frac{ml \cdot kg^{-1} \cdot min^{-1}}{steps \cdot min^{-1}} \right)$$

For example, if a person is stepping 30 times per minute on a 10-cm bench, then the $\dot{V}O_2$ in ml $\cdot$ kg^{-1} $\cdot$ min^{-1} = (0.1 m $\cdot$ step^{-1} $\times$ 30 steps $\cdot$ min^{-1} $\times$ 2.4 ml $\cdot$ kg^{-1} $\cdot$ min^{-1}/m $\cdot$ min^{-1} + (30 steps $\cdot$ min^{-1} $\times$ 0.35 ml $\cdot$ kg^{-1} $\cdot$ min^{-1}/steps $\cdot$ min^{-1}) = 17.68 ml $\cdot$ kg^{-1} $\cdot$ min^{-1} $\cdot$ METs = 17.68 ml $\cdot$ kg^{-1} $\cdot$ min^{-1}/3.5 ml $\cdot$ kg^{-1} $\cdot$ min^{-1} = 5 METs.

Because 1 MET = 1 kcal $\cdot$ kg^{-1} $\cdot$ hour^{-1}, energy expenditure in kcal $\cdot$ min^{-1} can be determined by multiplying the MET value by the body weight of the person in kilograms, and then dividing by 60 minutes per hour. For example, for a person weighing 65 kg,

$$5 \text{ METs} = 5 \text{ kcal} \cdot kg^{-1} \cdot hour^{-1}$$
$$= 5 \text{ kcal} \cdot kg^{-1} \cdot hour^{-1} \times 65 \text{ kg} \cdot hour^{-1}$$
$$= 325 \text{ kcal} \cdot hour^{-1}$$
$$\text{or} \quad 5.4 \text{ kcal} \cdot min^{-1}$$

$\dot{V}O_{2max}$
$$= 15.1 + (21.8 \times speed)$$
$$- (0.327 \times heart\ rate) - (0.263 \times speed \times age)$$
$$+ (0.00504 \times \text{eart rate} \times age) + (5.98 \times gender)$$

[speed is treadmill speed in mph; gender = 0 for females, 1 for males]

For example, if a 45-year-old male walks at 3.0 mph up a 5% grade at a heart rate of 145 bpm, his $\dot{V}O_{2max}$ would be estimated as

$\dot{V}O_{2max}$
$$= 15.1 + (21.8 \times 3\ mph)$$
$$- (0.327 \times 145\ bpm) - (0.263 \times 3\ mph \times 45\ yr)$$
$$+ (0.00504 \times 145\ bpm \times 45\ yr) + (5.98 \times 1)$$
$$= 36.4\ ml \cdot kg^{-1} \cdot min^{-1}$$

This equation is fairly valid; 95% of the time, values are within $\pm 4.85\ ml \cdot kg^{-1} \cdot min^{-1}$ of actual $\dot{V}O_{2max}$.[57]

Cycle Ergometer Submaximal Laboratory Tests

Before discussing submaximal cycle ergometer tests, a comparison of the advantages and disadvantages of treadmills versus bicycles is helpful.[18] (See Box 4.2.) The most commonly used submaximal cycle ergometer tests include the multistage physical work capacity test developed by Sjostrand[64] and a single-stage test by Astrand and Rhyming.[56] Both tests assume that because heart rate and $\dot{V}O_2$ are linearly related over a broad range, the submaximal heart rate at a certain workload can predict $\dot{V}O_{2max}$. The YMCA has adopted these tests for use in their nationwide testing program.

A Description of Cycle Ergometers

A few facts on cycle ergometers include the following:[53]

- There are two major types of bicycle ergometers—mechanically braked and electronically braked (see Figure 4.12). The mechanically braked cycle ergometers are very accurate in workload adjustment and are not as expensive as the electronic versions. The mechanically braked cycle ergometers have a front flywheel braked by a belt running around the rim, attached to a weighted pendulum. The workload is adjusted by tightening or loosening the brake belt. The pedaling rate has to be maintained by the person being tested, in time to a metronome. The electronically braked ergometers use an electromagnetic braking force to adjust the workload (the resistance is variable, in relation to the pedaling rate, so that a constant work output in watts is maintained). (*Note:*

Box 4.2

Treadmills versus Cycle Ergometers

In general, both treadmills and cycle ergometers have their place in exercise testing facilities.

Advantages of Treadmills

1. Walking, jogging, or running are the most natural forms of locomotion. Most Americans are unaccustomed to bicycling (the treadmill was invented in the United States, the cycle ergometer in Europe).

2. In general, subjects reach higher $\dot{V}O_{2max}$ values during treadmill tests than they do with the cycle. $\dot{V}O_{2max}$ is usually 5 to 25% lower with cycle tests than with treadmill tests, depending on the participant's conditioning and leg strength. Only elite cyclists can achieve $\dot{V}O_{2max}$ values on cycles that equal treadmill values.

Disadvantages of Treadmills

1. Treadmills are more expensive than most cycle ergometers.

2. The treadmill is less portable than the cycle, requires more space, is heavy, and makes more noise.

3. The power (workload) of the treadmill cannot be measured directly in $kgm \cdot min^{-1}$ or watts, so it must be calculated.

4. The workload on the treadmill depends on body weight. In longitudinal studies with body weight changes, the workload changes. The body weight has a much smaller effect on cycle ergometer performance.

5. The danger of a fall is greater while running on a treadmill than while cycling on the cycle ergometer.

6. Measurement of heart rate and blood pressure is more difficult when a person is exercising on a treadmill than when on a cycle.

Because of the high expense of the electronically braked ergometer, the rest of this discussion focuses on mechanically braked cycle ergometers.)

- The mechanically braked cycle ergometer should be accurate, easily calibrated, have constant torque, and have a range of 0–2100 kilogram-meters per minute.

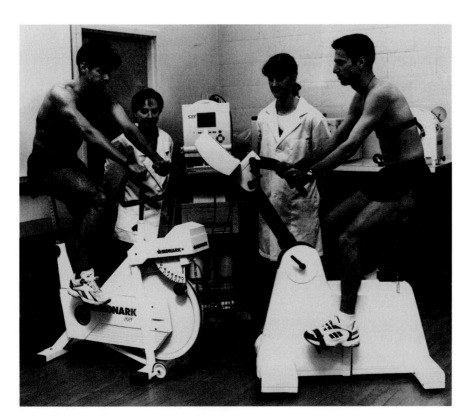

Figure 4.12 Mechanically braked cycle ergometers such as the Monark model pictured here have a front flywheel braked by a belt running around the rim attached to a weighted pendulum. The workload is adjusted by tightening or loosening the brake belt. The pedaling rate has to be maintained by the exerciser in time to a metronome. Good mechanically braked models cost between $750 and $1,000. The electronically braked ergometer uses an electromagnetic braking force to adjust the workload. The resistance is variable in relation to the pedaling rate, so that a constant work output in watts is maintained. However, electronically braked ergometers cost over $2,500.

Several ergometers meet these specifications. (See the equipment list in Appendix B.)

- The calibration of the cycle should always be checked before testing. If using the Monark, be sure the red line on the pendulum weight is reading 0 on the workload scale. An adjusting wing nut easily corrects malalignments. The calibration of the cycle itself is done precisely at the factory and unless the adjusting screw on the pendulum weight has been tampered with, there is seldom a need for recalibration. The calibration can be checked by hanging a known 2- or 4-kilogram weight on the part of the strap that moves the pendulum weight. The pendulum weight should read exactly 2 or 4 kg. If the numbers don't agree, the adjusting screw on the pendulum weight should be adjusted.

- The seat height of the ergometer should be set to the leg length of the rider. With the pedal in its lowest position, if the heel of the foot is put onto the pedal, the leg should be straight. When the ball of the foot is put onto the pedal (as should be done during cycling), a slight bend of the leg at the knee should be apparent.

- The workload on the Monark or other mechanically braked bicycles is usually expressed in *kilogram-meters per minute* (kg · m · min^{-1}) or in *watts* (1 watt =

6 kg · m · min^{-1}). The equation $W = F \times D$ (W = work in kg · m · min^{-1}; F = the force or resistance in kilograms; D = the distance traveled by the flywheel rim per pedal revolution) applies to the Monark cycle ergometers. On a Monark, the flywheel travels 6 meters per pedal revolution. If the resistance is set with the front handwheel knob (which sets the weighted pendulum at 1 kilopond or 1 kilogram, 2 kiloponds, etc.), the workload is easily figured out. If, for example, the cycling rate is 50 revolutions per minute with the weighted pendulum set at 2 kilograms, then the workload is

work = 2 kg × 6 m · rpm^{-1} × 50 rpm
= 600 kg · m · min^{-1} (100 watts)

The YMCA Submaximal Cycle Test

Following is a step-by-step approach in conducting the YMCA's popular submaximal cycle ergometer test:[53]

- For the YMCA test, set the metronome at 100 beats per minute, for a rate of 50 rpm (one beat for each foot down). Let the person being tested get used to the cadence, warming up for about 3 to 5 minutes.

- Next, set the workload, using Figure 4.13. The initial workload is set at 150 kg · m · min^{-1}.

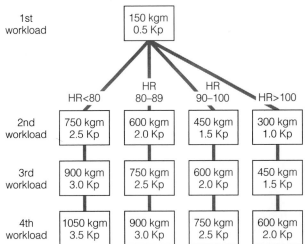

Directions:
1. Set the first workload at 150 kgm/min (0.5 Kp).
2. If the HR in the third minute is
   - less than (<) 80, set the second load at 750 kgm (2.5 Kp);
   - 80 to 89, set the second load at 600 kgm (2.0 Kp);
   - 90 to 100, set the second load at 450 kgm (1.5 Kp);
   - greater than (>) 100, set the second load at 300 kgm (1.0 Kp).
3. Set the third and fourth (if required) loads according to the loads in the columns below the second loads.

Figure 4.13 Guide to setting workloads for males on the YMCA's submaximal cycle ergometer test.
Source: Reprinted from *Y's Way to Physical Fitness* (3rd ed.) with permission of the YMCA of the U.S.A., 101 N. Wacker Drive, Chicago, IL 60606.

The person cycles at the first workload for 3 minutes, then stops, with the heart rate counted immediately, using either a stethoscope for 10 seconds (and then multiplying by 6) or a heart rate monitor. If there is doubt as to the accuracy of the heart rate, let the subject cycle another minute at the same workload, and try again. The objective is to get a steady-state heart rate at this particular workload.

- Check Figure 4.13 to decide on the next workload setting. Workloads are adjusted on the basis of heart rate response.

- Regularly check the workload setting on the cycle ergometer during each workload period. As the friction belt gets hot, the workload creeps upward, so continual readjustment during the early stages is necessary.

- Again check the pulse after 3 or 4 minutes of cycling at the new workload. Determine the steady-state pulse rate, and check Figure 4.13 to determine the third and final workload. (*Note:* If the first workload produced a heart rate greater than 110 bpm, the third workload is not necessary.)

- Throughout the test, watch for exertional intolerance or other signs of undue fatigue or unusual response. Explain to the participant that the rating of perceived exertion should be between 3 and 5 on the Borg scale.[65] (See Figure 4.14.)

- The objective of the YMCA submaximal bicycle test is to obtain two heart rates between 110 and 150 bpm. There is a linear relationship between heart rate and workload between these two rates for most people. When the heart rate is less than 110, many external

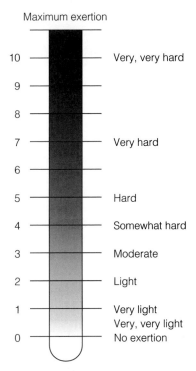

Figure 4.14 Borg scale rating of perceived exertion. During exercise heart rates of 110–115, exercise for most people will feel "3—Moderate" to "5—Hard." If the exercise feels harder than this, the workload should be reassessed. *Source:* Noble B, Borg GAV, Jacobs I, Ceci R, Kaiser P. A category ratio perceived exertion scale: Relationship to blood and muscle lactates and heart rate. *Med Sci Sports Exerc* 15:523–528, 1983.

stimuli can affect the rate (talking, laughter, nervousness). Once the heart rate climbs between 110 and 150 external stimuli should no longer affect the rate, and there is a linear relationship. If the heart rate climbs above 150, the relationship becomes curvilinear. So the objective of this test is to obtain two heart rates between 110 and 150 bpm (steady state) at two different workloads, to establish linearity between heart rate and workload for the person being tested.

- To establish the line, two points are needed. It is important that the heart rates taken be true steady-state values. To ensure this, it is better to let participants cycle beyond 3 minutes, especially during the second workload (the heart rate takes longer to plateau when the workload is harder).

- Once the test is completed, the two steady-state heart rates should be plotted against the respective workload in Figure 4.15. A straight line is drawn through the two points and extended to that participant's predicted maximal heart rate (220 − age). The point at which the diagonal line intersects the horizontal predicted maximal heart rate line represents the maximal working capacity for that participant. A perpendicular line should be dropped from this point to the baseline where the maximal physical workload capacity can be read in $kg \cdot m \cdot min^{-1}$.

- The maximal physical workload capacity in $kg \cdot m \cdot min^{-1}$ can then be used to predict a person's maximum oxygen uptake. These values are listed at the bottom of the graph. Use the norms in Appendix A (Tables 23 and 24) for interpretation. Remember that these results are predictions or estimates, not direct measurements, and are thus open to error (but usually within 15% of the actual value).

Cycling Equations

The American College of Sports Medicine has developed a formula to estimate the MET cost of cycle ergometry.[18] Box 4.3 describes the use of the formula.

An equation has also been developed for estimating VO_2 during outdoor bicycling on a level surface.[66]

$$\dot{V}O_2 \, (L \cdot min^{-1}) = -4.5 + (0.17 \times rider \; kmh)$$
$$+ (0.052 \times wind \; kmh)$$
$$+ (0.022 \times weight, \, kg)$$

For example, if a 70-kg bicyclist is cycling at 30 kmh (kilometers per hour) with no head wind in his face, his oxygen consumption would be

$$\dot{V}O_2 = -4.5 + (0.17 \times 30) + (0.052 \times 0) + (0.022 \times 70)$$
$$= 2.14 \, L \cdot min^{-1}$$
$$or \quad 30.6 \, ml \cdot kg^{-1} \cdot min^{-1} \, [(2.14 / 70) \times 1000]$$

Drafting (riding closely behind another cyclist) reduces the oxygen consumption by 18–39% depending on speed and the formation and number of riders being drafted.[66]

MAXIMAL LABORATORY TESTS

The graded exercise test (GXT) to exhaustion, with ECG monitoring, is considered the best substitute for the gold-standard test (direct $\dot{V}O_{2max}$ determination). This diagnostic, functional capacity test is mandatory for all people in the high-risk category who want to start an exercise program.[18]

The maximal graded exercise test (usually done with a treadmill or cycle ergometer) with ECG serves several purposes:[1,5,18,67]

- To diagnose overt or latent heart disease
- To evaluate cardiorespiratory functional capacity (heart and lung endurance)
- To evaluate responses to conditioning or cardiac-rehabilitation programs
- To increase individual motivation for entering and adhering to exercise programs

Maximal Graded Exercise Treadmill Test Protocols

When deciding on a test modality, the treadmill should be considered for most individuals because it tends to produce the best test outcomes. For example, among one group of triathletes, $\dot{V}O_{2max}$ from tethered swimming or cycle ergometry was 13–18% and 3–6% lower, respectively, than values obtained from treadmill running.[68]

Figures 4.16 and 4.17 describe the most commonly used maximal treadmill protocols.[29,69–71] There are many other protocols, many of which have been developed for cardiac patients or athletes.[71] For example, in the Naughton protocol, high-risk patients first go through a 4-minute warm-up, with the speed then set at 2 mph and the grade increased 3.5% every 2 minutes until maximal effort is reached.[72] In the Costill and Fox protocol for the athlete, following a 10-minute warm-up, the speed is set at 8.9 mph, with the grade increasing 2% every 2 minutes until exhaustion.[73] Of the treadmill protocols, the Bruce (Figure 4.16) is by far the most popular, followed by the Balke (Figure 4.17). The Bruce has relatively large, abrupt increases in workload every 3 minutes (8.5 $ml \cdot kg^{-1} \cdot min^{-1}$ each stage), and some have criticized the test for this. Nonetheless, excellent maximal data can be obtained, and because the test is so widely used, there is an abundance of comparative data. (See Appendix A, Table 23.)

The main criticism of the Balke test is its duration (nearly twice as long as the Bruce). In testing large numbers

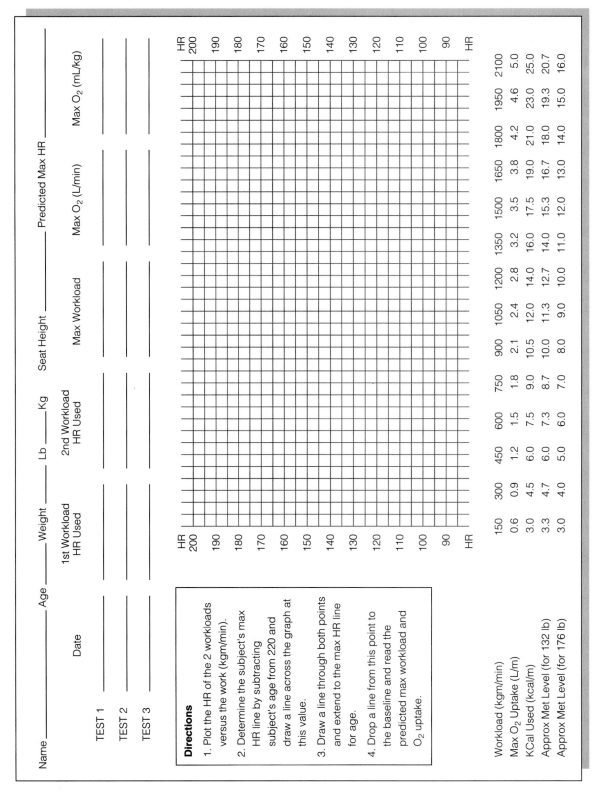

Figure 4.15 Graph for determining $\dot{V}O_{2max}$ from submaximal heart rates obtained during the YMCA's submaximal cycle test. *Source:* Reprinted from *Y's Way to Physical Fitness* (3rd ed.), with permission of the YMCA of the U.S.A., 101 N. Wacker Drive, Chicago, IL 60606.

Box 4.3

Estimated Oxygen Demand Formula for Cycle Ergometry[9]

The ACSM formula for estimating oxygen demands for cycle ergometer exercise is

$$\dot{V}O_2 \, ml \cdot min^{-1} = \left(\frac{kg \cdot m}{min} \times \frac{2 \, ml}{kg \cdot m} \right) + (3.5 \, ml \cdot kg^{-1} \cdot min^{-1} \times kg)$$

To get $\dot{V}O_2$ in $ml \cdot kg^{-1} \cdot min^{-1}$, divide final answer by body weight in kilograms.

For example, if a 70-kg man cycles at a work rate of 900 kg · m · min⁻¹, the $\dot{V}O_2$ in ml · min⁻¹ = [(900 kg · m · min⁻¹ × 2 ml · kgm⁻¹) + 245 ml · min⁻¹] = 2045 ml · min⁻¹.

To get $\dot{V}O_2$ in ml · kg⁻¹ · min⁻¹, divide by body weight of 70 kg, which is 2045 ml · min⁻¹ / 70 kg = 29.2 ml · kg⁻¹ · min⁻¹ or 8.3 METs.

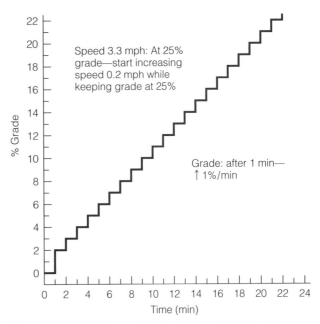

Figure 4.17 The Balke maximal graded exercise test protocol. *Source:* Balke B, Ware RW. An experimental study of "physical fitness" of Air Force personnel. *U.S. Armed Forces Medical Journal* 10(6): 675–688, 1959.

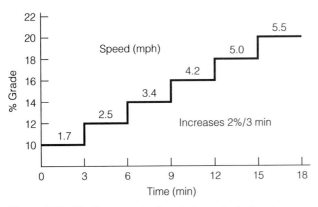

Figure 4.16 The Bruce maximal graded exercise test protocol. *Source:* Bruce RA, Kusumi F, Hosmer D. Maximal oxygen intake and nomographic assessment of functional aerobic impairment in cardiovascular disease. *Am Heart J* 85:546–562, 1973.

of people, the length of time needed for the Balke makes its use prohibitive. Ken Cooper uses the Balke protocol at the Aerobics Center in Dallas because he feels the Balke allows for a more gradual warm-up and is therefore safer.[29] The Balke is basically an uphill walking test, whereas the Bruce starts out as an uphill walking test and then in Stage 4 becomes an uphill running test.

In general, $\dot{V}O_{2max}$ can be estimated accurately from performance time on the treadmill (Figure 4.18). Maximal treadmill tests using performance time show very high correlations with laboratory-determined $\dot{V}O_{2max}$.[71] Thus, actual

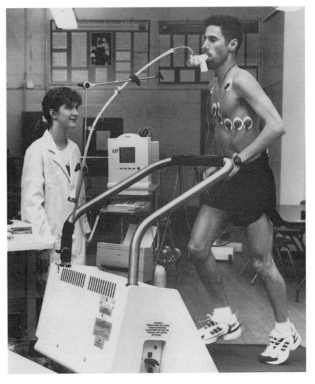

Figure 4.18 $\dot{V}O_{2max}$ can be estimated accurately from performance time on the treadmill if the subject is taken to a "true max" and does *not* hold on to the treadmill bar.

measurement of $\dot{V}O_{2max}$ is not always necessary if the person is taken to a "true max," which means

- The person is allowed to practice one time before the maximal test to become "habituated" to the treadmill

- Testers give verbal support to urge on the subject until exhaustion is reached

- When the subject is "maxed-out," there is no additional increase in heart rate despite an increase in workload, signs of exertional intolerance (fatigue, staggering, inability to keep up with the workload, facial pallor), and a maximal rating of perceived exertion is given (Figure 4.14).

- During the test, the subject is not allowed to hold onto the treadmill bar, except for the tips of two fingers, to maintain balance when needed.[74]

To ensure valid and reliable $\dot{V}O_{2max}$ values, the testing protocol should be very specific to the type of exercise the person is accustomed to. The laboratory environment should be 20–23°C, 50% humidity, and if follow-up testing is conducted, tests should be repeated at the same time of the day, using the exact same procedures.[75]

Treadmill Equations for Predicting $\dot{V}O_{2max}$

When the participant is allowed to exercise to maximal capacity in this way, $\dot{V}O_{2max}$ can be estimated very precisely. Appendix A (Table 23) contains a table that accurately estimates $\dot{V}O_{2max}$ based on length of time until exhaustion with the Bruce or Balke protocol.[76] Appendix A (Tables 24 and 25) also contains norms for classifying $\dot{V}O_{2max}$.

Formulas have been developed for predicting $\dot{V}O_{2max}$ from maximal treadmill tests.[3,70,77,78] These are summarized in Table 4.9. The critical measurement is time to exhaustion, with subjects not holding onto the bar or being aided in any way.

Maximal Treadmill Test for College Students

A maximal treadmill graded exercise test for college students has been developed by researchers at Arizona State University, which (a) allows the participant to select a comfortable walking–jogging speed, (b) is time-efficient, and (c) is relatively accurate in estimating $\dot{V}O_{2max}$.[79] The test protocol is as follows:

TABLE 4.9 Equations for Estimating $\dot{V}O_{2max}$ from Maximal Treadmill Tests

Protocol	Equation
Bruce[78]	$\dot{V}O_{2max}$ (ml · kg^{-1} · min^{-1}) = 14.76 − (1.379 × time) + (0.451 × time²) − (0.012 × time³)
Balke[77]	$\dot{V}O_{2max}$ (ml · kg^{-1} · min^{-1}) = 11.12 + (1.51 × time)

- Stage 1—Participant walks up a 5% grade at a self-selected, brisk pace for 3 minutes.

- Stage 2—Participant has the option to either continue walking briskly on a 5% grade, or self-select a comfortable jogging pace on a 0% grade for 3 minutes. The first two stages are considered a warm-up.

- Stages 3 to maximum—Starting at 0% grade, increase treadmill grade by 1.5% each minute while keeping the speed constant until participants are unable to continue despite verbal encouragement. Note ending speed in miles per hour (mph) and the final treadmill percent grade that the participant is able to sustain for close to 1 minute.

$\dot{V}O_{2max}$ in ml · kg^{-1} · min^{-1} is estimated from this formula:[79]

$$\dot{V}O_{2max} \text{ ml} \cdot \text{kg}^{-1} \cdot \text{min}^{-1}$$
$$= 4.702 − (0.0924 \times \text{kg}) + (6.191 \times \text{mph})$$
$$+ (1.311 \times \% \text{ grade}) + (2.674 \times \text{sex})$$

For sex, males are given 1, females 0. For example, if a 70-kg male chooses a jogging speed of 5.4 mph, and is "maxed out" after the treadmill grade reaches 10%, the estimated $\dot{V}O_{2max}$ is

$$4.702 − (0.0924 \times 70) + (6.191 \times 5.4)$$
$$+ (1.311 \times 10) + (2.674 \times 1)$$
$$= 47.4 \text{.ml} \cdot \text{kg}^{-1} \cdot \text{min}^{-1}$$

The standard error of estimate is 2.1 ml · kg^{-1} · min^{-1}.

ACSM Equations for Estimating $\dot{V}O_2$ for Walking and Running

The American College of Sports Medicine has developed steady-state $\dot{V}O_2$ formulas for running outdoors and on the treadmill, and also for walking (Box 4.4).[18] The formula for graded treadmill exercise has been validated with a large number of people and found to be accurate for adults.[80] Once again, these data are *steady-state* values, which means that if they are used to predict $\dot{V}O_{2max}$, data 2 to 4 minutes from the endpoint should be used. *Note:* 1 mph = 26.8 m · min^{-1} = 1.6 kmh.

Maximal Graded Exercise Cycle Test Protocols

There are two recommended maximal graded exercise cycle test protocols: the Astrand and the Storer-Davis.[71,81]

The Astrand Maximal Cycle Protocol

For the Astrand maximal cycle test, the initial workload is 300 kg · m · min^{-1} (50 watts) (1 kp at 50 rpm) for women, and 600 kg · m · min^{-1} (100 watts) (2 kp at 50 rpm) for men.[71] (See Figure 4.19.) After 2 minutes at this initial workload,

Box 4.4

ACSM Energy Requirements Formulas

The American College of Sports Medicine formulas for these data are as follows:

Walking

$\dot{V}O_2$ ml · kg^{-1} · min^{-1}

$\qquad$ = speed m · min^{-1}
$\qquad\qquad$ × 0.1 ml · kg^{-1} · min^{-1}/m · min^{-1}
$\qquad\qquad$ + 3.5 ml · kg^{-1} · min^{-1}

Example: For 80 m · min^{-1} (3 mph):

80 m · min^{-1} × 0.1 ml · kg^{-1} · min^{-1}/m · min^{-1}
+ 3.5 ml · kg^{-1} · min^{-1}
$\qquad$ = 11.5 ml · kg^{-1} · min^{-1} (METs = 11.5/3.5 = 3.3)

Graded Walking

Use preceding equation plus:

$\dot{V}O_2$ ml · kg^{-1} · min^{-1}

$\qquad$ = percent grade × speed m · min^{-1}
$\qquad\qquad$ × 1.8 ml · kg · min^{-1}/m · min^{-1}

Example: If person walks at 80 m · min^{-1} up 13% grade, then $\dot{V}O_2$ is equal to 11.5 ml · kg^{-1} · min^{-1} (see above) plus:

0.13 × 80 m · min^{-1} × 1.8 ml · kg · min^{-1}/m · min^{-1}
$\qquad$ = 18.72 = 11.5 + 18.72 = 30.22 ml · kg^{-1} · min^{-1}
$\qquad$ (8.64 METs)

Jogging and Running (speeds over 5 mph)

$\dot{V}O_2$ ml · kg^{-1} · min^{-1}

$\qquad$ = speed m · min^{-1}
$\qquad\qquad$ × 0.2 ml · kg^{-1} · min^{-1}/m · min^{-1}
$\qquad\qquad$ + 3.5 ml · kg^{-1} · min^{-1}

Example: For 200 m · min^{-1} (7.5 mph):

$\dot{V}O_2$ ml · kg^{-1} · min^{-1}
$\qquad$ = 200 m · min^{-1} × 0.2 ml · kg^{-1} · min^{-1}/m · min^{-1}
$\qquad\qquad$ + 3.5 ml · kg^{-1} · min^{-1}
$\qquad$ = 43.5   (METs = 43.5/3.5 = 12.4)

Note: For speeds in units of kmh, the MET requirement is approximately equal to the speed (10 kmh = 10 METs; 16 kmh = 16 METs).

Inclined Running

Use the equation for running, plus:

On treadmill: $\dot{V}O_2$ ml · kg^{-1} · min^{-1}
$\qquad$ = speed in m · min^{-1} × percent grade
$\qquad\qquad$ × 1.8 ml · kg · min^{-1}/m · min^{-1} × 0.5

Note: Because the oxygen cost of graded running off the treadmill (running outdoors up hills) may not be reliably predicted, the equation does not apply to this activity.

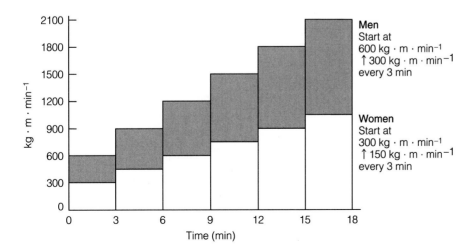

Figure 4.19 The Astrand maximal graded cycle exercise test protocol. The metronome should be set at 100, with a cycling rate of 50 rpm (one foot down with each click of the metronome). With the pedaling speed at 50 rpm, 300 kg · m/min is achieved with the cycle ergometer belt tension set at 1 kg, 600 kg · m/min at 2 kg, 900 kg · m/min at 3 kg, etc. *Source:* Astrand PO. *Work Tests with the Bicycle Ergometer.* Varberg, Sweden: AB Cykelfabriken Monark, 1965.

Men
Start at
600 kg · m · min^{-1}
↑ 300 kg · m · min^{-1}
every 3 min

Women
Start at
300 kg · m · min^{-1}
↑ 150 kg · m · min^{-1}
every 3 min

the workload is increased every 2 to 3 minutes in increments of 150 kg · m · min⁻¹ (25 watts, or ½ kp) for women, and 300 kg · m · min⁻¹ (50 watts, or 1 kp) for men. The test is continued until the participant is exhausted or can no longer maintain the pedaling frequency of 50 rpm. A metronome should be used, with the tester carefully ensuring that the proper cadence is maintained.

The $\dot{V}O_{2max}$ for most people (except for elite cyclists) will be lower when derived from the maximal cycle test than when derived from the Bruce's treadmill protocol.

Caution should be used with estimating $\dot{V}O_{2max}$ from the ACSM cycle formula. The ACSM cycle formula assumes that a steady state has been achieved, and for the normal population, it has been shown that $\dot{V}O_2$ often plateaus 1 to 3 minutes before the test is completed (if the participant is taken to a "true max"). Steady-state $\dot{V}O_2$ tables will thus overpredict $\dot{V}O_{2max}$, unless steady-state values 2 to 4 minutes from the endpoint are used. In addition, the ACSM formulas may not be accurate for workloads over 200 watts. For people with high fitness levels, direct measurement of $\dot{V}O_{2max}$ is necessary.

The Storer-Davis Maximal Cycle Protocol

The Storer-Davis equation was developed to make maximal cycle ergometer testing more practical and accurate and to provide a valid method for estimating $\dot{V}O_{2max}$. This equation was developed after testing 115 males and 116 females, ages 20 to 70.[81] After a 4-minute warm-up at 0 watts, the workload is increased by 15 watts per minute, with a recommended rate of 60 rpm. On a mechanically braked ergometer, the kp setting should be increased ¼ kp each minute (see Figure 4.20).

The equation uses the final workload in watts:

Males

$\dot{V}O_{2max}$ (ml · min⁻¹)

$$= (10.51 \times watts) + (6.35 \times kg) - (10.49 \times age) + 519.3 \text{ ml} \cdot \text{min}^{-1}$$

Females

$\dot{V}O_{2max}$ (ml · min⁻¹)

$$= (9.39 \times watts) + (7.7 \times kg) - (5.88 \times age) + 136.7 \text{ ml} \cdot \text{min}^{-1}$$

For males, the correlation with measured oxygen consumption is very high ($r = 0.94$). The standard error of estimate (SEE) is low for both males (± 212 ml · min⁻¹) and females (± 145 ml · min⁻¹) ($r = 0.93$). These SEEs are lower than they are with the Bruce treadmill equation.

The Wingate Anaerobic Test

The maximal treadmill and cycle protocols described thus far test cardiorespiratory capacity. A different type of test has been developed to test maximal anaerobic power. *Anaerobic power* is the ability to exercise for a short time at high power levels and is important for various sports where sprinting and power movements are common (e.g., football).

The Wingate anaerobic test (WAnT) was developed during the 1970s at the Department of Research and Sport Medicine of the Wingate Institute for Physical Education and Sport in Israel.[82,83] The impetus for the development of the WAnT was the lack of interest in anaerobic performance as a component of fitness, and the scarcity of appropriate, easily administered laboratory tests. Various other tests for anaerobic power and capacity have been promoted at various times, including the vertical jump, the Margaria step–running test, high-velocity treadmill running, and leg

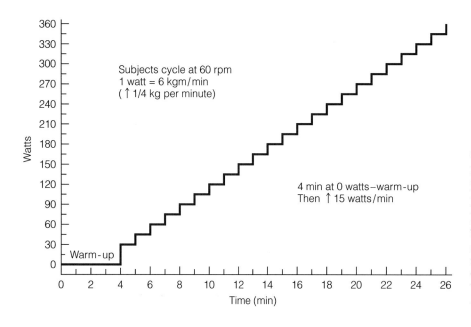

Figure 4.20 The Storer-Davis maximal cycle protocol. In the protocol, subjects cycle for 4 min at 0 watts to warm up. The workload is then increased 15 watts per min, at a recommended rate of 60 rpm. On a mechanically braked ergometer, the kg setting should be increased ¼ kg each minute. *Source:* Storer TW, Davis JA, Caiozzo, VJ. Accurate prediction of $\dot{V}O_{2max}$ in cycle ergometry. *Med Sci Sports Exerc* 22:704–712, 1990.

extensor force, but none of them have achieved the prominence and acceptance of the WAnT.

The WAnT requires pedaling or arm cranking on a cycle ergometer for 30 seconds at maximal speed against a constant force (with 5 minutes of both warm-up and cool-down recommended).[82,83] Power in watts is determined by counting pedal revolutions (watts = kp × rpm) or by using computerized equipment (Figure 4.21).[84]

Three indices are measured: (1) peak power (the highest mechanical power in watts elicited during the test, usually within the first 5 seconds); (2) mean power (the average power sustained throughout the 30-second period); (3) rate of fatigue (peak power minus the lowest power, divided by the peak power).

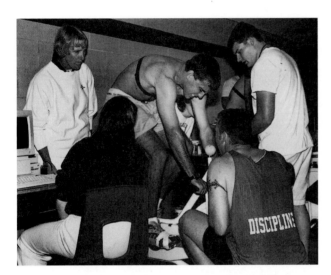

Figure 4.21 The Wingate anaerobic test requires pedaling for 30 seconds at maximal speed against a constant force. Verbal encouragement is recommended throughout the test.

A predetermined force is used to ensure that a supramaximal effort is given. As a general guideline, with the Monark ergometer, a force of 0.090 kp/kg body weight should be used with adult nonathletes and of 0.100 kp/kg with adult athletes. The Monark cycle ergometer, however, is limited to athletes weighing less than 95 kg unless it is mechanically adapted. The use of toe stirrups increases performance by 5–12%. Some tentative norms have been developed[82] (see Table 4.10).

When to Terminate the Maximal GXT-ECG Test

As emphasized in Chapter 3, maximal exercise testing, with precautions, is a relatively safe procedure.[18] ACSM has stated that the death rate in clinical exercise laboratories is about 1 per 20,000 exercise tests.[18] The death rate is even lower in preventive medicine clinics, suggesting that the rate of complications during exercise testing is higher in coronary-prone individuals.

To safely conduct a maximal GXT-ECG test, various criteria should be carefully adhered to, and emergency drugs and equipment, along with an attending physician, should be available.[18]

In a maximum graded exercise stress test, the exercise usually continues until the participant voluntarily terminates the test because of exhaustion. However, if the exercise technician and attending physician notice any of the signs or symptoms listed under the "absolute indications" in Table 4.11, the test should be stopped immediately.[18] (*Note:* Interpretation of most of the stress test termination points listed in Table 4.11 should be made by a physician. Exercise technicians are not expected to be able to diagnose these problems.)

TABLE 4.10 Young Adult (Ages 18–25) Norms for the Wingate Anaerobic Test

Classification	Males		Females	
	Peak Power (watts/kg)	Mean Power (watts/kg)	Peak Power (watts/kg)	Mean Power (watts/kg)
Very poor	5.4–6.8	5.1–6.0	6.3–7.3	4.3–4.9
Poor	6.8–7.5	6.0–6.4	7.3–7.8	4.9–5.2
Below average	7.5–8.2	6.4–6.9	7.8–8.3	5.2–5.5
Average	8.2–8.8	6.9–7.3	8.3–8.8	5.5–5.8
Good	8.8–9.5	7.3–7.7	8.8–9.3	5.8–6.1
Very good	9.5–10.2	7.7–8.2	9.3–9.8	6.1–6.4
Excellent	10.2–11.6	8.2–9.0	9.8–10.8	6.4–7.0
Elite sprinters/jumpers	11.0–12.2	8.5–9.5		
Elite rowers	11.2–12.2	9.9–10.9		

Source: Inbar O, Bar-Or O, Skinner JS. *The Wingate Anaerobic Test.* Champaign, IL: Human Kinetics, 1996. Reprinted with permission.

Emergency Procedures

The American College of Sports Medicine advises the following:[18]

1. All personnel concerned with an exercise testing program should be trained in cardiopulmonary resuscitation (CPR).

2. When possible, the exercise program director or laboratory supervisor should be trained in Advanced Cardiac Life Support.

3. Emergency equipment and drugs must be available in the immediate areas where maximal exercise testing is conducted.

4. Telephone numbers for emergency assistance should be clearly posted at all telephones.

5. Evacuation plans should be established and posted.

Every staff person should be thoroughly familiar with all specific duties and evacuation procedures required in an emergency.

6. Procedures (code-team drills) should be practiced on a regularly scheduled basis.

Personnel

It is advised that ACSM-certified personnel administer the graded exercise test (see Chapter 3). When low-risk, young adult participants are being tested, a physician need not be in attendance (but a qualified physician should be the overall director of any testing program and should be consulted concerning protocols and emergency procedures). When testing people classified as high risk, the test should be physician supervised.[18]

TABLE 4.11 Absolute and Relative Indications for Termination of an Exercise Test

Following are the absolute and the relative indications for terminating an exercise test.

Absolute indications

1. Acute myocardial infarction or suspicion of a myocardial infarction
2. Onset of moderate-to-severe angina
3. Drop in systolic blood pressure with increasing workload, accompanied by signs or symptoms or drop below standing resting pressure
4. Serious arrhythmias (e.g., second- or third-degree atrioventricular block, sustained ventricular tachycardia or increasing premature ventricular contractions, atrial fibrillation with fast ventricular response)
5. Signs of poor perfusion, including pallor, cyanosis, or cold and clammy skin
6. Unusual or severe shortness of breath
7. Central nervous system symptoms, including ataxia, visual vertigo, gait problems, or confusion
8. Technical inability to monitor the ECG
9. Patient's request

Relative indications

1. Pronounced ECG changes from baseline [>2mm of horizontal or downsloping ST segment depression, or >2mm of ST segment elevation (except in aVR)]
2. Any chest pain that is increasing
3. Physical or verbal manifestations of severe fatigue or shortness of breath
4. Wheezing
5. Leg cramps or intermittent claudication (grade 3 on 4-point scale)
6. Hypertensive response (systolic blood pressure >260 mm Hg; diastolic blood pressure >115 mm Hg)
7. Less serious arrhythmias such as supraventricular tachycardia
8. Exercise-induced bundle branch block that cannot be distinguished from ventricular tachycardia

Source: American College of Sports Medicine. *ACSM's Guidelines for Exercise Testing and Prescription* (5th ed.). Baltimore: Williams & Wilkins, 1995. Used with permission.

SPORTS MEDICINE INSIGHT

Administering the Electrocardiogram

Learning to interpret the electrocardiogram (ECG) takes special training under the guidance of experienced health professionals. Nevertheless, many experts feel that health and fitness leaders should be familiar with basic ECG principles. In addition, treadmill or cycle ergometer operators are expected to be able to know when abnormal ECG patterns appear on the oscilloscope (and to call the attending physician, or if necessary terminate the test). The following description should be reviewed with an instructor familiar with ECG interpretation.

THE ECG

The *ECG* presents a visible record of the heart's electrical activity, by means of a stylus that traces the activity on a continuously moving strip of special heat-sensitive paper.[85] All heartbeats appear as a similar pattern, equally spaced, and consist of three major units (see Figure 4.22):

- *P wave* (transmission of electrical impulse through the atria)
- *QRS complex* (impulse through the ventricles)
- *T wave* (electrical recovery or repolarization of the ventricles)

Heart cells are charged or *polarized* in the resting state (negative ions inside the cell, positive outside), but when electrically stimulated, they depolarize (positive ions go inside the heart cell, negative ions go outside) and contract. Thus, when the heart is stimulated, a wave of depolarization passes through the heart (an advancing wave of positive charges within the cells). As the positive wave of depolarization within the heart cells moves toward a positive skin electrode, there is a positive upward deflection recorded on the ECG.

The P wave (atrial wave) begins in the SA node (the normal physiological pacemaker) located near the top of the atrium. The impulse reaches the AV node located in the superior aspect of the ventricles. There is a $^1/_{10}$-second pause, allowing blood to enter the ventricles from the contracting atria (see Figure 4.23).

The QRS complex (ventricular wave) begins in the AV node. After the $^1/_{10}$-second pause, the AV node is stimulated, initiating an electrical impulse that starts down the AV bundle, called the *bundle of HIS* into the *bundle branches* and finally into the *Purkinje fibers*. The neuromuscular conduction system of the ventricles is composed of specialized nervous material that transmits the electrical impulse from the AV node into the ventricular heart cells.

The ECG is recorded on ruled paper. The smallest divisions are 1-millimeter squares. On the horizontal line, 1 small block represents 0.04 second (1 large block of 5 small blocks is 0.20 second). On the vertical axis, 1 small

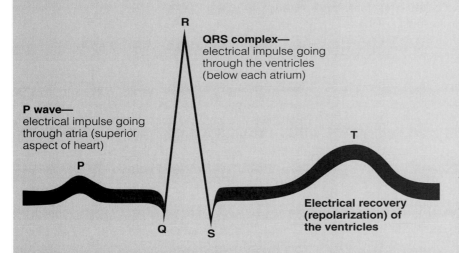

P wave—
electrical impulse going
through atria (superior
aspect of heart)

P

R

QRS complex—
electrical impulse going
through the ventricles
(below each atrium)

Q   **S**

T

**Electrical recovery
(repolarization) of
the ventricles**

Figure 4.22 Normal single heartbeat. All heartbeats consist of three major units, the P wave, the QRS complex, and the T wave, which represent the transmission of electrical impulses through the heart.

(continued)

Administering the Electrocardiogram (continued)

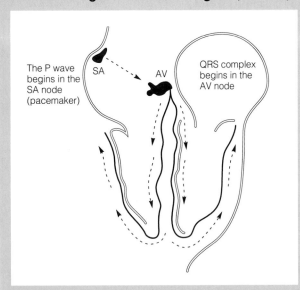

Figure 4.23 Normal electrical pathway. The P wave (atrial wave) begins in the SA node (normal physiological pacemaker) located near the top of the atrium. The QRS complex (ventricular wave) begins in the AV node.

block represents $1/10$ of a millivolt (10 small blocks vertically or 2 large blocks is 1 millivolt). (See Figure 4.24.)

The standard ECG is composed of 12 separate leads:

Limb leads: Lead 1, Lead 2, Lead 3

Augmented unipolar leads: aVR, aVL, aVF

Chest leads: V_1, V_2, V_3, V_4, V_5, V_6

An *ECG lead* is a pair of electrodes placed on the body and connected to an ECG recorder. An axis is an imaginary line connecting the two electrodes. The electrodes for the three limb leads are placed on the right arm, left arm, and left leg. The ground electrode is placed on the right leg. This is electronically equivalent to placing the electrodes at the two shoulders and the symphysis pubis. From these three electrodes (plus the ground), the ECG recorder can make certain electrodes positive and others negative to produce six leads (1, 2, 3, aVR, aVL, aVF). (See Figure 4.25.)

It is not the purpose of this book to give details on how to interpret the ECG. The exercise technician can administer the resting 12-lead ECG, but a qualified physician (especially cardiologists and internists) should interpret the results.[67] The resting 12-lead ECG should be administered to high-risk patients before the treadmill ECG to help screen out those with various contraindications to exercise.

EXERCISE TEST ELECTRODE PLACEMENT

The diagnostic GXT should be performed with a multiple-lead electrocardiographic system. The best possible GXT-ECG test is one in which all 12 leads are monitored. The *Mason-Likar* 12-lead exercise ECG system should be used, in which the six precordial electrodes are placed in their usual positions: the right and left arm electrodes are placed on the shoulders at the distal ends of the clavicles; and the right and left leg electrodes are positioned at the base of the torso, just medial to the anterior iliac crests.[18,86] (See Figure 4.25.)

However, the majority of abnormal ECG responses to exercise can be picked up by lead V_5 alone.[56] When only V_5 is monitored, the CM5 electrode placement system is generally used, in which the second electrode (the negative) is placed on the top third of the sternum (RA electrode), and the third electrode (the ground) is placed on the right side of the chest in the V_5 position (RL electrode).[18,86] The V_5 electrode (LA) is put in its normal position.

All leads should be continuously monitored by oscilloscope and recordings taken at the end of each minute of exercise or when significant ECG changes or abnormalities are noted on the screen. During recovery, this should continue every 1 to 2 minutes for the 8-minute postexercise test.

During the early part of the recovery period, the participant should exercise at low intensity (2 mph, 0% grade on the treadmill). The ECG and blood pressure should be recorded every 1 to 2 minutes for at least 8 minutes of recovery (or longer if there are abnormalities). The participant should not be allowed to stand still or sit still immediately following the exercise test. After approximately 2 minutes of cool-down, the subject can sit down and continue to move her or his feet for several more minutes. Disposable electrodes (available for about 25 cents each) stick on the body very well despite the accumulation of sweat, and they conduct the electrical impulses from the body to the electrocardiograph with little or no movement-artifact interference. Proper skin

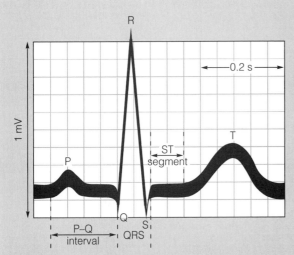

Figure 4.24 On the horizontal line, one small block represents 0.04 second or 1 millimeter. One large block of five small blocks is 0.20 second. On the vertical axis, one small block represents ¹⁄₁₀ of a millivolt. Ten small blocks vertically or two large blocks is 1 millivolt.

preparation is essential for the best ECG recordings. The resistance of the skin should be lowered by first cleansing thoroughly with an alcohol-saturated gauze pad and then removing the superficial layer of the skin by rubbing vigorously. Shaving of the skin is not necessary.

BASIC PRINCIPLES IN ARRHYTHMIA DETERMINATION

An *arrhythmia* is any disturbance of rate, rhythm, or conduction of electrical impulses in the heart.[74] The following criteria should be systematically analyzed for each ECG strip (while watching the oscilloscope), until the ability to pick out abnormal ECGs becomes automatic.

1. *R to R intervals*—evenly spaced (maximum allowable difference between R waves is 3 small squares)

2. *P waves*—
   a. within the 3 × 3 small square box
   b. positive
   c. same consistent, rounded shape

3. *P-R interval*—3 to 5 small squares (0.12 to 0.20 second)

4. *P to QRS ratio*—always 1:1 ratio

5. *QRS duration*—less than 2½ small squares (0.10 second)

The exercise technician should be (a) able to monitor the screen and pick out any abnormal PQRST wave complex, and (b) alert to call the supervising physician for an interpretation. However, the exercise technician does not necessarily need to know how to interpret abnormal ECGs during exercise. (One of the most common ECG abnormalities during the exercise test is the premature ventricular contraction (PVC). (See Figure 4.26 for examples of PVCs.)

One of the major purposes in giving a treadmill ECG stress test is to load the heart muscle beyond normal demands, to see whether any obstruction to blood flow in the coronary arteries can be picked up on the ECG.[18] During the maximal exercise test, coronary blood flow increases fivefold. If the coronary blood vessel is restricted approximately two thirds, the ST segment of the PQRST wave complex may be depressed.

ST segment depression is determined if all the following criteria are present (see Figure 4.26 for examples):

- 1 mm or more depressed (below baseline)
- at least 0.08 second (2 small squares) in length
- flat or downsloping
- three or more consecutive complexes

When ST segment depression is recorded, this is a "positive" test for coronary heart disease (CHD). When ST segment depression is not present, the test is called "negative."

The supervising physician should know that the specificity, sensitivity, and diagnostic accuracy of the test can vary considerably, according to the prevalence of CHD in the population being tested (Bayes theorem) and according to criteria used.[18,86] Ischemic chest pain induced by the exercise test is strongly predictive of CHD and is even more predictive with ST segment depression.[1,86] Severity of CHD is also related to the time of appearance of ST segment depression, with changes occurring early translating to a poor prognosis and increased risk of multivessel disease. The probability and severity of CHD are also directly related to the amount of ST segment depression and the downslope.[56]

(continued)

Administering the Electrocardiogram *(continued)*

Standard or bipolar limb leads	Electrodes connected	Marketing code
Lead 1	LA & RA	.
Lead 2	LL & RA	..
Lead 3	LL & LA	...
Augmented unipolar limb leads		
a VR	RA & (LA-LL)	—
a VL	LA & (RA-LL)	— —
a VF	LL (RA-LA)	— — —
Chest or precordial leads		
V	C & (LA-RA-LL)	(see data on right)

Recommended positions for multiple chest leads
(Line art illustration of chest positions)

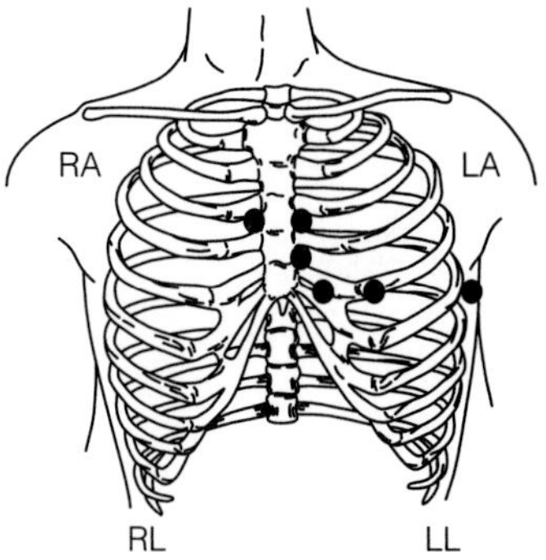

V_1	Fourth intercostal space at right margin of sternum	— .
V_2	Fourth intercostal space at left margin of sternum	— ..
V_3	Midway between position 2 and position 4	— ...
V_4	Fifth intercostal space at junction of left midclavicular line	— ....
V_5	At horizontal level of position 4 at left anterior axillary line	— .....
V_6	At horizontal level of position 4 at left midaxillary line	— ......

Figure 4.25   Ten electrode positions form 12 leads for the routine electrocardiogram. Electrodes should be placed in the exact anatomical position noted, so that the physician can compare the ECG with appropriate standards.

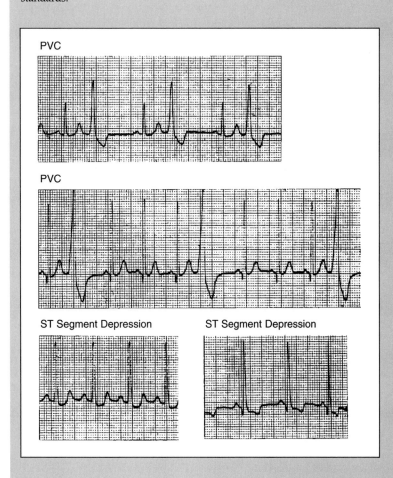

PVC

PVC

ST Segment Depression   ST Segment Depression

Figure 4.26   One of the most common arrhythmias is the premature ventricular contraction (PVC). ST segment depression may occur when coronary blood vessels are partially restricted, decreasing blood flow during exercise.

SUMMARY

1. While the direct measurement of $\dot{V}O_{2max}$ is the best estimate of heart and lung endurance, for various practical reasons, other tests have been developed as substitutes. These include field tests (mainly running tests), step tests (YMCA 3-minute step test, Canadian Home Fitness Step Test), submaximal laboratory tests (YMCA submaximal cycle test), and maximal laboratory tests (both cycle and treadmill).

2. This chapter provided a detailed description of these tests. Maximal treadmill testing with ECG is explained in detail because of its great value in diagnosing overt or latent heart disease, evaluating cardiorespiratory functional capacity, evaluating responses to conditioning or cardiac rehabilitation programs, and increasing individual motivation for entering and adhering to exercise programs.

3. Resting and exercise blood pressure and heart rate determination are reviewed. The diagnosis of adult hypertension is confirmed when the average of two or more measurements on at least two separate visits are 140/90 mm Hg or higher.

4. Principles for taking blood pressure measurements are listed. At rest, diastolic blood pressure equals the disappearance of the pulse sound (fifth Korotkoff sound).

5. Heart rate can be determined through several methods, including the use of heart rate rulers, auscultation with a stethoscope, and heart rate monitors.

6. A number of performance tests, such as maximal endurance runs on a track have been devised for testing large groups in field situations. Equations for predicting $\dot{V}O_{2max}$ from one's ability to run various distances at maximal speed have been developed. A 1-mile walk test has been developed to more safely test adults.

7. Both maximal and submaximal step tests have been developed for predicting $\dot{V}O_{2max}$. Of these, the Canadian Aerobic Fitness Test and the YMCA's 3-minute step test have been most widely used.

8. The American College of Sports Medicine has developed equations for predicting oxygen consumption during bench stepping, cycling, walking, and running. Two important terms are used by the American College of Sports Medicine in their equations and calculations—"METs" and kcal · min⁻¹. One MET is equal to 3.5 ml · kg⁻¹ · min⁻¹, or the oxygen consumption during rest. One MET is also equal to 1 kcal · kg⁻¹ · hour⁻¹.

9. Both treadmill and cycle ergometers are used in testing cardiorespiratory fitness. In the United States, most facilities use treadmills for exercise testing because walking, jogging, and running are more familiar to Americans, who generally are unaccustomed to cycling. In addition, most people reach higher $\dot{V}O_{2max}$ values during treadmill tests than they do with the cycle.

10. A complete description of cycle ergometers is presented. The workload on the Monark or other mechanically braked cycles is usually expressed in kilogram-meters per minute (kg · m · min⁻¹) or in watts (1 watt = 6 kg · m · min⁻¹). Work = kg setting × 6 m · rpm⁻¹ × rpm = kg · m · min⁻¹.

11. One of the best submaximal cycle protocols is the one used by the YMCA in its testing program. The objective of the YMCA submaximal cycle test is to obtain two heart rates between 110 and 150 bpm and then extrapolate these to an estimated maximal oxygen consumption.

12. The most commonly used maximal treadmill protocols are the Bruce and the Balke. $\dot{V}O_{2max}$ can be estimated accurately from performance time to exhaustion during these protocols.

13. There are two recommended maximal graded exercise cycle test protocols: the Astrand and the Storer-Davis.

14. The maximal treadmill and cycle protocols described herein test maximal cardiorespiratory capacity. A different type of test, the Wingate anaerobic test (WAnT), has been developed to test maximal anaerobic power. The WAnT requires pedaling or arm cranking on a cycle ergometer for 30 seconds at maximal speed against a constant force.

15. The Sports Medicine Insight reviewed basic principles for administering electrocardiograms.

REFERENCES

1. Fletcher GF, Balady G, Froelicher VF, Hartley LH, Haskell WL, Pollock ML. Exercise standards: A statement for healthcare professionals from the American Heart Association. *Circulation* 91:580–615, 1995.

2. Wilmore JH, Costill DL. *Physiology of Sport and Exercise.* Champaign, IL: Human Kinetics, 1994.

3. Maud PJ, Foster C. *Physiological Assessment of Human Fitness.* Champaign, IL: Human Kinetics, 1995.

4. Bassett DR, Howley ET. Maximal oxygen uptake: "Classical" versus "contemporary" viewpoints. *Med Sci Sports Exerc* 29: 591–603, 1997.

5. American College of Sports Medicine. *Resource Manual for Guidelines for Exercise Testing and Prescription* (3rd ed.). Baltimore: Williams & Wilkins, 1998.

6. Melanson EL, Freedson PS, Hendelman D, Debold E. Reliability and validity of a portable metabolic measurement system. *Can J Appl Physiol* 21:109–119, 1996.

7. Vanderburgh PM, Katch FI. Ratio scaling of $\dot{V}O_{2max}$ penalizes women with larger percent body fat, not lean body mass. *Med Sci Sports Exerc* 28:1204–1208, 1996.

8. Howley ET, Bassett DR, Welch HG. Criteria for maximal oxygen uptake: Review and commentary. *Med Sci Sports Exerc* 27: 1292–1301, 1995.

9. Duncan GE, Howley ET, Johnson BN. Applicability of $\dot{V}O_{2max}$ criteria: Discontinuous versus continuous protocols. *Med Sci Sports Exerc* 29:273–278, 1997.

10. National High Blood Pressure Education Program. *The Sixth Report of the Joint National Committee on Detection, Evaluation, and Treatment of High Blood Pressure.* National Heart, Lung, and Blood Institute, National Institutes of Health, NIH Publication No. 98-4080. Bethesda, MD: National Institutes of Health, 1997.

11. Burt VL, Cutler JA, Higgins M, Horan MJ, Labarthe D, Whelton P, Brown C, Roccella EJ. Trends in the prevalence, awareness, treatment, and control of hypertension in the adult US population: Data from the Health Examination Surveys, 1960 to 1991. *Hypertension* 26:60–69, 1995.

12. American Society of Hypertension Public Policy Position Paper. Recommendations for routine blood pressure measurement by indirect cuff sphygmomanometry. *Am J Hypertension* 5:207–209, 1992.

13. Reeves RA. Does this patient have hypertension? How to measure blood pressure. *JAMA* 273:1211–1218, 1995.

14. Perloff D, Grim C, Flack J, et al. Human blood pressure determination by sphygmomanometry. *Circulation* 88:2460–2470, 1993.

15. Griffin SE, Robergs RA, Heyward VH. Blood pressure measurement during exercise: A review. *Med Sci Sports Exerc* 29: 149–159, 1997.

16. Lightfoot JT, Tuller B, Williams DF. Ambient noise interferes with auscultatory blood pressure measurement during exercise. *Med Sci Sports Exerc* 28:502–508, 1996.

17. Daida H, Allison TG, Squires RW, Miller TD, Gau GT. Peak exercise blood pressure stratified by age and gender in apparently healthy subjects. *Mayo Clinic Proc* 71:445–452, 1996.

18. American College of Sports Medicine. *ACSM's Guidelines for Exercise Testing and Prescription* (5th ed.). Baltimore: Williams & Wilkins, 1995.

19. Gillum RF. Epidemiology of resting pulse rate of persons ages 25–74: Data from NHANES 1971–74. *Pub Health Rep* 107: 193–201, 1992.

20. Jackson AS, Blair SN, Mahar MT, Wier LT, Ross RM, Stuteville JE. Prediction of functional aerobic capacity without exercise testing. *Med Sci Sports Exerc* 22:863–870, 1990.

21. Heil DP, Freedson PS, Ahlquist LE, Price J, Rippe JM. Nonexercise regression models to estimate peak oxygen consumption. *Med Sci Sports Exerc* 27:599–606, 1995.

22. Williford HN, Scharff-Olson M, Wang N, Blessing DL, Smith FH, Duey WJ. Cross-validation of non-exercise predictions of $\dot{V}O_{2peak}$ in women. *Med Sci Sports Exerc* 28:926–930, 1996.

23. Whaley MH, Kaminsky LA, Dwyer GB, Getchell LH. Failure of predicted $\dot{V}O_{2peak}$ to discriminate physical fitness in epidemiological studies. *Med Sci Sports Exerc* 27:85–91, 1995.

24. George JD, Stone WJ, Burkett LN. Non-exercise $\dot{V}O_{2max}$ estimation for physically active college students. *Med Sci Sports Exerc* 29:415–423, 1997.

25. Cardinal BJ. Predicting cardiorespiratory fitness without exercise testing in epidemiologic studies: A concurrent validity study. *J Epidemiol* 6:31–35, 1996.

26. Cureton KJ, Sloniger MA, O'Bannon JP, Black DM, McCormack WP. A generalized equation for prediction of $\dot{V}O_{2peak}$ from 1-mile run/walk performance. *Med Sci Sports Exerc* 27:445–451, 1995.

27. Draper DO, Jones GL. The 1.5-mile run revisited: An update in women's times. *JOPERD*, September 1990, 78–80.

28. George JD, Vehrs PR, Allsen PE, Fellingham GW, Fisher AG. $\dot{V}O_{2max}$ estimation from a submaximal 1-mile track jog for fit college-age individuals. *Med Sci Sports Exerc* 25:401–406, 1993.

29. American Alliance for Health, Physical Education, Recreation, and Dance. *AAHPERD Norms for College Students: Health Related Physical Fitness Test.* Reston, VA: Author, 1985.

30. Conley DS, Cureton KJ, Hinson BT, Higbie EJ, Weyand PG. Validation of the 12-minute swim as a field test of peak aerobic power in young women. *Res Quart Exerc Sport* 63:153–161, 1992.

31. Conley DS, Cureton KJ, Dengel DR, Weyand PG. Validation of the 12-minute swim as a field test of peak aerobic power in young men. *Med Sci Sports Exerc* 23:766–773, 1991.

32. Cooper KH. *The Aerobics Way.* New York: M. Evans and Co., 1977.

33. Zwiren LD, Freedson PS, Ward A, Wilke S, Rippe JM. Estimation of $\dot{V}O_{2max}$: A comparative analysis of five exercise tests. *Res Quart Exerc Sport* 62:73–78, 1991.

34. McCutcheon MC, Sticha SA, Giese MD, Nagle FJ. A further analysis of the 12-minute run prediction of maximal aerobic power. *Res Quart Exerc Sport* 61:280–283, 1990.

35. Tokmakidis SP, Leger L, Mercier D, Peronnet F, Thibault G. New approaches to predict $\dot{V}O_{2max}$ and endurance from running performance. *J Sports Med* 27:401–409, 1987.

36. Laukkanen POR, Pasanen M, Tyry T, Vuori I. A 2-km walking test for assessing the cardiorespiratory fitness of healthy adults. *Int J Sports Med* 12:356–362, 1991.

37. Kline GM, Porcari JP, Hintermeister R, et al. Estimation of $\dot{V}O_{2max}$ from a one-mile track walk, gender, age, and body weight. *Med Sci Sports Exerc* 19:253–259, 1987.

38. Widrick J, Ward A, Ebbeling C, Clemente E, Rippe JM. Treadmill validation of an over-ground walking test to predict peak oxygen consumption. *Eur J Appl Physiol* 64:304–308, 1992.

39. Jeukendrup A, Saris WHM, Brouns F, Kester ADM. A new validated endurance performance test. *Med Sci Sports Exerc* 28: 266–270, 1996.

40. Grant S, Corbett K, Amjad AM, Wilson J, Aitchison T. A comparison of methods of predicting maximum oxygen uptake. *Br J Sports Med* 29:147–152, 1995.

41. Berthon P, Fellmann N, Bedu M, Beaune B, Dabonneville M, Coudert J, Chamoux A. A 5-minute field test as a measurement of maximal aerobic velocity. *Eur J Appl Physiol* 75:233–238, 1997.

42. Warren BJ, Dotson RG, Nieman DC, Butterworth DE. Validation of a one-mile walk test in elderly women. *J Aging Phys Act* 1:13–21, 1993.

43. Montoye HJ, Ayen T, Washbum RA. The estimation of $\dot{V}O_{2max}$ from maximal and sub-maximal measurements in males, age 10–39. *Res Quart Exerc Sport* 57:250–253, 1986.

44. Cavanagh PR, Kram R. The efficiency of human movement: A statement of the problem. *Med Sci Sport Exerc* 17:303–308, 1985.

45. Thomas SG, Weller IMR, Cox MH. Sources of variation in oxygen consumption during a stepping task. *Med Sci Sports Exerc* 25:139–144, 1993.

46. Nagle FS, Balke B, Naughton JP. Gradational step tests for assessing work capacity. *J Appl Physiol* 20:745–748, 1965.

47. Ellestad MH, Blomqvist CG, Naughton JP. Standards for adults exercise testing laboratories. *Circulation* 59:421A–430A, 1979.

48. Shephard RJ, Thomas S, Weller I. The Canadian Home Fitness Test: 1991 update. *Sports Med* 11:358–366, 1991.

49. Shephard RJ. Current status of the step test in field evaluations of aerobic fitness: The Canadian Home Fitness Test and its analogues. *Sports Med Training Rehab* 6:29–41, 1995.

50. Jette M, Mongeon J, Shephard RJ. Demonstration of a training response by the Canadian Home Fitness Test. *Eur J Appl Physiol* 49:143–150, 1982.

51. Weller IM, Thomas SG, Gledhill N, Paterson D, Quinney A. A study to validate the modified Canadian Aerobic Fitness Test. *Can J Appl Physiol* 20:211–221, 1995.

52. Canadian Society for Exercise Physiology. *The Canadian Physical Activity, Fitness & Lifestyle Appraisal.* Ottawa, Ontario: Author, 1996.

53. Golding LA, Myers CR, Sinning WE. *Y's Way to Physical Fitness: The Complete Guide to Fitness Testing and Instruction* (4th ed.). Champaign, IL: Human Kinetics, 1998.

54. McArdle WD, Katch FI, Katch VL. *Exercise Physiology: Energy, Nutrition, and Human Performance.* Philadelphia: Lea & Febiger, 1991.

55. Brouha L. The step test: A simple method of measuring physical fitness for muscular work in young men. *Res Quart* 14:31–36, 1943.

56. Astrand PO, Rhyming I. A nomogram for calculation of aerobic capacity (physical fitness) from pulse rate during submaximal work. *J Appl Physiol* 7:218–221, 1954.

57. Ebbeling CB, Ward A, Puleo EM, Widrick J, Rippe JM. Development of a single-stage submaximal treadmill walking test. *Med Sci Sports Exerc* 23:966–973, 1991.

58. Foster C, Crowe AJ, Daines E, et al. Predicting functional capacity during treadmill testing independent of exercise protocol. *Med Sci Sports Exerc* 28:752–756, 1996.

59. George JD, Vehrs PR, Allsen PE, Fellingham GW, Fisher AG. Development of a submaximal treadmill jogging test for fit college-aged individuals. *Med Sci Sports Exerc* 25:643–647, 1993.

60. Hermiston RT, Faulkner JA. Prediction of maximal oxygen uptake by a stepwise regression technique. *J Appl Physiol* 30:833–837, 1971.

61. Metz KF, Alexander JF. Estimation of maximal oxygen intake from submaximal work parameters. *Res Quart Exerc Sport* 42:187–193, 1971.

62. Town GP, Golding LA. Treadmill test to predict maximum aerobic capacity. *J Phys Ed* 74:6–8, 1977.

63. Wilmore JH, Roby FB, Stanforth PR, et al. Ratings of perceived exertion, heart rate, and treadmill speed in the prediction of maximal oxygen uptake during submaximal treadmill exercise. *J Cardio Rehab* 5:540–546, 1985.

64. Sjostrand T. Changes in respiratory organs of workmen at an ore melting works. *Acta Med Scand* 196(suppl):687–695, 1947.

65. Noble B, Borg GAV, Jacobs I, Ceci R, Kaiser P. A category ratio perceived exertion scale: Relationship to blood and muscle lactates and heart rate. *Med Sci Sports Exerc* 15:523–528, 1983.

66. McCole SD, Claney K, Conte JC, Anderson R, Hagberg JM. Energy expenditure during bicycling. *J Appl Physiol* 68:748–753, 1990.

67. Gibbons RJ, Balady GJ, Beasley JW, et al. ACC/AHA guidelines for exercise testing: Executive summary. A report of the American College of Cardiology/American Heart Association Task Force on Practice Guidelines (Committee on Exercise Testing). *Circulation* 96:345–354, 1997.

68. O'Toole ML, Douglas PS, Hiller WDB. Applied physiology of a triathlon. *Sports Med* 8:201–225, 1989.

69. Bruce RA, Kusumi F, Hosmer D. Maximal oxygen intake and nomographic assessment of functional aerobic impairment in cardiovascular disease. *Am Heart J* 85:546–562, 1973.

70. Balke B, Ware RW. An experimental study of "physical fitness" of Air Force personnel. *U.S. Armed Forces Med J* 10(6):675–688, 1959.

71. Heyward VH. *Advanced Fitness Assessment & Exercise Prescription* (3rd ed.). Champaign, IL: Human Kinetics, 1998.

72. Naughton J, Balke B, Nagle F. Refinement in methods of evaluation and physical conditioning before and after myocardial infarction. *Am J Cardiol* 14:837–842, 1964.

73. Costill DL, Fox EL. Energetics of marathon running. *Med Sci Sports Exerc* 1:81–86, 1969.

74. Manfre MJ, Yu GH, Varma AA, Mallis GI, Kearney K, Karageorgia MA. The effect of limited handrail support on total treadmill time and the prediction of $\dot{V}O_{2max}$. *Clin Cardiol* 17:445–450, 1994.

75. McConnell TR. Practical considerations in the testing of $\dot{V}O_{2max}$ in runners. *Sports Med* 5:57–68, 1988.

76. Pollock ML, Wilmore JH, Fox SM. *Exercise in Health and Disease.* Philadelphia: W. B. Saunders Co., 1984.

77. Froelicher VF, Lancaster MC. The prediction of maximal oxygen consumption from a continuous exercise treadmill protocol. *Am Heart J* 87:445–450, 1974.

78. Foster C, Jackson AS, Pollock ML, et al. Generalized equations for predicting functional capacity from treadmill performance. *Am Heart J* 108:1229–1234, 1984.

79. George JD. Alternative approach to maximal exercise testing and $\dot{V}O_{2max}$ prediction in college students. *Res Quart Exerc Sport* 67:452–457, 1996.

80. Montoye HJ, Ayen T, Nagle F, Howley ET. The oxygen requirement for horizontal and grade walking on a motor-driven treadmill. *Med Sci Sports Exerc* 17:640–645, 1985.

81. Storer TW, Davis JA, Caiozzo VJ. Accurate prediction of $\dot{V}O_{2max}$ in cycle ergometry. *Med Sci Sports Exerc* 22:704–712, 1990.

82. Inbar O, Bar-Or O, Skinner JS. *The Wingate Anaerobic Test.* Champaign, IL: Human Kinetics, 1996.

83. Bar-Or O. The Wingate Anaerobic Test: An update on methodology, reliability, and validity. *Sports Med* 4:381–394, 1987.

84. Mcklin RC, O'Bryant HS, Zehnbauer TM, Collins MA. A computerized method for assessing anaerobic power and work capacity using maximal cycle ergometry. *J Appl Sports Sci Res* 4:135–140, 1990.

85. Dubin D. *Rapid Interpretation of EKGs.* Tampa: Cover Publishing Co., 1974.

86. Evans CH. *Exercise Testing: Current Applications for Patient Management.* Philadelphia: W. B. Saunders Co., 1994.

PHYSICAL FITNESS ACTIVITY 4.1

Practical Use of the ACSM Equations

The American College of Sports Medicine equations presented in this chapter are highly useful for health and fitness instructors. However, the use of these equations can be initially confusing to some students. It is highly recommended that prospective instructors practice using the equations many times over, applying them to varying situations to gain a full understanding of them. In the ACSM Health / Fitness Instructor Certification program, the ACSM equations are an integral part of the process.

Here are some sample questions to help you learn how to use the equations. Correct answers are noted with an asterisk (*). Consult your instructor to help clarify use of the equations. However, all the information you need to solve these problems is in this chapter.

1. If a person is cycling at 60 rpm with the bicycle ergometer set at 2 kp, the workload in watts is

   a. 200

   b. *120

   c. 150

   d. 180

   e. none of the above

2. If a 60-kg man runs 9 mph for 45 minutes, how many Calories will he expend?

   a. 750

   b. 857

   c. 1142

   d. *665

   e. 443

3. If a 100-kg man is expending 5 METs during exercise, how many Calories / min is this?

   a. 7.5

   b. 4.8

   c. 5.8

   d. 6.2

   e. *8.3

4. If a 60-kg woman is cycling at a work rate of 600 kgm · min^{-1}, the energy expenditure in METs is

   a. *6.7

   b. 6.2

   c. 7.0

   d. 5.3

   e. 4.0

5. If a person walks at 5.0 mph, what is the energy expenditure in METs?

  a. 2.3

  b. *4.8

  c. 5.3

  d. 3.0

  e. 6.9

6. If the person in the previous question is a male weighing 70 kg, how many Calories would he burn if he walked for 30 minutes?

  a. 100

  b. 284

  c. 154

  d. *168

  e. 220

7. The oxygen cost of running on the level at 300 meters / min would be about

  a. 6 METs

  b. 8 METs

  c. 10.5 METs

  d. 12.5 METs

  e. *18.1 METs

8. If a person is cycling at 50 rpm with the cycle ergometer set at 4 kp, the workload in kgm $\cdot$ min^{-1} is

  a. 200

  b. *1,200

  c. 1,500

  d. 2,200

  e. none of the above

9. If a 50-kg man is expending 10 METs during exercise, how many Calories per hour is this?

  a. *500

  b. 600

  c. 650

  d. 750

  e. none of the above

10. If a 72-kg man is cycling at a work rate of 600 kgm $\cdot$ min^{-1}, the energy expenditure in ml $\cdot$ kg^{-1} $\cdot$ min^{-1} is

  a. 15

  b. *20.2

  c. 34

  d. 48

  e. none of the above

11. If an 80-kg person walks at 2.0 mph, how many Calories will be expended after 2 hours?

   a. *405

   b. 502

   c. 609

   d. 650

   e. none of the above

12. The oxygen cost in $ml \cdot kg^{-1} \cdot min^{-1}$ of running on the level at 8 mph would be

   a. 34.2

   b. *46.4

   c. 53.9

   d. 56.7

   e. 65.0

Questions 13 to 18 apply to Mr. Smith's graded exercise test on a cycle ergometer (3-min stages, 80 rpm). This was conducted without a physician present because Mr. Smith is an athlete training for national competition, is 22 years old, weighs 65 kg, and is apparently healthy.

Stage	Work Rate	Heart Rate	Blood Pressure	RPE
1	50 watts	100	125/70	2
2	100 watts	135	140/72	3
3	150 watts	150	150/70	4
4	200 watts	164	160/73	5
5	250 watts	178	172/70	6
6	300 watts	190	185/73	8
7	350 watts	200	190/72	9
8	400 watts	205	195/75	10

13. The final workload in kilogram-meters per minute is approximately

   a. 1,200

   b. *2,400

   c. 1,500

   d. 3,500

   e. none of the above

14. What was the final approximate "kg" setting (if test was conducted on a Monark mechanically braked cycle)?

   a. *5.0

   b. 3.5

   c. 4.4

   d. 6.4

   e. none of the above

15. What was the energy expenditure in METs during Stage 7 (assume he reached close to a steady state)?

    a. 15.6

    b. 17.4

    c. *19.5

    d. 20.2

    e. none of the above

16. What is his energy expenditure in kcal · min⁻¹ during Stage 5?

    a. *15.4

    b. 10.4

    c. 11.5

    d. 8.6

    e. none of the above

17. What is his energy expenditure in METs during Stage 3?

    a. 5.4

    b. *8.9

    c. 9.5

    d. 10.8

    e. 12.4

18. What is his energy expenditure in L · min during Stage 6?

    a. *3.83

    b. 4.23

    c. 5.67

    d. 5.8

    e. none of the above

PHYSICAL FITNESS ACTIVITY 4.2

Cardiorespiratory Endurance Testing

In this chapter, detailed information is given for several tests of cardiorespiratory endurance ($\dot{V}O_{2max}$), including the following:

- 1-mile run
- YMCA 3-minute step test
- Canadian aerobic fitness test
- YMCA submaximal cycle test
- Storer-Davis maximal cycle test
- Bruce maximal treadmill test

Under the supervision of your instructor or a local fitness center director, using the directions outlined in the chapter and the norms outlined in Appendix A, take each of these six tests and fill in the cardiorespiratory test worksheet. Be sure to follow the precautions outlined in this chapter. If you are not categorized as "apparently healthy" using the ACSM guidelines, these tests should not be taken unless under the direct supervision of a physician. (See Chapter 3.)

After taking these tests, answer the following questions.

1. Did the estimated $\dot{V}O_{2max}$ vary widely for the six different tests? (Define "widely" as more than 25% from the Bruce treadmill maximal test result.)

   a. Yes

   b. No

2. If you answered "yes" on Question #1, list at least five reasons as to why you feel $\dot{V}O_{2max}$ varied so widely.

   a. _____

   b. _____

   c. _____

   d. _____

   e. _____

Assessment of Cardiorespiratory Endurance Testing

Test	Your Score	Classification
1-mile run		
YMCA 3-minute step test		
Canadian aerobic fitness test		
YMCA submaximal cycle test		
Storer-Davis maximal cycle test		
Bruce maximal treadmill test		

Note: Record all scores in ml · kg^{-1} · min^{-1}, except for the YMCA 3-minute step test. Use $\dot{V}O_{2max}$ norms from Appendix A for classification. For the 1-mile run, use the estimating equation from Table 4.4. For the YMCA 3-minute step test, record 60-second recovery pulse, and then use norms in Appendix A (Table 22). For the Canadian aerobic fitness test, use the aerobic fitness score described in the text. For the YMCA submaximal cycle test, use Figure 4.15. For the Storer-Davis maximal cycle test, use equations from the text. For the Bruce maximal treadmill, use the equation described in Table 4.9.

5

Body Composition

Fat is a chronic preoccupation of much of the adult population, though possibly for different reasons in different places. In most parts of the world, fat is regarded as aesthetically undesirable when it becomes superficially evident. There is the more compelling reason for concern over excess fat for its adverse influence on longevity and, more specifically, on the degenerative diseases.

—Dr. William E. Siri, 1956

Interest in measurement of body composition has grown tremendously since the early 1970s. Elite athletes, people seeking to reach or maintain optimal body weight, and patients in hospitals have all benefited from the increased popularity and accuracy of body composition measurement.[1–3]

Research to establish ways of determining body composition through indirect methods began during the 1940s. Since then, a wide variety of methods have been developed. These methods are described here, with emphasis on the most practical techniques.

Most body composition analyses are based on seeing the body as consisting of two separate components: fat and fat-free.[3] Thus, *body composition* is often defined as the ratio of fat to fat-free mass. Common terms used in the study of body composition include those defined in Table 5.1.[1]

To study body composition, the body mass is subdivided into two or more components. The classic two-component model divides the body mass into fat and fat-free mass (Figure 5.1a). The *fat mass* contains all extractable lipids, and the *fat-free mass* includes water, protein, and mineral components (Figure 5.1b). In 1963, Brozek and colleagues dissected three white male cadavers and measured the density of body fat at 0.901 grams per cubic centimeter (g/cc), and the density of the fat-free mass as 1.10 g/cc. The Brozek et al.[4] equation estimated percent body fat as follows:

percent body fat = [(4.57/body density) − 4.142] × 100

TABLE 5.1   Definition of Terms Used in Body Composition

Term	Definition
Obesity	An excessive amount of total body fat for a given body weight
Fat mass	All extractable lipids from adipose and other tissues in the body
Fat-free mass	All residual, lipid-free chemicals and tissues, including water, muscle, bone, connective tissue, and internal organs
Relative body fat	Also called percent body fat; fat mass, expressed as a percentage of total body mass
Total body density	Total body mass, expressed relative to total body volume

Source: Heyward VH, Stolarczyk LM. *Applied Body Composition Assessment.* Champaign, IL: Human Kinetics, 1996. Reprinted with permission.

This was similar to an equation published 2 years earlier by Siri[5]

percent body fat = [(4.95/body density) − 4.50] × 100

Since the 1960s, these two formulas have been used to estimate percent body fat from the body density obtained from hydrostatic or underwater weighing, once considered

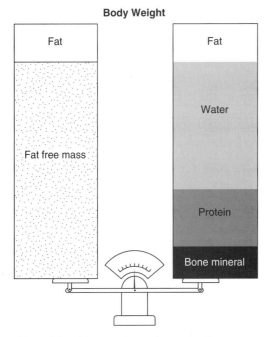

Body Weight

Figure 5.1a There are two body composition models currently in use: the two-component model (fat-free mass and fat) and the four-component model (bone mineral, protein, water, and fat).

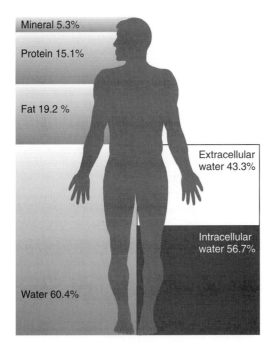

Figure 5.1b Body composition on the molecular level for the 70-kg reference man. The "reference man" is about 60% water, with the rest composed of fat, bone mineral, and protein.

the "gold standard" method. (This method of measuring body composition is described in detail later on in this chapter). However, recent technological advances for measuring water (isotope dilution), mineral (dual-energy x-ray absorptiometry, DEXA), and protein (neutron activation analysis) have shown that the fat-free mass varies widely among groups because of age, sex, ethnicity, level of body fatness, and physical activity level. Because the fat-free mass varies among people, the two-component model equations of Brozek et al.[4] and Siri[5] can either under- or overestimate the actual percent body fat. Table 5.2 summarizes the fat-free mass densities recently measured for different groups of people, using multicomponent models that take into account variations in the water and mineral components.[1] For these various subgroups, the estimated body density from underwater weighing, skinfold equations, and bioelectrical equations can be converted to percent body fat by using the conversion formulas listed in Table 5.2. These population-specific conversion formulas were calculated by Heyward, using multicomponent model estimates of fat-free mass density obtained from the literature.[1]

Before exploring the various methods of measuring body composition (skinfold techniques, underwater weighing, bioelectrical impedance, DEXA, and other new techniques), this chapter discusses height and weight tables and the use of various height-to-weight ratios.

HEIGHT AND WEIGHT MEASUREMENTS

Weight measurement alone cannot accurately determine the body fat status of a person (Figure 5.2). Weight measurement does not differentiate between fat-free mass and fat mass. In other words, some people with *mesomorphic* or athletic, muscular body types (such as bodybuilders) can have normal or low body fat even though they are overweight according to standard charts. Some people who are *ectomorphic* (or lean, thin, and linear) with low amounts of fat-free mass can be underweight according to the weight charts and extremely low in body fat as well (endurance athlete). The *endomorphic* (heavy, big, soft) individual is overweight from large amounts of both fat-free and fat mass (e.g., football lineman).[2]

Figure 5.3 summarizes the effect of body type (or somatype) on fat mass and body weight. Body type is strongly affected by genetics but little by lifestyle and exercise habits. Most people are a mixture of the three body types, with tendencies toward one. Only 5% of the population are "pure" ectomorphs or "pure" mesomorphs. Because total body weight is so strongly related to somatype, body composition (i.e., the ratio of fat to fat-free mass) is a much better indication of ideal body weight than is the total weight obtained from stepping on a weight scale.

TABLE 5.2 Population-Specific Fat-Free Mass Density and Formulas for Conversion of Body Density to Percent Body Fat

Population	Age (yr)	Gender	Fat-Free Mass Density (g/cc)	Percent Fat Formula
White	7–12	Male	1.084	$(5.30/Db) - 4.89$
		Female	1.082	$(5.35/Db) - 4.95$
	13–16	Male	1.094	$(5.07/Db) - 4.64$
		Female	1.093	$(5.10/Db) - 4.66$
	17–19	Male	1.098	$(4.99/Db) - 4.55$
		Female	1.095	$(5.05/Db) - 4.62$
	20–80	Male	1.10	$(4.95/Db) - 4.50$
		Female	1.097	$(5.01/Db) - 4.57$
Black	18–32	Male	1.113	$(4.37/Db) - 3.93$
	24–79	Female	1.106	$(4.85/Db) - 4.39$
American Indian	18–60	Female	1.108	$(4.81/Db) - 4.34$
Hispanic	20–40	Female	1.105	$(4.87/Db) - 4.41$
Japanese native	18–48	Male	1.099	$(4.97/Db) - 4.52$
	18–48	Female	1.111	$(4.76/Db) - 4.28$
	61–78	Male	1.105	$(4.87/Db) - 4.41$
	61–78	Female	1.100	$(4.95/Db) - 4.50$
Obese	17–62	Female	1.098	$(5.00/Db) - 4.56$
Anorexic	15–30	Female	1.087	$(5.26/Db) - 4.83$

Sources: Heyward VH. Evaluation of body composition: Current issues. *Sports Med* 22:146–156, 1996. Heyward VH, Stolarczyk LM. *Applied Body Composition Assessment.* Champaign, IL: Human Kinetics, 1996. Used with permission.

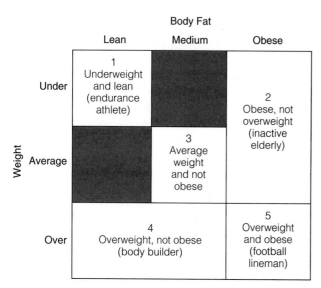

Figure 5.2 The relationship among three categories of body weight and body fat can be described in five different ways. Weight measurement alone cannot accurately determine the body fat status of a person.

This chapter emphasizes skinfold measurements and underwater weighing in assessing body composition prior to estimation of ideal body weight. Because of the widespread use of height–weight tables, however, a brief review of this methodology is given first.

Historical Review of Height–Weight Tables

Since the 1940s, tables have been developed by the Metropolitan Life Insurance Company for "ideal" and "desirable" weights.[6–9] They were derived from the 1959 Build and Blood Pressure Study, based on the combined experience of 26 life insurance companies in the United States and Canada from 1935 to 1954, involving observation of nearly 5 million insured people for periods of up to 20 years. Height and weight were measured with street shoes and indoor clothing. The study excluded those with heart disease, cancer, or diabetes. In the resulting 1959 Metropolitan Life Insurance Co. "Desirable Weights for Men and Women," "desirable weights" were those associated with the lowest mortality.[7]

These 1959 tables set forth weight ranges for small-, medium-, and large-frame men and women of differing heights. Unfortunately, the method of determining frame size was not given.[6,8]

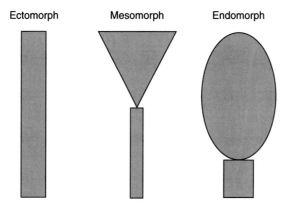

	Ectomorph	Mesomorph	Endomorph
Fat mass	Low or normal	Low or normal	High
Fat-free mass	Low	High	High
Total body weight	Underweight	Overweight	Overweight

Figure 5.3 Somatypes. Body type or somatype has a strong influence on total body weight.

TABLE 5.3 **1983 Metropolitan Height–Weight Tables**

(In Pounds by Height and Frame in Indoor Clothing, Men—5 lbs, 1-Inch Heel; Women—3 lbs, 1-Inch Heel)

Men				Women			
Height (inches)	Small	Medium	Large	Height (inches)	Small	Medium	Large
62	128–134	131–141	138–150	58	102–111	109–121	118–131
63	130–136	133–143	140–153	59	103–113	111–123	120–134
64	132–138	135–145	142–156	60	104–115	113–126	122–137
65	134–140	137–148	144–160	61	106–118	115–129	125–140
66	136–142	139–151	146–164	62	108–121	118–132	128–143
67	138–145	142–154	149–168	63	111–124	121–135	131–147
68	140–148	145–157	152–172	64	114–127	124–138	135–151
69	142–151	148–160	155–176	65	117–130	127–141	137–155
70	144–154	151–163	158–180	66	120–133	130–144	140–159
71	146–157	154–166	161–184	67	123–136	133–147	143–163
72	149–160	157–170	164–188	68	126–139	136–150	146–167
73	152–164	160–174	168–192	69	129–142	139–153	149–170
74	155–168	164–178	172–197	70	132–145	142–156	152–173
75	158–172	167–182	176–202	71	135–148	145–159	155–176
76	162–176	171–187	181–207	72	138–151	148–162	158–179

Source: Reprinted with permission from the Metropolitan Life Insurance Company, New York.

On March 1, 1983, the Metropolitan Life Insurance Company issued new height–weight tables derived from the 1979 Build Study[8] (see Table 5.3). It utilized data from 25 insurance companies reporting the U.S. and Canadian mortality experience from 1954 to 1972 for more than 4 million insured, again excluding applicants with major diseases.

In these most recent tables, weights associated with lowest mortality are no longer called "desirable" or "ideal." Also, this time, a method for determining *frame size* by utilizing elbow breadth measurement was included (see Table 5.4). These frame size measurements were based on the National Health and Nutrition Examination Survey (NHANES I and II) data and were so devised that 50% of the population fell within the medium-frame area, 25% within the small-frame area, and 25% within the large-frame area.[10]

There are several considerations to bear in mind in using the 1983 weight tables.[7–10]

- The 1983 weight tables present weight ranges that are 2–13% higher than the 1959 tables.[7,8] These up ward revisions, however, are not uniformly distrib-

TABLE 5.4   Height and Elbow Breadth

	Height (inches, no shoes)	Elbow Breadth (in inches)		
		Small Frame	Medium Frame	Large Frame
Men	61–62	$<2\frac{1}{2}$	$2\frac{1}{2}$–$2\frac{7}{8}$	$>2\frac{7}{8}$
	63–66	$<2\frac{5}{8}$	$2\frac{5}{8}$–$2\frac{7}{8}$	$>2\frac{7}{8}$
	67–70	$<2\frac{3}{4}$	$2\frac{3}{4}$–3	>3
	71–74	$<2\frac{3}{4}$	$2\frac{3}{4}$–$3\frac{1}{8}$	$>3\frac{1}{8}$
	75	$<2\frac{7}{8}$	$2\frac{7}{8}$–$3\frac{1}{4}$	$>3\frac{1}{4}$
Women	57–58	$<2\frac{1}{4}$	$2\frac{1}{4}$–$2\frac{1}{2}$	$>2\frac{1}{2}$
	59–62	$<2\frac{1}{4}$	$2\frac{1}{4}$–$2\frac{1}{2}$	$>2\frac{1}{2}$
	63–66	$<2\frac{3}{8}$	$2\frac{3}{8}$–$2\frac{5}{8}$	$>2\frac{5}{8}$
	67–70	$<2\frac{3}{8}$	$2\frac{3}{8}$–$2\frac{5}{8}$	$>2\frac{5}{8}$
	71	$2\frac{1}{2}$	$2\frac{1}{2}$–$2\frac{3}{4}$	$>2\frac{3}{4}$

Note: Tables adapted to represent height without shoes. To measure the elbow breadth, extend the arm, and then bend the forearm upward at a 90-degree angle, fingers straight up, palm turned toward the body. Measure with a sliding caliper the width between the two prominent bones on either side of the elbow (measure the widest point). Make sure that the arm is positioned correctly and that the upper arm is parallel to the ground. The elbow breadth frame gauge ($5) is available from Metropolitan Life Insurance Company, Health and Safety Education Division, One Madison, New York, NY 10010.

Source: Reprinted with permission from Metropolitan Life Insurance Company, New York.

uted throughout the height categories; the largest increases are for the shorter men and women.

- The tables are based on specific populations that are not representative of the whole population. The data for the 1983 tables were drawn from people who were able to purchase nongroup insurance (excluding those who purchased group insurance) and who were 25–59 years of age (excluding the elderly). Thus insurees were predominantly white, middle-class adults. Blacks, Asians, and low-income and other population groups were not represented proportionally. Also, people with serious chronic diseases or acute illnesses were not included.

- No consideration was made for cigarette smoking. Cigarette smoking is associated with lower weight and shorter life span. Including smokers in the data thus skewed the "ideal weights" upward.[11]

- The height–weight tables were based on the lowest mortality, and did not take into account the health problems often associated with obesity. Such disease conditions as cardiovascular disease, cancer, hypertension, high blood cholesterol levels, and many other health problems are more prevalent among the obese. For these reasons, the American Heart Association and others have urged the populace to use the weight tables as a "mere gross estimate."[7]

- Only initial weights were used in the determination of ideal weight. People taking out insurance policies had their weights measured, but no further data were collected on weight or development of disease after the policy was initially purchased. If weight changed between issuance of the policy and death, this was not taken into account.[7]

- Finally, weight tables do not provide information on actual body composition. As stated previously, what really matters is the quality of the weight, not the quantity. "Ideal body weight" is not ideal for everyone at a given height because of bone and muscle differences. Thus, height–weight tables are merely gross estimates, and other methods, such as anthropometric measures, should be used to refine the estimate of proper weight.

In 1990, the U.S. Department of Agriculture (USDA) published a new table of "Suggested Weight for Adults."[12] There were two unique features of the USDA table:

1. One weight range was given for *both* men and women.

2. A separate weight range for a given height was listed for people 35 years and over. Men or any individual with more muscle and bone than normal were urged to use the upper end of the weight range for their height.

It was the second feature that caused the most controversy among scientists because older people were allowed to be 10–18 pounds heavier than their younger counterparts.[13,14]

While some researchers felt that this amount of weight gain after age 35 was normal and posed no risk to health, others felt that risk of coronary heart disease, hypertension, diabetes, and other obesity-related diseases was increased.

Researchers from the Framingham Heart Study and the Harvard Medical School were foremost in urging that the weight tables be changed.[14] There was a growing consensus that "the present standards are too permissive," and that there is "no biological rationale for recommending that people increase their weight as they grow older."[14]

In response to these concerns, the Dietary Guidelines Advisory Committee of the USDA submitted an updated height–weight table in 1995 (Table 5.5).[15] The updated table listed one healthy weight range for a given height for men and women of all ages. In the words of the committee, "The health risks due to excess weight appear to be the same for older adults as for younger adults. Based on published data, there appears to be no justification for the establishment of a cut point that increases with age."[15] Weight ranges were given in the table "because people of the same height may have equal amounts of body fat but different amounts of muscle and bone. However, the ranges do not mean that it is healthy to gain weight, even within the same weight range. The higher weights in the healthiest weight range apply to people with more muscle and bone."[15] A figure was supplied with the table (Figure 5.4), giving zones to depict moderate and severe overweight. A body mass index of 25 was used as the upper boundary of healthy weight (see the section on body mass index starting on page 127 in this chapter).

TABLE 5.5   1995 USDA Healthy Weight Ranges for Men and Women

Height (no shoes)	Weight (in pounds) (without clothes)
4'10"	91–119
4'11"	94–124
5'0"	97–128
5'1"	101–132
5'2"	104–137
5'3"	107–141
5'4"	111–146
5'5"	114–150
5'6"	118–155
5'7"	121–160
5'8"	125–164
5'9"	129–169
5'10"	132–174
5'11"	136–179
6'0"	140–184
6'1"	144–189
6'2"	148–195
6'3"	152–200
6'4"	156–205
6'5"	160–211
6'6"	164–216

Source: USDA. *1995 Dietary Guidelines for Americans.*

Relative Weight

Obesity has been defined as being 20% or more overweight, using the concept of relative weight. *Relative weight* uses the ratio or percentage of actual weight to desirable weight. Most researchers use as the point of reference the midpoint value of the weight range for the subject's height. A man who is 70 inches tall and weighs 180 pounds, for example, would have the following relative weight, using the midpoint value of the range given in the 1995 USDA tables (Table 5.5).

$$\text{relative weight} = \left[\frac{\text{body weight}}{\text{midpoint value of weight range}} \right] \times 100$$

$$= \left[\frac{180}{153} \right] \times 100 = 117.6\%$$

In other words, this person is 17.6% overweight. Standards for relative weight are given in Table 5.6. As with any value taken from a height–weight table, these standards can be inaccurate for people with higher than normal amounts of muscle and bone.

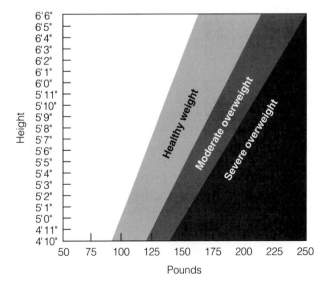

Are you overweight?

Figure 5.4   USDA height–weight chart: Are you overweight?   *Source:* USDA. *1995 Dietary Guidelines for Americans.*

TABLE 5.6 Standards for Relative Weight

<90%	Underweight
90–110%	Desirable
111–119%	Overweight
120–139%	Mild obesity
140–199%	Moderate obesity
≥200%	Severe obesity

Measuring Body Weight

Body weight should be measured on a physician's balance-beam scale, with minimal clothing, preferably shorts and light T-shirt, and no shoes, or better yet, a disposable paper gown[16] (see Figure 5.5). The beam scale should have movable weights, with the scale readable from both sides. Balance-beam scales are available from various companies (see Appendix B).

The scale should be positioned on a level, solid floor (not carpet), so that the measurer can stand behind the beam, facing the person being measured, and can move the beam weights without reaching around. The scale should be calibrated each time before use by putting the beam weight on zero, and seeing whether the beam scale balances out. If not, a screwdriver can be used on the movable tare weight to adjust the beam weight. The weight should be read to the nearest 0.25 pound.

If the objective is to assess changes in weight, great care should be taken to repeat measurement of weight under the same conditions and at the same time of day.[17] The weight of an average adult varies approximately 4 to 5 pounds (2 kg) within a day.

Measuring Height

The measurement of height (or stature) requires a vertical ruler with a horizontal headboard that can be brought into contact with the highest point on the head.[16] The headboard and ruler taken together are called a *stadiometer*.

When measuring height, have the person stand without shoes, heels together, back as straight as possible, heels, buttocks, shoulders, and head touching the wall, and looking straight ahead. Weight should be distributed evenly on both feet, arms hanging freely by the sides of the body. Just before measurement, the person being measured should inhale deeply, and hold the breath, while the headboard is brought onto the highest point on the head, with sufficient pressure to compress the hair.[16,17] Fixed and portable stadiometers are available from various companies (see Appendix B).

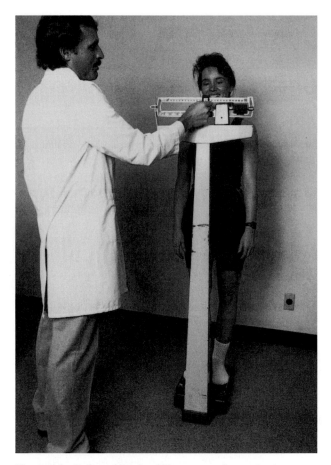

Figure 5.5 Body weight should be measured on a physician's balance-beam scale, with minimal clothing.

If a professional stadiometer is not available, a ruler should be affixed to the wall, and a right angle measuring block (such as a clipboard on edge) used, measuring straight back from the crown of the head. A wall should be chosen that does not have a baseboard, and a floor without a carpet should be used (see Figure 5.6). Measurement of height while standing on a physician balance-beam scale is *not* recommended—it invites substantial error.

Measuring Frame Size

As discussed previously, frame size is most commonly determined by measuring the width of the elbow. Other measures have been proposed as estimates of frame size, including bony chest diameter and wrist circumference, but national norms are not yet available for these measurements.[18]

When measuring the width of the elbow, the person being measured should stand erect, with the right arm extended forward perpendicular to the body. The arm is then flexed until the elbow forms a 90-degree angle, with fingers up, palm facing inward[19] (see Figure 5.7). The measurer

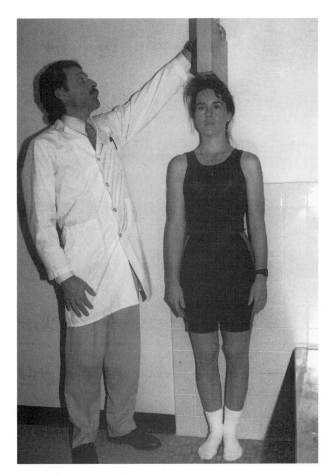

Figure 5.6 Height should be measured while standing erect, with heels, buttocks, back of shoulders, and head touching the vertical ruler. A right-angle object should be brought into contact with the highest point on the head after a deep inhalation and holding of breath.

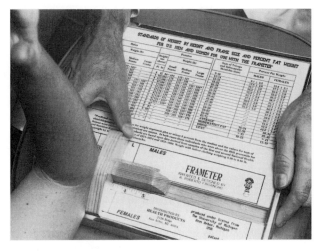

Figure 5.7 The elbow breadth measurement is used for determining frame size. With the arm in this position, the sliding caliper is used to measure the widest point at the elbow.

should first feel for the widest bony width of the elbow, and put the caliper heads at those points.

A sliding caliper should be used[17] (Figure 5.7), with pressure firm enough to compress soft tissue over the bone. Table 5.4 summarizes how the data are used to determine frame size. Sliding calipers are available from various companies (see Appendix B).

Body Mass Index

In large population studies of obesity, a commonly used measure of obesity is the *body mass index*.[20,21] A number of body mass indices (BMI) have been developed, all derived from body weight and height measurements. The more popular BMIs include the weight–height ratio W/H, Quetelet index W/H^2, and Khosla-Lowe index W/H^3. These indices represent different attempts to adjust body weight for height to derive a height-free measure of obesity.[21] These BMIs are widely used in large population studies because of their simplicity of measurement and calculation, and their low cost.

The *Quetelet index* or kg/m^2 (body weight in kilograms, divided by height in meters squared) is the most widely accepted BMI. This measure was an attempt by the nineteenth-century mathematician Lambert Adolphe Jacques Quetelet to describe the relation between body weight and stature in humans. Studies have shown that the Quetelet index correlates rather well ($r = 0.70$) with actual measurement of body fat from hydrostatic weighing.[1–3] However, the SEE is 5% body fat, which means that if a person is 15% fat, the Quetelet index would predict a percent body fat ranging from 10 to 20%.[1–3]

The following example can be used to learn how to calculate the Quetelet index. For example, a man weighing 154 pounds (or 70 kilograms—divide weight in pounds by 2.2), standing 68 inches tall (or 1.727 meters tall—multiply height in inches by 0.0254) has a Quetelet index of

$$\text{Quetelet index} = \frac{70\ kg}{(1.727\ m)^2} = \frac{70}{2.98} = 23.5\ kg/m^2$$

Another simpler method uses this formula:

$$\text{Quetelet index} = \text{weight in pounds}$$
$$\div \text{ height in inches}$$
$$\div \text{ height in inches} \div 0.0014192$$

Using our subject:

$$154 \div 68 \div 68 \div 0.0014192 = 23.5\ kg/m^2$$

The Quetelet index of 23.5 puts this man in the normal range (see standards in Figure 5.8). Figure 5.8 makes calculation of the Quetelet index easy, through use of a nomogram. Figure 5.9 depicts the average Quetelet Index for American males and females throughout the life cycle.[17]

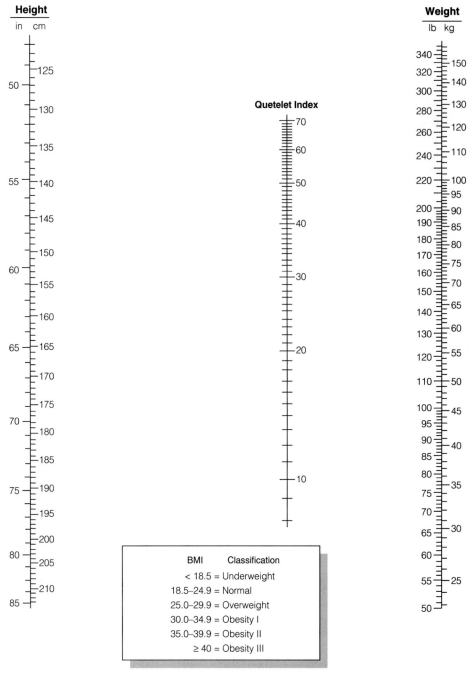

Figure 5.8 The Quetelet index (kg/m²) is calculated from this nomogram by reading the central scale after a straight edge is placed between height and body weight.

Some experts feel that the major limitation of the body mass index is that it is difficult both to interpret to patients, and to relate to needed weight loss.[10] It does have the advantage of being more precise than weight tables, and of permitting comparison of populations. Also, many studies have confirmed that the health risks associated with obesity begin in the range of 25–30 kg/m².[22] (See Chapter 11.) Thus,

the body mass index has proven to be a useful marker of disease status.

However, various studies have shown that the Quetelet Index can be somewhat insensitive in detecting obesity or leanness for individuals with extremes of fat-free mass.[21] For example, someone with a large fat-free mass (e.g., a football player) would be classified by the Quetelet index

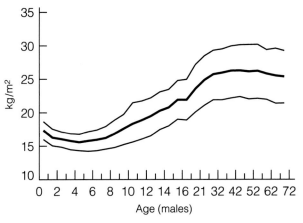 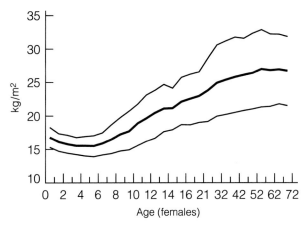

Figure 5.9 The average body mass index (kg/m²) of American males (left) and females (right) is shown for all ages. The area around the mean represents the fifteenth to eighty-fifth percentiles (or middle 70%) taken from a large national sample of Americans.[15] Data based on combined NHANES I and NHANES II.

as obese. It is recommended that skinfold testing be used for these types of individuals.

SKINFOLD MEASUREMENTS

The most widely used and practical method for determining obesity is based on the thickness of skinfolds. *Skinfold measurements* have several advantages:

1. The necessary equipment is inexpensive and needs little space.
2. The measures can be obtained quickly and easily.
3. When performed correctly the measures have a high correlation ($r \geq .80$) with body density from underwater weighing. Skinfold variables provide more accurate estimates of body fat than the various height–weight ratios do.[1–3,23–25]

Rules for Taking Skinfolds

Many researchers in the United States (including those performing the large national surveys of the U.S. population that form the basis for normative data worldwide) take skinfold measurements on the right side of the body.[24] European investigators, on the other hand, tend to take measurements on the left side of the body. Most research, however, reveals that it matters little on which side measurements are taken.[24] It is the opinion of this author, however, that students in the United States should be taught to take all skinfold measurements on the right side, to coincide with the efforts of most U.S. researchers.

1. As a general rule, those with little experience in skinfold measurement should mark the site to be measured with a black felt pen. Use a flexible steel tape with sites when you need to locate a body midpoint. With experience, however, you can locate the sites without marking.[24]
2. Feel the site prior to measurement to prepare yourself and the subject.
3. Firmly grasp the skinfold with the thumb and index finger of your left hand, and pull away from the subject's body. While this is usually easy with thin people, it is much harder with the obese and can be somewhat uncomfortable for the person being tested. The amount of tissue pinched up must be enough to form a fold with approximately parallel sides (Figure 5.10). The thicker the fat layer under the skin, the wider the necessary fold (and the more separation needed between thumb and index finger).
4. Hold the caliper in your right hand, perpendicular to the skinfold and with the skinfold dial facing up and easily readable. Place the caliper heads ¼–½ inch away from the fingers holding the skinfold, so that the pressure of the caliper will not be affected.
5. Do not place the skinfold caliper too deep into the skinfold or too far away on the tip of the skinfold. Try to visualize where a true double fold of skin thickness is, and place the caliper heads there. It is good practice to position the caliper arms one at a time—first the fixed arm on one side, and then the lever arm on the other.
6. Read the dial approximately 4 seconds after the pressure from your hand has been released on the lever arm of the caliper jaw.
7. Take a minimum of two measurements at each site. Measurements should be at least 15 seconds apart,

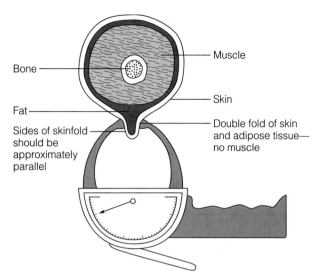

Figure 5.10   The double fold of skin and subcutaneous adipose tissue grasped by the thumb and index finger of the left hand should be large enough to form approximately parallel sides. Care should be taken to elevate only skin and adipose tissue.   *Source:* Lee RD, Nieman DC. *Nutritional Assessment.* Dubuque, IA: Wm. C. Brown Communications, Inc., 1993. Copyright © 1993 Wm. C. Brown Communications, Inc. All rights reserved. Used with permission.

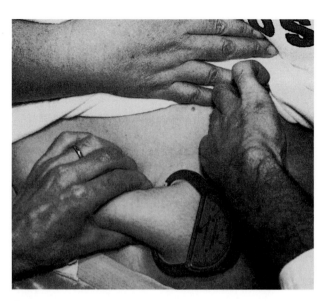

Figure 5.11   Skinfold measurement is very difficult with obese subjects and requires experience to know just where the caliper heads should be placed.

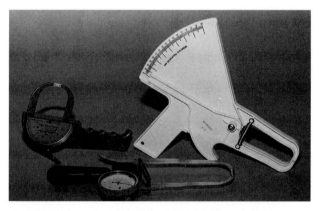

Figure 5.12   Pictured are the Lange, Harpenden, and Slim Guide skinfold calipers.

to allow the skinfold site to return to normal. If consecutive measurements vary by more than 10%, take more until there is consistency.

8. Maintain the pressure with the thumb and forefinger throughout each measurement.

9. When measuring the obese, it may be impossible to elevate a skinfold with parallel sides, particularly over the abdomen (Figure 5.11). In this situation, try using both hands to pull the skinfold away, while a partner attempts to measure the width. If the skinfold is too wide for the calipers, you will have to use underwater weighing or another technique.

10. Do not take measurements when the subject's skin is moist because there is a tendency to grasp extra skin, obtaining inaccurately large values. Also do not take measurements immediately after exercise or when the person being measured is overheated because the shift of body fluid to the skin will inflate normal skinfold size.

11. It takes practice to be able to grasp the same amount of skinfold consistently at the same location every time. Accuracy can be tested by having several technicians take the same measurements and comparing results. It may take up to 20–50 practice sessions to become proficient.

Calipers should be accurately calibrated and have a constant pressure of 10 g/mm² throughout the full measurement range[1-3,24] (see Figure 5.12). (See Appendix B for a listing of companies that sell skinfold calipers.) Box 5.1 provides a summary of the major skinfold calipers and their approximate prices.

The accuracy of skinfold measurements can be reduced by many factors, including measurement at the wrong sites, inconsistencies among different calipers and testers, and the use of inconsistent equations.[24] However, when testers practice together and take care to standardize their testing procedures, inconsistencies among testers can usually be held under 1%. The largest source of error is the nonstandardization of site selection.[1-3,24]

Eight skinfold sites are described here next. They are in accordance with the Airlie Consensus Conference that resulted in the publication of the *Anthropometric Standardization Reference Manual.*[24]

Box 5.1

Description of Skinfold Calipers

The following is a brief description of the major types of skinfold calipers, listed in order of decreasing retail price.

1. *Skyndex 1.* This unique caliper has a built-in computer, which calculates and displays percent body fat directly on its LCD (liquid-crystal display) digital readout, thus eliminating the necessity to add the skinfold readings and compute the percent body fat from formulas or tables. Available with Durnin, Jackson–Pollock, and Slaughter–Lohman formulas. Only one program is in each caliper, and the desired formula needs to be specified when ordering. $350

2. *Harpenden.* This has been a standard research caliper for many years. Some skinfold equations in use today are based on studies done using the Harpenden. It is accurate to within ±0.2 mm. Some researchers have provided data that the Harpenden skinfold calipers provide smaller values, when compared to the Lange skinfold calipers. $290

3. *Skyndex 11.* This is basically the same as the Skyndex 1, except that it does not have the built-in computer. It has an easy-to-read digital readout and a "hold" feature. When the user is satisfied with the reading, the hold button can be pushed, and this will lock the reading on the digital display until it can be written down. A second push on the hold button returns the caliper to "0." $200

4. *Lange.* This is the best selling of the high-priced calipers. Jackson–Pollock skinfold data were obtained using the Lange skinfold calipers. It has been manufactured since 1962 and is widely used in schools, colleges, fitness centers, etc. $180

5. *Baseline or Jamar or TEC.* This is a copy of the Lange but is made in Korea and sold under several different names. It appears to be identical to the Lange, even to the paint color. However, its internal quality is not as high, and repair has been reported to be a problem. $170

6. *Trimmeter.* This is the newest of the professional calipers. It has a bright, easy-to-read, LED (light-emitting diode) digital readout, and a comfortable, easy-to-use design, with a symmetrical shape for right- or left-hand use. The Trimmeter has the largest jaw opening (over 90 mm) of any of the calipers, allowing easier measurement of skinfold from obese subjects and measurement of elbow width. It has the lowest price of the professional calipers. $150

7. *Slim Guide.* Much lower priced than any of the aforementioned calipers yet will produce results that are almost as accurate. This is the only low-cost caliper accurate enough to be used for professional measurements and is the most widely used professional caliper. Its primary disadvantage is that it does not look professional. The caliper is easy to use, with convenient pistol grip and trigger. It is very durable. $25

8. *Fat-O-Meter.* A low-priced economy caliper. The caliper is small and lightweight and can be conveniently carried in a pocket. Although not as accurate as other calipers, it will provide reasonable estimates of body fat if correct procedures are carefully followed. $13

Each of these calipers is available through Creative Health Products, 5148 Saddle Ridge Road, Plymouth, MI 48170; 800-742-4478

To reduce error, skinfold sites should be precisely determined and verified by a trained instructor before measurement. The measurements should be made carefully, in a quiet room, and without undue haste. (Figures 5.13 to 5.22 depict the correct site marking and method of measurement for each site.)

- *Chest.* The chest or pectoral skinfold is measured using a skinfold with its long axis directed to the nipple. The skinfold is picked up just next to the anterior axillary fold (front of armpit line) (Figure 5.13). The measurement is taken ½ inch from the fingers.

The site is approximately 1 inch from the anterior axillary line toward the nipple. The measurement is the same for both men and women.

- *Abdomen.* A horizontal fold is picked up slightly more than 1 inch (3 cm) to the side of and ½ inch below the naval (Figure 5.14).

- *Thigh.* Pick up a vertical fold on the front of the thigh, midway between the hip (inguinal crease) and the nearest border of the patella or kneecap (Figures 5.15 and 5.16). The person being tested should first flex the hip to make it easier to locate the inguinal crease.

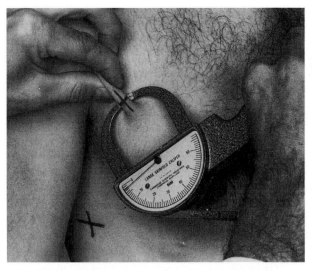

Figure 5.13   Measurement of the chest or pectoral skinfold.

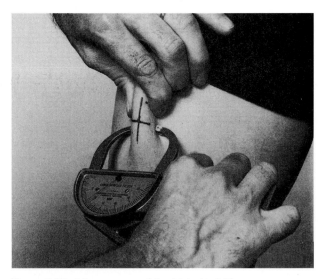

Figure 5.15   Measurement of the thigh skinfold.

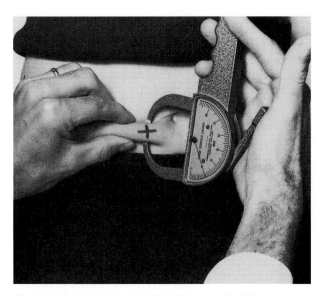

Figure 5.14   Measurement of the abdominal skinfold.

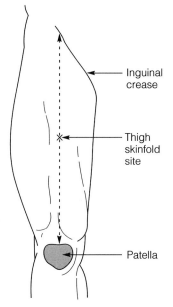

Figure 5.16   The thigh skinfold site lies along the anterior midline of the thigh halfway between the inguinal crease and the proximal border of the patella.   *Source:* Lee RD, Nieman DC. *Nutritional Assessment.* Dubuque, IA: Wm. C. Brown Communications, Inc., 1993. Copyright © 1993 Wm. C. Brown Communications, Inc. All rights reserved. Used with permission.

Be sure to pick a spot on the hip crease that is exactly above the midpoint of the front of the thigh. The closest border of the kneecap should be located while the knee is extended. When measuring the thigh skinfold, the body weight should be shifted to the other foot while the leg on the side of the measurement is relaxed, with the knee slightly flexed and the foot flat on the floor.

- *Triceps.* Measure a vertical fold on the rear midline of the upper arm, halfway between the lateral projection of the acromion process of the scapula (bump on back side of shoulder) and the inferior part of the olecranon process (the elbow) (Figure 5.17a and b).

The site should first be marked by measuring the distance between the lateral projection of the acromial process and the lower border of the olecranon process of the ulna, using a tape measure, with the elbow flexed to 90°. The midpoint is marked on the lateral side of the arm. The skinfold is measured with the arm hanging loosely at the side. The measurer stands behind the person being measured and picks

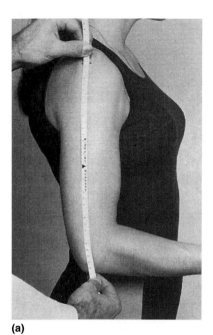

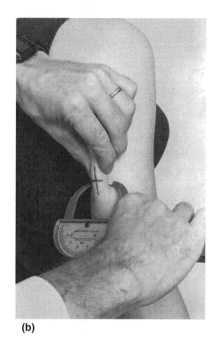

(a) **(b)**

Figure 5.17a and b Measurement of the triceps skinfold.

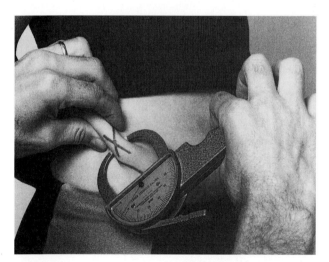

Figure 5.18 Measurement of the suprailiac skinfold.

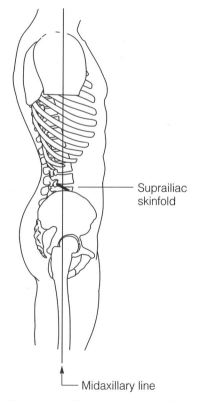

Suprailiac skinfold

Midaxillary line

up the skinfold site on the back of the arm, with the thumb and index finger directed down toward the feet. The triceps skinfold is picked up with the left thumb and index finger, approximately ½ inch above the marked level where the tips of the caliper are applied.

- *Suprailiac.* Measure a diagonal fold above the crest of the ilium at the spot where an imaginary line would come down from the midaxillary line (Figures 5.18 and 5.19). The person being measured should stand erect, with feet together. The arms should hang by the sides but can be moved slightly to improve access to the site. A diagonal fold should be grasped

Figure 5.19 The suprailiac skinfold is measured just above the iliac crest at the midaxillary line. The long axis of the skinfold follows the natural cleavage lines of the skin. *Source:* Lee RD, Nieman DC. *Nutritional Assessment.* Dubuque, IA: Wm. C. Brown Communications, Inc., 1993. Copyright © 1993 Wm. C. Brown Communications, Inc. All rights reserved. Used with permission.

just to the rear of the midaxillary line, following the natural cleavage lines of the skin. The skinfold caliper jaws should be applied about ½ inch from the fingers.

- *Midaxillary.* Measure a horizontal fold on the midaxillary line at the level of the xiphi-sternal junction (bottom of the sternum, where the xiphoid process begins) (Figure 5.20). The arm of the person being measured can be moved slightly backward during measurement to allow easy access to the site.

- *Subscapular.* The site is just below the lowest angle of the scapula (Figure 5.21). A fold is taken on a diagonal line directed at a 45-degree angle toward the right side. To locate the site, the measurer should feel for the bottom of the scapula. In some cases, it helps to place the arm of the person being measured behind his or her back.

- *Medial calf.* For the measurement of the medial calf skinfold, the person being measured sits with his or her right knee flexed to about 90 degrees, sole of the foot on the floor. The level of the maximum calf circumference is marked on the inside (medial) of the calf (Figure 5.22). Facing from the front, the measurer raises a vertical skinfold and measures at the marked site.

One-Site Skinfold Test

The triceps skinfold site has been used most often in large population group studies. The average triceps skinfold

thicknesses (in millimeters) for various age groups are given in Figure 5.23. The data were derived from the first and second National Health and Examination Surveys (NHANES I and II) for 1971–1974 and 1976–1980.[17] (See Appendix A, Table 27.)

Care should be taken when classifying obesity with the use of just one skinfold site. No equations for body fat estimation have been developed using just the triceps skinfold, and individual values must therefore be compared to tables developed from national norms. Some people have a higher proportion of their body fat distributed on the backs of their upper arms than others, which could lead to an overestimation of their degree of obesity. Therefore, the single-site skinfold test should only be used as a rough approximation of obesity.

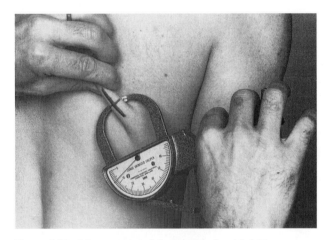

Figure 5.21 Measurement of the subscapular skinfold.

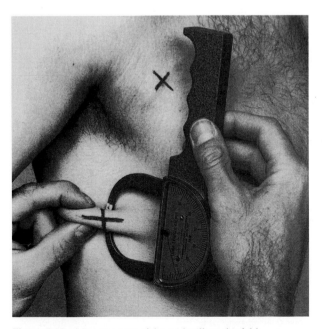

Figure 5.20 Measurement of the midaxillary skinfold.

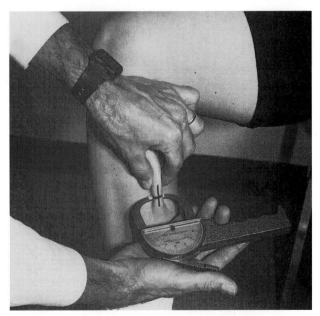

Figure 5.22 Measurement of the medial calf skinfold.

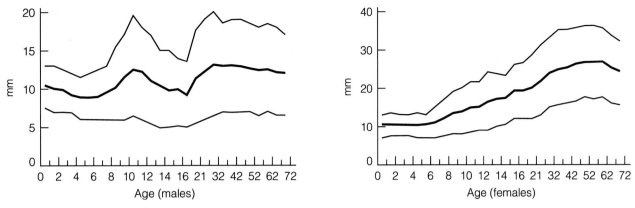

Figure 5.23   Average triceps skinfold of American males (left) and females (right). The area around the mean represents the fifteenth and eighty-fifth percentiles of a national sample of individuals of all ages.[15]

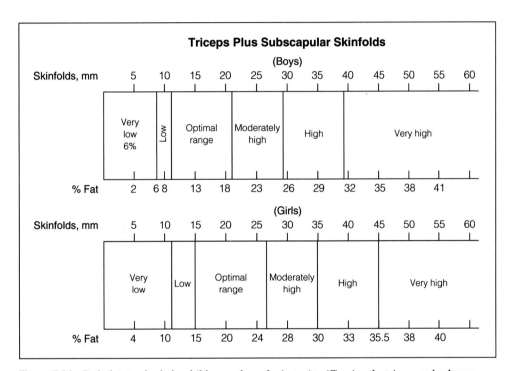

Figure 5.24   Body fat standards for children and youths (ages 6 to 17) using the triceps and subscapular skinfolds.   *Source:* Lohman TG. The use of skinfold to estimate body fatness on children and youth. *JOPERD,* November/December, 1987, 98–102. Reprinted with permission from the Journal of Physical Education, Recreation & Dance, a publication of the American Alliance for Health, Physical Education, Recreation, and Dance, 1900 Association Drive, Reston, VA 22091.

Two-Site Skinfold Test for Children, Youths, and College-Age Adults

The two-site skinfold test, using the triceps and subscapular sites, has been the most commonly used body composition test for young people ages 6 through 22.[26–28] Norms utilizing the sum of triceps and subscapula or triceps and medial calf skinfolds have been developed and are found in Ap-

pendix A (Tables 1, 2, 11, 12, 13) and in Figures 5.24 and 5.25.[29–31]

The choice of the triceps and subscapular sites over other commonly measured sites (medial calf, abdomen, supra-iliac, thigh, etc.) was originally made for several reasons:[32]

- Correlations between these sites and other measures of body fat have been consistently among the highest in many studies.

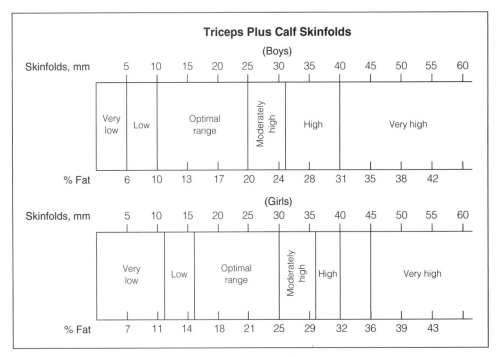

Figure 5.25 Body fat standards for children and youths (ages 6 to 17) using the triceps and medial calf skinfolds. *Source:* Lohman TG. The use of skinfold to estimate body fatness on children and youth. *JOPERD,* November/December, 1987, 98–102. Reprinted with permission from the Journal of Physical Education, Recreation, & Dance, a publication of the American Alliance for Health, Physical Education, Recreation, and Dance, 1900 Association Drive, Reston, VA 22091.

- These sites are more reliably and objectively measured than most other sites.
- There are available national norms for these sites.

Recently, however, use of the subscapular site has been questioned.[30] Some parents of school-age children are concerned that the modesty of their children is infringed upon when the physical educator raises the shirt of the child to gain access to the subscapular site. The medial calf skinfold site is more easily accessible, and studies have found it to be valid and reliable.[30]

Unfortunately, many public school physical educators do not support skinfold testing, often because they feel inadequately trained to conduct it or to interpret results accurately.[33]

To assist educators in making accurate skinfold measurements, an audiovisual tape has been developed by the American Alliance for Health, Physical Education, Recreation, and Dance with Human Kinetics. (Write to Human Kinetics, Box 5076, Champaign, IL 61825.)

Teachers are also encouraged to attend workshops where training is offered on the skinfold-measurement technique. It is recommended that skinfold measurements be taken for all children at least once a year, with records kept to track children from year to year.

Equations to estimate percent body fat of children and youths from the sum of triceps and calf skinfolds are as follows:[3]

Males 6 to 17 years

% body fat = (0.735 × sum of skinfolds) + 1.0

Females 6 to 17 years

% body fat = (0.610 × sum of skinfolds) + 5.0

Computer software is available from Human Kinetics to calculate body composition of children, using these equations and others.[3]

Multiple Skinfold Tests for Adults

Since 1951, more than 100 body composition regression equations using anthropometric techniques (skinfold measurements and circumference and diameter measures) have been published.[23] Most of these equations have been developed for specific types of people (athletes or young men or elderly women, etc.) and are thus limited to the groups they were developed for.[25]

The more recent trend has been to develop generalized, rather than population-specific equations. These equations

TABLE 5.7   Generalized Body Composition Equations

Males

7-Site Formula

> **Body Density** = 1.11200000 − 0.00043499 (*Sum of Seven Skinfolds*) + 0.00000055 (*Sum of Seven Skinfolds*)^2 − 0.00028826 (*Age*)
> (chest, midaxillary, triceps, subscapular, abdomen, suprailiac, thigh)

4-Site Formula

> **Percent Body Fat** = 0.29288 (*Sum of Four Skinfolds*) − 0.0005 (*Sum of Four Skinfolds*)^2 + 0.15845 (*Age*) − 5.76377
> (abdomen, suprailiac, tricep, thigh)

3-Site Formula

> **Body Density** = 1.1093800 − 0.0008267 (*Sum of Three Skinfolds*) + 0.0000016 (*Sum of Three Skinfolds*)^2 − 0.0002574 (*Age*)
> (chest, abdomen, thigh)

> **Body Density** = 1.1125025 − 0.0013125 (*Sum of Three Skinfolds*) + 0.0000055 (*Sum of Three Skinfolds*)^2 − 0.0002440 (*Age*)
> (chest, triceps, subscapular)

> **Percent Body Fat** = 0.39287 (*Sum of Three Skinfolds*) − 0.00105 (*Sum of Three Skinfolds*)^2 + 0.15772 (*Age*) − 5.18845
> (abdomen, suprailiac, triceps)

Females

7-Site Formula

> **Body Density** = 1.0970 − 0.00046971 (*Sum of Seven Skinfolds*) + 0.00000056 (*Sum of Seven Skinfolds*)^2 − 0.00012828 (*Age*)
> (chest, midaxillary, triceps, subscapular, abdomen, suprailiac, thigh)

4-Site Formula

> **Percent Body Fat** = 0.29669 (*Sum of Four Skinfolds*) − 0.00043 (*Sum of Four Skinfolds*)^2 + 0.02963 (*Age*) + 1.4072
> (abdomen, suprailiac, tricep, thigh)

3-Site Formula

> **Percent Body Fat** = 0.41563 (*Sum of Three Skinfolds*) − 0.00112 (*Sum of Three Skinfolds*)^2 + 0.03661 (*Age*) + 4.03653
> (triceps, abdomen, suprailiac)

> **Body Density** = 1.0994921 − 0.0009929 (*Sum of Three Skinfolds*) + 0.0000023 (*Sum of Three Skinfolds*)^2 − 0.0001392 (*Age*)
> (triceps, suprailiac, thigh)

Note: The researchers who developed these equations used vertical instead of horizontal skinfolds at the abdominal and midaxillary sites.

Sources: Jackson AS, Pollock ML. Practical assessment of body composition. *Phys Sportsmed* 13:76–90, 1985. Golding LA, Myers CR, Sinning WE. *The Y's Way to Physical Fitness* (3rd ed.), 1989. Champaign, IL: Human Kinetics, Inc.

have been developed using regression models that take into account data from many different research projects. The main advantage is that one generalized equation replaces several population-specific equations without a loss in prediction accuracy for a wide range of people.[23]

Jackson and Pollock have published generalized equations for adult men and women[23,25,32,34,35] (see Table 5.7). The three-site equations utilizing triceps, suprailiac, and abdomen skinfolds for adult females, and chest, abdomen, and thigh skinfolds for adult males have been most widely used.

Notice that the equations in Table 5.7 predict either percent body fat or body density. The body density formulas require an additional step to estimate percent body fat, using the formulas summarized earlier in this chapter in Table 5.2. For ease of determination, a nomogram has been developed to calculate percent body fat using age and the sum of three skinfolds for both men and women[36] (see Figure 5.26).

The nomogram is based on the three-site skinfold equations listed in Table 5.7, which use the chest, abdomen, and thigh sites for males, and the triceps, suprailiac, and thigh skinfolds for women. However, this nomogram is based on the Brozek equation, which is applicable only for white male and female adults.

Table 5.8 summarizes equations from Durnin and Womersley,[37] which have been used by many researchers, and which vary according to the age of the subject. The equations are based on the logarithm of the sum of four skinfolds (biceps, triceps, subscapular, and suprailiac). The biceps skinfold is defined as a vertical fold on the anterior aspect of the upper arm, directly opposite the triceps skinfold site.

Table 5.2 summarizes age- and sex-specific constants for conversion of body density (derived from equations in Table 5.7) to percent body fat in children and youths.[1] These

Skinfold Measurements

Name _____ Date _____

Age _____ Sex _____ Height _____ Weight _____

MEASUREMENTS (mm)

_____ Chest   _____ Suprailiac

_____ Abdominal   _____ Midaxillary

_____ Thigh   _____ Subscapular

_____ Tricepts   _____ Medial Calf

CALCULATIONS
(Use appropriate formula)

_____ Total skinfolds (mm)

_____ Body fat percent

_____ Pounds of fat
(Total wt × body fat %)

_____ Pounds of lean body weight
(Total wt − fat wt)

_____ Classification
(see norms)

_____ Ideal body weight
[LBW / (100% − desired fat %)]

Figure 5.26 To use the nomogram, place a straight edge connecting the age and sum of three skinfolds. The percent body fat is read at the point where the straight edge crosses the line representing the gender of the subject. *Source:* Baun WB, Baun MR, Raven PB. A nomogram for the estimate of percent body fat from generalized equation. *Res Quart Exerc Sport* 52:380–384, 1981. Used with the permission of Dr. W. B. Baun.

constants are necessary, in that the density of the fat-free mass is lower in children than in adults, because of less bone mineral and more water, proportionately. Thus, use of "adult" skinfold equations (Table 5.7) to predict body density generally *overestimates* percent body fat in children and youths.[38] To determine percent body fat from body density for an 11-year-old boy, using the fat-free mass density of 1.084, the equation would be (Table 5.2)

$$\% \text{ body fat} = \left(\frac{5.30}{\text{body density}} - 4.89 \right) \times 100$$

A sample skinfold testing form is outlined in Figure 5.27. In making the calculations for fat, lean body weight (fat-free mass), and ideal body weight, the following formulas should be used:

pounds of fat = total weight × % body fat

lean body weight = total weight − fat weight

$$\text{ideal body weight} = \frac{\text{present lean body weight}}{100\% - \text{desired fat }\%}$$

For example, if a subject weighs 200 pounds, has 25% body fat, and desires to have 15% body fat,

body fat = 200 × 0.25 = 50 pounds

lean body weight = 200 − 50 = 150 pounds

$$\text{ideal body weight} = \frac{150}{0.85} = 176 \text{ pounds}$$

The ideal weight formula assumes that the lean body weight stays the same during weight loss. Excess body weight, however, has been determined to be 75% body fat and 25% lean body weight (fat-free mass). For some people, therefore, a reduction in lean body weight is actually

TABLE 5.8   **Calculation* of Body Density According to the Method of Durnin and Womersley**

Equations for Men		Equations for Women	
Age range		**Age range**	
17–19	$D = 1.1620 - 0.0630 \times (\log \Sigma)$	17–19	$D = 1.1549 - 0.0678 \times (\log \Sigma)$
20–29	$D = 1.1631 - 0.0632 \times (\log \Sigma)$	20–29	$D = 1.1599 - 0.0717 \times (\log \Sigma)$
30–39	$D = 1.1422 - 0.0544 \times (\log \Sigma)$	30–39	$D = 1.1423 - 0.0632 \times (\log \Sigma)$
40–49	$D = 1.1620 - 0.0700 \times (\log \Sigma)$	40–49	$D = 1.1333 - 0.0612 \times (\log \Sigma)$
50+	$D = 1.1715 - 0.0779 \times (\log \Sigma)$	50+	$D = 1.1339 - 0.0645 \times (\log \Sigma)$

*Based on 4 skinfolds: biceps, triceps, subscapula, and suprailiac. Sum and calculate logarithm.

Note: To calculate percent body fat, use the percent fat equations summarized in Table 5.2.

Source: See reference 37.

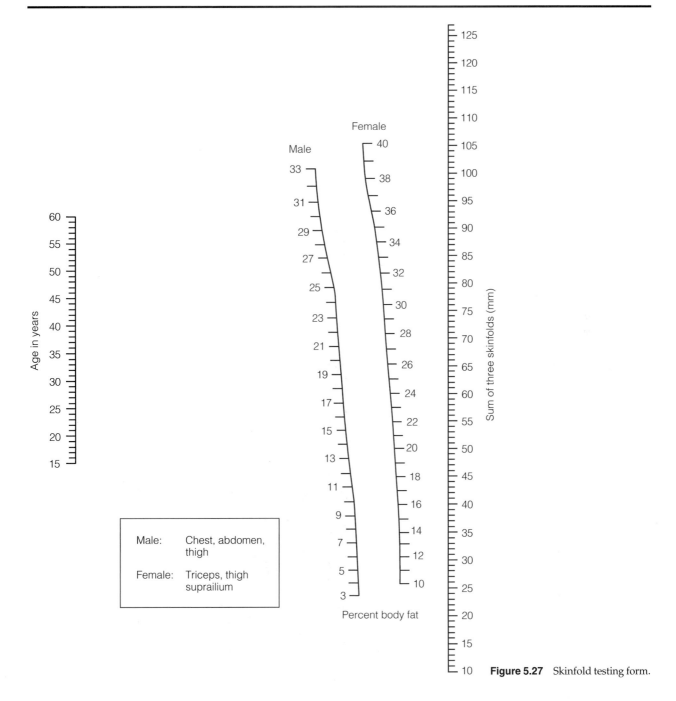

Figure 5.27   Skinfold testing form.

TABLE 5.9   Body Fat Ranges for Ages 18 and Older

Classification	Male	Female
Unhealthy range (too low)	≤5%	8% and below
Acceptable range (lower end)	6–15%	9–23%
Acceptable range (higher end)	16–24%	24–31%
Unhealthy range (too high)	25% and above	32% and above
Average Body Fat Ranges for Elite Athletes		
Long-distance runners	4–9%	6–15%
Wrestlers	4–10%	—
Gymnasts	4–10%	10–17%
Body builders	6–10%	10–17%
Swimmers	5–11%	14–24%
Basketball athletes	7–11%	18–27%
Cross-country skiers	7–13%	15–23%
Baseball athletes	11–15%	—
Canoers / kayakers	11–15%	18–24%
Tennis players	14–17%	19–22%
Shot-putters / discus throwers	15–20%	25–28%
Football linemen	15–20%	—

Source: Lohman, T. G. 1992. *Advances in Body Composition Assessment: Current Issues in Exercise Science,* Monograph Number 3. Champaign, IL: Human Kinetics Publishers.

desirable and should be represented in the equation by subtracting 25% of the excess weight (e.g., 25% of 12 excess pounds, or 3 pounds) from the present lean body weight.

Norms for body fat are listed in Table 5.9. Athletes involved in sports where the body weight is supported, such as canoeing, kayaking, and swimming, tend to have higher body fat values than athletes involved in sports such as running, which are very anaerobic (sprinting) or very aerobic (marathoning).[39,40] An extensive listing of the relative body fat of male and female athletes from a variety of sports is given in Appendix A, Table 28.

It is important to recognize that every measurement method has defined sources of error. Researchers have estimated that the standard error of estimate (SEE) for percent body fat when using the underwater weighing technique (with residual volume measured accurately) is 2.7%.[1,3] Generalized equations using skinfolds add only about 1% to this measurement error.[3] In other words, if on the basis of the seven-site skinfold equation, a person is calculated to have 15% body fat, two thirds of the time the actual percent body fat will range within ±4% of that estimated 15% (11–19% body fat).

UNDERWATER WEIGHING

The most widely used laboratory procedure for measuring body density is *underwater weighing.* In this procedure, whole-body density is calculated from body volume, ac-

cording to Archimedes' Principle of Displacement, which states that an object submerged in water is buoyed up by the weight of the water displaced.[1,3]

The protocol requires weighing a person underwater, as well as on land. The densities of bone and muscle tissues are higher than that of water, while fat is less dense than water. Thus a person with more bone and muscle mass will weigh more in water and thus have a higher body density and lower percentage of body fat.

By using a standard formula, the volume of the body is calculated and the individual's body density determined. From body density, percent body fat can be calculated using the formulas described in Table 5.2.

To determine body density from underwater weighing, the following equation has been developed:[1,3]

$$\text{body density} = \frac{Wa}{\dfrac{(Wa - Ww)}{Dw} - (RV + 100\ \text{ml})}$$

(Wa = body weight out of water; Ww = weight in water; Dw = density of water; RV = residual volume. 100 ml is the estimated air volume of the gastrointestinal tract.)

Equipment

The equipment is simple and relatively inexpensive (see Figure 5.28). In some new systems, the chair seat rests on load cells that are directly connected to a computer for instant analysis and feedback (but these systems are expensive and are no more accurate when used by experienced technicians). The scale and chair can be suspended from a diving board or an overhead beam into a pool, small tank,

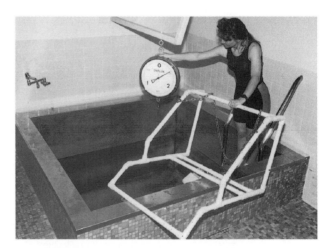

Figure 5.28   Equipment for underwater weighing includes a tank of sufficient size and shape for total human submersion, an accurate scale for measuring weight with 15–25 g divisions, a method of measuring water temperature so that water density can be corrected, and a chair that has been weighted to prevent flotation.

or hot tub that is 4–5 feet deep. The water should be warm enough to be comfortable (85–92° F) and undisturbed by wind or the motions of other people during the time of the test. The water should be filtered and chlorinated. Use a 9-kilogram autopsy scale with 15–25 g divisions.

The chair can be constructed of ¾–1 inch plastic pipe, which can be cut and assembled easily. The direct cost is only about $30 in materials (the plastic pipe and glue). Figure 5.28 gives an example of one type of underwater weighing chair. A simple cradle can also be used.[1]

The back height of the chair in Figure 5.28 is 24 inches, the width 32 inches. Other joints and dimensions need not be precise and can be estimated from the figure. It is important that the chair be assembled so that the person being weighed can sit underwater with legs slightly bent, and the water at shoulder level. Very small or large people will have to adapt their sitting position.

Holes should be drilled in the plastic pipe to avoid air entrapment. The chair should be weighed down with skin-diving weights or barbell weights to ensure that the weight of the chair underwater (tare weight) is at least 3 kg for normal-weight people being weighed, and 4–6 kg for obese people.

Procedures

1. Obtain basic data (name, date, age, sex, height, weight). The form in Figure 5.29 can be used to record these data. Weight should be taken wearing only a swimsuit and after an opportunity to go to the bathroom. The person being weighed should not eat or smoke for 2–3 hours before the test and should try to avoid foods that can cause excessive

---

Body Composition Worksheet

Name_____ Date_____

Age_____ Sex_____ Height (shoes off)_____

SKINFOLDS (mm)

Male	Female
_____ Chest	Suprailiac _____
_____ Abdominal	Midaxillary _____
_____ Thigh	Subscapular _____
_____ TOTAL _____	

HYDROSTATIC MEASUREMENTS

_____ Body weight in air (pounds)
_____ Net body weight in water (kg) (subtract tare from gross weight)
   _____ Gross weight in water (kg)
   _____ Tare weight (weight of appartus – kg)
_____ H$_2$O density (see norms)   _____ _____ _____
_____ Residual volume (L)   _____ _____ _____
_____ (use equation or measure directly) (take 4–6 determinations until steady)

CALCULATIONS

_____ Body fat % = (495/density) – 450

Density = dry wt./$\left[\left(\dfrac{\text{dry wt.} - \text{net underwater wt.}}{\text{Density water}}\right) - (RV + 100\text{ml})\right]$

_____ Fat weight (pounds) (dry body weight × fat %)
_____ Lean body weight (pounds) (dry body weight – fat weight)
_____ Fat % classification (see norms)

RECOMMENDATIONS

_____ Estimated ideal weight weight [LBW/(100% – desired fat %)]

   _____ _____ _____

_____ Pounds of fat you need to lose
_____ Pounds of lean body weight you need to gain

Figure 5.29 Body composition worksheet.

amounts of intestinal gas. Care should be taken to expel any trapped air from the swimsuit.

2. Take skinfolds. Because some people have difficulty in blowing out all the air from their lungs underwater, it is a good idea to have skinfold data to help verify the results.

3. Give basic instructions.

   a. How to sit in chair. Sit in the chair with seat on the back bars, feet on the forward bar in the corners, legs slightly bent, hands gripping the lower side bars (see Figure 5.30).

   b. Underwater position. After making a full exhalation of air from the lungs, slowly lean forward until the head is underwater. Continue to press all air out of the lungs. When all air is out, count for 5–7 seconds, then come up (see Figure 5.31). The test will be repeated 4–10 times until a consistent reading is obtained.

   Note: When the person goes under water, keep one hand on the scale to steady it. Try to keep the water as calm as possible to get a good reading on the scale needle. The person being weighed should be as still as possible underwater during the 5–7 second count.

4. Record the consistent underwater weight. The underwater weight should be recorded as the "gross weight in water (kg)," then the tare weight (weight of chair apparatus alone) should be subtracted from it to obtain the "net body weight in water." It is important to be exact in determining the gross underwater weight. A 100-gram error can result in close to a 1% body fat error.

   Many testers have trouble with the oscillations of the scale needle. To minimize this, use a small tank, keep the water as calm as possible, and teach the person being tested to move as slowly as possible. Testers should practice reading the scale with known weights attached.

5. Determine the water density. Measure the temperature of the water, and then consult Table 5.10 for the water density.

6. Determine the residual volume. The residual volume is the amount of air left in the lungs after a maximal expiration. The residual volume can be

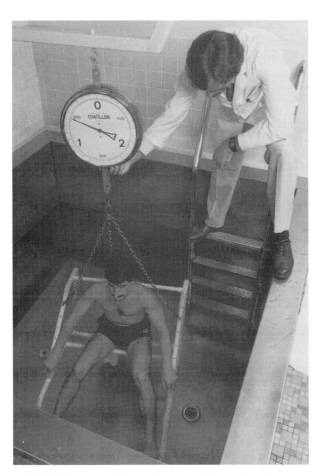

Figure 5.30   The position of the person being weighed, before underwater weighing.

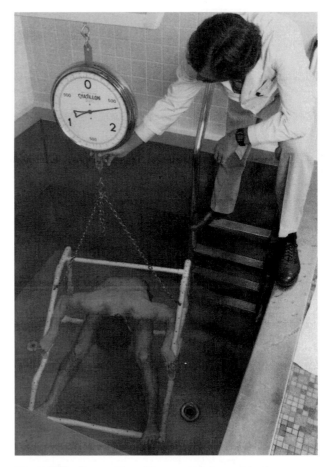

Figure 5.31   The position of the person being weighed, during underwater weighing.

TABLE 5.10 Density of Water at Different Temperatures

Water Temp (°C)	Density H_2O	Water Temp (°C)	Density H_2O
23	.997569	31	.995372
24	.997327	32	.995057
25	.997075	33	.994734
26	.996814	34	.994403
27	.996544	35	.994063
28	.996264	36	.993716
29	.995976	37	.993360
30	.995678		

Source: Handbook of Chemistry and Physics. Cleveland: Chemical Rubber Company, 1967. Reprinted with permission from CRC Press, Inc., Boca Raton, FL 33431.

measured or estimated. Measurement of residual volume can be conducted using nitrogen washout, helium dilution, or oxygen dilution. Controversy exists regarding whether measurement of residual volume should take place while the person being weighed is in or outside the tank.[1,3,41–43] When possible, it appears desirable to measure residual volume when the subject is in the tank, but this is not always practical with some modern automated equipment.

Whenever possible, residual volume should be measured directly. When residual volume is estimated, hydrostatically determined percent body fat is no more accurate than when measured with skinfolds because of the large amount of error in residual volume estimation formulas.[41]

When necessary, the following formulas can be used to estimate residual volume (RV) in liters:[44]

Males

$$RV = (0.017 \times \text{age in years}) + (0.06858 \times \text{height in inches}) - 3.447$$

Females

$$RV = (0.009 \times \text{age in years}) + (0.08128 \times \text{height in inches}) - 3.9$$

7. Calculate percent body fat. Following is an example of how to use the formula:

$$\text{body density} = \frac{\text{body weight}}{\text{body volume}}$$

$$\text{body volume} = \left(\frac{\text{body wt kg} - \text{underwater wt kg}}{\text{density of } H_2O}\right) - (RV + 100 \text{ ml})$$

$$\text{relative fat percent}^* = \left(\frac{495}{\text{density}}\right) - 450$$

$$\text{fat weight} = \text{body weight} \times \text{relative fat percent}$$

$$\text{lean weight} = \text{body weight} - \text{fat weight}$$

$$\text{ideal weight} = \frac{\text{present lean body weight}}{(100\% - \text{desired fat }\%)}$$

Example: Male, 18 years of age, weighs 180 lb (81.8 kg), has a net underwater weight of 3.8 kg. Estimated RV is 1.660 (adding 100 ml for gastrointestinal trapped air = 1.760), based on his height of 70 inches, age, and sex. The density of the water is 0.995678 based on a water temperature of 30°C.

$$\text{body volume} = \left(\frac{81.8 - 3.8}{0.995678}\right) - 1.760 = 76.579$$

$$\text{body density} = \frac{81.8}{76.579} = 1.0682$$

$$\text{relative fat }\% = \left(\frac{495}{1.0682}\right) - 450 = 13.4\%$$

$$\text{fat weight} = (180 \text{ lb} \times 0.134) = 24.1 \text{ lb}$$

$$\text{lean body weight} = 180 - 24.1 = 155.9$$

ideal weight if the person wants to get to 10% body fat (often for athletic reasons)

$$= \frac{155.9}{(100\% - 10\%)} = \frac{155.9}{0.9}$$

$$= 173.2 \text{ lb (needs to lose 9 lb fat)}$$

BIOELECTRICAL IMPEDANCE

A large number of publications is available evaluating the effectiveness of bioelectrical impedance analysis (BIA) (impedance plethysmography).[1–3,45–52] BIA was developed in the 1960s and has emerged as one of the most popular methods for estimating relative body fat. A harmless 50 kHz current (800 microamps maximum) is generated and passed through the person being measured (see Figure 5.32). The measurement of electrical impedance is detected as the resistance to electrical current. Electrical impedance is greatest in fat tissue (14–22% water) because the conductive pathway is directly related to the percentage of water (which is greatest in the fat-free tissue, averaging 73%).

The total body water can be detected, therefore, as shifts in total body impedance. Total body water is accurately measured using bioelectrical impedance analysis from the following equation:[3]

*This is the Siri equation, which applies only to white male and female adults. See Table 5.2 to choose the appropriate formula for other individuals.

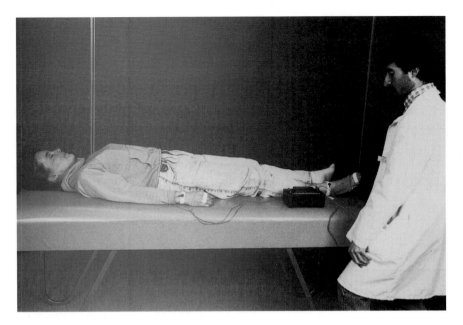

Figure 5.32 Bioelectrical impedance procedures are relatively simple. The person lies on a table with limbs not touching his or her body. Electrodes are placed on the right hand and right foot, and a harmless 50 kHz current (800 microamps maximum) is passed through him or her. The measurement of electrical conductance (or impedance) is detected as the resistance to electrical current.

total body water (kg)

$$= \left(0.593 \times \frac{\text{height, cm}^2}{\text{whole-body resistance, ohm}}\right) + (0.065 \times \text{body weight, kg})$$

For example, a person weighing 70 kg and standing 170 cm tall, with a 470 ohm resistance (measured through bioelectrical impedance) would have a total body water of 41.0 kg or 58.6% of total body weight.

There is a wide variety of BIA equations available for predicting fat-free mass and percent body fat. Table 5.11 summarizes several of them that have been developed for specific population groups.[1] In general, it is best not to use the fat-free mass and percent body fat estimates obtained directly from the BIA analyzer unless the equations are known to apply directly to the subjects being measured.[1]

There are several sources of measurement error with the BIA method, which need to be controlled as much as possible to improve accuracy and reliability:[1,3,50]

Instrumentation. BIA analyzers differ greatly from one company to another and can be a source of substantial error. To control for this error, the same instrument should be used when monitoring body composition changes in clients (and research subjects) over time.

Subject and Environmental Factors. The client's state of hydration can greatly affect the BIA process. Factors such as eating, drinking, voiding of fluids, and exercising can affect hydration state and therefore introduce error. Cool, ambient temperatures cause a drop in skin temperature that results in an underestimation of fat-free mass. Client and environmental guidelines prior to BIA measurements include the following:

1. No eating or drinking within 4 hours of the test
2. No exercise within 12 hours of the test
3. Urinate within 30 minutes of the test
4. No alcohol consumption within 48 hours of the test
5. No diuretic medications within 7 days of the test
6. No testing of female clients who perceive they are retaining water during that stage of their menstrual cycle
7. BIA measurements made in a room with normal ambient temperature

Technician Skill. The BIA technician should ensure that the client is lying in a supine position with arms and legs comfortably apart, at about a 45° angle to each other (see Figure 5.32). BIA measures are taken on the right side of the body. Electrodes need to be correctly positioned at the wrist and ankle, according to manufacturer guidelines. The sensor (proximal) electrodes should be placed on the dorsal surface of the wrist so that the upper border of the electrode bisects the head of the ulna and placed on the dorsal surface of the ankle so that the upper border of the electrode bisects the medial and lateral malleoli. The source (distal) electrodes should be placed at the base of the second or third metacarpal–phalangeal joints of the hand and foot. There should be at least 5 centimeters between the proximal and distal electrodes. A new leg-to-leg BIA system, combined with a digital scale that employs stainless-steel pressure-contact foot-pad electrodes for standing impedance and body weight measurements,

TABLE 5.11   BIA Prediction Equations for Specific Populations

White, boys and girls, 6–10 years	TBW (1)^a = 0.593 (HT^2/R) + 0.065 (BW) + 0.04
White, boys and girls, 10–19 years	FFM (kg) = 0.61 (HT^2/R) + 0.25 (BW) + 1.31
Women, 18–29 years	FFM (kg) = 0.4764 (HT^2/R) + 0.295 (BW) + 5.49
Women, 30–49 years	FFM (kg) = 0.493 (HT^2/R) + 0.141 (BW) + 11.59
Women, 50–70 years	FFM (kg) = 0.474 (HT^2/R) + 0.180 (BW) + 7.3
Women, 65–94 years	FFM (kg) = 0.28 (HT^2/R) + 0.27 (BW) + 0.31 (thigh C) − 1.732
Men, 18–29 years	FFM (kg) = 0.485 (HT^2/R) + 0.338 (BW) + 5.32
Men, 17–62 years, <20% body fat	FFM (kg) = 0.00066360 (HT^2) − 0.02117 (R) + 0.62854 (BW) − 0.12380 (age) + 9.33285
Men, 17–62 years, ≥20% body fat	FFM (kg) = 0.00088580 (HT^2) − 0.02999 (R) + 0.42688 (BW) − 0.07002 (age) + 14.52435
Men, 50–70 years	FFM (kg) = 0.600 (HT^2/R) + 0.186 (BW) + 0.226 (X$_c$) − 10.9
Men, 65–94 years	FFM (kg) = 0.28 (HT^2/R) + 0.27 (BW) + 0.31 (thigh C) − 2.768

^{a}To convert TBW to FFM, use the following age–gender hydration constants:

Boys	5–6 years FFM (kg) = TBW / 0.77	**Girls**	5–6 years FFM (kg) = TBW / 0.78
	7–8 years FFM (kg) = TBW / 0.768		7–8 years FFM (kg) = TBW / 0.776
	9–10 years FFM (kg) = TBW / 0.762		9–10 years FFM (kg) = TBW / 0.77

Note: FFM = fat-free mass; BW = body weight (kg); HT = height (cm); R = resistance in ohms; X$_c$ = reactance; thigh C = thigh circumference (cm).

Source: Heyward VH, Stolarczyk LM. *Applied Body Composition Assessment.* Champaign, IL: Human Kinetics, 1996. Used with permission.

has been developed by the Tanita Corporation (see Figure 5.33).[49] This system has been found to perform as well as the conventional arm-to-leg gel-electrode BIA system but is much quicker and easier to use.

When the appropriate BIA equation is used, and the sources of measurement error are controlled, estimation of fat-free mass and relative body fat through the BIA method has been found to have about the same accuracy as the skinfold method. The BIA method, however, may be more preferable in some settings than the skinfold method because it does not require a high degree of technician skill, and it is more comfortable and less intrusive. There is still debate over whether BIA accurately predicts changes in body composition during a weight-loss program.[1,51] Published studies are mixed, with some supporting the accuracy of BIA in detecting fat-free mass and body composition changes, while others claim there is substantial over- or underestimation when compared to the underwater weighing method.

NEAR-INFRARED LIGHT INTERACTANCE

Near-infrared (NIR) light interactance has been used by the USDA since the 1960s, to measure the protein, fat, and water content of agricultural products.[1] In 1984, researchers

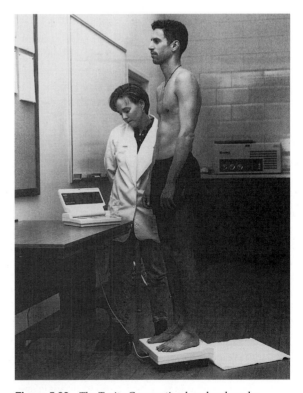

Figure 5.33   The Tanita Corporation has developed a BIA system using stainless-steel pressure-contact foot-pad electrodes.

first applied this technology to study human body composition. During the late 1980s, a commercial NIR analyzer was developed (the FUTREX-5000) and marketed as a fast, accurate, and easy method for analyzing human body composition. Three models are now available, the most expensive one costing $4,000 and allowing measurement of children, adults, and high school wrestlers (FUTREX-5000A/WL).

The FUTREX-5000 emits near-infrared light at two frequencies (938nm and 948nm) into the biceps area of the dominant arm. At these frequencies, body fat absorbs the light, while the lean body mass reflects the light. A light wand measures the amount of light emitted and reflected back, providing an estimate of the distribution of body fat and fat-free mass in the biceps area. FUTREX Inc. claims that years of research have shown that taking measurements of other anatomical sites does not significantly improve the accuracy of the estimation of relative body fat.

There are several advantages in using the FUTREX-5000 over other methods of estimating body fat percentage: Fasting is not required, there is no need for disrobing, measurements can be made before or after exercise, there is no need for voiding, and women can take measurements during any day of the menstrual cycle.

However, numerous researchers have reported unacceptable prediction errors (SEE = 3.7–6.3% body fat).[1–3,53–56] The manufacturer's equation—which incorporates body weight, height, gender, exercise level, and optical density measurements—has been found to systematically underestimate body fat percentage by as much as 2–10% with the underestimation especially apparent with obese clients. At this time, most experts recommend that more research is needed to substantiate the validity, accuracy, and applicability of the NIR method for body composition assessment.[1–3]

TOPOGRAPHY OF THE HUMAN BODY

The male *android* (or apple shape) type of obesity is characterized by a predominance of body fat in the upper half of the body. In contrast, the female *gynoid* (or pear shape) form of obesity is characterized by excess body fat in the lower half of the body, especially the hips, buttocks, and thighs (see Figure 5.34). The third type of obesity is the intermediate form, characterized by both upper- and lower-body fat predominance.

The male type of obesity, which can occur in both genders, is associated with many of the health problems of obesity, including hypertension, high serum cholesterol levels, cardiovascular disease, and diabetes.[57]

Many different methods have been used to estimate android obesity, including the waist-to-hip circumference ratio, various skinfold ratios (e.g., subscapular-to-triceps ratio and trunk-to-peripheral skinfold ratios), and sophisticated

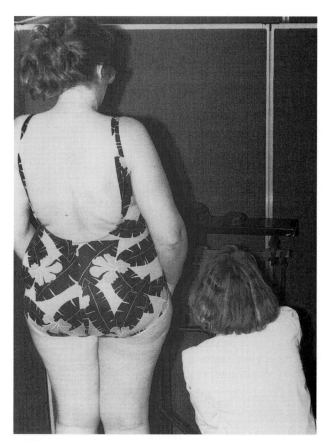

Figure 5.34 This subject has gynoid obesity, characterized by excess body fat in the lower half of the body.

imaging techniques such as computed tomography (CT) or DEXA, or magnetic resonance imaging (MRI).[3] These imaging techniques (see the Sports Medicine Insight at end of chapter) allow a precise measurement of the amount of deep abdominal or visceral fat, versus subcutaneous fat.

It is the visceral fat that appears to be most strongly related to various negative health consequences; these cells release and take in fat more readily than other cells (e.g., fat cells in the gluteal and femoral regions), which leads to increased risk of disease. Abdominal fat cells release their fatty acids straight to the liver, which appears to be a factor in the increased risk of metabolic disorders.

Some researchers have found that the *ratio of waist-to-hip circumference* (WHR) is a simple and convenient method of determining the type of obesity present. Circumferences should be measured while wearing only nonrestrictive briefs or underwear, or a light smock over the underwear.

Waist or abdominal circumference is defined as the smallest waist circumference below the rib cage and above the umbilicus, while standing with abdominal muscles relaxed (not pulled in).[24] The measurer faces the person being measured and places an inelastic tape in a horizontal plane, at the level of the natural waist (the narrowest part of the torso, as seen from the rear). If there appears to be no

TABLE 5.12 Disease Risk Associated with Body Mass Index and Waist Circumference

| Classification | Obesity Class | BMI (kg/m²) | Disease Risk Relative to Normal Weight and Waist Circumference* | |
			Men ≤40 in Women ≤35 in	>40 in >35 in
Underweight		<18.5	—	—
Normal		18.5–24.9	—	—
Overweight		25.0–29.9	increased	high
Obesity	I	30.0–34.9	high	very high
	II	35.0–39.9	very high	very high
Extreme obesity	III	≥40	extremely high	extremely high

*Disease risk for type 2 diabetes, hypertension, and cardiovascular disease.

Source: NHLBI Obesity Education Initiative Expert Panel (1998). *Clinical Guidelines on the Identification, Evaluation, and Treatment of Overweight and Obesity in Adults.* National Heart, Lung, and Blood Institute: www.nhlbi.nih.gov/nhlbi/.

"smallest" area around the waist, the measurement should be made at the level of the navel.

Hip or gluteal circumference is defined as the largest circumference of the buttocks–hip area while the person is standing.[24] The measurer should squat at the person's side, to see where the buttocks circumference is the greatest, and should place an inelastic tape around the buttocks and hips in a horizontal plane at that point, without compressing the skin. An assistant is needed to help position the tape on the opposite side of the body.

The WHR is calculated by dividing the waist circumference by the hip circumference. For example, the idealized beauty contest female with a waist of 24 inches and hips of 36 inches would have a WHR of 0.67. In one study of 44,820 women who were members of TOPS Clubs, Inc. (Take Off Pounds Sensibly), the WHR varied between 0.39 and 1.45.[58] Women with higher WHRs were at greater risk for diabetes, hypertension, gallbladder disease, and oligomenorrhea (irregular menses).

More research is needed to establish precise norms for the WHR. At present, the risk of disease increases steeply when the WHR of men rises above 0.9, and of women, above 0.8.[57] A nomogram for determining the WHR is given in Figure 5.35.[59]

The WHR has been criticized for misclassifying people, due to factors unrelated to visceral fat, including frame size and gluteal muscle mass.[60] There is some evidence that the waist circumference alone correlates highly with visceral fat and is associated with increased risk of disease.[60,61] In one study conducted by researchers at Laval University in Quebec, a waist circumference exceeding 37.5 inches was related to both high levels of visceral fat and risk factors for disease.[60] The researchers concluded that the waist circum-

ference was a stronger correlate of visceral adipose tissue than was the WHR, and it was also easier to use. In 1998, the National Heart, Lung, and Blood Institute (NHLBI) expert panel on obesity concluded that the waist circumference was more highly associated with disease risk than the WHR. As summarized in Table 5.12, a high waist circumference (defined as >40 inches in men and >35 inches in women) combined with a BMI >25 predicts increased disease risk. At BMIs ≥35, waist circumference has little added predictive power of disease risk beyond that of BMI.

Various prediction equations have been developed to estimate body fat levels of military personnel.[1,62] These equations use various combinations of body weight, height, neck, abdomen, hip, thigh, arm, forearm, and wrist circumferences to predict either fat-free mass or percent body fat. However, these prediction equations have yielded large and unacceptable errors (SEE = 3.7–5.2% body fat).[1] Most experts do not recommend the use of these anthropometry equations in determining to dismiss personnel from the armed services when their body fat percentage exceeds military standards.[1,62]

One equation for predicting body composition of men from girth measurements has been developed, and has a relatively low SEE of 3.6%.[63] The regression equation is as follows:

$$\begin{aligned}
\% \text{ body fat} &= -47.371817 + (0.57914807 \times \text{abdomen}) \\
&+ (0.25189114 \times \text{hips}) + (0.21366088 \times \text{iliac}) \\
&- (0.35595404 \times \text{weight kg})
\end{aligned}$$

The abdomen and hip circumferences were described earlier in this section. The iliac circumference is taken between the abdomen and hip circumference levels, at the iliac crest.

SPORTS MEDICINE INSIGHT

Other Methods of Determining Body Composition

This chapter has reviewed some of the more practical and standard methods for determining body composition, for which the present standard is hydrostatic weighing. However, it requires relatively expensive equipment and requires direct measurement of residual volume for optimum accuracy. In contrast, Quetelet's Index is a simple and practical measurement of degree of overweight, but it is insensitive to individuals with low or high amounts of muscle and bone. Skinfold measurements can give an accurate assessment of body fat levels when conducted by experienced health professionals. Bioelectrical impedance analysis and near-infrared interactance (FUTREX-5000) are highly convenient methods but are also less accurate in estimating fatness of lean or obese than of normal-weight individuals. For regional fat distribution, calculations using waist and hip circumferences are useful, but they do not accurately assess the deep abdominal fat.

Table 5.13 summarizes the relative costs, ease of use, and accuracy of these and other techniques. This section reviews several of the newer and more promising methods for assessing body fat.

DEXA

The advent of dual-energy x-ray absorptiometry (DEXA) in 1987 has created much excitement among body composition researchers because this method allows simultaneous measurement of bone mineral, fat, and nonbone lean tissue.[1-3,64-72] DEXA is safe (low radiation dose) and quick (10–20 min), requires virtually no cooperation from the subject, and makes study of the elderly, young, and diseased much easier than with other methods (see Figure 5.36).

Manufacturers of DEXA machines have designed software that allows personnel with minimal training to operate the scanners. In the near future, DEXA may become a "gold standard" reference method for estimation of body composition, but much more research is needed to understand potential limitations. Most studies thus far have concluded that DEXA is a precise method and correlates highly with results from underwater weighing.[64-72]

DEXA uses a stable x-ray generator and two energy levels as the radiation source. A series of transverse scans are made of the subject, from head to toe, at 1-cm intervals, with bone mineral and soft tissue composition determined from the differential attenuation of the two energy photon beams. After passing through the subject, the attenuated beam is detected by a sodium-iodide detector. DEXA is based on a three-component model of composition (bone, fat, and lean soft tissue) and can therefore provide accurate assessments of fat and lean tissue in individuals with below- and above-average bone mineral.

Some researchers have found differences between body composition results from DEXA and those from underwater weighing because of variation in bone mineral content between subjects and the use of a constant fat-

TABLE 5.13 Comparison among Body Composition Methods: Cost, Ease of Use, and Accuracy in Estimating Body Fat

Method	Cost	Ease of Use	Accuracy
Quetelet index	low	easy	low
Three- to seven-site skinfold tests	low	moderate	moderate
Hydrostatic weighing	moderate	difficult	high
Bioelectrical impedance	moderate	easy	moderate
TOBEC (total body electrical conductivity)	very high	easy	high
DEXA	high	easy	high
Computed tomography	very high	difficult	moderate
Near-infrared light interactance	moderate	easy	moderate
Magnetic resonance imaging	very high	difficult	moderate

Sources: See references 1, 2, 3.

Other Methods of Determining Body Composition *(continued)*

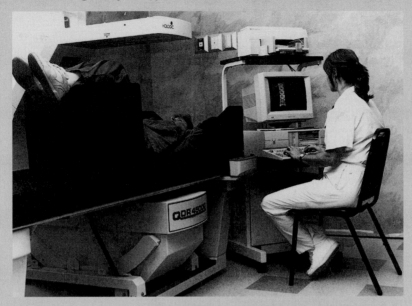

Figure 5.36 Originally developed for assessing bone mineral, recent technology has enabled estimates of fat and lean tissue via DEXA.

free mass density factor in the Siri equation.[72] In other words, underwater weighing may be the confusing factor and may actually be too inaccurate to furnish a comparison for DEXA results. Obviously the search for a "gold standard" reference method will continue and may lie in a combination of several techniques.[3]

MAGNETIC RESONANCE IMAGING (MRI)

In MRI, the hydrogen nuclei of water and lipid molecules are excited by electromagnetic radiation in the presence of a magnetic field, resulting in a detectable signal, which is measured. The amount of water and lipid, and their freedom of motion, define the signal size, permitting discrimination between these tissues.

Subjects lie in the magnet, with arms placed above the head. For the entire body, transverse slices (10 mm thickness) are acquired every 50 mm, from head to toe. Computers outline edges of the body and areas of adipose and nonfatty tissues, and calculate volumes. MRI uses no ionizing radiation and is therefore safe for all types of individuals.

High-quality images of the body tissues are provided, allowing study of the amount and distribution of fat. MRI accurately quantifies adipose tissue in pigs and has proven to be a reliable and valid measure of subcutaneous and visceral fat distribution in humans.[73-77] MRI

is relatively rapid (about 30 minutes), and subjects need only lie still. Drawbacks of the method are its restricted availability and high cost. Its greatest usefulness may be for measurement of visceral fat distribution.

TOTAL BODY ELECTRICAL CONDUCTIVITY (TOBEC)

Lean tissues conduct electricity much better than fat does. TOBEC operates on the principle that an object placed in an electromagnetic field will perturb the field, and the degree of perturbation depends on the quantity of conducting material (primarily electrolytes in lean body mass). Since 1971, the lean tissues of farm animals have been measured by putting them in a box that emits electrical impulses and measures responses.

The TOBEC system for human use consists of a large solenoid coil into which the person being measured is slid on a stretcher. The coil (driven by a 5 mHz radio frequency current) induces a current within the person's body in proportion to the mass of the conductive tissues. The instrument measures 10 total body conductivity readings in about 10 seconds. Studies show a very high correlation with hydrostatic weighing ($r = 0.93$).[78-80] TOBEC has also been found to be very sensitive to small changes in lean body mass and total body water. The major limitation of this technique is the high cost of the equipment.

(continued)

Other Methods of Determining Body Composition (continued)

COMPUTED TOMOGRAPHY (CT)

With this method, a computed tomography (CT) scanner is used to produce a cross-sectional image of the distribution of x-ray transmission. The person being measured is placed next to an x-ray tube, which directs a collimated beam of x-ray photons toward a scintillation detector.

Computed tomography can readily distinguish adipose tissue from adjacent skin, muscles, bones, vascular structures, and intra-abdominal and pelvic organs because fat transmits poorly. The cross-sectional CT images can be obtained at any level within the body. Computed tomography can thus noninvasively quantify body fat distribution at various sites—particularly useful is CT's ability to give a ratio of intra-abdominal to extra-abdominal fat.[81-84] The potential for using CT in assessing body composition is limited by problems of radiation exposure, high cost, and low availability.

PLETHYSMOGRAPHY

A new air-displacement plethysmograph, referred to as the Bod Pod® Body Composition System (Life Measurement Instruments, Concord, CA) has been developed to measure human body composition.[85] The system determines body volume through an air-displacement method. A volume-perturbing element (movable diaphragm) is mounted on the wall separating the front and rear chambers of the dual-chambered plethysmograph. When this diaphragm is oscillated under computer control, it produces complementary volume perturbations in the two chambers (equal in magnitude but opposite in sign). These volume perturbations produce very small pressure fluctuations that are analyzed to yield chamber air volume. The process is repeated with the subject inside the chamber. In one study of 68 subjects, reliability and validity were found to be excellent.[85] The mean difference in percent body fat with hydrostatic weighing was only 0.3%, with a 95% confidence interval of −0.6 to 0% fat. This new method has several advantages over hydrostatic weighing, in that it is quick (about 5 minutes), relatively simple to operate, and can accommodate special populations such as the obese, the elderly, and the disabled. Limited demands are made on the subjects, and instructions are minimal. The Bod Pod is mobile, so that it can be moved from one location to another. Minimal training is needed to operate the Bod Pod, due to the menu-driven software and the small number of tasks required to reliably and accurately operate the system.

SUMMARY

1. This chapter discussed the various methods of measuring obesity, starting with the least precise and progressing toward the more accurate (weight tables, body mass index, skinfolds, underwater weighing). The chapter ended with a brief discussion of some of the newer laboratory methods of evaluating body composition.

2. In general, in light of the various factors, validity, reliability, economy, and good norms, the various skinfold tests are probably most practical and useful. With proper training and practice, testers can learn to assess body composition quickly and accurately. However, careful selection of specific anatomic sites and observance of rules for measuring are important.

3. Height–weight tables only provide a rough estimate of ideal weight. Frame size can be determined by measuring the width of the elbow. Use of the Quetelet Index (kg/m^2) produces a higher correlation with actual body composition than does use of the height–weight tables.

4. Underwater weighing remains the laboratory standard, but the time, expense, and expertise needed is prohibitive for many clinical settings.

5. More research is needed to develop some of the newer techniques. As better equations are developed, bioelectrical impedance should prove to be a convenient, safe, accurate, and rapid method of body composition analysis.

6. Fat distribution on the body has been shown to be an important predictor of the health consequences of obesity. A number of the researchers have found that the ratio of waist-to-hip circumference (WHR) is an accurate and convenient method for determining type of obesity. When the ratio is above 0.9 for men and 0.8 for women, obesity-associated risks rise sharply.

REFERENCES

1. Heyward VH, Stolarczyk LM. *Applied Body Composition Assessment*. Champaign, IL: Human Kinetics, 1996.

2. Maud PJ, Foster C. *Physiological Assessment of Human Fitness*. Champaign, IL: Human Kinetics, 1995.

3. Lohman TG. *Advances in Body Composition Assessment: Current Issues in Exercise Science, Monograph Number 3*. Champaign, IL: Human Kinetics, 1992.

4. Brozek J, Grande F, Anderson IT, Kemp A. Densiometric analysis of body composition: Revision of some quantitative assumptions. *Ann New York Academy Sciences* 110:113–140, 1963.

5. Siri WE. Body composition from fluid spaces and density: Analysis of methods. In Brozek J, Henschel A (eds), *Techniques for Measuring Body Composition*. Washington, DC: National Academy of Sciences, 1961.

6. Weigley ES. Average? Ideal? Desirable? A brief overview of height–weight tables in the United States. *J Am Diet Assoc* 84:417, 1984.

7. Robinette-Weiss N. The Metropolitan Height–Weight Tables: Perspectives for use. *J Am Diet Assoc* 84:1480–1481, 1984.

8. Abraham S. Height–weight tables: Their sources and development. *Clin Consult Nutr Support* 3:5–8, 1983. Reprinted in Shils ME, Young VR (eds.), *Modern Nutrition in Health and Disease*. Philadelphia: Lea & Febiger, 1988, 1509–1513.

9. Simopoulos AP. Obesity and body weight standards. *Ann Rev Public Health* 7:481–492, 1986.

10. National Institutes of Health. Consensus development conference statement: Health implications of obesity. *Ann Intern Med* 103:981–1077, 1985.

11. Garrison RJ. Cigarette smoking as a confounder of the relationship between relative weight and long term mortality. *JAMA* 249:2199–2203, 1983.

12. U.S. Department of Agriculture, U.S. Department of Health and Human Services. *Nutrition and Your Health: Dietary Guidelines for Americans* (3rd ed.). Washington, DC: U.S. Government Printing Office, 1990.

13. Willett WC, Stampfer M, Manson J, Van Itallie T. New weight guidelines for Americans: Justified or injudicious? *Am J Clin Nutr* 53:1102–1103, 1991.

14. Marwick C. Obesity experts say less weight still best. *JAMA* 269:2617–2618, 1993.

15. U.S. Department of Agriculture, Agricultural Research Service, Dietary Guidelines Advisory Committee, 1995. *Report of the Dietary Guidelines Advisory Committee on the dietary guidelines for Americans, 1995, to the Secretary of Health and Human Services and the Secretary of Agriculture*. Washington, DC: Author, 1995.

16. Gordon CC, Chumlea WC, Roche AF. Stature, recumbent length, and weight. In Lohman TG, Roche AF, Martorell R (eds), *Anthropometric Standardization Reference Manual*. Champaign, IL: Human Kinetics, 1988.

17. Frisancho RA. *Anthropometric Standards for the Assessment of Growth and Nutritional Status*. Ann Arbor: University of Michigan Press, 1990.

18. Himes JH, Frisancho RA. Estimating frame size. In Lohman TG, Roche AF, Martorell R (eds), *Anthropometric Standardization Reference Manual*. Champaign, IL: Human Kinetics, 1988.

19. Wilmore JH, Frisancho RA, Gordon CC, Himes JH, Martin AD, Martorell R, Seefeldt VD. Body breadth equipment and measurement techniques. In Lohman TG, Roche AF, Martorell R (eds), *Anthropometric Standardization Reference Manual*. Champaign, IL: Human Kinetics, 1988.

20. Revicki DA, Israel RG. Relationship between body mass indices and measures of body adiposity. *Am J Public Health* 76:992–994, 1986.

21. Smalley KJ, Knerr AN, Kendrick ZU, et al. Reassessment of body mass indices. *Am J Clin Nutr* 52:405–408, 1990.

22. Jequier E. Energy, obesity, and body weight standards. *Am J Clin Nutr* 45:1035–1047, 1987.

23. Jackson AS, Pollock ML. Practical assessment of body composition. *Physician Sportsmed* 13:76–90, 1985.

24. Lohman TG, Roche AF, Martorell R. *Anthropometric Standardization Reference Manual*. Champaign, IL: Human Kinetics, 1988.

25. Jackson AS. Practical methods of measuring body composition. In Storlie J, Jordan HA (eds), *Evaluation and Treatment of Obesity*. New York: Medical and Scientific Books, Spectrum Publications, Inc., 1984.

26. AAHPERD. *Health-Related Physical Fitness Test Manual*. Reston, VA: Author, 1980.

27. AAHPERD. *Norms for College Students: Health-Related Physical Fitness Test*. Reston, VA: Author, 1985.

28. Public Health Service. Summary of findings from National Children and Youth Fitness Study. *JOPERD*, January 1985, 44–90.

29. Ross JG, Pate RR, Delpy LA, Gold RS, Svilar M. New health-related fitness norms. *JOPERD*, November/December, 1987, 66–70.

30. Lohman TG. The use of skinfold to estimate body fatness on children and youth. *JOPERD*, November/December, 1987, 98–102.

31. American Alliance Physical Fitness Education & Assessment Program. *Physical Best*. Reston, VA: Author, 1988.

32. AAHPERD. *Technical Manual: Health-Related Physical Fitness*. Reston, VA: Author, 1984.

33. Riley JH. A critique of skinfold tests from the public school level. *JOPERD*, October 1990, 71–73.

34. Jackson AS, Pollock ML, Ward A. Generalized equations for predicting body density of women. *Med Sci Sport Exerc* 12:175–182, 1980.

35. Jackson AS, Pollock ML. Generalized equations for predicting body density of men. *Br J Nutr* 40:497–504, 1978.

36. Baun WB, Baun MR, Raven PB. A nomogram for the estimate of percent body fat from generalized equation. *Res Quart Exerc Sport* 52:380–384, 1981.

37. Durnin JVGA, Womersley J. Body fat assessment from total body density and its estimation from skinfold thickness: Measurements on 481 men and women aged 16 to 72 years. *Br J Nutr* 32:77–97, 1974.

38. Lohman TG. Applicability of body composition techniques and constants for children and youth. *Ex Sport Sci Rev* 14:325–357, 1986.

39. Fleck SJ. Body composition of elite American athletes. *Am J Sports Med* 11:398, 1983.

40. Wilmore JH. *The Physiological Basis of the Conditioning Process*. Boston: Allyn and Bacon, Inc., 1982.

41. Morrow JR, Jackson AS, Bradley PW, Hartung GH. Accuracy of measured and predicted residual lung volume on body density measurement. *Med Sci Sports Exerc* 18:647–652, 1986.

42. Weltman A, Katch V. Comparison of hydrostatic weighing at residual volume and total lung capacity. *Med Sci Sports Exerc* 13:210–213, 1981.

43. Nelson AG, Stuart DW, Fisher AG. The effect of hydrostatic weighing protocols on body density measurement. *Med Sci Sports Exerc* 17:246, 1985.

44. Goldman HI, Becklake MR. Respiratory function tests. *Am Rev Tuberc Pulm Dis* 79:457–467, 1959.

45. Stolarczyk LM, Heyward VH, Van Loan MD, Hicks VL, Wilson WL, Reano LM. The fatness-specific bioelectrical impedance analysis equations of Segal et al: Are they generalizable and practical? *Am J Clin Nutr* 66:8–17, 1997.

46. Heymsfield SB, Wang ZM, Visser M, Gallagher D, Pierson RN. Techniques used in the measurement of body composition: An overview with emphasis on bioelectrical impedance analysis. *Am J Clin Nutr* 64(suppl):478S–484S, 1996.

47. Kotler DP, Burastero S, Wang J, Pierson RN. Prediction of body cell mass, fat-free mass, and total body water with bioelectrical impedance analysis: Effects of race, sex, and disease. *Am J Clin Nutr* 64(suppl):489S–497S, 1996.

48. Houtkooper LB, Lohman TG, Going SB, Howell WH. Why bioelectrical impedance analysis should be used for estimating adiposity. *Am J Clin Nutr* 64(suppl):436S–448S, 1996.

49. Nunez C, Gallagher D, Visser M, Pi-Sunyer FX, Wang Z, Heymsfield SB. Bioimpedance analysis: Evaluation of leg-to-leg system based on pressure contact foot-pad electrodes. *Med Sci Sports Exerc* 29:524–531, 1997.

50. NIH. Bioelectrical impedance analysis in body composition measurement: National Institutes of Health Technology Assessment Conference statement. *Am J Clin Nutr* 64(suppl): 524S–532S, 1996.

51. Carella MJ, Rodgers CD, Anderson D, Gossain VV. Serial measurements of body composition in obese subjects during a very-low-energy diet (VLED) comparing bioelectrical impedance with hydrodensitometry. *Obes Res* 5:250–256, 1997.

52. Chumlea WC, Guo SS. Bioelectrical impedance and body composition: Present status and future directions. *Nutr Rev* 52: 123–131, 1994.

53. Heyward VH. Evaluation of body composition: Current issues. *Sports Med* 22:146–156, 1996.

54. McLean KP, Skinner JS. Validity of FUTREX-5000 for body composition determination. *Med Sci Sports Exerc* 24:253–258, 1992.

55. Heyward VH, Cook KL, Hicks VL, et al. Predictive accuracy of three field methods for estimating relative body fatness of non-obese and obese women. *Int J Sport Nutr* 2:75–86, 1992.

56. Hortobagyi T, Israel RG, Houmard JA, et al. Comparison of four methods to assess body composition in black and white athletes. *Int J Sport Nutr* 2:60–74, 1992.

57. Van Itallie TB. Topography of body fat: Relationship to risk of cardiovascular and other diseases. In Lohman TG, Roche AF, Martorell R (eds), *Anthropometric Standardization Reference Manual*. Champaign, IL: Human Kinetics, 1988.

58. Rimm AA, Hartz AJ, Fischer ME. A weight shape index for assessing risk of disease in 44,820 women. *J Clin Epidemiol* 41: 459–465, 1988.

59. Bray GA, Gray DS. Obesity: Part 1. Pathogenesis. *West J Med* 149:429–441, 1988.

60. Lemieux S, Prud'homme D, Bouchard C, Tremblay A, Despres J-P. A single threshold value of waist girth identifies normal-weight and overweight subjects with excess visceral adipose tissue. *Am J Clin Nutr* 64:685–693, 1996.

61. Goodman-Gruen D, Barrett-Connor E. Sex differences in measures of body fat and body fat distribution in the elderly. *Am J Epidemiol* 143:898–906, 1996.

62. Bathalon GP, Hughes VA, Campbell WW, Fiatarone MA, Evans WJ. Military body fat standards and equations applied to middle-aged women. *Med Sci Sports Exerc* 27:1079–1085, 1995.

63. Tran ZV, Weltman A. Predicting body composition of men from girth measurements. *Human Biol* 60:167–175, 1988.

64. Ogle GD, Allen JR, Humphries IRJ, et al. Body-composition assessment by dual-energy x-ray absorptiometry in subjects aged 4–26 y. *Am J Clin Nutr* 61:746–753, 1995.

65. Tataranni PA, Ravussin E. Use of dual-energy x-ray absorptiometry in obese individuals. *Am J Clin Nutr* 62:730–734, 1995.

66. Kohrt WM. Body composition by DXA: Tried and true? *Med Sci Sports Exerc* 27:1349–1353, 1995.

67. Bracco D, Thiebaud D, Chiolero RL, Landry M, Burckhardt P, Schutz Y. Segmental body composition assessed by bioelectrical impedance analysis and DEXA in humans. *J Appl Physiol* 81:2580–2587, 1996.

68. Clasey JL, Hartman ML, Kanaley J, Wideman L, Teates CD, Bouchard C, Weltman A. Body composition by DEXA in older adults: Accuracy and influence of scan mode. *Med Sci Sports Exerc* 29:560–567, 1997.

69. Roubenoff R, Kehayias JJ, Dawson-Hughes B, Heymsfield SB. Use of dual-energy x-ray absorptiometry in body composition studies: Not yet a "gold standard." *Am J Clin Nutr* 58:589–591, 1993.

70. Svendsen OL, Haarbo J, Hassager C, Christiansen C. Accuracy of measurements of body composition by dual energy x-ray absorptiometry in vivo. *Am J Clin Nutr* 57:605–608, 1993.

71. Wellens R, Chumlea WC, Guo S, Roche AF, Reo NV, Siervogel RM. Body composition in white adults by dual-energy x-ray absorptiometry, densitometry, and total body water. *Am J Clin Nutr* 59:547–555, 1994.

72. Clark RR, Kuta JM, Sullivan JC. Prediction of percent body fat in adult males using dual energy x-ray absorptiometry, skinfolds, and hydrostatic weighing. *Med Sci Sports Exerc* 25: 528–535, 1993.

73. Fowler PA, Fuller MF, Glasbey CA, et al. Validation of the in vivo measurement of adipose tissue by magnetic resonance imaging of lean and obese pigs. *Am J Clin Nutr* 56:7–13, 1992.

74. Ross R, Shaw KD, Rissanen J, Martel Y, deGuise J, Avruch L. Sex differences in lean and adipose tissue distribution by magnetic resonance imaging: Anthropometric relationships. *Am J Clin Nutr* 59:1277–1285, 1994.

75. Ross R, Shaw KD, Martel Y, et al. Adipose tissue distribution measured by magnetic resonance imaging in obese women. *Am J Clin Nutr* 57:470–475, 1993.

76. Abate N, Garg A, Coleman R, Grundy SM, Peshock RM. Prediction of total subcutaneous abdominal, intraperitoneal, and retroperitoneal adipose tissue masses in men by a single axial magnetic resonance imaging slice. *Am J Clin Nutr* 65:403–408, 1997.

77. Schreiner PJ, Terry JG, Evans GW, Hinson WH, Crouse JR, Heiss G. Sex-specific associations of magnetic resonance imaging-derived intra-abdominal and subcutaneous fat areas with conventional anthropometric indices. *Am J Epidemiol* 144:335–345, 1996.

78. Van Loan MD, Belko AZ, Mayclin PL, Barbieri TF. Use of total-body electrical conductivity for monitoring body composition changes during weight reduction. *Am J Clin Nutr* 46:5–8, 1987.

79. Cochran WJ, Wong WW, Fiorotto ML, et al. Total body water estimated by measuring total-body electrical conductivity. *Am J Clin Nutr* 48:946–950, 1988.

80. de Bruin NC, van Velthoven KAM, Stijnen T, Juttmann RE, Degenhart HJ, Visser HKA. Body fat and fat-free mass in infants: New and classic anthropometric indexes and prediction equations compared with total-body electrical conductivity. *Am J Clin Nutr* 61:1195–1205, 1995.

81. Grauer WO. Quantification of body fat distribution in the abdomen using computed tomography. *Am J Clin Nutr* 39:631–637, 1984.

82. Jensen MD, Kanaley JA, Reed JE, Sheedy PF. Measurement of abdominal and visceral fat with computed tomography and dual-energy x-ray absorptiometry. *Am J Clin Nutr* 61:274–278, 1995.

83. Wang Z-M, Gallagher D, Nelson ME, Matthews DE, Heymsfield SB. Total-body skeletal muscle mass: Evaluation of 24-h urinary creatinine excretion by computerized axial tomography. *Am J Clin Nutr* 63:863–869, 1996.

84. Orphanidou C, McCargar L, Birmingham L, Mathieson J, Goldner E. Accuracy of subcutaneous fat measurement: Comparison of skinfold calipers, ultrasound, and computed tomography. *J Am Diet Assoc* 94:855–858, 1994.

85. McCrory MA, Gomez TD, Bernauer EM, Mole PA. Evaluation of a new air displacement plethysmograph for measuring human body composition. *Med Sci Sports Exerc* 27:1686–1691, 1995.

PHYSICAL FITNESS ACTIVITY 5.1

Measurement of Body Composition

In this activity, you will be measuring the body composition of at least one individual, using several different methods. It is highly recommended that you duplicate the worksheet from this activity and measure three or more individuals.

The body composition methods for this activity have been fully described in this chapter, and you should review each description before administering the test. Ideally, you should first learn the techniques while in a class laboratory under experienced supervision. Misclassification of the body composition status of an individual can lead to undue anxiety.

Body Composition Measurement

Name _____ Date _____

Age _____ Sex _____ Height _____ Weight _____

Skinfolds and BIA Measurements

_____ Chest   _____ Suprailiac

_____ Abdominal   _____ Midaxillary

_____ Thigh   _____ Subscapular

_____ Triceps   _____ Total (mm)

_____ Impedance (BIA)

Hydrostatic Measurements

_____ Net weight in water (kg)   (Gross wt = _____)

                                                        (Tare wt = _____)

            _____

            _____   _____

            _____   _____

_____ Water density

_____ Residual volume (L) (measured)

Client and environmental guidelines prior to BIA measurements include the following:

☐ 1. No eating or drinking within 4 hours of the test.

☐ 2. No exercise within 12 hours of the test.

☐ 3. Urinate within 30 minutes of the test.

☐ 4. No alcohol consumption within 48 hours of the test.

☐ 5. No diuretic medications within 7 days of the test.

☐ 6. No testing of female clients who perceive they are retaining water during that stage of their menstrual cycle.

☐ 7. BIA measurements should be made in a room with normal ambient temperature.

Calculations		Classification
_____	Frame size (mm)	_____
_____	Body mass index (kg/m²)	_____
_____	Relative weight (%)	_____
_____	Skinfold body fat %	_____
_____	BIA body fat %	_____
_____	Hydrostatic body fat %	_____
_____	Fat weight (lb) (*total weight* ×	
_____	*fat%*)	
_____	Fat-free weight (lb) (*total weight − fat weight*)	
	Ideal body weight (lb) (*fat-free weight/(100% − desired fat%)*)	

Body Composition Classification Tables

1995 USDA Healthy Weight Ranges

Height (no shoes)	Frame (mm) (medium) M	F	Weight (pounds) (without clothes) Range	Midpoint
4'10"		57–64	91–119	105
4'11"		57–64	94–124	109
5'0"		57–64	97–128	112.5
5'1"	64–73	57–64	101–132	116.5
5'2"	64–73	57–64	104–137	120.5
5'3"	67–73	60–67	107–141	124
5'4"	67–73	60–67	111–146	128.5
5'5"	67–73	60–67	114–150	132
5'6"	67–73	60–67	118–155	136.5
5'7"	70–76	60–67	121–160	140.5
5'8"	70–76	60–67	125–164	144.5
5'9"	70–76	60–67	129–169	149
5'10"	70–76	60–67	132–174	153
5'11"	70–79	64–70	136–179	157.5
6'0"	70–79	64–70	140–184	162
6'1"	70–79	64–70	144–189	166.5
6'2"	70–79	64–70	148–195	171.5
6'3"	73–83	64–70	152–200	176
6'4"	73–83		156–205	180.5
6'5"	73–83		160–211	185.5
6'6"	73–83		164–216	190

Weight ranges are for men and women. People with low muscle and bone mass should use low end of weight range, and vice versa. For same size, values below the range are rated "small" and above, "large."

Percent Body Fat Norms

Classification	Male	Female
Unhealthy range (too low)	5%	<8%
Acceptable range (lower end)	6–15%	9–23%
Acceptable range (higher end)	16–24%	24–31%
Unhealthy range (too high)	≥25%	≥32%

Body Mass Index Norms (M & F)

Underweight	<18.5 kg/m²
Normal	18.5–24.9 kg/m²
Overweight	25–29.9 kg/m²
Obesity I	30–34.9 kg/m²
Obesity II	35–39.9 kg/m²
Obesity III	≥40 kg/m²

Relative Body Weight Norms (M & F)

Underweight	<90%
Desirable	90–110%
Overweight	111–119%
Mild obesity	120–139%
Moderate obesity	140–199%
Severe obesity	>200%

PHYSICAL FITNESS ACTIVITY 5.2

Case Study: Providing Body Composition Counseling for a Female Track and Field Athlete

The track and field coach refers a female collegiate shotput athlete to your body composition lab for testing. She is 70 inches tall, weighs 245 pounds, has a waist circumference of 37 inches, a BMI of 35.2, and a percent body fat of 32% (determined by underwater weighing). Although this athlete has been very successful in competition, the body composition data indicates she is at very high disease risk if she continues to carry this fat mass throughout adulthood (see Table 5.12). What advice would you give this athlete and her coach?

_____

_____

_____

_____

_____

_____

Author comments: Coaches often feel that field athletes must carry a lot of weight to be successful. However, this female athlete is carrying too much fat mass (both from athletic and health perspectives). This athlete should attempt to decrease her fat mass while increasing her fat-free mass through proper dietary habits and resistance training. Once her competitive days are over, she should attain a healthy BMI and waist circumference to ensure long-term health.

CHAPTER
6

Musculoskeletal Fitness

At the Institute for Aerobics Research, we're learning more every day about the importance of strong muscles and bones. We think there's a definite connection between adequate muscle strength and endurance, and quality of life.

—Dr. Kenneth H. Cooper

As outlined in Chapter 2, musculoskeletal fitness has three elements:

1. *Muscular strength*—the maximal one-effort force that can be exerted against a resistance
2. *Muscular endurance*—the ability of the muscles to apply a submaximal force repeatedly or to sustain a muscular contraction for a certain period of time
3. *Flexibility*—the functional capacity of the joints to move through a full range of movement

The purpose of this chapter is to describe the various types of tests that measure each of these three elements, concentrating on the tests that were outlined in the testing batteries at the end of Chapter 3.

Elaborate and expensive musculoskeletal fitness testing equipment is available, and many books have been written describing it, including the use of isokinetic equipment for testing muscular strength and endurance.[1,2,3] The purpose of both this book and this chapter, however, is to concentrate more on the physical fitness tests that are widely available, inexpensive (yet valid and reliable), and health-related.

HEALTH-RELATED BENEFITS OF MUSCULOSKELETAL FITNESS

Various systems of resistance training for developing muscular strength and endurance are reviewed in Chapter 8. In this chapter, we discuss some of the benefits of musculoskeletal fitness, as well as some means for enhancing it. For one thing, the American College of Sports Medicine,[4] the American Heart Association,[5] and the surgeon general's report on physical activity and health[6] have each acknowledged the importance of strength training as a key component of physical fitness and quality of life (especially in old age). These organizations have recommended performing one set of 8–12 repetitions of 8–10 exercises two to three times per week, for persons under 50–60 years of age and the same regimen using 10–15 repetitions for persons over 50–60 years of age.[7] This is a basic program, however, and greater gains in muscular strength and power can be experienced using a higher intensity (fewer repetitions with greater weight) with multiple sets.[8,9]

Development of muscular strength and endurance has been associated with several important health-related benefits, including increased bone density and connective tissue strength, lean body mass and muscle strength, anaerobic power and capacity, and self-esteem.[7–11] Between the ages of 30 and 70, muscle mass and strength decrease by an average of 30%, much of this due to inactivity. The weakness and frailty of old age is often attributed to this loss of muscular strength and has been shown in several studies to be in part reversible through resistance training.[11–16]

Although there are some indications that high-volume resistance training may lead to reduced resting heart rate and blood pressure, improvements in the blood lipid profile and insulin sensitivity, and an increase in aerobic power, results of studies have been inconclusive, with reported changes small at best when compared to aerobic endurance training (see Table 6.1).[7,10,16–20]

Oxygen uptake during heavy resistance exercise using large muscle groups seldom exceeds 60% of maximal aerobic power, even though heart rates of up to 170 beats per minute and blood pressures exceeding 400/300 mm Hg have been recorded during the last repetitions of a set to volitional fatigue. Most studies have shown that during weight training exercise at a measured percent heart rate maximum, the aerobic demand or percent $\dot{V}O_{2max}$ is less than for endurance exercise. While mean heart rates are usually between 60% and 100% of maximum during weight lifting, oxygen consumption averages 35–60% of aerobic power.[9]

Although the mechanism underlying the higher heart rate of weight training exercise compared to endurance exercise at the same oxygen consumption is unknown, it may be related in part to enhanced sympathetic activity. The net result is that skeletal muscle oxidative capacity in resistance-trained individuals is lacking and aerobic power is not enhanced to a significant degree (Table 6.1).[7]

The American College of Sports Medicine (ACSM) maintains that "optimal musculoskeletal function requires that an adequate range of motion be maintained in all joints. Of particular importance is maintenance of flexibility in the lower back and posterior thigh regions. Lack of flexibility in this area may be associated with an increased risk for development of chronic lower back pain."[21] ACSM recommends static stretching at least three times a week, that an active warm-up precede vigorous stretching, and that each session involve at least four repetitions of each stretching exercise, sustained for 10 to 30 seconds.

Although many sports-medicine specialists agree that participation in a regular flexibility program will help a person maintain good joint mobility, increase resistance to muscle injury and soreness, prevent low-back and other spinal column problems, improve and maintain good postural alignment, enhance proper and graceful body movement, improve personal appearance and self-image, facilitate the development and maintenance of motor skills throughout life, and reduce neuromuscular tension and stress, there are limited scientific data to support these beliefs.[22–24]

PREVENTION AND TREATMENT OF LOW-BACK PAIN

Low-back pain is a common ailment among modern-day men and women.[25–29] At some point in their lives, 60–80% of all Americans and Europeans will experience a bout of low-back pain, ranging from a dull, annoying ache to intense and prolonged pain. After headaches, low-back pain is the second most common ailment in the United States and is topped only by colds and flus in time lost from work. Next to arthritis, low-back pain is the most frequently reported disability.

A nationwide government survey revealed that back pain lasting for at least a week is reported by 18% of the working population each year.[30] Of these, about half attributed the cause of the back pain to a work-related activity or injury, with the proportion much higher among workers in farming, forestry, or fishing occupations. This problem is not unique to the civilian population, in that back pain accounts for at least 20% of all medical discharges from the U.S. Army.

Low-back pain commonly affects people in their most productive years, resulting in a substantial economic cost to society. When all the costs connected with low-back pain are added up—job absenteeism, medical and legal fees, social security disability payments, worker's compensation, long-term disability insurance—the bill to business, industry, and the government has been estimated to range from 16 to 50 billion dollars per year.[25,31]

Males and females appear to be affected equally, with most cases of low-back pain occurring between the ages of 25 and 60 years, with a peak at about 40 years of age.[25] The first attack often occurs early in life, however, with up to one third of adolescents reporting they have experienced at least one bout of low-back pain.[32] A 25-year study of schoolchildren in Denmark showed that low-back pain during the growth period is an important risk factor for low-back pain later in life.[33] Because of this, preventive measures should start within elementary schools.

Fortunately, most low-back pain is self-limiting.[25,31] Without treatment, 60% of back pain sufferers go back to work within a week, and nearly 90% return within 6 weeks. A significant proportion (at least one third) of those experiencing low-back pain once have recurrent episodes. Pain remains for up to 5–10% of patients, creating a chronic con-

TABLE 6.1 Health and Fitness Benefits of Aerobic Compared to Strength Training

Variable	Aerobic Exercise	Resistance Exercise
Resting blood pressure	↓↓	↔↓
Serum HDL cholesterol	↑↑	↔↑
Insulin sensitivity	↑↑	↑
Percent body fat	↓↓	↓
Bone mineral density	↑	↑↑↑
Strength	↔↑	↑↑↑
Physical function in old age	↑↑	↑↑↑
$\dot{V}O_{2max}$	↑↑↑	↔↑

Source: Pollock ML, Vincent ML. Resistance training for health. *The President's Council on Physical Fitness and Sports Research Digest* (Series 2, No. 8). December, 1996.

dition. About 70–90% of the total costs related to back pain are borne by these patients.

The spine is composed of 24 vertebrae, 23 discs, 31 pairs of spinal nerves, 140 attaching muscles, plus a large number of ligaments and tendons (see Figure 6.1). Though humans are born with 33 separate vertebrae (the bones that form the spine), by adulthood, most people have only 24. The 9 vertebrae at the base of the spine grow together. Of these, 5 form the sacrum, while the lowest 4 form the coccyx. Seven cervical vertebrae (C1 to C7) support and provide movement for the head, while 12 thoracic vertebrae (T1 to T12) join with and are supported by the ribs. The 5 lumbar vertebrae (L1 to L5) are most frequently involved in back pain because they carry most of the body's stress. Anatomically, the term *low-back-pain syndrome* is applied to pain experienced in the lumbosacral region (L1 to S1 vertebrae). The most commonly indicated site of low-back pain is the L4–L5 lumbar segment.

Risk Factors for Low-Back Pain

Various risk factors for low-back pain have been advanced[25,26,33–43] (See Box 6.1 for a self-quiz for estimating risk of low-back pain).[34] Many cases of low-back pain appear to be due to unusual stresses on the muscles and ligaments that support the spine of susceptible individuals. When the body is in poor shape, for example, weak spinal and abdominal muscles may be unable to support the spine properly during certain types of lifting or physical activities.

Nonetheless, even hardy occupational workers or athletes who exercise beyond their tolerance are susceptible. Rowers, triathletes, professional golfers and tennis players, wrestlers, and gymnasts, for example, have all been reported to have high rates of back injury (up to 30% in golfers and football players, for example).[44–46] Among athletes,

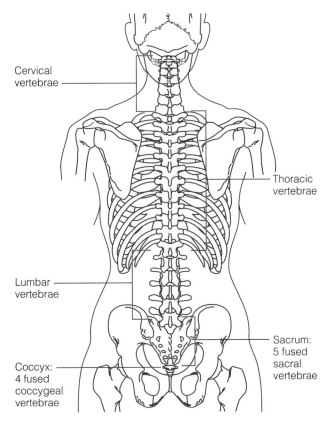

Cervical vertebrae

Thoracic vertebrae

Lumbar vertebrae

Sacrum: 5 fused sacral vertebrae

Coccyx: 4 fused coccygeal vertebrae

Figure 6.1   The human spine is made up of 24 vertebrae divided into five distinct regions. Low-back pain is most commonly experienced at the L4–L5 lumbar segment.[18,22]

Box 6.1

A Self-Quiz for Estimating Risk of Low-Back Pain

Take the following quiz, to evaluate your own risk for low-back pain.

1. _____ Am I overweight?
2. _____ Does my stomach stick out?
3. _____ Do I smoke, especially heavily?
4. _____ Does my work require a lot of sitting, especially without breaks?
5. _____ Is my chair at work comfortable?
6. _____ Does my work entail repetitive pushing and pulling movements or lifting while bending or twisting? (This applies whether you're working at home, in an office, in a warehouse, or outdoors.)
7. _____ Does my work require me to use power tools or heavy moving equipment or to drive a lot?
8. _____ Is my bed comfortable?
9. _____ Do I stand in one place a lot when I work, at home or on the job?
10. _____ Do I slouch most of the time?
11. _____ Is my car seat comfortable for me?
12. _____ Do I engage in any kind of exercise or sport regularly?
13. _____ Does stress in my daily life make my back pain worse?
14. _____ Do I get enough calcium in my diet, especially if I'm over 50?

Source: YMCA of the USA. *YMCA Healthy Back Book.* Champaign, IL: Human Kinetics, 1994. Used with permission of the YMCA of the USA, 101 N. Wacker Drive, Chicago, IL 60606.

back pain and degenerative changes of the spine later on in life are most prevalent among those who experience extreme loading and twisting as a regular part of their training (e.g., weight lifters, track and field power athletes, and gymnasts).[45] Jobs that involve bending and twisting, or lifting heavy objects repeatedly—especially when the loads are beyond a worker's strength—are a chief cause of low-back pain.[40,41]

Certain occupations—such as truck or bus driving, firefighting, or nursing—are particularly hard on the back.[31,38] The truck driver, for example, sits for long periods of time in a vibrating truck and then often helps to unload the truck, lifting and straining at the end of the day. This explains why truck driving ranks first in worker's compensation cases for low-back pain. Firefighters also have a high incidence of low-back pain, which has been related to such high-risk activities as operating charged water hoses, climbing ladders, breaking windows, and lifting heavy objects.[47]

In general, for all workers, occupational risk factors include heavy lifting; lifting with bending and twisting motions; pushing and pulling; slipping, tripping, or falling; and long periods of sitting or driving, especially with vibrations. Individual risk factors may include obesity, smoking, poor posture, psychological stress and anxiety, minimal physical activity level, and reduced degree of muscular strength and joint flexibility.[33–43]

Prevention of low-back pain has typically involved several recommendations:[31,33–43]

- Exercise regularly to strengthen back and abdominal muscles.
- Lose weight, if necessary, to lessen strain on the back. Most studies have shown that obese people are at greater risk for developing low-back pain.
- Avoid smoking. Studies have consistently shown that smokers have a risk of low-back pain 1.5 to 2.5 times that of nonsmokers. Smoking appears to increase degenerative changes of the spine.
- Lift by bending at the knees, rather than the waist, using leg muscles to do most of the work.
- Receive objects from others or from platforms near to the body, and avoid twisting or bending at the waist while handling or transferring the objects.
- Avoid sitting, standing, or working in any one position for too long.
- Maintain a correct posture (sit with shoulders back and feet flat on the floor, or on a footstool or chair rung. Stand with head and chest high, neck straight, stomach and buttocks held in, and pelvis forward).
- Use a comfortable, supportive seat while driving.

- Use a firm mattress, and sleep either on the side, with knees drawn up, or on the back, with a pillow under bent knees.
- Try to reduce emotional stress that causes muscle tension.
- Be thoroughly warmed up before engaging in vigorous exercise or sports.
- Undergo a gradual progression when attempting to improve strength or athletic ability.

Education is the most common back pain prevention strategy used in industry. There are many different types of programs, including comprehensive "back school" programs, which provide information on how the back works, preferred lifting techniques, optimal posture, exercises to prevent back pain, and management of stress and pain.

Despite the numerous causes and risk factors that have been related to low-back pain, most attention has been directed toward viewing low-back pain as a by-product of deficient musculoskeletal fitness.[25] Many researchers feel that the combination of a weak back and a back-straining occupation greatly increases the risk of low-back pain. In particular, emphasis has been placed on the relationship of low-back pain to weak abdominal and back muscles, and poor flexibility of lower back and hamstring muscle groups. Low-back pain has been described as a disease of the sedentary lifestyle, and most fitness testing batteries from professional organizations include some version of a sit-up to evaluate abdominal strength/endurance and the sit-and-reach test to evaluate low-back and hamstring flexibility.

Theoretically, weak muscles that are easily fatigued cannot support the spine in proper alignment. When standing, weak abdominals and inflexible posterior thigh muscles allow the pelvis to tilt forward, causing a curvature in the lower back (called *lordosis*). This places increased stress on the spine and a greater load on other muscles, leading to their fatigue. The tight hamstring muscles and lower back muscles, combined with the weak abdominals, can lead to the low-back pain syndrome.

A study in Japan, for example, showed that subjects with a prior history of low-back pain had weaker trunk muscle strength and a "generalized muscular weakness" when compared to those who had not experienced low-back pain.[48] A study of youths in Finland found that a low level of physical activity and decreased spinal and abdominal muscle strength characterized those who developed low-back pain.[39] Many other studies have reported that low-back-pain patients have low trunk muscle strength, reducing support and stabilization of the spine.[25,26,37]

The evidence is far from conclusive, however, that poor musculoskeletal fitness predicts low-back pain among the general population.[41,42,49–52] For example, in one study of 119 nurses, performance on fitness and back-related isometric strength tests did not effectively predict low-back pain during an 18-month period.[50] A 10-year study of 654 people in Finland failed to demonstrate any relationship between muscle function at baseline and the development of low-back pain.[52] In both adolescents and adults, flexibility measurements have been reported to have a low predictive value for low-back pain.[49,51] Regarding prevention, most experts feel that (a) exercise interventions may be mildly protective against back pain, but (b) evidence is limited to support the contention that exercises to strengthen back or abdominal muscles and to improve overall fitness can decrease the incidence and duration of low-back pain episodes.[28,43]

There is some indication, however, that low levels of musculoskeletal fitness are predictive of recurrent low-back pain.[25] In other words, when an individual of any age suffers a low-back problem and then, as a reaction, engages in very little exercise, the likelihood of further episodes is enhanced. This can set up a vicious cycle, leading to chronic back problems.

For years, the 1-minute timed bent-knee sit-up has been used for measurement of abdominal strength/endurance, while the sit-and-reach test has been touted as a measure of low-back and hamstring flexibility. Unfortunately, there is no evidence that people who score low on both tests are at increased risk of low-back pain in the future. Andrew Jackson, working with researchers at the Cooper Institute for Aerobics Research in Dallas, Texas, studied the effect of low scores on the sit-up and sit-and-reach tests on future low-back pain: Nearly 3,000 adults were followed for 7 years—those who scored low on these tests were not at increased risk for the development of low-back pain.[53]

Treatment of Low-Back Pain with Exercise

Treatment of low-back pain has proven to be complex and frustrating.[28] The optimal management of low-back pain is still under debate.[54-70] Many nonsurgical treatments are available for patients with low-back pain, but few have been proven effective or clearly superior to others.

Nonsurgical treatments include physical therapy (with exercise), strict and extended bed rest, trigger-point injections, spinal manipulation, epidural steroid injections, conventional traction, corsets, and transcutaneous electrical stimulation. Many treatments have been added to the list of ineffective treatments, with little guidance as to the clearly effective ones.[28]

Even physicians are confused. Back pain is one of the most common symptoms that lead people to visit a physician,[71] yet according to a national survey, physicians vary widely in their beliefs regarding treatment of low-back

pain.[72] Results of the survey showed that there was poor correspondence between the treatments physicians believed were effective and those that have been found effective by well-designed studies. For example, a significant proportion of the physicians advocated strict and extended bed rest and traction to treat low-back pain, yet there is now strong evidence that these treatments are ineffective.[72]

Physical therapy with exercise is recommended by physicians more than any other nonsurgical treatment for low-back pain (both acute and chronic),[72] yet, according to most experts, the role of exercise in treatment of low-back pain remains controversial. A recent review, for example, reported that only one of four well-designed studies has found a positive effect of exercise therapy in low-back-pain patients.[67] In one of the earliest studies, Kraus and Raab used musculoskeletal exercises to treat 3,000 adult patients with chronic and acute back pain, and they reported "good" improvement in 65% and "fair" improvement in 26% of the patients, while only 9.2% had poor improvement.[60] In this study, however, no control group was used for determining whether patients engaging in no exercise at all would have experienced similar improvement.

Some researchers advocate an intensive back-muscle-strengthening exercise program to treat low-back pain.[54,56] Patients cannot exercise strenuously at first, but after various pain control measures are initiated, patients are gradually progressed through an increasingly difficult series of resistance exercises to improve back muscle strength. In one study of 105 low-back-pain patients in Denmark, 30 sessions of intense back extensor exercises, over a 3-month period, led to significant improvement, relative to groups exercising less intensely.[54] Other studies have shown that lumbar extension strength training over a 2- to 3-month period is associated with decreased low-back and leg pain and an improved ability to perform daily activities. These researchers have urged that strengthening the entire trunk area over an extended period of time is critical to treating low-back pain.[73] This approach, however, is not accepted by all low-back-pain experts, and it is time-consuming and costly, requiring trained staff and hospital resources.

A study of 186 civil workers who sought treatment for acute low-back pain in Helsinki, Finland, has provided some of the best data to date regarding the relative merits of bed rest, exercise, and ordinary activity in the treatment of acute back pain.[68] The patients were randomized to one of three groups: bed rest (for 2 days), exercise (back extension and side bending movements), and normal activity (continue normal day routines within the limits permitted by the back pain).

As shown in Figure 6.2, after 3 weeks, those patients who maintained normal activities were significantly better off than those who had either rested in bed or exercised. Their back pain was less intense and did not last as long, and they had missed fewer days on the job and felt better

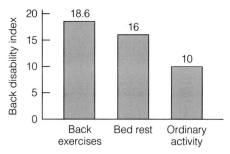

Figure 6.2 Treatment of acute low-back pain: Ordinary activity is superior to bed rest or back exercises. In this study of Finnish civil workers, those who maintained normal activities had better recovery from low-back pain than did those resting in bed or engaging in back exercises. *Source:* Data from Malmivaara A, Häkkinen U, Aro T, et al. The treatment of acute low back pain: Bed rest, exercises, or ordinary activity? *N Engl J Med* 332:351–355, 1995.

able to work. Recovery was slowest for the bed-rest patients. The researchers concluded that avoiding bed rest and maintaining ordinary activity, as tolerated, led to the most rapid recovery.

Most experts now feel that low-back pain should be treated as a benign, self-limiting condition that usually requires little medical intervention.[28] In a large study of close to 1,000 patients in Norway, researchers reported that light and normal activity, combined with information and instruction designed to increase activity and reduce fear associated with the condition, had a significantly better effect on sickness leave than did ordinary medical practice.[66]

This conclusion is similar to that reached by a panel of 23 experts sponsored by the U.S. Agency for Health Care Policy and Research, which reviewed nearly 4,000 studies on back pain. Among the agency's recommendations:[28]

- Engage in low-stress activities such as walking, biking, or swimming during the first 2 weeks after symptoms begin, even if the activities make the symptoms a little worse. "The most important goal," the panel concludes, "is to return to your normal activities as soon as it is safe."

- Bed rest usually is not necessary and should not last longer than 2–4 days. More than 4 days of rest can weaken muscles and delay recovery.

- Nonprescription pain relievers such as aspirin and ibuprofen work as well as prescription painkillers and muscle relaxants and cause fewer side effects.

- Among treatments not recommended, due to lack of evidence that they work, are traction, acupuncture, massage, ultrasound, and transcutaneous electrical nerve stimulation.

- Diagnostic tests such as x-rays and CT scans are rarely useful during the first month of symptoms, so they should be avoided during that time.

- Surgery helps only 1 in 100 people with acute low-back problems. It should be done during the first 3 months of symptoms only when a serious underlying condition, such as a fracture or a dislocation, is suspected.

- Spinal manipulation by a chiropractor or other therapist can be helpful when symptoms begin, but patients should be reevaluated if they have not improved after 4 weeks of treatment.

TESTS FOR MUSCULAR ENDURANCE AND STRENGTH

Although low-back pain has prompted great interest in abdominal, back, and thigh muscle strength, fitness instructors must maintain interest in all muscle groups. Because muscular strength and endurance are specific to each muscle group,[1] no single test can be used to evaluate total body muscle strength and endurance. It is recommended that the selected strength/endurance battery include measures for the upper body, midbody, and lower body.

In this chapter, the emphasis is on field tests for musculoskeletal fitness used in physical fitness testing batteries from the most popular programs: Cooper Institute for Aerobics Research, FITNESSGRAM®[74] and FITCHECK®;[75] President's Council on Physical Fitness and Sports, "President's Challenge" program;[76] Chrysler Fund–Amateur Athletic Union, "Physical Fitness Program";[77] YMCA, "Physical Fitness Program";[78] and the Canadian "Physical Activity, Fitness & Lifestyle Appraisal" program.[79]

Abdominal Tests: Bent-Knee Sit-Ups and Partial Curl-Ups

Abdominal exercises are used for a variety of reasons, including improved posture and appearance, enhanced sports performance, and the prevention and treatment of low-back pain. As discussed earlier in this chapter, although abdominal and back strength have been linked to diminished low-back pain, the data are far from consistent. The Sports Medicine Insight at the end of this chapter summarizes current understanding regarding the appropriate exercises for abdominal fitness.

During the 1950s and 1960s, straight-leg sit-ups were commonly used in physical fitness testing batteries for children and youths.[80] After concerns were raised about lower back strain and the reliance on hip flexor muscles during the straight-leg sit-up, the bent-leg sit-up test (knees bent to 90°) with the hands clenched behind the neck became the test of choice during the 1970s and 1980s. However, researchers soon reported that stress was still placed on the lower back, due to anterior pelvic tilt, and that the hip flexor muscles became dominant in the late stage of the test after the spine had been fully flexed by the abdominal muscles.[80-83] Support at the feet while performing the sit-up was found to increase hip flexor activity and decrease rectus abdominis muscular activity.

Nonetheless, some testing batteries still use the bent-knee sit-up but alter the position of the hands; these include the Cooper Institute for Aerobics Research FITCHECK®[75] (arms crossed on chest), the YMCA[78] (fingers next to ears), and the President's Council on Physical Fitness and Sports "President's Challenge"[76] (arms crossed on chest). In the original Canadian "Standardized Test of Fitness," the 1-minute bent-knee sit-up test was included[84] (fingers over the ears), but in the revised Canadian Physical Activity, Fitness & Lifestyle Appraisal program, this test has been replaced with the partial curl-up test.[79] The YMCA[78] also includes the partial curl-up test in its testing battery, as does the Cooper Institute for Aerobics Research FITNESSGRAM®.[74]

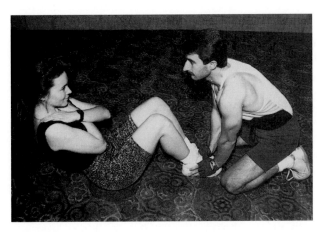

Figure 6.3 The 1-minute timed bent-knee sit-up test. The purpose of this test is to evaluate abdominal muscle strength and endurance.

Partial curl-ups (also called "abdominal crunches" or "half sit-ups"), in which the spine is flexed less than 30°, do not cause strong recruitment of the hip flexor muscles and appear to place less strain on the lower back.[85] Performing the partial curl-up with the feet unsupported and the knees flexed has been reported to maximize abdominal muscle activity.

To perform the 1-minute bent-knee sit-up with the arms crossed over the chest, follow these instructions (Figure 6.3):[75,84]

- Start on the back, with knees flexed, feet on floor, with the heels 12–18 inches from the buttocks.
- The arms are crossed on the chest, with the hands on the opposite shoulders. The arms must be folded across and flat against the chest.
- The feet are held by the partner, to keep them firmly on the ground.
- During the sit-up, arm contact with the chest must be maintained. This is critically important. Another important rule is that the buttocks must remain on the mat, no more than 18 inches from the heels.
- In the up position, the elbow and forearm must touch the thighs (without the arms pulling away from the chest).
- In the down position, the midback makes contact with the floor.
- The number of correctly executed sit-ups performed in 60 seconds is the score. See Appendix A for norms for all age groups (Tables 5, 6, 15, 20, 29, 35). Figure 6.4 represents normative data from the Canadian Fitness Survey.

The protocol used for the partial curl-up test in the Canadian Physical Activity, Fitness & Lifestyle Appraisal program is as follows (see Figure 6.5):[79]

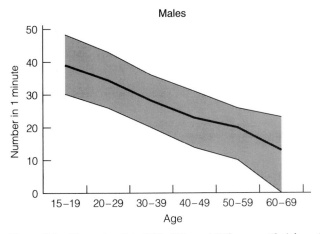

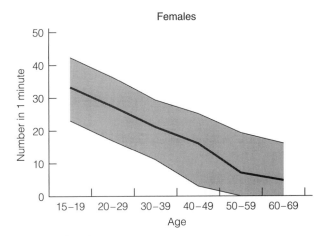

Figure 6.4 Normative data (15th, 50th, and 85th percentiles) from Canada on the bent-knee, 1-minute timed sit-ups in males (left) and females (right).[42] *Source:* Data based on the Canada Fitness Survey, 1981.

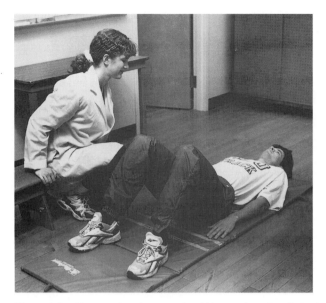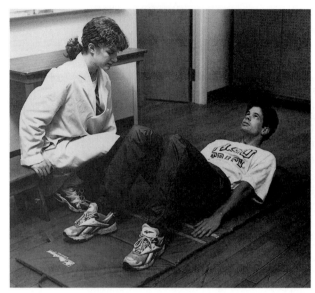

Figure 6.5 The partial curl-up test should be conducted with the feet unsupported.

- Apply masking tape and string across a gym mat in two parallel lines, 10 cm apart.

- The individual to be tested should lie in a supine position, with the head resting on the mat, arms straight and fully extended at the sides and parallel to the trunk, palms of the hands in contact with the mat, and the middle fingertip of both hands at the 0 mark line. The knees should be bent at a 90° angle. The heels must stay in contact with the mat, and the test is performed with the shoes on.

- Set a metronome to a cadence of 50 beats per minute. The subject performs as many consecutive curl-ups as possible, without pausing, at a rate of 25 per minute. The test is terminated after 1 minute. During each curl-up, the upper spine should be curled up so that the middle fingertips of both hands reach the 10-cm mark. During the curl-up the palms and heels must remain in contact with the mat. Anchoring of the feet is not permitted. On the return, the shoulder blades and head must contact the mat, and the fingertips of both hands must touch the 0 mark. The movement is performed in a slow, controlled manner at a rate of 25 per minute.

- The test is terminated before 1 minute if subjects experience undue discomfort, are unable to maintain the required cadence, or are unable to maintain the proper curl-up technique (e.g., heels come off the floor) over two consecutive repetitions, despite cautions by the test supervisor.

Norms for the Canadian partial curl-up test appear in Table 32 of Appendix A. FITNESSGRAM® standards for the partial curl-up are in Table 19 of Appendix A.[74] The FITNESSGRAM® partial curl-up protocol is slightly different from that of the Canadian test.[74] The parallel strips on the mat are placed 3 inches apart for grades kindergarten through four, and 4½ inches apart for older children and youths. The knees are at a 140° angle, and the curl-up is performed at a cadence of 20 per minute. The student continues without pausing until the technique can no longer be followed or 75 curl-ups have been conducted.

Pull-Ups

The purpose of this test is to measure the muscular strength and endurance of the arms and shoulder girdle.[86]

The Traditional Pull-Up

The traditional pull-up requires the following procedures (Figure 6.6):

- The person being tested starts in a hanging position, with arms straight, hands in an *overhand* position (palms away).

- The body is pulled upward until the chin is over the bar.

- After each pull-up, the person returns to a fully extended hanging position.

- Swinging and snap-up movements are to be avoided.

- A partner should hold an extended arm across the front of the person's thighs to prevent swinging. The knees should stay straight during the entire test.

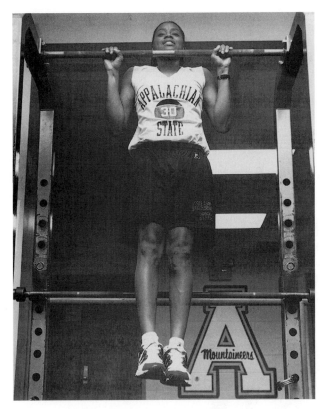

Figure 6.6 Traditional pull-ups. The purpose of this test is to measure the muscular strength and endurance of the arms and shoulder girdle in pulling the body upward.

- The score is the total number of pull-ups until exhaustion. (See norms in Appendix A, Tables 3, 4, 18, 19, 39.)

The Modified Pull-Up

Experience has revealed certain problems with the traditional pull-up and the flexed-arm hang.[87–90] Performance is markedly affected by body weight, and a large proportion of children are incapable of doing even one pull-up.

In 1985, the President's Council on Physical Fitness and the Sports School Population Fitness Survey revealed that 70% of all girls (ages 6–17) tested could not do more than one pull-up, with 55% not being able to do even one.[91] Forty percent of boys ages 6 to 12 could not do more than one pull-up, and 25% could not do any. Fifty-five percent of all girls could not hold their chins over a raised bar for more than 10 seconds. Forty-five percent of boys 6 to 14 could not hold their chins over a raised bar for more than 10 seconds.

A better test of upper-body muscular strength/endurance may be a modification of the traditional pull-up. This modified pull-up was used in the National Children and Youth Fitness Study II for children ages 6 to 9, but it can be used for all age groups.[87,89] In the FITNESSGRAM® testing program, the modified pull-up test is recommended for all students, especially those who cannot do one traditional pull-up[74] (see Appendix A, Table 19).

- The subject is positioned on the back, with shoulders directly below a bar that is set at a height 1 or 2 inches beyond reach.
- An elastic band is suspended across the uprights parallel to and 7–8 inches below the bar.
- In the start position, the subject is suspended holding onto the bar, buttocks off the floor, arms and legs straight, and only heels in contact with the floor.
- The bar is held with an overhand grip (palm away from the body), with thumbs around the bar.
- A pull-up is completed when the chin is hooked over the elastic band. The movement should be accomplished using only the arms, with the body kept rigid and straight. The body is then lowered to starting position and the pull-up repeated as many times as possible.

Flexed-Arm Hang

The purpose of the flexed-arm hang is to assess forearm and upper-arm flexor strength and endurance, and it is included in many fitness testing programs for children and youths.[74,76,91]

- The height of the bar should be adjusted so that it is slightly higher than the subject's standing height.
- The subject (both boys and girls) should use an overhand grip.
- With the assistance of two spotters, the subject is raised to a position with the chin above the bar (not touching), arms flexed, chest close to the bar.
- Spotters then release their support and start a stopwatch, with the subject trying to keep the chin above the bar as long as possible without extraneous body movement.
- The watch is stopped when the chin touches the bar or falls below the level of the bar.
- Total seconds are recorded and can be compared with norms (Appendix A, Table 19).

Push-Ups

The purpose of the push-up test is to assess upper-body (triceps, anterior deltoids, and pectoralis major) muscle strength and endurance and is used in many testing batteries. It is administered differently to males and females in some testing batteries, but not all.[74–76,79]

Males

- The person being tested assumes the standard position for a push-up, with the body rigid and straight, toes tucked under, and hands approximately shoulder-width apart and straight under the shoulders.

- A partner places a fist on the floor beneath the person's chest, who lowers himself until his chest touches the fist, keeping his back perfectly straight; he then raises himself back up to the starting position (see Figure 6.7).
- The most common performance error is not keeping the back rigid and straight throughout the entire push-up.
- Rest is allowed in the up position only.
- The score is the total number of push-ups to exhaustion. (See norms in Appendix A, Tables 30, 34.)

Females

- Everything is the same as for the males, except that the test is performed from the bent-knee position

(see Figure 6.7). In addition, the person being tested should make sure that her hands are slightly ahead of her shoulders in the up position, so that her hands are directly under her shoulders in the down position.

- A common error for females also is not keeping the back rigid.
- The score is the total number of push-ups to exhaustion. (See norms in Appendix A, Tables 30, 34.) Figure 6.8 shows normative data from the Canadian Fitness Survey.[79]

Grip Strength Test with Hand Dynamometer

The grip strength test is used in the Canadian Physical Activity, Fitness & Lifestyle Appraisal program.[79] Both the

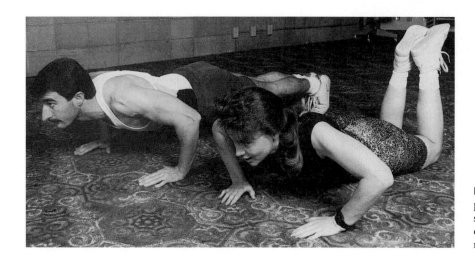

Figure 6.7 Push-ups. The purpose of the push-up test is to assess upper-body (triceps, anterior deltoids, and pectoralis major) muscle strength and endurance.

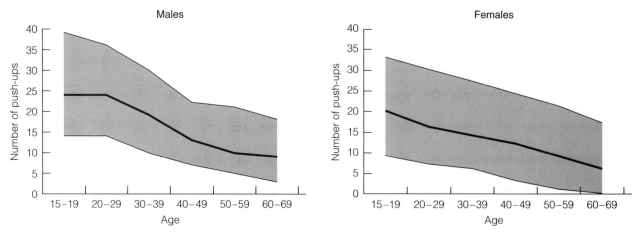

Figure 6.8 Normative data (15th, 50th, and 85th percentiles) from Canada on push-ups for males (left) and females (right).[79] *Source:* Data based on the Canada Fitness Survey, 1981.

right and left hands should be measured. (See norms in Appendix A, Table 31.)

The hand-grip *dynamometer* should be adjustable for any hand size.[92] A maximum reading pointer should be available to hold the reading until it is manually reset (see Appendix B for a list of suppliers).

The purpose of the hand-grip dynamometer test is to measure the static strength of the grip squeezing muscles.[92-98] The hand-grip test is easy to administer, relatively inexpensive, portable, and highly reliable. There is some concern, however, that the hand-grip strength test does not correlate well with muscle mass.[98] Hand-grip strength tends to be higher in taller and heavier people.[95]

To perform the test (Figure 6.9),[92-98]

- The person being tested should first dry and chalk both hands.

- The dynamometer should be adjusted and placed comfortably in the hand to be tested. The second joint of the hand should fit snugly under the handle, which should be gripped between the fingers and the palm at the base of the thumb.

- The person should assume a slightly bent forward position, with the hand to be tested out in front of her or his body. The person's hand and arm should be free of the body, not touching anything. The arm can be slightly bent.

- The test involves an all-out gripping effort for 2–3 seconds. No swinging or pumping of the arm is allowed. The dial can be visible for motivational purposes.

- The score is the sum of the test of both hands, based on the best of 2–4 trials for each. The scale is read in kilograms.

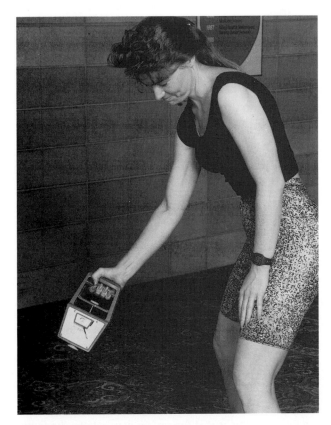

Figure 6.9 Grip strength test with hand dynamometer. Both the right and the left hands should be measured. The purpose of the hand-grip dynamometer test is to measure the static strength of the grip squeezing muscles.

Figure 6.10 shows normative data from the Canadian Fitness Survey.[79] Hand-grip strength diminishes with age and has been used as a risk factor for early death and disability.[96,97]

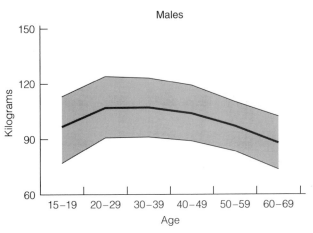

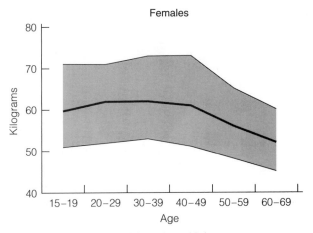

Figure 6.10 Normative data (15th, 50th, and 85th percentiles) from Canada on the grip strength of the right and left hands (combined) for males (left) and females (right).[79] *Source:* Data based on the Canada Fitness Survey, 1981.

Bench-Press Strength and Endurance Tests

The two bench-press tests discussed in this chapter are the 1-RM test for strength and the YMCA test for muscular endurance.

Bench-Press 1-RM Test for Strength

The muscular strength of the major muscle groups can be measured with the one-repetition maximum test (1-RM) (the greatest weight that can be lifted once for a muscle group).[21,75,86,99] The objective of the 1-RM bench-press test is to test the strength of the muscles involved in arm extension (triceps, pectoralis major, anterior deltoid).

The test is performed as follows (see Figure 6.11):

- The person being tested should first be allowed to become familiar with the bench-press test by practicing a few lifts with light weights. For the test, the person lies on her or his back on a bench, with arms extended and hands gripping the bar, approximately shoulder-width apart. The bar is lowered until it touches the chest and then is pushed straight up, with maximum effort, until the arms are locked once again. The person breathes in as the weight is being lowered, and breathes out during the weight-lifting phase. (This helps to prevent the *Valsalva's Maneuver*—the high buildup of blood pressure and decrease of blood flow to the brain, owing to the high pressures that are built up in the chest during weight lifting.)

- Free weights can be used with a spotter, but the use of machine weights allows for safer and easier test-

ing sessions, especially when a series of trials is necessary to determine a true 1-RM.

- As many trials are allowed as it takes to achieve a true maximum effort. Each trial requires maximum effort for one repetition. Allow 1–3 minutes between trials.

- The best lifting score is divided by the person's weight, to derive a ratio. (See Appendix A, Table 36 for the norms.) Norms for strength-to-body-weight ratios are also available for the arm curl, lat pull-down, leg press, leg extension, and leg curl.[1] The Cooper Institute for Aerobic Research has published detailed norms for both men and women for the 1-RM bench-press and leg-press tests.[21,75] (See Appendix A, Tables 36, 37.)

YMCA Bench-Press Test for Muscular Endurance

There are several types of weight-lifting tests used to test muscular endurance. One test of muscular endurance uses a fixed percentage of the person's body weight as the resistance, with the test score being the number of times this weight can be lifted.

Another method uses a fixed percentage (preferably 70%) of 1-RM or absolute strength for the resistance. Good norms have yet to be established, however, for these types of tests. On the basis of limited data, 12–15 repetitions at 70% of 1-RM appear optimal for most people; athletes should aim for 20–25 repetitions.

The YMCA has developed a bench-press test for muscular strength and endurance using an absolute weight. The advantage of this is that for certain occupations (firefight-

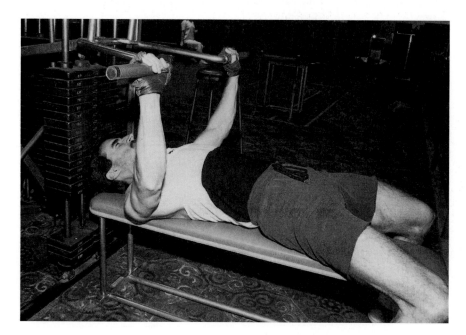

Figure 6.11 Bench-press 1-RM test for strength. Muscular strength can be measured with the one-repetition maximum test (1-RM).

ing, construction, etc.), being able to work with absolute weights is very important. The disadvantage of such a test is that it discriminates against lighter people.

The YMCA bench-press test uses the following steps (Figure 6.12):[78]

- Use a 35-pound barbell for women and an 80-pound barbell for men.

- Set a metronome for 60 beats per minute.

- The person being tested lies on a bench, with feet on the floor.

- A spotter hands the weight to the person. The down position is the starting position (elbows flexed, hands shoulder-width apart, hands gripping the barbell, palms facing up).

- The person presses the barbell upward using free weights (with careful spotting) to fully extend the elbows. After each extension, the barbell is returned to the original down position, the bar touching the chest. The rhythm is kept by the metronome, each click representing a movement up or down (30 lifts per minute).

- The score is the number of successful repetitions. (See Appendix A, Table 38 for the norms.) The test is terminated when the person is unable to reach full extension of the elbows or breaks cadence and cannot keep up with the rhythm of the metronome. Emphasize *proper breathing technique* (breathe in as weight comes down to chest, breathe out as weight is pushed up).

Parallel Bar Dips

This test is for measuring the muscular strength and endurance of the arms and shoulder girdle (triceps, deltoid, and pectoralis major and minor).

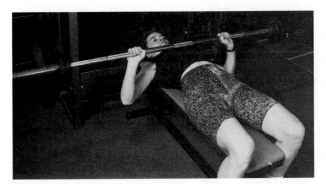

Figure 6.12 YMCA bench-press test for muscular endurance. The YMCA has developed a bench-press test for muscular strength and endurance using an absolute weight (35 pounds for females, 80 pounds for males).

To perform the test, follow these steps[86] (see Figure 6.13):

- The person being tested should assume a straight-arm support position between parallel bars, with legs straight.

- The body should be lowered until the elbows form a right angle, with the upper arm (humerus) parallel to the floor. The tester should indicate to the person when the proper position is attained.

- The person should then push back up to a straight-arm support and continue the exercise for as many repetitions as possible.

- Rest is permitted in the up position. No swinging or kicking is allowed during the test.

- The score is the total number of bar dips until exhaustion. (Excellent is ≥25; good is 18–24, average is 9–17, fair is 4–8, and poor ≤3.)

FLEXIBILITY TESTING

As stated in Chapter 2, flexibility is the capacity of a joint to move fluidly through its full range of motion.[1] The major

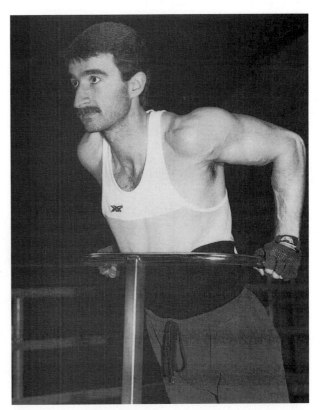

Figure 6.13 Parallel bar dip. This test is for measuring the muscular strength and endurance of the arms and shoulder girdle (triceps, deltoid, and pectoralis major and minor).

limitation to joint flexibility is tightness of soft tissue structures (joint capsule, muscles, tendons, ligaments). The muscle is the most important and modifiable structure in terms of improving flexibility.[100]

Flexibility is related to age and physical activity.[100] As a person ages, flexibility decreases, although this is due more to inactivity than to the aging process itself. Exercises to increase flexibility are discussed in Chapter 8.

Nearly all health-related physical fitness testing batteries now use the sit-and-reach test for a measure of flexibility. The sit-and-reach test is singled out because it has been noted in some clinical settings that people with low-back problems often have a restricted range of motion in the hamstring muscles and the lower back.

However, as noted earlier in this chapter, there are limited scientific data to back the assertion that people with poor flexibility are more likely to develop low-back pain in the future.[53] There is also some doubt as to whether the sit-and-reach test (all forms, including the modified test or the "back saver" test using one leg at a time) actually measures lower-back flexibility because studies have concluded it is actually a better measure of hamstring flexibility.[101–105] There probably is no test of flexibility that will discriminate between those who will develop low-back pain and those who will not.[105] Hip joint flexibility, however, is important for sports performance, and for this reason, the sit-and-reach test will probably remain as a component of most fitness test batteries.

Some researchers also feel that subjects with longer arms or shorter legs receive better ratings from the sit-and-reach test than those with shorter arms or longer legs, even though they may not have better lower-back and hamstring flexibility.

A modified sit-and-reach test has been proposed to deal with this problem.[106,107] In the modified protocol, subjects first sit with head, back, and hips against a wall; legs straight; and feet flat against a 12-inch box. While maintaining contact with the wall (including the head), the subject reaches as far forward as possible to determine a zero point and then conducts the typical sit-and-reach test, using this zero point as the reference. Norms for this modified test are available, but the test has not yet been adopted for use in national testing.[106,107]

Figure 6.14 shows the flexibility testing box that can be purchased or constructed before administering the test. It is 12 inches high and has an overlap in front, so that minus readings can be obtained when the person being tested is unable to reach her or his feet. The various testing batteries use different measuring-scale settings at the footline. For standardization purposes, the footline can be set at zero, with plus or minus readings in inches or centimeters, measured from the zero line. (See norms in Appendix A, Tables 7, 8, 18, 19, 33.)

If a box is not available, a 12-inch bench with a ruler taped onto it can be used.

To perform the sit-and-reach test for flexibility (Figure 6.14),[79]

- The person being tested should first warm up, using static stretching exercises (discussed in Chapter 8). A brisk walking or cycling warm-up is also advisable (on a treadmill or ergometer, if available). Warm muscles can stretch more safely.

- To start, the persons being tested remove their shoes and sit facing the flexibility box, with knees fully extended, feet 4 inches apart. The feet should be flat, heels touching, against the end board.

- To perform the test, the arms are extended straight forward, with the hands placed on top of each other, fingertips perfectly even. The person reaches directly

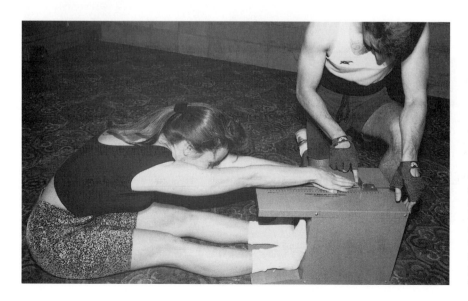

Figure 6.14 The purpose of the sit-and-reach flexibility test is to evaluate the flexibility of the lower back and posterior leg muscles. A flexibility box is required, which is 12 inches high and has an overlap toward the person being tested; it can be purchased or constructed.

forward, palms down, as far as possible along the measuring scale, extending forward maximally four times, and then holds the position of maximum reach for 1–2 seconds.

- The score is the most distant point reached on the fourth trial, measured to the nearest centimeter (or quarter of an inch). The test administrator should remain close to the scale and note the most distant line touched by the fingertips of both hands. If the hands reach unevenly, the test should be readministered. The tester should place one hand lightly on the person's knees, to ensure that they remain locked. Figure 6.15 shows normative data from the Canadian Fitness Survey.[79]

Many other methods are used in addition to the sit-and-reach test for measuring flexibility.[1] Flexibility of one joint does not necessarily indicate flexibility in other joints, and there is no general flexibility test for the whole body.[108] Other flexibility tests used for the general population include the shoulder rotation test, total body rotation test, and the shoulder flexibility test.[1,9,74,75] In the shoulder flexibility test, the subject stands and places the right hand over the right shoulder, palm against the back, reaching down as far as possible. At the same time, the left hand is placed behind the back at the waistline, back of the hand against the back, reaching up as high as possible. A partner measures the overlap distance between the tips of the right and left middle fingers (value is negative if they don't touch). Positions of right and left hands can then be reversed. Try both ways. Overlapping by 1 inch or more is considered good.[75]

Various tests have been devised to measure the range of motion of each major body joint using the goniometer (a protractor-like device with arms that are attached to body segments using the joint as a fulcrum) and Leighton flexometer (360-degree dial with weighted pointer).[1]

VERTICAL JUMP

The vertical jump is a simple yet effective test for measuring muscular power and has been used as an index of sports training.[9,79] For example, in one large study of 774 Finnish males and females, vertical jumping height was found to be highest in those engaging in a variety of sports, compared to those who practiced aerobic training alone (e.g., running, cycling, or swimming) or who largely avoided all forms of exercise.[109]

The vertical jump test is included in the Canadian Physical Activity, Fitness & Lifestyle Appraisal (CPAFLA), and it can be scored in two ways: as a straight height jumped, and in terms of leg power.[79] In the test, clients take a standing position facing sideways to a wall on which a measuring tape has been attached. Special equipment for measuring vertical jump can also be used, as shown in Figure 6.16. Standing erect with the feet flat on the floor, the client reaches as high as possible on the tape, with the arm and fingers fully extended and the palm toward the wall. This is recorded as the beginning height. Standing about a foot away from the wall, the individual brings the arms downward and backward, while bending the knees to a balanced semisquat position, and then jumps as high as possible, with the arms moving forward and upward. The tape should be touched at the peak height of the jump with the fingers of the arm facing the wall. Record the highest jump from three trials, with a rest period of 10–15 seconds between trials. Subtract the beginning height from the peak height to determine the height jumped in centimeters.

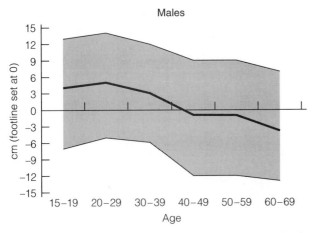

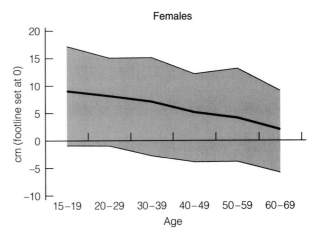

Figure 6.15 Normative data (15th, 50th, and 85th percentiles) from Canada on the sit-and-reach test (in centimeters) for males (left) and females (right).[79] *Source:* Data based on the Canada Fitness Survey, 1981.

TABLE 6.2 **Age Group and Gender Classifications for Leg Power (kgm/second) from Vertical Jump**

Age	Excellent	Very Good	Good	Fair	Needs Improvement
15–19					
Male	≥ 104	88–103	73–87	61–72	≤ 60
Female	≥ 74	67–73	58–66	51–57	≤ 50
20–29					
Male	≥ 121	102–120	89–101	74–88	≤ 73
Female	≥ 78	65–77	56–64	52–55	≤ 51
30–39					
Male	≥ 120	102–119	87–101	70–86	≤ 69
Female	≥ 74	64–73	56–63	51–55	≤ 50
40–49					
Male	≥ 113	96–112	81–95	73–80	≤ 72
Female	≥ 72	60–71	56–59	52–55	≤ 51
50–59					
Male	≥ 105	93–104	76–92	68–75	≤ 67
Female	≥ 71	63–70	57–62	54–56	≤ 53
60–69					
Male	≥ 98	84–97	75–83	67–74	≤ 66
Female	≥ 64	56–63	53–55	49–52	≤ 48

Source: Canadian Society for Exercise Physiology. *The Canadian Physical Activity, Fitness & Lifestyle Appraisal:* CSEP's Plan for Healthy Active Living. Ottawa, Ontario: Canadian Society for Exercise Physiology, 1996. Used with permission.

Leg power can be calculated through use of this equation:[79]

leg power (kgm/second)
$$= 2.21 \times \text{weight kg} \times \sqrt{\text{vertical jump meters}}$$

For example, if a 22-year-old female weighing 60 kg vertical jumps 0.35 meters, then her leg power would be calculated as follows:

$$\text{leg power} = 2.21 \times 60 \times \sqrt{0.35} = 78.4 \text{ kgm/second}$$

According to the CPAFLA, leg power can be classified using the age and gender group standards presented in Table 6.2.[79] For example, this 22-year-old female with a leg power of 78.4 kgm/second would be given an "excellent" rating by the CPAFLA.

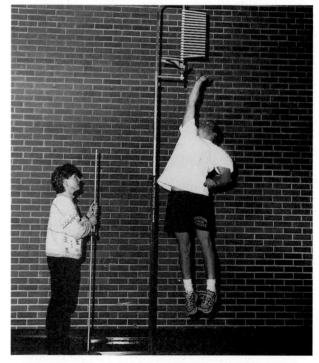

Figure 6.16 The vertical jump is a simple yet effective test for measuring the muscular power of the legs.

SPORTS MEDICINE INSIGHT

Searching for the Safest Abdominal Exercise Challenge

Abdominal exercises are used to improve appearance and posture, develop abdominal strength for sports performance (e.g., gymnastics and wrestling), and prevent and treat low-back pain. A wide variety of abdominal exercises and equipment have been used to maximize abdominal muscle strength and endurance. Concerns, however, have been raised regarding the safety of some abdominal exercises, especially in regard to compressive forces on the lumbar spine. As discussed earlier in this chapter, partial curl-ups (also called "abdominal crunches") have become popular because they appear to optimize abdominal muscle contraction without causing stress to the lower back.

Researchers at the University of Waterloo in Waterloo, Ontario, Canada, have published a series of studies in which they have tried to identify the safer and more effective exercises to train the abdominal muscles.[85,110] Twelve different abdominal exercises have been compared, while abdominal muscular action was measured with electromyographic (EMG) equipment and lumbar spinal compression was measured with specialized equipment. The 12 different abdominal exercises are depicted in Figure 6.17 and can be described as follows.[85]

a. *Straight-leg sit-up*—with the feet anchored and legs straight, and arms positioned with the fingers touching the ears, raising the torso to a vertical position and then returning to the starting position

b. *Bent-leg sit-up*—similar to the straight-leg sit-up, except that the knees are bent to a 90° angle

c. *Partial curl-up* (with feet anchored)—similar to bent-leg sit-up, except that the arms are straight at the sides of the torso, with the hands flat on the mat, the hands slide forward 10 cm, with the head, shoulders, and torso lifted off the mat

d. *Partial curl-up* (with feet unanchored)—similar to "c," except that the feet are not anchored

e. *Quarter sit-up*—similar to partial curl-up, except that both the knees and the hips are bent at a 90° angle (with legs and feet parallel to the ground), and the fingers touch the ears

f. *Straight-leg raise*—while lying supine, put the hands under the lumbar region, raising both legs to a 90° angle off the mat

g. *Bent-leg raise*—similar to the straight-leg raise except that the knees are bent at a 90° angle, and the bent legs are raised until the hips achieve a 90° flexion

h. *Dynamic cross-knee curl-up*—similar to the quarter sit-up except that the torso is twisted to bring one elbow toward the opposite knee (contact of the elbow to the knee is not recommended)

i. *Static cross-knee curl-up*—similar to the dynamic cross-knee curl-up except that the hand is brought up and over to the opposite knee and then pushed against the knee for 3 seconds

j. *Hanging straight-leg raise*—while hanging from the hands on a chin-up bar, lift the straight legs to a horizontal position (avoid pelvic rotation)

k. *Hanging bent-leg raise*—similar to the hanging straight-leg raise except that the knees are bent to a 90° angle

l. *Isometric side support*—raise the torso and legs off the mat, supported by only the right foot, right elbow, and right forearm

The researchers found that no single abdominal exercise best recruited all of the abdominal muscles simultaneously, primarily because the obliques and the rectus abdominis have different functions.[85] Sit-ups with feet unanchored, legs elevated, or twists of the torso did not significantly increase the level of abdominal activity. Contrary to popular belief, no differences in lumbar spine compression or utilization of the hip flexor muscles (psoas) were observed in sit-ups performed with the legs bent versus with the legs straight. No sit-up exercise was considered ideal (defined as high abdominal activity with low lumbar spine compression), although the partial curl-ups came closest. Figure 6.18 shows that it is not possible to recommend just one type of abdominal exercise for all individuals. Several exercises are required to train the entire abdominal muscle area, and different exercises may best suit certain individuals based on their fitness level, training goals, injury history, and other personal characteristics. Several abdominal exercises are not recommended because of their high lumbar compression effects, including the supine straight- or bent-leg raises (f and g), the static cross-knee curl-up (i), and the hanging bent-leg raise (k).

(continued)

Searching for the Safest Abdominal Exercise Challenge *(continued)*

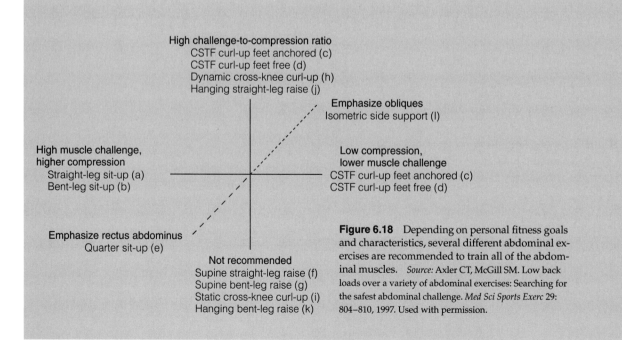

(a) Straight-leg sit-up　(b) Bent-leg sit-up　(c) CSTF curl-up (feet fixed)　(d) CSTF curl-up (feet free)

(e) Quarter sit-up　(f) Straight-leg raise　(g) Bent-leg raise　(h) Dynamic cross-knee curl-up

(i) Static cross-knee curl-up　(j) Hanging straight-leg raise　(k) Hanging bent-leg raise　(l) Isometric side support

Figure 6.17 Twelve different abdominal exercises (see text for description). *Source:* Axler CT, McGill SM. Low back loads over a variety of abdominal exercises: Searching for the safest abdominal challenge. *Med Sci Sports Exerc* 29: 804–810, 1997. Used with permission.

High challenge-to-compression ratio
CSTF curl-up feet anchored (c)
CSTF curl-up feet free (d)
Dynamic cross-knee curl-up (h)
Hanging straight-leg raise (j)

Emphasize obliques
Isometric side support (l)

High muscle challenge,
higher compression
Straight-leg sit-up (a)
Bent-leg sit-up (b)

Low compression,
lower muscle challenge
CSTF curl-up feet anchored (c)
CSTF curl-up feet free (d)

Emphasize rectus abdominus
Quarter sit-up (e)

Not recommended
Supine straight-leg raise (f)
Supine bent-leg raise (g)
Static cross-knee curl-up (i)
Hanging bent-leg raise (k)

Figure 6.18 Depending on personal fitness goals and characteristics, several different abdominal exercises are recommended to train all of the abdominal muscles. *Source:* Axler CT, McGill SM. Low back loads over a variety of abdominal exercises: Searching for the safest abdominal challenge. *Med Sci Sports Exerc* 29: 804–810, 1997. Used with permission.

SUMMARY

1. This chapter focused on the various musculoskeletal tests that are economical in terms of time, money, and ease of administration, and that are effectively health related. Musculoskeletal testing centers around the flexibility of the lower back and the muscular strength and endurance of the abdominals because of the widespread prevalence of low-back pain in the United States. Although more research is needed, exercises that can improve the musculoskeletal fitness of the lower trunk area in particular may sometimes help in the rehabilitation of low-back pain.

2. The musculoskeletal tests described in this chapter are based on the testing batteries outlined in Chapter 3, with the norms listed in Appendix A.

3. The 1-minute timed bent-knee sit-up test has been traditionally used to evaluate abdominal muscle strength and endurance. However, there has been, and still is, dissatisfaction with it. Although research has indicated that the abdominals (spinal flexors) are active during a sit-up, hip flexor muscles are also involved. The use of the hip flexor muscles during the sit-up is potentially harmful to the lower back, especially when the feet are held down. Bending the knees does not appear to avoid this problem. Trunk curling exercises are helpful in increasing the strength and endurance of the abdominal muscles, and a new test using a curl-up motion has been developed.

4. The pull-up is used to measure the muscular strength and endurance of the arms and shoulder girdle. Because many children and youths cannot do a pull-up, a modified pull-up test has been developed.

5. Push-ups are used to assess upper-body muscle strength and endurance; separate tests have been developed for men and women.

6. The grip strength test with the hand dynamometer measures the static strength of the grip squeezing muscles. However, because strength is specific to each muscle group, it is recommended that additional strength tests be administered.

7. The bench-press exercise can be used for a test either of *strength* (greatest amount of weight that can be lifted just once) or *endurance* (number of successful repetitions using an absolute weight).

8. The sit-and-reach test has been developed to measure the flexibility of the low-back and posterior leg muscles. However, it appears to be a better measure of hamstring rather than lower-back flexibility.

REFERENCES

1. Heyward VH. *Advanced Fitness Assessment and Exercise Prescription* (3rd ed.). Champaign, IL: Human Kinetics, 1998.

2. Maud PJ, Foster C. *Physiological Assessment of Human Fitness.* Champaign, IL: Human Kinetics, 1995.

3. Davies GJ. *A Compendium of Isokinetics in Clinical Usage and Rehabilitation Techniques* (3rd ed.). Onalaska, Wisconsin: S & S Publishers, 1987.

4. American College of Sports Medicine, Position Stand. The recommended quantity and quality of exercise for developing and maintaining cardiorespiratory and muscular fitness in healthy adults. *Med Sci Sports Exerc* 22:265–274, 1990; *Med Sci Sports Exerc* 30:975–991, 1998.

5. Fletcher GF, Balady G, Froelicher VF, Hartley LH, Haskell WL, Pollock ML. Exercise standards: A statement for healthcare professionals from the American Heart Association. *Circulation* 91:580–615, 1995.

6. U.S. Department of Health and Human Services. *Physical Activity and Health: A Report of the Surgeon General.* Atlanta, GA: U.S. Department of Health and Human Services, Centers for Disease Control and Prevention, National Center for Chronic Disease Prevention and Health Promotion, 1996.

7. Pollock ML, Vincent ML. *Resistance Training for Health: The President's Council on Physical Fitness and Sports Research Digest* (Series 2, No. 8). December, 1996.

8. Fleck SJ, Kraemer WJ. *Designing Resistance Training Programs.* Champaign, IL: Human Kinetics, 1987.

9. Baechle TR. *Essentials of Strength Training and Conditioning.* Champaign, IL: Human Kinetics, 1994.

10. Stone MH, Fleck SJ, Triplett NT, Kraemer WJ. Health- and performance-related potential of resistance training. *Sports Med* 11:210–231, 1991.

11. Braith RW, Mills RM, Welsch MA, Keller JW, Pollock ML. Resistance training restores bone mineral density in heart transplant recipients. *J Am Coll Cardiol* 28:1471–1477, 1996.

12. Israel S. Age-related changes in strength and special groups. In Komi PV (ed), *Strength and Power in Sport: The Encyclopædia of Sports Medicine.* Oxford: Blackwell Scientific Publications, 1992.

13. Grimby G, Aniansson A, Hedberg M, et al. Training can improve muscle strength and endurance in 78- to 84-yr-old men. *J Appl Physiol* 73:2517–2523, 1992.

14. Aoyagi Y, Shephard RJ. Aging and muscle function. *Sports Med* 14:376–396, 1992.

15. Morey MC, Pieper CF, Sullivan RJ, Crowley GM, Cowper PA, Robbins MS. Five-year performance trends for older exercisers: A hierarchical model of endurance, strength, and flexibility. *J Am Geriatr Soc* 44:1226–1231, 1996.

16. Vuori I. Exercise and physical health: Musculoskeletal health and functional capabilities. *Res Quart Exerc Sport* 66:276–285, 1995.

17. Hurley BF, Kokkinos PF. Effects of weight training on risk factors for coronary heart disease. *Sports Med* 4:231–238, 1987.

18. Tesch PA. Training for bodybuilding. In Komi PV (ed), *Strength and Power in Sport: The Encyclopædia of Sports Medicine.* Oxford: Blackwell Scientific Publications, 1992.

19. Fleck SJ. Cardiovascular response to strength training. In Komi PV (ed), *Strength and Power in Sport: The Encyclopædia of Sports Medicine.* Oxford: Blackwell Scientific Publications, 1992.

20. Tucker LA, Silvester LJ. Strength training and hypercholesterolemia: An epidemiologic study of 8499 employed men. *Am J Health Promot* 11:35–41, 1996.

21. American College of Sports Medicine. *ACSM's Guidelines for Exercise Testing and Prescription* (5th ed.). Baltimore: Williams & Wilkins, 1995.

22. Alter MJ. *Science of Flexibility* (2nd ed.). Champaign, IL: Human Kinetics, 1996.

23. Hoeger WWK, Hopkins DR. Assessing muscular flexibility. *Fitness Management,* February, 1990, 34–42.

24. Worrell T, Perrin D, Gansneder B, Gieck J. Comparison of isokinetic strength and flexibility measures between injured and noninjured athletes. *J Orthop Sports Phys Ther* 13:118–125, 1991.

25. Plowman SA. Physical activity, physical fitness, and low back pain. *Exerc Sport Sci Rev* 20:221–242, 1992.

26. Biering-Sorensen F, Bendix T, Jorgensen K, Manniche C, Nielsen H. Physical activity, fitness and back pain. In Bouchard C, Shephard RJ (eds), *Exercise, Fitness, and Health: A Consensus of Current Knowledge.* Champaign, IL: Human Kinetics, 1994.

27. Deyo R, Cherkin D, Conrad D, Volinn E. Cost, controversy, crisis: Low back pain and the health of the public. *Ann Rev Pub Health* 12:141–156, 1991.

28. Agency for Health Care Policy and Research. *Clinical Practice Guideline: Acute Low Back Problems in Adults.* Silver Spring, MD: Publications Clearinghouse, 1994.

29. Papageorigiou AC, Croft PR, Ferry S, Jayson MIV, Silman AJ. Estimating the prevalence of low back pain in the general population. *Spine* 20:1889–1894, 1995.

30. Park C, Wagener D. *Health Conditions among the Currently Employed: United States, 1988.* National Center for Health Statistics, (PHS) 93-1412. Washington, DC: Government Printing Office, 1993.

31. Zammula E. Back talk: Advice for suffering spines. *FDA Consumer,* April, 1989, 28–35.

32. Olsen TL, Anderson RL, Dearwater SR, et al. The epidemiology of low back pain in an adolescent population. *Am J Public Health* 82:606–608, 1992.

33. Harreby M, Neergaard K, Hesseisoe G, Kjer J. Are radiologic changes in the thoracic and lumbar spine of adolescents risk factors for low back pain in adults. *Spine* 20:2298–2302, 1995.

34. YMCA of the USA. *YMCA Healthy Back Book.* Champaign, IL: Human Kinetics, 1994.

35. Toroptsova NV, Benevolenskaya LI, Karyakin AN, Sergeev IL, Erdesz S. Cross-sectional study of low back pain among workers at an industrial enterprise in Russia. *Spine* 20:328–332, 1995.

36. Croft PR, Papageorgiou AC, Ferry S, Thomas E, Jayson MIV, Silman AJ. Psychologic distress and low back pain. *Spine* 20:2731–2737, 1996.

37. Takemasa R, Yamamoto H, Tani T. Trunk muscle strength in and effect of trunk muscle exercises for patients with chronic low back pain. *Spine* 20:2522–2530, 1995.

38. Liira JP, Shannon HS, Chambers LW, Haines TA. Long-term back problems and physical work exposures in the 1990 Ontario Health Survey. *Am J Public Health* 86:382–387, 1996.

39. Salminen JJ, Erkinalo M, Laine M, Pentti J. Low back pain in the young: A prospective three-year follow-up study of subjects with and without low back pain. *Spine* 19:2101–2108, 1994.

40. Macfarlane GJ, Thomas E, Papageorgiou AC, Croft PR, Jayson MIV, Silman AJ. Employment and physical work activities as predictors of future low back pain. *Spine* 22:1143–1149, 1997.

41. Kujala UM, Taimela S, Viljanen T, Jutila H, Viitasalo JT, Videman T, Battié MC. Physical loading and performance as predictors of back pain in healthy adults: A 5-year prospective study. *Eur J Appl Physiol* 73:452–458, 1996.

42. Gibbons LE, Videman T, Battié MC. Isokinetic and psychophysical lifting strength, static back muscle endurance, and magnetic resonance imaging of the paraspinal muscles as predictors of low back pain in men. *Scand J Rehabil Med* 29:187–191, 1997.

43. Campello M, Nordin M, Weiser S. Physical exercise and low back pain. *Scand J Med Sci Sports* 6:63–72, 1996.

44. Dreisinger TE, Nelson B. Management of back pain in athletes. *Sports Med* 21:313–319, 1996.

45. Videman T, Sarna S, Battié MC, Koskinen S, Gill K, Paananen H, Gibbons L. The long-term effects of physical loading and exercise lifestyles on back-related symptoms, disability, and spinal pathology among men. *Spine* 20:699–709, 1995.

46. Kujala UM, Taimela S, Erkintalo M, Salminen JJ, Kaprio J. Low-back pain in adolescent athletes. *Med Sci Sports Exerc* 28:165–170, 1996.

47. Nuwayhid IA, Stewart W, Johnson JV. Work activities and the onset of first-time low back pain among New York City fire fighters. *Am J Epidemiol* 137:539–548, 1993.

48. Lee J-H, Ooi Y, Nakamura K. Measurement of muscle strength of the trunk and the lower extremities in subjects with history of low back pain. *Spine* 20:1994–1996, 1995.

49. Kujala UM, Salminen JJ, Taimela S, et al. Subject characteristics and low back pain in young athletes and nonathletes. *Med Sci Sports Exerc* 24:627–632, 1992.

50. Ready AE, Boreskie SL, Law SA, Russell R. Fitness and lifestyle parameters fail to predict back injuries in nurses. *Can J Appl Physiol* 18:80–90, 1993.

51. Battié MC, Bigos SJ, Fisher LS, et al. The role of spinal flexibility in back pain complaints within industry. *Spine* 15:768–773, 1990.

52. Leino P, Aro S, Hasan J. Trunk muscle function and low back disorders: A ten-year follow-up study. *J Chron Dis* 40:289–296, 1987.

53. Jackson AW, Morrow JR, Brill P, Kohl HW, Gordon NF, Blair SN. Relationships of fitness tests to low back pain in adults: A prospective study. *Med Sci Sports Exerc* 27:S211, 1995.

54. Manniche C, Hesselsoe G, Bentzen L, Christensen I, Lundberg E. Clinical trial of intensive muscle training for chronic low back pain. *Lancet,* December 24/31:1473–1476, 1988.

55. Jarvikoski A, Mellin G, Estlander AM, et al. Outcome of two multimodal back treatment programs with and without intensive physical training. *J Spinal Disord* 6(2):93–98, 1993.

56. Manniche C, Asmussen K, Lauritsen B, et al. Intensive dynamic back exercises with or without hyperextension in chronic back pain after surgery for lumbar disc protrusion: A clinical trial. *Spine* 18(5):587–594, 1993.

57. Risch SV, Norvell NK, Pollock ML, Risch ED, et al. Lumbar strengthening in chronic low back pain patients: Physiologic and psychological benefits. *Spine* 18(2):232–238, 1993.

58. Hansen FR, Bendix T, Skov P, et al. Intensive, dynamic back-muscle exercises, conventional physiotherapy, or placebo-control treatment of low-back pain: A randomized observer-blind trial. *Spine* 18(1):98–108, 1993.

59. Lindstrom I, Ohlund C, Eek C, et al. The effect of graded activity on patients with subacute low back pain: A randomized prospective clinical study with an operant-conditioning behavioral approach. *Phys Ther* 72:279–290, 1992.

60. Kraus H, Raab W. *Hypokinetic Disease*. Springfield, IL: Charles C. Thomas, 1961.

61. Gundewall B, Liljeqvist M, Hansson T. Primary prevention of back symptoms and absence from work: A prospective randomized study among hospital employees. *Spine* 18(5): 587–594, 1993.

62. Carey TS, Garrett J, Jackman A, McLaughlin C, Fryer J, Smucker DR. The outcomes and costs of care for acute low back pain among patients seen by primary care practitioners, chiropractors, and orthopedic surgeons. *N Engl J Med* 333: 913–917, 1995.

63. Twomey L, Taylor J. Spine update: Exercise and spinal manipulation in the treatment of low back pain. *Spine* 20:615–619, 1995.

64. Faas A, van Eijk JTM, Chevannes AW, Gubbels JW. A randomized trial of exercise therapy in patients with acute low back pain. *Spine* 20:941–947, 1995.

65. Dettori JR, Bullock SH, Sutlive TG, Franklin RJ, Patience T. The effects of spinal flexion and extension exercises and their associated postures in patients with acute low back pain. *Spine* 20:2303–2312, 1995.

66. Indahl A, Velund L, Reikeraas O. Good prognosis for low back pain when left untampered: A randomized clinical trial. *Spine* 20:473–477, 1995

67. Lahad A, Malter AD, Berg AO, Deyo RA. The effectiveness of four interventions for the prevention of low back pain. *JAMA* 272:1286–1291, 1994.

68. Malmivaara A, Häkkinen U, Aro T, et al. The treatment of acute low back pain: Bed rest, exercises, or ordinary activity? *N Engl J Med* 332:351–355, 1995.

69. Scheer SJ, Watanabe TK, Radack KL. Randomized controlled trials in industrial low back pain: Part 3. Subacute/chronic pain interventions. *Arch Phys Med Rehabil* 78:414–423, 1997.

70. Faas A. Exercises: Which ones are worth trying, for which patients, and when? *Spine* 21:2874–2878, 1996.

71. Hart LG, Deyo RA, Cherkin DC. Physician office visits for low back pain. *Spine* 20:11–19, 1995.

72. Cherkin DC, Deyo RA, Wheeler K, Ciol MA. Physician views about treating low back pain: The results of a national survey. *Spine* 20:1–10, 1995.

73. Nelson BE, O'Reilly E, Miller M. The clinical effects of intensive, specific exercise on chronic low-back pain: A controlled study of 895 consecutive patients with one year follow-up. *Orthopedics* 18:971–981, 1995.

74. Cooper Institute for Aerobics Research. *The Prudential FITNESSGRAM Test Administration Manual*. Dallas: Author, 1992.

75. Cooper Institute for Aerobics Research. *The Strength Connection*. Dallas, TX: Author, 1990.

76. The President's Council on Physical Fitness and Sports. *Get Fit: A Handbook for Youth Ages 6–17*. Washington, DC: Author, 1993.

77. Chrysler Fund–Amateur Athletic Union. *Physical Fitness Program*. Bloomington, IN: Author, 1987.

78. Golding LA, Myers CR, Sinning WE. *The Y's Way to Physical Fitness* (4th ed.) Champaign, IL: Human Kinetics, 1998.

79. Canadian Society for Exercise Physiology. *The Canadian Physical Activity, Fitness & Lifestyle Appraisal*. Ottawa, Ontario: Author, 1996.

80. Diener MH, Golding LA, Diener D. Validity and reliability of a one-minute half sit-up test of abdominal strength and endurance. *Sports Med Train Rehab* 6:105–119, 1995.

81. Robertson LD, Magnusdottir H. Evaluation of criteria associated with abdominal fitness testing. *Res Quart Exerc Sport* 58: 355–359, 1987.

82. Hall GL, Hetzler RK, Perrin D, Weltman A. Relationship of timed sit-up tests to isokinetic abdominal strength. *Res Quart Exerc Sport* 63:80–84, 1992.

83. Faulkner RA, Sprigings EJ, McQuarrie A, Bell RD. A partial curl-up protocol for adults based on an analysis of two procedures. *Can J Sport Sci* 14:135–141, 1989.

84. Minister of State, Fitness and Amateur Sport. *Canadian Standardized Test of Fitness (CSTF) Operations Manual* (3rd ed.). Ottawa, Ontario, Canada: Author, 1987.

85. Axler CT, McGill SM. Low back loads over a variety of abdominal exercises: Searching for the safest abdominal challenge. *Med Sci Sports Exerc* 29:804–810, 1997.

86. Johnson BL, Nelson JK. *Practical Measurements for Evaluation in Physical Education*. Minneapolis: Burgess Publishing Co., 1979.

87. Pate RR, Ross JG, Baumgartner TA, Sparks RE. The National Children and Youth Fitness Study II: The modified pull-up test. *JOPERD* November/December, 1987, 71–73.

88. Cotten DJ. An analysis of the NCYFS II modified pull-up test. *Res Quart Exerc Sport* 61:272–274, 1990.

89. Pate RR, Burgess ML, Woods JA, Ross JG, Baumgartner TA. Validity of field tests of upper body muscular strength. *Res Quart Exerc Sport* 64:17–24, 1993.

90. Rutherford WJ, Corbin CB. Validation of criterion-referenced standards for tests of arm and shoulder girdle strength and endurance. *Res Quart Exerc Sport* 65:110–119, 1994.

91. Reiff GG, Dixon WR, Jacoby D, Ye GX, Spain CC, Hunsicker PA. *The President's Council on Physical Fitness and Sports 1985: National School Population Fitness Survey*. HHS-Office of the Assistant Secretary for Health, Research Project 282-82-0086, University of Michigan, 1986.

92. Phillips DA, Hornak JE. *Measurement and Evaluation in Physical Education*. New York: John Wiley & Sons, 1979.

93. Larson LA, International Committee for the Standardization of Physical Fitness Tests. *Fitness, Health, and Work Capacity: International Standards for Assessment*. New York: Macmillan Publishing Co., Inc., 1974.

94. Fiutko R. The comparison study of grip strength in male populations of Kuwait and Poland. *J Sports Med* 27:497–500, 1987.

95. Chatterjee S, Chowdhuri BJ. Comparison of grip strength and isometric endurance between the right and left hands of men and their relationship with age and other physical parameters. *J Hum Ergol* (Tokyo) 20:41–50, 1991.

96. Hughes S, Gibbs J, Dunlop D, Edelman P, Singer R, Change RW. Predictors of decline in manual performance in older adults. *J Am Geriatr Soc* 45:905–910, 1997.

97. Laukkanen P, Heikkinen E, Kauppinen M. Muscle strength and mobility as predictors of survival in 75 84-year-old people. *Age Ageing* 24:468–473, 1995.

98. Johnson MJ, Friedl KE, Frykman PN, Moore RJ. Loss of muscle mass is poorly reflected in grip strength performance in healthy young men. *Med Sci Sports Exerc* 26:235–240, 1994.

99. Brzycki M. Strength testing: Predicting a one-rep max from reps-to-fatigue. *JOPERD* January, 1993, 88–90.

100. Hein V, Jurimae T. Measurement and evaluation of trunk forward flexibility. *Sports Med Train Rehab* 7:1–6, 1996.

101. Jackson AW, Baker AA. The relationship of the sit and reach test to criterion measures of hamstring and back flexibility in young females. *Res Quart Exerc Sport* 57:183–186, 1986.

102. Jackson AW, Langford NJ. The criterion-related validity of the sit and reach test: Replication and extension of previous findings. *Res Quart Exerc Sport* 60:384–387, 1989.

103. Magnusson SP, Simonsen EB, Aagaard P, Boesen J, Johannsen F, Kjaer M. Determinants of musculoskeletal flexibility: Viscoelastic properties, cross-sectional area, EMG and stretch tolerance. *Scand J Med Sci Sports* 7:195–202, 1997.

104. Minkler S, Patterson P. The validity of the modified sit-and-reach test in college-age students. *Res Quart Exerc Sport* 65:189–192, 1994.

105. Patterson P, Wiksten DL, Ray L, Flanders C, Sanphy D. The validity and reliability of the back saver sit-and-reach test in middle school girls and boys. *Res Quart Exerc Sport* 67:448–451, 1996.

106. Hoeger WWK, Hopkins DR. A comparison of the sit and reach and the modified sit and reach in the measurement of flexibility in women. *Res Quart Exerc Sport* 63:191–195, 1992.

107. Hoeger WWK. *Principles and Labs for Physical Fitness and Wellness.* Englewood, CO: Morton Publishing, 1991.

108. Shephard RJ, Berridge M, Montelpare W. On the generality of the "sit and reach" test: An analysis of flexibility data for an aging population. *Res Quart Exerc Sport* 61:326–330, 1990.

109. Kujala UM, Viljanen T, Taimela S, Viitasalo JT. Physical activity, $\dot{V}O_{2max}$, and jumping height in an urban population. *Med Sci Sports Exerc* 26:889–895, 1994.

110. McGill SM. The mechanics of torso flexion: Sit-ups and standing dynamic flexion maneuvers. *Clin Biochem* 10:184–192, 1995.

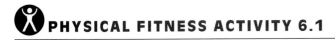**PHYSICAL FITNESS ACTIVITY 6.1**

Musculoskeletal Fitness Testing

Select a partner from class, and conduct the following musculoskeletal tests on each other. Use the procedures outlined in this chapter, being careful to follow each detail. After taking each test, record your score, and then use the norms in Appendix A to classify your results.

Assessment of Musculoskeletal Fitness

Test	Your Score	Classification
1-minute sit-up test		
Traditional pull-up test		
Push-up test		
1-RM bench-press test		
Parallel bars dip test (males)		
Sit-and-reach flexibility test		
YMCA bench-press endurance test		
Grip strength test		

PART III

Conditioning for Physical Fitness

7

The Acute and Chronic Effects of Exercise

In the process of training, the getting wind, as it is called, is largely a gradual increase in the capability of the heart. . . . The large heart of athletes may be due to the prolonged use of their muscles, but no man becomes a great runner or oarsman who has not naturally a capable if not a large heart.

—W. Osler, M.D., 1892[1]

You are reading this textbook, and suddenly you notice black smoke rising from your friend's apartment complex, 1 mile away. If you were to run to your friend's aid, you would notice several immediate changes in body function.

Your breathing rate would quicken, as you take in larger quantities of air with each breath, supplying more vital oxygen to your body. You might observe that your heart is pounding faster as it pumps more blood to your active leg muscles. If your pace is too quick, you may feel a burning sensation in your legs as the lactic acid concentration increases. These sudden, temporary changes in body function caused by exercise are called *acute responses to exercise*, and they disappear shortly after the exercise period is finished.

On the other hand, if you were to run 1 or 2 miles at a hard pace every day, after a few weeks, you might discern some changes in the way your body functioned during both rest and exercise. You might notice that your heart beats more slowly while you sit and study, as well as during your run. The amount of air you breathe in during each mile of your run might decrease, and you might feel less of a burning sensation in your legs. These persistent changes in the structure and function of your body following regular exercise training are called *chronic adaptations to exercise*—changes that enable the body to respond more easily to exercise.

This chapter includes a brief description of the acute and chronic effects of exercise. Only the very basic and important material is covered. For a deeper discussion of exercise physiology, the reader is referred to the excellent textbooks available on this topic.[2–9] In addition, see Appendix D for diagrams of the various body systems and Chapter 9 for a discussion of energy metabolism.

PHYSIOLOGICAL RESPONSES TO ACUTE EXERCISE

The acute responses to exercise are influenced by a number of factors, including the level of training or the fitness status of the participant, ambient temperature and humidity, time of day, sufficiency of sleep, coffee and food intake, use of alcohol and tobacco, menstrual cycle, and general anxiety.[7,8] For example, a person who is anxious about the treadmill test can have higher than normal heart rates during the first and second stages. Those who are fit usually have lower acute responses to certain levels of exercise than those who are unfit. These factors must be considered when interpreting the following discussion of acute effects.

Increase of Heart Rate

Figure 7.1 summarizes several important points relative to the way heart rate responds to increasing levels of exercise, such as during a graded treadmill exercise test (e.g., the Bruce protocol).

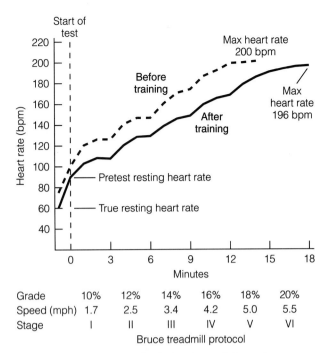

Figure 7.1   Heart rate results during the graded exercise test of a 20-year-old before and after exercise training. Notice that his pretest exercise heart rate is much higher than his true resting heart rate. The exercise heart rate increases in a linear fashion with increase in workload until the maximal heart rate is reached, when it plateaus.

- The pre-exercise heart rate may be elevated, owing to the *anticipatory response*. In my own study of nearly 1,000 college students (unpublished data), the average resting heart rate, measured in the student's dorm rooms upon waking for three mornings in a row and then averaged, was 67 beats per minute. However, when sitting before a treadmill before a maximal graded exercise test, the average "resting" heart rate of these same students was 95. (This pre-exercise increase is mediated through release of the neurotransmitter norepinephrine from the sympathetic nervous system, and the hormone epinephrine from the adrenal gland.)

- During the graded exercise test, heart rate will increase in direct proportion to the intensity of the exercise. In other words, the heart rate rises in a linear fashion with increasing workload.

- At exhaustion, the rise in heart rate will flatten out. This is called the *maximal heart rate*. When the heart rate increases little if at all after a stage change during a graded exercise test, this is a good indication that the maximal heart rate has been reached.

  The average maximal heart rate is equal to 220 minus the person's age (in years). This equation, however, is the average found in large groups of people. People for a given age vary widely, with a

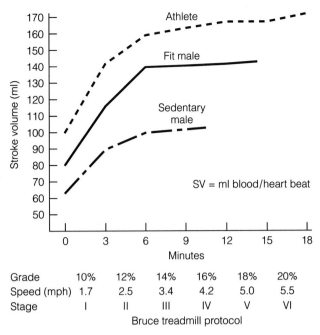

Figure 7.2   Stroke volume represents the amount of blood pumped per beat of the heart. Instead of rising linearly with increase in workload, stroke volume increases strongly up to a workload of 40–60% of $\dot{V}O_{2max}$. There is little change beyond this level, despite increasing workload.

standard deviation of ±10–12 beats per minute. In other words, the average maximal heart rate for a 20-year-old person is 220 − 20, or 200 beats per minute. However, two thirds of the people this age vary between 190 and 210 beats per minute, and 95% vary between 180 and 220 beats per minute. (See Chapter 8 for a more detailed discussion.)

- At submaximal levels of exercise, when the workload is held steady, the heart rate will increase for 1 to 3 minutes and then level off at a steady-state value. The harder the submaximal workload, the longer the heart rate will take to level off. For example, as you look at Figure 7.1, notice that in Stages 1 and 2, the heart rate plateaus relatively early in the stage, whereas in Stage 5, a more difficult stage, there is little indication of a plateau even after 3 minutes.

Increase of Stroke Volume

The *stroke volume* is the quantity of blood pumped out of the heart per heartbeat.[7] Stroke volume is regulated by several factors, including the amount of venous blood that is returned to the heart, the capacity to enlarge the ventricle, the force of contraction of the heart muscle, arterial pressure, and sympathetic nervous stimulation. Figure 7.2 summarizes several important points regarding the change in stroke volume from rest to exercise exhaustion.

- The change in stroke volume during graded exercise does not follow the pattern of change in the heart rate. Instead of rising linearly with increase in workload, stroke volume increases strongly only up to a workload of 40–60% of $\dot{V}O_{2max}$. Beyond this intensity level, increasing workload brings only small increases in stroke volume.[2,7,8] Highly trained athletes appear capable of increasing their stroke volume after exceeding 40–60% of $\dot{V}O_{2max}$ a bit more than untrained subjects.

- Resting stroke volume values for sedentary people range between 60 and 70 ml of blood per heartbeat. Those who are highly trained may have resting stroke volume values as high as 100–120 ml.[7,8] Submaximal and maximal stroke volumes are also much higher for fit than for sedentary people. Stroke volumes of elite world-class runners have been measured as high as 200 ml per heart beat.[7]

- When changing positions from lying down to standing, there is an immediate drop in the stroke volume because of the influence of gravity and a corresponding increase in heart rate to maintain the flow of blood out of the heart (i.e., cardiac output, which equals stroke volume times heart rate). When exercise is performed in a horizontal position (as in swimming), the stroke volume is larger, and the heart rate lower than when the same level of upright exercise is performed (as in running). Therefore, heart rate during exercises such as swimming will be lower for a given percentage of $\dot{V}O_{2max}$ than for running. Exercise training heart rates should thus be adjusted downward about 10–15 beats per minute when exercising in a horizontal position.[9]

Increase in Cardiac Output

Cardiac output (also designated "$\dot{Q}$" by exercise physiologists) is equal to the stroke volume (SV) times the heart rate (HR) ($\dot{Q} = SV \times HR$). In other words, cardiac output represents the quantity of blood pumped out of the heart each minute. At rest, average cardiac output is approximately 5 liters per minute; it can rise to 20–40 liters per minute during maximal exercise, the amount depending on individual fitness status and size[7,8] (see Figure 7.3).

Figure 7.3 demonstrates that

- Cardiac output rises linearly with increasing workload and plateaus slightly at exercise exhaustion.

- During the initial stages of exercise, the increase in cardiac output is due to increases in both heart rate and stroke volume. During upright exercise, when the intensity reaches 40–60% of $\dot{V}O_{2max}$, any further increase in cardiac output is due primarily to an increase in heart rate.

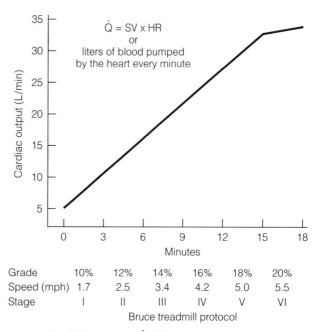

Grade	10%	12%	14%	16%	18%	20%
Speed (mph)	1.7	2.5	3.4	4.2	5.0	5.5
Stage	I	II	III	IV	V	VI

Bruce treadmill protocol

Figure 7.3 Cardiac output ($\dot{Q}$) follows a pattern similar to that of the heart rate. With increasing workload, cardiac output rises linearly and plateaus slightly at exercise exhaustion.

Increased Arteriovenous Oxygen Difference

The *arteriovenous oxygen difference* (a − $\bar{v}O_2$) is the difference between the amount of oxygen carried in the arterial blood and the amount in the mixed venous blood. Thus the a − $\bar{v}O_2$ reflects the amount of oxygen extracted by the tissues of the body.[7]

- At rest, the oxygen content of arterial blood is approximately 20 ml of oxygen per 100 ml of blood, compared to an oxygen content of 14 ml / 100 ml blood for the mixed venous blood. Thus the resting a − $\bar{v}O_2$ is 6 ml / 100 ml blood.

- During very intense exercise, the venous oxygen content can drop to 2–4 ml / 100 ml blood. Thus the a − $\bar{v}O_2$ can increase nearly threefold to 16–18 ml / 100 ml blood.

Increase in $\dot{V}O_2$

The maximal oxygen uptake $\dot{V}O_{2max}$ can be defined as the "maximal rate at which oxygen can be taken up, distributed, and used by the body in the performance of exercise that utilizes a large muscle mass."[8] In other words, $\dot{V}O_{2max}$ is the highest rate of oxygen consumption attainable during maximal or exhaustive exercise. $\dot{V}O_{2max}$ is usually expressed in terms of milliliters of oxygen consumed per kilogram of body weight per minute (ml $\cdot$ kg^{-1} $\cdot$ min^{-1}). With this allowance for body weight, the $\dot{V}O_{2max}$ of people of varying size

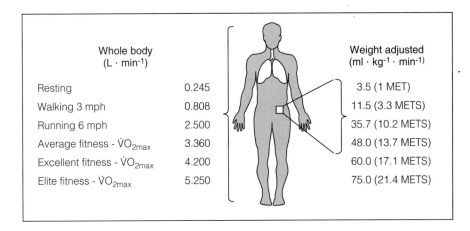

Figure 7.4 Oxygen consumption ($\dot{V}O_2$) can be expressed in units of $L \cdot min^{-1}$ for the entire body, or in units of $ml \cdot kg^{-1} \cdot min^{-1}$ to represent the oxygen consumption for each kilogram of body weight. The example shows the oxygen consumption in a 70-kg male (25 years old).

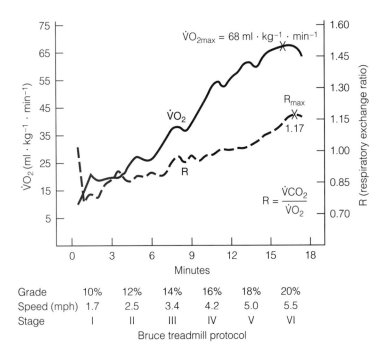

Figure 7.5 With increasing workload, oxygen consumption increases up to the last stage of exercise. At this point, $\dot{V}O_2$ plateaus and is called the $\dot{V}O_{2max}$.

and in different environments can be compared. $\dot{V}O_{2max}$ can also be expressed as liters per minute, representing the oxygen consumption of the entire body (see Figure 7.4).

During graded exercise, active muscle tissue needs more and more oxygen to burn the carbohydrates and fats needed for energy production. For every liter of oxygen the body consumes during exercise, approximately 5 kilocalories of energy are produced. Figures 7.5, 7.6, and 7.7 demonstrate that[2,7]

- With increasing workload, oxygen consumption increases up to the last stage of exercise. At this point, $\dot{V}O_2$ plateaus, and is called the $\dot{V}O_{2max}$. If the person being tested is willing to push hard enough, a small decrease in $\dot{V}O_2$ can be seen just prior to exhaustion

(as demonstrated in Figure 7.5). Many people, however, do not achieve a true $\dot{V}O_2$ plateau, and for this reason, some exercise physiologists prefer the term "peak $\dot{V}O_2$." $\dot{V}O_{2max}$ values are greatly influenced by size, age, heredity, sex, and level of fitness. (See next section.)

- Figure 7.6 shows that if the cardiac output and $a - \bar{v}O_2$ are known, oxygen consumption can be calculated using the formula, $\dot{V}O_2 = \dot{Q} \times a - \bar{v}O_2$. In other words, if measurement of arterial and mixed venous blood shows that for every liter of blood passing through the tissues, 150 milliliters of oxygen are being consumed, and that 20 liters of blood / minute are passing through those tissues, total oxygen consumption is easily determined by multiplying

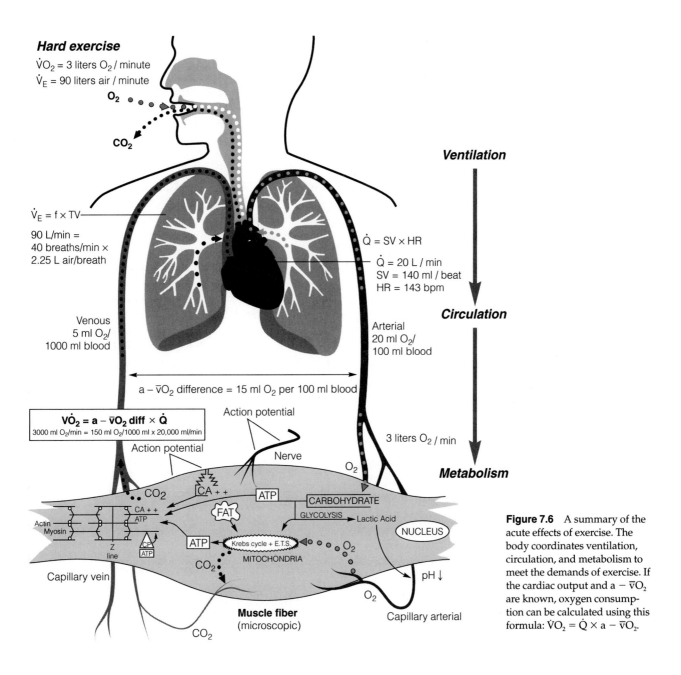

Hard exercise

$\dot{V}O_2 = 3$ liters O_2 / minute

$\dot{V}_E = 90$ liters air / minute

O_2

CO_2

Ventilation

$\dot{V}_E = f \times TV$

90 L/min =
40 breaths/min ×
2.25 L air/breath

$\dot{Q} = SV \times HR$

$\dot{Q} = 20$ L / min
SV = 140 ml / beat
HR = 143 bpm

Circulation

Venous
5 ml O_2/
1000 ml blood

Arterial
20 ml O_2/
100 ml blood

a − $\bar{v}O_2$ difference = 15 ml O_2 per 100 ml blood

$\boxed{\dot{V}O_2 = a - \bar{v}O_2 \text{ diff} \times \dot{Q}}$
3000 ml O_2/min = 150 ml O_2/1000 ml x 20,000 ml/min

3 liters O_2 / min

Metabolism

Action potential

Action potential

Nerve

O_2

CO_2

$CA + +$

ATP

CARBOHYDRATE

FAT

GLYCOLYSIS

Lactic Acid

$CA + +$
ATP

Actin
Myosin

Z line

CP
ATP

ATP

Krebs cycle + E.T.S.
MITOCHONDRIA

O_2

NUCLEUS

CO_2

Capillary vein

pH ↓

O_2

Muscle fiber
(microscopic)

CO_2

Capillary arterial

Figure 7.6 A summary of the acute effects of exercise. The body coordinates ventilation, circulation, and metabolism to meet the demands of exercise. If the cardiac output and a − $\bar{v}O_2$ are known, oxygen consumption can be calculated using this formula: $\dot{V}O_2 = \dot{Q} \times a - \bar{v}O_2$.

150 ml $O_2 \cdot$ liter^{-1} by 20 liters $\cdot$ min^{-1}, which equals 3,000 ml $O_2 \cdot$ min^{-1}.

- *Oxygen debt* refers to the volume of oxygen consumed during the recovery period following exercise, in excess of the volume normally consumed at rest (see Figure 7.7). This debt pays back the *oxygen deficit* built up during the initial minutes of exercise, on account of the body adjusting to the exercise, plus other metabolic factors built up during the exercise bout itself.

For example, if you were to start running at a 7-minute-per-mile pace, approximately 3.46 liters of oxygen per minute would be required immediately. However, because

your body takes approximately 2 to 3 minutes to adjust to this workload, anaerobic sources of ATP (stored ATP and glycolysis) are utilized, building up an oxygen deficit. During recovery, you will breathe harder than during rest, to help restore this deficit and allow your body systems to return to normal.

Increased Systolic BP; Diastolic BP Unchanged

Blood pressure (BP) response during exercise was reviewed in Chapter 4, with an emphasis on accurate measurement (see Figure 4.4). Important concepts include[7]

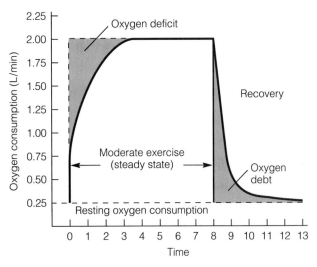

Figure 7.7 *Oxygen debt* refers to the volume of oxygen consumed during the recovery period following exercise, in excess of the volume normally consumed at rest.

- The systolic blood pressure increases in direct proportion to the increase in aerobic exercise intensity, with resting values of 120 mm Hg, often rising to 200 mm Hg or greater at exhaustion.

- The diastolic blood pressure changes little if any during aerobic exercise.

- The exercise-induced increase in systolic blood pressure is related to the increase in cardiac output. The increase in blood pressure would be much higher except that arterial blood vessels in the active muscles dilate, reducing peripheral resistance. *Total peripheral resistance* is the sum of all the forces that oppose blood flow in the body's blood vessel system. During exercise, total peripheral resistance decreases because the blood vessels in the active muscles dilate.

- Cycling with arms (arm ergometry) increases systolic and diastolic blood pressures 15%, compared to cycling with legs. This probably occurs because of the smaller muscle mass in the arms, which offers a greater resistance to blood flow than the larger muscles in the legs.

- Weight lifting or isometric contractions cause large increases in both systolic and diastolic blood pressures. This is discussed in more detail in Chapter 8.

- Some researchers like to report the *mean arterial pressure*. This represents the average pressure exerted by the blood against the inner walls of the arteries. An estimate of mean arterial pressure is obtained by using this equation:[8]

Mean arterial pressure
$$= \tfrac{1}{3}\,(\text{systolic pressure} - \text{diastolic pressure})$$
$$+ \text{diastolic pressure}$$

For example, if during Stage 3 of the Bruce treadmill test, the systolic blood pressure is 150 mm Hg and the diastolic blood pressure is 80 mm Hg, then the mean arterial pressure equals one third of the difference between systolic and diastolic blood pressures (0.33×70 mm Hg), or 23 mm Hg, plus the diastolic blood pressure ($23 + 80$), or 103 mm Hg. Maximal exercise mean arterial pressures approximate 130 mm Hg.[8]

Increase in Minute Ventilation

Minute ventilation is the volume of air that is breathed into the body each minute. Minute ventilation is usually determined by measuring the volume of air breathed out or expired ($\dot{V}_E$), and then correcting this for *BTPS*, the volume of air at the temperature and pressure of the body, and 100% water vapor saturation (as in the human lung). The minute ventilation is equal to the tidal volume (TV) times the frequency (f) of breaths. At rest, the *tidal volume* is usually 0.5 liter of air per breath, and the *frequency* is about 12 breaths per minute, resulting in a minute ventilation of 6 liters of air per minute.[7,8]

Figure 7.8 gives the various terms used by respiratory and exercise physiologists when reporting research or clinical findings. The TV is the amount of air breathed into or out of the lung while at rest. The TV usually ranges between 0.4 and 1.0 liter of air per breath. *Inspiratory reserve volume* (IRV) is the amount of air that can be breathed into the lung on top of a resting inspired tidal volume (2.5–3.5 liters). *Expiratory reserve volume* (ERV) is the amount of air that can be pushed out of the lung following an expired resting tidal volume (1.0–1.5 liters). *Residual volume* (RV) is the amount of air left in the lung after the expiratory reserve volume (1–2 liters). *Functional residual capacity* (FRC) is the combined expiratory reserve volume and residual volume. *Forced vital capacity* (FVC) is the total amount of air that can be breathed into the lung on top of the residual volume (usually 3–4 liters for women, 4–5 liters for men). The *total lung capacity* (TLC) represents the total amount of air in the lung.

Figure 7.9 summarizes changes in minute ventilation during graded exercise testing.[3,7,8]

- During graded exercise, minute ventilation increases in a curvilinear pattern from a resting value of 6 liters · min^{-1} to 60–120 liters · min^{-1} for females and 100–200 liters · min^{-1} for males, depending on size and fitness status. Below 50% of $\dot{V}O_{2max}$, minute ventilation increases in a linear fashion with increasing workload. At higher intensities, however, the relationship is curvilinear, with ventilation rising strongly relative to the workload.

- The insert in Figure 7.9 shows that at higher intensities, an increase in minute ventilation is produced

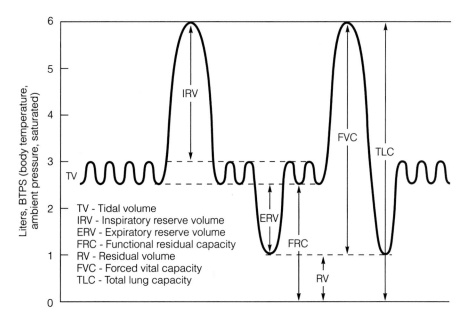

Figure 7.8 Terms used to represent the dynamic lung volumes and capacities.

TV - Tidal volume
IRV - Inspiratory reserve volume
ERV - Expiratory reserve volume
FRC - Functional residual capacity
RV - Residual volume
FVC - Forced vital capacity
TLC - Total lung capacity

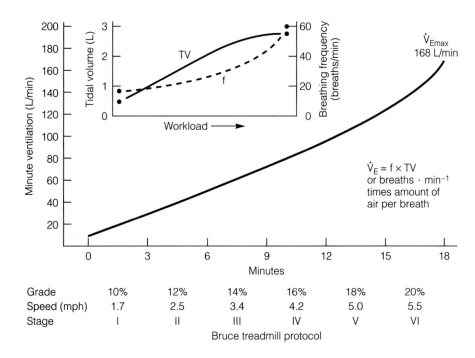

$$\dot{V}_E = f \times TV$$
or breaths $\cdot$ min^{-1}
times amount of
air per breath

$\dot{V}_{Emax}$
168 L/min

Figure 7.9 Minute ventilation increases in a curvilinear fashion during graded maximal exercise. The frequency of breathing also follows this pattern, while tidal volume plateaus during intense exercise.

Grade	10%	12%	14%	16%	18%	20%
Speed (mph)	1.7	2.5	3.4	4.2	5.0	5.5
Stage	I	II	III	IV	V	VI

Bruce treadmill protocol

primarily from increased breathing rates. The tidal volume tends to plateau at higher intensities.

- During graded exercise, the residual volume increases slightly, with the vital capacity decreasing slightly, keeping the overall total lung volume the same.

- The movement of air in and out of the lung during exercise requires considerable amounts of energy for the respiratory muscles. At rest, the energy cost of ventilation is 1 ml of oxygen per liter of air breathed, or 2% of the total oxygen being consumed at rest. During maximal exercise this can rise to 10%.

- *Lung diffusion* refers to the rate at which gases diffuse from the lung air sacs (*alveoli*) to the blood in the pulmonary capillaries. Diffusion capacity during exercise can increase threefold from a resting value of 25 ml O$_2$ $\cdot$ min^{-1} $\cdot$ mm Hg^{-1} to 75 ml O$_2$ $\cdot$ min^{-1} $\cdot$ mm Hg^{-1} at maximum.

Increased Blood Flow to Active Muscle Areas

- During exercise, blood is redirected away from areas where it is not needed (e.g., organs) and to the muscles. At rest, only 21% of the cardiac output goes to the muscles, compared with as much as 88% during exhaustive exercise (see Table 7.1).[2]

- As the body heats up, an increasing amount of blood is directed to the skin, to conduct heat away from the body core. The primary means by which the body loses heat during exercise is through evaporation of sweat on the skin (see Chapter 9). The sweat glands will use fluid from the cells and from the blood to produce the sweat, which can reach 2 to 3 liters per hour during hard exercise in humid heat. If the sweat rate is high, blood volume will decrease, ultimately to the point of heat injury.

- During endurance exercise, plasma volume shifts to the muscles. During graded exercise testing, 12–16% of the plasma volume leaves the blood and enters the active muscle tissue.[10] This plasma volume shift, combined with the fluid loss from sweating, leads to an increase in the thickness of blood called *hemoconcentration*.

Changes in Respiratory Exchange Ratio

During exercise the muscles use oxygen (O_2) to burn carbohydrates and fats, producing carbon dioxide (CO_2) and ATP. Ventilation increases to help bring in more O_2 and to expel CO_2. Exercise physiologists use the *respiratory exchange ratio* (R) to help determine the type of fuel (primarily fat and carbohydrate) being used by the muscles. The respiratory exchange ratio is the ratio between the amount of carbon dioxide produced and the amount of oxygen consumed by the body during exercise ($R = \dot{V}CO_2 / \dot{V}C_2$).[7]

The R value will vary, depending on what fuel the muscles are using. When only fats are being used, R = 0.71; when only carbohydrates are being used, R = 1.0.

With hard exercise, the R value approaches 1.0 because carbohydrate is the preferred fuel with heavy exercise. At rest, the R value is usually 0.75 to 0.81. Just prior to exercise, the R value can rise above 1.0, due to pretest anxiety, which causes hyperventilation (which "blows off" CO_2). During recovery, the R value can rise above 1.5, due to the buffering of lactic acid and carbon dioxide production. When R values rise to 1.15 or greater during exercise, this is usually a sign of maximal exertion, with the body relying on anaerobic metabolism.

- Figure 7.5 shows that as the intensity of exercise increases, R increases, meaning that more and more CO_2 is being produced, relative to the O_2 being consumed. This indicates that more and more carbohydrate is being used by the muscles as the intensity of exercise increases.

- At rest, the blood pH is 7.4. When the exercise intensity of unconditioned people rises above 50% $\dot{V}O_{2max}$, or above 70–90% for conditioned people, the pH will drop, owing to lactic acid buildup. Blood pH values can drop to 7.0 with maximal exercise; tissue pH levels can drop to 6.5. Blood lactate levels range from 10 mg/100 ml at rest (1.1 millimole per liter of blood) to 200 mg/100 ml (22 millimoles per liter blood) within 5 minutes following exhaustive short-term exercise. Typical lactate values immediately postexercise range from 7.5 to 9.0 mmol/L, with the highest values reached in trained endurance athletes.

TABLE 7.1   Distribution of Cardiac Output During Rest and Light, Moderate, and Maximal Exercise

Vascular Region	Cardiac Output (ml · min⁻¹)			
	At Rest (6%)	Light Exercise (30%)	Heavy Exercise (75%)	Maximal Exercise (100%)
Cardiac output	6,000	12,000	24,000	30,000
Cerebral	720 (12%)	720 (6%)	720 (3%)	720 (2%)
Myocardial	240 (4%)	480 (4%)	960 (4%)	1,200 (4%)
Muscle	1,260 (21%)	5,760 (48%)	17,280 (72%)	26,400 (88%)
Renal	1,320 (22%)	1,200 (10%)	720 (3%)	300 (1%)
Hepatosplanchnic	1,560 (26%)	1,440 (12%)	960 (4%)	300 (1%)
Skin	540 (9%)	1,920 (16%)	2,640 (11%)	900 (3%)
Other	360 (6%)	480 (4%)	720 (3%)	180 (<1%)

Source: Data from Shephard RJ, Astrand P-O. *Endurance in Sport: The Encyclopædia of Sports Medicine* (Volume II). Oxford: Blackwell Scientific Publications, 1992.

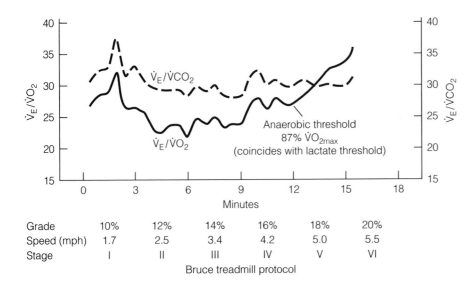

Figure 7.10 Anaerobic threshold in an elite woman masters runner. Anaerobic threshold represents the point at which lactic acid begins to build up in the blood. This can be measured indirectly by looking at the rise in $\dot{V}_E / \dot{V}O_2$ relative to $\dot{V}_E / \dot{V}CO_2$.

- During graded maximal exercise, the *anaerobic threshold* is the point at which blood lactate concentrations start to rise above resting values.[11–14] The anaerobic threshold can be expressed as a percentage of $\dot{V}O_{2max}$. Some of the best athletes in the world have anaerobic thresholds of between 80 and 90% of $\dot{V}O_{2max}$; unfit people average 40–60% of $\dot{V}O_{2max}$.

Although a discussion of the measurement of anaerobic threshold is beyond the scope of this book, Figure 7.10 shows that anaerobic threshold can be estimated when the ratio of minute ventilation to oxygen consumption ($\dot{V}_E / \dot{V}O_2$) rises sharply, while the ratio of minute ventilation to carbon dioxide consumption ($\dot{V}_E / \dot{V}CO_2$) remains constant.[13,15] Figure 7.10 reflects the measurement of an elite woman masters runner who holds several world records for ultra-marathon distances. Her anaerobic threshold of 87% of $\dot{V}O_{2max}$ is very high, thus allowing her to run at an intensity close to her capacity without danger of the lactic acid buildup. (See Sports Medicine Insight at the end of this chapter.)

CHRONIC ADAPTATIONS TO REGULAR EXERCISE

As discussed earlier in this chapter, the persistent changes in the structure and function of the body following regular exercise training are called chronic adaptations to exercise.[2–8]

What quantity of exercise training is necessary to produce chronic adaptations? Do different body systems adapt to exercise training at different rates?

Several of the cardiorespiratory and metabolic responses of exercise appear to adapt very rapidly to exercise training.[16–17] Within the first 1–3 weeks of intensive cardiorespiratory training by young healthy college students, for example (40–60 minutes per session, six sessions per week, 70–90% $\dot{V}O_{2max}$), significant improvements in $\dot{V}O_{2max}$, submaximal exercise heart rate and lactate responses, and ventilation can already be measured. Some adaptations to aerobic exercise, however, take longer. For example, the increase in number of capillaries per muscle fiber may take several months or years.[17]

Interestingly, exercise-induced changes are lost just as rapidly as they are gained. This (the effects of inactivity or detraining) is discussed later in this chapter.

The magnitude of the chronic adaptations of regular exercise training depends on the frequency, intensity, and duration of training, the mode of activity, and the initial fitness status. For example, overweight middle-aged people who have been inactive for many years have the potential for dramatic improvements in cardiorespiratory fitness (e.g., a 100% increase in $\dot{V}O_{2max}$) with weight loss and a few months of regular aerobic exercise. Relatively active college students, on the other hand, can expect smaller improvements (e.g., a 10–20% increase in $\dot{V}O_{2max}$).

Changes That Occur in Skeletal Muscles as a Result of Aerobic Training

Exercise physiologists have had an ongoing debate for several decades regarding the relative importance of "central" versus "peripheral" adaptations to regular cardiorespiratory exercise. Figure 7.6 shows that ventilation and circulation (central elements) work closely with the muscle cells (peripheral elements) to allow physical activity to take place. While most researchers have reported that the circulation, specifically the stroke volume and cardiac output, is the primary limiting factor during intense exercise, some feel that factors within the muscle cells are more important.[18–24] There is a growing consensus that during *acute* intense endurance exercise, the cardiovascular system is limiting (i.e., the ability to deliver oxygen to the muscles), while improvement in $\dot{V}O_{2max}$ with *chronic* exercise training is largely dependent on peripheral changes in the muscles (especially increase in capillary surface area).[18]

In response to regular aerobic training, many significant changes take place in the muscle cells.[2–8]

- An increase in *myoglobin* content (Myoglobin aids in the delivery of oxygen from the blood to the *mitochondria* (organelles in the muscle cell that produce ATP for energy; see Figure 7.6.)

- An increase in the number and size of mitochondria

- An increase in the concentration of important enzymes in the mitochondria, specifically those of the Krebs cycle and the electron transport system (These enzymes are involved in the production of ATP from aerobic metabolism.)

- An increase in both the amount of glycogen stored in the muscle and the maximal capacity to oxidize carbohydrates

- An increased capacity to oxidize fat (from both muscle fat and adipose tissue stores)[25,26] (The trained person thus oxidizes more fat and less carbohydrate during cardiorespiratory exercise [at an absolute workload], which means less glycogen depletion, less lactic acid accumulation, and therefore less muscle fatigue and greater endurance.)

- An increase in the area of slow-twitch fibers (The *aerobic-type muscle fibers* are called Type I [red, tonic, *slow twitch*]; the *anaerobic-type fibers* are called Type II [white, glycolytic, *fast twitch*]. People vary widely in their proportions of slow-twitch and fast-twitch fibers. This proportion is set at birth and remains constant throughout life.)

The fast-twitch muscle cells are capable of producing high amounts of ATP through *glycolysis*, a process that does not require oxygen (anaerobic). Fast-twitch muscle cells are important in activities that require sprinting and jumping. Slow-twitch muscle cells generate ATP in the presence of oxygen (aerobically) and have high numbers of mitochondria and a good capillary supply.

Endurance athletes usually have a high proportion of slow-twitch muscle fibers, sprinters a high proportion of fast-twitch muscle fibers. For example, trained endurance athletes average 60–80% slow-twitch fibers, while sprinters average only 35–40% slow-twitch fibers[2] (see Figure 7.11).

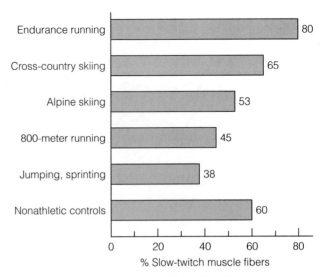

Figure 7.11 Slow-twitch muscle fibers (Type I) among successful endurance competitors. Endurance athletes tend to have a greater proportion of slow-twitch muscle fibers than do jumpers and sprinters. *Source:* Data from Shephard RJ, Astrand P-O. *Endurance in Sport: The Encyclopædia of Sports Medicine* (Volume II). Oxford: Blackwell Scientific Publications, 1992.

Blacks have been found to have a higher percentage of fast-twitch fibers than Caucasians, helping to explain why they excel in sports requiring sprinting and jumping.[27]

With regular aerobic training, the size of the slow-twitch fibers can be increased. Some researchers have reported that some fast-twitch muscle cells can be changed into slow-twitch muscle cells through regular aerobic training over a long time period.[28,29] However, fiber transformation appears to be of minor importance, relative to the increase in fiber size.

Major Cardiorespiratory Changes from Exercise Training When at Rest

Several major cardiorespiratory changes at rest follow exercise training:

- An increase in heart size.[1] The size of the left and right ventricular cavities increases, with proportional increases in the thicknesses of the heart muscle walls and septum.[30] These changes occur gradually over months or years of training.[8]

- A decrease in resting heart rate. The resting heart rate decreases approximately one beat per minute for every 1 to 2 weeks of aerobic training for about 10 to 20 weeks. Further decreases are possible if training volume and intensity are increased. Some of the best endurance athletes in the world have resting heart rates below 40 bpm.

In my own study of nearly 1,000 college students (unpublished data), the average college male's resting heart rate decreased from 67 bpm to 60 bpm after 7 weeks of regular aerobic training (5 sessions per week, 30 minutes per session, 70–80% of $\dot{V}O_{2max}$). Female college students on the same program decreased their resting heart rates from 69 bpm to 62 bpm after 7 weeks.

The decrease in resting heart rate is attributable to an increase in *parasympathetic* control (through the vagus nerve, which slows the heart rate).[8] Other aerobic training effects on resting physiologic variables include[7,8]

- An increase in stroke volume, with more blood pumped per beat, with a corresponding decrease in rate. For example, sedentary people have stroke volumes at rest of about 60 ml, whereas those of athletes often measure greater than 100 ml.

- Resting cardiac output. The resting cardiac output stays about the same (about 5 liters per minute).

- An increase in the total blood volume from about 5 liters in sedentary people to 6 or 7 liters in athletes. The 20–25% increase in blood volume is evident in males and females of all ages.[31–33] Although both plasma volume and hemoglobin increase, the increase in plasma volume is greater, leading to a slightly decreased *hematocrit*, red blood cell proportion per 100 ml of blood. This increase in the plasma volume is directly linked to the increase in stroke volume. This adaptation is gained after only a few bouts of exercise and is quickly reversed when training ceases.[32]

- An increase in capillary density. Untrained human muscle has about 1.5 to 2.0 capillaries per muscle fiber, whereas elite endurance athletes have 2 to 3 times this number.[28,34]

In general, pulmonary function characteristics (total lung capacity, forced vital capacity residual volume) are not changed by training.[35] Some individuals may experience a slight increase in vital capacity and a slight decrease in residual volume.[7] Resting minute ventilation is not affected by training.

Major Cardiorespiratory Changes during Submaximal Exercise

What cardiorespiratory changes during submaximal exercise can be expected following exercise training? Tables 7.2 and 7.3 summarize data from a study I conducted.[36] This study was conducted on 20 males, 9 of whom were sedentary and 11 experienced runners. All were tested in the laboratory using the Balke maximal graded exercise test, with cardiorespiratory variables measured every 5 minutes to complete exhaustion. During the 3 previous years, the athletes had averaged 42.5 ± 4.0 miles per week of running, with an average personal marathon record of 3.1 ± 0.1 hours.

Maximal oxygen uptake and ventilation were 63% and 39% higher, respectively, for the athletes than for the nonathletes, with percent body fat nearly 50% lower.

Important differences in submaximal exercise parameters between the sedentary and trained males can be summarized as follows:

- There were no significant differences in oxygen consumption during any of the three submaximal workloads. When adjusted for weight changes, training does not appear to decrease oxygen consumption during submaximal exercise. However, among individuals, the amount of oxygen utilized during any given workload can vary widely. Notice in Table 7.3 that oxygen consumption varied 16–36% depending on the workload (see ranges for each workload).

- Heart rates of the trained males were significantly lower than those of the sedentary males. This has

TABLE 7.2   Differences between Sedentary and Trained Males during a Balke Treadmill Graded Exercise Test (Resting and Maximal Exercise Parameters)

Parameter	Sedentary Males ($n = 9$)	Trained Males ($n = 11$)
Age (years)	44.2	42.7
Weight (lb)	185	171
Percent body fat (%)	24.5	12.5
Resting heart rate (bpm)	66.8	52.5
$\dot{V}O_{2max}$ (ml · kg^{-1} · min^{-1})	33.3	54.2
Ventilation, max (L · min^{-1})	119	165
Heart rate, max (bpm)	188	177

Source: Data from Nieman DC, et al. Complement and immunoglobulin levels in athletes and sedentary controls. *Int J Sports Med* 10:124–128, 1989.

TABLE 7.3 Differences between Sedentary versus Trained Males during a Balke Treadmill Graded Exercise Test (Mean [Range])

	Time Speed Grade	5 min 3.3 mph 5%	10 min 3.3 mph 10%	15 min 3.3 mph 15%
$\dot{V}O_2$ (ml $\cdot$ kg^{-1} $\cdot$ min^{-1})				
Sedentary males		18.4	24.8	32.1
		(16.0–21.8)	(22.4–28.2)	(29.6–34.4)
Trained males		19.7	26.7	34.0
		(17.2–22.8)	(25.1–30.1)	(31.3–38.5)
Heart rate (bpm)				
Sedentary males		123	152	177
		(100–139)	(128–175)	(164–197)
Trained males		88	107	126
		(77–96)	(98–120)	(112–138)
Ventilation (L $\cdot$ min^{-1})				
Sedentary males		42	63	88
		(35–54)	(47–88)	(62–106)
Trained males		37	52	66
		(30–47)	(44–64)	(57–85)
Respiratory exchange ratio				
Sedentary males		0.95	1.08	1.24
		(0.90–1.09)	(1.01–1.23)	(1.12–1.46)
Trained males		0.87	0.95	0.99
		(0.78–1.00)	(0.87–1.02)	(0.92–1.06)

Source: Data from Nieman DC, et al. Complement and immunoglobulin levels in athletes and sedentary controls. *Int J Sports Med* 10:124–128, 1989.

been shown by others to be due to a higher stroke volume. The cardiac output at a certain absolute workload does not appear to be affected by exercise training[37] (see also Figures 7.1 and 7.2).

- Ventilation was significantly lower for the trained males than it was for the sedentary males during each stage. They ventilated less air while achieving the same oxygen consumption.

  The trained body is much more efficient in the transport and utilization of oxygen. The $a - \bar{v}O_2$ difference is slightly higher, meaning that the muscle cells are extracting more oxygen. The heightened extraction of oxygen is due to the increased capillary density around each muscle cell.[7,8]

- The respiratory exchange ratio (R) was much lower for the athletes. As discussed earlier, a lower R indicates that the muscle cells are utilizing more fat and less glycogen for fuel. This decreases the concentration of lactic acid, increasing the anaerobic threshold. This allows one to exercise at a higher intensity without interference from lactic acid. (These benefits result primarily from the exercise-training-induced increase in the number and size of mitochondria.)

Major Cardiorespiratory Changes during Maximal Exercise

During maximal graded exercise testing, subjects are taken to complete exhaustion. What changes during maximal exercise can be expected after regular exercise training? Table 7.2 shows the following differences:

- Training provides a significantly higher maximal aerobic power ($\dot{V}O_{2max}$). This means that a greater amount of oxygen can be consumed during maximal exercise. Figure 7.4 outlines some of the increases in $\dot{V}O_{2max}$ that can be expected in response to increasing levels of training. Figure 7.12 compares $\dot{V}O_{2max}$ among different athletes.[38] Cross-country skiers generally have the highest $\dot{V}O_{2max}$ because almost all the major muscle groups in the body are activated.[39] One of the highest $\dot{V}O_{2max}$ values ever measured was in a Scandinavian cross-country skier (93 ml $\cdot$ kg^{-1} $\cdot$ min^{-1}).

In my own study of nearly 1,000 college students (unpublished findings), male students had an average $\dot{V}O_{2max}$ of 49.0 ml $\cdot$ kg^{-1} $\cdot$ min^{-1} before and 55.0 ml $\cdot$ kg^{-1} $\cdot$ min^{-1} after

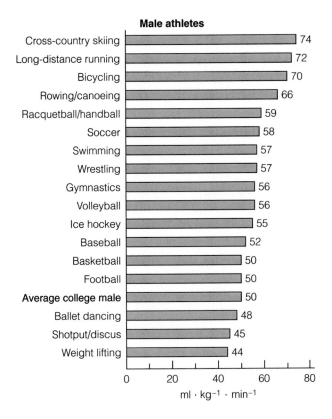

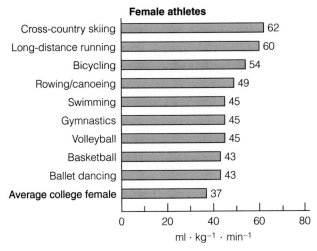

Figure 7.12 Maximal oxygen uptake. Endurance athletes have the highest $\dot{V}O_{2max}$ values for both males and females. *Source:* National Center for Health Statistics. Drury EF (ed), *Assessing Physical Fitness and Physical Activity in Population-Based Surveys.* DHHS Pub. No. (PHS) 89-1253. Public Health Service. Washington, DC: U.S. Government Printing Office, 1989.

7 weeks of regular aerobic exercise (5 sessions per week, 30 minutes per session, 70–80% of $\dot{V}O_{2max}$). Female college students averaged 36.0 ml $\cdot$ kg^{-1} $\cdot$ min^{-1} before training and 41.0 ml $\cdot$ kg^{-1} $\cdot$ min^{-1} after training.

The 12–14% increase in $\dot{V}O_{2max}$ realized by these young adults after 7 weeks of training is typical.[7] The 36% differ-ence in $\dot{V}O_{2max}$ between genders has also been reported by others.[40] (See section on gender differences.)

- The increase in $\dot{V}O_{2max}$ is primarily attributable to a greater cardiac output and a greater oxygen extrac-tion by the muscle cells. Maximal cardiac output is only about 20 liters per minute in the untrained, whereas athletes may have maximal outputs ranging between 30 and 40 liters per minute.[7] Maximal stroke volumes can increase from 100–120 ml/beat to 180–200 ml/beat, and the max a − $\overline{v}O_2$ difference from 14.5 ml/100 ml to 16.0 ml/100 ml.

The major limiting factor to performance according to many studies is cardiac output and the ability to achieve a large stroke volume.[19,22,41] The single biggest difference be-tween endurance-trained and untrained individuals is the size of stroke volume.

- Trained athletes have a higher maximal ventilation. This means that trained people can ventilate more air during maximal exercise. Their maximal tidal vol-ume and frequency are also higher. Large, highly trained endurance athletes such as rowers can have maximal ventilation rates of more than 240 L/min, which are twice the rates of untrained individuals. Lung diffusion capacity also improves with training, meaning that oxygen can diffuse from the lung alve-oli to the blood more readily.

- Maximum heart rate usually changes little with training. The maximum heart rate of adults under age 30 may decrease a few beats per minute with ex-ercise training, but more research is needed to estab-lish this relationship.

Other changes that occur during maximal exercise with training include

- An increase of blood flow to the active muscles, with better constriction of blood vessels in inactive areas and vasodilatation in active muscle areas[42]

- An increased ability to tolerate higher lactic acid lev-els at max

Table 7.4 summarizes the changes in cardiorespiratory parameters that occur during rest, submaximal exercise, and maximal exercise following endurance training. Table 7.5 compares typical values in sedentary, trained, and elite individuals.

Other Physiological Changes with Aerobic Exercise

Other changes that occur in response to regular cardiores-piratory exercise include

- A small decrease in total body fat and a slight in-crease in lean body weight (see Chapter 11)

TABLE 7.4   Summary of Changes in Cardiorespiratory Parameters with Endurance Training

Cardiovascular Parameter	Resting	Submax Exercise	Maximal Exercise
Oxygen consumption	No change	No change	Increase
Heart rate	Decrease	Decrease	No/slight change
Stroke volume	Increase	Increase	Increase
Cardiac output	No change	No change	Increase
Active muscle blood flow	No change	Increase	Increase
Ventilation	No change	Decrease	Increase
$a - \bar{v}O_2$ difference	No change	Slight increase	Increase
Lactic acid levels	No change	Decrease	Increase

TABLE 7.5   Comparison of Hypothetical Physiological and Body Composition Changes from an Endurance Training Program for a Sedentary, Normal Person and a World-Class Endurance Runner of the Same Age

Variable	Sedentary Normal Pre-*	Sedentary Normal Post-*	World-Class Athlete
Cardiovascular			
Resting HR (bpm)	71	59	36
Max HR (bpm)	185	183	174
Resting SV (ml)	65	80	125
Max SV (ml)	120	140	200
Resting $\dot{Q}$ (L/min)	4.6	4.7	4.5
Max $\dot{Q}$ (L/min)	22.2	25.6	34.8
Heart volume (ml)	750	820	1,200
Blood volume (L)	4.7	5.1	6.0
Resting systolic BP (mm Hg)	135	130	110
Resting diastolic BP (mm Hg)	78	76	70
Respiratory			
Resting $\dot{V}_E$ (L/min)	7	6	6
Max $\dot{V}_E$ (L/min)	110	135	195
Resting F (breaths/min)	14	12	12
Max F (breaths/min)	40	45	55
Resting TV (L/breath)	0.5	0.5	0.5
Max TV (L/breath)	2.75	3.0	3.5
Vital capacity (L)	5.8	6.0	6.2
Residual volume (L)	1.4	1.2	1.2
Metabolic			
$a - \bar{v}O_2$ difference (ml/dL)	6.0	6.0	6.0
Max $a - \bar{v}O_2$ difference (ml/dL)	14.5	15.0	16.0
$\dot{V}O_{2max}$ (ml·kg^{-1}·min^{-1})	40.5	49.8	76.7
Max lactate (mmol/L)	7.5	8.5	9.0
Body composition			
Weight (lb)	175	170	150
Fat weight (lb)	28	21.3	11.3
Lean weight (lb)	147	148.7	138.7
Relative fat (%)	16.0	12.5	7.5

* = six-month training program, jogging 3–4 times per week, 30 min/day, at 75% $\dot{V}O_{2max}$. HR = heart rate; SV = stroke volume; $\dot{Q}$ = cardiac output; BP = blood pressure; $\dot{V}_E$ = ventilation; F = frequency; TV = tidal volume.

Source: Wilmore JH, Norton AC. *The Heart and Lungs at Work.* Schiller Park, IL: Beckman Instruments, 1974. Used with permission of Sensor Medics Corporation, 1630 South State College Blvd., Anaheim, CA 92806.

- An increase in HDL cholesterol, a decrease in triglycerides, but little or no change in total serum or LDL cholesterol (see Chapter 10)

- A greater ability to exercise in the heat (see Chapter 9)

- An increase in the density and breaking strength of bone, ligaments, and tendons, and an increase in the thickness of cartilage in the joints (see Chapter 12)

Changes That Occur in Muscles Due to Strength Training

What changes in the skeletal muscle occur in response to strength training (Figure 7.13)?[43–53] (See Figure 7.14 for an overview of the structure of muscle.)

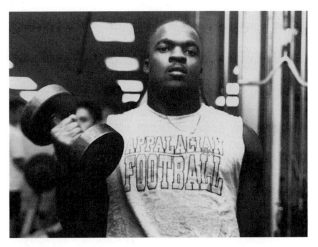

Figure 7.13 Strength training increases the size of muscle fibers and is associated with a better recruitment pattern and synchronization of motor units.

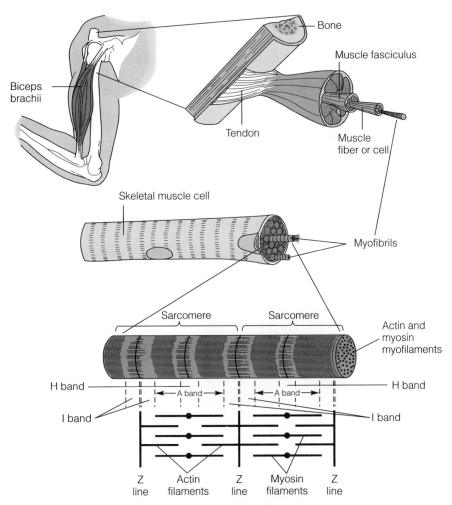

Figure 7.14 The structure of skeletal muscle. *Skeletal muscle* is composed of parallel cells (also called fibers). The number and type of muscle cells (slow-twitch) is set at birth. Each muscle cell contains groups of *actin* and *myosin* protein *myofilaments* called *myofibrils*. Skeletal muscle cells have alternating dark and light bands, caused by the overlap of the myosin and actin myofilaments, the basic contractile proteins of skeletal muscle. The smallest functional skeletal muscle subunit capable of contraction is the *sarcomere*, which extends from Z-line to Z-line. Skeletal muscle contraction takes place as the myofilaments slide past each other, and the actin and myosin form and re-form bonds.

- Regarding *hypertrophy* (increase in size) of muscle cells, especially the fast-twitch fibers,[46] the fibers of untrained muscle vary considerably in diameter, but strength training brings the smaller muscle fibers up to the size of the larger ones. This hypertrophy is caused by an increase in the number and size of myofibrils per muscle cell, increased total protein (especially myosin), and increased amounts and strength of connective, tendinous, and ligamentous tissues. When a pronounced hypertrophy of muscle fibers occurs after high-load, low-repetition resistance training, the capillary density tends to decrease. A training regimen emphasizing moderately high-load, high-repetition exercise as performed by bodybuilders, however, may induce some new capillary growth.[46]

- There is growing evidence that training leads to a small increase in the number of muscle cells. Similarly, there is some support for the theory that extensive weight training may result in some muscle fiber conversions. However, even if hyperplasia and muscle-fiber conversion do take place, the overall effect on the cross-sectional area of the muscle appears to be minor.[43–45,48]

- There is a selective hypertrophy of fast-twitch fibers with an associated increase in the ratio of fast-twitch to slow-twitch muscle fiber area.[46] Therefore, people born with a high percentage of fast-twitch fibers can "bulk up" more easily than those with a high percentage of slow-twitch fibers.

- The normal inhibitory nervous impulses from the brain are lessened. During the first 3–5 weeks of strength training, substantial gains in strength occur without concomitant increases in muscle mass.[47,50]

The nervous system adapts to regular weight training, resulting in a *disinhibition* of the muscle. With these adaptations, more *motor units* (motor nerve and attached muscle cells) can be activated, and there is a better recruitment pattern and synchronization of motor units. Thus, the increase in strength is not due to an increase in size of muscle cells alone.

- The biochemical changes are small and inconsistent. Traditional weight training programs do not appear to improve either oxidative or glycolytic enzyme activity.[46]

- Most studies have shown that weight training programs will increase lean body mass and decrease the percentage of body fat.[50] Weight training programs of 7–24 weeks generally increase the lean body mass by between 0.5 and 3.0%.

- $\dot{V}O_{2max}$ is not effectively increased by strength training programs.[43,50,53] There may be small increases in cardiorespiratory fitness after *circuit resistance training* (weight lifting with little pause between a series of different stations). However, these improvements are relatively minor (5–8%) compared to those typical in aerobic programs (see Figure 7.15).

- The heart adapts to the stresses (especially the rise in blood pressure) imposed during weight training by increasing the thickness of the left ventricle wall without an increase in the volume.[43,51]

Interestingly, weight training to increase leg strength has been shown to improve short-term (4–8 min) cycling or running endurance, and long-term cycling, but not long-term running endurance.[52,53] It appears that the increase in leg strength improves endurance performance (despite no

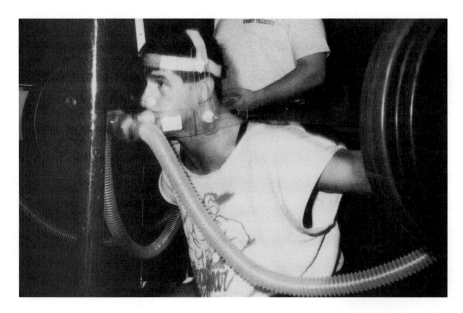

Figure 7.15 Studies show that $\dot{V}O_{2max}$ is not effectively increased by strength training.

improvement in $\dot{V}O_{2max}$) by reducing the rate of fast-twitch fiber recruitment and increasing the lactate threshold.

The Effects of Gender, Age, and Heredity

Do females adapt to regular exercise differently than males? Do middle-aged and elderly people adjust differently than younger adults? Are there special considerations for children and teenagers? How much is the ability to improve $\dot{V}O_{2max}$ due to heredity?

The Influence of Gender

Not long ago, women were thought to be too fragile to compete in athletics. Women were first allowed to participate in the 1912 Olympics, and some events, such as the women's marathon, were only added in 1984. Today, more and more sports are available to women, and there is a push worldwide to ensure equity for women in sport. The Atlanta Olympic Games, for example, included a record number of women (3,779, including 280 on the U.S. team) and sports for women (21).

Women are also proving that they are capable of feats once thought impossible for the "weaker sex." At the 1984 Olympic Games in Los Angeles, Joan Benoit-Samuelson won the gold medal in the first-ever Olympic marathon race event for women. Her time was 2 hours and 24 minutes, a standard that would have won 11 of the previous 20 men's Olympic marathons. In 1988, Paula Newby-Fraser completed the Hawaiian Ironman triathlon—comprising a 2.4-mile sea swim, a 111-mile cycle ride, and a 26-mile run—in 9 hours and 1 minute, just 30 minutes (6%) slower than the male winner. Only 10 men were ahead of her that year. During the 1990s, women runners and swimmers from China have stunned the world with their dominating performances. For example, Wang Junxia set a world record for the 10,000-meter race in September of 1993 by running a time of 29 minutes and 31 seconds, shattering the old record by 42 seconds. Wang's time was better than the times of all male runners prior to 1949.

The gap between the best men and the best women athletes has shrunk sharply since the early 1970s. In the Boston marathon, for example, the difference in winning times for men and women has diminished from 54 minutes in 1972 to about 16 minutes in 1995. The gender performance gap in many endurance events has now stabilized, however, largely because the quick gains following the loosening of social restraints have run their course. Figure 7.16 summarizes world record times in the 5,000-meter run for men and women. Notice that women started late in racing 5,000 meters, quickly began to narrow the gender gap, but then stalled during the mid-1980s.

Can women get as fit as men?[6,54–58] At puberty, testosterone secretion in males increases, leading to larger bones and increased muscle mass. In females, estrogen secretion increases, broadening the pelvis, stimulating breast development, and increasing the amount of fat in the thigh and hip areas. These unique sex differences continue into adulthood and largely explain why men and women differ in size, strength, and athletic performance.[6]

When the top female runners in the world are compared with their male counterparts, race times are 9–15% slower over all distances. This gap is not expected to decrease, largely because males and females differ in at least two important areas related to physical fitness.

1. *Heart and lung fitness.* Women have less hemoglobin in their blood than men do, thereby reducing the amount of oxygen that can be delivered to working muscles.[6] Women also tend to have more body fat, less skeletal muscle, and smaller lungs and hearts.[54–57] Together, these factors mean that women have a lower $\dot{V}O_{2max}$ than men (25% lower on average, when comparing nonathletes), and they tend to perform at a lower level in aerobic sports such as

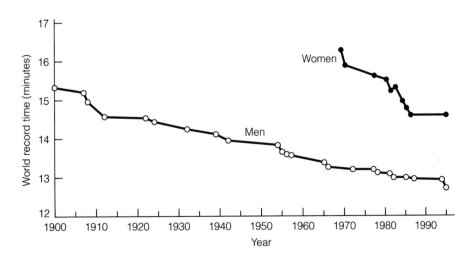

Figure 7.16 Comparison between men and women: progress in the 5,000-meter run. The gender gap in performance has stabilized in the 5,000-meter run and other endurance events.

running, cycling, swimming, and rowing. When women and men train at the same intensity, duration, and frequency, both show expected improvements in $\dot{V}O_{2max}$. Men, however, usually start and end at higher levels. Elite female athletes have $\dot{V}O_{2max}$ values that exceed those of most men but still fall 8–12% below those of elite male athletes.

2. *Muscle strength and size.* The average woman has about half the upper-body strength of men, and one fourth the lower-body strength.[6] In the weight room, women can experience strength gains with regular training, but increase in muscle size is less than what is seen in most men. Of course, some female bodybuilders have more muscle size and definition than most untrained men. There are few such women, however, and the best female bodybuilders cannot compare in muscle mass to the best male bodybuilders. In general, women have less muscle and more fat than men, and this is an important reason for the gap in performance times between the sexes.[6]

The issue of whether too much exercise can be harmful to women is explored in Chapter 16. For some female athletes, the pressure to keep body weight low and to be successful can lead to heavy training and disordered eating, loss of the menstrual period, and thinning of the bones, a syndrome called the *female athlete triad*.[59]

Do different phases of the menstrual cycle affect a woman's ability to exercise? Although some women report that premenstrual symptoms interfere with ability to exercise, researchers have been unable to link this with actual changes in the body.[6,60] In surveys, between one third and two thirds of female athletes report that their ability to exercise is *not* negatively affected during any phase of the menstrual cycle.[6] Up to one fourth report that performance is hindered during the premenstrual phase and the first few days of menstrual flow, with an improvement during the immediate postmenstrual days. Many women link premenstrual symptoms (PMS) such as fluid retention, weight gain, and mood changes with decreases in ability to exercise.

Scientists have studied whether there are actual physiological explanations for these reports by women athletes. Changes in many body functions do occur throughout the normal menstrual cycle, but researchers have been unable to associate menstrual cycle phase with problems in athletic performance.[60] Also, female athletes report that they can rise above their feelings when necessary to compete, and experts point out that world records have been set during all phases of the menstrual cycle. Joan Benoit-Samuelson's period was due the day of the 1984 Olympic marathon, and she won the gold medal.

The Influence of Age

The influence of the aging process on chronic adaptations to exercise is covered in more detail in Chapter 12. With aging, the ability to engage intensively in physical exercise declines, with a reduction of maximal aerobic power.[61–63] Aerobic power normally decreases 8–10% per decade after 30 years of age. Data suggest that the overall rate of loss is similar for active and inactive people, but that at any given age, the active conserve more function. Most researchers have shown that the cardiorespiratory trainability of the elderly does not differ greatly from that of younger adults when groups are compared on a percentage but not an absolute basis.[61] Between the ages of 30 and 70 years, muscle mass and strength decreased on average about 30%.[43] The aging process appears to account for only a small portion of this loss, with inactivity having the major influence.

Do children and youths respond to aerobic exercise programs in a similar fashion to adults? Most researchers have reported that the cardiorespiratory systems of children and youths respond to regular aerobic exercise in a fashion somewhat similar to that seen in adults.[6,64–70] There are a few differences, however.

Studies have shown that children can improve aerobic fitness after training, but that the increase is less than that found for adults.[64] In one study of 37 boys and girls, ages 11 to 13 years, 12 weeks of regular aerobic training improved $\dot{V}O_{2max}$ by 6.5%, about half what adults typically experience.[64] The researchers concluded that several factors may be responsible for this difference: (a) Children often have high aerobic fitness levels to begin with; (b) adults may train more effectively than children; and (c) the bodies of children may lack the ability to adapt and respond fully to regular exercise.

There are some other important differences between children and adults. Children have smaller hearts, lungs, and blood volumes.[6] The heart of a child cannot pump out as much blood per minute of exercise as an adult heart can, resulting in a lower oxygen delivery to the child's working muscles. $\dot{V}O_{2max}$ does not fully develop until late adolescence.

Children have a larger body surface area than adults do, when calculated per unit of body mass.[6] As a result, the smaller the child, the greater is the risk of excessive heat loss. This is particularly important when the child exercises in water, which can draw the body heat from the child very quickly, leading to *hypothermia* (i.e., low body temperature). To prevent hypothermia, children who swim or play in the water should be encouraged to leave the water periodically and to avoid cold lakes and streams.

Children, when compared to adults, have a less well developed sweating capacity.[6] They also produce more heat during activities such as running or vigorous sports play, and they can experience a faster increase in body temperature when dehydrated. These differences put children at risk for heat-related illness during long-term exercise in the heat. Researchers strongly recommend that children drink fluids frequently and avoid excessive exercise in the heat.

In 1993, an international group of experts sponsored by 13 scientific, medical, and governmental organizations submitted guidelines on physical activity for teenagers.[65] Two guidelines were recommended:

1. All adolescents should be physically active nearly every day. The activity can be a part of play, games, sports, work, transportation, recreation, physical education classes, or planned exercise with the family or community. Adolescents should engage in a variety of physical activities, and these should be enjoyable and involve most of the major muscle groups. The experts agreed that this would help reduce the risk of obesity and would promote the development of healthy bones. According to the conference report, "This is consistent with adult recommendations to engage in 30 minutes of daily activities of moderate intensity."[65] Studies show that most adolescents meet this guidelines, getting about 60 minutes per day of some type of physical activity, most of this outside of school. Unfortunately, during adolescence, time spent by both girls and boys in physical activity declines, continuing into adulthood.

2. Teenagers should pursue vigorous exercise for 20 minutes or more each session, at least three times a week. Among adolescents, only about two thirds of males and one half of females meet this guideline. Examples of activities that are recommended include brisk walking, jogging, stair climbing, basketball, racquet sports, soccer, dance, swimming laps, skating, weight training, lawn mowing, cross-country skiing, and cycling. The consensus was that the more vigorous exercise should enhance psychological health, increase HDL cholesterol, and increase cardiorespiratory fitness.

Is it safe for children and youths to lift weights?[67-70] For many years, weight training was not recommended for children and adolescents for two reasons: (1) Heavy weight lifting was thought to interfere with bone growth and to promote bone and joint injury; (2) it was claimed that weight training was not effective in children before the time of puberty. Most studies now support weight training as both safe and effective for children and youths.[69] Still, the American Academy of Pediatrics has cautioned that children and adolescents should avoid intensive weight lifting, power lifting, and bodybuilding until they are about 15 years of age.[67] Moderate weight lifting by children should be under adult supervision to decrease the risk of injury. Weight training is recommended two or three times a week for 20 to 30 minutes a session and should be part of an overall comprehensive program designed to increase total fitness.

According to most experts, children can improve strength with appropriate weight training by about 15–30%.[67-70] The rise in strength is not usually related to any measurable increase in muscle size, however. Instead, improvements in nerve and muscle cell interactions occur, augmenting strength.[70]

The Influence of Heredity

Studies reporting the influence of heredity on aerobic performance have had conflicting results.[71-77] Several twin studies have suggested that $\dot{V}O_{2max}$ and work capacity were almost entirely inherited, whereas others have reported little genetic effect. Many of these studies have failed to control for age, sex and other factors.

These various factors were controlled in a large study of 42 brothers, 66 dizygotic twins of both sexes, and 106 monozygotic twins of both sexes.[73] They were given various exercise performance tests, including maximal bicycle tests and tests of total work output during a 90-minute, high-intensity bicycle test. The magnitude of the genetic effect was determined to be 40% for $\dot{V}O_{2max}$, 50% for maximal heart rate, 60% for maximal ventilation, and 70% for 90-minute work output. When $\dot{V}O_{2max}$ was expressed per kilogram of fat-free weight, the genetic effect was found to be only 25%.[77] These results are in sharp contrast with those of other twin studies, in which it was reported that the heritability of $\dot{V}O_{2max}$ was about 90% of the total variance.

Researchers have also shown that sensitivity of $\dot{V}O_{2max}$ improvement to exercise training is in part dependent on heredity.[72,74-77] In one study of 10 pairs of monozygotic twins, results showed a large variety of responses to the exercise program (a range of 0–41% $\dot{V}O_{2max}$ improvement, with all subjects cycling 40 minutes, four to five times per week, at 80% of $\dot{V}O_{2max}$), but the members of each twin pair reacted approximately the same way to the exercise program.[72] In other words, some genotypes appear to be more sensitive to exercise training than others.[76]

Prior endowment and an adequate training program will produce exceptionally high performance. From a practical point of view, because of heredity, it is almost impossible to accurately predict an individual response to a given training program. Nonetheless, most Olympic winners appear to be genetically selected for their events, and then train long and hard to gain the extra advantage needed for success[2] (see Figure 7.17).

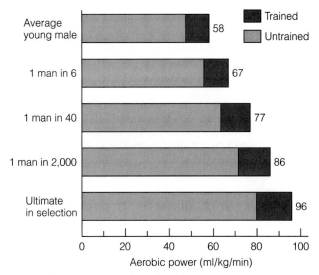

Assumption is that peak effect of training is 20% increase in aerobic power.

Figure 7.17 Relative importance of inherited athletic selection and rigorous training. Few people are genetically selected for athletic success and a high aerobic power. Even among those selected for a high $\dot{V}O_{2max}$, intense training may improve aerobic power only an additional 20%. *Source:* Data from Shephard RJ, Astrand P-O. *Endurance in Sport: The Encyclopædia of Sports Medicine* (Volume II). Oxford: Blackwell Scientific Publications, 1992.

THE EFFECTS OF INACTIVITY

Prolonged inactivity has many detrimental effects on the muscles, bones, and cardiovascular system of the human body.[78-80] Disuse adversely affects all body tissues and all body functions. For example, bed rest leads to a muscle protein loss of 8 grams per day, a bone calcium loss of 1.54 grams per week, a decrease in $\dot{V}O_{2max}$ of 0.8% per day, and a 10–15% decrease in plasma volume within several days.[79,80]

Few humans undergo prolonged bed rest. However, nearly all people have exercised for a certain period of time and then for various reasons reduced or terminated formal exercise while continuing normal day-to-day activities. This period of *detraining* leads to many changes in physiological function.[80-91]

Edward Coyle, from the University of Texas at Austin, has been a leading researcher on the physiological effects of detraining. In one study, Coyle studied the effects of 84 days of no formal exercise on athletes who had been training hard for 10 years.[82,83]

During this long detraining period, the various systems of the body reacted differently. In the first 3 weeks after training ceased, runners quickly lost most of their cardiovascular conditioning, primarily due to a rapid decline in stroke volume. The maximal stroke volume declined 10–14% below the trained level in just 12 days and dropped to a

level no different from sedentary controls by the end of the study. $\dot{V}O_{2max}$ declined 7% in the first 21 days and stabilized after 56 days at a level 16% below the trained level. At the end of 8 weeks, the oxidative enzyme levels in the muscles had dropped 40% from the trained levels.

Other researchers have also found that the activities of mitochondrial enzymes are markedly reduced with the cessation of physical training.[84]

Muscle capillarization, however, dropped only 7% below trained levels after 84 days. Although maximal cardiac output and stroke volume declined to untrained levels, $\dot{V}O_{2max}$ levels in the detrained athletes remained 17% above untrained levels, primarily because of an elevation of maximal a − $\bar{v}O_2$ difference.

Eighty-four days of detraining also affected responses to submaximal exercise (74% $\dot{V}O_{2max}$, trained state).[83] Within 8 weeks, most of the negative adaptations occurred, including an 18% increase in oxygen consumption (using the same workload), a 17% increase in heart rate (158 when trained vs. 185 when detrained), a 24% increase in ventilation, a 6% increase in the respiratory exchange ratio, and a 34% increase in the rating of perceived exertion (as measured on the Borg scale). Within 8 weeks, the rise in lactate in response to the same workload was nearly sixfold. Other researchers have shown that running or cycling endurance performance (e.g., running races or cycling time trials) is negatively affected early in the detraining period.[85-88]

Even after detraining for 12 weeks, however, the athletes still had high muscle capillary densities and a mitochondrial enzyme level 50% above that of the sedentary controls. These represent persistent adaptations resulting from many years of hard training and helped to partially preserve their exercise performance ability.

These studies support the argument that physical activity must be continued on a regular basis if one is to retain the benefits. As noted previously, when athletes detrain after many years of intense training, they display large reductions in cardiorespiratory fitness during the first 12–21 days of inactivity. The decline in stroke volume appears to be largely a result of reduced plasma volume, which also drops 12% within 12–21 days.[81] Interestingly, Coyle has shown that if an athlete who has detrained for 2–4 weeks expands the blood volume back to that of the trained state, using 6% dextran solution in saline, stroke volume and $\dot{V}O_{2max}$ can be increased to within 2–4% of trained values.[80,81]

Researchers have shown that the rise in aerobic power with training is just as rapid as its fall without it. Studies show that most of the improvements in $\dot{V}O_{2max}$ occur within 3 weeks of beginning intense cardiorespiratory training. In addition, once the desired $\dot{V}O_{2max}$ is achieved, it is possible to maintain it by reducing the frequency while maintaining the intensity of training.[92,93]

In one study, 12 participants bicycled and ran for 40 minutes, 6 days per week, following an intensive interval training regimen.[92] After 10 weeks, they continued to train at the same intensity and daily duration, but the frequency was lowered to 2 days per week for half of them, 4 days for the others. After 5 weeks, the $\dot{V}O_{2max}$ in both groups remained at the 25% improved level attained at the end of the first 10 weeks of training. Among distance runners, if training volume is decreased by more than half during a 3-week period while intensity is maintained, no decrement in 5-K running performance has been measured.[87]

In other words, it appears to take more energy expenditure to increase $\dot{V}O_{2max}$ than to maintain it. It also appears that training intensity is an essential requirement for maintaining the increased $\dot{V}O_{2max}$ and performance ability gained from hard aerobic training. Detraining also has a strong effect in reducing muscle strength and size.[89-91] Muscular strength returns to control levels within 4–12 weeks of detraining but can be maintained if weight training frequency is just one or two sessions per week.

SPORTS MEDICINE INSIGHT
Factors Affecting Performance

If a group of people are asked to run 10 kilometers or cycle 40 kilometers as fast as possible, would it be possible to predict the top finishers? What factors are most important in cardiorespiratory endurance performance? Three major physiological factors affect cardiorespiratory endurance performance:[94-109]

1. $\dot{V}O_{2max}$
2. Anaerobic threshold
3. Exercise oxygen economy

If a group of people varying widely in activity patterns (sedentary to elite athlete) were examined in the laboratory, $\dot{V}O_{2max}$ would be the most important variable predicting ability to engage in cardiorespiratory endurance events. However, among a homogeneous group of elite endurance athletes, the anaerobic threshold and exercise oxygen economy would be better indicators of performance ability.

Although important, $\dot{V}O_{2max}$ is only one of several factors that determine success in endurance events. There can be a large variation in performance among athletes of equal $\dot{V}O_{2max}$.[94] Relatively low $\dot{V}O_{2max}$ values have been reported among some top-class marathon runners. Derek Clayton, former world-record holder in the marathon (2:08.33), had a $\dot{V}O_{2max}$ of only 66.8 ml · kg^{-1} · min^{-1}, while Frank Shorter, an Olympic gold medalist in the marathon, measured only 72 ml · kg^{-1} · min^{-1}. Stahl, formerly one of the best master runners in the world, had a $\dot{V}O_{2max}$ of only 66.8 ml · kg^{-1} · min^{-1}.

Joan Benoit-Samuelson, one of the best female marathon runners in history (2:21), had a $\dot{V}O_{2max}$ of 78 ml · kg^{-1} · min^{-1}, a value much higher than Clayton's, Shorter's, and Stahl's, yet her marathon time was much

slower. Obviously, other factors play an important role in cardiorespiratory endurance performance.

Exercise oxygen economy is the oxygen cost of exercise, usually expressed as $\dot{V}O_2$ at a certain running or exercise pace.[104] It is a well-established fact that $\dot{V}O_2$ at a certain workload or running speed can vary considerably among different athletes[94,95,106] (see Figure 7.18). Some of the best performers have low oxygen requirements at specific running velocities. While it is not possible to explain this variation precisely, biomechanical, physiological, psy-

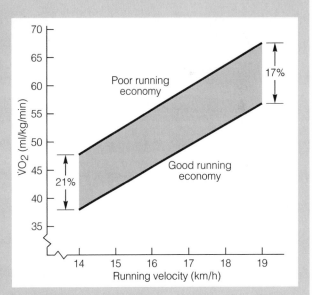

Figure 7.18 Oxygen economy. The shaded area represents the entire range in the oxygen cost of running at different velocities for good and elite runners. *Source:* Adapted from Sjodin B, Svedenhag H, and J. R. Brotherhood. Applied physiology of marathon running. *Sports Med* 2:83–99, 1985. Used with permission by ADIS Press Limited, Auckland, New Zealand.

(continued)

Factors Affecting Performance *(continued)*

chological, and biochemical factors probably all play a part. There is good evidence that athletes with a high percentage of slow-twitch fibers have the best exercise oxygen economy.[103,106]

Another important factor influencing athletic performance is the anaerobic threshold. Anaerobic threshold is highly correlated with endurance performance ($r = 0.94$ to 0.98).[11-15,94] If a performer can exercise at a high percentage of $\dot{V}O_{2max}$ before lactic acid builds up in the bloodstream, that capacity provides a great advantage. Such a capacity is built up through long years of training, with an emphasis on interval training (see Figure 7.19).

Other factors, nonphysiological in nature, also play an important role in cardiorespiratory endurance capac-

ity. In one study of 4,358 runners, the most important predictors of 16-K race time, in order, were weekly training distance, age, body mass index, years of regular running, and weekly training frequency.[101] Other studies have also consistently shown weekly training distance to provide the highest correlation with endurance race performance.[94] Although elite athletes often average only 60–65% of $\dot{V}O_{2max}$ intensity during training, most have two or three sessions per week where they run intervals at 5-K and 10-K race pace to improve $\dot{V}O_{2max}$ and the anaerobic threshold.[107-109]

Table 7.6 summarizes the physical and physiological characteristics of different categories of endurance runners.[94]

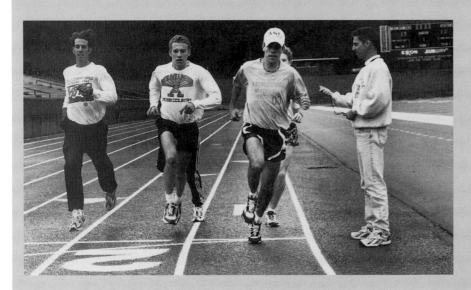

Figure 7.19 The anaerobic threshold is built up through long years of training, with an emphasis on interval training.

TABLE 7.6 Physical and Physiological Characteristics of Different Categories of Endurance Runners

	Elite Runners	Good Runners	Slow Runners
Age (years)	26	30	36
Weight (kg)	66	67	71
Type I fibers (%)	76	64	56
Years of training	7	4	2
Average weekly distance (km)	145	115	57
$\dot{V}O_{2max}$ (ml · kg^{-1} · min^{-1})	72	66	59
$\dot{V}O_2$ at 15 km/hr	45	49	51
Lactate threshold*	88	88	85

*Percent $\dot{V}O_{2max}$ when lactic acid is a concentration of 4 mmol/L.

Source: Adapted from: Sjodin B, Svedenhag J., and J. R. Brotherhood. Applied physiology of marathon running. *Sports Med* 2:83–99, 1985.

SUMMARY

1. This chapter summarized the acute responses and chronic adaptations that occur with exercise.

2. The acute responses include increases of heart rate, stroke volume, cardiac output, blood flow to active muscles, systolic blood pressure, arteriovenous oxygen difference, ventilation, lung diffusion capacity, oxygen uptake, and a decrease in blood pH and plasma volume (red blood cell count rises).

3. Chronic adaptations include biochemical changes in skeletal muscles (increased myoglobin, mitochondria, enzymes, fuels, slow-twitch fiber area); resting cardiorespiratory changes (increase in heart size, stroke volume, blood volume, and capillary density, with a decrease in resting heart rate); submaximal exercise changes (increase in anaerobic threshold and stroke volume, with a decrease in lactic acid production, heart rate, and cardiac output); maximal exercise changes (increase in $\dot{V}O_{2max}$, stroke volume, blood flow to active muscles, ability to tolerate higher lactic acid levels, ventilation, and lung diffusion capacity, plus a variable effect on maximal heart rate); and other assorted changes (decrease in total body fat, blood lipids, and recovery heart rate, with an increase in heat acclimatization and the density and strength of bone and connective tissues).

4. The performance gap between the sexes occurs because of important differences between men and women. Women have less hemoglobin, more body fat, less skeletal muscle, smaller lungs and heart, a lower $\dot{V}O_{2max}$, and less strength than their male counterparts at all similar levels of fitness (sedentary to elite status). Most researchers have shown that cardiorespiratory trainability of the elderly does not differ greatly from that of younger adults when groups are compared on a percentage (not absolute) basis.

For children and teenagers, researchers have in general concluded that when programs satisfy adult-related criteria for intensity and duration, children demonstrate a similar physiological training effect.

5. The genetic effect has been determined as 25% for $\dot{V}O_{2max}$. There is large variability in trainability, and researchers have concluded that the sensitivity of $\dot{V}O_{2max}$ improvement to exercise training depends in part on hereditary factors. Therefore, an exceptionally high performance level will be the result of prior endowment, an adequate training program, and genetic characteristics associated with the status of a high responder to training.

6. Inactivity (through bed rest) affects virtually every physiological system. Early responses involve the fluid, electrolyte, and blood pressure control systems, with significant muscular atrophy and decreases in bone density occurring somewhat later.

7. *Detraining* (termination of exercise training, but not bed rest) affects the different systems variously, with stroke volume being affected quickly (decreasing to control levels within 1 month), and muscle capillarization dropping only 7% after 84 days of detraining. The respiratory capacity of trained muscles (mitochondrial enzymes) decreases by 50% after 1 week of inactivity. To prevent these detraining effects, it is more important to maintain the intensity of exercise than the frequency of exercise.

8. Factors affecting performance include $\dot{V}O_{2max}$, anaerobic threshold, and exercise oxygen economy. While $\dot{V}O_{2max}$ is most important when evaluating the performance ability of a heterogeneous group, the anaerobic threshold and exercise oxygen economy are most important when comparing athletes of similar ability.

REFERENCES

1. Huston TP, Puffer JC, Rodney WM. The athletic heart syndrome. *N Engl J Med* 313:24–31, 1985.

2. Shephard RJ, Astrand P-O. *Endurance in Sport: The Encyclopædia of Sports Medicine* (Volume II). Oxford: Blackwell Scientific Publications, 1992.

3. Bouchard C, Shephard RJ, Stephens T. *Physical Activity, Fitness, and Health: International Proceedings and Consensus Statement.* Champaign, IL: Human Kinetics, 1994.

4. Komi PV (ed). *Strength and Power in Sport: The Encyclopædia of Sports Medicine.* Oxford: Blackwell Scientific Publications, 1992.

5. Baechle TR. *Essentials of Strength Training and Conditioning.* Champaign, IL: Human Kinetics, 1994.

6. Wilmore JH, Costill DL. *Physiology of Sports and Exercise.* Champaign, IL: Human Kinetics, 1994.

7. Brooks GA, Fahey TD, White TP. *Exercise Physiology: Human Bioenergetics and Its Applications* (2nd ed.). Mountain View, CA: Mayfield Publishing Company, 1996.

8. American College of Sports Medicine. *Resource Manual for Guidelines for Exercise Testing and Prescription* (2nd ed.). Philadelphia: Lea & Febiger, 1993.

9. Di Carlo LJ, Sparling PB, Millard-Stafford ML, Rupp JC. Peak heart rates during maximal running and swimming: Implications for exercise prescription. *Int J Sports Med* 12:309–312, 1991.

10. Senay LC, Pivarnik JM. Fluid shifts during exercise. *Exerc Sport Sci Rev* 13:335–387, 1985.

11. Brooks GA. Current concepts in lactate exchange. *Med Sci Sports Exerc* 23:895–906, 1991.

12. McLellan TM, Cheung KSY. A comparative evaluation of the

individual anaerobic threshold and the critical power. *Med Sci Sports Exerc* 24:543–550, 1992.

13. Davis JA. Anaerobic threshold: Review of the concept and directions for future research. *Med Sci Sports Exerc* 17:6–18, 1985.

14. Londeree BR. Effect of training on lactate/ventilatory thresholds: A meta-analysis. *Med Sci Sports Exerc* 29:837–843, 1997.

15. Loat CER, Rhodes EC. Relationship between the lactate and ventilatory thresholds during prolonged exercise. *Sports Med* 15:104–115, 1993.

16. Rogers MA, Yamamoto C, Hagberg JM, et al. Effect of 6 d of exercise training on responses to maximal and sub-maximal exercise in middle-aged men. *Med Sci Sports Exerc* 20:260–264, 1988.

17. Hickson RC. Time course of the adaptive responses of aerobic power and heart rate to training. *Med Sci Sports Exerc* 13: 17–20, 1981.

18. Wagner PD. Central and peripheral aspects of oxygen transport and adaptations with exercise. *Sports Medicine* 11:133–142, 1991.

19. Blomqvist CG, Saltin B. Cardiovascular adaptations to physical training. *Ann Rev Physiol* 45:169–189, 1983.

20. Moore RL, Thacker EM, Kelley GA, et al. Effect of training/detraining on submaximal exercise responses in humans. *J Appl Physiol* 63:1719–1724, 1987.

21. Sutton JR. $\dot{V}O_{2max}$—New concepts on an old theme. *Med Sci Sports Exerc* 24:26–29, 1992.

22. Saltin B, Strange S. Maximal oxygen uptake: "Old" and "new" arguments for a cardiovascular limitation. *Med Sci Sports Exerc* 24:30–37, 1992.

23. Green HJ, Patla AE. Maximal aerobic power: Neuromuscular and metabolic considerations. *Med Sci Sports Exerc* 24:38–46, 1992.

24. Wagner PD. Gas exchange and peripheral diffusion limitation. *Med Sci Sports Exerc* 24:54–58, 1992.

25. Spina RJ, Chi MMY, Hopkins MG, Nemeth PM, Lowry OH, Holloszy JO. Mitochondrial enzymes increase in muscle in response to 7–10 days of cycle exercise. *J Appl Physiol* 80: 2250–2254, 1996.

26. Jansson E, Kaijser L. Substrate utilization and enzymes in skeletal muscle of extremely endurance-trained men. *J Appl Physiol* 62:999–1005, 1987.

27. Ama PFM, Simoneau JA, Boulay MR, et al. Skeletal muscle characteristics in sedentary black and Caucasian males. *J Appl Physiol* 61:1758–1761, 1986.

28. Pette D. Activity-induced fast to slow transitions in mammalian muscle. *Med Sci Sports* Exerc 16:517–528, 1984.

29. Howard H, Hoppeler H, Cloassen H, et al. Influences of endurance training on the ultrastructural composition of the different muscle fiber types in humans. *Pflugers Arch* 403: 369–376, 1985.

30. Cohen JL, Segal KR. Left ventricular hypertrophy in athletes: An exercise-echocardiographic study. *Med Sci Sports Exerc* 17: 695–700, 1985.

31. Convertino VA. Blood volume: Its adaptation to endurance training. *Med Sci Sports Exerc* 23:1338–1348, 1991.

32. Hopper MK, Coggan AR, Coyle EF. Exercise stroke volume relative to plasma-volume expansion. *J Appl Physiol* 64:404–408, 1988.

33. Nadel ER. Physiological adaptations to aerobic training. *American Scientist* 73:334–343, 1985.

34. Costill DL, Fink WJ, Flynn M, Kirwan J. Muscle fiber composition and enzyme activities in elite female distance runners. *Int J Sports Med* 8(suppl):103–106, 1987.

35. Martin DE, May DF. Pulmonary function characteristics in elite women distance runners. *Int J Sports Med* 8(suppl):84–90, 1987.

36. Nieman DC, Tan SA, Lee JW, Berk LS. Complement and immunoglobulin levels in athletes and sedentary controls. *Int J Sports Med* 10:124–128, 1989.

37. Pate RR, Sparling PB, Wilson GE, Cureton KJ, Miller BJ. Cardiorespiratory and metabolic responses to submaximal and maximal exercise in elite women distance runners. *Int J Sports Med* 8(suppl):91–95, 1987.

38. National Center for Health Statistics, Drury EF (ed). *Assessing Physical Fitness and Physical Activity in Population-Based Surveys*. DHHS Pub. No. (PHS) 89-1253. Public Health Service. Washington, DC: U.S. Government Printing Office, 1989.

39. Rusko HK. Development of aerobic power in relation to age and training in cross-country skiers. *Med Sci Sports Exerc* 24: 1040–1047, 1992.

40. Vogel JA, Patton JF, Mello RP, Daniels WL. An analysis of aerobic capacity in a large United States population. *J Appl Physiol* 60:494–500, 1986.

41. Hammond HK, Froelicher VF. The physiologic sequelae of chronic dynamic exercise. *Med Clinics N Amer* 69:21–39, 1985.

42. Martin WH, Montgomery J, Snell PG, et al. Cardiovascular adaptations to intense swim training in sedentary middle-aged men and women. *Circulation* 75:323–330, 1987.

43. Komi PV (ed). *Strength and Power in Sport: The Encyclopædia of Sports Medicine*. Oxford: Blackwell Scientific Publications, 1992.

44. Abernethy PJ, Jürimäe J, Logan PA, Taylor AW, Thayer RE. Acute and chronic response of skeletal muscle to resistance exercise. *Sports Med* 17:22–38, 1994.

45. Kelley G. Mechanical overload and skeletal muscle fiber hyperplasia: A meta-analysis. *J Appl Physiol* 81:1584–1588, 1996.

46. Tesch PA. Skeletal muscle adaptations consequent to long-term heavy resistance exercise. *Med Sci Sports Exerc* 20(suppl): S132–S134, 1988.

47. Sale DG. Neural adaptation to resistance training. *Med Sci Sports Exerc* 20(suppl):S135–S145, 1988.

48. McCall GE, Byrnes WC, Dickinson A, Pattany PM, Fleck SJ. Muscle fiber hypertrophy, hyperplasia, and capillary density in college men after resistance training. *J Appl Physiol* 81: 2004–2012, 1996.

49. Taylor NAS, Wilkinson JG. Exercise-induced skeletal muscle growth: Hypertrophy or hyperplasia? *Sports Med* 3:190–200, 1986.

50. Kraemer WJ, Deschenes MR, Fleck SJ. Physiological adaptations to resistance exercise: Implications for athletic conditioning. *Sports Med* 6:246–256, 1988.

51. Fleck SJ, Pattany PM, Stone MH, Kraemer WJ, Thrush J, Wong K. Magnetic resonance imaging determination of left ventricular mass: Junior Olympic weightlifters. *Med Sci Sports Exerc* 25:522–527, 1993.

52. Hickson RC, Dvorak BA, Gorostiaga EM, Kurowski TT, Foster C. Potential for strength and endurance training to amplify endurance performance. *J Appl Physiol* 65:2285–2290, 1988.

53. Marcinik EJ, Potts J, Schlabach G, Will S, Dawson P, Hurley BF. Effects of strength training on lactate threshold and endurance performance. *Med Sci Sports Exerc* 23:739–743, 1991.

54. Hutchinson PL, Cureton KJ, Outz H, Wilson G. Relationship of cardiac size to maximal oxygen uptake and body size in men and women. *Int J Sports Med* 12:369–373, 1991.

55. Suetta C, Kanstrup IL, Fogh-Andersen N. Hematological status in elite long-distance runners: Influence of body composition. *Clin Physiol* 16:563–574, 1996.

56. Graves JE, Pollock ML, Sparling PB. Body compositions of elite female distance runners. *Int J Sports Med* 8(suppl): 96–102, 1987.

57. Pate RR, Sparling PB, Wilon GE, Cureton KJ, Miller BJ. Cardiorespiratory and metabolic responses to submaximal and maximal exercise in elite women distance runners. *Int J Sports Med* 8(suppl):91–95, 1987.

58. Bam J, Noakes TD, Juritz J, Dennis SC. Could women outrun men in ultramarathon races? *Med Sci Sports Exerc* 29:244–247, 1997.

59. American College of Sports Medicine. The female athlete triad. *Med Sci Sports Exerc* 29:i–ix, 1997.

60. Lebrun CM, McKenzie DC, Prior JC, Taunton JE. Effect of menstrual cycle phase on athletic performance. *Med Sci Sports Exerc* 27:437–444, 1995.

61. Green JS, Crouse SF. The effects of endurance training on functional capacity in the elderly: A meta-analysis. *Med Sci Sports Exerc* 27:920–926, 1995.

62. Jackson AS, Beard EF, Wier LT, et al. Changes in aerobic power in men, ages 25–70 yr. *Med Sci Sports Exerc* 27:113–120, 1995.

63. Jackson AS, Wier LT, Ayers GW, Beard EF, Stuteville JE, Blair SN. Changes in aerobic power of women, ages 20–64 yr. *Med Sci Sports Exerc* 28:884–891, 1996.

64. Rowland TW, Boyajian A. Aerobic response to endurance exercise training in children. *Pediatrics* 96:654–658, 1995.

65. Sallis JF, Patrick K. Physical activity guidelines for adolescents: Consensus statement. *Pediatric Exerc Sci* 6:302–314, 1994.

66. Turley KR, Wilmore JH. Cardiovascular responses to treadmill and cycle ergometer exercise in children and adults. *J Appl Physiol* 83:948–957, 1997.

67. Committee on Sports Medicine. Strength training, weight and power lifting, and bodybuilding by children and adolescents. *Pediatrics* 86:801–803, 1990.

68. Blimkie CJR. Resistance training during preadolescence: Issues and controversies. *Sports Med* 15:389–407, 1993.

69. Falk B, Tenenbaum G. The effectiveness of resistance training in children: A meta-analysis. *Sports Med* 22:176–186, 1996.

70. Ozmun JC, Mikesky AE, Surburg PR. Neuromuscular adaptations following prepubescent strength training. *Med Sci Sports Exerc* 26:510–514, 1994.

71. Bouchard C, Lortie G. Heredity and endurance performance. *Sports Med* 1:38–64, 1984.

72. Prud'homme D, Bouchard C, et al. Sensitivity of maximal aerobic power to training is genotype-dependent. *Med Sci Sports Exerc* 16:489–493, 1984.

73. Bouchard C, Lesage R, Lortie G, et al. Aerobic performance in brothers, dizygotic and monozygotic twins. *Med Sci Sports Exerc* 18:639–646, 1986.

74. Hamel P, Simoneau JA, Lortie G, Boulay MR, Bouchard C. Heredity and muscle adaptation to endurance training. *Med Sci Sports Exerc* 18:690–696, 1986.

75. Bouchard C, Boulay MR, Simoneau JA, Lortie G, Pérusse L. Heredity and trainability of aerobic and anaerobic performances: An update. *Sports Med* 5:69–73, 1988.

76. Dionne FT, Turcotte L, Thibault M-C, Boulay MR, Skinner JS, Bouchard C. Mitochondrial DNA sequence polymorphism, $\dot{V}O_{2max}$, and response to endurance training. *Med Sci Sports Exerc* 23:177–185, 1991.

77. Bouchard C, Dionne FT, Simoneau J-A, Boulay MR. Genetics of aerobic and anaerobic performances. *Exerc Sport Sci Rev* 20: 27–58, 1992.

78. Tipton CM, Hargens A. Physiological adaptations and countermeasures associated with long-duration spaceflights. *Med Sci Sports Exerc* 28:974–976, 1996.

79. Bortz WM. The disuse syndrome. *West J Med* 141:691–694, 1984.

80. Bloomfield SA, Coyle EF. Bed rest, detraining, and retention of training-induced adaptations. In American College of Sports Medicine, *Resource Manual for Guidelines for Exercise Testing and Prescription*. Philadelphia: Lea & Febiger, 1988, 83–89.

81. Coyle EF, Hemmert MK, Coggan AR. Effects of detraining on cardiovascular responses to exercise: Role of blood volume. *J Appl Physiol* 60:95–99, 1986.

82. Coyle EF, Martin WH, Sinacore DR, et al. Time course of loss of adaptations after stopping prolonged intense endurance training. *J Appl Physiol* 57:1857–1864, 1984.

83. Coyle EF, Martin WH, Bloomfield SA, et al. Effects of detraining on responses to submaximal exercise. *J Appl Physiol* 59: 853–859, 1985.

84. Costill DL. Metabolic characteristics of skeletal muscle during detraining from competitive swimming. *Med Sci Sports Exerc* 17:339–343, 1985.

85. Houmard JA, Hortobagyi T, Johns RA, et al. Effect of short-term training cessation on performance measures in distance runners. *Int J Sports Med* 13:572–576, 1992.

86. Madsen K, Pedersen PK, Djurhuus MS, Klitgaard NA. Effects of detraining on endurance capacity and metabolic changes during prolonged exhaustive exercise. *J Appl Physiol* 75: 1444–1451, 1993.

87. Houmard JA. Impact of reduced training on performance in endurance athletes. *Sports Med* 12:380–393, 1991.

88. McConell GK, Costill DL, Widrick JJ, Hickey MS, Tanaka H, Gastin PB. Reduced training volume and intensity maintain aerobic capacity but not performance in distance runners. *Int J Sports Med* 14:33–37, 1993.

89. Hortobagyi T, Houmard JA, Stevenson JR, Fraser DD, Johns RA, Israel RG. The effects of detraining on power athletes. *Med Sci Sports Exerc* 25:929–935, 1993.

90. Colliander EB, Tesch PA. Effects of detraining following short term resistance training on eccentric and concentric muscle strength. *Acta Physiol Scand* 144:23–29, 1992.

91. Graves JE, Pollock ML, Leggett SH, Braith RW, Carpenter DM, Bishop LE. Effect of reduced training frequency on muscular strength. *Int J Sports Med* 9:316–319, 1988.

92. Hickson RC, Rosenkoetter MA. Reduced training frequencies and maintenance of increased aerobic power. *Med Sci Sports Exerc* 13:13–16, 1981.

93. Hickson RC, et al. Reduced training intensities and loss of aerobic power, endurance, and cardiac growth. *J Appl Physiol* 58:492–499, 1985.

94. Sjodin B, Svedenhag J. Applied physiology of marathon running. *Sports Med* 2:83–99, 1985.

95. Sleivert GC, Rowlands DS. Physical and physiological factors associated with success in the triathlon. *Sports Med* 22:8–18, 1996.

96. Van Ingen Schenau GJ, De Koning JJ, Bakker FC, de Groot G. Performance-influencing factors in homogenous groups of top athletes: A cross-sectional study. *Med Sci Sports Exerc* 28: 1305–1310, 1996.

97. Anderson T. Biomechanics and running economy. *Sports Med* 22:76–89, 1996.

98. Keul J, Konig D, Huonker M, Halle M, Wohlfahrt B, Berg A. Adaptation to training and performance in elite athletes. *Res Quart Exerc Sport* 67(suppl):S29–S36, 1996.

99. Pereira MA, Freedson PS. Intraindividual variation of running economy in highly trained and moderately trained males. *Int J Sports Med* 18:118–124, 1997.

100. Billat LV. Use of blood lactate measurements for prediction of exercise performance and for control of training. *Sports Med* 22:157–175, 1996.

101. Marti B, Abelin T, Minder CE. Relationship of training and life-style to 16-km running time of 4000 joggers: The '84 Berne "Grand-Prix" study. *Int J Sports Med* 9:85–91, 1988.

102. Pate RR, Macera CA, Bailey SP, Bartoli WP, Powell KE. Physiological, anthropometric, and training correlates of running economy. *Med Sci Sports Exerc* 24:1128–1133, 1992.

103. Coyle EF, Feltner ME, Kautz SA, et al. Physiological and biomechanical factors associated with elite endurance cycling performance. *Med Sci Sports Exerc* 23:93–107, 1991.

104. Morgan DW, Bransford DR, Costill DL, Daniels JT, Howley ET, Krahenbuhl GS. Variation in the aerobic demand of running among trained and untrained subjects. *Med Sci Sports Exerc* 27:404–409, 1995.

105. Barbeau P, Serresse O, Boulay MR. Using maximal and submaximal aerobic variables to monitor elite cyclists during a season. *Med Sci Sports Exerc* 25:1062–1069, 1993.

106. Coyle EF, Sidossis LS, Horowitz JF, Beltz JD. Cycling efficiency is related to the percentage of Type I muscle fibers. *Med Sci Sports Exerc* 24:782–788, 1992.

107. Pate RR, Branch JD. Training for endurance sport. *Med Sci Sports Exerc* 24(suppl):S340–S343, 1992.

108. Robinson DM, Robinson SM, Hume PA, Hopkins WG. Training intensity of elite male distance runners. *Med Sci Sports Exerc* 23:1078–1082, 1991.

109. Anderson O. The perfect pace. *Runner's World,* May 1992, 43–50.

PHYSICAL FITNESS ACTIVITY 7.1

Labeling Figures That Depict Acute and Chronic Responses to Exercise

The figure below illustrates eight different resting dynamic lung volumes, and acute and chronic changes associated with exercise. As explained in this chapter, the *acute responses to exercise* are the sudden, temporary changes in body function caused by exercise, which disappear shortly after the exercise period is finished. The *chronic adaptations to exercise* are the persistent changes in the structure and function of your body following regular exercise training, which apparently enable the body to respond more easily to subsequent exercise bouts.

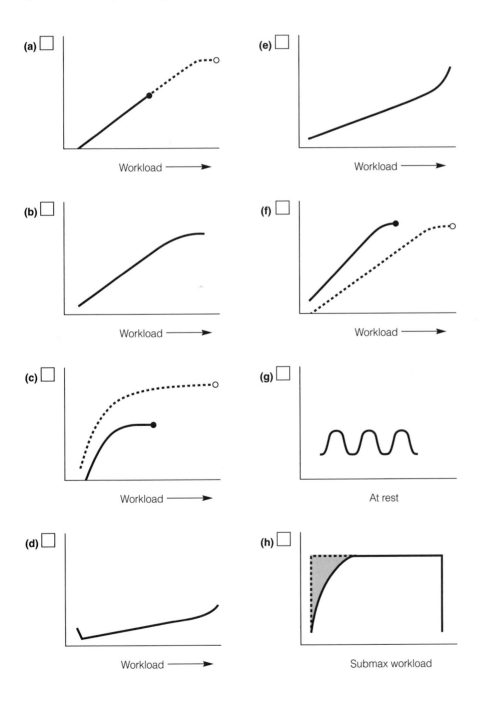

(a) ☐   Workload ⟶

(b) ☐   Workload ⟶

(c) ☐   Workload ⟶

(d) ☐   Workload ⟶

(e) ☐   Workload ⟶

(f) ☐   Workload ⟶

(g) ☐   At rest

(h) ☐   Submax workload

Your assignment is to label each illustration with one of the following listings. In some of the illustrations, the solid line represents the response of an untrained person; the dashed line represents the response of a trained person.

Match these answers with the appropriate illustration (A through H).

1. Respiratory exchange ratio

2. $\dot{V}O_{2max}$

3. Minute ventilation

4. Heart rate differences of trained and untrained people

5. Tidal volume

6. Stroke volume differences of trained and untrained people

7. Oxygen deficit

8. Cardiac-output differences of trained and untrained people

CHAPTER

8

Exercise Prescription

Significant health benefits can be obtained by including a moderate amount of physical activity (e.g., 30 minutes of brisk walking or raking leaves, 15 minutes of running, or 45 minutes of playing volleyball) on most, if not all, days of the week. Through a modest increase in daily activity, most Americans can improve their health and quality of life. Additional health benefits can be gained through greater amounts of physical activity. People who can maintain a regular regimen of activity that is of longer duration or of more vigorous intensity are likely to derive greater benefit.

—*Physical Activity and Health: A Report of the Surgeon General*, 1996

According to the American College of Sports Medicine (ACSM), exercise prescription is the process of designing a regimen of physical activity in a systematic and individualized manner.[1,2] Each exercise prescription has five essential components:

1. Frequency
2. Duration
3. Intensity
4. Mode
5. Progression

These five components should be used when developing an exercise prescription for individuals of all ages and all fitness and health levels. This chapter places emphasis on exercise prescription principles for apparently healthy individuals, with attention given to a comprehensive fitness approach (both cardiorespiratory and musculoskeletal). In other chapters of this book, guidelines for adapting the basic exercise prescription for children and adolescents (Chapter 7), the elderly (Chapter 15), obese individuals (Chapter 13), cardiac patients (Chapter 10), diabetics (Chapter 12), cancer patients (Chapter 11), asthmatics (Chapter 16), arthritis patients (Chapter 15), and pregnant women (Chapter 16) are outlined. ACSM has published a textbook, *Exercise Management for Persons with Chronic Diseases and Disabilities*, which provides additional physical activity guidelines for a wide variety of patients, including those

with pulmonary disease, anemia, acquired immune deficiency syndrome (AIDS), chronic fatigue syndrome, stroke, spinal cord injury, epilepsy, cerebral palsy, mental retardation, visual impairment, and other diseases and disabilities[3] (see Box 8.1).

The major objective of exercise prescription is to facilitate positive changes in a client's personal physical activity habits.[1-10] According to the ACSM, "the art of exercise prescription is the successful integration of exercise science with behavioral techniques that result in long-term program compliance and attainment of the individual's goals."[2] This chapter reviews basic theories of health-behavior change. Chapter 1 summarized the strategies for increasing physical activity at both the population and individual levels, and the reader is invited to review that chapter once again.

According to the U.S. Surgeon General's report on physical activity and health, despite common knowledge that physical activity is healthful, more than 60% of American adults are not regularly active, and 25% of adults are not active at all (see Chapter 1).[11] Although a significant proportion of people have enthusiastically embarked on vigorous exercise programs at one time or another, most do not sustain that participation. These statistics have led to recent changes in recommendations for physical activity among various governmental and professional groups.

The first position statement from the ACSM on exercise prescription was published in 1978[12] (see Table 8.1). These

Box 8.1

Exercise Prescription Guidelines for People with Chronic Ailments

People who suffer from chronic ailments need to take special precautions when planning and following an exercise regimen.

Special Safety Tips

Coronary heart disease and hypertension

People with coronary disease

- Keep heart rate well below level where abnormalities appeared on stress test.
- Don't exercise near busy roads.
- Exercise with a companion.
- Carry nitroglycerin when you exercise. Take it if you experience chest pain; then see a doctor as soon as possible. (Or take nitroglycerin before workout instead.)

People with hypertension

- Keep heart rate below 70% of its maximum rate (220 − your age).

People on beta-blockers

- Beta-blockers slow heart rate, so gauge exercise intensity by perceived exertion, not by heart rate method. To stay in safe range, exercise should feel somewhat hard but should not make breathing or talking difficult.

Diabetes

- Take exercise stress test before starting exercise program, to rule out coronary disease.
- Keep heart rate below 70% of its maximum rate (220 − your age).
- To prevent excessive absorption of injected insulin, inject it into muscle that won't be exercised, then wait at least 1 hour before exercising.
- Wait at least 1 hour after meals before exercising.
- Check blood sugar levels before and after workout; if necessary, adjust diet or insulin dosage to prevent excessive drop in sugar.
- Carry sugar packets during workout, in case you feel symptoms of low blood sugar.

Arthritis

- Do only stretching when pain or inflammation is worse than usual.
- Try aerobic exercise only if you can do easier exercises, such as stretching or light strength training, without pain.
- Choose maximum intensity that causes no significant discomfort, including pain during workout and aches that persist for more than about 24 hours after workout.
- Consider doing calisthenics (in a heated pool) or tai chi, which can safely stretch and strengthen all major joints.

Osteoporosis

- Avoid strength training maneuvers that stress the back, since they can fracture vertebrae.
- Choose maximum intensity that causes no significant discomfort, including pain during workout and aches that persist for more than about 24 hours after workout.
- Be wary of exercises that involve any risk of falling.
- Choose weight-bearing exercises over activities such as swimming and biking, which put too little pressure on the hips and spine.

Asthma

- Drink water before, during, and after workout, even in cool weather, to moisten airways.
- If exercise triggers asthma attacks, take medication before workout and carry it during workout.
- Don't exercise near busy roads.
- Cover mouth with mask or scarf when exercising in cold, to heat and humidify air.
- For aerobic exercise, consider swimming because high humidity near water helps prevent attacks.

Benefits of Taking Precautions

	Warm up	Cool down	Watch the weather	Avoid high-impact exercise	Strength train safely
Precautions (general)	Do light calisthenics, march in place, or gently go through motions of exercise you're about to perform, for about 5 minutes.	After workout, walk slowly until heart rate is just 10 to 15 beats higher than resting rate. After cool-down, stretch.	Exercise indoors if weather is unfavorable for people with your disease (see below). Be particularly careful to drink plenty of water before, during, and after workout if it's hot or you sweat a lot.	Don't do activities that jar joints or require jumping, such as running, basketball, or certain aerobic-dance routines. Reduce impact by wearing well-padded shoes and exercising on soft surfaces.	Exhale during exertion phase of maneuver; inhale during other half of maneuver. Use elastic bands or weight machines, no free weights, if strength or balance has declined significantly.

Disease

	Warm up	Cool down	Watch the weather	Avoid high-impact exercise	Strength train safely
Coronary disease or hypertension	Prevents sudden rise in blood pressure and provides heart muscle with enough oxygen-bearing blood to meet initial demands of exercise.	Helps prevent sudden, potentially dangerous drop in blood pressure.	Fluid loss from heavy sweating can cause potentially dangerous drop in blood pressure and increases risk of potentially dangerous blood clots. Cold constricts blood vessels, raising blood pressure and forcing heart to pump harder. Polluted air reduces amount of oxygen reaching heart muscle.	High-impact exercise is generally strenuous; that can cause excessive rise in blood pressure or place excessive demands on heart.	Straining to lift excessive weight or holding breath during exertion can cause potentially dangerous rise in blood pressure.
Diabetes	By boosting blood flow, warming up partially compensates for the poor circulation in some diabetics.	Helps prevent sudden, dangerous drops in blood pressure, which are particularly likely in diabetics due to impaired blood-vessel constriction.	Poor circulation and impaired nerve function increase the likelihood of numbness in feet; cold further increases that likelihood, which can lead to foot injury during exercise. Neurologic problems may also impair sense of thirst, making dehydration more likely; rarely, such problems inhibit sweating, increasing risk of heat stroke.	Can break blood vessels in diseased eye or injure foot that is permanently numb due to nerve damage.	Straining and holding breath can break blood vessels in diseased eye.
Arthritis	Warms and loosens stiff muscles and joints.	Stretching after each workout helps maintain joint mobility by keeping muscles from contracting.	Cold stiffens joints and muscles.	Can damage arthritic joints.	Pushing past range of motion can injure joints.
Osteoporosis	No special warning.	No special warning.	Ice can cause bone-breaking falls.	Can crack thin bones.	Free weights can cause bone-breaking falls, if strength or balance is poor.
Asthma	Warming up warms the air entering lungs, reducing risk of asthma attacks.	Stopping abruptly can trigger attack.	Cold or polluted air, especially when dry, can trigger or worsen attack.	No special warning.	No special warning.

Source: Consumer Reports on Health, January, 1997. Copyright © 1997 by Consumers Union of U.S., Inc., Yonkers, NY 10703-1057. Reprinted by permission from *Consumer Reports,* January 1997. For more information, see American College of Sports Medicine, *ACSM's Exercise Management for Persons with Chronic Diseases and Disabilities.* Champaign, IL: Human Kinetics, 1997.

TABLE 8.1 Exercise Prescription Recommendations

	Intensity ($\%\dot{V}O_{2max}$)	Duration (minutes)	Frequency (days/week)	Purpose
ACSM, 1978	50–85%	15–60	3–5	Develop, maintain fitness, body composition
ACSM, 1990, 1998	50–85%	20–60	3–5	Develop, maintain fitness, body composition[a]
CDC–ACSM, 1995	Moderate/hard	30 or more in bouts of at least 8–10 min	Near daily	Health promotion[b]
AHA, 1996	40–75%	30–60	3–6	Health promotion and cardiovascular disease prevention[a]
NIH, 1996	Moderate/hard	30 or more	Near daily	Cardiovascular disease prevention for adults and children[b]
Surgeon General, 1996	Moderate/hard	30 or more	Near daily	Health promotion, disease prevention[b]

[a]Also includes recommendations for developing and maintaining muscular strength and endurance (at least one set of 8–12 repetitions of 8–10 exercises that condition the major muscle groups at least 2 days a week).
[b]Also recommends regular participation in physical activities that develop and maintain muscular strength.

guidelines recommended an exercise training frequency of 3–5 days per week, an intensity of 60–90% of maximal heart rate (50–85% of maximal oxygen uptake or heart rate reserve), a duration of 15–60 minutes per session, and an exercise mode that used large muscle groups, such as running, walking, swimming, bicycling, rowing, cross-country skiing, and rope skipping. These recommendations addressed only cardiorespiratory fitness and body composition, and did not provide guidelines for musculoskeletal fitness, or link physical activity patterns to health promotion and disease prevention.

In 1990 (confirmed again in 1998), the ACSM revised the 1978 exercise prescription guidelines by adding the development of musculoskeletal fitness as a major objective[2] (see Table 8.1). ACSM advised that people engage in resistance training at least 2–3 days a week (minimum of one set of 8–12 repetitions of 8–10 different exercises). The 1990 recommendations also noted that "it is now clear that lower levels of physical activity than recommended by this position statement may reduce the risk for certain chronic degenerative diseases and yet may not be of sufficient quantity or quality to improve maximal oxygen uptake."[2] Recommendations on frequency, intensity, and exercise mode remained similar, but the duration was increased slightly to 20–60 minutes per session.

Epidemiological research since the mid-1970s has shown that health-related benefits are linked to physical activity and fitness in a dose–response manner[4,5,9–11] (see Chapters 10 through 15). The greatest difference in death rates for coronary heart disease and certain forms of cancer has been observed between the least physically active or most unfit and the next higher category.[10] In other words, the most significant public health benefits are experienced when the most sedentary individuals become moderately active. Many of the epidemiological studies used physical activity indexes that counted all activities conducted throughout the day. Exercise training studies have also indicated that middle-aged and older persons, obese patients, and individuals with low aerobic fitness can improve both disease risk factors and cardiorespiratory fitness at exercise intensity levels below the 50% threshold urged by the ACSM.[11] A few controlled studies compared single-session bouts of exercise to multiple bouts spread throughout the day, and reported similar improvements in fitness and risk factors.[13–15]

In response to these research findings, the Centers for Disease Control and Prevention and ACSM (CDC–ACSM) released their most recent physical activity guidelines in 1993 (published in 1995), recommending that all adults perform 30 or more minutes of moderate-intensity physical activity on most, and preferably all, days, either in a single session or accumulated throughout the day in multiple bouts (each lasting 8–10 minutes)[16] (Figure 8.1, Table 8.1). This recommendation differed from the 1978 and 1990 ACSM statements on three points:

1. The minimum starting exercise intensity was lowered to 40% for patients or individuals with very low fitness.

2. The frequency of exercise sessions was increased from 3–5 days per week to 5–7 days per week.

3. An option was included for allowing people to accumulate the minimum of 30 minutes per day in multiple sessions lasting at least 8–10 minutes.

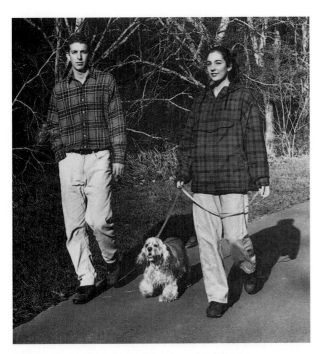

Figure 8.1 ACSM has urged that for public health benefits, every American adult should accumulate 30 minutes or more of moderate-intensity physical activity over the course of most days of the week.[3]

In 1998, ACSM revised their position stand on the recommended quantity and quality of exercise, stating that the minimal training intensity threshold for $\dot{V}O_{2max}$ is 40–50% of heart rate reserve, especially for the unfit. "The ACSM recognizes the potential health benefits of regular exercise performed more frequently and for a longer duration but at a lower intensity than recommended in the previous editions of this position stand, i.e. 40–49% of maximum $\dot{V}O_2$ reserve and heart rate reserve or 55–65% of maximum heart rate.... Thus, the ACSM now views exercise/physical activity for health and fitness in the context of an exercise dose continuum. That is, there is a dose response to exercise by which benefits are derived through varying quantities of physical activity ranging from approximately 700–2,000 plus kilocalories of effort per week."[2]

Other professional and governmental groups have responded by issuing similar reports. In 1992, the American Heart Association (AHA) published a statement identifying physical inactivity as a fourth major risk factor for coronary heart disease (along with smoking, high blood pressure, and high blood cholesterol).[17] The AHA published a second report in 1996 confirming the role of physical inactivity as a risk factor for heart disease and urging that people follow exercise guidelines similar to those released by the CDC–ACSM[18] (see Table 8.1). The AHA also advised that people pay attention to joint flexibility and muscle strength, especially as they age. A consensus statement from the 1993 International Consensus Conference on Physical Activity

Guidelines for Adolescents emphasized that youths should be physically active every day, as part of their general lifestyle activities and that they should engage in three or more 20-minute sessions of moderate-to-vigorous exercise each week[19] (see Chapter 7). In 1996, the American Cancer Society listed physical inactivity as a major risk factor for certain forms of cancer (see Chapter 15).[20] That same year, the U.S. Preventive Services Task Force recommended that healthcare providers counsel patients regarding the importance of incorporating physical activities into their daily routines to prevent coronary heart disease, hypertension, obesity, and diabetes.[21] The National Institutes of Health Consensus Development Panel on Physical Activity and Cardiovascular Health released a statement in 1995 (published in 1996; see Table 8.1) that encouraged all Americans to

> engage in regular physical activity at a level appropriate to their capacity, needs, and interest. Children and adults alike should set a goal of accumulating at least 30 minutes of moderate-intensity physical activity on most, and preferably all, days of the week.... Intermittent or shorter bouts of activity (at least 10 minutes), including occupational, nonoccupational, or tasks of daily living, also have similar cardiovascular and health benefits if performed at a level of moderate intensity (such as brisk walking, cycling, swimming, home repair, and yard work) with an accumulated duration of at least 30 minutes per day. People who currently meet the recommended minimal standards may derive additional health and fitness benefits from becoming more physically active or including more vigorous activity.... Developing muscular strength and joint flexibility is also important for an overall activity program to improve one's ability to perform tasks and to reduce the potential for injury.[22]

The surgeon general's report on physical activity and health was released in 1996[11] (see Chapter 1). This landmark report concluded that both the traditional, structured approach to exercise described by the ACSM in 1990 and the lifestyle approach recommended by the CDC–ACSM in 1993 and by the NIH in 1995 can be beneficial and that individual interests and opportunities should determine which is used. Five major recommendations were given[11] (see Table 8.1):

1. All people over the age of 2 years should accumulate at least 30 minutes of endurance-type physical activity, of at least moderate intensity, on most—preferably all—days of the week.

2. Additional health and functional benefits of physical activity can be achieved by adding more time in moderate-intensity activity, or by substituting more vigorous activity.

3. Persons with symptomatic cardiovascular disease, diabetes, or other chronic health problems who would like to increase their physical activity should be evaluated by a physician and provided an exercise program appropriate for their clinical status.

4. Previously inactive men over age 40, women over age 50, and people at high risk for cardiovascular disease should first consult a physician before embarking on a program of vigorous physical activity to which they are unaccustomed.

5. Strength-developing activities (resistance training) should be performed at least twice per week. At least 8–10 strength-developing exercises that use the major muscle groups of the legs, trunk, arms, and shoulders should be performed at each session, with one or two sets of 8–12 repetitions of each exercise.

This chapter describes in detail the traditional, structured exercise prescription guidelines published by the ACSM in 1990/1998.[2] However, as urged in the 1996 surgeon general's report, individual interests, goals, and opportunities should determine whether the structured or the lifestyle approach is used.[11] Even when the lifestyle approach is used, however, education on the five components of the structured exercise prescription (frequency, duration, intensity, mode, progression) should be given to the individual desiring to increase physical activity patterns. (See Physical Fitness Activities 8.1 and 8.2 for the two approaches in exercise prescription.)

THE INDIVIDUALIZED APPROACH

People vary widely in their health and fitness status, motivation, goals, occupation, age, needs, desires, and education.[1] Thus, to give an *exercise prescription* that best meets a person's needs in a safe and effective manner requires a clear understanding of that person.[1]

Part 2 of this book highlighted the need for obtaining medical, health, and physical fitness information for each participant to be given an exercise prescription. This cannot be emphasized enough. An exercise prescription should not be written before this information is available. In addition, it is a good idea to sit down with the person and discuss interests, felt needs, future goals, reasons for starting an exercise program, and feelings about the results of the physical fitness tests. (See Physical Fitness Activity 8.1.) (See Figure 8.2.) Once these preliminary requirements have been met, then the participant can be educated about the principles of exercise and given adequate leadership and direction through the use of an exercise prescription.

The focus since the late 1970s has been to use a comprehensive physical fitness approach. During the boom years of the aerobic movement in the 1970s and 1980s, cardiores-

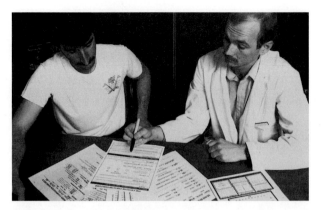

Figure 8.2 A clear understanding of the individual to be given the exercise prescription can be gained by reviewing medical, health, and physical fitness test information.

piratory conditioning was often the only type of exercise for many, leaving out exercises for flexibility and muscular strength and endurance. This was the reverse of what happened during the 1950s and 1960s, when muscular strength was preeminent, to the detriment of exercises for the heart and lungs. The comprehensive approach that has emerged gives attention to both cardiorespiratory and musculoskeletal fitness. On the other hand, cardiorespiratory training is still the foundation of any exercise prescription because most of the health benefits related to physical activity are associated with dynamic, whole-body, continuous, sustained activity.[4,5,11]

Figure 8.3 summarizes the comprehensive approach to physical fitness, emphasizing a five-step approach (i.e., warm-up, aerobic session, warm-down, flexibility exercises, muscular strength and endurance exercises). Each step, in the order given, is considered important for the development of "total fitness." The rest of this chapter focuses on describing these five steps.

Before discussing this conditioning format, an important point needs to be made. In order to realize the full benefits of regular exercise and physical activity, the development of physical fitness must be seen as one of several components contributing to wellness and health. Other components include adequate rest, a proper diet, management of stress, wholesome social and family influences, sufficient sunshine, pure air and water, sanitation, and a nurturing sense of spirituality. All these factors work together to promote health, happiness, and "good feelings."

CARDIORESPIRATORY ENDURANCE/ BODY COMPOSITION

Warm-Up

A *warm-up* is defined as a group of exercises performed immediately before an activity, which provides the body

THE EXERCISE PRESCRIPTION FORM

STAGE ONE—CARDIORESPIRATORY / BODY COMPOSITION

1. WARM-UP _____

   Purpose: To slowly elevate the pulse and body temperature to an aerobic level by engaging in 5–10 min of slow aerobic activity.

2. THE AEROBIC SESSION

   Purpose: To improve the cardiorespiratory system of the body by exercising vigorously for at least 20–30 min, 3 times/wk, on a regular basis.

		FITNESS STATUS	
F.I.T. GUIDELINES	Low	Average	High
F Frequency (sessions/wk)	3	3–4	≥5
I Intensity (% heart rate reserve)	40–60%	60–75%	70–85%
T Time (min/session)	10–20	20–30	30–60

   MODE SELECTION (your personal)_____

   TRAINING HR = [(MAX HR − RHR)× 40–85%]+ RHR

   _____ = _____ − _____ × _____ + _____

   DAYS OF WEEK AND TIME OF EXERCISE SESSIONS

   Sun_____ Mon_____ Tue_____ Wed_____ Thu_____ Fri_____ Sat_____

3. WARM-DOWN

   Purpose: To slowly decrease the heart rate and body temperature by engaging in slow aerobic activity for at least 5 min

STAGE TWO—MUSCULOSKELETAL FITNESS

1. FLEXIBILITY EXERCISES _____

   _____

   Purpose: To stretch the major muscles and joints, especially those involved in the aerobic session, using static stretching techniques.

2. MUSCULAR STRENGTH AND ENDURANCE EXERCISES _____

   _____

   Purpose: To build muscular endurance and strength, especially in the muscles not developed in the aerobic session, using appropriate weight-training and calisthenic exercises.

Figure 8.3 This exercise prescription form can be used to organize the exercise prescription process.

with a period of adjustment from rest to exercise.[23] Warm-up can take two forms:[23,24]

1. *Passive*—use of a warming agent to increase body temperature (e.g., hot baths, infrared light, ultrasound, or sauna)

2. *Active*—consisting of body movements to moderately increase the heart rate and body temperature; may include light calisthenics, jogging, stationary cycling, or exercises that provide a rehearsal for the actual performance activity (e.g., throwing a ball, swinging a bat, ballet or gymnastic movements)

The extent of the warm-up depends on individual needs, clothing, air temperature, and the intensity of the exercise to follow, but in general, the warm-up should be intense enough to increase the body's core temperature and cause some sweating.[22] However, the warm-up should not be so intense as to cause fatigue or reduce muscle glycogen stores.[24] Generally, warm-ups should take 5–20 minutes, depending on the sport and the environmental conditions.

There has been some debate as to whether *flexibility exercises* (i.e., exercises that are used to increase joint range of motion) should be included within the warm-up routine.[23–27] Some fitness leaders have advocated flexibility exercises prior to light aerobic warm-up activities,[25] while others urge that these exercises be conducted only after the body temperature has been elevated.[23] For instance, the textbook *Science of Flexibility* asserts that "flexibility exercises should always be preceded by a set of mild warm-up exercises, because the increase in the tissue temperature produced by the warm-up exercise will make the stretching both safer and more productive."[23] The ACSM has "recommended that an active warm-up precede vigorous stretching exercises."[1]

Holding *static flexibility* positions before the muscle becomes warm can be potentially injurious.[23] A good plan for athletes would be to exercise moderately for 5–10 minutes, then stretch, compete, cool down, and then stretch again. International-class gymnasts have long prepared for performances by running lightly (or engaging in other slow aerobic exercise) to raise body temperature, inducing a light perspiration, and then engaging in flexibility exercises.[28]

The physiological benefits of the warm-up are listed in Box 8.2.[23–36] In general, a thorough warm-up (meaning an elevation in body temperature) before hard aerobic exercise will enhance the activity of enzymes in the working muscles, reduce the viscosity of muscle, improve the mechanical efficiency and power of the moving muscles, facilitate the transmission speed of nervous impulses augmenting coordination, increase muscle blood flow and thus improve delivery of necessary fuel substrates, increase the level of free fatty acids in the blood, help prevent injuries to the muscles and various supporting connective tissues, and allow the heart muscle to adequately prepare itself for aerobic exercise.

For these reasons, researchers advise that the warm-up consist of the specific exercise that will be engaged in during the aerobic session, but at moderate intensity, allowing for a gradual increase in body temperature.[23] This not only warms the body, but also provides a slight rehearsal of the event that is to take place. Flexibility exercises should not be undertaken until the body is warm. Muscle, tendon, and ligament elasticity depends on blood saturation. Cold connective tissues, which have a low blood saturation, can be more susceptible to damage and do not stretch as readily.

For athletes, the best plan is to stretch just after the warm-up and just after the warm-down. Recreational exercisers can concentrate on flexibility exercises after the aerobic session is over. Stretching at this time has the special advantage of allowing one to stretch warm muscles that have been contracting forcibly during aerobic exercise. It makes sense that muscles that have been continually contracting and shortening should be lengthened after the session is over. This is safer, helps ease the aftereffects of the aerobic exercise, and allows greater stretching because the muscle is warm.

For example, a jogger would start the exercise session by walking for a minute or so, then jogging easily for 2–4 more minutes, and then finally building up speed to elevate

---

Box 8.2

Beneficial Effects of Warm-Up before Strenuous Exercise

1. Increases breakdown of oxyhemoglobin, allowing greater delivery of oxygen to the working muscle.

2. Increases the release of oxygen from myoglobin.

3. Decreases the activation energy for vital cellular metabolic chemical reactions.

4. Decreases muscle viscosity, improving mechanical efficiency and power.

5. Increases speed of nervous impulses and augments sensitivity of nerve receptors.

6. Increases blood flow to the muscles.

7. Decreases number of injuries to muscles, tendons, ligaments, and other connective tissues.

8. Improves the cardiovascular response to sudden, strenuous exercise (especially heart muscle blood flow).

9. Leads to earlier sweating, which reduces risk of high body temperature during exercise.

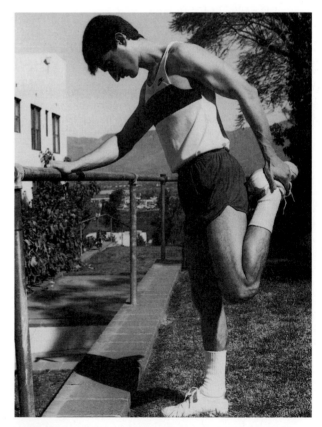

Figure 8.4 Flexibility exercises are best conducted when the body is warm from aerobic activity.

the pulse to the training-level intensity. After a warm-down with jogging/walking for several minutes (reversing the warm-up), static flexibility exercises can be performed for at least 5 minutes, emphasizing the posterior leg, lower back, and upper-front chest areas (muscles that are shortened during running). (See Figure 8.4.) The same would be true for swimmers or cyclers, except that flexibility exercises would be directed more toward shoulder and thigh areas, respectively.

The Aerobic Session

To be most effective, an exercise prescription must give specific written instructions for the frequency, intensity, and time of exercise. These are known as the F.I.T. criteria of cardiorespiratory endurance training. Figure 8.3 outlines the basic guidelines for aerobic exercise prescription, and Figure 8.5 puts this in graphic form. Improvement in $\dot{V}O_{2max}$ is directly related to the F.I.T. criteria followed in training. Depending on the quantity and quality of training, improvement in $\dot{V}O_{2max}$ ranges from 5 to 30%.[1,2] Greater improvement may be found for those with a very low initial level of fitness due to obesity or cardiac disease. Many articles have been written on exercise prescription.[2,6–8,12,16–19] A discussion of the major criteria follows.

Frequency

Frequency of exercise refers to the number of exercise sessions per week in the exercise program. In order both to improve cardiorespiratory endurance and keep body fat at optimal levels, most reviewers have concluded that it is necessary to exercise at least three times weekly with no more than 2 days between workouts.[1,2,6] Some studies have shown some cardiorespiratory improvements with an exercise frequency of less than 3 days per week, but such improvements are at most minimal to modest and result in little or no body fat loss.

When a person is initiating an aerobic exercise program, conditioning every other day is recommended. This is especially true for running programs with those who are unfit and have been previously sedentary. For such people, the musculoskeletal system is unable to adapt quickly to hard daily exercise, and it will lead to muscle soreness, fatigue, and injury. If those starting a running program want to exercise more frequently than 3 days per week, jogging days should be mixed with days of walking, bicycling, or swimming, which are easier on the musculoskeletal system.

ACSM recommends that patients with a low functional capacity (<3 METs) may benefit from multiple short exercise sessions (of about 3–5 minutes each) spread throughout each day.[1] As fitness improves to 3–5 METs, one to two short sessions each day are appropriate, before moving to longer sessions of 20–30 minutes, 3–5 days a week.

In the lifestyle approach advocated by the CDC–ACSM, individuals are urged to accumulate at least 30 minutes of moderate-intensity physical activity on most, preferably all, days of the week.[16] This recommendation emphasizes the benefits of moderate-intensity physical activity and of physical activity that can be accumulated in multiple short bouts. According to the CDC–ACSM, the recommended 30 minutes of activity can be accumulated by frequently walking up the stairs instead of taking the elevator, walking instead of driving short distances, doing calisthenics, or pedaling a stationary cycle while watching television.[16] Gardening, housework, raking leaves, dancing, and playing actively with children can also contribute to the 30-minute-per-day total, urges the CDC–ACSM, if performed at an intensity corresponding to brisk walking. Research from Finland has demonstrated that people who walk or cycle to work gain substantial health and fitness benefits.[37]

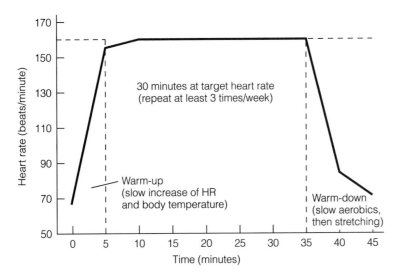

Figure 8.5 The aerobic exercise session: Exercise heart rates and time for average college student. The aerobic session has three phases (warm-up, exercising at the target heart rate, and warm-down).

Several experimental studies have addressed the effects of continuous versus intermittent activity on fitness. In one study conducted at Stanford University, three daily 10-minute bouts of moderate-to-vigorous activity were found to have a similar effect on fitness improvement, as compared to a single 30-minute daily period of exercise.[13] In Japan, a study showed that one, two, or three running sessions a day had comparable effects on fitness improvement when intensity and running distance were equalized.[14] Another study at the University of Pittsburgh showed that multiple short bouts improved exercise adherence during a 20-week period and was as effective as long single bouts in improving fitness.[15] More research in this area is needed to confirm both the fitness and the health benefits of multiple short bouts of exercise spread throughout the day. In the University of Pittsburgh study, the researchers reported that the subjects preferred exercising in durations of approximately 15 minutes and were unable to maintain four exercise bouts per day, as was prescribed.[15] Thus, two or three 15-minute exercise sessions per day may be preferable for adherence, rather than several 10-minute bouts.

Athletic endeavor requires a high frequency and intensity of training, as discussed in Chapter 7.[38] Many athletes put in double workouts each day for many years to improve aerobic power, anaerobic threshold, and economy of movement. (See the section on systems of training, later on in this chapter).

Intensity

As described previously in Chapter 4, the *maximum heart rate* (HR_{max}) represents the maximum attainable heart rate at the point of exhaustion from all-out exertion. During a graded treadmill test, the ECG heart rate recorder measures the maximum heart rate when the person reaches total exhaustion. If the oxygen uptake is measured at this same point, the $\dot{V}O_{2max}$ can be determined ($ml \cdot kg^{-1} \cdot min^{-1}$). (See Figure 8.6.)

For healthy adults to develop and maintain cardiorespiratory fitness and proper body composition, the American College of Sports Medicine and others have emphasized that the *intensity of exercise* needs to be between 50 and 85% of *maximum heart rate reserve,* which is approximately the same as 50–85% of maximum oxygen uptake reserve.[1,2] Maximum heart rate reserve (HRR) and maximum $\dot{V}O_2$ reserve ($\dot{V}O_2$ R) are calculated from the difference between resting and maximum heart rate and resting and maximum $\dot{V}O_2$, respectively. To estimate training intensity, a percentage of this value is added to the resting heart rate and/or resting $\dot{V}O_2$ and is expressed as a percentage of HRR or $\dot{V}O_2R$.[2] As emphasized earlier in this chapter, when improved health and lowered disease risk are the goals, intensity of exercise can drop to 40%, with duration and frequency becoming the more important standards.[1] These recommendations are based on substantial evidence that

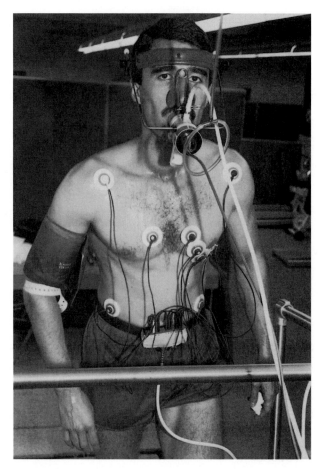

Figure 8.6 Although not required, the process of exercise prescription is enhanced when maximal heart rate and $\dot{V}O_{2max}$ are measured during graded exercise testing.

low-to-moderate levels of physical activity can reduce risk of heart disease and other chronic conditions, even though they do not produce significant changes in $\dot{V}O_{2max}$, and that long-term adherence to exercise regimens goes down when intensity rises above moderate levels.[11,16,39–41] However, as noted in the NIH[22] and surgeon general[11] reports,[11] the greatest fitness and health benefits are experienced by individuals who are capable of sustained, high-intensity exercise on a regular basis.[42,43]

For athletes, the greatest improvements in aerobic power occur when intensity is high (90–100% $\dot{V}O_2R$).[38,44] When exercise duration exceeds 30–45 minutes, training intensity can be reduced to 70–80% $\dot{V}O_2R$ and training effects will be similar to those from training at higher intensities for shorter durations. Athletes need to balance this information with the consistent finding that high-intensity exercise increases the risk of injury.

As explained in Chapter 7, top athletes do interval training (mixing race-pace-intensity exercise with recovery) to improve fitness for competition.[38] Even with two or three intense sessions a week, however, elite athletes (when fol-

TABLE 8.2   MET Values for Various Physical Activities

Physical Activity	MET Range	Physical Activity	MET Range
Archery	3–4	Running	
Backpacking	5–11	12 min per mile	8.7
Badminton	4–9+	11 min per mile	9.4
Basketball		10 min per mile	10.2
Nongame	3–9	9 min per mile	11.2
Game play	7–12+	8 min per mile	12.5
Bicycle		7 min per mile	14.1
Pleasure	3–8+	6 min per mile	16.3
10 mph	7	Sailing	2–5
Bowling	2–4	Scuba diving	5–10
Canoeing, rowing, kayaking	3–8	Skating, ice and roller	5–8
Calisthenics	3–8+	Skiing, snow	
Dancing		Downhill	5–8
Social and square	3–7	Cross-country	6–12+
Aerobic	6–9	Skiing, water	5–7
Fencing	6–10+	Sledding, tobogganing	4–8
Fishing		Snowshoeing	7–14
Bank, boat, or ice	2–4	Squash	8–12+
Stream, wading	5–6	Soccer	5–12+
Football (touch)	6–10	Stair climbing	4–8
Golf		Swimming	4–8+
Power cart	2–3	Table tennis	3–5
Walking, carrying bag or pulling cart	4–7	Tennis	4–9+
Handball	8–12+	Volleyball	3–6
Hiking, cross-country	3–7	Walking	
Horseback riding	3–8	1.7 mph	2.3
Horseshoe pitching	2–3	2.0 mph	2.4
Hunting, walking		2.5 mph	2.9
Small game (walking, carrying light load)	3–7	3.0 mph	3.3
Big game (dragging carcass, walking)	3–14	3.4 mph	3.6
Mountain climbing	5–10+	Uphill	5–10+
Music playing	2–3		
Paddleball, racquetball	8–12		
Rope jumping	9–12		

+ = MET level may be higher than indicated, depending on how vigorously the exercise is engaged in.

Source: American College of Sports Medicine. *ACSM's Guidelines for Exercise Testing and Prescription* (5th ed.). Baltimore: Williams & Wilkins, 1995. Used with permission.

lowed for 6–8 weeks with heart rate monitors) have been found to average 60–65% $\dot{V}O_2R$ during training when all sessions are included.[45]

Calculating Exercise Intensity   Exercise intensity can be assessed using the results of the graded exercise test. Based on the length of time the participant stays on the treadmill, $\dot{V}O_{2max}$ can be estimated. (See Chapter 4.) This $\dot{V}O_{2max}$ can be expressed in METs ($3.5 \text{ ml} \cdot \text{kg}^{-1} \cdot \text{min}^{-1} = 1$ MET). If the subject desires to exercise at 70% of $\dot{V}O_{2max}$, then the MET value is simply multiplied by 70%. For example, if a participant has a $\dot{V}O_{2max}$ of 10 METs, then 70% times 10 METs is

7 METs. Tables 8.2 and 8.3 can then be consulted to determine the types of activities that represent the 7-MET level.[1] Also consult Appendix E for a full compendium of the MET values of physical activities.[46]

However, using a set MET level for exercise can have some disadvantages. Various environmental factors such as wind, hills, sand, snow, heat, cold, humidity, altitude, pollution, and bulky or restrictive clothing, can increase or decrease the amount of actual work being accomplished during a given activity.[1] Also, as the person improves in fitness, different MET levels will be needed to ensure an adequate training stimulus.

TABLE 8.3   Occupation Activities and MET Values

MET	Occupational Activities
1.5–2	Desk work, driving auto, electric calculating machine operation, light housework—polishing furniture or washing clothes
2–3	Auto repair, radio and TV repair, janitorial work, riding lawn mower, light woodworking
3–4	Brick laying, plastering, wheelbarrow (100 lb load), machine assembly, welding, cleaning windows, mopping floors, vacuuming
4–5	Painting, masonry, paperhanging, light carpentry, raking leaves
5–6	Digging garden, shoveling light earth
6–7	Shoveling 10 times/min (10 lb), splitting wood, snow shoveling
7–8	Digging ditches, carrying 36 kg or 80 lb, sawing hardwood
8–9	Shoveling 10 times/min (14 lb)
10+	Shoveling 10 times/min (16 lb)

Note: Since 1 MET = 1 kcal $\cdot$ kg^{-1} $\cdot$ hour^1, multiply the MET value by the body weight of the person in kg, and divide by 60 min per hour to obtain the energy expenditure in kcal $\cdot$ min^{-1}. Example for a 65-kg person playing golf while carrying his or her clubs: 5 METs = 5 kcal $\cdot$ kg^{-1} $\cdot$ hour^1 $\cdot$ (5 kcal $\cdot$ hour^{-1} $\times$ 65 kg)/60 min $\cdot$ hr^{-1} = 5.4 kcal $\cdot$ min^{-1}.

Source: Fox SM, et al. Physical activity and cardiovascular health. *Mod Concepts Cardiovasc Dis* 41:25–30, 1972. Used with permission of the American Heart Association, Inc.

For these reasons, either the training heart rate or the rating of perceived exertion (RPE) is often used instead as an indicator of exercise intensity. The heart rate and the RPE are indicators of exercise intensity that adjust for environmental factors and improvement in fitness.

There are several methods of determining the *training heart rate*. The first method used by researchers is to plot the slope of the line between a person's exercise heart rates and the exercise workload in METs or $\dot{V}O_2$.[1] (See Chapter 4.) From this relationship, the exercise heart rate pertaining to a given percent of $\dot{V}O_{2max}$ can be obtained.

A second method for determining the exercise heart rate for training is to calculate a given percentage of the maximum heart rate (MHR).[1] However, this method is not the same as using the heart rate reserve or $\dot{V}O_{2max}$[1] and will result in an underestimation of the training heart rate unless an upward adjustment is made. ACSM recommends that 60–90% of maximum heart rate gives training heart rates similar to 50–85% of HRR or $\dot{V}O_2$R.[2]

The relationship between percent HR$_{max}$, percent $\dot{V}O_2$R, and percent HRR is summarized in Table 8.4. Various regression equations have been developed to express the relationship between percent HR$_{max}$ and percent $\dot{V}O_{2max}$, and they vary according to exercise mode, as shown in Table 8.5.[47] In general, exercise modes that are upright and weight bearing (e.g., walking/running and stair climbing) affect the percent HR$_{max}$ and percent $\dot{V}O_{2max}$ relationship differ-

TABLE 8.4   Classification of Physical Activity Intensity, Based on Physical Activity Lasting up to 60 Minutes

Intensity	Endurance-Type Activity							Strength-Type Exercise
	Relative Intensity			Absolute Intensity (METs) in Healthy Adults (age in years)				Relative Intensity[a]
	Maximum $\dot{V}O_2$ Reserve; Heart Rate Reserve (%)	Maximal Heart Rate (%)	RPE[b]	Young (20–39)	Middle-aged (40–64)	Old (65–79)	Very Old (80+)	Maximal Voluntary Contraction (%)
Very light	<20	<35	<10	<2.4	<2.0	<1.6	≤1.0	<30
Light	20–39	33–54	10–11	2.4–4.7	2.0–3.9	1.6–3.1	1.1–1.9	30–49
Moderate	40–59	55–69	12–13	4.8–7.1	4.0–5.9	3.2–4.7	2.0–2.9	50–69
Hard	60–84	70–89	14–16	7.2–10.1	6.0–8.4	4.8–6.7	3.0–4.25	70–84
Very hard	≥85	≥90	17–19	≥10.2	≥8.5	≥6.8	≥4.25	>85
Maximal[c]	100	100	20	12.0	10.0	8.0	5.0	100

[a]Based on 8–12 repetitions for persons under age 50–60 years and 10–15 repetitions for persons age 50–60 years and older.
[b]Borg rating of relative perceived exertion (RPE) 6–20 scale.
[c]Maximal values are mean values achieved during maximal exercise by healthy adults. Absolute intensity values (METs) are approximate mean values for men. Mean values for women are approximately 1–2 METs lower than those for men.

Sources: U.S. Department of Health and Human Services. *Physical Activity and Health: A Report of the Surgeon General.* Atlanta, GA: U.S. Department of Health and Human Services, Centers for Disease Control and Prevention, National Center for Chronic Disease Prevention and Health Promotion, 1996; American College of Sports Medicine. The recommended quantity and quality of exercise for developing and maintaining cardiorespiratory and muscular fitness, and flexibility in healthy adults. *Med Sci Sports Exerc* 30:975–991, 1998.

TABLE 8.5 Regression Equations for Estimating Percent $\dot{V}O_{2max}$ from Percent HR_{max} for Different Exercise Modes

Exercise Mode	Estimating Equation for $\dot{V}O_{2max}$	At 70% HR_{max}
Treadmill walking/running	% $\dot{V}O_{2max}$ = (1.303 × %HR_{max}) − 34.5	56.7%
Cycle ergometer	% $\dot{V}O_{2max}$ = (1.408 × %HR_{max}) − 45.1	53.5%
Cross-country ski simulator	% $\dot{V}O_{2max}$ = (1.271 × %HR_{max}) − 34.4	54.6%
Stair-climber ergometer	% $\dot{V}O_{2max}$ = (1.224 × %HR_{max}) − 28.4	57.3%
Rowing erometer	% VO_{2max} = (1.182 × %HR_{max}) − 21.0	61.7%
Combined average	% VO_{2max} = (1.273 × %HR_{max}) − 31.8	57.3%

Source: Londeree BR, Thomas TR, Ziogas G, Smith TD, Zhang Q. %$\dot{V}O_{2max}$ versus %HR_{max} regressions for six modes of exercise. *Med Sci Sports Exerc* 27:458–461, 1995.

ently than weight-supported modes (e.g., cycling and rowing). The relationship between percent HR_{max} and percent $\dot{V}O_{2max}$ can be expressed with this equation:

$$\% \dot{V}O_{2max} = (1.273 \times \%HR_{max}) - 31.8$$

For example, at a percent HR_{max} of 80, percent $\dot{V}O_{2max}$ would be estimated with this equation to be 70, a 10% difference. At a percent HR_{max} of 90, percent $\dot{V}O_{2max}$ would be estimated to be 83, a 7% difference.

The third method for determining training heart rate was developed in Scandinavia.[48,49] The *Karvonen formula* attempts to calculate the training heart rate using a percentage of the HRR, which is the difference between the maximum and resting heart rates. (See Figure 8.7.)

Training heart rate
$$= [(MHR - RHR) \times 40\text{–}85\%] + RHR$$

(MHR = maximum heart rate; RHR = resting heart rate.) The intensity range of 40–85% of heart rate reserve is approximately equal to 40–85% of $\dot{V}O_2R$.

Investigators from Old Dominion University have shown that a sizeable error exists in the relationship between percent HRR and percent $\dot{V}O_{2max}$ at low exercise intensity, especially for relatively unfit subjects.[50] Researchers from the University of Florida have shown that percent heart rate reserve was less than percent $\dot{V}O_{2max}$ at various exercise intensities for elderly subjects, and that the percent HR_{max} more closely represented percent $\dot{V}O_{2max}$ in this age group.[51] In 1998, ACSM began relating HRR to $\dot{V}O_2R$ rather than a percentage of $\dot{V}O_{2max}$.[2,48–51] Using $\dot{V}O_2R$ improves the accuracy of the relationship, particularly at the lower end of the intensity scale. It is incorrect, according to ACSM, to relate HRR to a level of $\dot{V}O_2$ that starts from zero rather than a resting level.[2] Table 8.6 summarizes recommendations for the appropriate intensity percentile to be used in the Karvonen formula.

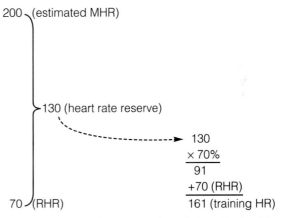

Figure 8.7 Use of the Karvonen formula for a 20-year-old man (average shape, RHR = 70 bpm). The Karvonen formula calculates the training heart rate using a percentage of the *heart rate reserve,* the difference between the maximum and resting heart rates.

TABLE 8.6 Criteria for Choosing Intensity Percentile for Karvonen Formula

Criteria	Intensity Range
Low fitness status and/or desiring lower intensity, longer duration program	40%–60%
Average fitness status	60%–75%
Excellent fitness status and/or an athlete desiring to improve fitness for competition	75%–85%

There are two methods of determining maximum heart rate. The most accurate way is to directly measure the maximum heart rate with an ECG recorder during graded exercise testing. The other way is to estimate MHR by using the simple formula:[1]

$$MHR = 220 - Age$$

The problem with using this formula is that it is based on population averages, with a standard deviation of ± 12 bpm. In other words, there is large variability. For example a 20-year-old would be estimated to have a MHR of 200 bpm, but two thirds of individuals of this age could actually have MHRs varying between 188 and 212 bpm. If estimations are used, the accuracy of the Karvonen formula is lessened. When the training heart rate is based on an estimated maximum heart rate, it should not be used as a precise measure and should be readjusted if the exercise participant complains that perceived exertion (using the Borg scale) is "very hard" or higher. Various attempts have been made to improve the accuracy of estimating MHR. One research group from Ball State University tested 2,010 men and women and found the following equations work better:[52]

Men

$$MHR = 203.9 - (0.812 \times age) + (0.276 \times RHR) - (0.084 \times kg) - (4.5 \times smoking\ code)$$

Women

$$MHR = 204.8 - (0.718 \times age) + (0.162 \times RHR) - (0.105 \times kg) - (6.2 \times smoking\ code)$$

(MHR = maximum heart rate; RHR = resting heart rate; kg = body weight in kilograms; smoking code: 1 = smoker; 0 = non-smoker.) These equations account for the fact that people with higher RHRs tend also to have higher MHRs, while smokers and heavyweight people tend to have lower MHRs. Also the "220 − age" equation has been found to underestimate MHR for many older people. For obese people (body fat >30%), this equation has been shown to estimate MHR quite accurately: $MHR = 200 - (0.5 \times age)$.[53]

To determine the resting heart rate, it is best to take one's pulse while in a sitting position, upon waking in the morning. This should be done three mornings in a row, and then the values are averaged. After waking, one should allow the heart to calm down, which might mean sitting quietly for a few minutes or emptying the bladder.

Resting heart rates taken prior to graded exercise testing are often elevated because of pretest apprehension. In such situations, it is best to estimate the resting heart rate based on the health and fitness history of the person. (See Appendix A, Table 21, for resting heart rate [RHR] norms.) Some people are in the habit of taking their RHRs on a periodic, regular basis, and if they are validated with careful questioning, these reported values can be used.

Based on the results of the graded exercise test or exercise history, and the exercise goals of the person, the intensity percentile used in the Karvonen formula can be varied, as summarized in Table 8.6.

To summarize with an example, the exercise training heart rate for a 20-year-old male of average cardiorespiratory fitness and a resting heart rate of 70 bpm would be calculated as follows (see Figure 8.7):

$$(MHR - RHR) \times intensity\ percentage + RHR = training\ heart\ rate$$

$$(200 - 70) \times 70\% + 70 = 161\ bpm$$

So this 20-year-old person of average fitness status would need to exercise at an intensity of 161 bpm, for 20–30 minutes, 3–5 days a week, to develop and maintain a healthy level of cardiorespiratory fitness and proper body composition. Figure 8.8 summarizes the training heart rate zone for people of various ages.

Assessment of Training Heart Rate   Training heart rate or intensity can be assessed by three methods:

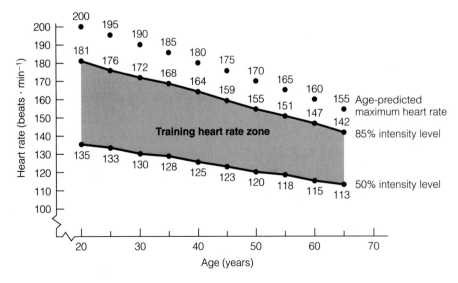

Figure 8.8 Training heart rate zone using the Karvonen formula. Maximal heart rates and the training heart rate zone for people of varying ages using the Karvonen formula. The resting heart rate is assumed to be 70 bpm.

1. The metabolic method (the use of METs or Calories per minute) (Tables 8.2, 8.3).

2. Measurement of the pulse for 10 seconds

3. The use of the Borg rating of perceived exertion scale[1]

To measure training heart rate during exercise, the participant should stop every 5 minutes or so during the initial days of the exercise program and count the pulse. It should be located quickly, within 1–2 seconds.

The pulse is best counted using the carotid pulse; when properly done, this method is safe and accurate.[54] When palpating the carotid pulse, two fingers of one hand should be placed lightly on one side of the neck adjacent to the larynx or voice box area. (See Figure 8.9.)

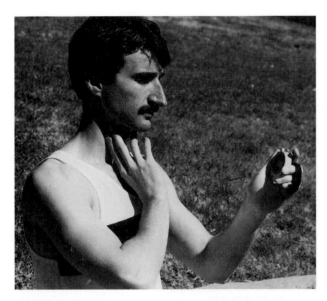

Figure 8.9 To measure the training heart rate during exercise, the participant should stop periodically and count the pulse, using the carotid artery.

TABLE 8.7 10-Second Pulse Count Values for Various Ages, Based on the Karvonen Formula for Average Fitness Status and RHR of 70 BPM

Age Range	10-Second Pulse Count
20–24	27
25–29	26
30–34	25–26
35–39	25
40–44	25
45–49	24–25
50–54	24
55–59	23–24
60–64	23
65–69	22–23

Beginners should compare resting heart rates taken by both carotid and radial palpations (the latter taken on the thumb side of the bottom of the wrist). If the carotid pulse rate is consistently lower than the radial count, it is advisable to use the radial count because some people's heart rates slow down when their carotid pulse is palpated, especially when excessive pressure is applied. However, during exercise, the radial pulse is more difficult to locate because it is smaller and lies among the tendons of the hand and finger flexors. So if possible, it is best to learn to take the carotid pulse properly (as lightly as possible).[55]

To estimate the pulse during an exercise bout, count for 10 seconds, and then multiply by six. Table 8.7 gives 10-second pulse count values for various age groups. These training heart rate values have been estimated using the Karvonen formula, assuming average fitness status and resting heart rates of 70 bpm.

Various heart rate monitors have been developed to aid the exerciser in counting the pulse. The best ones use chest-strap transmitters that wirelessly signal the heart rate to a monitor on the wrist. These types of heart rate monitors have been found to agree within one or two heart beats per minute with ECG recordings. (See Figure 8.10; see Appendix B for a listing of companies that sell these monitors.)

Although monitoring exercise heart rates with the 10-second carotid pulse count or heart rate monitors has been popular and generally satisfactory, errors do occur, arising from mistakes in counting, difficulty in finding the palpation site, taking too long (and thereby measuring an altered rate), or slippage of the chest-strap transmitter. Various medications can also affect the exercise heart rate (see Table 8.8). Heart rate monitors are also expensive (about $100–$500). In addition, some participants do not like to

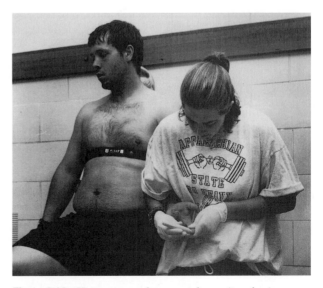

Figure 8.10 Heart rates can be accurately monitored using chest-strap transmitters that wirelessly signal the heart rate to a monitor on the wrist.

TABLE 8.8   Effects of Medications on the Exercise Heart Rate and Blood Pressure

Medication	Exercise Heart Rate	Exercise Blood Pressure
Beta blockers	↓	↓
Nitrates	↑ or ↔	↓ or ↔
Calcium channel blockers		
Felodopine, isradipine, nicardipine, nifedipine	↑ or ↔	↓
Bepridil, diltiazem, verapamil	↓	↓
Digitalis	↓ or ↔	↔
Diuretics	↔	↓ or ↔
Vasodilators		
Nonadrenergic	↑ or ↔	↓
ACE inhibitors	↔	↓
Alpha-adrenergic blockers	↔	↓
Antiarrhythmic agents		
Quinidine, disopyramide	↑ or ↔	↔
Bronchodilators		
Anticholinergic agents	↔	↔
Methylxanthines	↑ or ↔	↔
Sympathomimetic agents	↑ or ↔	↔ ↓ ↑
Cromolyn sodium, corticosteroids	↔	↔
Hyperlipidemic agents		
Clofibrate, nicotinic acid, probucol, others	↔	↔
Psychotropic medications		
Antidepressants, major tranquilizers	↑ or ↔	↓ or ↔
Lithium	↔	↔
Antihistamines	↔	↔
Cold medications	↑ or ↔	↔ ↓ ↑
Thyroid medications	↑	↑
Insulin, oral hypoglycemic agents	↔	↔
Anticoagulants	↔	↔
Antigout medications	↔	↔
Antiplatelet medications	↔	↔

Source: American College of Sports Medicine. *ACSM's Guidelines for Exercise Testing and Prescription* (5th ed.). Baltimore: Williams & Wilkins, 1995. Used with permission.

worry about taking their heart rates or feel that it is unnecessary.

To counter these problems, Gunnar Borg, a professor of psychology in Sweden, developed the rating (R) of perceived (P) exertion (E) scale (RPE) in the 1960s.[56] Two types of RPE scales are most commonly used (see Table 8.9). The RPE scale is very easy to use. After some basic instructions on what the numbers mean and the importance of being honest, the people exercising are asked, "How hard do you feel it to be?" Exercisers then give a number from the RPE scale to indicate how the exercise feels to them at that moment. In the original RPE scale, the numbers ranged from 6 to 20 and corresponded roughly to a heart rate range of 60 to 200 beats / min.

Borg's original RPE scale was convenient for indirectly tracking heart rate and oxygen consumption, which increase linearly with increased workload. This scale did not account for variables such as lactic acid and excessive ventilation, which rise in a nonlinear fashion. Consequently, a category scale with ratio properties was developed.[57] The ratio scale uses verbal expressions, which are simple to understand and more accurately describe sensations such as aches and pain. Both scales have been used to rate effort signals from the entire body during exercise.

TABLE 8.9   Perceived Exertion Category Scales

Fifteen-Category RPE Scale		Category-Ratio RPE Scale	
6	No exertion at all	0	Nothing at all
7	Extremely light	0.5	Very, very weak (just noticeable)
8			
9	Very light	1	Very weak
10		2	Weak (light)
11	Light	3	Moderate
12		4	Somewhat strong
13	Somewhat hard	5	Strong (heavy)
14		6	
15	Hard (heavy)	7	Very strong
16		8	
17	Very hard	9	
18		10	Very, very strong (almost max)
19	Extremely hard	●	Maximal
20	Maximal exertion		

Sources: Borg GAV. *Med Sci Sports Exerc* 14:377–387, 1982; Noble B, Borg GAV, Jacobs I, Ceci R, Kaiser P. *Med Sci Sports Exerc* 15:523–528, 1983.

There is widespread consensus that perception of effort during aerobic exercise is determined by a combination of sensory inputs from local factors (sensations of strain or discomfort in the exercising muscles and joints) and central factors (sensations related to rapid heart beat and breathing rates).[58] The RPE scale is often used during graded exercise testing to indicate perceived exertion (see Figure 8.11).

Available evidence suggests that RPE independently or in combination with pulse rate can be effectively used for prescribing exercise intensity.[58-60] Indeed, an RPE of "somewhat hard or strong" may be more effective for some people than heart rate in estimating the percentage of $\dot{V}O_{2max}$ necessary to elicit a training effect.

Trained and untrained men and women have been found to perceive the exercise intensity at the lactate threshold (intensity at which lactate begins to accumulate in the blood) as "somewhat hard or strong" (13 to 14 on the original RPE Borg scale, 4 on the category-ratio, 10-point scale).[59] In other words, despite gender or state of cardiorespiratory fitness, the "somewhat hard" level correlates with exercising at the lactate threshold, a point that is recommended as the ideal exercise intensity.

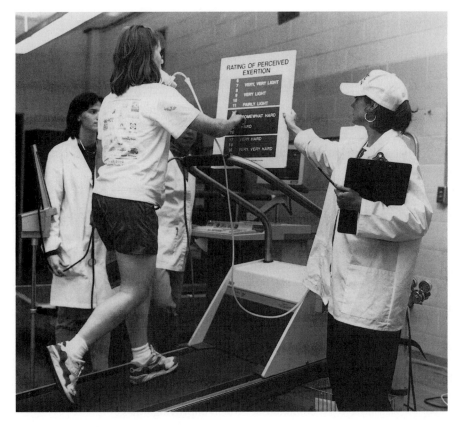

Figure 8.11   The RPE scale is commonly used during graded exercise testing to indicate progress toward maximal exertion.

When exercising at the "somewhat hard" level, one can think, talk intermittently with a partner, look around and enjoy the scenery, and engage in prolonged endurance activity. When exercising at a "very hard" level, the pulse is too high, and it is difficult to talk or exercise for prolonged periods of time. When exercising below "somewhat hard," the exercise stimulus is not adequate to develop cardiorespiratory endurance. The level of training intensity that can be tolerated depends on several factors, such as age, experience, fitness status, health, and motivation.[1] Long-distance runners are capable of running 26.2-mile marathons at 80% $\dot{V}O_{2max}$, while most beginners cannot tolerate this level for more than 5–15 minutes. For this reason, beginners should choose a lower intensity level, near 40–60% of heart rate reserve. The intensity percentage can gradually be increased during the ensuing weeks of training.

In summary, the RPE has several advantages:[56-65]

- Simple to use, takes only a few seconds, and costs little

- Good correlation to blood lactate and oxygen consumption measures

- For people on certain types of medications, better than the heart rate in determining the proper exercise training zone

- Teaches people to "listen" to their bodies during exercise

There are some problems, however, with the RPE method:[56-65]

- The RPE scale may not give an accurate indication of exercise intensity in children and elderly subjects, and the obese.

- People who were depressed, neurotic, or anxious tend to give high RPE numbers, while extroverts tend to give low numbers. Thus, psychological factors and mood state can affect RPE responses.

- The RPE is less reliable at low versus high workloads.

- Feelings in the legs and the chest both influence the RPE, but depending on the intensity and mode of activity, the most potent sensation determines what RPE number is given. Thus, different exercise modes (running versus cycling, for example) may give different RPE responses despite similar percent $\dot{V}O_{2max}$ levels.

- In the heat, people tend to give RPE numbers that are too high for the effort.

- In the lab, RPE indications tend to differ from those at the same level of effort outside in pleasant surroundings.

- During long exercise bouts (for example, greater than 1 hour), the RPE tends to increase despite no change in the percent $\dot{V}O_{2max}$.

Because of weaknesses and strengths in both the heart rate and the RPE methods, most authorities recommend that exercisers learn to use both. As explained by Borg,

> The aches and the strain we feel may be very important indicators of the real degree of strain, taking all physiological and psychological factors together. We should not rigidly keep to a certain heart rate, e.g., 130 or 150 beats/minute. On one occasion this might be a suitable intensity level. Another day when he or she has a slight infection, has been working hard for many days and been subjected to a very heavy physical and emotional stress, to exercise at 150 beats/minute may feel very hard and stressful. The extra strain he/she then feels in comparison to the usual feeling is most probably an important symptom and a good reason to take it a bit easier.[62]

Time

Time of exercise refers to the duration of time in minutes that the proper intensity level should be maintained to develop $\dot{V}O_{2max}$. Beginners should start with 10–20 minutes of aerobic activity, those in average shape should go for 20–30 minutes, and highly fit people can exercise for 30–60 minutes.[1,2]

In 1998, ACSM advised that "duration is dependent on the intensity of the activity; thus lower-intensity activity should be conducted over a longer period of time (30 minutes or more), and, conversely, individuals training at higher levels of intensity should train at least 20 minutes or longer. Because of the importance of "total fitness" and that it is more readily attained with exercise sessions of longer duration and because of the potential hazards and adherence problems associated with high-intensity activity, moderate-intensity activity of longer duration is recommended for adults not training for athletic competition."[2]

For health benefits, ACSM recommends accumulating 30 minutes or more of moderate-intensity physical activity during most days.[3] As discussed earlier, this is based on growing evidence that even when fitness is the goal, splitting up the exercise session to several different times of the day is just about as beneficial as doing it all at once.[11,13-16] Two studies from Finland have shown, for example, that intermittent stair climbing spread throughout the day improves fitness as well as more formal training regimens,[66,67] while an 8-week study from Stanford found that three 10-minute running sessions were about as effective as one 30-minute session in improving fitness.[13]

An important factor in cardiorespiratory endurance improvement is expending 200–400 Calories (or 4 Calories/kg of body weight) a day in exercise at an intensity of 40–60% HRR or higher several times a week.[1,2] While this is a minimum threshold for health and fitness gains, for the athlete, training long and frequently is critical in order to perform successfully at competitive levels (Chapter 7).

It appears that body fitness and health respond fruitfully to 4–5 days per week of aerobic exercise, with sessions lasting 20–30 minutes. Most of the psychological, cardiorespiratory, and heart disease benefits from physical activity appear to be positively affected within this exercise range.

The proper balance between exercise risks and benefits is hotly debated and is discussed in Chapter 16. Athletes, in their attempts to enhance performance as much as possible, are continuously challenging the delicate balance between training and overtraining. Chapter 16 discusses two terms in more detail:[68]

1. *Overreaching*—an accumulation of training or nontraining stress, resulting in a short-term decrement in performance capacity, with or without related physiological and psychological signs and symptoms of overtraining, in which restoration of performance capacity may take from several days to several weeks.

2. *Overtraining*—an accumulation of training or nontraining stress, resulting in long-term decrement in performance capacity, with or without related physiological and psychological signs and symptoms of overtraining, in which restoration of performance capacity may take several weeks or months.

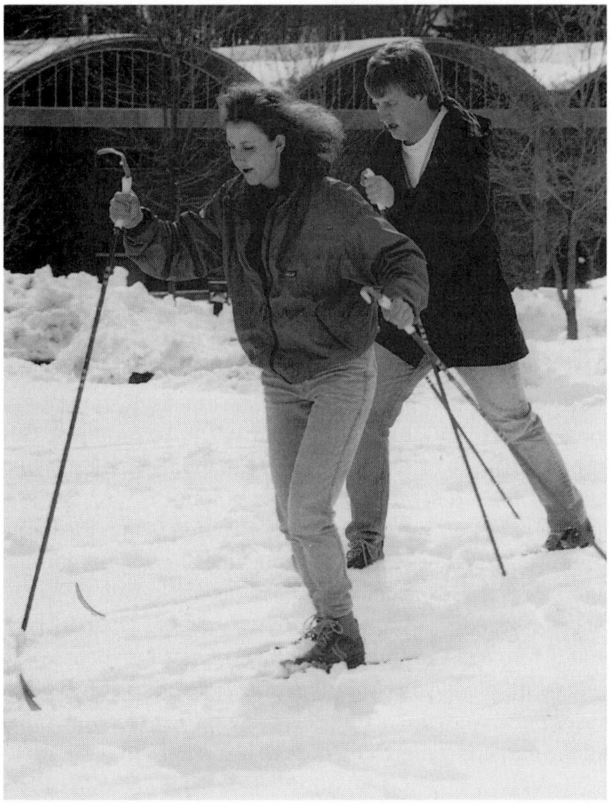

Mode of Exercise

If frequency, intensity, and duration of training are similar, and a minimum of 200–400 Calories are expended during the session, the training result appears to be independent of the *mode* of aerobic activity.[1,2] Activities should thus be selected on the basis of individual functional capacity, interests, time availability, equipment and facilities, and personal goals and objectives. Exercisers can use any activity that uses large-muscle groups, can be maintained continuously, and is rhythmical and cardiorespiratory in nature. Common examples include running/jogging, walking/hiking, swimming, skating, bicycling, rowing, cross-country skiing, rope skipping, and various endurance sports (see Figures 8.12 and 8.13). Table 8.10 lists some of the better modes for developing cardiorespiratory endurance.

One of the trends since the late 1980s has been an emphasis on *cross-training* participation in a variety of aerobic

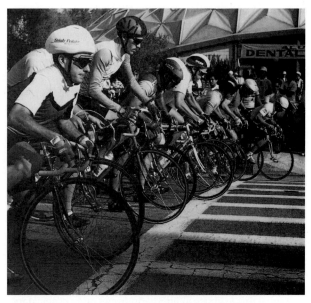

Figure 8.12 Cross-country skiing involves both upper- and lower-body muscles and provides an excellent total body conditioning effect, in addition to a high $\dot{V}O_{2max}$.

Figure 8.13 Outdoor bicycling causes less trauma to the joints and muscles than running, but high speeds are required for a training effect. Safety is thus a concern unless bicycle paths are available and helmets are worn.

TABLE 8.10   Activities That Rate High in Cardiorespiratory Benefits and Their Approximate Energy Requirements

Summarized are some of the better cardiorespiratory exercises and the number of Calories expended per hour of the exercise. An important concept is to select several of these activities that are enjoyable, and to use them in such a way that scheduled exercise sessions are looked forward to, not dreaded.

Caloric expenditure is based on a 150-lb person. There is a 10% increase in caloric expenditure for each 15 lbs over this weight and a 10% decrease for each 15 lbs under.

Activity	Calories per Hour	Activity	Calories per Hour
Badminton, competitive singles	480	Skating, ice or roller, rapid	700
Basketball	360–660	Skiing, downhill, vigorous	600
Bicycling		Skiing, cross-country	
10 mph	420	2.5 mph	560
11 mph	480	4 mph	600
12 mph	600	5 mph	700
13 mph	660	8 mph	1,020
Calisthenics, heavy	600	Swimming, 25–50 yards per min	360–750
Handball, competitive	660	Walking	
Rope skipping, vigorous	800	Level road, 4 mph (fast)	420
Rowing machine	840	Upstairs	600–1,080
Running		Uphill, 3.5 mph	480–900
5 mph	600	Additional activities	
6 mph	750	Gardening, with much lifting, stooping, digging	500
7 mph	870	Mowing, pushing hand mower	450
8 mph	1,020	Sawing hardwood	600
9 mph	1,130	Shoveling, heavy	660
10 mph	1,285	Wood chopping	560

Source: Wynder EL. *The Book of Health: The American Health Foundation.* New York: Franklin Watts, Inc., 1981. Used with permission.

activities, rather than intense concentration on one sport. Cross-training has several benefits, including decreased risk of overuse injury, reduced boredom, increased compliance, and increased overall fitness.[69]

Rating the Cardiorespiratory Exercises   As emphasized in Chapter 2, "total fitness" is equated with the development of each of the major exercise components (cardiorespiratory and muscular fitness) through a well-rounded exercise program. Some individuals weight train to develop muscular strength and endurance but pay little attention to aerobic exercise for their cardiorespiratory system. Some runners rank high in heart and lung fitness, but low in upper-body strength. Some modes of exercise even do it all; for instance, rowing, cross-country skiing, swimming, and aerobic dance train both the upper- and lower-body musculature while giving the heart and lung system a good workout (see Figure 8.12). Table 8.11 rates various activities according to their overall potential for developing total fitness.

The 1996 surgeon general's report on physical activity and health emphasized a lifestyle approach to physical activity, urging that people accumulate at least 30 minutes of physical activity on a near-daily basis.[11] According to this report, "People can select activities that they enjoy and that fit into their daily lives. Because amount of activity is a function of duration, intensity, and frequency, the same amount of activity can be obtained in longer sessions of moderately intense activities (such as brisk walking) as in shorter sessions of more strenuous activities (such as running)." Box 8.3 summarizes different ways that people can engage in physical activity, burning a minimum of 150 Calories per day, or 1,000 Calories per week, as recommended in the surgeon general's report.[11]

Brisk Walking   As emphasized in the surgeon general's report,[11] moderate-intensity activities of longer duration are more acceptable to the masses, increasing the likelihood of a permanent change in lifestyle. Also, the musculoskeletal

TABLE 8.11   Rating Physical Activities for Total Fitness Benefits

Physical Activity	Aerobic Fitness and Body Composition	Muscular Strength and Endurance
Aerobic dance, moderate-to-hard[a]	4	4
Basketball, game play	4	2
Bicycling, fast pace	5	3
Canoeing, rowing, hard pace[a]	5	4
Circuit weight training	3	5
Handball, game play	4	3
Golf, walking, carrying bag	3	2
Lawn mowing, power push	3	3
Racquetball, squash, game play	4	3
Rope jumping, moderate-to-hard	4	3
Running, brisk pace	5	2
In-line or ice skating	4	3
Shoveling dirt, digging[a]	4	4
Skiing, downhill	2	3
Skiing, cross-country[a]	5	4
Soccer	4	3
Splitting wood[a]	4	4
Stair climbing	5	3
Swimming[a]	5	4
Tennis, game play	3	3
Volleyball, game play	3	3
Walking, briskly	3	2
Weight training	1	5

Note: Activities are rated on a 5-point scale in terms of their capacity to develop aerobic fitness/body composition (grouped together because they both deal with energy expenditure), or muscular strength/endurance. 1 = not at all; 2 = somewhat or just a little; 3 = moderately; 4 = strongly; 5 = very strongly. For muscular strength and endurance, the activity is rated high if both upper- and lower-body musculature is improved. In general, activities that rank high in aerobic fitness/body composition would also rank high in prevention of chronic disease.
[a]Best overall modes of physical activity for total fitness.

risk is less, and studies show that health benefits are still realized, especially when total energy expenditure averages at least 1,000 Calories per week.[70–77]

Brisk walking for exercise is now one of the fastest growing activities in the United States. (See Chapter 1.) From a public health viewpoint, brisk walking is probably the best overall exercise for the majority of American adults.[70–72] Walking has been found to have a higher compliance rate than other physical activities because it can easily be incorporated into a busy time schedule, does not require any special skills, equipment, or facility, is companionable, and is much less apt to cause injuries.

Several studies have shown that brisk walking can be used to improve aerobic capacity.[70–77] In most of these walking studies, a walking pace equal to 60% $\dot{V}O_{2max}$ has been found to increase the $\dot{V}O_{2max}$ of previously sedentary adults 10–20% within 5–20 weeks. In one study of people ages 30–69, more than 90% of the women and 67% of the men were able to reach the training zone by walking.[72] With visual feedback from heart rate monitors, all participants with high $\dot{V}O_{2max}$ values were able to maintain appropriate training heart rates if the walking pace was appropriately adjusted.[72] The researchers concluded that fast walking offers an adequate aerobic training stimulus for nearly all adults. The $\dot{V}O_{2max}$ of competitive race walkers averages 63 ml $\cdot$ kg^{-1} $\cdot$ min^{-1}, which is an excellent cardiorespiratory fitness level.[24] In one study, most exercise walkers were found to self-select a walking pace that ranged from 40 to 65% of $\dot{V}O_{2max}$, demonstrating that most walkers fall within ACSM guidelines.[77]

While walking burns fewer calories than running, its energy cost can be increased by carrying weights. Many studies have verified that hand/wrist weights increase the energy expenditure of walking significantly more than ankle weights.[78–82] The use of 3-pound hand/wrist weights increases the oxygen cost of walking by 1 MET, with an associated 7–13 beat per minute increase in exercise heart rate.[78,79] The hand/wrist weights also tend to improve upper-body muscular endurance.

Aerobic Dance   Aerobic dance traces its origins to Jacki Sorenson, the wife of a naval pilot, who began conducting exercise classes at a U.S. Navy base in Puerto Rico in 1969.[83] The original aerobic-dance programs consisted of an eclectic combination of dance forms, including ballet, modern jazz, disco, and folk, as well as calisthenic-type exercises.

More recent innovations include water aerobics (done in a swimming pool), nonimpact or low-impact aerobics (one foot on the ground at all times), specific dance aerobics, step aerobics, and "assisted" aerobics with weights on the wrists and/or ankles.

Several studies have shown that when aerobic dancers follow the F.I.T. criteria, aerobic dancing is similar to other aerobic activities in improving the cardiorespiratory system.[83–91] Aerobic dancing also builds the muscular endurance of upper-body muscles, enhancing musculoskeletal fitness.

One cause of concern for the aerobic-dance movement has been the alarming number of reported injuries.[83] This is discussed in greater detail in Chapter 15. *Low-impact aerobics* has been growing in popularity to help reduce the

Box 8.3

As the following examples show, a moderate amount of physical activity[a] can be achieved in a variety of ways. People can select activities that they enjoy and that fit into their daily lives. Because amount of activity is a function of duration, intensity, and frequency, the same amount of activity can be obtained in longer sessions of moderately intense activities (such as brisk walking) as in shorter sessions of more strenuous activities (such as running).[b]

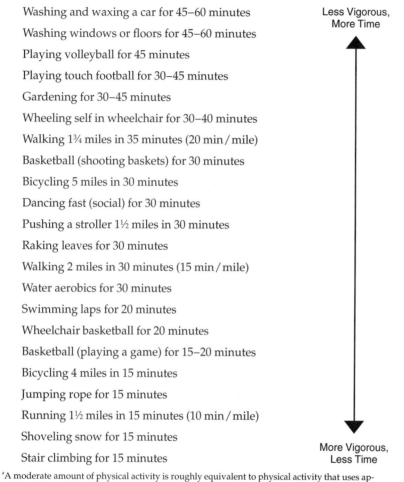

Washing and waxing a car for 45–60 minutes

Washing windows or floors for 45–60 minutes

Playing volleyball for 45 minutes

Playing touch football for 30–45 minutes

Gardening for 30–45 minutes

Wheeling self in wheelchair for 30–40 minutes

Walking 1¾ miles in 35 minutes (20 min / mile)

Basketball (shooting baskets) for 30 minutes

Bicycling 5 miles in 30 minutes

Dancing fast (social) for 30 minutes

Pushing a stroller 1½ miles in 30 minutes

Raking leaves for 30 minutes

Walking 2 miles in 30 minutes (15 min / mile)

Water aerobics for 30 minutes

Swimming laps for 20 minutes

Wheelchair basketball for 20 minutes

Basketball (playing a game) for 15–20 minutes

Bicycling 4 miles in 15 minutes

Jumping rope for 15 minutes

Running 1½ miles in 15 minutes (10 min / mile)

Shoveling snow for 15 minutes

Stair climbing for 15 minutes

Less Vigorous, More Time

More Vigorous, Less Time

[a]A moderate amount of physical activity is roughly equivalent to physical activity that uses approximately 150 Calories (kcal) of energy per day, or 1,000 Calories per week.
[b]Some activities can be performed at various intensities; the suggested durations correspond to expected intensity of effort.

Source: U.S. Department of Health and Human Services. *Physical Activity and Health: A Report of the Surgeon General.* Atlanta, GA: U.S. Department of Health and Human Services, Centers for Disease Control and Prevention, National Center for Chronic Disease Prevention and Health Promotion, 1996.

number of injuries.[90] At least one foot touches the floor throughout the aerobic portion. Movements are not ballistic, but focus on large upper-body movements, combined with leg kicks and high-powered steps and lunges. However, to achieve appropriate intensity, low-impact aerobics must be performed at a high rate. Ankle and wrist weights or steps are often used to increase the intensity of exercise.

Aerobic dance in the water uses many of the same upper-body movements practiced on the aerobic dance floor, but without the associated stress on the legs and feet.[91]

These *aquacize* programs are especially beneficial for the obese, elderly, and those with physical disabilities such as arthritis.

Racquet Sports   Many people do not like the structure and monotony of the continuous aerobic exercises such as running, swimming, and cycling. A large number have found *racquet sports* such as racquetball, squash, and tennis to be more attractive. The competitive and social aspects of these sports make them enjoyable for many, and they help promote long-lasting compliance.

When played at appropriate intensity levels, racquet sports provide an adequate cardiorespiratory stimulus.[92–97] (See Figure 8.14.) Racquetball participants of intermediate ability expend an average of 600 Calories per hour, playing at 50% $\dot{V}O_{2max}$.[94] Tennis players of intermediate ability average 60% of their heart rate reserve during singles matches, but only 33% playing doubles.[92,95]

Other Modes of Activity   Some people find vigorous work activities more satisfying. Tables 8.3 and 8.10 show that various occupational activities (e.g., wood chopping, heavy shoveling and gardening, using a hand mower for mowing grass, or sawing hardwood) can lead to an energy expenditure of close to 300 Calories in 30 minutes (the recommended amount). In addition, the upper body is given a good workout along with the heart and lungs (and a direct, purposeful task is accomplished).

Some have wondered whether *circuit weight training programs*, which involve 8–12 repetitions with various weight machines at 7–14 stations while moving quickly

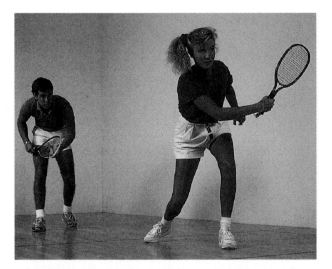

Figure 8.14   Racquetball participants of intermediate ability have been found to expend an average of 600 Calories per hour of play, which provides an adequate stimulus for cardio-respiratory improvement. (© Bill Bachmann / PhotoEdit)

from one station to the next, develop cardiorespiratory endurance. Most studies have concluded that there is little or no cardiorespiratory improvement (at most a 6% increase in $\dot{V}O_{2max}$) with such regimens.[24,98–102] Nonetheless, circuit weight lifting tends to elevate the heart rate substantially, with average heart rates of 150 (80% of maximum heart rate) reported.[100] However, actual oxygen uptake is relatively low—about 40% of $\dot{V}O_{2max}$. The heavy muscle exertion increases the heart rate through sympathetic nervous system stimulation, but because the involved muscle mass is small, the blood flow and oxygen uptake are low. Caloric expenditure is also modest, averaging 8 Calories for every 1,000 pounds lifted in the weight room.[103]

Such weight-lifting circuits, however, should not be confused with circuit training systems such as the *parcourse*, which emphasize running between stations, each of which calls for various calisthenics or weight-lifting maneuvers. Outdoor circuit training systems of this sort have been shown to burn 400 Calories in 30 minutes and contribute to high improvement in cardiorespiratory endurance.[104]

For some, the convenience of indoor aerobic-exercise equipment is important, and there is a wide variety of such equipment available today. (See Appendix B for a list of equipment, including company addresses.) However, expensive indoor equipment is not needed for a good aerobic workout. Such forms of indoor, home exercise as rope skipping, stationary running, or aerobic step dancing have all been shown to be beneficial to the cardiorespiratory system.[105–108]

There are certainly good reasons for preferring home to outdoor exercise—including unpleasant weather, environmental pollution, darkness, and safety concerns. Home exercise equipment can help make exercising convenient. The concern is that such devices will quickly lose their appeal because of lack of motivation and boredom.

Popular equipment includes stationary bicycles, rowing machines, motorized treadmills, stair climbers, and simulated cross-country skiing machines, each of which has been studied extensively and shown to elicit excellent training responses.[109–114] (See Appendix B.) Rowing and cross-country skiing equipment are especially valuable because they give the entire body musculature a workout, along with the cardiorespiratory system.[110,111] Several studies have shown that people tend to expend more energy on treadmills, compared to other equipment[113,114] (see Figure 8.15).

Rate of Progression

Appropriate progression in an exercise conditioning program depends on a person's fitness status, health status, age, needs or goals, family support, and many other factors (see Box 8.4 and Box 8.5). The American College of Sports Medicine defines three progression stages for the aerobic

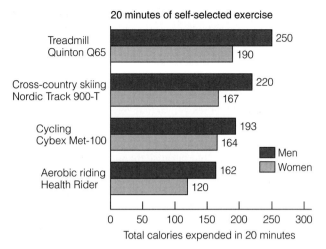

Figure 8.15 Total energy expenditure when using different indoor exercise equipment: 20 minutes of self-selected exercise. At self-selected exercise intensities, both men and women burn more Calories when using a treadmill, compared to other indoor exercise equipment. *Source:* Kravitz L, Robergs RA, Heyward VH, Wagner DR, Powers K. Exercise mode and gender comparisons of energy expenditure at self-selected intensities. *Med Sci Sports Exerc* 29:1028–1035, 1997.

phase of the exercise prescription for apparently healthy people:[1]

- *Initial conditioning stage.* This stage typically lasts 4–6 weeks but depends on the adaptation of the participant to the program. ACSM suggests that exercise intensity be 40–60% $\dot{V}O_{2max}$ to help avoid muscle soreness, injury, discomfort, and discouragement. It is best to be conservative when starting an exercise program and then gradually progress. Participants can start at 12 minutes and slowly work up to 20 minutes of exercise during this stage. ACSM recommends that individuals who are starting a conditioning program exercise three times per week on nonconsecutive days.[1]

- *Improvement conditioning stage.* This stage usually lasts 4–5 months and the rate of progression is more rapid. The exercise intensity is increased to 50–85% of $\dot{V}O_{2max}$, and the duration of exercise can be increased every 2–3 weeks until participants are able to exercise nonstop for 20–30 minutes. The degree and frequency of progression during this stage depend largely on the age of the participant and her or his ability to adapt to the exercise program. For each decade of life after age 30, it takes approximately 1 week longer for the body to adapt to a higher conditioning stimulus. Participants should strive to burn 300 Calories per session (usually accomplished in 30 minutes), and 1,000 Calories per week (at least

three sessions per week). An energy expenditure of 2,000 Calories per week is considered optimal for fitness and health benefits.[1]

- *Maintenance conditioning stage.* Once the desired level of fitness is reached, the person enters the maintenance stage of the exercise program. This stage usually begins 6 months after the start of training and continues on a regular, long-term basis (lifetime commitment). Here particularly, it is important both to select aerobic exercises that are enjoyable and to establish long-term goals.

Systems of Cardiorespiratory Training

There are several systems of cardiorespiratory training.[24–26,38]

- *Continuous training.* This involves continuous exercise such as jogging, swimming, walking, or cycling, at "somewhat hard to hard" intensities without rest intervals. The prescribed exercise intensity is maintained consistently throughout the exercise session.

- *Interval training.* This involves a repeated series of exercise work bouts, interspersed with rest periods. Higher intensities can be used during the exercise to overload the cardiorespiratory system because the exercise is discontinuous. A miler training for competition, for example, could use an interval regimen where one lap (400 meters) is run at slightly faster than the race-pace goal, followed by 1 minute of rest or walking, with the cycle repeated 5–20 times. In time, the "rest" interval of walking can gradually be increased in intensity, until the miler can run at a high intensity for four full laps.

  Interval training is necessary for athletes who wish to compete.[38] A good endurance base (at least 1–2 months of regular aerobic training) and a 10-minute warm-up are prerequisites to interval training. In addition, the first interval training sessions should be moderate, with gradual transitions to higher intensity levels. Interval sessions should not number more than one or two per week. Above all, hard anaerobic workouts should not be conducted on consecutive days.

- *Fartlek training.* This is like interval training, but it is a free form of training done out on trails or roads. People who abhor track running can do Fartlek training on roads, golf courses, or trails. The exercise–rest cycle is not systematic or precisely timed and measured but is based on the feelings of the participant.

- *Circuit training.* As noted previously, this training involves 10–20 stations of varying calisthenic and weight-lifting exercises, interspersed with running. The parcourse is a good example.

Box 8.4

Case History of a Typical Middle-Age American Female

Data from Medical/Health Questionnaire

Age: 45 years; *height:* 64 inches; *weight:* 154 pounds; *desired weight:* 130 pounds

Smoking status: quit 5 years ago

Exercise habits: sedentary both at work and during leisure for all of adult life

Family history of disease: father died of coronary heart disease at age 52 years

Personal history of disease: negative

Signs or symptoms suggestive of cardiopulmonary or metabolic disease: negative

Dietary habits: fruit/vegetables, 2 servings/day (low); cereals/grains, 5/day (low and refined)

Personal goals: lose weight, improve appearance and muscle tone, decrease risk of heart disease

Preferred modes of aerobic exercise: brisk walking, stationary bicycling

Data from Physical Fitness Testing Session (Physician's Office and Fitness Center)

Resting heart rate: 79 bpm (poor)

Resting blood pressure: 142/93 mm Hg (mild hypertension) (from 2 measurements on 2 days)

Serum cholesterol: 247 mg/dl (high risk)

HDL cholesterol: 33 mg/dl (low)

Cholesterol-to-HDL-cholesterol ratio: 7.5 (high risk)

Percent body fat: 35% (obese)

$\dot{V}O_{2max}$: estimated from Bruce treadmill test with EKG—23 ml/kg/min (low); EKG, negative

Sit-and-reach flexibility test: −2 inches from footline (fair)

Hand-grip dynamometer (sum of right and left hands): 55 kg (below average)

Comments

Using the medical/health questionnaire and laboratory data from recent testing, this client was classified as an "individual at increased risk," using ACSM criteria. This classification was given because she has two or more major coronary risk factors (family history, hypertension, hypercholesterolemia, sedentary lifestyle). Due to the number of risk factors, especially the family history of coronary heart disease, and the client's desire to engage in moderate-to-vigorous exercise, a medical exam and diagnostic exercise test were recommended. The treadmill-ECG test was negative (no evidence of ischemia or arrhythmias), and physician clearance was given for the client to begin a moderate exercise program, with gradual progression. Additional physical fitness tests were conducted at a fitness center to determine body composition and musculoskeletal fitness.

Recommended Exercise Program

A home-based program, using brisk walking and indoor stationary bicycling, supported with calisthenics for general muscle toning is recommended. During the first month, have the client warm up with range-of-motion calisthenics and walking for 5–10 minutes, followed by 15 minutes of brisk walking or stationary cycling at 50–60% heart rate reserve, 3 days per week. After warming down, the client should engage in static stretching activities for 5–10 minutes, followed by toning calisthenics for 10–15 minutes.

After the first month has passed, gradually increase the duration of brisk walking or cycling to 30–45 minutes per session, and the frequency to 5–6 days per week. The intensity of exercise can also be gradually increased to 70% of heart rate reserve. These increases, along with careful control of dietary habits, will help ensure a steady weight loss of about 1 pound per week. Because the client has 24 pounds of body fat to lose, ideal body weight should be attained after 24–30 weeks of training. This degree of weight loss, combined with improvements in physical fitness, should help to bring both hypertension and hypercholesterolemia under control if improvements in dietary quality are made (i.e., less saturated fat and cholesterol, more fruits, vegetables, and whole grains, less sodium and alcohol). The client has a high risk of coronary heart disease, and it is imperative that the risk factors be brought under control through weight loss and dietary and exercise lifestyle changes. Enlist the services of a dietitian to ensure adherence to an antiatherogenic diet.

Retest every 3 months to help ensure motivation and attainment of goals. Long-term compliance can be enhanced by encouraging family support, setting goals and contracting for their achievement, establishing rewards for attainment of goals, and combating time obstacles.

Box 8.5

Case History of a 30-Year-Old Male

Data from Medical/Health Questionnaire

Age: 30 years; *height:* 70 inches; *weight:* 160 pounds; *desired weight:* 175 pounds

Smoking status: never smoked

Exercise habits: plays golf on the weekends, but no other formal exercise; desk job at work

Family history of disease: negative

Personal history of disease: negative

Signs or symptoms suggestive of cardiopulmonary or metabolic disease: negative

Dietary habits: has a healthy diet and tries to follow Food Pyramid guidelines

Personal goals: increase muscle weight through weight training program; improve aerobic fitness moderately

Preferred modes of aerobic exercise: indoor equipment, especially rowing machine and stationary bicycle

Data from Physical Fitness Testing Session (Fitness Center)

Resting heart rate: 67 bpm (average)

Resting blood pressure: 123 / 82 mm Hg (normal) (from 2 measurements on 2 days)

Serum cholesterol: 195 mg / dl (within desirable range)

HDL cholesterol: 46 mg / dl (average)

Cholesterol-to-HDL-cholesterol ratio: 4.2 (average, but above optimal ratio of 3.5)

Percent body fat: 14% (desirable)

$\dot{V}O_{2max}$: estimated from timed Bruce treadmill test—43 ml / kg / min (average)

Sit-and-reach flexibility test: +2 inches from footline (average)

Hand-grip dynamometer (sum of right and left hands): 110 kg (average)

1-RM bench-press test: 95% of body weight (average)

Pull-ups: 7 (fair)

Push-ups: 25 (above average)

Timed (1 minute) bent-knee sit-ups: 32 (above average)

Comments

This client has no major risk factors for disease and is therefore classified as "apparently healthy," using ACSM guidelines. According to ACSM, a medical exam or diagnostic exercise test is not needed prior to initiating a vigorous exercise program for this type of client. Although the client has a normal percentage of body fat his body weight is somewhat low for his height, and he desires to gain 15 pounds through a weight training program while moderately improving his aerobic fitness. He is especially interested in adding muscle bulk to improve his golf game, which is his weekend passion.

Recommended Exercise Program

The client desires an intensive weight training program at the fitness center, 3 days per week, with a moderate aerobic program 2 days a week. Because the client has never lifted weights seriously, a gradual, progressive resistance program should be established. During the first month, a one-set, 10-repetition maximum (RM) program of 10 different exercises will allow the client to adapt to the weight training program without undue fatigue and soreness (which would interfere with his weekend golf game). Over the next 2–3 months, gradually increase the sets to three, with the RM lowered to 6–8.

On 2 days of the week, after 5 minutes of warm-up, the client can use the rowing machine or bicycle for 20–30 minutes at 60–75% of heart rate reserve. On weight-lifting days, it is recommended that the client warm up for 10 minutes, prior to lifting, by rowing or cycling. This will allow additional aerobic training and will help warm up the muscles and joints to allow safe and effective weight lifting.

Establish 1-RM weight-lifting goals for each of the 10 exercises, and retest every 3 months. Also retest aerobic fitness and body composition every 3 months. To facilitate a healthy gain in body weight, consult with a dietitian to provide nutrient and energy analysis of the diet every 3 months. The dietitian can also give recommendations to improve the energy density of the diet.

The Question of Supervision

- *Unsupervised exercise programs.* Apparently healthy individuals can usually exercise safely in an unsupervised conditioning program.[1] Participant safety and compliance can be improved by individualizing the exercise prescription and educating participants on signs of overexertion, effects of heat and humidity, and so on. Some people find it more enjoyable to exercise alone at home; some like the group support of a community exercise class.

- *Supervised exercise programs.* Exercise should be supervised for symptomatic and cardiorespiratory disease patients who are considered to be clinically stable and for others who desire instruction in proper exercise techniques. ACSM recommends that people with two or more coronary artery disease risk factors, known heart disease, or a functional capacity of less than 8 METs exercise under supervision.[1] These programs should be under the combined guidance of a trained ACSM-certified professional and a physician (see Chapter 3). Direct supervision of each session by a physician is, however, not required.

Warm-Down (Cool-Down)

The purpose of the *warm-down* (cool-down) is to slowly decrease the pulse rate and to lower the body temperature, both of which have been elevated during the aerobic phase. This is effectively and safely done by keeping the feet and legs moving, such as via walking, light jogging, slow swimming, or bicycling. In other words, the warm-down is the warm-up in reverse.

There are at least three important physiological reasons for it:[24–26,115–117]

1. By moving during recovery for about 5–10 minutes (more or less, depending on fitness status, state of fatigue, and environmental factors), muscle and blood lactic acid levels decrease more rapidly than if the exerciser completely rests. In other words, moving during the warm-down promotes faster recovery from fatigue.

2. Mild activity following heavy aerobic exercise keeps the leg muscle "pumps" going and thus prevents the blood from pooling in the legs. The leg muscles promote venous return by the "milking" action of the contraction and relaxation cycle. Preventing the pooling of the blood reduces the possibility of delayed muscular stiffness, and also reduces any tendency toward fainting and dizziness.

3. Following very hard aerobic exercise, there is an increase of catecholamines in the blood. Among high-risk people, this can adversely affect the heart, causing cardiac irregularities. The majority of severe cardiac irregularities that can be dangerous appear to occur following exercise, not during it. Although such exercise-related irregularities of the heart are relatively rare, a careful warm-down is only prudent.

MUSCULOSKELETAL CONDITIONING

Musculoskeletal conditioning includes flexibility exercises and exercises for muscular strength and endurance.

Flexibility Exercises

The major reason for performing flexibility exercises after the aerobic phase is to more safely and effectively stretch the warm muscle groups and joints that were involved in the aerobic exercise.[23,29,32] Appendix C contains pictures and descriptions of eight common flexibility exercises. The *ACSM Fitness Book* describes 22 flexibility exercises for all of the major joints of the body.[18]

A *flexibility program* is defined as a planned, deliberate, and regular program of exercises that can progressively increase the range of motion of a joint or set of joints over a period of time.[23] In 1998, ACSM included recommendations for flexibility exercise in their position stand for the first time based on growing evidence that flexibility can improve joint range of motion and function, and enhance muscular performance.[2] ACSM recommends that a basic stretching program be followed at least 2–3 days a week and involve at least four repetitions of several static stretches that are held 10–30 seconds at a position of mild discomfort.[1,2] ACSM also recommends that major emphasis be placed on the lower back and thigh areas, and all other major muscle/tendon groups.[2]

One study of 238 athletes participating in a wide variety of sports showed that nearly all the athletes pursued a stretching program of some kind, but their practices varied greatly.[119] Only 39% of the athletes stretched daily, 37% stretched before activity, and 33% stretched both before and after exercise. In a study of 2,310 Los Angeles marathon runners, 26% reported that they usually did not stretch, with 10% stretching after running, 24% before, and 40% both before and after running. (See Figure 8.16.)

It is commonly accepted that flexibility is an important factor in reducing the potential for injury and in improving

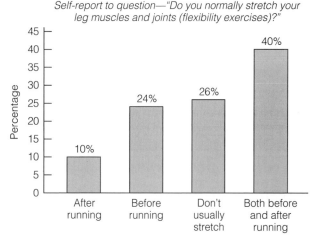

Self-report to question—"Do you normally stretch your leg muscles and joints (flexibility exercises)?"

Figure 8.16 Stretching habits of 2,310 Los Angeles marathon runners: Self-report to question—"Do you normally stretch your leg muscles and joints (flexibility exercises)?" Stretching habits of marathon runners vary widely. *Source:* Unpublished observations of the author.

performance, and it serves as an important component of overall physical fitness.[23]

In the textbook *Science of Flexibility,* several benefits of a flexibility training program are advanced:[23,120–125]

- Relaxation of stress and tension
- Muscular relaxation
- Improved body fitness, posture, and symmetry
- Relief of muscular cramps
- Relief of muscular soreness
- Injury prevention

There is still much debate as to whether improved flexibility is related to injury prevention. When questioned, the majority of sports-medicine specialists support the use of flexibility training in injury prevention but also readily admit that there is little scientific support for it.[126] Some studies have provided convincing evidence that flexibility training prevents injuries[23,120,127] while others have not.[128–131] Researchers have also published results showing that greater flexibility predicts more injury.[132,133] Part of the problem is that flexibility is a complex characteristic that is highly specific to the type of sport being investigated.[23,134] Most athletic endeavors involve dynamic flexibility or the ability to use a range of joint movement in the performance of a physical activity at either normal or rapid speed. Flexibility is very specific to the type and speed of movement and to the involved joint.[23] Some sports require unique types of flexibility, including Olympic weight lifting, ballet dancing, gymnastics, swimming, and wrestling. Therefore, flexibility training is adapted by trainers to the special needs of the athlete or individual. When researchers attempt to study the relationship between flexibility and injury prevention, they often use static range-of-motion measures that may not translate to the specific dynamic flexibility demands of the sport.

Four types of stretching techniques have been developed by athletes, dancers, and physical therapists.[23,121,122,125,135–142] *Ballistic methods,* commonly referred to as "bouncing" stretches, use the momentum of the moving body segment to produce the stretch. *Slow movements* often used by dancers are a second method, in which muscle stretching occurs as the movement progresses gradually from one body position to another and then smoothly returns to the starting point. However, the two other techniques—static stretching and proprioceptive neuromuscular facilitation—discussed here are considered best for developing flexibility.

Static Stretching

Static stretching involves slowly applying stretch to the muscle and then holding it in a lengthened position for a period of 10–30 seconds.[23,121,139] During this easily held stretch, one relaxes, focusing attention on the muscles being stretched. The feeling of slight tension in the stretching muscle should slowly subside. Then one stretches a bit further, until the mild tension is again felt (never any pain), and one holds this position for 30–60 seconds. The tension should again slowly subside. One should be breathing easily and feel relaxed.

Each major joint and muscle group of the body should be stretched. Appendix C contains pictures of eight common static stretching exercises.

Proprioceptive Neuromuscular Facilitation

Studies have shown that proprioceptive neuromuscular facilitation (PNF) flexibility techniques are more effective than conventional stretching methods for increasing joint range of motion.[23,135–137] Muscle relaxation using PNF is first induced by a contraction of the muscle to be stretched, followed by a static stretching of the same muscle group. There are two ways to do PNF:

1. *Contract–relax.* An isometric contraction of the muscle group being stretched precedes the slow, static stretching (relaxation) of the same muscle group. Theoretically, the isometric contraction of the muscles to be stretched induces a reflex relaxation.

2. *Contract–relax with agonist contraction.* This is the same as the contract–relax technique, except that at the same time the muscle is stretched, the opposing muscle group is submaximally contracted. This is supposed to facilitate even more relaxation in the stretched muscles.

PNF is usually done with a partner. The following steps are recommended:

1. Stretch the muscle group by moving the joint to the end of its range of motion.

2. Have a partner provide resistance as the same muscle group is statically contracted (for example, in a sit-and-reach stretch, after the person stretching has extended his or her reach forward, the partner will push on his or her back as he or she strives to lean back).

3. Have the partner apply pressure to aid in a slow, static stretch of the muscle group, while the person stretching contracts the opposing muscle group (for example, in the sit-and-reach, the partner pushes down on the person's back while the person tries to relax the hamstrings and contract the quadriceps).

PNF appears to produce the largest gains in flexibility.[23] However, it is associated with more pain and muscle stiffness, requires a partner, and takes more time. For these reasons, the static stretching method is often the most practical one. Risk of injury and pain is low with static stretching, and it requires little time and assistance.

Muscular Strength and Endurance Exercises

The fifth and final stage of the comprehensive or total fitness workout involves the development of muscular strength and endurance. This stage can follow the warmdown, or as many people do, it can be alternated with an aerobic program on separate days.

There are a wide variety of training programs available, depending on the goals and preferences of the individual. Table 8.12 and Box 8.6 summarize some of them.[1,2,143–146]

The American College of Sports Medicine and the surgeon general's report recommend that at least 2–3 days per week, people engage in a minimum of one set of 8–12 repetitions of 8–10 different exercises that condition all of the major muscle groups. (See Box 8.7).[1,2] This strength training guideline has also been recommended for elderly people and cardiac patients, except that lighter loads and more repetitions are advised.[144,147–149]

ACSM feels that this is a minimum and basic program that many Americans will have time for.[1,2] Another reason is that most of the strength gains appear to be experienced during the first set.[147–150] This has caused considerable controversy, but ACSM has been careful to describe these as minimum standards. The Institute for Aerobics Research has chosen to provide three different programs, which differ according to the number of sets.[146] Box 8.6 shows that athletes go way beyond the recommendations given for the general population, with systems varying according to the sport.[143,145]

Principles of Weight Training

When appropriate weight training principles are followed, average strength improvement during the first 6 months of training is about 25–30%.[143,145] The effect of exercise training is very specific, however, to the area of the body and training methods utilized and heavily dependent on overloading the muscle groups.[143–160] Although much of the early gain in strength is from neural adaptations, significant hypertrophy of muscle cells can be measured within 2 months.[143–145]

There are three major principles of weight training:[143–160]

1. *Overload principle.* Strength and endurance development is based on what is known as the *overload*

TABLE 8.12 Recommendations for Improving Muscular Strength and Endurance for the General Adult Population[a]

	Number of Sets	Number of Reps[b]	Sessions/ Week	Number of Exercises	Overall Purpose
ACSM[1,2]	1	8–12	2–3	8–10[c]	Basic development and maintenance of the fat-free mass
Surgeon General[11]	1–2	8–12	2	8–10	Basic muscular strength and endurance
Cooper Institute for Aerobics Research[146]					
Minimum	1	8–12	2	10	Strength maintenance
Recommended	2	8–12	2	10	Strength improvement
Optimal	3	8–12	2	10	Noticeable gains in strength

[a]Recommendations for older people (50–60 years of age and above) and cardiac patients are similar, except that lighter weights and more repetitions (10–15) are recommended.[144,147–149]

[b]In all examples listed, repetitions represent maximal weight lifted to fatigue.

[c]Minimum of one exercise per major muscle group (e.g., chest press, shoulder press, triceps extension, biceps curl, pull-down, lower-back extension, abdominal crunch/curl-up, quadriceps extension, leg curls, calf raise).

Box 8.6

Systems of Resistance Training

1. *Single-set system.* Each weight-lifting exercise is performed for one set, 8–12-RM. Although improvement is not as good as with a multiple-set system, this system may be appropriate for those with little time to dedicate to weight training.

2. *Multiple-set system.* A minimum of three sets, 4–6-RM, are performed.

3. *Light-to-heavy system.* As the name implies, the light-to-heavy system entails progressing from light to heavy resistances. A set of 3–5 reps is performed with a relatively light weight. Five pounds are then added to the bar, and another set, 3–5 reps, performed. This is continued until only one repetition can be executed.

4. *Heavy-to-light system.* This is a reversal of the light-to-heavy system. The research suggests that this produces better strength gains than the light-to-heavy system.

5. *The triangle program.* This consists of the light-to-heavy system followed immediately by the heavy-to-light system. It is used by many power lifters.

6. *Super-set system.* This is used by bodybuilders. Two types are used. In one, multiple sets of two exercises for the same body part but opposing muscle groups (biceps vs. triceps, for example) are performed without any rest in between. The second type of super setting uses one set of several exercises in rapid succession for the same muscle group or body part. Both types of super setting involve many sets of 8–10 reps, with little or no rest between sets or exercises.

7. *Circuit program.* Circuit programs consist of a series of resistance training exercises performed one after the other, with minimal rest (15–30 seconds) between exercises. Approximately 10–15 reps of each exercise are performed per circuit, at a resistance of 40–60% RM. Cardiorespiratory endurance can increase about 5% with such programs.

8. *Split-routine system.* Many bodybuilders use a split-routine system. Bodybuilders like to perform many sets and many types of exercises for each body part, to cause hypertrophy. This is a time-consuming process, and not all parts of the body can be exercised in a single session. A typical split-routine system may entail the training of arms, legs, and abdomen on Monday, Wednesday, and Friday, and chest, shoulders, and back on Tuesday, Thursday, and Sunday.

Source: Fleck SJ, Kraemer WJ. *Designing Resistance Training Programs.* Champaign, IL: Human Kinetics, 1987.

---

principle, which states that the strength, endurance, and size of a muscle will increase only when the muscle performs for a given period of time at its maximal strength and endurance capacity (against workloads that are above those normally encountered). Muscle endurance and strength will improve best when muscle groups are brought to a state of fatigue.

2. *Progressive resistance principle.* The resistance (pounds of weight) against which the muscle works should be increased periodically, as gains in strength and endurance are made, until the desired state is reached.

3. *Principle of specificity.* The development of muscular fitness is specific to the muscle group that is exer-

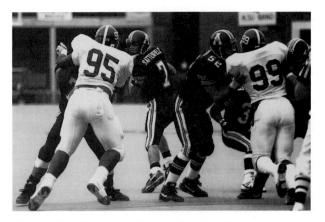

Figure 8.17 Gains in muscle strength and endurance are specific to the type, speed, and intensity of weight-lifting exercises utilized in training. The movement pattern involved in the sports skill should be simulated as closely as possible in the weight room.

cised, its type of contraction, and the training intensity. In other words, weight-resistance training appears to be motor-skill specific. Thus, weight training programs should exercise the muscle groups actually used in the sport or activity the person is training for, and they should simulate as closely as possible the movement patterns involved in that activity. (See Figure 8.17).

Research has also shown that training should be conducted at high speeds because gains in strength and endurance are specific to the speed of training, with maximal gains for activities at velocities equal to or slower, but not faster, than the training velocity.

Systems of Muscular Strength and Endurance Training

Weight-lifting centers around five different variables which can be manipulated according to specific goals.[143,145]

1. *Repetitions to fatigue.* When repetitions are low (3–5) they build greater strength; when high (15–25), they promote endurance.

2. *Sets.* One set is fine for beginners, but three to five are optimal for strength and muscle size gains.

3. *Rest between sets.* Bodybuilders have a short rest interval (<1 minute); 1–2 minutes is typical, and >2 minutes is practiced by Olympic and power lifters.

4. *Order of exercises.* Some lifters exercise the large-muscle groups first, while others start out with small-muscle groups. Bodybuilders emphasize working out the front and back of arms and legs.

5. *Type of exercise.* The lift can involve a single joint (e.g., arm curls) or multiple joints (e.g., leg squat). Multiple joint, large-muscle-mass lifts burn more calories.

There are three classifications of muscle contractions: isometric, isotonic (concentric), and isotonic (eccentric).[24–26]

Isometric   In *isometrics,* the muscle group contracts against a fixed, immovable resistance. For example, the hands could be placed under a desk while sitting in a chair with arms at a 90° angle. The biceps are then contracted, but there is no movement as the hands attempt to push up on the heavy desk.

Maximum gains in strength appear to come from 5–10, 6-second isometric contractions at 100% of maximal strength, repeated at three different points in the full range of motion. Isometric exercises are easy to perform, can be done nearly anywhere, and require little time or expense. It is important to do each exercise at several different angles for each joint because strength gain is specific to the angle at which the isometric exercise is performed.

Isotonic   Traditionally, *isotonic training* has involved the use of weights in the form of barbells, dumbbells, and pulleys, or heavy calisthenics such as push-ups, sit-ups, leg squats, etc. Appendix C summarizes the more common calisthenics used to develop muscular endurance and strength.

Isotonic muscular contractions take two forms: *concentric,* muscle contraction with shortening, and *eccentric,* muscular contraction with lengthening. For example, when a heavy weight is lowered, there is eccentric muscle contraction resisting the downward movement of the weight. Running downhill involves eccentric muscle contraction.

A muscle can maximally produce 40% more tension eccentrically than concentrically. However, training with eccentric contractions produces no greater increases in strength than isotonic programs. In fact, at the same relative power level, people performing concentric work will experience greater increases in muscle size and strength than when training with eccentric contractions.[161] However, gains in strength after concentric or eccentric training depend on the muscle action used for training and should be directed toward specific performance goals.[161,162] The major problem with eccentric contraction is its association with muscle soreness. (See Figure 8.18; this is discussed in more detail in Chapter 16.)

As emphasized earlier, isotonic muscle movement usually centers around *sets* and *repetitions.* A *repetition* is defined as one particular weight-lifting or calisthenic movement, with a *set* defined as a certain number of these repetitions. *One-repetition maximum* (1-RM) is defined as the maximal load a muscle or muscle group can lift just once. Six-repetitions maximum (6-RM), for example, is the greatest amount of weight that can be lifted six times. Box 8.6 summarizes the large number of different combinations that are possible.

The isotonic weight training program should be conducted according to personal goals, with caution given for overtraining.[153] Chronic fatigue can develop from daily training. Some athletes will focus on the upper body one day, and then the lower body the next, allowing 48 hours for exercised muscle groups to recover.

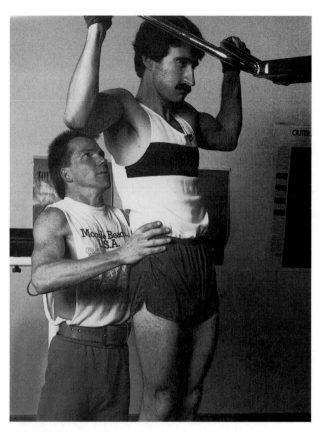

Figure 8.18   *Eccentric muscle contractions* involve muscle lengthening as it develops tension. For example, when at the top of a pull-up, if a partner pulls you down, as you attempt to resist the downward action, eccentric muscle contraction will take place. Eccentric muscle contraction is associated with muscle soreness.

Bodybuilding is a unique activity in which competitors work to develop the mass, definition, and symmetry of their muscles, rather than the strength, skill, or endurance required for traditional athletic events.[155,158] In one study of 31 competitive bodybuilders (15 female, 16 male) who were free of steroids, subjects averaged four to six 90-minute weight training workouts each week. Particular muscle groups were generally exercised twice a week, using several different exercises for each muscle group. Each exercise was performed to the point of muscle failure, using a resistance that achieved this effect with 8–15 repetitions. Exercises were repeated for 5–8 sets.[155]

Box 8.8 summarizes some of the more common weight-lifting exercises, with a description of technique, overall benefits, and the specific muscle groups improved. (Figures 8.19 through 8.23 illustrate these exercises.) Consult Appendix D for identification of the muscles involved.

Isokinetic   This type of muscular training is relatively new. In joint motion, the muscles controlling the movement

---

Box 8.8

Common Weight-Lifting Exercises

The following exercises are commonly used for bodybuilding.

1. *Bench press* (Figure 8.19). Lie down on the bench, with shoulders just in back of the bar. Space the hands evenly on the bar. Let the bar down to the chest, and then forcefully push the bar back up to a straight-arm position. Breathe in as the bar is lowered, and exhale as you raise the bar.

   Overall benefit: Builds up the front of the chest and back of upper arms.

   Muscles involved: Forearm extensors (triceps), arm flexors (pectoralis major, anterior deltoid).

2. *Lat pull* (Figure 8.20). Kneel directly below the handle, with your hands grasping it, arms straight. Forcefully pull the bar down behind the head.

   Overall benefit: Develops the "lats," which helps give the back the "V-shaped look."

   Muscles involved: Forearm flexors (biceps brachii, brachialis); arm extensors and abductors (latissimus dorsi, posterior deltoid, pectoralis major, teres major).

3. *Two-arm curl* (Figure 8.21). Grasp the bar with palms up and away from body. Standing straight, forcefully raise hands to chest. Try not to arch the lower back or let the elbows drive backward during the lift.

   Overall benefit: Develops the biceps, a muscle important for carrying objects when arms are bent at a 90° angle.

   Muscles involved: Forearm flexors (biceps brachii, brachialis).

4. *Military press* (Figure 8.22). Grasp the bar with hands shoulder-width apart, arms down, and palms toward body. Raise the bar to shoulder height, and then press hands straight up above body.

   Overall benefit: Develops the shoulder area and firms back of arm.

   Muscles involved: Arm abductors (deltoid, supraspinatus), forearm extensor (triceps).

5. *Leg squats* (Figure 8.23). A partner places the bar on the shoulders behind the head. Squat down so that the legs are at a 90° angle (to a bench), and then stand back up.

   Overall benefit: Develops the front of the thigh, giving better strength for climbing stairs and hills, bicycling, and kicking in various sports; also firms the buttock muscles.

   Muscles involved: Knee extensors (quadriceps—rectus femoris and vastus lateralis, medialis, and intermedius), thigh extensors (gluteus maximus, adductor magnus, posterior part).

---

have points at which strength is greater and points where it is less. For example, the greatest tension or strength of the elbow flexors (biceps, brachialis) is at 120°, with the least tension and strength at 30°. In true isokinetic exercise, the resistance adjusts so that it is exactly matched to the force applied by the muscle throughout the full range of joint motion. This means that the muscle can apply maximal tension during the entire lift. This is accomplished by controlling the speed of the movement (*iso* = same, *kinetic* = motion) with specialized equipment. (See Figure 8.24.)

Figure 8.25 demonstrates use of an isokinetic device that allows the exercising limb to work at a fixed speed,

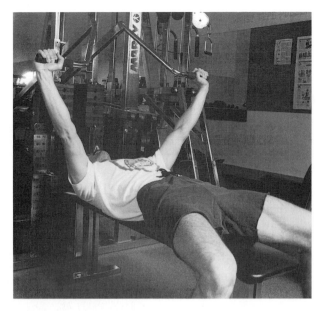

Figure 8.19 Bench press.

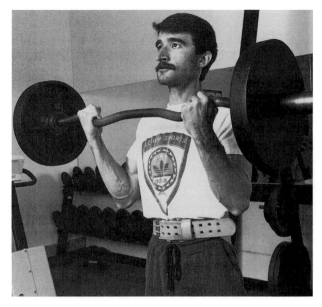

Figure 8.21 Two-arm curl.

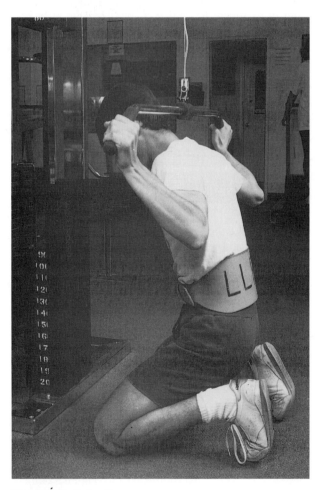

Figure 8.20 Lat pull.

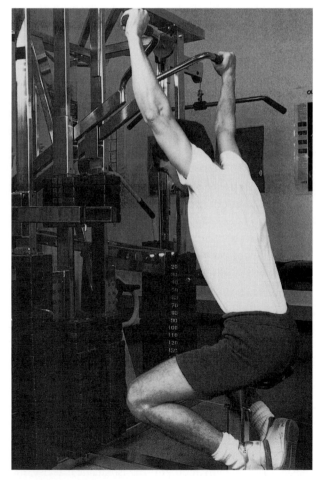

Figure 8.22 Military press.

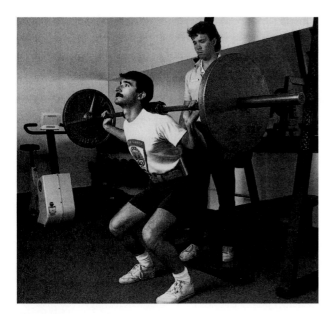

Figure 8.23 Leg squats.

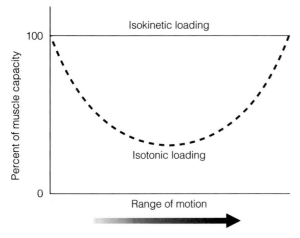

Figure 8.24 Isokinetic versus isotonic exercise. During isotonic muscle contraction, the amount of weight that can be utilized must be adjusted to the weakest point of the lift. Thus the muscle is not operating at 100% capacity during all parts of the lift. With isokinetic exercise, the specialized equipment allows the muscle to contract maximally throughout the entire range of motion.

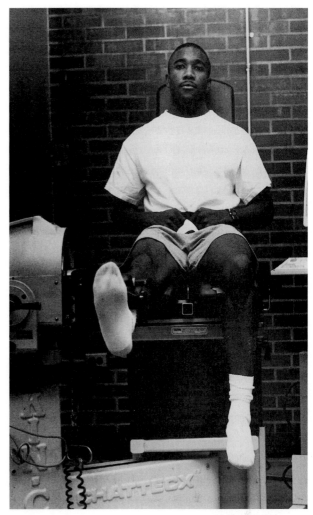

Figure 8.25 The Kincom allows *isokinetic exercise,* keeping all movement at a specific speed while varying the resistance to allow maximal effort throughout the range of motion.

with a variable resistance that is totally accommodating to the individual throughout the entire range of motion.[154]

In comparing the different systems, there are several advantages and disadvantages with each.[154] Motivation is generally superior with isotonic exercises because they are self-testing in nature. Also, if heavy calisthenics instead of weight lifting are used for isotonic training, no special equipment is needed (see Appendix C).

Isometrics can also be performed without equipment and can be done anywhere, but gains in strength are joint-angle specific (within 20°), and care must be taken to exercise at several angles. As for isokinetics, studies show that muscular strength and endurance development is somewhat better with such programs, but the specialized, expensive equipment makes this type of training impractical for most people.

It should be noted that Nautilus and similar equipment are not isokinetic in concept (fixed speed, accommodating resistance) but actually isotonic equipment that attempts imperfectly to vary the resistance using various devices to work around the weak points of each lift.

SPORTS MEDICINE INSIGHT

Understanding and Promoting Physical Activity

Only 15% of U.S. adults engage regularly (three times a week for at least 20 minutes each time) in vigorous physical activity during their leisure time.[11] About 25% of adults report no physical activity. Many people have started exercise programs, only to drop out when various barriers present themselves (e.g., time problems, bad weather, family emergencies).[163,164]

Chapter 1 discussed some strategies for promoting physical activity at the population level. Emphasis was placed on four targets of change: (1) the person; (2) organizations; (3) the environment; and (4) public policies. This Sports Medicine Insight discusses models of extensive behavior change in individuals. Lifestyle behaviors do not occur in a vacuum but are affected by many complex factors, including personal beliefs, attitudes, self-esteem, education, ethnicity, income, environment, and culture.

As explained in the surgeon general's report, "as the benefits of moderate, regular physical activity have become more widely recognized, the need has increased for interventions that can promote this healthful behavior."[11] Numerous theories and models have been used to help people improve health behavior and physical activity patterns. These are summarized in Table 8.13.[11]

The transtheoretical model developed by psychologists James O. Prochaska and Carlos C. DiClemente is one of the most effective approaches to health behavior change and to improvement in physical activity habits.[165] This model has been adopted by the Canadian Society of Exercise Physiology in their *Canadian Physical Activity, Fitness & Lifestyle Appraisal* program.[166] Although originally developed for smokers, it has since been applied to other health behavior, including physical activity.

In the transtheoretical model, behavior change is described as a five-stage process:

1. *Precontemplation*—not intending to make changes
2. *Contemplation*—considering a change
3. *Preparation*—making small changes or ready to change in the very near future
4. *Action*—actively engaging in the new behavior
5. *Maintenance*—sticking with the behavior change

During the first three stages, people experience different processes of knowing and valuing. These include *consciousness raising* (increasing awareness of the problem in order to reduce defensiveness toward any intention to change), *dramatic relief* (expressing a strong emotional reaction to anything associated with the be-

havioral target), *social liberation* (being aware of enabling conditions in the immediate environment, which support the target behavior), *self-reevaluation* (reappraising personally relevant consequences associated with changing the target behavior), and *environmental reevaluation* (considering how the target behavior affects the social and physical environment).

During the last two stages, people experience certain behavioral processes of change, which include *self-liberation* (choosing and committing to implementation of the target behavior), *counterconditioning* (substituting an alternative behavior to replace a problem behavior that interferes with the desired change), *stimulus control* (removing cues or avoiding situations that trigger the problem behavior), *reinforcement management* (being rewarded by oneself or others for fully changing the target behavior), and *helping relationships* (trusting, accepting, and utilizing the support of caring others in the process of establishing the target behavior).

The amount of confidence people have in their ability to maintain a regular fitness program (self-efficacy) is related to their current stage. People in the early stages have less belief in their ability than those in later stages. Success has a powerful effect on self-efficacy. People often slip, however, and have to recycle through earlier stages.

According to the surgeon general's report, consistent influences on physical activity patterns among adults and young people include[11]

- Confidence in one's ability to engage in regular physical activity (self-efficacy)
- Enjoyment of physical activity
- Support from others
- Positive beliefs concerning the benefits of physical activity
- Lack of perceived barriers to being physically active

In working with people, long-term interest, enthusiasm, and compliance to an exercise program can be promoted by several strategies, including the following:[6]

- Encourage group participation or exercising with a partner.
- Emphasize variety and enjoyment in the exercise program.
- Minimize musculoskeletal injuries with a moderate exercise intensity and rate of progression.

TABLE 8.13   Summary of Theories and Models Used in Physical Activity Research

Theory/Model	Level	Key Concepts
Classic learning theories	Individual	Reinforcement Cues Shaping
Health-belief model	Individual	Perceived susceptibility Perceived severity Perceived benefits Perceived barriers Cues to action Self-efficacy
Transtheoretical model	Individual	Precontemplation Contemplation Preparation Action Maintenance
Relapse prevention	Individual	Skills training Cognitive reframing Lifestyle rebalancing
Social-cognitive theory	Interpersonal	Reciprocal determinism Behavioral capability Self-efficacy Outcome expectations Observational learning Reinforcement

Theory of planned behavior	Interpersonal	Attitude toward the behavior
		    Outcome expectations
		    Value of outcome expectations
		Subjective norm
		    Beliefs of others
		    Motive to comply with others
		Perceived behavioral control

Social support	Interpersonal	Instrumental support Informational support Emotional support Appraisal support

Ecological perspective	Environmental	Multiple levels of influence
		    Intrapersonal
		    Interpersonal
		    Institutional
		    Community
		    Public policy

Source: U.S. Department of Health and Human Services. *Physical Activity and Health: A Report of the Surgeon General.* Atlanta, GA: U.S. Department of Health and Human Services, Centers for Disease Control and Prevention, National Center for Chronic Disease Prevention and Health Promotion, 1996.

- Help the client draw up reasonable goals and highlight these in a contract the client signs.

- Recruit the client's spouse or significant other for support.

- Provide progress charts to document achievement of goals.

- Recognize accomplishments through a system of rewards.

- Maximize convenience in terms of time, travel, and disruptions in family relationships.

- Complement fitness activities with nutrition education, stress management, and other health-promotion activities to improve the overall health of the client.

SUMMARY

A comprehensive approach to exercise prescription should be used to provide all of the elements of physical fitness:

Warm-up. Engage in slow aerobic activity for several minutes, to gradually elevate the pulse and body temperature for hard aerobic activity. This will prepare the body by elevating the pulse, warming the body, and increasing blood flow. Flexibility exercises should not be done before the muscles and joints are warm.

Frequency. Start with 3 days per week and gradually build up to 5 or more days. Less than 3 days per week of aerobic activity does not build adequate fitness or help keep body fat under control. More than 5 days per week brings fewer fitness returns for the time and effort invested.

Intensity. Exercise at 40–85% of maximal capacity, depending on fitness status. The Karvonen formula is helpful for determining the training heart rate. The heart rate should be periodically counted (10-second pulse count) during exercise.

Time. The duration of an aerobic workout should be 20–60 minutes, depending on fitness status, intensity of exercise, and age. Time and intensity are interrelated and can be adjusted, as long as 4 Calories/kg of body weight is expended. Informal exercise for 1 hour a day is advised, to complement the formal exercise program.

Mode. If frequency, intensity, and duration of training are similar, and a minimum of 4 Calories/kg are expended during the session, the training result is independent of the mode of exercise. Aerobic activities that are enjoyable should be utilized. A variety of exercises will enhance compliance.

Warm-down. The purpose is to slowly decrease the pulse rate and body temperature, which were elevated during the aerobic phase by engaging in slow aerobics. This will enhance recovery by reducing the muscle and blood lactic acid levels and promoting venous return to the heart.

Flexibility. Engage in flexibility exercises after the aerobic session, to stretch warm muscle groups that have been especially involved in the aerobic activities. Static stretching is advised, with each specific position held for two sets of about 15–30 seconds each.

Conditioning exercises for muscular endurance and strength. Strength, size, and endurance of muscle tissue is enhanced when the muscle performs for a period of time at its maximal strength and endurance capacity, against workloads above those normally encountered. The resistance should be gradually increased until the desired state is achieved. Isometric, isotonic, and isokinetic muscle training systems have been developed.

REFERENCES

1. American College of Sports Medicine. *ACSM's Guidelines for Exercise Testing and Prescription* (5th ed.). Baltimore: Williams & Wilkins, 1995.

2. American College of Sports Medicine. The recommended quantity and quality of exercise for developing and maintaining cardiorespiratory and muscular fitness in healthy adults. *Med Sci Sports Exerc* 22:265–274, 1990; *Med Sci Sports Exerc* 30:975–991, 1998.

3. American College of Sports Medicine. *ACSM's Exercise Management for Persons with Chronic Diseases and Disabilities.* Champaign, IL: Human Kinetics, 1997.

4. Haskell WL. Health consequences of physical activity: Understanding and challenges regarding dose–response. *Med Sci Sports Exerc* 26:649–660, 1994.

5. Haskell WL. Physical activity, sport, and health: Toward the next century. *Res Quart Exerc Sport* 67(suppl):S37–S47, 1996.

6. Nieman DC. Programming for the healthy adult. In Cotton RT (ed), *Personal Trainer Manual.* San Diego: American Council on Exercise, 1996.

7. King CN, Senn MD. Exercise testing and prescription: Practical recommendations for the sedentary. *Sports Med* 21:326–336, 1996.

8. Phillips WT, Pruitt LA, King AC. Lifestyle activity: Current recommendations. *Sports Med* 22:1–7, 1996.

9. Oja P. Descriptive epidemiology of health-related physical activity and fitness. *Res Quart Exerc Sport* 66:303–312, 1995.

10. Blair SN, Booth M, Gyarfas I, Iwane H, Marti B, Matsudo V, Morrow MS, Noakes T, Shephard R. Development of public policy and physical activity initiatives internationally. *Sports Med* 21:157–163, 1996.

11. U.S. Department of Health and Human Services. *Physical Activity and Health: A Report of the Surgeon General.* Atlanta, GA: U.S. Department of Health and Human Services, Centers for Disease Control and Prevention, National Center for Chronic Disease Prevention and Health Promotion, 1996.

12. American College of Sports Medicine. The recommended quantity and quality of exercise for developing and maintaining fitness in healthy adults. *Med Sci Sports Exerc* 10:vii–x, 1978.

13. DeBusk RF, Stenestrand U, Sheehan M, et al. Training effects of long versus short bouts of exercise in healthy subjects. *Am J Cardiol* 65:1010–1013, 1990.

14. Ebisu T. Splitting the distance of endurance running: On cardiovascular endurance and blood lipids. *Jap J Phys Educ* 30:37–43, 1985.

15. Jakicic JM, Wing RR, Butler BA, Robertson RJ. Prescribing exercise in multiple short bouts versus one continuous bout: Effects on adherence, cardiorespiratory fitness, and weight loss in overweight women. *Int J Obesity* 19:893–901, 1995.

16. Pate RR, Pratt M, Blair SN, et al. Physical activity and public health: A recommendation from the Centers for Disease Control and Prevention and the American College of Sports Medicine. *JAMA* 273:402–407, 1995.

17. Fletcher GF, Blair SN, Blumenthal J, et al. Benefits and recommendations for physical activity programs for all Americans: A statement for health professionals by the Committee on Exercise and Cardiac Rehabilitation of the Council on Clinical Cardiology, American Heart Association. *Circulation* 86: 340–344, 1992.

18. Fletcher GF, Balady G, Blair SN, et al. Benefits and recommendations for physical activity programs for all Americans: A statement for health professionals by the Committee on Exercise and Cardiac Rehabilitation of the Council on Clinical Cardiology, American Heart Association. *Circulation* 94:857–862, 1996.

19. Sallis JF, Patrick K. Physical activity guidelines for adolescents: Consensus statement. *Pediatric Exerc Sci* 6:302–314, 1994.

20. American Cancer Society. *Cancer Facts & Figures—1996*. Atlanta: American Cancer Society, 1996.

21. U.S. Preventive Services Task Force. *Guide to Clinical Preventive Services* (2nd ed.). Alexandria, VA: International Medical Publishing, 1996.

22. NIH Consensus Development Panel on Physical Activity and Cardiovascular Health. Physical activity and cardiovascular health. *JAMA* 276:241–246, 1996.

23. Alter MJ. *Science of Flexibility* (2nd ed.). Champaign, IL: Human Kinetics, 1996.

24. McCardle WD, Katch FI, Katch VL. *Exercise Physiology: Energy, Nutrition, and Human Performance* (4th ed.). Baltimore: Williams & Wilkins, 1996.

25. Wilmore JH, Costill DL. *Physiology of Sports and Exercise*. Champaign, IL: Human Kinetics, 1994.

26. Brooks GA, Fahey TD, White TP. *Exercise Physiology: Human Bioenergetics and Its Applications* (2nd ed). Mountain View, CA: Mayfield Publishing Company, 1996.

27. Institute for Aerobics Research. *The Strength Connection*. Dallas: Author, 1990.

28. Maddux GT. *Men's Gymnastics*. Pacific Palisades, CA: Goodyear Publishing Co., Inc., 1970.

29. Shellock FG. Physiological benefits of warm-up. *Physician Sportsmed* 11:134–139, 1983.

30. Hetzler RK, Knowlton RG, Kaminsky LA, Kamimori GH. Effect of warm-up on plasma free fatty acid responses and substrate utilization during submaximal exercise. *Res Quart Exerc Sport* 57:223–228, 1986.

31. Wiktorsson-Möller M, Oberg B, Ekstrand J, Gillquist J. Effects of warming up, massage, and stretching on range of motion and muscle strength in the lower extremity. *Am J Sports Med* 11:249–252, 1983.

32. Shellock FG, Prentice WE. Warming-up and stretching for improved physical performance and prevention of sports-related injuries. *Sports Med* 2:267–278, 1985.

33. Strickler T, Malone T, Garrett WE. The effects of passive warming on muscle injury. *Am J Sports Med* 18:141–145, 1990.

34. Houmard JA, Johns RA, Smith LL, Wells JM, Kobe RW, McGoogan SA. The effect of warm-up on responses to intense exercise. *Int J Sports Med* 12:480–483, 1991.

35. Moneta-Chivalbinska J, Hänninen O. Effect of active warming-up on thermoregulatory, circulatory, and metabolic responses to incremental exercise in endurance-trained athletes. *Int J Sports Med* 10:25–29, 1989.

36. Lund RJ, Guthrie AJ, Mostert HJ, Travers CW, Nurton JP, Adamson DJ. Effect of three different warm-up regimens on heat balance and oxygen consumption of thoroughbred horses. *J Appl Physiol* 80:2190–2197, 1996.

37. Vuori IM, Oja P, Paronen O. Physically active community to work—testing its potential for exercise promotion. *Med Sci Sports Exerc* 26:844–850, 1994.

38. Pate RR, Branch JD. Training for endurance sport. *Med Sci Sports Exerc* 24(suppl):S340–S343, 1992.

39. Caspersen CJ, Bloemberg BPM, Saris WHM, Merritt RK, Kromhout D. The prevalence of selected physical activities and their relation with coronary heart disease risk factors in elderly men: The Zutphen study, 1985. *Am J Epidemiol* 133: 1078–1092, 1991.

40. Sallis JF, Hovell MF. Determinants of exercise behavior. *Exerc Sport Sci Review* 18:307–336, 1990.

41. King AC, Blair SN, Bild DE, et al. Determinants of physical activity and interventions in adults. *Med Sci Sports Exerc* 24(suppl):S221–S236, 1992.

42. Mensink GBM, Heerstrass DW, Neppelenbroek SE, Schuit AJ, Bellach BM. Intensity, duration, and frequency of physical activity and coronary risk factors. *Med Sci Sports Exerc* 29: 1192–1198, 1997.

43. Barinaga M. How much pain for cardiac gain? *Science* 276: 1324–1327, 1997.

44. Lindsay FH, Hawley JA, Myburgh KH, Schomer HH, Noakes TD, Dennis SC. Improved athletic performance in highly training cyclists after interval training. *Med Sci Sports Exerc* 28: 1427–1434, 1996.

45. Robinson DM, Robinson SM, Hume PA, Hopkins WG. Training intensity of elite male distance runners. *Med Sci Sports Exerc* 23:1078–1082, 1991.

46. Ainsworth BE, Haskell WL, Leon AS, Jacobs DR, Montoye HJ, Sallis JF, Paffenbarger RS. Compendium of physical activities: Classification of energy costs of human physical activities. *Med Sci Sports Exerc* 25:71–80, 1993.

47. Londeree BR, Thomas TR, Ziogas G, Smith TD, Zhang Q. %$\dot{V}O_{2max}$ versus %HR_{max} regressions for six modes of exercise. *Med Sci Sports Exerc* 27:458–461, 1995.

48. Karvonen M, Kentala E, Mustala O. The effects of training on heart rate: A longitudinal study. *Ann Med Exp Biol Fenn* 35: 307–315, 1957.

49. Davis JA, Convertino VA. A comparison of heart rate methods for predicting endurance training intensity. *Med Sci Sports* 7: 295–298, 1975.

50. Swain DP, Leutholtz BC. Heart rate reserve is equivalent to %$\dot{V}O_2$ reserve, not to %$\dot{V}O_{2max}$. *Med Sci Sports Exerc* 29:410–414, 1997. (See also *Med Sci Sports Exec* 30:318–321, 1998.)

51. Panton LB, Graves JE, Pollock ML, Garzarella L, Carroll JF, Leggett SH, Lowenthal DT, Guillen GJ. Relative heart rate, heart rate reserve, and $\dot{V}O_2$ during submaximal exercise in the elderly. *J Gerontol A Biol Sci Med Sci* 51:M165–M171, 1996.

52. Whaley MH, Kaminsky LA, Dwyer GB, Getchell LH, Norton JA. Predictors of over- and underachievement of age-predicted maximal heart rate. *Med Sci Sports Exerc* 24:1173–1179, 1992.

53. Miller WC, Wallace JP, Eggert KE. Predicting Max HR and the HR–V̇O₂ relationship for exercise prescription in obesity. *Med Sci Sports Exerc* 25:1077–1081, 1993.

54. Couldry W, Corbin CB, Wilcox A. Carotid vs radial pulse counts. *Physician Sportsmed* 10:67–72, 1982.

55. Boone T, Frentz KL, Boyd NR. Carotid palpation at two exercise intensities. *Med Sci Sports Exerc* 17:705–709, 1985.

56. Borg G. Perceived exertion as indicator of somatic stress. *Scand J Rehabil Med* 2:92–98, 1970.

57. Noble BJ, Borg GAV, Jacobs I., Ceci R., Kaiser P. A category-ratio perceived exertion scale: Relationship to blood and muscle lactates and heart rate. *Med Sci Sports Exerc* 15:523–528, 1983.

58. Robertson RJ, Noble BJ. Perception of physical exertion: Methods, mediators, and applications. *Exerc Sport Sci Rev* 25:407–452, 1997.

59. Demello JJ, Cureton KJ, Boineau RE, et al. Ratings of perceived exertion at the lactate threshold in trained and untrained men and women. *Med Sci Sports Exerc* 19:354–362, 1987.

60. Stoudemire NM, Wideman L, Pass KA, McGinnes CL, Gaesser GA, Weltman A. The validity of regulating blood lactate concentration during running by ratings of perceived exertion. *Med Sci Sports Exerc* 28:490–495, 1996.

61. Whaley MH, Woodall T, Kaminsky LA, Emmett JD. Reliability of perceived exertion during graded exercise testing in apparently healthy adults. *J Cardiopulm Rehabil* 17:37–42, 1997.

62. Borg G. *An Introduction to Borg's RPE-Scale.* Ithaca, NY: Movement Publications, 1985.

63. Potteiger JA, Weber SF. Rating of perceived exertion and heart rate as indicators of exercise intensity in different environmental temperatures. *Med Sci Sports Exerc* 26:791–796, 1994.

64. Ueda T, Kurokawa T. Relationships between perceived exertion and physiological variables during swimming. *Int J Sports Med* 16:385–389, 1995.

65. Glass SC, Knowlton RG, Becque MD. Perception of effort during high-intensity exercise at low, moderate, and high wet bulb globe temperatures. *Eur J Appl Physiol* 68:519–524, 1994.

66. Ilmarinen J, Ilmarinen R, Koskela A, Korhonen O, et al. Training effects of stair-climbing during office hours on female employees. *Ergonomics* 22:507–516, 1979.

67. Ilmarinen J, Rutenfranz J, Knauth P, Ahrens M, et al. The effect of an on the job training program, stairclimbing, on the physical working capacity of employees. *Eur J Appl Physiol* 38:25–40, 1978.

68. Kuipers H. How much is too much? Performance aspects of overtraining. *Res Quart Exerc Sport* 67(suppl):S65–S69, 1996.

69. Loy SF, Hoffmann JJ, Holland GJ. Benefits and practical use of cross-training in sports. *Sports Med* 19:1–8, 1996.

70. Porcari JP, Ebbeling CB, Ward A, Freedson PS, Rippe JM. Walking for exercise testing and training. *Sports Med* 8:189–200, 1989.

71. Morris JN, Hardman AE. Walking to health. *Sports Med* 23:306–332, 1997.

72. Porcari J, McCarron R, Kline G, et al. Is fast walking an adequate aerobic training stimulus for 30- to 69-year-old men and women. *Physician Sportsmed* 15(2):119–129, 1987.

73. Davison RCR, Grant S. Is walking sufficient exercise for health? *Sports Med* 16:369–373, 1993.

74. Nieman DC, Haig JL, De Guia ED, Dizon GP, Register UD. Reducing diet and exercise training effects on resting metabolic rates in mildly obese women. *J Sports Med* 28:79–88, 1988.

75. Warren BJ, Nieman DC, Dotson RG, Adkins CH, O'Donnell KA, Haddock BL, Butterworth DE. Cardiorespiratory responses to exercise training in septuagenarian women. *Int J Sports Med* 14:60–65, 1993.

76. Stensel DJ, Brooke-Wavell K, Hardman AE, Jones PRM, Norgan NG. The influence of a 1-year program of brisk walking on endurance fitness and body composition in previously sedentary men aged 42–59 years. *Eur J Appl Physiol* 68:531–537, 1994.

77. Spelman CC, Pate RR, Macera CA, Ward DS. Self-selected exercise intensity of habitual walkers. *Med Sci Sports Exerc* 25:1174–1179, 1993.

78. Graves JE, Pollock ML, Montain SJ, et al. The effect of hand-held weights on the physiological responses to walking exercise. *Med Sci Sports Exerc* 19:260–265, 1987.

79. Graves JE, Martin AD, Miltenberger LA, Pollock ML. Physiological responses to walking with hand weights, wrist weights, and ankle weights. *Med Sci Sports Exerc* 20:265–271, 1988.

80. Auble TE, Schwartz L. Physiological effects of exercising with handweights. *Sports Med* 11:244–256, 1991.

81. Miller JF, Stamford BA. Intensity and energy cost of weighted walking vs. running for men and women. *J Appl Physiol* 62:1497–1501, 1987.

82. Claremont AD, Hall SJ. Effects of extremity loading upon energy expenditure and running mechanics. *Med Sci Sports Exerc* 20:167–171, 1988.

83. Garrick JG, Requa RK. Aerobic dance: A review. *Sports Med* 6:169–179, 1988.

84. Watterson VV. The effects of aerobic dance on cardiovascular fitness. *Physician Sportsmed* 10:138–145, 1984.

85. Milburn S, Butts NK. A comparison of the training responses to aerobic dance and jogging in college females. *Med Sci Sports Exerc* 15:510–513, 1983.

86. McMurray RG, Hackney AC, Guion WK, Katz VL. Metabolic and hormonal responses to low-impact aerobic dance during pregnancy. *Med Sci Sports Exerc* 28:41–46, 1996.

87. Noreau L, Moffet H, Drolet M, Parent E. Dance-based exercise program in rheumatoid arthritis: Feasibility in individuals with American College of Rheumatology Functional Class III disease. *Am J Phys Med Rehabil* 76:109–113, 1997.

88. Nelson DJ, Pels AE, Geenen DL, White TP. Cardiac frequency and caloric cost of aerobic dancing in young women. *Res Quart Exerc Sport* 59:229–233, 1988.

89. Williford HN, Blessing DL, Barksdale JM, Smith FH. The effects of aerobic dance training on serum lipids, lipoproteins and cardiopulmonary function. *J Sports Med* 28:151–157, 1988.

90. Koszuta LE. Low-impact aerobics: Better than traditional aerobic dance? *Physician Sportsmed* 14(7):156, 1986.

91. Koszuta LE. Water exercise causes ripples. *Physician Sportsmed* 14(10):163–167, 1986.

92. Jétte M, Landry F, Tiemann B, Blümchen G. Ambulatory blood pressure and Holter monitoring during tennis play. *Can J Spt Sci* 16:40–44, 1991.

93. Bartoli WP, Slentz CA, Murdoch SD, Pate RR, Davis JM, Durstine JL. Effects of a 12-week racquetball program on maximal oxygen consumption, body composition and blood lipoproteins. *Sports Med Train Rehab* 5:157–164, 1994.

94. Montpetit RR, Beauchamp L, Léger L. Energy requirements of

squash and racquetball. *Physician Sportsmed* 15(8):106–112, 1987.

95. Morgans LF, Jordan DL, Baeyens DA, Franciosa JA. Heart rate responses during singles and doubles tennis competition. *Physician Sportsmed* 15(7):67–74, 1987.

96. Locke S, Colquhoun D, Briner M, Ellis L, O'Brien M, Wollstein J, Allen G. Squash racquets: A review of physiology and medicine. *Sports Med* 23:130–138, 1997.

97. Loftin M, Anderson P, Lytton L, Pittman P, Warren B. Heart rate response during handball singles match-play and selected physical fitness components of experienced male handball players. *J Sports Med Phys Fitness* 36:95–99, 1996.

98. Hurley BF. Effects of high-intensity strength training on cardiovascular function. *Med Sci Sports Exerc* 16:483–488, 1984.

99. Gettman LR, Ayres JJ, Pollock ML, Jackson A. The effect of circuit weight training on strength, cardiorespiratory function, and body composition of adult men. *Med Sci Sports Exerc* 10:171–176, 1978.

100. Ballor DL, Becque MD, Katch VL. Metabolic responses during hydraulic resistance exercise. *Med Sci Sports Exerc* 19:363–367, 1987.

101. Harris KA, Holly RG. Physiological response to circuit weight training in borderline hypertensive subjects. *Med Sci Sports Exerc* 19:246–252, 1987.

102. Dudley GA, Fleck SJ. Strength and endurance training: Are they mutually exclusive? *Sports Med* 4:79–85, 1987.

103. Kuehl K, Elliot DL, Goldberg L. Predicting caloric expenditure during multi-station resistance exercise. *J Appl Sport Sci Res* 4(5):63–66, 1990.

104. Sleamaker RH. Caloric cost of performing the Perrier Parcourse Fitness Circuit. *Med Sci Sports Exerc* 16:283–286, 1984.

105. Berry MJ, Cline CC, Berry CB, Davis M. A comparison between two forms of aerobic dance and treadmill running. *Med Sci Sports Exerc* 24:946–951, 1992.

106. Olson MS, Williford HN, Blessing DL, Greathouse R. The cardiovascular and metabolic effects of bench stepping exercise in females. *Med Sci Sports Exerc* 23:1311–1318, 1991.

107. Quirk JE, Sinning WE. Anaerobic and aerobic responses of males and females to rope skipping. *Med Sci Sports Exerc* 14:26–29, 1982.

108. Town GP, Sol N, Sinning WE. The effect of rope skipping rate on energy expenditure of males and females. *Med Sci Sports Exerc* 12:295–298, 1980.

109. Mahler DA, Andrea BE, Ward JL. Comparison of exercise performance on rowing and cycle ergometers. *Res Quart Exerc Sport* 58:41–46, 1987.

110. Hagerman FC, Lawrence RA, Mansfield MC. A comparison of energy expenditure during rowing and cycling ergometry. *Med Sci Sports Exerc* 20:479–488, 1988.

111. Secher NH. Physiological and biomechanical aspects of rowing: Implications for training. *Sports Med* 15:24–42, 1993.

112. Howley ET, Colacino DL, Swensen TC. Factors affecting the oxygen cost of stepping on an electronic stepping ergometer. *Med Sci Sports Exerc* 24:1055–1058, 1992.

113. Zeni AI, Hoffman MD, Clifford PS. Energy expenditure with indoor exercise machines. *JAMA* 275:1424–1427, 1996.

114. Kravitz L, Robergs RA, Heyward VH, Wagner DR, Powers K. Exercise mode and gender comparisons of energy expenditure at self-selected intensities. *Med Sci Sports Exerc* 29:1028–1035, 1997.

115. Dimsdale JE, Hartley LH, Guiney T, et al. Postexercise peril: Plasma catecholamines and exercise. *JAMA* 251:630–632, 1984.

116. Ahmaidi S, Granier P, Taoutaou Z, Mercier J, Dubouchaud H, Prefaut C. Effects of active recovery on plasma lactate and anaerobic power following repeated intensive exercise. *Med Sci Sports Exerc* 28:450–456, 1996.

117. El-Sayed M, Rattu AJM, Lin X, Reilly T. Effects of active warm-down and carbohydrate feeding on free fatty acid concentrations after prolonged submaximal exercise. *Int J Sport Nutr* 6:337–347, 1996.

118. American College of Sports Medicine. *ACSM Fitness Book* (2nd ed.). Champaign, IL: Human Kinetics, 1998.

119. Levine M, Lombardo J, McNeeley J, Anderson T. An analysis of individual stretching programs of intercollegiate athletes. *Physician Sportsmed* 15(3):130–137, 1987.

120. Krivickas LS. Anatomical factors associated with overuse sports injuries. *Sports Med* 24:132–146, 1997.

121. Bandy WD, Irion JM. The effect of time on static stretch on the flexibility of the hamstring muscles. *Phys Ther* 74:845–852, 1994.

122. Webright WG, Randolph BJ, Perrin DH. Comparison of non-ballistic active knee extension in neural slump position and static stretch techniques on hamstring flexibility. *J Orthop Sports Phys Ther* 26:7–13, 1997.

123. Rodenburg JB, Steenbeek D, Schiereck Bar PR. Warm-up, stretching and massage diminish harmful effects of eccentric exercise. *Int J Sport Med* 15:414–419, 1994.

124. Halbertsma JPK, Goeken LNH. Stretching exercises: Effect on passive extensibility and stiffness in short hamstring of healthy subjects. *Arch Phys Med Rehabil* 75:976–981, 1994.

125. Sullivan MK, Dejulia JJ, Worrell TW. Effect of pelvic position and stretching method on hamstring muscle flexibility. *Med Sci Sports Exerc* 24:1383–1389, 1992.

126. Higdon H. True or false? *Runner's World,* April, 1997, 100–105.

127. Krivickas LS, Feinberg JH. Lower extremity injuries in college athletes: Relation between ligamentous laxity and lower extremity muscle tightness. *Arch Phys Med Rehabil* 77:1139–1143, 1996.

128. Ekstrand J, Gillquist J. The frequency of muscle tightness and injuries in soccer players. *Am J Sports Med* 10:75–78, 1982.

129. Worrell T, Perrin D, Gansneder B, Gieck J. Comparison of isokinetic strength and flexibility measures between injured and noninjured athletes. *J Orthop Sports Phys Ther* 13:118–125, 1991.

130. Wiesler ER, Hunter DM, Martin DF, Curl WW, Hoen H. Ankle flexibility and injury patterns in dancers. *Am J Sports Med* 24:754–757, 1996.

131. Twellaar M, Verstappen FT, Huson A, van Mechelen W. Physical characteristics as risk factors for sports injuries: A four year prospective study. *Int J Sports Med* 18:66–71, 1997.

132. Kirby RL, Simms FC, Symingtom VJ, Garner JB. Flexibility and musculoskeletal symptomatology in female gymnasts and age-matched controls. *Am J Sports Med* 9:160–164, 1981.

133. Bennell KL, Crossley K. Musculoskeletal injuries in track and field: Incidence, distribution and risk factors. *Aust J Sci Med Sport* 28:69–75, 1996.

134. Craib MW, Mitchell VA, Fields KB, Cooper TR, Hopewell R, Morgan DW. The association between flexibility and running economy in sub-elite male distance runners. *Med Sci Sports Exerc* 28:737–743, 1996.

135. Etnyre BR, Lee JA. Chronic and acute flexibility of men and women using three different stretching techniques. *Res Quart Exerc Sport* 59:222–228, 1988.

136. Etnyre BR, Abraham LD. Antagonist muscle activity during stretching: A paradox re-assessed. *Med Sci Sports Exerc* 20: 285–289, 1988.

137. Cornelius WL, Craft-Hamm K. Proprioceptive neuromuscular facilitation flexibility techniques: Acute effects on arterial blood pressure. *Physician Sportsmed* 16(4):152–161, 1988.

138. Hutton RS. Neuromuscular basis of stretching exercises. In Komi PV (ed), *Strength and Power in Sport: The Encyclopædia of Sports Medicine*. Oxford: Blackwell Scientific Publications, 1992.

139. Anderson B. *Stretching*. Bolinas, CA: Shelter Publications, 1980.

140. Godges JJ, MacRae H, Longdon C, Tinberg C, MacRae P. The effects of two stretching procedures on hip range of motion and gait economy. *J Orthop Sports Phys Ther* 10:350–357, 1989.

141. Sady JP, Wortman M, Blanke D. Flexibility training: Ballistic, static, or PNF? *Arch Phys Med Rehabil* 63:261–263, 1982.

142. Osternig LR, Robertson RN, Troxel RK, Hansen P. Differential responses to proprioceptive neuromuscular facilitation (PNF) stretch techniques. *Med Sci Sports Exerc* 22:106–111, 1990.

143. Baechle TR. *Essentials of Strength Training and Conditioning*. Champaign, IL: Human Kinetics, 1994.

144. Feigenbaum MS, Pollock ML. Strength training: Rationale for current guidelines for adult fitness programs. *Physician Sportsmed* 25(2):45–64, 1997.

145. Fleck SJ, Kraemer WJ. *Designing Resistance Training Programs*. Champaign, IL: Human Kinetics, 1987.

146. Institute for Aerobics Research. *The Strength Connection*. Dallas: Author, 1990.

147. Pollock ML, Graves JE, Swart DL, et al. Exercise training and prescription for the elderly. *South Med J* 87:S88–S95, 1994.

148. American Association of Cardiovascular and Pulmonary Rehabilitation. *Guidelines for Cardiac Rehabilitation Programs* (2nd ed.). Champaign, IL: Human Kinetics, 1995.

149. Fletcher GF, Balady G, Froelicher VE, et al. Exercise standards: A statement for healthcare professionals from the American Heart Association. *Circulation* 91:580–615, 1995.

150. Starkey DB, Pollock ML, Ishida Y, Welsch MA, Brechue WF, Graves JE, Feigenbaum MS. Effect of resistance training volume on strength and muscle thickness. *Med Sci Sports Exerc* 28:1311–1320, 1996.

151. Morrissey MC, Harman EA, Johnson MJ. Resistance training modes: Specificity and effectiveness. *Med Sci Sports Exerc* 27: 648–660, 1995.

152. Rooney KJ, Herbert RD, Balnave RJ. Fatigue contributes to the strength training stimulus. *Med Sci Sports Exerc* 26:1160–1164, 1994.

153. Fry AC, Kraemer WJ. Resistance exercise overtraining and overreaching: Neuroendocrine responses. *Sports Med* 23: 106–129, 1997.

154. Davies GJ. *A Compendium of Isokinetics in Clinical Usage*. S & S Publishers, 1707 Jennifer Court, Onalaska, Wisconsin 54650, 1987.

155. Elliot DL, Goldberg L, Kuehl KS, Catlin DH. Characteristics of anabolic–androgenic steroid-free competitive male and female bodybuilders. *Physician Sportsmed* 15(6):169–180, 1987.

156. Braith RW, Graves JE, Pollock ML, Leggett SL, Carpenter DM, Colvin AB. Comparison of 2 vs 3 days / week of variable resistance training during 10- and 18-week programs. *Int J Sports Med* 10:450–454, 1989.

157. Kraemer WJ, Deschenes MR, Fleck SJ. Physiological adaptations to resistance exercise: Implications for athletic conditioning. *Sports Med* 6:246–256, 1988.

158. Tesch PA. Training for bodybuilding. In Komi PV (ed), *Strength and Power in Sport: The Encyclopædia of Sports Medicine*. Oxford: Blackwell Scientific Publications, 1992.

159. Sale DG. Neural adaptation to resistance training. *Med Sci Sports Exerc* 20(suppl):S135–S145, 1988.

160. Tesch PA. Skeletal muscle adaptations consequent to long-term heavy resistance exercise. *Med Sci Sports Exerc* 20(suppl): S132–S134, 1988.

161. Mayhew TP, Rothstein JM, Finucane SD, Lamb RL. Muscular adaptation to concentric and eccentric exercise at equal power levels. *Med Sci Sports Exerc* 27:868–873, 1995.

162. Higbie EJ, Cureton KJ, Warren GL, Prior BM. Effects of concentric and eccentric training on muscle strength, cross-sectional area, and neural activation. *J Appl Physiol* 81:2173–2181, 1996.

163. Franklin BA. Program factors that influence exercise adherence: Practical adherence skills for the clinical staff. In Dishman RK (ed), *Exercise Adherence*. Champaign, IL: Human Kinetics, 1988.

164. Robison JI, Rogers MA. Adherence to exercise programs: Recommendations. *Sports Med* 17:39–52, 1994.

165. Prochaska JO, DiClemente CC, Norcross JC. In search of how people change: Applications to addictive behaviors. *Am Psychol* 47:1102–1114, 1992.

166. Canadian Society for Exercise Physiology. *The Canadian Physical Activity, Fitness & Lifestyle Appraisal*. Ottawa, Ontario: Canadian Society for Exercise Physiology, 1996.

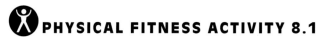

PHYSICAL FITNESS ACTIVITY 8.1

Writing the Exercise Prescription

In this physical fitness activity, you will be writing an exercise prescription for someone needing your guidance (choose a fellow student, family member, or friend). There are several steps that you should follow:

1. Have the client you are writing the exercise prescription for fill out the medical/health questionnaire (see Chapter 3). Review this questionnaire with the client, to gain a complete picture of background, present health status, and future goals. Next classify the client according to the American College of Sports Medicine criteria listed in Chapter 3 (apparently healthy, individual at higher risk, or patient with disease). Make an appropriate judgment as to the need for further testing with physician supervision. (Review Chapter 3.)

2. Review physical fitness testing results. It is preferable to have test results indicating the cardiorespiratory, body composition, and musculoskeletal status of the client you are counseling. Make sure the client understands the test results and their ranking within the norm tables.

3. Now that you have a better understanding of the medical, health, and physical fitness status of the client, start the exercise prescription process by reviewing the preferred mode of exercise. Using Table 8.11, have the person mark at least two cardiorespiratory endurance activities that have been enjoyed in the past or can be utilized in present circumstances.

4. Using the form in Figure 8.3, go step-by-step through each stage of the exercise prescription, explaining the basic concepts involved. It is a good idea to have the client fill in the blanks, to facilitate acceptance of the information. Important concepts to keep in mind with each stage of the exercise prescription include the following:

   Cardiorespiratory warm-up. Emphasize the importance of elevating body temperature through slow aerobic activity, preferably the aerobic activity that will be utilized in the workout session. Explain that flexibility exercises are best done when the body is warm, after the aerobic session.

   Cardiorespiratory/body composition, aerobic session. Circle the appropriate F.I.T. criteria, based on the fitness status of the client. Help the client determine the training heart rate, using the Karvonen formula, and fill in the appropriate blanks. Explain how to measure the training heart rate, and fill in the blank for the 10-second pulse count. Review the concept of rating of perceived exertion, explaining that an RPE of "somewhat hard" appears appropriate for most people. Caution against overexertion. Fill in the mode selected by the client. Discuss the concept of informal exercise and the importance of using the stairs when possible, walking during work breaks, and so on. Finally, have the client mark the appropriate blanks indicating the time and days of the week for which the exercise sessions will be planned.

   Cardiorespiratory, warm-down. Explain that this is basically the warm-up in reverse, to help the body through the transition from hard aerobic exercise to rest.

   Musculoskeletal, flexibility. Using the exercises pictured in Appendix C, review the principles of flexibility calisthenics and the particular importance of stretching the muscles utilized in the aerobic session.

Musculoskeletal, muscular strength and endurance. First find out whether your client has access to a weight training facility. If so, discuss both the principles of weight training and the basic lifts summarized in Table 8.11. If not, review the calisthenics pictured in Appendix C.

Before starting the exercise prescription process with your clients, a few concepts about counseling are helpful for providing better service. It is important to understand that no one person can motivate another. One can only create a climate that will facilitate others to motivate themselves. In other words, motivation comes from within. People tend to be motivated by challenge, growth, achievement, promotion, and recognition. Emphasis should be placed on providing a proper environment for self-growth by challenging clients, giving responsibility, encouraging, and giving full range to individual strength. The effective exercise counselor develops warm personal relationships with each participant and regards each as worthy of his or her genuine concern and attention.

Traits of a good counselor include

- *Empathy*—ability to climb into the world of the client and communicate feelings of understanding
- *Respect*—a deep and genuine appreciation for the worth of the client, separate and apart from his or her behavior, particularly acknowledging the strength and ability of the client to overcome obstacles and adjust to situations
- *Warmth*—communication of concern and appropriate affection
- *Genuineness*—being freely and deeply one's self, congruent, not just playing a role
- *Concreteness*—ferreting out essential ideas and elements
- *Self-disclosure*—revelations about self, for the benefit of the client, at the appropriate time
- *Potency and self-actualization*—dynamic, in command, conveying feelings of trust and warmth; competent, inner directed, creative, sensitive, nonjudgmental, productive, serene, satisfied—and able to convey this to the client in a helpful way

PHYSICAL FITNESS ACTIVITY 8.2

The Activity Pyramid

To help people better understand the new physical activity recommendations from the CDC–ACSM, the Health Education Center of the Institute for Research and Education, HealthSystem Minnesota, developed the activity pyramid (see Figure 8.26). Like the U.S. Department of Agriculture's food guide pyramid, the activity pyramid illustrates a balanced approach to physical activity.

This physical fitness activity is used to assess a person's position on the activity pyramid. Fill out each assessment, marking the statements that most closely apply to your (or your client's) personal situation. Then add up your scores at the bottom of each quiz and on the overall assessment at the end, to see where you stand and where you can begin to improve.

The activity pyramid can be ordered from

Park Nicollet HealthSource
3800 Park Nicollet Boulevard
Minneapolis, MN 55416
800-372-7776

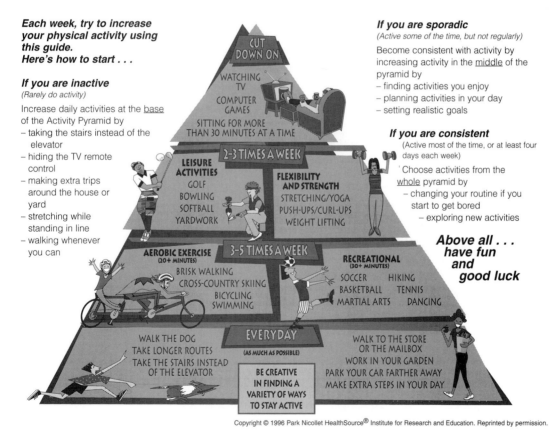

Each week, try to increase your physical activity using this guide. Here's how to start . . .

If you are inactive
(Rarely do activity)

Increase daily activities at the <u>base</u> of the Activity Pyramid by
– taking the stairs instead of the elevator
– hiding the TV remote control
– making extra trips around the house or yard
– stretching while standing in line
– walking whenever you can

If you are sporadic
(Active some of the time, but not regularly)

Become consistent with activity by increasing activity in the <u>middle</u> of the pyramid by
– finding activities you enjoy
– planning activities in your day
– setting realistic goals

If you are consistent
(Active most of the time, or at least four days each week)

Choose activities from the <u>whole</u> pyramid by
– changing your routine if you start to get bored
– exploring new activities

Above all . . . have fun and good luck

CUT DOWN ON
WATCHING TV
COMPUTER GAMES
SITTING FOR MORE THAN 30 MINUTES AT A TIME

2-3 TIMES A WEEK

LEISURE ACTIVITIES
GOLF
BOWLING
SOFTBALL
YARDWORK

FLEXIBILITY AND STRENGTH
STRETCHING/YOGA
PUSH-UPS/CURL-UPS
WEIGHT LIFTING

3-5 TIMES A WEEK

AEROBIC EXERCISE (20+ MINUTES)
BRISK WALKING
CROSS-COUNTRY SKIING
BICYCLING
SWIMMING

RECREATIONAL (30+ MINUTES)
SOCCER   HIKING
BASKETBALL   TENNIS
MARTIAL ARTS DANCING

EVERYDAY
(AS MUCH AS POSSIBLE)

WALK THE DOG
TAKE LONGER ROUTES
TAKE THE STAIRS INSTEAD OF THE ELEVATOR

BE CREATIVE IN FINDING A VARIETY OF WAYS TO STAY ACTIVE

WALK TO THE STORE OR THE MAILBOX
WORK IN YOUR GARDEN
PARK YOUR CAR FARTHER AWAY
MAKE EXTRA STEPS IN YOUR DAY

Figure 8.26 Each week, try to increase your physical activity using this guide.

For each of the following sets of items, mark the statements that most closely apply to you. Then add up your scores at the bottom of each quiz and on the overall assessment at the end, to see where you stand and where you can begin to improve.

Your Readiness for Building a Pyramid: *Personal Motivation*
Mark the one box in each row that most closely reflects your answer.

Column 1	*Column 2*	*Column 3*
❑ I have all the energy I need to perform my daily tasks and recreational activities.	❑ By the end of the day, I'm often too tired to do anything active.	❑ I am usually sluggish or physically drained, even during the day.
❑ I am already active and committed to regular physical activity.	❑ I plan to become more physically active within the next month.	❑ I have no plans for becoming more physically active.
❑ I make time for exercise each week.	❑ I fit exercise into my schedule when I can.	❑ I rarely plan when I will exercise.
❑ When it comes to exercise, such things as bad weather or finding a place to exercise don't get in the way.	❑ Occasionally, such things as weather or inconvenient exercise facilities make it difficult to exercise.	❑ More often than not, it is really inconvenient to get some exercise.
❑ I have all the proper shoes, workout clothes or other equipment I need to exercise.	❑ I make do with what I have.	❑ I don't have any exercise shoes, clothes, or equipment.
Number of Column 1 responses = 1 point each	*Number of Column 2 responses = 2 points each*	*Number of Column 3 responses = 3 points each*
Column 1 points _____	Column 2 points _____	Column 3 points _____

Add your points from columns 1, 2, and 3, to arrive at your "Readiness Points" total, and enter it here.

_____
READINESS POINTS

Your finding:

6 or less: Solid Pyramid
7 to 10: Pyramid under Construction
10 or more: Get Building!

The Base of the Pyramid: *Adding Steps to Your Day*

Mark the one box in each row that most closely reflects your answer.

Column 1	*Column 2*	*Column 3*
❑ I rarely ride when I have an opportunity to walk or bike.	❑ I occasionally use walking or biking as a form of transportation.	❑ I rarely walk or bike anywhere when I have an opportunity to ride.
❑ I usually seek out the stairs instead of using elevators or escalators.	❑ I park a distance from my destination if it is convenient at the time.	❑ I routinely park as close as I can to my destination.
❑ I have a very active job that keeps me moving, walking, or lifting for two or more hours a day.	❑ My job involves occasional physical activity and moving around for up to two hours a day.	❑ My job involves sitting or standing in one place most of the day.
❑ I always take extra steps in my day.	❑ I sometimes take extra steps in my day.	❑ I rarely take extra steps in my day.
Number of Column 1 responses = 1 point each	*Number of Column 2 responses = 2 points each*	*Number of Column 3 responses = 3 points each*
Column 1 points _____	Column 2 points _____	Column 3 points _____

Add your points from columns 1, 2, and 3, to arrive at your total, and enter it here.

_____

ADD STEPS TO
YOUR DAY

Your finding:

6 or less: Solid Pyramid
7 to 10: Pyramid under Construction
10 or more: Get Building!

The Second Level of the Pyramid: *Aerobics and Recreation*

Mark the one box in each row that most closely reflects your answer.

Column 1

❑ I can choose from a variety of recreational* sports activities that I enjoy.

❑ I can choose from a variety of aerobic** activities that I enjoy.

❑ I participate in aerobic or recreational sports activities at least three to five times a week.

❑ I set realistic physical activity goals and stick with them.

❑ I can walk a mile in 15 minutes or less.

Number of Column 1 responses = 1 point each

Column 1 points _____

Column 2

❑ I enjoy only one or two recreational sports activities.

❑ I enjoy only one or two aerobic activities.

❑ I usually participate in aerobic activities or recreational sports activities one to three times a week.

❑ I sometimes lose sight of my goals, but usually get back on track.

❑ It takes me 15 to 20 minutes to walk a mile.

Number of Column 2 responses = 2 points each

Column 2 points _____

Column 3

❑ I have not found any recreational sports activities that I enjoy.

❑ I have not found any aerobic activities that I enjoy.

❑ I rarely or never participate in aerobic or recreational sports activities.

❑ I rarely set activity-related goals.

❑ It takes me more than 20 minutes to walk a mile.

Number of Column 3 responses = 3 points each

Column 3 points _____

Add your points from columns 1, 2, and 3, to arrive at your "Aerobics & Recreation" total, and enter it here.

Examples of recreational sports activities include tennis, basketball, volleyball, racquetball, soccer, hockey, or skiing.

**Aerobic activities include exercise such as "aerobics" classes, jogging, brisk walking, cross-country skiing, skating, swimming, or bicycling for 20 minutes or more per session.*

_____

AEROBICS & RECREATION

Your finding:

6 or less: Solid Pyramid
7 to 10: Pyramid under Construction
10 or more: Get Building!

The Third Level of the Pyramid: *Flexibility, Strength, and Leisure*

Mark the one box in each row that most closely reflects your answer.

Column 1	*Column 2*	*Column 3*
❑ I know stretching and strengthening exercises for each of the major muscle groups.	❑ I know a few strengthening and stretching exercises but not for each of the major muscle groups.	❑ I don't know any stretching or strengthening exercises.
❑ I have a warm-up and cool-down routine that includes good stretching exercises	❑ I sometimes stretch before and after exercising.	❑ I don't do any stretching exercises.
❑ I regularly include muscle-strengthening exercises (calisthenics, or weight lifting) as part of my exercise routine.	❑ I occasionally include muscle-strengthening exercises in my routine.	❑ I almost never do muscle-strengthening exercises.
❑ My job, hobbies, or work I do at home regularly require lifting or stooping.	❑ My job, hobbies, or work I do at home occasionally require lifting or stooping.	❑ I rarely do hobbies or work at home that requires lifting or stooping.
❑ I participate in leisure physical activities* one to two times a week.	❑ I only sporadically participate in leisure physical activities.	❑ I rarely or never participate in leisure physical activities.
Number of Column 1 responses = 1 point each	*Number of Column 2 responses = 2 points each*	*Number of Column 3 responses = 3 points each*
Column 1 points _____	Column 2 points _____	Column 3 points _____

Add your points from columns 1, 2, and 3, to arrive at your "Flexibility, Strength & Leisure" total, and enter it here.

*Examples of leisure physical activities are golf, bowling, and softball.

———
FLEXBILITY, STRENGTH
& LEISURE

Your finding:

6 or less: Solid Pyramid
7 to 10: Pyramid under Construction
10 or more: Get Building!

The Peak of the Pyramid: *Cut Down on Sitting*

Mark the one box in each row that most closely reflects your answer.

Column 1	Column 2	Column 3
❏ I'm the type of person who rarely sits still for any length of time.	❏ I often sit for extended periods, but I'm trying to get up and move more often.	❏ My work life or home life involves a lot of sitting.
❏ Many of my friends or colleagues enjoy physical activities or sports.	❏ I have only a few friends or colleagues who enjoy physical activities or sports.	❏ None of my friends enjoy talking about or doing physical activities.
❏ When I exercise, I can choose from a variety of activities.	❏ I have limited exercise activities to choose from.	❏ I can't think of any exercise activities that suit me.
❏ Getting regular physical exercise is a priority in my life.	❏ I exercise when I can, but it competes with other priorities.	❏ I have too many other priorities to exercise regularly.
Number of Column 1 responses = 1 point each	*Number of Column 2 responses = 2 points each*	*Number of Column 3 responses = 3 points each*
Column 1 points _____	Column 2 points _____	Column 3 points _____

Add your points from columns 1, 2, and 3, to arrive at your "Cut Down on Sitting" total, and enter it here.

_____

CUT DOWN ON SITTING

Your finding:

5 or 6: Solid Pyramid
7 to 10: Pyramid under Construction
10 or more: Get Building!

The Strength of Your Pyramid

To evaluate how your pyramid is stacking up, add your findings from the pyramid level checklists. Then read the guidelines that follow:

Your Scores

_____ Readiness Points

_____ Adding Steps to Your Day

_____ Aerobics and Recreation

_____ Flexibility, Strength, and Leisure

_____ Cut Down on Sitting

The Strength of Your Overall Pyramid

_____ 30 or less: Solid Pyramid

_____ 31 to 46: Pyramid under Construction (shaky, swaying)

_____ 47 or more: Get Building! (toppling, decaying, falling)

Solid Pyramid

If your findings indicate that you have built a solid pyramid, it is very likely that you not only lead an active, healthy life, but you also actively seek a variety of opportunities to improve your fitness level. Keep it up—now and in the future—and continue to seek opportunities to enhance your active lifestyle.

Pyramid under Construction

For the best results, physical activity should be done consistently. Your score indicates that you enjoy a fair amount of activity, but you remain inconsistent. By building on your activity level, you can develop a fitness program that is ongoing, more active, and, most important, lifelong.

Get Building!

A "Get Building!" score probably indicates that your daily habits are more supportive of a sedentary existence than an active lifestyle. Remaining physically inactive not only threatens your future well-being, but also can impede your ability to continue to do the activities you enjoy today. Getting back into shape starts with your conviction that remaining sedentary is not a choice you are willing to accept.

Source: Copyright © 1996 Park Nicollet HealthSource® Institute for Research and Education. Reprinted by permission.

CHAPTER
9

Nutrition
and Performance

Aside from the limits imposed by heredity and the physical improvements associated with training, no factor plays a bigger role in exercise performance than does nutrition.

—David Costill[1]

Since the time of the ancient Greeks, athletes and their coaches have practiced special dietary regimens to improve performance and gain a competitive edge over their competitors. Paul Anderson, who once raised 6,270 pounds, the greatest weight ever lifted by a human, had a special drink he used while in training. Using his bare hands, he would squeeze the blood from two pounds of raw hamburger into a glass of tomato juice, and then drink the mixture.[2]

Milo of Crotona, legendary wrestler of the ancient Greeks who was never once brought to his knees over five Olympiads (532–516 B.C.), ate gargantuan amounts of meat, as did the Roman gladiators.[3] Swimmer Jim Montgomery, winner of four gold medals in the 1976 Olympics, normally ate a breakfast consisting of eight eggs, a pound of bacon, a loaf of bread, and a quart of orange juice. Don Kardong, Olympic marathon runner, proudly boasted of his huge intake of ice cream, soda pop, cookies, pastries, and beer.[4] Olympic marathoner Cathy O'Brien skipped breakfast, consumed only 1,300 Calories a day, and had a weakness for Pepsi and whole milk.[5]

On the other hand, many fine athletes are very meticulous about their diets. Nancy Ditz, once America's top ranked female marathoner, emphasized carbohydrates, which averaged 65–75% of her daily energy intake.[5] Dave Scott, former world-record holder in the Ironman triathlon, ate a diet high in complex carbohydrates—74% of total Calories, consisting of brown rice, tofu, low-fat dairy products, and up to 20 pieces of fruit and vegetables per day.[6] Former Olympic marathoner Margaret Groos also emphasized a high-carbohydrate diet (over 60% of total energy intake),

eating foods such as English muffins, rice cakes, fruit, pasta, high-carbohydrate drinks, and low-fat dairy products.[5]

These examples point out the obvious: Among our top athletes, dietary practices cover a wide range. Questions that naturally arise are

1. Could athletes or fitness enthusiasts improve their ability to train and perform by optimizing their diet?

2. What is the optimal diet for people who exercise regularly or compete athletically?

3. Can regular exercise protect one from the effects of a bad diet (e.g., high blood cholesterol, high blood pressure, and heart disease)?

4. Are the nutritional stresses imposed by hard training greater than can be met by ordinary foods, without protein, vitamin, or mineral supplementation?

5. Do weight lifters need protein supplements to maximize muscle strength and size?

6. Are there special nutrient aids or supplements that can improve performance beyond that attainable on a normal diet?

This chapter answers these and other questions through a discussion of 10 cardinal sports-nutrition principles. This listing represents a summary of the most recent and important research in this area. These principles apply to both the basic fitness exerciser and, even more importantly, the competitive endurance athlete.

Before reviewing these principles, it is important to realize that the ability to exercise hard and perform well depends on much more than diet. In fact, most sports-nutrition experts feel that proper nutrition ranks third, behind *talent* and *training* as factors affecting athletic accomplishment.[1]

However, researchers have also shown that athletes can *maximize* this talent and training by putting into practice the 10 sports-nutrition principles listed in this chapter. You cannot eat your way to Olympic gold, but a prudent diet can definitely improve your chances. On the other hand, don't expect to run your fastest 10-K right after improving your diet, unless you also improve the quality of your training program. What you can expect is that a good diet will help you feel better from day to day, allowing you to train harder.

A major emphasis of this chapter is that the most important sports-nutrition principles for those who exercise long and hard are to consume optimal amounts of carbohydrate and of water.

PRINCIPLE 1: PRUDENT DIET IS THE CORNERSTONE

For all Americans, whether physically active or inactive, a "prudent diet" is recommended for general health and prevention of disease.[7,8] The prudent diet is defined in this chapter as the diet adhering to the 1989 National Research Council "Diet and Health"[9] and the 1995 U.S. Department of Agriculture's (USDA) "Dietary Guidelines for Americans."[10]

This diet is advocated for fitness enthusiasts (those exercising 3–5 days per week, 20–30 minutes per session) and nearly all athletes, including those in most individual, dual, and team sports, and power events (weight lifting, track and field) (see Table 9.1). For the competitive endurance athlete (who trains more than 90 minutes a day in such sports as running, swimming, and cycling), several adaptations beyond the prudent diet are beneficial, including a

higher percentage of carbohydrate, less fat, and more water; for those who are at risk, close attention to iron status is also important.

Americans tend to eat too much food energy (Calories) in the form of fat (especially the hard saturated fat common in animal products), and excess amounts of cholesterol (found only in animal products) and sodium. They also have diets too low in complex carbohydrates (starch) and fiber (found only in plant foods). Such dietary indiscretions are a major reason why Americans have high rates of obesity, heart disease, high blood pressure, stroke, diabetes, and some forms of cancer. As noted in the final principle of this chapter, Principle 10, even the athlete must be concerned about diet–disease relationships, because hard exercise does not appear to negate the increased disease risk associated with poor diets.

Diseases caused by vitamin and mineral deficiencies are rare in this and other developed nations, where malnutrition is generally not a problem. Tables 9.2 and 9.3 summarize the recommended dietary allowances (RDA) for important vitamins and minerals. Of practical importance to most people is that when guidelines for a low-fat, high-carbohydrate diet are followed, intake of these vitamins and minerals is usually assured.

These guidelines have been summarized by several organizations, including the National Research Council, the American Heart Association, the American Cancer Society, and the U.S. Department of Agriculture.[8–12] Their recommendations are for all healthy Americans age 2 and over— not for younger children and infants, whose dietary needs differ (see Tables 9.2 and 9.3). The guidelines reflect recommendations of nutrition authorities, who agree that enough is known about diet's effect on health to encourage certain dietary practices for Americans.

There are seven major dietary guidelines:[9,10]

1. Eat a variety of foods.
2. Balance the food eaten with physical activity. Maintain or improve weight.
3. Choose a diet with plenty of grain products, vegetables, and fruits.

TABLE 9.1   The Energy and Quality of Diet Recommended for People Who Exercise

	Calories[a]		% of Total Energy Intake		
	Males	Females	Carbohydrate	Fat	Protein
Average American	2,500	1,600	51	33	16
Fitness enthusiasts	2,900	2,000	55	30	15
Endurance athletes	3,500	2,600	60–70	15–25	15
Team/power athletes	4,000	3,000	55	30	15

[a]Energy intake can vary widely, depending on body size and amount of exercise.

TABLE 9.2 Food and Nutrition Board, Institute of Medicine–National Academy of Sciences Dietary Reference Intakes: Recommended Levels for Individual Intake

Life-Stage Group	Calcium (mg/d)	Phosphorus (mg/d)	Magnesium (mg/d)	D (μg/d)[a,b]	Fluoride (mg/d)	Thiamin (mg/d)	Riboflavin (mg/d)	Niacin (mg/d)[c]	B$_6$ (mg/d)	Folate (μg/d)[d]	B$_{12}$ (μg/d)	Pantothenic Acid (mg/d)	Biotin (μg/d)	Choline[e] (mg/d)
Infants														
0–5 mo	210*	110*	30*	5*	0.01*	0.2*	0.3*	2*	0.1*	65*	0.4*	1.7*	5*	125*
6–11 mo	270*	275*	75*	5*	0.5*	0.3*	0.4*	3*	0.3*	80*	0.5*	1.8*	6*	150*
Children														
1–3 yr	500*	**460**	**80**	5*	0.7*	**0.5**	**0.5**	**6**	**0.5**	**150**	**0.9**	2*	8*	200*
4–8 yr	800*	**500**	**130**	5*	1*	**0.6**	**0.6**	**8**	**0.6**	**200**	**1.2**	3*	12*	250*
Males														
9–13 yr	1,300*	**1,250**	**240**	5*	2*	**0.9**	**0.9**	**12**	**1.0**	**300**	**1.8**	4*	20*	375*
14–18 yr	1,300*	**1,250**	**410**	5*	3*	**1.2**	**1.3**	**16**	**1.3**	**400**	**2.4**	5*	25*	550*
19–30 yr	1,000*	**700**	**400**	5*	4*	**1.2**	**1.3**	**16**	**1.3**	**400**	**2.4**	5*	30*	550*
31–50 yr	1,000*	**700**	**420**	5*	4*	**1.2**	**1.3**	**16**	**1.3**	**400**	**2.4**	5*	30*	550*
51–70 yr	1,200*	**700**	**420**	10*	4*	**1.2**	**1.3**	**16**	**1.7**	**400**	**2.4**[f]	5*	30*	550*
> 70 yr	1,200*	**700**	**420**	15*	4*	**1.2**	**1.3**	**16**	**1.7**	**400**	**2.4**[f]	5*	30*	550*
Females														
9–13 yr	1,300*	**1,250**	**240**	5*	2*	**0.9**	**0.9**	**12**	**1.0**	**300**	**1.8**	4*	20*	375*
14–18 yr	1,300*	**1,250**	**360**	5*	3*	**1.0**	**1.0**	**14**	**1.2**	**400**[g]	**2.4**	5*	25*	400*
19–30 yr	1,000*	**700**	**310**	5*	3*	**1.1**	**1.1**	**14**	**1.3**	**400**[g]	**2.4**	5*	30*	425*
31–50 yr	1,000*	**700**	**320**	5*	3*	**1.1**	**1.1**	**14**	**1.3**	**400**[g]	**2.4**	5*	30*	425*
51–70 yr	1,200*	**700**	**320**	10*	3*	**1.1**	**1.1**	**14**	**1.5**	**400**[g]	**2.4**[f]	5*	30*	425*
> 70 yr	1,200*	**700**	**320**	15*	3*	**1.1**	**1.1**	**14**	**1.5**	**400**	**2.4**[f]	5*	30*	425*
Pregnancy														
≤ 18 yr	1,300*	**1,250**	**400**	5*	3*	**1.4**	**1.4**	**18**	**1.9**	**600**[h]	**2.6**	6*	30*	450*
19–30 yr	1,000*	**700**	**350**	5*	3*	**1.4**	**1.4**	**18**	**1.9**	**600**[h]	**2.6**	6*	30*	450*
31–50 yr	1,000*	**700**	**360**	5*	3*	**1.4**	**1.4**	**18**	**1.9**	**600**[h]	**2.6**	6*	30*	450*
Lactation														
≤ 18 yr	1,300*	**1,250**	**360**	5*	3*	**1.5**	**1.6**	**17**	**2.0**	**500**	**2.8**	7*	35*	550*
19–30 yr	1,000*	**700**	**310**	5*	3*	**1.5**	**1.6**	**17**	**2.0**	**500**	**2.8**	7*	35*	550*
31–50 yr	1,000*	**700**	**320**	5*	3*	**1.5**	**1.6**	**17**	**2.0**	**500**	**2.8**	7*	35*	550*

Note: This table presents Recommended Dietary Allowances (RDAs) in bold type and Adequate Intakes (AIs) in ordinary type followed by an asterisk (*). RDAs and AIs may both be used as goals for individual intake. RDAs are set to meet the needs of almost all (97 to 98 percent) individuals in a group. For healthy breastfed infants, the AI is the mean intake. The AI for other life-stage groups is believed to cover their needs, but lack of data or uncertainty in the data prevent clear specification of this coverage.

[a] As cholecalciferol. 1 μg cholecalciferol = 40 IU vitamin D.
[b] In the absence of adequate exposure to sunlight.
[c] As niacin equivalents. 1 mg of niacin = 60 mg of tryptophan.
[d] As dietary folate equivalents (DFE). 1 DFE = 1 μg food folate = 0.6 μg of folic acid (from fortified food or supplement) consumed with food = 0.5 μg of synthetic (supplemental) folic acid taken on an empty stomach.
[e] Although AIs have been set for choline, there are few data to assess whether a dietary supply of choline is needed at all stages of the life cycle, and it may be that the choline requirement can be met by endogenous synthesis at some of these stages.
[f] Since 10 to 30 percent of older people may malabsorb food-bound B$_{12}$, it is advisable for those older than 50 years to meet their RDA mainly by consuming foods fortified with B$_{12}$ or a B$_{12}$-containing supplement.
[g] In view of evidence linking folate intake with neural tube defects in the fetus, it is recommended that all women capable of becoming pregnant consume 400 μg of synthetic folic acid from fortified foods and/or supplements in addition to intake of food folate from a varied diet.
[h] It is assumed that women will continue consuming 400 μg of folic acid until their pregnancy is confirmed and they enter prenatal care, which ordinarily occurs after the end of the periconceptual period—the critical time for formation of the neural tube.

TABLE 9.3 **Food and Nutrition Board, National Academy of Sciences–National Research Council Recommended Dietary Allowances,**[a] **Revised 1989 (Abridged)**

Designed for the maintenance of good nutrition of practically all healthy people in the United States

Category	Age (year) or Condition	Weight[b] (kg)	Weight[b] (lb)	Height[b] (cm)	Height[b] (in)	Protein (g)	Vitamin A (μg RE)[c]	Vitamin E (mg α-TE)[d]	Vitamin K (μg)	Vitamin C (mg)	Iron (mg)	Zinc (mg)	Iodine (μg)	Selenium (μg)
Infant	0.0–0.5	6	13	60	24	13	375	3	5	30	6	5	40	10
	0.5–1.0	9	20	71	28	14	375	4	10	35	10	5	50	15
Children	1–3	13	29	90	35	16	400	6	15	40	10	10	70	20
	4–6	20	44	112	44	24	500	7	20	45	10	10	90	20
	7–10	28	62	132	52	28	700	7	30	45	10	10	120	30
Males	11–14	45	99	157	62	45	1,000	10	45	50	12	15	150	40
	15–18	66	145	176	69	59	1,000	10	65	60	12	15	150	50
	19–24	72	160	177	70	58	1,000	10	70	60	10	15	150	70
	25–50	79	174	176	70	63	1,000	10	80	60	10	15	150	70
	51+	77	170	173	68	63	1,000	10	80	60	10	15	150	70
Females	11–14	46	101	157	62	46	800	8	45	50	15	12	150	45
	15–18	55	120	163	64	44	800	8	55	60	15	12	150	50
	19–24	58	128	164	65	46	800	8	60	60	15	12	150	55
	25–50	63	138	163	64	50	800	8	65	60	15	12	150	55
	51+	65	143	160	63	50	800	8	65	60	10	12	150	55
Pregnant						60	800	10	65	70	30	15	175	65
Lactating	1st 6 months					65	1,300	12	65	95	15	19	200	75
	2nd 6 months					62	1,200	11	65	90	15	16	200	75

Note: This table does not include nutrients for which Dietary Reference Intakes have recently been established (see *Dietary Reference Intakes for Calcium, Phosphorus, Magnesium, Vitamin D, and Fluoride,* 1997 and *Dietary Reference Intakes for Thiamin, Riboflavin, Niacin, Vitamin B₆, Folate, Vitamin B₁₂, Pantothenic Acid, Biotin, and Choline,* 1998).

[a]The allowances, expressed as average daily intakes over time, are intended to provide for individual variations among most normal persons as they live in the United States under usual environmental stresses. Diets should be based on a variety of common foods in order to provide other nutrients for which human requirements have been less well defined. See text for detailed discussion of allowances and of nutrients not tabulated.
[b]Weights and heights of Reference Adults are actual medians for the U.S. population of the designated age, as reported by NHANES II. The use of these figures does not imply that the height-to-weight ratios are ideal.
[c]Retinol equivalents. 1 retinol equivalent = 1 μg retinol or 6 μg β-carotene.
[d]α-Tocopherol equivalents. 1 mg d-α tocopherol = 1 α-TE.

4. Select a diet low in fat, saturated fat, and cholesterol.

5. Pick a diet moderate in sugars.

6. Choose a diet moderate in salt and sodium.

7. Drink alcoholic beverages in moderation, if at all.

Variety of Foods

More than 40 different nutrients, classified into six groups (protein, carbohydrate, fat, vitamin, mineral, and water), are needed for good health.[7] (See the RDAs in Tables 9.2 and 9.3, for some of these.) These nutrients should come from a variety of foods, not from a few highly fortified foods or supplements. (See Tables 9.4 and 9.5 for a summary of the major food sources of vitamins and minerals.) According to the 1995 USDA Dietary Guidelines for Americans, "No single food can supply all nutrients in the amounts needed."[10] (A copy of this report can be downloaded via the World Wide Web at http://www.nal.usda.gov/fnic/dga/dga95.html.)

Supplements of some nutrients taken regularly in large amounts can be harmful, due to direct toxicity or interference with the absorption of other nutrients (see Principle 6 on vitamin and mineral supplements). Some people use

TABLE 9.4 Functions and Food Sources for Vitamins

Vitamins	Adult RDA	Role in Body and Good Food Sources
Fat soluble		
Vitamin A	800–1,000 µg R.E.	Assists in the formation and maintenance of healthy skin, hair, and mucous membranes; aids in the ability to see in dim light (night vision); essential for proper bone growth, tooth development, and reproduction. *Food:* deep yellow/orange and dark green vegetables and fruits (carrots, broccoli, spinach, cantaloupe, sweet potatoes); cheese, milk, and fortified margarines.
Vitamin D	5–15 µg	Aids in the formation and maintenance of bones and teeth; assists in the absorption and use of calcium and phosphorus. *Food:* milks fortified with vitamin D; tuna, salmon, or cod liver oil. Also made in the skin when exposed to sunlight.
Vitamin E	8–10 mg α-TE	Protects vitamin A and essential fatty acids from oxidation; prevents cell membrane damage. *Food:* vegetable oils and margarine, nuts, wheat germ and whole-grain breads and cereals, green leafy vegetables.
Vitamin K	60–80 µg	Aids in synthesis of substances needed for clotting of blood; helps maintain normal bone metabolism. *Food:* green leafy vegetables, cabbage, and cauliflower. Also made by bacteria in intestines of humans, except for newborns.
Water Soluble		
Vitamin C	60 mg	Important in forming collagen, a protein that gives structure to bones, cartilage, muscle, and vascular tissue; helps maintain capillaries, bones, and teeth; aids in absorption of iron; helps protect other vitamins from oxidation. *Food:* citrus fruits, berries, melons, dark green vegetables, tomatoes, green peppers, cabbage, and potatoes.
Thiamin	1.1–1.2 mg	Helps in release of energy from carbohydrates; promotes normal functioning of nervous system. *Food:* whole-grain products, dried beans and peas, sunflower seeds, nuts.
Riboflavin	1.1–1.3 mg	Helps body transform carbohydrate, protein, and fat into energy. *Food:* nuts, yogurt, milk, whole-grain products, cheese, poultry, leafy green vegetables.
Niacin	14–16 mg N.E.	Helps body transform carbohydrate, protein, and fat into energy. *Food:* nuts, poultry, fish, whole-grain products, dried fruit, leafy greens, beans. Can be formed in the body from tryptophan, an essential amino acid found in protein.
Vitamin B_6	1.3–1.7 mg	Aids in the use of fats and amino acids; aids in the formation of protein. *Food:* sunflower seeds, beans, poultry, nuts, leafy green vegetables, bananas, dried fruit.
Folate acid	400 µg	Aids in the formation of hemoglobin in red blood cells; aids in the formation of genetic material. *Food:* dark green leafy vegetables, nuts, beans, whole-grain products, fruit juices.
Pantothenic acid	5 mg	Aids in the formation of hormones and certain nerve-regulating substances; helps in the metabolism of carbohydrate, protein, and fat. *Food:* nuts, beans, seeds, dark green leafy vegetables, poultry, dried fruit, milk.
Biotin	30 µg	Aids in the formation of fatty acids; helps in the release of energy from carbohydrate. *Food:* occurs widely in foods, especially eggs. Made by bacteria in the human intestine.
Vitamin B_{12}	2.4 µg	Aids in the formation of red blood cells and genetic material; helps the functioning of the nervous system. *Food:* milk, yogurt, cheese, fish, poultry, and eggs. Not found in plant foods unless fortified (such as in some breakfast cereals).

Source: Nieman DC, Butterworth DE, Nieman CN. *Nutrition.* Dubuque, IA: W. C. Brown Publishers, 1992.

supplements to cover up their poor dietary habits—something that cannot be done with pills and capsules. As a general rule, most Americans do not need supplements for good health.[9–13]

The RDAs have been published since 1941, by the National Academy of Sciences.[13] The *RDA* is defined as the daily dietary intake level that is sufficient to meet the nutrient requirements of nearly all (97%) individuals in a certain age and gender group. The Food and Nutrition Board, Institute of Medicine, and National Academy of Sciences,

with the involvement of Health Canada, are currently revising the RDAs. New reference values called Dietary Reference Intakes (DRIs) are being established, which will replace the RDAs and be used for planning and assessing diets for healthy populations[14] (available via the World Wide Web at http://www.nap.edu). Unlike the RDAs, the DRIs will consider both nutrient adequacy for proper body function and optimal intake for reduction of disease risk; this will result in increased intake recommendations for some nutrients. The current calcium RDA, for example, is

TABLE 9.5   Functions and Food Sources for Minerals

Major Minerals	Adult RDA[a] M	F	Role in Body and Good Food Sources
Calcium	1,000–1,200 mg	1,000–1,200 mg	Used for building bones and teeth and maintaining bone strength; also involved in muscle contraction, blood clotting, and maintenance of cell membranes. *Food:* all dairy products, dark green leafy vegetables, beans, nuts, sunflower seeds, dried fruit, molasses, canned fish.
Phosphorus	700 mg	700 mg	Used to build bones and teeth; release energy from carbohydrate, proteins, and fats; and form genetic material, cell membranes, and many enzymes. *Food:* beans, sunflower seeds, milk, cheese, nuts, poultry, fish, lean meats.
Magnesium	400–420 mg	310–320 mg	Used to build bones, produce proteins, release energy from muscle carbohydrate stores (glycogen), and regulate body temperature. *Food:* sunflower and pumpkin seeds, nuts, whole-grain products, beans, dark green vegetables, dried fruit, lean meats.
Sodium	500 mg	500 mg	Regulates body fluid volume and blood acidity; aids in transmission of nerve impulses. *Food:* most of the sodium in the American diet is added to food as salt (sodium chloride) in cooking, at the table, or in commercial processing. Animal products contain some natural sodium.
Chloride	750 mg	750 mg	Is a component of gastric juice and aids in acid–base balance. *Food:* table salt, seafood, milk, eggs, meats.
Potassium	2,000 mg	2,000 mg	Assists in muscle contraction, the maintenance of fluid and electrolyte balance in the cells, and the transmission of nerve impulses. Also aids in the release of energy from carbohydrate, proteins, and fats. *Food:* widely distributed in foods, especially fruits and vegetables, beans, nuts, seeds, and lean meats.
Minor Minerals			
Iron	10 mg	15 mg	Involved in the formation of hemoglobin in the red blood cells of the blood and myoglobin in muscles. Also a part of several enzymes and proteins. *Food:* molasses, seeds, whole-grain products, fortified breakfast cereals, nuts, dried fruits, beans, poultry, fish, lean meats.
Zinc	15 mg	12 mg	Involved in the formation of protein (growth of all tissues), wound healing, and prevention of anemia. A component of many enzymes. *Food:* whole-grain products, seeds, nuts, poultry, fish, beans, lean meats.
Iodine	150 µg	150 µg	Integral component of thyroid hormones. *Food:* table salt (fortified), dairy products, shellfish, and fish.
Fluoride	4 mg	3 mg	Maintenance of bone and tooth structure. *Food:* fluoridated drinking water is the best source. Also found in tea, fish, wheat germ, kale, cottage cheese, soybeans, almonds, onions, milk.
Copper	1.5–3.0 mg	1.5–3.0 mg	Vital to enzyme systems and in manufacturing red blood cells. Needed for utilization of iron. *Food:* nuts, oysters, seeds, crab, wheat germ, dried fruit, whole grains, legumes.
Selenium	70 µg	55 µg	Functions in association with vitamin E and may assist in protecting tissues and cell membranes from oxidative damage. May also aid in preventing cancer. *Food:* nuts, whole grains, lean pork, cottage cheese, milk, molasses, squash.
Chromium	50–200 µg	50–200 µg	Required for maintaining normal glucose metabolism. May assist insulin function. *Food:* nuts, prunes, vegetable oils, green peas, corn, whole grains, orange juice, dark green vegetables, legumes.
Manganese	2.0–5.0 mg	2.0–5.0 mg	Needed for normal bone structure, reproduction, and the normal functioning of the central nervous system. Is a component of many enzyme systems. *Food:* whole grains, nuts, seeds, pineapple, berries, legumes, dark green vegetables, tea.
Molybdenum	75–250 µg	75–250 µg	Component of enzymes and may help prevent dental caries. *Food:* tomatoes, wheat germ, lean pork, legumes, whole grains, strawberries, winter squash, milk, dark green vegetables, carrots.

[a]Instead of RDA, "safe and adequate" daily dietary intake range is given for copper, chromium, manganese, and molybdenum. Estimated minimum requirements are given for sodium, chloride, and potassium. It is recommended that sodium intake be limited to 2,400 mg per day.

Source: Nieman DC, Butterworth DE, Nieman CN. *Nutrition.* Dubuque, IA: W. C. Brown Publishers, 1992.

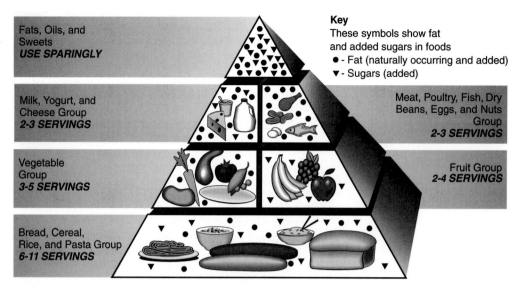

Figure 9.1 Food guide pyramid: A guide to healthy food choices. The food guide pyramid emphasizes that bread, cereals, rice, and pasta be included with each meal, and should form the foundation of a healthy diet. At least five servings of fruit and vegetables each day are recommended, supplemented with low-fat choices of dairy and meat products. *Source:* United States Department of Agriculture, The Food Guide Pyramid. *Home and Garden Bulletin* 252, 1992.

800 mg/day for male and female adults 25 years of age and older. The calcium DRI has been set at 1,000 mg/day for adults 19–50 years of age, and 1,200 mg/day for those older than 50. The increased DRI values reflect new research data that have established a link between high dietary calcium intakes and decreased risk of osteoporosis.

Diet variety is probably the single most important nutrition principle. The U.S. Department of Agriculture urges that all people try to follow the recommendations of the "Food Guide Pyramid," choosing at least the lower number of servings suggested from each food group[9,10,15] (see Figure 9.1). (The food guide pyramid is available via the World Wide Web at http://www.nalusda.gov/fnic.html.) Grains and cereals should form the basis of each meal, supplemented with liberal servings of vegetables and fruits and with low-fat servings of dairy and meat products. Typical serving sizes are one slice of bread or ½ cup of pasta; ½ cup of cooked vegetables; one medium apple, banana, or other fruit; 1 cup of milk or yogurt; and 2–3 ounces of cooked lean meat, poultry, or fish. Box 9.1 summarizes information on the recommended number and size of servings for each of the food groups in the food guide pyramid.[15]

Unfortunately, Americans fall short of following the dietary guidelines shown in the food pyramid. According to the USDA, less than one third of American adults consume five or more servings of fruits and vegetables each day, and intake of nutrient-packed dark green and deep yellow vegetables is much lower than recommended[16–19] (see Figure

9.2). Consumption of grain-based products is rising, but much of that increase can be traced to less-than-nutritious snack foods, such as corn chips, crackers, popcorn, and pretzels, instead of more healthful whole-grain breads, cereals, and rice.[17] Whole grains, which are rich in dietary fiber, compose only 17% of intake from the bread and cereal food group.[17] Data from the National Cancer Institute show that the situation is even worse among children and adolescents.[20] Only one in five children eats five or more servings of fruits and vegetables a day, and when children do eat vegetables, one quarter of them are french fries. This is disturbing, in that many experts feel that a high fruit and vegetable intake is one of the best ways to keep cancer at bay and to decrease risk of cardiovascular disease.[11,12,21–24]

Balance of Food Intake with Physical Activity Output

Being overweight is common in the United States (33% of adults and 22% of adolescents) and is linked with high blood pressure, heart disease, stroke, diabetes, certain cancers, arthritis, and other types of illness.[9,10] (See Chapter 13.) A healthy weight can be maintained by being physically active and consuming a variety of foods low in calories and fat, such as fruits, vegetables, whole grains, nonfat dairy products, and baked fish or poultry. Calories can be restricted by limiting serving sizes, particularly of high-fat

Box 9.1

Food Guide Pyramid: What Is a Serving?

	Sedentary Women, Some Older Adults	Children, Teenage Girls, Active Women, Sedentary Men	Teenage Boys, Active Men
Calories[a]	About 1,600	About 2,000	About 2,800
Breads, cereals, rice, and pastas group	6	9	11
Vegetable group	3	4	5
Fruit group	2	3	4
Milk, yogurt, and cheese group[b]	2–3	2–3	2–3
Meat, poultry, fish, dry beans, eggs, and nuts group	2 (5 oz total)	2 (6 oz total)	3 (7 oz total)
Total fat (g)	53	73	93
Added sugar (tsp)	6	12	18

[a]Assumes mostly low-fat and low-calorie food choices.
[b]Women who are pregnant or lactating, teenagers, and young adults to age 24 need three servings.

Source: U.S. Department of Agriculture, *Home and Garden Bulletin* 252 (1992):9.

KEY: Nutrient Density
A Foods generally highest in nutrient density (preferable first choice).
B Foods moderate in nutrient density (reasonable second choice).
C Foods lowest in nutrient density (limit selections).

Bread, Cereal, Rice, and Pasta Group

These foods contribute complex carbohydrates and fiber, plus riboflavin, thiamin, niacin, iron, protein, magnesium, and other nutrients.

6–11 servings per day.

Serving = 1 slice bread; ½ c cooked cereal, rice, or pasta; 1 oz ready-to-eat cereal; ½ bun, bagel, or English muffin; 1 small roll, biscuit, or muffin; 3–4 small or 2 large crackers.

A Whole grains (wheat, oats, barley, millet, rye, bulgur), enriched breads, rolls, tortillas, cereals, bagels, rice, pastas (macaroni, spaghetti)

B Pancakes, muffins, cornbread, crackers, low-fat cookies, biscuits, presweetened cereals, granola
C Croissants, fried rice, doughnuts, pastries, sweet rolls

Vegetable Group

These foods contribute fiber, vitamin A, vitamin C, folate, potassium, and magnesium.

3–5 servings per day (use dark green, leafy vegetables and legumes several times a week).

Serving = ½ c cooked or raw vegetables; 1 c leafy raw vegetables; ½ c cooked legumes; ¾ c vegetable juice.

A Bean sprouts, broccoli, brussels sprouts, cabbage, carrots, cauliflower, cucumbers, green beans, green peas, leafy greens (spinach, mustard, and collard greens), legumes, lettuce, mushrooms, summer and winter squash, tomatoes, sweet potatoes, yams
B Corn, potatoes
C French fries, olives, tempura vegetables

(continued)

Food Guide Pyramid: What Is a Serving? *(continued)*

Fruit Group

These foods contribute fiber, vitamin A, vitamin C, and potassium.

> 2–4 servings per day.
>
> Serving = typical portion (such as 1 medium apple, banana, or orange; ½ grapefruit; 1 melon wedge; ¾ c juice; ½ c berries; ½ c diced, cooked, or canned fruit; ¼ c dried fruit.

A Apricots, cantaloupe, grapefruit, oranges, peaches, strawberries, apples, bananas, pears
B Canned or frozen fruit; fruit juices; dried fruit
C Avocados

Meat, Poultry, Fish, Dry Beans, Eggs, and Nuts

These foods contribute protein, phosphorus, vitamin B_6, vitamin B_{12}, zinc, magnesium, iron, niacin, and thiamin.

> 2–3 servings per day.
>
> Serving = 2–3 oz lean, cooked meat, poultry, or fish (total 5–7 oz per day); count 1 egg, ½ c cooked legumes, or 2 tbs peanut butter as 1 oz meat (or about ⅓ serving).

A Poultry, fish, lean meat, legumes, egg whites, tofu, nuts, seeds
B Fat-trimmed beef, lamb, pork; refried beans; egg yolks, tempeh
C Hot dogs, luncheon meats, peanut butter, sausage, bacon, fried fish or poultry, duck

Milk, Yogurt, and Cheese

These foods contribute calcium, riboflavin, protein, vitamin B_{12}, and, when fortified, vitamin D and vitamin A.

> 2 servings per day.
>
> 3 servings per day for teenagers and young adults, pregnant/lactating women, and women past menopause.
>
> 4 servings per day for pregnant/lactating teenagers.
>
> Serving = 1 c milk or yogurt; 2 oz processed cheese food; 1½ oz cheese.

A Nonfat and 1% low-fat milk (and nonfat products such as buttermilk, cottage cheese, cheese, yogurt); fortified soy milk
B 2% low-fat milk (and low-fat products such as yogurt, cheese, cottage cheese); sherbet; ice milk
C Whole milk (and whole-milk products such as cheese, yogurt, cottage cheese); custard; milk shakes; pudding; ice cream

Fats, Oils, and Sweets

These foods contribute sugar, fat, alcohol, and food energy (calories). Their consumption should be limited because these foods provide few nutrients. Alcoholic beverages are not classed as foods on the pyramid; they contribute few nutrients, but they do contribute calories and so are mentioned here.

> Foods high in fat include butter, margarine, salad dressings, oils, mayonnaise, cream, sour cream, cream cheese, gravy, and sauces.
>
> Foods high in sugar include candy fruit rolls, other candies, soft drinks, fruit drinks, jelly, syrup, gelatin, desserts, sugar, and honey.
>
> Alcoholic beverages include wine, beer, and liquor.

---

foods. However, it is important to recognize that many fat-free cakes, cookies, snack foods, and frozen and other desserts remain high in Calories.

Current caloric intake among Americans is about 9% higher than it was in the late 1970s (now about 2,500 and 1,600 calories/day for men and women, respectively).[17] (See Table 9.6 for a summary of current American adult dietary intake.) At the same time, as reviewed in Chapter 1, more than 75% of American adults are not regularly physically active. In fact, 25% of all adults are not active at all. It is obvious that the increase in prevalence of obesity has occurred because many people eat more calories than they expend.

It should be noted that the 1995 USDA Dietary Guidelines for Americans included physical activity as a key ingredient of their recommendations for the first time.[10] In 1990, the guideline read "maintain healthy weight"; in 1995, this was switched to "balance the food you eat with physical activity; maintain or improve your weight."

Diet Including Plenty of Grain Products, Vegetables, and Fruits

As outlined in discussing Principle 1, people should eat more servings of grain products at each meal than any other

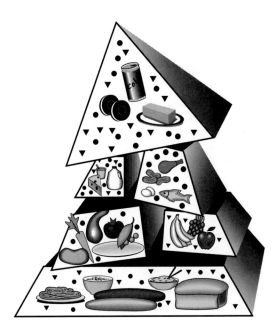

Figure 9.2 Actual consumption pyramid. Actual U.S. diets make a top-heavy pyramid, compared with the USDA–HHS food guide pyramid. The latter recommends these daily intakes: 6–11 servings of bread, cereal, rice, pasta; 3–5 servings of vegetables; 2–4 servings of fruits; 2–3 servings of milk, yogurt, cheese; 2–3 servings of meat, poultry, fish, dry beans, eggs, nuts; and only sparing use of fats, oils, and sweets. American diets come up particularly short in the vegetable and fruit groups. *Source: Eating in America Today,* Edition II, A Dietary Pattern and Intake Report commissioned by the National Live Stock and Meat Board.

TABLE 9.6 **Current American Adult (Age 20 and over) Dietary Intake, Compared to Recommended Levels**

	Males	Females	Recommended
Energy (kilocalories)	2,470	1,633	Varies[a]
Carbohydrate (% total energy)	49.2	51.6	55–60
Fat (% total energy)	33.5	32.5	<30
Saturated fat (% total energy)	11.2	10.8	<10
Protein (% total energy)	16.0	16.1	~15
Dietary fiber (gm)	18.5	13.7	20–35
Cholesterol (mg)	337	217	<300
Sodium (mg)[b]	4,114	2,748	<2,400
Antioxidants[c]			
Vitamin A (μg RE)	1,161	951	M: 1,000; F: 800
Vitamin C (mg)	111	89	60
Vitamin E (mg α-TE)	10.0	7.1	M: 10; F: 8
Vitamin B$_6$ (mg)	2.2	1.51	M: 1.3–1.7; F: 1.3–1.5
Folate (μg)	300	224	400
Calcium (mg)	891	647	1,000; >50 yrs, 1,200[d]
Iron (mg)	18.5	12.9	M: 10; F: 15
Zinc (mg)	14.1	9.2	M: 15; F: 12

[a]Energy needs vary according to body size and physical activity, with RDA average set at 2,900 kilocalories for males, and 2,200 for females. There is evidence that energy intake is underestimated in national surveys. Nonetheless, obesity prevalence is increasing, which means that Americans tend to take in more energy than they expend.
[b]Includes sodium in food only. Does not represent salt added at the table.
[c]High dietary intake of antioxidants has been associated with reduced risk of cancer and heart disease.
[d]Calcium requirement reflects new DRI (dietary reference intake).

Source: Wilson JW, Enns CW, Goldman JD, et al. *Data Tables: Combined Results from USDA's 1994 and 1995 Continuing Survey of Food Intakes by Individuals and Diet and Health Knowledge Survey.* Riverdale, MD: Food Surveys Research Group, Beltsville Human Nutrition Research Center, Agricultural Research Service, U.S. Department of Agriculture, 1997 (can be downloaded via the World Wide Web at http://www.barc.usda.gov/bhnrc/foodsurvey/home.htm).

type of food, followed by fruits and vegetables. Grains (e.g., pasta, rice, wheat, cereals) should form the center of most meals. By choosing more whole-grain products, fruits, and vegetables, total carbohydrate and fiber intake will increase, while total fat, saturated fat, and cholesterol intake will decrease.[9,10]

The American Cancer Society recommends that most of the foods people eat should come from plant sources, and that the following practices be adopted:[21]

- Include grain products, fruits, or vegetables in every meal.
- Choose fruits and vegetables for snacks.
- Choose beans as an alternative to meat.
- Choose whole grains in preference to processed (refined) grains.

Most authorities advise that at least 55% of calories come from carbohydrate.[9,10] For an individual eating 2,000 calories a day, this amount would be 1,100 calories (275 grams of carbohydrate; 1,100 ÷ 4, the number of calories per gram of carbohydrate). American male and female adults consume an average of 49% and 52% of calories from carbohydrate, respectively (Table 9.6).[17] Also, much of this carbohydrate is in the form of processed sugar instead of the preferable starch (also called complex carbohydrate).

Dietary fiber is primarily from the storage and cell wall carbohydrates of plants, which cannot be hydrolyzed or digested by human digestive enzymes.[21–26] There are two primary types of dietary fiber: (1) *soluble fiber,* the fraction of the total fiber that is suspended in water during analysis; and (2) *insoluble fiber,* the fraction of the total fiber that is not water soluble.[25] About two thirds to three fourths of the dietary fiber in typical mixed-food diets is water insoluble. The "Nutrition Facts" food label, now required on all packaged foods, lists the total amount of dietary fiber found in a normal serving size[10] (see Figure 9.3).

The American Dietetic Association recommends that people eat 20–35 grams of dietary fiber each day (i.e., 10–13 grams/1,000 Calories).[25] As summarized in Table 9.6, current intake of dietary fiber is about 14 grams/day for females, and 18.5 grams/day for males, well below the recommended intake levels.[17] Most popular American foods are not high in dietary fiber. Dietary fiber is found solely in plant foods (none in animal-based foods, including meats, eggs, and dairy products) and is abundant in legumes, nuts and seeds, whole grains, fresh and dried fruits, and vegetables. Table 9.7 summarizes the amounts of soluble and total fiber in selected plant foods.

A high dietary fiber intake has been associated with lower risks of colon cancer and heart disease and is an important component of the diet used to help control blood glucose levels in diabetics (see Chapters 10–12).[9,10,22–27] Risk of colorectal cancer could be reduced by one third if fiber

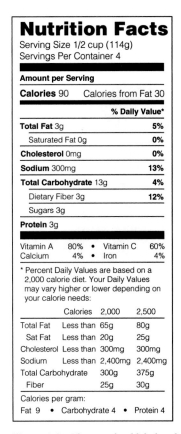

Figure 9.3 The new food label makes it much easier to count fat grams and to choose foods lower in saturated fat and cholesterol.

intake from food sources were increased by an average of 13 grams/day.[25] Fiber may also protect against breast and colon cancers.[21]

Some types of dietary fiber, called water-soluble fibers, have a role in the treatment of diabetes because they slow the absorption of glucose from the small intestine.[25] Water-soluble fibers delay transit through the stomach and small intestine and are rapidly broken down or fermented by bacteria in the large intestine. Water-soluble fibers appear to slow the absorption of glucose from the small intestine and thus help diabetics maintain better glucose control.

Water-soluble fibers also serve other healthful functions. Blood cholesterol levels are typically decreased by 5% in people who add significant amounts of water-soluble fibers to their diet, with larger decreases reported in individuals with high initial blood cholesterol levels.[25] Water-soluble fibers appear to bind bile acids and pull them down to the colon, causing the liver to make new bile acids by using cholesterol. By-products from the action of colonic bacteria on water-soluble fiber (i.e., fermentation) improve the health of colon-lining cells and travel through the blood to the liver, to decrease cholesterol production. Water-

TABLE 9.7 **Selected Sources and Amounts of Dietary Fiber**

Food	Amount	Soluble Fiber, g	Total Fiber, g
Legumes (cooked)			
Black beans	$1/2$ cup	2.1	7.5
Kidney beans	$1/2$ cup	2.3	5.7
Pinto beans	$1/2$ cup	2.7	7.4
Vegetables (cooked)			
Green peas	$1/2$ cup	1.2	4.4
Buternut winter squash	$1/2$ cup	0.4	3.4
Brussels sprouts	$1/2$ cup	1.3	2.9
Broccoli	$1/2$ cup	1.1	2.3
Zucchini	$1/2$ cup	0.3	2.3
Corn	$1/2$ cup	0.1	2.2
Spinach	$1/2$ cup	0.6	2.2
Green beans	$1/2$ cup	0.8	2.0
Potato	$1/2$ cup	0.2	0.9
Fruits (raw)			
Apple	1 medium	1.4	3.7
Orange	1 medium	2.1	3.1
Prunes	$1/4$ cup	1.3	3.0
Banana	1 medium	1.0	2.8
Blueberries	$1/2$ cup	0.6	2.0
Raisins	$1/4$ cup	0.5	1.7
Strawberries	$1/2$ cup	0.6	1.7
Mango slices	$1/2$ cup	0.9	1.5
Grapefruit	$1/2$ medium	0.8	1.3
Grapes	1 cup	0.1	0.8
Grains			
Oat bran (dry)	$1/3$ cup	2.0	4.4
Raisin bran (dry)	$1/2$ cup	0.5	3.6
Grape-Nuts (dry)	$1/3$ cup	2.0	3.6
Oatmeal (cooked)	$1/2$ cup	1.2	2.0
Whole-wheat bread	1 slice	0.4	1.9
Brown rice (cooked)	$1/2$ cup	0.2	1.8
Nuts and Seeds			
Dry roasted almonds	1 ounce	0.4	3.9
Dry roasted sunflower seeds	1 ounce	1.0	3.1
Dry roasted peanuts	1 ounce	0.6	2.3

Note: Within each category, the foods are listed from high to low in total fiber.

Source: The Food Processor, v. 7.0. Salem, OR: ESHA Research, 1997.

insoluble fibers, on the other hand, are not easily fermented and increase the bulk of the colon stool mass, shortening colonic transit time and decreasing the concentration of certain carcinogens such as secondary bile acids. For all these reasons, people who take in a high number of servings of vegetables, fruits, and whole grains tend to have less heart disease and cancer than those who largely avoid these foods.[21–27]

Plant-based foods are also rich sources of antioxidant nutrients, phytochemicals, and folic acid, each of which have been related to decreased risk of chronic disease.[27–37] There is increasing evidence that heavy exertion produces an oxidative stress that leads to the generation of oxygen-free radicals and to lipid peroxidation.[38–41] (See Principle 6, on vitamins and minerals, in this chapter.) Antioxidant enzymes within the body provide the first line of defense, with antioxidant nutrients from the diet such as vitamins E, C, and A providing a second line of defense. Chronic physical training augments the physiological antioxidant defenses in several tissues. People who exercise regularly and intensely are urged to ingest foods rich in antioxidants, and those who have a high intake of fruit, vegetables, and whole grains are at a special advantage.[38] The role of antioxidant supplements is still controversial, and until more is known, the safest source of antioxidant nutrients is plant-based foods.[28-34] Vegetables and fruits are complex foods containing more than 100 beneficial vitamins, minerals, fiber, and other substances, and no pill has captured their protective effects against chronic diseases.

A diet rich in plant foods provides a wide variety of *phytochemicals,* nonnutritive substances in plants, which possess health-protective effects.[35-37] Nuts, whole grains, fruits, and vegetables contain an abundance of phenolic compounds, terpenoids, pigments, and other natural antioxidants that have been associated with protection from heart disease, cancer, diabetes, and high blood pressure.[36] The foods and herbs with the highest anticancer activity include garlic, soybeans, cabbage, ginger, and umbelliferous vegetables (carrots, celery, cilantro, parsley, and parsnips). Other foods with anticancer activity include onions, citrus fruits, cruciferous vegetables (broccoli, brussels sprouts, cabbage, and cauliflower), tomatoes, peppers, brown rice, and whole wheat.[36]

There is increasing evidence that elevated blood levels of the amino acid homocysteine are linked to risk of cardiovascular disease.[11, 42] Plasma homocysteine levels are strongly influenced by the diet, with the greatest effects from folic acid and vitamins B_6 and B_{12}. For folic acid, optimal dietary intake levels are approximately 400 µg/day (higher than the RDA).[42] The American Heart Association advises a healthy balanced diet and the use of supplements only when the diet is not adequate to achieve these intakes.[11] Good sources of folic acid are citrus fruits, tomatoes, vegetables, and grain products. In January 1998, wheat flour was first fortified with folic acid, to add an estimated 100 µg/day to the average diet.[42]

Diet Low in Fat, Saturated Fat, and Cholesterol

According to the National Research Council, "a large and convincing body of evidence from studies in humans and laboratory animals shows that diets low in saturated fatty acids and cholesterol are associated with low risk and rates of cardiovascular disease."[9,10] High-fat diets have also been related to some types of cancer and are a major factor explaining human obesity.

Fats contain both saturated and unsaturated (monounsaturated and polyunsaturated) fatty acids[10] (see Chapter 10). The fats from meat, milk, and milk products are the main sources of saturated fats in most diets. Saturated fats tend to raise blood cholesterol levels and have been linked to an increased risk of cardiovascular disease. Olive and canola oils are particularly high in monounsaturated fats; most other vegetable oils, nuts, and high-fat fish are good sources of polyunsaturated fats. Both kinds of unsaturated fats reduce blood cholesterol when they replace saturated fats in the diet.[11]

Total dietary fat intake should be less than 30% of calories, with saturated fat less than 10% of calories.[10] For example, at 2,000 calories per day, the suggested upper limit for total fat is 600 calories (2,000 × 0.30). This is equal to 67 grams of fat (600 ÷ 9, the number of calories each gram of fat provides). For saturated fat, no more than 200 out of 2,000 calories should be ingested, which is 22 grams (200 ÷ 9). American male adults average 33.5% total calories as fat, and female adults, 32.4%[17] (see Table 9.6). For saturated fat, both male and female adults average 11% in their diets. Only one third of Americans keep their intake under 30% of total energy intake. Americans are making some positive changes in the quality of their diets, but much more work is needed until the majority of individuals are following recommended dietary practices. The "Nutrition Facts" food label lists the total amount of fat and saturated fat found in a typical serving size (see Figure 9.3).[10]

To limit intake of high-fat foods, especially those containing high amounts of saturated fat, the American Cancer Society recommends the following:[21]

- Replace fat-rich foods with fruits, vegetables, grains, and beans.
- Eat smaller portions of high-fat foods.
- Choose baked and broiled foods instead of fried foods.
- Select nonfat and low-fat milk and dairy products.
- When eating meat, pick lean cuts ("select" or "choice" USDA grade).
- Eat smaller portions of meats.
- Choose beans, seafood, and poultry as an alternative to beef, pork, and lamb.
- Select baked and broiled meats, seafood, and poultry, rather than fried.

Cholesterol intake should be below 300 mg/day. Women, whose average intake is 217 mg/day, consume cholesterol below this level. Men, however, take in an average of 337 mg/day, which exceeds the desired level[17] (see Table 9.6). Animal products are the source of all dietary cholesterol, egg yolks being one of the richest sources, with each containing about 220 mg of cholesterol. Chapter 10 contains more information on the fat, saturated fat, and cholesterol content of various foods.

There has been some concern about *trans fatty acids,* which contain at least one double bond in the trans chemical configuration.[11,43] The carbon/carbon double bonds of fatty acids can exist in either the cis or the trans configuration. The presence of a trans double bond results in fatty acids that can pack together more tightly. Trans double bonds do occur in meat and dairy products, resulting from the anaerobic bacterial fermentation in ruminant animals. More commonly, however, trans fatty acids are formed during the hydrogenation of either vegetable or fish oils.[43] Oils are hydrogenated to increase their plasticity and chemical stability. Most studies have shown that consumption of trans fatty acids results in higher blood cholesterol levels than consumption of cis fatty acids or of naturally occurring oils (but not to the same extent as the hard saturated fats).[11,43] Thus far, no consistent link between consumption of trans fatty acids and cardiovascular disease has been established. Nonetheless, the American Heart Association advises that it is prudent at this point to use unhydrogenated oil when possible and to substitute unhydrogenated oil for hydrogenated or saturated fat in processed food.[43] Also, softer versus harder margarines and cooking fats are recommended.

Diet Moderate in Sugars

Sugars are usually classified as *simple carbohydrates,* while starch and fiber are defined as *complex carbohydrates.*[9,10] During digestion, all carbohydrates except fibers break down into sugars. Sugars and starches occur naturally in many foods, including milk, fruits, some vegetables, bread, cereals, and grains. These foods also supply many other important nutrients.

Sugars and many foods that contain them in large amounts (e.g., soft drinks, desserts) supply calories but are limited in nutrients. The USDA has located such foods at the top of the food guide pyramid, urging that they be used only moderately.[10] On the food label, sugars are listed by many different names, including brown sugar, corn sweetener, corn syrup, fructose, fruit juice concentrate, glucose or dextrose, high-fructose corn syrup, honey, invert sugar, lactose, maltose, molasses, raw sugar, table sugar (sucrose), and syrup. For very physically active people, sugars can be an additional source of energy. However, because maintaining a nutritious diet and a healthy weight is very important, sugars should be used only in moderation by most healthy people and sparingly by people with low calorie needs.[10]

Sugars and starches can both promote tooth decay. The more often foods that contain sugars and starches are eaten, and the longer these foods are in the mouth before the teeth are brushed, the greater the risk for tooth decay.[9,10]

Sugar substitutes such as sorbitol, saccharin, and aspartame are ingredients in many foods, and they have been shown to be safe by many different research teams and professional organizations.[9,10] Most of the sugar substitutes do not provide significant calories and can be useful in the diets of people trying to lose weight. Foods containing sugar substitutes, however, may not always be lower in calories than similar products that contain sugars. Thus, the food label should be checked carefully.

Despite widespread concerns, intake of sugar has not been associated with increased risk of heart disease, cancer, diabetes, or abnormal behavior.[9,10,44,45] In a small proportion of people, diets containing large amounts of sugar can increase plasma triglyceride levels.[44] However, for most people, sugar consumption does not influence blood cholesterol or fat levels. Many parents feel that sugar affects the behavior of their children. Researchers from Vanderbilt University closely examined results from 23 studies and concluded that there is no scientific support for the belief that sugar causes hyperactivity, impairment in cognitive performance, or abnormal behavior in children.[45]

Diet Moderate in Salt and Sodium

Sodium and sodium chloride (table salt) occur naturally in foods, usually in small amounts. Although some people add salt to their food at the table, most salt comes from foods to which salt has already been added during processing or preparation.[9,10] Table salt is 40% sodium, with 1 teaspoon of salt containing approximately 2,000 mg of sodium. The USDA recommends that people take in less than 2,400 mg of sodium or 6,000 mg of salt per day to lower their risk of developing high blood pressure. Most people eat more salt and sodium than they need, averaging 4,000–6,000 mg of sodium a day.[17] The richest sources of sodium are sauces, salad dressings, cheeses, processed meats, soups, and grain and cereal products. The food label identifies the sodium content of packaged foods (see Figure 9.3).

Studies suggest that eating foods high in potassium (e.g., fruits and vegetables) helps to counter some of the effects of high salt consumption on blood pressure.[9,10,11] The relationship among sodium, potassium, and high blood pressure is discussed in greater detail in Chapter 10.

Moderate Consumption of Alcoholic Beverages

Alcoholic beverages supply calories but few or no nutrients. Drinking them has no net health benefit and is linked with many health problems, as well as birth defects, accidents, violent crimes, and addiction. While moderate amounts of alcohol do lower the risk of coronary heart disease, they increase the risk of several forms of cancer.[9,10] The USDA has identified several groups of people who should not drink alcoholic beverages at all:[10]

- Children and adolescents
- Individuals of any age who cannot restrict their drinking to moderate levels, a special concern for recovering alcoholics and people whose family members have alcohol problems
- Women who are trying to conceive or who are pregnant (Major birth defects, including fetal alcohol syndrome, have been attributed to heavy drinking by the mother when she was pregnant. No safe level of alcohol intake during pregnancy has been established.)
- Individuals who plan to drive or take part in activities that require attention or skill (Most people retain some alcohol in the blood up to 2–3 hours after a single drink.)
- Individuals using prescription and over-the-counter medications (Alcohol may alter the effectiveness or toxicity of medicines.)

If adults elect to drink alcoholic beverages, they should consume them in moderate amounts, which is defined as no more than two drinks a day for men, and one drink a day for women.[9,10] One drink is defined as 12 ounces of regular beer (150 Calories), 5 ounces of wine (100 Calories), or 1.5 ounces of 80-proof distilled spirits (100 Calories), each of which contains 0.5 ounce of pure ethanol.

Put simply, these guidelines stress the need for many Americans to eat more plant foods (fruits, vegetables, and whole grains), while eating fewer high-fat dairy products and meats. These guidelines call for moderation—avoiding extremes in diet. The moderate use of sugars, salt, and, if used at all, alcoholic beverages is emphasized.

For the endurance athlete, these guidelines become even more important. As time spent in endurance activity increases, the percentage of the diet represented by fat should be reduced, and the percentage of dietary carbohydrate increased. This is best accomplished by consuming smaller amounts of visible fats (margarine, oil, salad dressing, mayonnaise, etc.), high-fat dairy products (most cheeses, whole milk, butter, cream cheese, etc.), and high-fat meats (fried meats, bacon, corned beef, ground beef, ham, sausages, processed meats, etc.), as well as larger amounts of grain products (pasta, bagels, breads, brown rice, cereals, etc.), tubers (potatoes, yams), legumes (kidney beans, pinto beans, etc.), dried fruits (raisins, dates, etc.), fresh fruits, and fresh vegetables. However, as is summarized in the next section, most athletes do not eat the recommended amounts of carbohydrate.

Dietary Practices of Athletes

A large number of studies have measured the dietary intake and eating behaviors of a wide variety of athletes.[46–81] Table 9.8 summarizes some of the cross-sectional studies that have evaluated dietary intakes by athletes.

Examination of Table 9.8 reveals that there is a wide range of energy intake among athletes. In general, however, athletes tend to be high energy consumers, with the size of the participant and the energy demands of the sport having much to do with the amount of calories each consumes. Very large athletes training intensively for several hours each day (e.g., football players in the early fall) have the highest caloric requirements. Smaller athletes who transport their body mass over long distances on a regular basis (e.g., cross-country skiers and distance runners) also have high caloric requirements. In some studies, energy intake of athletes falls below expected levels which may be related to underreporting by the athlete during the food-recording process.[47–51]

Athletes who purposely keep their body weights below natural weight for competition (e.g., wrestlers, gymnasts, bodybuilders, runners, and ballet dancers) tend to have reported caloric intakes that appear to fall way below calculated energy expenditure. Several researchers have reported that athletes in sports that emphasize leanness are exceptionally preoccupied with weight, tend to use unhealthy methods for weight control, tend toward eating disorders, and demonstrate poor nutrition practices.[68–82]

The desire of the highly competitive wrestler to alter body weight without medical supervision has caused much concern among sports-medicine professionals. A high percentage induce dehydration, utilizing sauna baths, fluid restriction, and rubber or plastic suits. Some also resort to laxatives, diuretics, and vomiting. Such practices may endanger health, adversely affect performance, and affect a young person's growth potential.[79–82]

As long as wrestling competition is organized by weight categories, the popular practice of competing at the lowest possible weight will probably continue. Some sort of control, such as limiting the amount of weight that can be lost or establishing a minimum body fat percentage level, may be necessary[82] (see Box 9.2).

As can be seen from Table 9.8, protein in athletes' diets, on average, accounts for about 13–17% of energy intake, but research has shown that the proportions among different athletes can vary from 10 to 36%. Protein intakes tend to be lower among endurance athletes and higher among some groups of power and strength athletes, who can consume more than 20% of their energy as protein.[53,54,57,74] Relative to body weight, protein intakes usually exceed 1.5 g/kg/day, and intakes exceeding 2.0 g/kg/day are common. Although the Recommended Dietary Allowance (RDA) is only 0.8 g/kg/day, athletes do not appear to be much different than the nonathletic population, who tend to consume nearly double the RDA.

Table 9.8 also shows that fat accounts for about 36% of athletes' energy intakes. This is above the 33% reported in

TABLE 9.8   Dietary Intakes by Athletes (Reported in Various Studies)

Sport	Daily Calories	Protein Grams/%	Fat Grams/%	Carbohydrate Grams/%
Aerobic				
Males				
Runner	2,500–4,000	120/16	107/32	390/52
Cross-country skier	3,500–5,500	150/13	215/38	600/49
Triathlete	3,600–6,400	130/13	125/28	560/59
Females				
Runner	1,700–3,000	80/16	70/32	260/52
Cross-country skier	2,400–4,000	115/14	145/41	330/42
Swimmer	2,030–4,000	100/15	110/38	310/47
Triathlete	1,500–3,500	80/13	85/31	350/56
Aerobic–Anaerobic				
Males				
Soccer	3,000–5,000	140/15	175/40	460/45
Football	2,000–11,000	200/16	215/40	540/44
Basketball	2,000–9,000	180/15	215/41	500/44
Wrestler	1,100–6,700	95/14	100/34	400/52
Females				
Basketball	1,900–3,900	110/14	145/40	380/46
Volleyball	1,100–3,200	100/16	95/34	315/50
Power				
Males				
Track/field	3,500–4,700	175/17	330/36	470/47
Bodybuilder	2,000–5,000	200/23	157/40	320/37
Females				
Track/field	1,500–2,800	95/17	95/38	260/45
Bodybuilder	1,000–4,000	100/20	70/30	250/50
Skill				
Males				
Gymnast	600–4,300	80/15	90/40	230/45
Ballet dancer	1,740–4,100	122/17	140/42	300/38
Females				
Gymnast	1,350–1,900	70/15	75/37	225/48
Ballet dancer	900–2,900	70/15	69/34	230/50

Sources: Data taken from references 46–81.

national diet surveys.[17] Again, the proportions for athletes vary and range from about 20% to more than 50%. Power and strength athletes tend to have higher fat intakes than endurance athletes, and these higher fat intakes are often associated with their higher protein intakes.

Carbohydrate provides about 46% of the energy consumed by athletes, slightly below the percentage for the average American. (See Table 9.6.) The range of percentages is wide, and intakes of 22–72% have been reported. Triathletes are unique, in that they tend to have higher carbohydrate intakes than other athletes.[58,63] Figure 9.4 compares

the percentage of total energy intake from carbohydrate, fat, and protein, consumed by a large group of runners with those of the general population.[78] In general, the diet quality of the runners was similar to that of the general population and fell short of the recommendations summarized in Table 9.1. Several studies have shown that in the days just before, during, and after prolonged endurance events, carbohydrate intake increases dramatically as the athlete attempts to "carbohydrate load."[46,47]

In most studies, the diets of athletes contain vitamins and minerals in excess of the RDA, in part because they eat

Box 9.2

American College of Sports Medicine Recommendations on Weight Loss in Wrestlers

1. Coaches and wrestlers should be educated about the adverse consequences of prolonged fasting and dehydration on physical performance and health. They

   a. Appear to adversely influence the wrestler's energy reserves and fluid and electrolyte balances, which may affect performance

   b. May alter hormonal status

   c. Diminish protein nutritional status

   d. Can impede normal growth and development

   e. May affect psychological state

   f. Can impair academic performance

   g. May have severe health consequences, such as pulmonary emboli, pancreatitis, and reduced immune function.

2. The use of rubber suits, steam rooms, hot boxes, saunas, laxatives, and diuretics for "making weight" should be discouraged.

3. New state or national legislation should be adopted, which would schedule weigh-ins immediately prior to competition.

4. Weigh-ins should be scheduled each day before and after practice, to monitor weight loss and dehydration. Weight lost during practice should be regained through adequate food and fluid intake.

5. The body composition of each wrestler should be assessed prior to the season, using valid techniques. Males 16 years of age and younger, with a body fat below 7% or those over 16 years of age with a body fat below 5% should be required to have medical clearance before being allowed to compete. Female wrestlers should be required to have a minimal body fat of 12–14%.

6. The need for daily caloric intake obtained from a balanced diet high in carbohydrates (>55% of Calories), low in fat (<30%), with adequate protein (1.0–1.5 grams/kg body weight) should be emphasized and determined on the basis of RDA guidelines and physical activity levels. The minimal caloric intake for wrestlers of high school and college age should range from 1,700 to 2,500 Calories/day, and rigorous training may increase the requirement up to an additional 1,000 Calories/day. Wrestlers should be discouraged by coaches, parents, school officials, and physicians from consuming less than their minimal daily needs.

Source: American College of Sports Medicine. Weight loss in wrestlers. *Med Sci Sports Exerc* 28:ix–xii, 1996. Reprinted with permission.

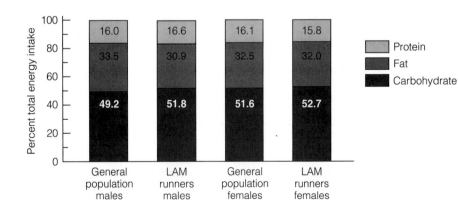

Figure 9.4 Los Angeles marathon (LAM) runners versus general population: Percentage of total energy intake—carbohydrate, fat, and proteins. The diets of Los Angeles marathon runners (N = 347) in this study tended to contain less fat and more carbohydrate than the diets of the general population. However, the percentage of total energy intake obtained from carbohydrate was lower than what is recommended for endurance runners. *Source:* Nieman DC, Butler JV, Pollett LM, Dietrich SJ, Lutz RD. Nutrient intake of marathon runners. *J Am Diet Assoc* 89:1273–1278, 1989.

more food than inactive people.[46,52,55,57,67,78] For example, in one study comparing highly conditioned and sedentary elderly women, the fit women had a higher energy intake, which was linked to a significantly greater intake of all major vitamins and minerals per kilogram of body weight (see Figure 9.5).[83] However, despite the adequacy of minerals and vitamins in their diets, athletes make widespread use of dietary supplements. (This is discussed further in the section on vitamins and minerals in this chapter.) Several large-scale studies have concluded that sports training does not have a negative effect on the nutritional status of athletes (as measured both by diet and biochemical methods), and that the use of supplements is generally unnecessary for the vast majority of athletes.[52,55,61,67,78]

Athletes in sports that emphasize leanness, however, have been found to consume insufficient quantities of vitamins and minerals, largely because of inadequate total food intake. Close to half of all gymnasts, wrestlers, and ballet dancers, for example, have been reported to consume less than two thirds the RDA for various important minerals and vitamins.[68–76]

In general, the quality of the diets of most athletes is somewhat similar to that of the general population, although some endurance athletes are making efforts to increase their carbohydrate intake. Some athletes eat more or less calories, depending on their sport, but usually energy intake increases with the demands of the training program. As a rule of thumb, athletes consume more calories per kilogram of body weight than the general population. Even though the dietary composition may be similar to those who exercise little, vitamin and mineral intake is usually sufficient for the athlete because they are eating more.

Athletes appear to snack more than inactive people to obtain these extra calories, and studies indicate snacks may contribute 25–35% of the total daily energy intake.[56,58,60,63] Figure 9.6 shows the results of one study of 347 marathon runners.[56] Time periods for breakfast (5:00–8:59 A.M.), lunch (11:00 A.M.–1:59 P.M.) and supper (4:00–7:59 P.M.) contributed 71.5% of total energy intake, while other time periods (defined as "snack times") represented 28.5% of intake. About half of energy intake occurred after 4:00 P.M. A "grazing" pattern was the rule, with 82% of the runners eating five or more times a day.

Do people who start moderate exercise programs improve the quality of their diets? Although this is an interesting hypothesis, most studies that have randomly divided sedentary subjects into exercise and nonexercise groups, and then followed them for several months while measuring their diets, have concluded that moderate exercise is an insufficient stimulus to cause people to make meaningful changes in their diets.[83–85] While some athletes may make dietary changes to enhance performance, nonathletes have little reason to make changes unless they are making a complete overhaul of their lifestyle when they initiate an exercise program. It should be noted that some cross-sectional studies report higher quality diets in physically active versus inactive subjects.[86,87] However, it is difficult to sort out whether the physical activity prompts improved dietary habits or whether other behavioral factors are involved.

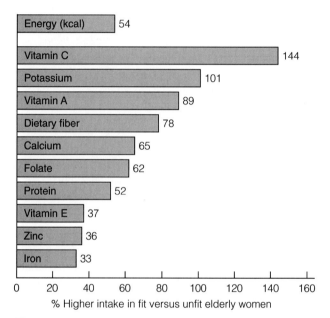

Figure 9.5 Nutrient intake in physically fit and unfit elderly women: Percentage difference in nutrient intake per kilogram of body weight. Physically fit elderly women eat more, improving nutrient intake.   *Source:* Butterworth DE, Nieman DC, Perkins R, Warren BJ, Dotson RG. Exercise training and nutrient intake in elderly women. *J Am Diet Assoc* 93:653–657, 1993.

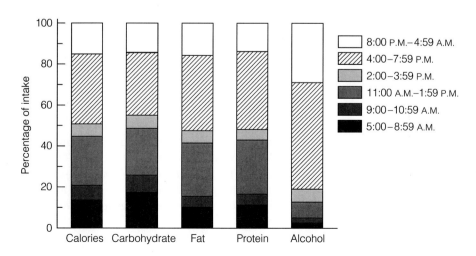

Figure 9.6 Food intake patterns of runners. In this study of 347 marathon runners, 28.5% of all Calories were eaten outside of traditional breakfast (5:00–8:59 A.M.), lunch (11:00 A.M.–1:59 P.M.), and supper (4:00–7:59 P.M.) time periods. Breakfast was highest in carbohydrate, while supper was higher in fat.   *Source:* Butterworth DE, Nieman DC, Butler JV, Herring JL. Feeding patterns of marathon runners. *Int J Sport Nutr* 4:1–7, 1994.

Nutrition Knowledge of Athletes and Coaches

Surveys conducted on the nutrition knowledge of athletes and coaches have shown, in general, that both are lacking in adequate nutrition knowledge.[88-92] Most studies have shown that few coaches have had formal nutrition education, yet they view themselves as adequately informed to dispense nutrition knowledge to athletes.

In one study of 70 female varsity athletes, scores on a nutritional knowledge test averaged 34%, which was no better than the average score of nonathletic female university students.[90]

In a large study of 430 college varsity athletes, nutrition information was, in rank order, obtained from popular magazines, trainers, friends, college courses, sport coaches, and parents.[91] Because coaches are in close contact with athletes, it is clear that it would be beneficial for them to receive nutrition education, to counter the popular sources of misinformation, particularly that given in popular magazines.

There are several excellent books written for the layperson, some especially for coaches and athletes. (See Box 9.3.)

PRINCIPLE 2: INCREASE TOTAL ENERGY INTAKE

If a person's body weight is normal, and she or he regularly engages in exercise, that person's energy consumption will need to be higher than that of the average sedentary individual to maintain body weight. Many athletes are high energy consumers because of their high working capacities and ability to train at high intensities for long periods of time. Body size is also an important determinant of caloric expenditure, with football players expending much more than gymnasts.[93-96] (See Tables 9.1 and 9.8.) In planning additional food consumption, the guidelines of the prudent diet will ensure a proper balance among the energy-providing nutrients.

Athletes Expend Large Amounts of Energy

The amount and intensity of training and body size are the chief determinants of the energy requirements of the athlete[93] (Table 9.8).

As physical activity increases, calories expended per kilogram of body weight steadily increase. Athletes are capable of amazingly high levels of energy output. A study from Great Britain reported that during a 24-hour cycling time trial in a human performance lab, one athlete cycled 430 miles, expending 20,166 Calories.[97] The athlete lost 1.19 kg of body weight because only 54% of energy needs were met through liquids and food.

Box 9.3
Sports-Nutrition Books

The following may be of interest to coaches, athletes, and fitness enthusiasts.

Clark N. *Nancy Clark's Sports Nutrition Guidebook.* Champaign, IL: Human Kinetics, 1997. (Slides are available.)

Coleman E, Nelson Steen S. *The Ultimate Sports Nutrition Handbook.* Palo Alto, CA: Bull Publishing, 1996.

Eisenman P. *Coaches' Guide to Nutrition and Weight Control.* Champaign, IL: Human Kinetics, 1990.

Peterson MS. *Eat to Compete.* St. Louis: Mosby, 1996.

Stainback R. *Alcohol and Sport.* Champaign, IL: Human Kinetics, 1997.

Tribole E. *Eating on the Run.* Champaign, IL: Human Kinetics, 1992.

University of Arizona. *Winning Sports Nutrition (VHS).* Champaign, IL: Human Kinetics, 1994.

In the 4,000 kilometer, 22-day Tour de France, cyclers ate an average of 6,000 Calories a day, half of those consumed while cycling.[98-100] Carbohydrate represented 62% of the Calories, with about a third supplied from various sport drinks that were 6–10% sugar.

Athletes are considered to be high energy expenders for two major reasons:[93-103]

1. *High working capacities.* As discussed in Chapter 7, one of the best indicators of fitness is the maximum amount of oxygen one can consume during maximal exercise ($\dot{V}O_{2max}$). Male athletes commonly have maximum oxygen uptakes exceeding 4.5 liters/min and some can achieve more than 6.0 liters/min. Female athletes, because of their smaller size, have $\dot{V}O_{2max}$ values about 30% lower. For every liter of oxygen consumed, approximately 5 Calories are expended, which for athletes with high maximal oxygen uptakes means high rates of energy expenditure (see Figure 9.7).

2. *Ability to work at high percentage of maximal capacity.* During competition and training, athletes often exercise at levels ranging from 70 to 90% of $\dot{V}O_{2max}$. With high $\dot{V}O_{2max}$ capacities to begin with, exercising at high percentages of $\dot{V}O_{2max}$ results in exceedingly high levels of energy expenditure (see Figure 9.7).

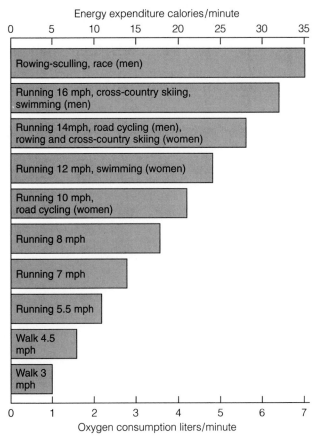

Figure 9.7 Energy-power chart. Some of the best endurance athletes in the world are capable of extremely high energy expenditure rates. *Source:* Data from Hagerman FC. Energy metabolism and fuel utilization. *Med Sci Sports Exerc* 24: S309–S314, 1992.

During periods of increased exercise or unusually heavy exertion, athletes tend to increase their caloric consumption to match energy expenditure, although periodic rest days improve the overall caloric balance.[99,101] In some studies, athletes have been reported to be eating far less than the caloric demands of their training program, but this appears to be due to underreporting of caloric intake by the athletes.[102] Measurement of nutrient intake is imprecise and difficult. Athletes must accurately record normal food intake over extended periods, a process that many subjects find onerous, leading to both dietary changes and underreporting.[8]

Athletes are not only high energy expenders, but they also have a unique pattern of energy utilization, which has important implications for the design of athletic diets. Although endurance athletes tend to expend amounts of energy comparable to those of workers in heavy-labor occupations, they expend a large quantity of their calories during short time periods—as much as 40% of the daily total in less than 2 hours. This has special nutritional implications for the athlete because of

- High utilization of glycogen (higher carbohydrate needs)
- High sweat rates (higher water needs)
- Musculoskeletal trauma (may effect protein and iron needs)
- Gastrointestinal disturbances (may effect iron balance)

Energy and ATP Production

The energy from food is transferred to the storage molecule called *adenosine triphosphate,* or *ATP.* Muscular contraction for any sport or physical activity is produced by movement within the muscle, powered by energy released from the separation of high-energy phosphate bonds from ATP.[94–96] (See Chapter 7.)

Although ATP is the immediate energy source for muscular contraction, the amount of ATP present in a muscle is so small (only about 85 grams) that it must be constantly replenished, or it will be depleted after several seconds of high-intensity exercise. ATP is replenished by two separate systems, the anaerobic system (which produces ATP in the absence of oxygen from the small ATP–CP stores and the lactate system) and the aerobic or oxygen system (see Figures 9.8 and 9.9).

The three sources from which ATP is supplied are

1. *ATP–CP stores.* The body stores a small amount of ATP and CP (creatine phosphate). The muscles can depend on these stores for up to 10 seconds (e.g., sprinting and weight lifting) before these stores are depleted.

2. *Lactate path.* ATP is produced at a high rate from carbohydrate (glycogen) stores within the muscle (see Chapter 7), during a process called *glycolysis.* Lactic acid is also produced. Because of the lactic acid by-product, which causes muscle fatigue, ATP production from the lactate system can empower intense exercise for only 1–3 minutes (for such sporting events as 400- to 800-meter runs, 100-meter swimming events, and boxing).

3. *Oxygen system.* This system, which can utilize fatty acids as well as carbohydrates, produces ATP at a slower rate than the other two energy systems. It represents an enormous potential source of energy—the body supply of fats and carbohydrates for exercise are more than enough for 5 continuous days of exercise. Oxygen is required, however, which is why the oxygen utilization capacity of the athlete becomes critically important. The oxygen system is the main provider of ATP in events lasting more than 3 minutes, and in such events as the 26.2-mile

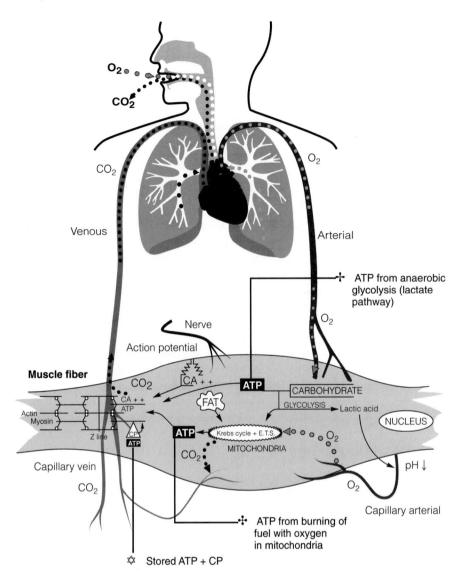

Figure 9.8 ATP is supplied via three pathways: (1) stored ATP and CP, (2) lactate pathway, and (3) mitochondrial oxygen system.

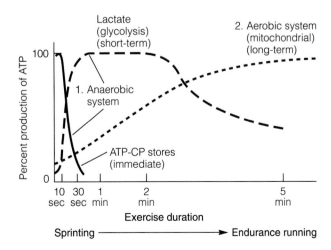

Figure 9.9 Contribution of the two energy systems during exercise of increasing duration. The anaerobic energy system provides ATP to the working myofilaments from ATP–CP stores and the lactate or glycolysis path. The aerobic system supplies ATP from mitochondria, which require oxygen to burn carbohydrates and fats.

marathon, this system becomes by far the main provider of ATP.

The aerobic and anaerobic systems work in tandem. When the exercise rate is pushed beyond the capability of the ventilation–circulation system to provide oxygen in sufficient amounts, the muscle cells rely more and more on the lactate system to provide ATP. When this reliance becomes too great, the accumulation of lactic acid may cause debilitating fatigue.

Figure 9.10 summarizes the anaerobic–aerobic continuum. In sports where both systems are utilized (such as in boxing), the training schedule should be designed to develop the capacities of both systems. (See Chapter 8.)

Fat and carbohydrate are the primary fuels for endurance exercise. As can be seen in Table 9.9, the body has relatively limited supplies of carbohydrate (1,880 Calories). These are generally distributed in the forms of blood glucose (80 Calories), and liver (350 Calories) and muscle

(1,450 Calories) glycogen. On the other hand, fat stores total 142,844 Calories.[94]

Three factors determine which primary fuel—fat or carbohydrate—will be utilized for ATP production.[94–96]

1. *Intensity and duration of exercise.* The high-intensity, low-duration events (for example, 200-meter sprinting), depend primarily on carbohydrate, through the anaerobic system. Carbohydrate is the only fuel that can be used anaerobically.

   As the intensity decreases and the duration increases (e.g., hiking), fat becomes the major preferred fuel source. Carbohydrate is still utilized, especially during the beginning portion of the exercise. Table 9.10 summarizes the utilization of meta-

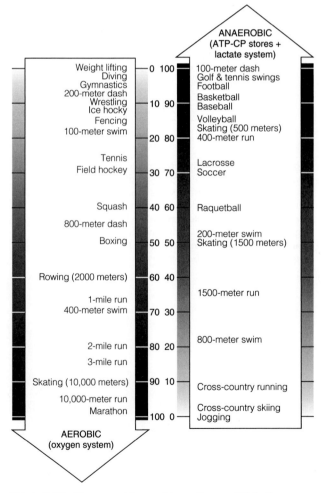

Figure 9.10 The anaerobic–aerobic continuum. While the 100-meter dash is considered a pure anaerobic event, and the marathon a pure aerobic event, most other activities use ATP from both systems. Athletes should train both systems in accordance with the demands of their sport.

TABLE 9.9 Substrate Stores of a "Normal Man"

Fuel	Weight (Kg)	Energy (Cal)
Circulating Fuels		
Glucose	0.020	80
Free fatty acids	0.0004	4
Triglycerides	0.004	40
Total		124
Tissue Stores		
Fat		
Adipose	15.0	140,000
Intramuscular	0.3	2,800
Protein (muscle)	10.0	41,000
Glycogen		
Liver	0.085	350
Muscle	0.350	1,450
Total		185,600

Source: Gollnick PD. Metabolism of substrates: Energy substrate metabolism during exercise and as modified by training. *Federation Proceedings* 44:353–357, 1985.

TABLE 9.10 How Intensity Affects Which Fuel the Muscle Uses

Exercise Intensity	Fuel Used by Muscle
< 30% $\dot{V}O_{2max}$ (easy walking)	Mainly muscle fat stores
40–60% $\dot{V}O_{2max}$ (jogging, brisk walking)	Fat and carbohydrate used evenly
75% $\dot{V}O_{2max}$ (running)	Mainly carbohydrate
≥ 80% $\dot{V}O_{2max}$ (hard running)	Nearly 100% carbohydrate

Source: Data from McCardle WD, Katch FI, Katch VL. *Exercise Physiology: Energy, Nutrition, and Human Performance* (4th ed.). Baltimore: Williams & Wilkins, 1996.

bolic fuels by muscles at different intensities of exercise.[94–96]

During prolonged exercise, the usage of carbohydrate is at first high. As the exercise continues, more and more fat is used to supply ATP for the working muscle (see Figures 9.11 and 9.12).[94–96,104,105]

2. *Fitness status.* With an improvement in aerobic fitness status, at any given workload there is an increase in the utilization of fat to produce ATP,

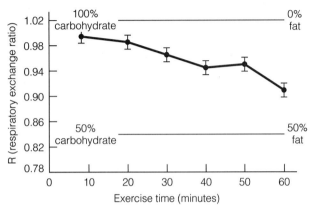

Figure 9.11 Change in use of fuel by muscle mitochondria during a 1-hour run at 70% $\dot{V}O_{2max}$. During a 1-hour run at 70% $\dot{V}O_{2max}$, the muscles gradually use more and more fat to produce ATP. *Source:* Data from Nieman DC, Carlson KA, Brandstater ME, et al. Running exhaustion in 27-h fasted humans. *J Appl Physiol* 63:2502–2509, 1987.

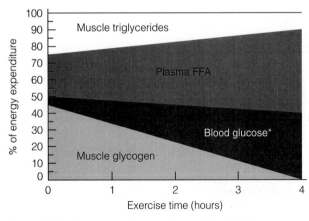

Figure 9.12 Percentage of energy derived from the four major substrates during prolonged exercise at 65–75% of maximal oxygen uptake. Initially, approximately half of the energy is derived each from carbohydrate and fat. As muscle glycogen concentration declines, blood glucose and fats become an increasingly important source of energy for muscle. After 2 hours of exercise, carbohydrate ingestion is needed to maintain blood glucose concentration and carbohydrate oxidation. *Source:* Coyle EF. Substrate utilization during exercise in active people. *Am J Clin Nutr* 61(suppl):968S–979S, 1995. © American Journal of Clinical Nutrition. American Society for Clinical Nutrition.

thereby preserving the limited carbohydrate stores and decreasing the lactate levels[1] (see Figure 9.13). This greater utilization of fat stores (which are relatively unlimited) enables the athlete to perform longer before muscle glycogen stores are depleted.

3. *Previous diet.* During the 1960s, it was discovered that when the pre-event diet was high in carbohydrate, relatively more carbohydrate was stored and available at any given workload for ATP production, and subjects could exercise much longer (Figure 9.14).[1,106] With a high-fat diet, relatively more fat was used, reducing the time of exercise to fatigue. The influence of diet is discussed fully in the following section.

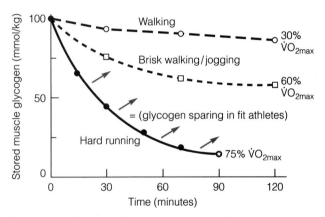

Figure 9.13 Relationship between intensity of exercise and fitness status and use of glycogen during exercise. With increasing intensity of exercise, more and more glycogen is utilized by the muscle. As the arrows depict, with aerobic training, fit athletes tend to use less glycogen during any given workload, sparing the glycogen. *Source:* Data from Costill DL. Carbohydrates for exercise: Dietary demands for optimal performance. *Int J Sports Med* 9:1–18, 1988.

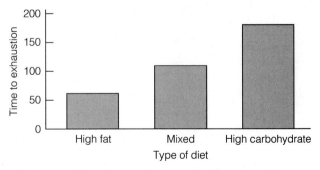

Figure 9.14 Effect of diet on duration of endurance exercise. High-carbohydrate diets allow athletes to perform endurance exercise longer. *Source:* Data from Bergstrom J, Hermansen L, Hultman E, et al. Diet, muscle glycogen and physical performance. *Acta Physiol Scand* 71:140–150, 1967.

PRINCIPLE 3: KEEP THE DIETARY CARBOHYDRATE INTAKE HIGH (55–70%) DURING TRAINING

A high-carbohydrate diet is probably the most important nutritional principle for both the fitness enthusiast and the endurance athlete. Body carbohydrate stores (glycogen) are critical because they are the primary fuel source for the working muscles. When muscle glycogen levels drop too low, the ability to exercise falls, and one feels more stale and tired and is more prone to injury. Athletes in heavy training may need more than 8 grams of carbohydrate per kilogram of body weight in their diet per day, which translates to approximately 55–70% of their total energy intake.

The Importance of Carbohydrate during Heavy Training

The story of carbohydrate (CHO) in endurance performance began in 1939, when Scandinavian researchers demonstrated the effect of exercise intensity on the fuel used by the muscle during exercise.[1,107,108] They found that as the intensity of the exercise increased, the relative contribution of CHO as muscular fuel increased.

The development of the biopsy needle in 1962 allowed researchers to extend these findings by measuring the actual amounts of glycogen in the muscle.[109] (See Figure 9.15.) A series of experiments by other Scandinavian investigators during the late 1960s demonstrated that the ability to exercise at a high intensity was related to the pre-exercise level of muscle glycogen.[1,110,111]

Several basic principles are now clear regarding the relationship between exercise and dietary carbohydrate, and muscle glycogen.[112–122]

- Body glycogen stores play an important role in hard exercise (70–85% of $\dot{V}O_{2max}$) that is either prolonged and continuous (e.g., running, swimming, cycling), or of an extended intermittent, mixed anaerobic–aerobic nature (e.g., soccer, basketball, ice hockey, repeated running intervals). The higher the intensity of exercise, the more dependent the working muscle is on glycogen (see Figure 9.13 and Table 9.10). For example, 2 hours of cycling at 30% of $\dot{V}O_{2max}$ will only reduce muscle glycogen by about 20%, whereas performing at 75% of $\dot{V}O_{2max}$ results in almost complete muscle glycogen depletion.[1]

- Because of limited CHO body stores (see Table 9.9), the body adapts in various ways to maximize its use of these stores. Endurance training leads to higher stored levels of muscle glycogen, nearly double those of untrained people.[94] Endurance training also leads to a greater utilization of fat at any given workload, sparing the glycogen.[123] In other words, aerobically fit people consume more fat at any given workload, sparing the glycogen (see Figure 9.13). For example, when fit and unfit people run together at a certain pace (e.g., 8 minutes/mile), the fit will use more fat and less carbohydrate per mile than the unfit. This is advantageous because muscle glycogen levels are spared, allowing the fit person to exercise longer.

- Exhaustion during prolonged, hard exercise is tied to low muscle glycogen levels. CHO stores are thus the

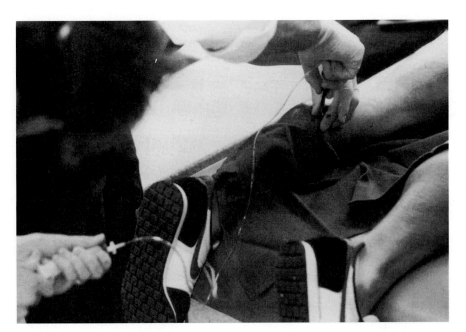

Figure 9.15 The needle biopsy allows researchers to obtain a small sample of muscle tissue to measure the amount of glycogen. A small incision is made in the muscle (after anesthetizing the area), the biopsy needle is inserted, suction pressure is applied, and a small piece of muscle is cut with a sliding knife device in the needle.

limiting factor in exercise bouts lasting longer than 60–90 minutes.[1,112–120] (See Figure 9.16.) Low glycogen levels are also limiting in various team sports that entail a lot of running. In soccer, for example, players with low glycogen levels have been found to run less and walk more than those with optimal levels.[121] In soccer, players cover an average of 10 kilometers, much of it at high sprinting speeds. Fatigue in shorter events is due to other factors, especially the buildup of metabolic by-products such as lactic acid and hydrogen ions within the muscle cells.

- When muscle and liver glycogen stores are low, a high work output cannot be maintained. Marathoners use the term "hitting the wall" to describe the fatigue and pain that is associated with reaching low glycogen levels. There is an apparent obligatory requirement of muscle and liver glycogen breakdown for intense exercise. The breakdown of fat cannot sustain metabolic rates during exercise at levels much above 50–65% of $\dot{V}O_{2max}$. In other words, when muscle glycogen levels are low, the exerciser will not be able to exercise at intensities above 50–65% of $\dot{V}O_{2max}$—which for many runners means a painful shuffle or jog.

For endurance cyclers, low initial glycogen levels have been shown to reduce power output during the end of the race.[122]

- During the first hour of hard exercise, most of the CHO and fat (triglycerides) come from within the muscle, which is a major depot of fuel (see Figures 9.12 and 9.17). As the exercise continues beyond 1 hour, more and more demands are placed upon adipose tissue fat fuel sources and blood glucose as muscle glycogen levels begin to be depleted. The longer the exercise period, the greater the need for glucose from the liver to keep pace with the increasing glucose demands of the glycogen-depleted working muscle.[1,112,114] As with muscle glycogen, trained individuals utilize less plasma glucose than the untrained, preserving liver glycogen, minimizing the possibility of hypoglycemia, and improving long-term endurance.[114]

- During strenuous training, muscle glycogen stores undergo rapid day-to-day fluctuation. Sedentary people on normal mixed diets have glycogen stores of only 70–110 mmol per kilogram wet muscle. Athletes on mixed diets, after 24 hours of rest, have glycogen levels of 130–135 mmol/kg wet muscle, and after 48 hours of rest with a high-carbohydrate diet, they have 140–230 mmol/kg.[1]

As Figure 9.18 shows, glycogen levels of athletes can be reduced 50% after a 2-hour workout.[124,125] If the carbohydrate content of the diet is low (about 40% of total Calories), little muscle glycogen is restored during the day, and with a 2-hour workout the next day the athlete will be less able to exercise intensely, or exercise will feel harder than nor-

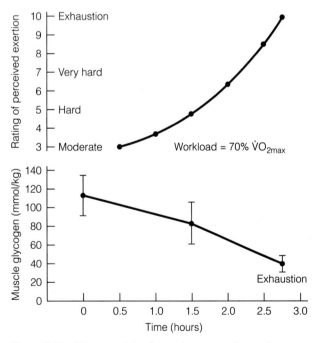

Figure 9.16 Nine experienced marathoners ran for nearly 3 hours on a treadmill at 70% $\dot{V}O_{2max}$. As the muscle glycogen levels fell, the rating of perceived exertion climbed strongly. Exhaustion was associated with low glycogen levels in the muscles of the runners. *Source:* Nieman DC, Carlson KA, Brandstater ME, et al. Running exhaustion in 27-h fasted humans. *J Appl Physiol* 63:2502–2509, 1987.

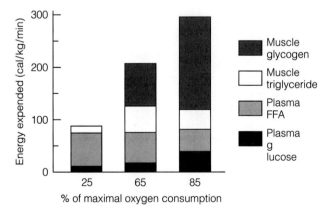

Figure 9.17 Contribution of the four major substrates to energy expenditure after 30 minutes of exercise at 25%, 65%, and 85% of maximal oxygen uptake when fasted. *Source:* Coyle EF. Substrate utilization during exercise in active people. *Am J Clin Nutr* 61(suppl): 968S–979S, 1995. Coyle EF. Perspectives in Exercise Science and Sports Medicine, *Recent Advances in the Science and Medicine of Sport,* Vol. 10. With permission from Cooper Publishing Group.

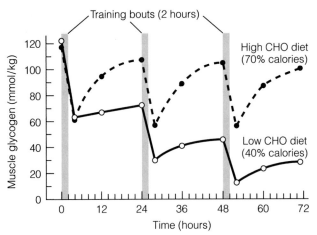

Figure 9.18 The importance of a high-carbohydrate diet during heavy training. Daily, 2-hour workouts deplete muscle glycogen stores by about 50%. A low-carbohydrate diet (40% of Calories) does not adequately restore this depleted glycogen, and there will be a progressive reduction in muscle glycogen as the daily workouts continue. A high-carbohydrate diet (70% of Calories) helps to keep muscle glycogen stores near normal despite heavy training, allowing the athlete to train harder with less effort. *Sources:* Data from Costill DL, Miller JM. Nutrition for endurance sports: Carbohydrate and fluid balance. *Int J Sports Med* 1:2–14, 1980; Costill DL, Bowers R, Branam G, Sparks K. Muscle glycogen utilization during prolonged exercise on successive days. *J Appl Physiol* 63:2388–2395, 1971.

mal.[1,113,118,124] This has been demonstrated in rowers, swimmers, and runners, leading most sports-nutrition experts to advise that endurance athletes adopt high-carbohydrate diets[113,115,120,126–128] (see Figure 9.19).

- Many endurance athletes compete or train repeatedly on the same day or on consecutive days, and thus the rapid restoration of muscle glycogen is essential. While earlier studies suggested that 48 hours or longer were required to replenish muscle glycogen stores after long endurance exercise, more recent investigations have shown that when 9–16 grams CHO/kg body weight are consumed soon after exercise, muscle glycogen stores can be normalized within 1 day, especially in highly trained individuals.[129–134] Carbohydrate-rich foods or fluids should be ingested soon after long-term exercise, until at least 8–10 grams CHO/kg (500–800 grams or 2,000–3,200 CHO Calories, depending on body size) are consumed.[119,129–134] There is some evidence that high-glycemic-index foods promote a greater glycogen storage rate.[131–135] (See Box 9.4.) This is also good advice for weight trainers. In one study, multiple sets of intense leg knee extensions decreased muscle glycogen by about 30%.[130] When subjects took in carbohydrate immediately after the session, most of the muscle glycogen was restored within 6 hours, while there was little change in subjects drinking only water (see Figure 9.20).

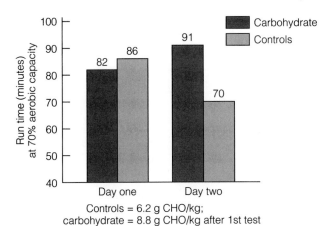

Figure 9.19 Carbohydrate intake and recovery from prolonged exercise. In this study, runners were able to run longer on Day 2 when they consumed nearly 9 grams CHO/kg after a hard bout of running the first day. *Source:* Data from Fallowfield JL, Williams C. Carbohydrate intake and recovery from prolonged exercise. *Int J Sport Nutr* 3:150–164, 1993.

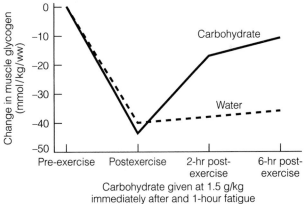

Figure 9.20 Glycogen resynthesis following resistance exercise: 9 sets of 6 reps, leg knee extensions, 70% 1–RM, to fatigue. Postexercise carbohydrate is important for weight trainers to restore muscle glycogen depleted during exercise. *Source:* Pascoe DD, Costill DL, Fink WJ, Robergs RA, Zachwieja JJ. Glycogen resynthesis in skeletal muscle following resistive exercise. *Med Sci Sports Exerc* 25:349–354, 1993.

Box 9.4

Should Athletes Be Concerned about the Glycemic Index?

Although most athletes know that they should consume liberal amounts of carbohydrate before, during, and after prolonged exercise, few are concerned about the types of carbohydrate foods to select. The glycemic index (GI) has been proposed as an important resource when selecting an ideal carbohydrate food to optimize glycogen storage rates.

The GI categorizes foods containing carbohydrates according to the blood glucose response they elicit. High-GI foods evoke the highest blood glucose response, while low glycemic foods produce a relatively low response. The GI was originally developed for diabetics to better control blood glucose levels. The GI is a percentage value, based on the area of the blood glucose response of 50 grams of carbohydrate in a reference food (typically white bread), multiplied by 100:

GI = (blood glucose area of test food)
    ÷ (blood glucose area of reference food) × 100

The GI approach has been criticized because some foods have been rated as good or bad simply on the basis of their GI. The GI was never intended to be used in isolation. Instead, the user must balance GI information with other measures of diet quality, including dietary fiber, vitamin and mineral content, and the amount of salt, cholesterol, and saturated fat.

Researchers from the University of British Columbia in Vancouver, Canada, have made these recommendations concerning exercise and the GI:

1. Athletes wishing to consume carbohydrates 30–60 minutes before exercise should be encouraged to ingest low-GI foods. This will decrease the likelihood of creating hyperglycemia and hyperinsulinemia at the onset of exercise, while providing exogenous carbohydrate throughout the early stages of exercise. Notice from the following list that low-GI foods include spaghetti, milk, fructose, some fruits and juices, and most legumes.

2. High-GI foods should be consumed during exercise to ensure rapid digestion and absorption, and elevated blood glucose levels. Notice from the following list that high-GI foods include instant rice, glucose, potatoes and other root vegetables, sucrose, bagels, and many types of breakfast cereals. Most sports drinks are a combination of glucose (high GI) and fructose (low GI), so the proportion should be checked carefully, with an emphasis on high-glucose sports drinks.

3. Postexercise meals should consist of high-GI carbohydrates, to enhance glycogen resynthesis.

Foods can be ranked as follows, according to their GI (with white bread used as the standard or a GI of 100):

High (GI >100)	GI	Moderate (GI = 60–100)	GI	Low (GI <60)	GI
Carrots	101	Muffin	88	Spaghetti	59
Bagels	103	Oatmeal	87	Apple juice	58
Honey	104	Ice cream	87	Tomato soup	54
Doughnut	108	Rice (white and brown)	80	Apple	52
Waffles	109	Oatmeal cookies	79	Yogurt, low fat	47
Sucrose	117	Corn	78	Dried apricots	44
Corn Chex	118	Banana	76	Kidney beans	42
Cornflakes	119	Orange juice	74	Peach, fresh	40
Baked potatoes	121	Chocolate	70	Whole milk	39
Crispix cereal	124	Lactose	65	Red lentils	36
Rice Chex	127	Orange	62	Fructose	32
Instant rice	128	Grapes	62	Soy beans	25
Glucose	138	All-bran cereal	60	Peanuts	21

Sources: Walton P, Rhodes EC. Glycemic index and optimal performance. *Sports Med* 23:164–172, 1997; Foster-Powell K, Miller JB. International tables of glycemic index. *Am J Clin Nutr* 62:871S–893S, 1995.

Practical Implications for Athletes

In general, glycogen synthesis increases in proportion to the amount of CHO consumed. About 8–10 grams of CHO are needed per kilogram of body weight (about 500–800 total grams) each day for the endurance athlete who is training for more than 60–90 minutes.[1,93,113,115] Athletes in heavy training should consume a diet of close to 70% CHO (525 grams per 3,000 Calories), which will restore muscle glycogen within 24 hours, enabling the athlete to continue heavy training. This is especially important after race events and long, intense training bouts.

This is more carbohydrate than most athletes would ordinarily choose, however, and they need to be educated to include this large amount. Athletes commonly underestimate their carbohydrate needs and are thus susceptible to feeling "stale" from glycogen depletion.

Table 9.11 is a sample listing of high-carbohydrate foods, in descending order of amount of the carbohydrate they contain (in grams per cup). Notice that foods high in simple sugars lead the list, followed by dried fruits, cereals, potatoes, rice, legumes, and fruit juices. While high-sugar foods such as honey, jams, and syrups provide high amounts of carbohydrate, too much simple sugar in the diet invites shortages of necessary vitamins and minerals. Although high- versus low-glycemic foods promote more rapid glycogen resynthesis, the athlete should choose foods that also promote nutritional health.

Table 9.12 outlines a sample menu for an athlete who is training more than 60–90 minutes a day aerobically. Notice that grain products and fruits predominate in this high-carbohydrate diet. The use of fatty meats and dairy products, nuts, olives, and oils should be limited, to ensure that sufficient carbohydrate is consumed to replete muscle glycogen stores. High-carbohydrate diets are healthy, supply more than 100% of the RDA for all nutrients, help prevent chronic disease, and can therefore be recommended on a daily basis. The process of "carbohydrate loading" before major events is discussed in Principle 8. Box 9.5 reviews the problems of the 40-30-30 diet or "Zone Diet."

PRINCIPLE 4: DRINK LARGE AMOUNTS OF FLUIDS DURING TRAINING AND THE EVENT

Probably the second most important dietary principle for those who exercise is to drink large quantities of fluids. As little as a 2% drop in body weight caused by water loss (primarily from sweat) can reduce exercise capacity. In other words, if an athlete weighs 150 pounds and loses

TABLE 9.11   High-Carbohydrate Foods—1-Cup Portions

Food	Grams Carbohydrate	Calories per Cup	% Carbohydrate Calories
Honey	272	1040	100
Pancake syrup	238	960	100
Jams/preserves	224	880	100
Molasses	176	720	100
Dates (chopped)	131	489	100
Raisins	115	434	100
Prunes	101	385	100
Grape-Nuts	94	407	92
Whole-wheat flour	85	400	85
Dried apricots (uncooked)	80	310	100
Sweet potato (boiled, mashed)	80	344	93
Sweetened applesauce	51	194	100
Brown rice	50	232	86
Prune juice	45	181	100
Kidney beans	42	230	73
Rolled wheat (cooked)	41	180	91
Macaroni (cooked)	39	190	82
Lentils (cooked)	39	210	74
Grape juice	38	155	98

Source: USDA Handbook No. 8 (revised).

TABLE 9.12 Sample Menu—3,500 Calories, High-Carbohydrate (79% Total Calories)

The foods listed here represent a 1-day sample of the type of diet recommended for the average male runner training for long endurance events. This type of diet is also recommended for "carbohydrate loading" during the 3-day period before a long endurance race. This sample diet meets the recommended dietary allowance (RDA) for all nutrients and follows the guidelines of the "prudent diet."

Portion	Food	Calories
Breakfast		
1 cup	Grape-Nuts	404
2 cups	2% lowfat milk	242
1 whole	banana	105
1/2 cup	seedless raisins	247
2 cups	orange juice	224
1 piece	whole-wheat bread	84
2 tsp	honey	43
Lunch		
1/2 whole	fresh tomato	12
1/2 cup	loose leaf lettuce	5
2 oz	cooked chicken	108
2 pieces	whole-wheat bread	168
1 tbs	low-cal dressing	35
2 cups	canned pineapple juice	278
Supper		
2 pieces	whole-wheat bread	168
1 tbs	peanut butter	96
2 whole	apple	162
2 cups	cooked brown rice	464
2 cups	mixed vegetables	105
1 tsp	seasonings	5
1 cup	low-fat yogurt	231
2 whole	bagels	330

Meal	Calories	Total CHO Grams	% CHO
Breakfast	1349	290	86
Lunch	606	108	71
Supper	1561	292	75
Totals	3516	690	79

Nutrients	Protein	Iron	Zinc	Calcium	Vit C	Vit A	Vit B_1
Day Totals	116 g	25 mg	18 mg	1578 mg	425 mg	15,009 IU	4.2 mg
% RDA	207%	250%	120%	197%	708%	300%	280%

3 pounds during an exercise bout, performance ability is reduced. A good habit is to measure body weight before and after each exercise session; each pound lost should be replaced with 1 pint (or 2 cups) of fluid.[136,137]

Thirst lags behind actual body needs. So before, during, and after the exercise bout, one should drink plenty of fluids, beyond the demands of thirst. A plan recommended by some sports-medicine experts is to drink 2 cups of water immediately before the exercise bout, 1 cup every 15 minutes during the exercise session, and then 2 more cups after the session. Whether to include carbohydrates and electrolytes in the exercise drink is important, and discussed on page 297. In general, when intense exercise lasts longer than 1 hour, carbohydrates (30–60 grams per hour) and sodium

Box 9.5

The Zone Diet

In 1995, Barry Sears wrote *Enter the Zone,* advancing a new dietary intake theory, called the "Zone Diet." The book soon became a best-seller and has been followed by other books, including *Mastering the Zone.* The zone diet is extremely popular among many Americans and has been recommended for weight loss, good health, and improved athletic performance.

Sears's theory centers around a "40-30-30" diet in which 40% of calories come from carbohydrates, 30% from protein, and 30% from fat. This diet is much higher in protein and lower in carbohydrate than has been recommended by most nutritional experts for health and endurance performance. Sears reasons that carbohydrates raise blood sugar levels, causing the release of insulin, a hormone that he claims causes high-carbohydrate foods to be stored as fat, rather than used as energy. "When a carbohydrate enters the blood too fast, the pancreas responds by secreting high levels of insulin," writes Sears. "While that brings the blood sugar level down, it also tells the body to store fat and keep it stored." The key to health, claims Sears, is to keep insulin within a relatively narrow zone by eating a 40-30-30 diet.

The zone diet is also promoted because it is associated, Sears claims, with "good" *eicosanoid* (a type of fatty acid) compounds, while decreasing "bad" eicosanoids. Good eicosanoids supposedly combat infections, allergies, and exposure to toxic substances, while bad eicosanoids contribute to heart disease, cancer, and immune-system diseases. Sears is the president of a company, Eicotech, that manufactures products that complement the zone diet.

The Center for Science in the Public Interest (CSPI) has strongly countered Sears's claims (see *Nutrition Action Newsletter,* July / August, 1996, and April, 1997). CSPI has reviewed the few studies used by Sears in support of his theories and have found them either flawed or misinterpreted. While carbohydrate intake does raise insulin, no research has been able to link meal-to-meal surges in insulin to obesity. Nearly all nutrition experts feel that surplus calories, not carbohydrates and insulin, cause increases in body fat.

The zone diet is too low in carbohydrate to promote athletic performance in endurance events lasting longer than 90 minutes. As reviewed in this chapter, one of the most important principles of sports nutrition is to consume a high-carbohydrate diet to maximize muscle glycogen stores. This concept has been supported by a wide variety of studies spanning more than 60 years. A few papers have been cited by Sears in support of his 40-30-30 diet for improved athletic performance, but these are considered flawed in research design and not representative of the consensus viewpoints established over many years of excellent research from the world's best human-performance laboratories. Three of the studies were sponsored by Bio-Foods, Inc., of Santa Barbara, which makes the Balance™ Bar and Balance Complete Nutritional Drink Mix, products that adhere to the 40-30-30 principle. Much of the evidence used by Sears is anecdotal. For example, the successful Stanford University men's and women's swim teams supposedly use both sports bars based on the 40-30-30 plan and fish-oil pills (to reduce bad eicosanoids), and they have been held up as evidence that the zone diet works. Barry Heyden, fitness coach for the New York Mets, touts the PR*Bar, offered by PR*Nutrition, in San Diego, as part of its 40-30-30™ Nutrition Program, claiming the players feel less sluggish than normal during baseball games. However, anecdotal data is highly suspect, is duly influenced by the placebo effect, and can be greatly affected by many confounders.

Thus far, there is insufficient evidence to support the zone diet for enhanced athletic performance, and the burden of proof lies with Sears and other proponents. It is highly doubtful that appropriate evidence will ever be produced.

(0.5–0.7 gram/liter of water) should be ingested to delay fatigue and promote fluid retention.[136,137]

The Importance of Water for Temperature Regulation during Exercise

As carbohydrate and fat are used by the working muscle to produce energy for movement, about 70–80% is transformed into heat (much like the engine in a car).[138–142] If this were retained by the body, body heat would potentially increase up to 1°C every 5 minutes resulting in serious heat injury (hyperthermia) within 20–30 minutes.[138,143]

During steady-state exercise at 75% of capacity, average heat loss from the body may range from 900 to 1,500 Calories/hour. An addition of up to 100–150 Calories/hour may be gained from the sun. The body heat is transferred from the warm muscle to the blood and then to the skin, where it is dissipated to the air by evaporation, radiation, or convection.[138,140] On a hot dry day at rest, 55% of

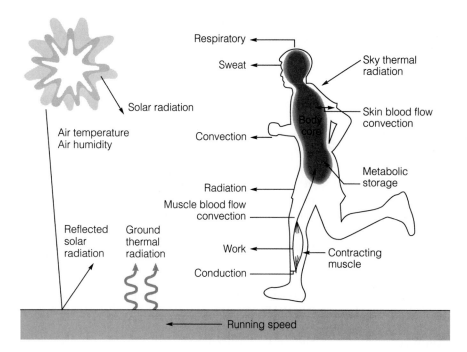

Figure 9.21   As the muscles contract during exercise, heat is produced, causing the core body temperature to rise. A small amount of heat is also gained by the body from the environment. The primary route for this heat to exit is sweat evaporation. Other routes include convection, radiation, conduction, and respiration. *Source:* Gisolfi CV, Wenger CB. Temperature regulation during exercise: Old concept, new ideas. In Terjung RL (ed), *Exercise and Sports Sciences Reviews,* Volume 12. Lexington: Collamore Press, 1984.

heat loss is by radiation and convection, 45% by sweat evaporation. During exercise, sweat evaporation becomes by far the major avenue of heat loss, accounting for greater than 80%. For every liter of sweat evaporated on the skin, close to 600 Calories are given off, preventing an increase in body temperature of a full 10°C. The body has 2–4 million sweat glands, and, on a hot but dry day, can secrete enough sweat to dissipate all of the heat generated by exercise.[141] For example, if an athlete sweats 1.8 liters/hour, 1,000 Calories of heat are removed from the body. Figure 9.21 shows the avenues of heat loss from the exercising human body.

The sweat glands draw fluid from stores between and within the body cells, and then from the plasma volume of the blood in the skin[137,144] (see Figure 9.22). However, the efficiency of sweat evaporation is greatly affected by humidity, especially if it rises above 70% (relative humidity).[136,137,145] If the humidity is so high that the sweat rolls off the skin without evaporation, little heat is given off, and body temperature rises. This can result in heat injury, including heat exhaustion and heat stroke (see Chapter 16). In heat stroke, the brain shuts off the sweat glands to protect blood fluid levels, resulting in dry, hot, and red skin and a deadly rise in body temperature.

Exercise in hot and humid weather can be dangerous. During the 1986 Pittsburgh marathon, for example, the temperature reached 87°F and the humidity 60%; as a result, half of the 2,879 runners were treated for heat injuries.[146] (The American College of Sports Medicine has established guidelines for race directors to follow to avoid this type of disaster; see Chapter 16.)

Figure 9.23 shows the effect of running pace and weather conditions on the sweat rate; rates become extremely high during fast running on hot and humid days.[142]

Sweat losses of 0.5 to 1.5 liters per hour are common in endurance sports.[136,137] Under extremely hot conditions, sweat rates (of fit participants) have been measured at over 2.5 liters per hour. During the 1984 Los Angeles Olympic Games, U.S. runner Alberto Salazar lost 12 pounds (8.1% of body weight) during the marathon, despite drinking nearly 2 liters of water during the race. Alberto's sweat rate was 3.7 liters per hour, one of the highest ever measured.[147] Sweat rates are influenced by fitness level, temperature and humidity, intensity of exercise, heat acclimation, hydration status, air velocity, and the type of clothing worn.[141] Sweat rates can be calculated using this formula:

(loss in body weight)
+ (fluids ingested during exercise)
− (urine excreted during exercise) = sweat loss

For example, if an athlete runs intensely for 1 hour and loses 0.5 kilogram of body weight, drinks 500 ml of fluid, and urinates 100 ml, the sweat rate = 1,100 g + 500 − 100 = 1,500 ml/hour.

The average 70-kilogram individual has 42 liters of body water (60% of body weight). The body water is divided into three components:[137]

1. Intracellular fluid (67%)

2. Interstitial (between cells) fluid (27%)

3. Plasma volume (6%)

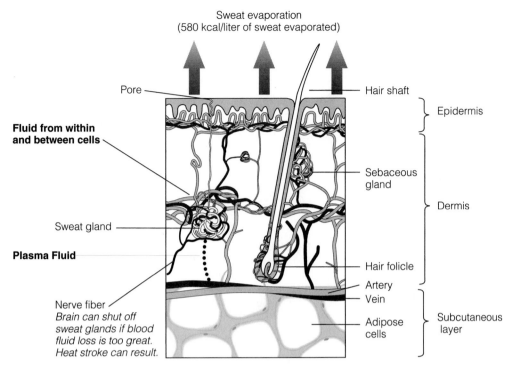

Figure 9.22   Sources of fluid for sweat production. The sweat glands draw fluids from between and within cells and from the blood, to produce sweat during exercise. If blood volume levels fall too low, the brain will shut off sweat gland activity. Continued exercise can then result in heat stroke.

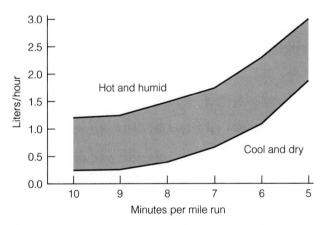

Figure 9.23   Sweat rates in runners. Sweat rates are affected by running pace and weather conditions. The specifics of measuring heat stress, including the relationship of heat and humidity, is described in Chapter 16.   *Source:* Data from Sawka MN. Physiological consequences of hypohydration: Exercise performance and thermoregulation. *Med Sci Sports Exerc* 24:657–670, 1992.

Loss of body water from sweating beyond 2% of body weight will significantly impair endurance capacity, through elevation of body temperature and decreased cardiac output. When sweat output exceeds water intake, both intracellular and extracellular water levels fall, and plasma volume decreases, resulting in an increase in body temperature, a decrease in the ability of the heart to pump blood, and a decrease in endurance performance. Even a slight amount of dehydration causes physiological consequences. For example, every liter (2.2 lbs) of water lost will cause heart rate to be elevated by about eight beats per minute, cardiac output to decline by 1 liter per minute, and core temperature to rise by 0.3°C when an individual participates in prolonged exercise in the heat.[137,138,141,148–153]

Table 9.13 outlines the adverse effects of dehydration.[149,150] Those most vulnerable to dehydration during exercise are obese, unfit, unacclimatized, overclothed people, who are exercising on hot, humid, sunny days. Early warning signals include clumsiness, stumbling, excessive sweat, cessation of sweating, headache, nausea, or dizziness.

People who are accustomed to exercising in the heat go through physiological changes that have been termed the "acclimatization process."[94–96,152,153] Acclimatization (using a gradual progression for safety) can occur within as few as 5–10 days of training in the heat. The acclimatized person has a higher plasma volume (400–700 ml increase) and sweat glands that produce more sweat earlier in the exercise session, with less loss of sodium. During exercise, the acclimatized person's body temperature and heart rate do not rise as strongly as those of unacclimatized people.

TABLE 9.13 Adverse Effects of Dehydration*

% Body Wt Loss	Symptoms
1.0	Thirst threshold
2.0	Stronger thirst, vague discomfort, loss of appetite
3.0	Increasing hemoconcentration, dry mouth, reduction in urine
4.0	Decrement of 20–30% in exercise capacity
5.0	Difficulty in concentrating, headache, impatience
6.0	Severe impairment in exercise temperature regulation, increased respiration, extremity numbness and tingling
7.0	Likely collapse if combined with heat and exercise

Physiological Responses to Dehydration

↑ Incidence of gastrointestinal distress	↓ Gastric emptying rate
↑ Plasma osmolality	↓ Splanchnic, renal blood flow
↑ Blood viscosity	↓ Plasma volume
↑ Heart rate	↓ Central blood volume
↑ Core temperature at which sweating begins	↓ Cardiac filling pressure
↑ Core temperature at which skin blood flow increases	↓ Stroke volume and cardiac output
↑ Core temperature at a given exercise intensity	↓ Sweat rate at a given core temperature
	↓ Maximal sweat rate
	↓ Maximal skin blood flow
	↓ Performance

*1% of body weight for a 150 lb. person would equal 3 cups of water (1 cup = 0.5 lb.).

Sources: Data from Greenleaf JE, Harrison MH. Water and electrolytes. In Layman DK (ed), *Nutrition and Aerobic Exercise.* Washington, DC: American Chemical Society, 1986; Murray R. Fluid needs in hot and cold environments. *Int J Sport Nutr* 5:S62–S73, 1995.

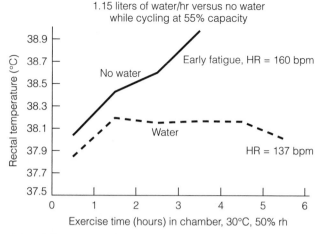

Figure 9.24 Fluid replacement during prolonged exercise: 1.15 liters of water / hr versus no water while cycling at 55% capacity. Drinking about 1.2 liters of water each hour during prolonged exercise in a moderately hot environment prevented dehydration, allowing subjects to exercise for 6 hours. *Source:* Barr SI, Costill DL, Fink WJ. Fluid replacement during prolonged exercise: Effects of water, saline, or no fluid. *Med Sci Sports Exerc* 23:811–817, 1991.

Fluid replacement during exercise reduces the adverse effects of dehydration by slowing the rise in core temperature, maintaining plasma volume and cardiac output, improving endurance, and lessening the risk of heat injury.[136,137,154–156]

During prolonged exercise, as the body loses water primarily through sweating, there tends to be a gradual decrease in heartstroke volume, and a corresponding increase in heart rate, making the exercise seem more difficult than normal. Drinking about 1 liter of fluid per hour helps prevent this "cardiovascular drift," making it easier to continue exercising.[151,156]

Figure 9.24 shows the results of one study where subjects cycled for 6 hours at 55% of $\dot{V}O_{2max}$ while either avoiding fluids or drinking enough to replace total body water loss (a little over 1 liter per hour in an environmental chamber set at 30°C and 50% relative humidity).[154] When fluids were restricted, subjects lost an average of 6.4% of their body weight (10 pounds), experienced high rectal temper-atures and heart rates, and found the exercise too difficult to complete, stopping 1.5 hours earlier than subjects who drank enough to maintain body water. These results demonstrate the deleterious effects of dehydration on exercise performance.

How much water should one drink during exercise to avoid dehydration? Figure 9.25 summarizes the water-balance needs of sedentary and physically active people. In general, most people sweat 0.5 to 1.5 liters per hour of exercise and need to replace this by drinking more fluids.[136,137] It is common for athletes to lose 2–4% of body weight during vigorous workouts. Marathoners can lose 6–8% of their body weight in water during the 26.2-mile event, with plasma volume decreasing 13–18%.[151,157] A 4% drop in body weight for a 150-pound person means a loss of 6 pounds, or about 3 quarts of water. It is not uncommon for such a person, if she or he were running in a hot environment, to lose half a pound per mile after the first hour. That would amount to a cup of water every mile, or every 6–8 minutes.

For most athletes, it is hard to drink this much water, mainly because such intake is beyond the demands of thirst. Exercise tends to blunt thirst, so a systematic plan should be followed for fluid consumption during exercise. In other words, when one is exercising, thirst provides a poor index of body needs, leading to what some researchers call "involuntary dehydration."[136,137,155] Most athletes are "reluctant" drinkers during exercise and do not drink enough to match body losses. Runners, for example, generally drink only 300–500 ml of fluids per hour of exercise.[151,155] Therefore, fluids need to be "forced down" during exercise.

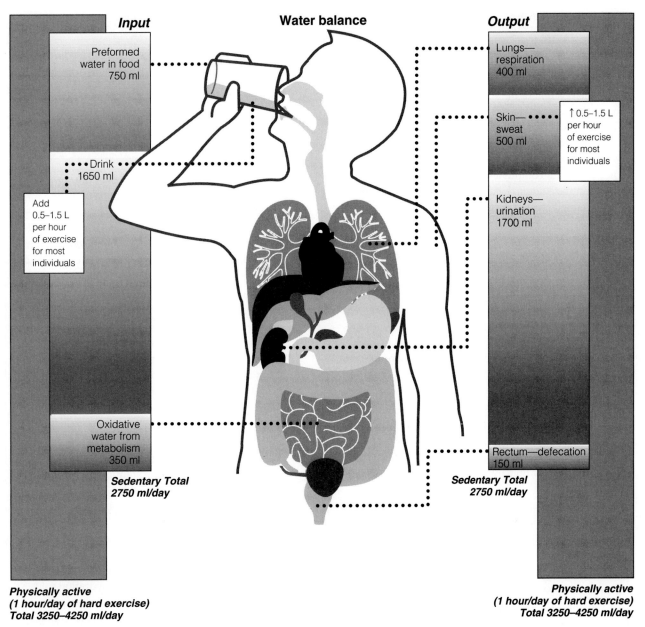

Figure 9.25   Water balance in a sedentary individual. Physically active people must increase fluid intake to match sweat rates that are typically between 0.5 and 1.5 liters/hour of exertion.

Box 9.6 summarizes information from the 1996 ACSM "Position Stand on Exercise and Fluid Replacement."[136] Notice several key points on fluid consumption:

- Emphasize fluid intake before exercise by drinking adequate fluids during the day before the event, and drink about 500 ml 2 hours before exercise.

Individuals who exercise heavily should make a conscious effort to ingest adequate volumes of fluid throughout the day. Often, the amount of fluid is beyond what is desired. For example, in one study of soccer players in Puerto Rico, players were randomly allocated to a week of voluntary hydration (2.7 liters of fluid per day) or a week of hyperhydration (4.6 liters per day).[158] Total body water was increased in the athletes forcing down extra fluids and was associated with improved sport performance. ACSM recommends that fluids be readily available during meal consumption because most people rehydrate during and after meals. To avoid or delay dehydration during exercise, ACSM recommends that about ½ liter of water be ingested 2 hours before exercise. The 2-hour limit allows the kidneys to adjust total body water stores at optimal pre-exercise levels. Individuals are urged to pay attention to the color, volume, and smell of their urine.[136,137,159] A well-hydrated

Box 9.6

ACSM Position Stand on Exercise and Fluid Replacement

It is the position of the American College of Sports Medicine that adequate fluid replacement helps maintain hydration and, therefore, promotes the health, safety, and optimal physical performance of individuals participating in regular physical activity. This position statement is based on a comprehensive review and interpretation of scientific literature concerning the influence of fluid replacement on exercise performance and the risk of thermal injury associated with dehydration and hyperthermia. Based on available evidence, the American College of Sports Medicine makes the following general recommendations on the amount and composition of fluid that should be ingested in preparation for, during, and after exercise or athletic competition:

1. It is recommended that individuals consume a nutritionally balanced diet and drink adequate fluids during the 24-hour period before an event, especially during the period that includes the meal prior to exercise, to promote proper hydration before exercise or competition.

2. It is recommended that individuals drink about 500 ml (about 17 ounces) of fluid about 2 hours before exercise to promote adequate hydration and allow time for excretion of excess ingested water.

3. During exercise, athletes should start drinking early and at regular intervals in an attempt to consume fluids at a rate sufficient to replace all the water lost through sweating (i.e., body weight loss), or consume the maximal amount that can be tolerated.

4. It is recommended that ingested fluids be cooler than ambient temperature (between 15° and 22°C [59° and 72°F]) and flavored to enhance palatability and promote fluid replacement. Fluids should be readily available and served in containers that allow adequate volumes to be ingested with ease and with minimal interruption of exercise.

5. Addition of proper amounts of carbohydrates and/or electrolytes to a fluid-replacement solution is recommended for exercise events of duration greater than 1 hour because it does not significantly impair water delivery to the body and may enhance performance. During exercise lasting less than 1 hour, there is little evidence of physiological or physical performance differences between consuming a carbohydrate–electrolyte drink and plain water.

6. During intense exercise lasting longer than 1 hour, it is recommended that carbohydrates be ingested at a rate of 30–60 grams per hour to maintain oxidation of carbohydrates and to delay fatigue. This rate of carbohydrate intake can be achieved without compromising fluid delivery by drinking 600–1,200 ml/hour of solutions containing 4–8% carbohydrates (g/100 ml). The carbohydrates can be sugars (glucose or sucrose) or starch (e.g., maltodextrin).

7. Inclusion of sodium (0.5–0.7 gram per liter of water) in the rehydration solution ingested during exercise lasting longer than 1 hour is recommended because it may be advantageous in enhancing palatability, promoting fluid retention, and possibly preventing hyponatremia in certain individuals who drink excessive quantities of fluid. There is little physiological basis for the presence of sodium in an oral rehydration solution for enhancing intestinal water absorption, as long as sodium is sufficiently available from the previous meal.

Source: American College of Sports Medicine. Position stand on exercise and fluid replacement. *Med Sci Sports Exerc* 28:i–vii, 1996. Reprinted with permission.

person excretes a good volume of urine that is light yellow in color and without a strong smell.[137]

- Athletes should start drinking early and at regular intervals during exercise, to replace nearly all the water lost through sweating.

Avoiding dehydration during exercise is critical. Without adequate fluid replacement during prolonged exercise, rectal temperature and heart rate are elevated above normal levels, impairing performance, and if continued long enough, leading to potentially life-threatening heat stroke.[136,137] Fluid intake must be above the thirst perception and must match body weight reduction in fluids (1 pint of fluid per pound of weight reduction). For most individuals, matching fluid intake with sweat loss can be accomplished by drinking 0.5 to 1 cup of water every 10–15 minutes of exercise. For sweat rates above 1.5 liters per minute, 1–2 cups of water should be ingested every 10 minutes.[137]

The rate at which the fluid leaves the stomach to be absorbed in the intestine depends on many factors, such as the exercise intensity and the temperature, volume, and composition of the ingested fluid. The most important factor influencing gastric emptying is the fluid volume in the stomach.[136] When gastric volume is maintained at 600 ml or more, most individuals can empty more than 1,000 ml per hour, even when the fluids contain 4–8% carbohydrate concentration. It is advantageous to maintain the largest volume of fluid that can be tolerated in the stomach during exercise (e.g., 400–600 ml).[160] Mild-to-moderate exercise appears to have little or no effect on gastric emptying, whereas heavy exercise at intensities above 80% of maximal capacity may slow gastric emptying.

- Ingested fluids should be cooler than ambient temperature and flavored to enhance palatability and promote fluid replacement.

ACSM recommends that fluid replacement beverages be sweetened, flavored, and cooled to between 15° and 21°C, to stimulate fluid intake.[136,161] Fluids and drinking containers should be readily available. Overall, several practical recommendations to encourage fluid intake include the following:[137]

- Do whatever it takes to make it easy to drink during physical activity (stash bottles in the bushes along a run course, have a friend on a bike hand you fluid on a long run, crush the top of a paper cup to form a small spout to make drinking easier during exercise, carry money to buy fluid, use a bottle belt to carry fluid, know where to find fluid from water fountains or convenience stores, practice drinking during exercise).
- Start prehydrating the day before a long race or training session.

- Make sure the urine is light-colored before exercising.
- Drink 8–16 fluid ounces (1–2 cups) in the 2 hours before exercise.
- Have plenty of fluid on hand during meals.
- Part of staying well-hydrated during exercise in the heat is to reduce sweat loss. Limit the intensity and duration of warm-up exercises, wear white, lightweight clothing, and get out of the sun when possible.
- During a race, make time to drink.
- Speed gastric emptying by drinking frequently, to keep a comfortably full stomach.

Can body temperature be controlled and dehydration prevented by wetting the head and skin during exercise? Although this may be psychologically pleasing, researchers have found that skin wetting does not reduce sweat rates or reduce core body temperature.[137,162] It is far better to drink the water.

Should Electrolytes and Carbohydrates Be Used during Exercise?

A wide variety of sports drinks are available, containing varying levels of electrolyte and carbohydrate. (See Table 9.14.) There are three reasons for using these drinks:[136,137,163–172]

1. To avoid dehydration
2. To counter the loss of electrolytes
3. To oppose the loss of body carbohydrate stores

Should electrolytes (sodium, potassium, and chloride) be added to the exercise drink? The electrolyte content of sweat is relatively very low. One liter of sweat has 400–1,000 mg of sodium, 500–1,500 mg of chloride, and 120–225 mg

TABLE 9.14 A Comparison of Sports Drinks (per Cup or 8 Fluid Ounces)

Sports Drink	Type of Carbohydrate	Carbohydrate Concentration	Sodium	Potassium	Calories
All sport	High fructose corn syrup	8%	55 mg	55 mg	70
Exceed	Glucose polymer / fructose	7%	50 mg	45 mg	70
Gatorade	Sucrose / glucose / fructose	6%	110 mg	30 mg	50
Hydra Fuel	Glucose polymer / glucose / fructose	7%	25 mg	50 mg	66
Power ade	High fructose corn syrup / glucose polymers	8%	55 mg	30 mg	70
10-K	Sucrose / fructose	6%	55 mg	30 mg	60
Orange juice	Fructose / sucrose / glucose	10%	6 mg	436 mg	104
Coca-Cola	High fructose corn syrup / sucrose	11%	6 mg	0 mg	103

of potassium.[172] Although sodium, chloride, potassium, magnesium, calcium, zinc, and some vitamins are excreted with the sweat, most studies have shown that such losses are rarely significant for properly nourished and acclimatized people. Electrolytes are very easily obtained in the diet—1 teaspoon of salt has 2,000 mg of sodium and 3,000 mg of chloride, while 1 cup of orange juice has 500 mg of potassium. In particular, athletes are very unlikely to develop sodium chloride deficiency, even with high sweat rates, because training develops adaptive mechanisms that conserve salt. The salt content of a trained athlete's sweat is one third that of an untrained person.

There are exceptions to this in extreme endurance events. Low levels of sodium (hyponatremia) have been measured in ultramarathoners and Ironman triathletes.[136,173] If large quantities of plain water are consumed during exercise exceeding 4–6 hours duration, low blood sodium levels (<130 mmol/L) become a concern. Symptoms include confusion, loss of coordination, extreme muscle weakness, and in severe cases, convulsions and coma. Therefore, athletes engaging in events lasting longer than 4 hours are urged to drink fluids containing electrolytes and to avoid overdrinking of plain water.

The addition of small amounts of sodium to a sports drink enhances palatability, helping people take more fluids during and after exercise. Also fluids with sodium in them lead to less urination than plain water and attenuates the decline in plasma volume during exercise.[136,167,174] Most sport drinks include small amounts of electrolytes for these reasons. (See Table 9.14.) Sodium does not enhance intestinal fluid absorption, however, or improve endurance performance. ACSM recommends that 0.5–0.7 gram of sodium be added to each liter of sports drink.[136] (See Box 9.6.)

Although the results of earlier studies suggested that solutions with more than 2.5% glucose slowed the rate of passage of the fluid through the stomach, recent gastric-emptying studies conducted during 2–4 hours of exercise show that 4–8% CHO solutions, regardless of CHO type, can be emptied from the stomach at rates similar to water.[136,137,168–171] Overall, the gastrointestinal tract appears capable of delivering up to 1.2 liters of fluid and 72 grams of carbohydrate each hour of exercise, enough to match the needs of most athletes.[165]

Beverages containing simple sugars or glucose polymers (4–6 glucose units) with small amounts of electrolytes minimize disturbances in temperature regulation and cardiovascular function as well as ordinary water, maintain blood glucose levels better than water, and enhance athletic performance more than water. Carbohydrate has been found to enhance performance in high-intensity endurance events lasting 1 hour or longer.[175–178] Sports drinks that contain 4–8% CHO of glucose polymer, glucose, or sucrose in volumes of 200–400 ml consumed every 15–20 minutes are preferable to plain water.[169] A total of 30–60 grams of car-

bohydrate (120–240 Calories) during each hour of exercise appears to be optimal and is found in 1 liter of most sports drinks.[136] Some research suggests that fructose can cause gastrointestinal distress and may compromise performance, so this type of sugar should be avoided. Fructose is absorbed more slowly than other sugars from the gut and then must be converted into glucose by the liver, limiting the amounts that can be absorbed and metabolized.[171,179]

Figure 9.26 summarizes this information. The importance of CHO in the drink solution lies in its ability to elevate blood glucose levels. Several studies have shown that even when muscle glycogen levels are low, ingestion of CHO solutions during long endurance exercise can counter the drop in blood glucose levels and prolong exercise by as much as 20–30%.[175–178,180,181] Apparently the elevated blood glucose levels from the CHO ingestion during exercise can support exercise even at 60–75% $\dot{V}O_{2max}$ levels.

Most athletes prefer to take in sports drinks throughout the event, and this has been shown to be highly effective in improving performance by maintaining blood glucose levels and sparing muscle glycogen levels.[181] Energy bars and gels are also popular sources of carbohydrate. Figure 9.27 shows the results of one study of cyclers where carbohydrate was consumed every 20 minutes of exercise, prolonging exercise by 1 hour.[105] Runners benefit, too, as shown in Figure 9.28. In this study, runners decreased their 30-kilometer race time by 3 minutes by drinking a 5% carbohydrate solution before and during the event.[180]

So in summary, when exercise exceeds 1 hour, the exerciser's fluid, electrolyte, and carbohydrate requirements can be met simultaneously by ingesting 600–1,200 ml per hour of a solution containing 4–8% CHO, and 0.5–0.7 gram of sodium per liter.[136] (See Box 9.6.)

PRINCIPLE 5: KEEP A CLOSE WATCH ON POSSIBLE IRON DEFICIENCY

A number of athletes, especially elite male and female endurance athletes, test positive for mild iron deficiency, best measured by evaluating serum ferritin levels. On the other hand, very few athletes reach a state of anemia, which is measured when the hemoglobin falls below 12 mg/dl for females and 13 mg/dl for males. In general, fitness enthusiasts do not usually need to be concerned with iron deficiency because moderate amounts of exercise have not been shown to cause any iron deficiency.

The Problem of Iron Deficiency

Several reports in the literature suggest that endurance athletes, especially females, may be prone to iron deficiency.[182–190]

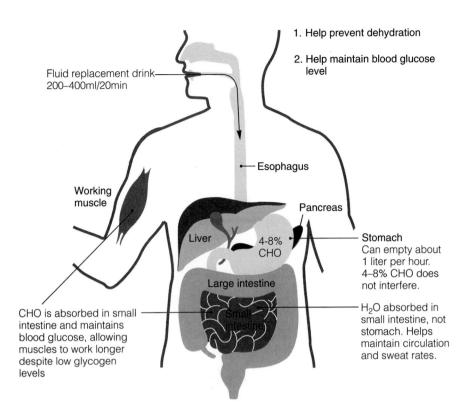

1. Help prevent dehydration

2. Help maintain blood glucose level

Fluid replacement drink—200–400ml/20min

Esophagus

Working muscle

Liver

Pancreas

4-8% CHO

Stomach
Can empty about 1 liter per hour. 4–8% CHO does not interfere.

Large intestine

Small intestine

CHO is absorbed in small intestine and maintains blood glucose, allowing muscles to work longer despite low glycogen levels

H_2O absorbed in small intestine, not stomach. Helps maintain circulation and sweat rates.

Figure 9.26 Two goals of fluid replacement drinks during exercise. There are two primary goals of fluid replacement during exercise: (1) to prevent dehydration; (2) to help maintain blood glucose levels.

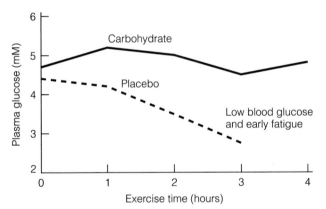

Figure 9.27 Sports drinks improve long-term endurance. Cyclers were able to prolong their exercise time by 1 hour by drinking fluids with sugar every 20 minutes during the event. *Source:* Coyle EF, Coggan AR, Hemmert MK, Ivy JL. Muscle glycogen utilization during prolonged strenuous exercise when fed carbohydrate. *J Appl Physiol* 61:165–172, 1986.

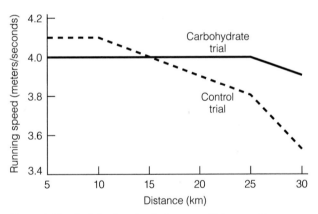

Figure 9.28 Carbohydrate intake improves 30-km race time: 250 ml 5% CHO prior to race, 150 ml / 5 km. Total race time: CHO trial = 128 ± 19.9; Control = 131.2 ± 18.7 min. Runners were able to maintain their race pace longer during a 30-km run by using a sports drink. *Source:* Tsintzas K, Liu R, Williams C, Campbell I, Gaitanos G. The effect of cabohydrate ingestion on performance during a 30-km race. *Int J Sport Nutr* 3:127–139, 1993.

Using serum ferritin levels as a criterion (less than 12 µg/liter), between 10% and 80% of female athletes, depending on the study, have been described as having mild iron deficiency. In one review, the prevalence of low serum ferritin concentration averaged 37% in female athletes, compared to 23% in untrained female controls.[183]

In nearly all studies, however, it is extremely rare to find that hemoglobin is low (an indication of anemia). Some elite athletes do tend to have hemoglobin levels that are somewhat low, but this appears to be due to their expanded plasma volumes and not because of depleted body iron stores.[191,192] Also, iron deficiency has not been a problem for

TABLE 9.15 Stages of Iron Deficiency

	Blood Indices[a] (values indicating deficiency)							
Stage	**SF** <12 μg/L	**FE** M <80 μg/dl F <60 μg/dl	**TIBC** Stage II >390 μg/dl Stage III >410 μg/dl	**SAT** <15%	**HGB** M <13 mg/dl F <12 mg/dl	**RBC**	**Bone Marrow FE**	**Iron Absorption**
I. Iron-deficient—mild	D	N	N	N	N	N	0	I
II. Iron-deficient erythropoiesis	D	D	I	D	N	N	0	I
III. Iron-deficient anemia	D	D	I	D	D	D[b]	0	I

[a]N = normal; D = decrease; I = increase; 0 = none; SF = serum ferritin; FE = serum iron; TIBC = total iron-binding capacity; SAT = transferrin saturation; HGB = hemoglobin; RBC = red blood cells.
[b]Red blood cells in iron-deficient anemia become small (microcytic) and less red (hypochromic). The amount of RBC protoporphyrin, a derivative of hemoglobin with one atom of iron deleted, increases (>1.24 μmol/L RBC).

Sources: Herbert V. Recommended dietary intakes (RDI) of iron in humans. *Am J Clin Nutr* 45:679–686, 1987; Expert Scientific Working Group. Summary of a report on assessment of the iron nutritional status of the United States population. *Am J Clin Nutr* 42:1318–1330, 1985.

fitness enthusiasts who exercise moderately (20–40 minutes per session, 3–5 sessions per week).[193,194]

Iron deficiency is commonly divided into three stages, which form a continuum, each shading gradually into the other (see Table 9.15).[195,196] The first stage is mild iron depletion, which is characterized by decreased or absent bone marrow iron stores and measured by a drop in plasma ferritin. There are usually 1,000 mg of iron in the bone marrow of male adults, and 300 mg in the marrow of female adults. At this stage, other indices of iron deficiency are normal. Serum ferritin levels below 12 μg/liter are associated with very low bone marrow iron stores.

Stage 2 follows the exhaustion of bone marrow iron stores and is characterized as a diminishing iron supply to the developing red cell. Iron-deficient *erythropoiesis* (formation of red blood cells) occurs and is measured by increased total iron-binding capacity and reduced serum iron and percent saturation (<15% is abnormal). The red blood cell *protoporphyrin* (a derivative of hemoglobin, which has an atom of iron deleted) increases above normal. The National Center for Health Statistics defines iron deficiency based on two of three abnormal tests of iron status: transferrin saturation less than 15%, serum ferritin less than 12 μg/liter, and erythrocyte protoporphyrin of greater than 1.24 μmol/liter red blood cells.[197] Based on these criteria, 11% of teenage and young adult women are iron deficient in the United States, but less than 1% of men are[197] (see Figure 9.29).

Stage 3 is iron-deficient anemia, characterized by a drop in hemoglobin. Hemoglobin levels below 12 mg/dl for females, and 13 mg/dl for males are considered anemic. The range of normal hemoglobin levels is 13–16 mg/dl for men and 12–16 mg/dl for women. During this stage, the bone

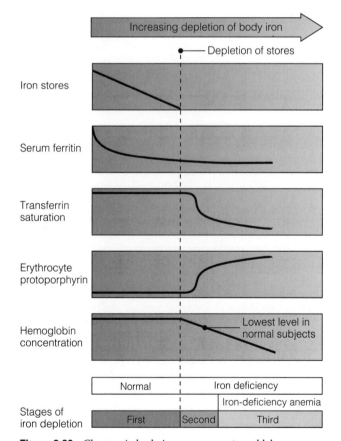

Figure 9.29 Changes in body iron components and laboratory assessments of iron status during the stages of iron depletion. *Source:* From Life Sciences Research Office, Federation of American Societies for Experimental Biology. *Nutrition Monitoring in the United States: An Update Report on Nutrition Monitoring.* Washington, DC: U.S. Government Printing Office, 1989.

marrow produces an increasing number of smaller and less brightly colored red blood cells. This is measured when the mean corpuscular volume (MCV) falls below 80 fl.

Anemia is generally acknowledged to be the most common single nutritional deficiency in both developing and developed countries. In the United States, 3–5% of female teenagers and young adults and less than 1% of males are anemic.[197] In one study of 85 female marathon runners, only 2% were anemic.[198] Another study of 111 runners and 65 inactive females found that 3% in each group were anemic (hemoglobin less than 12 mg/dl).[186] These studies show that anemia is extremely rare among athletes (see Figure 9.30).

Iron is an essential constituent of hemoglobin, myoglobin, and several iron-containing respiratory enzymes, and it plays a vital role in energy production. Relatively small decreases in hemoglobin (1–2 g/dl) have been shown to impair physical performance.[199,200] There is a very close association between the hemoglobin content of the blood and $\dot{V}O_{2max}$.

Although anemia does impair exercise performance, researchers disagree as to whether iron deficiency without anemia is a hindrance. There is a growing consensus, however, that although a significant proportion of athletes have iron deficiency, it has little or no meaningful impact on health or performance.[191,192,201–203] In several studies, for example, when iron-deficient subjects are put on iron therapy, plasma ferritin concentrations rise, but exercise performance is not affected.[204–208] Nonetheless, the high prevalence of iron deficiency among female athletes has led to a large number of investigations seeking to determine the causes.[184,209–217] Three major factors have been researched:

1. *Inadequate dietary iron.* The average Western diet supplies about 7–8 mg of iron per 1,000 Calories

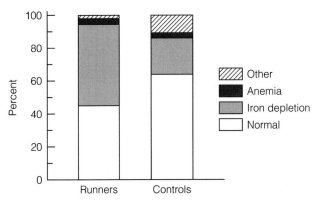

Figure 9.30 Iron status in female runners versus controls. Although female runners tend to have a higher prevalence of iron deficiency compared to inactive controls, anemia is rare. *Source:* Pate RR, Miller BJ, Davis JM, Slentz CA, Klingshirn LA. Iron status of female runners. *Int J Sport Nutr* 3:222–231, 1993.

(see Table 9.6). Several studies measuring the diets of female athletes have shown that a significant proportion consume less than the RDA of 15 mg.[184] In the general population, only one in four teenagers and young adult women meet 100% of the iron RDA.[16] Also, some female athletes are very conscious of their weight and eat too few calories or avoid red meat (a rich source of iron), putting themselves at risk for iron deficiency.[184,191] This may be one of the most important reasons for the high prevalence of iron deficiency among female athletes.

2. *Increased hemolysis.* Several studies suggest that exercise causes an accelerated destruction of red blood cells.[210,211,215] There is some evidence that the life span of red blood cells in runners is significantly less than that of these cells in nonrunners, which may be sufficient to precipitate iron deficiency when dietary intake is low.[215] The breakdown of red blood cells inside the capillaries (measured by a decrease in blood haptoglobin), together with kidney excretion of hemoglobin may contribute to the low iron states reported among athletes. Some researchers have attributed this to the mechanical trauma imposed on the capillaries of the feet from running.[211] Other factors may include elevated body temperatures, increased blood flow, acidosis, and the effects of catecholamines. However, only trace amounts of iron can be lost through this route, and it cannot be considered a major factor of iron deficiency.[191]

3. *Increased iron loss in sweat and feces.* Some iron is lost in sweat, about 0.13–0.42 mg/liter.[184,212] Running (especially when racing) has been found to induce some gastrointestinal bleeding, which can be measured in the feces.[184,213,214] One study showed that of 24 runners, 21 had an increase of fecal hemoglobin after racing (10K–42.2K).[214] Iron loss from sweat and through the gastrointestinal tract may be as high as 2 mg/day. Absorption rates of dietary iron are usually 5–10%. If dietary iron intake is low, some athletes may lose more than they absorb.[184]

In the general population, bleeding from the gastrointestinal tract is widely believed to be the most common cause of iron deficiency for patients without an obvious source of blood loss.[216] A thorough examination of the GI tract, especially the colon, is standard practice and may be recommended for some athletes with unexplained anemia.

Practical Implications for Athletes

The so-called "sports anemia" is for most athletes a false anemia, in that their expanded plasma volumes dilute the blood, lowering hemoglobulin concentrations. A very small percentage of athletes develop true anemia when iron losses exceed iron intake and absorption. Also, a significant proportion have iron deficiency without anemia, which probably has little effect on performance but still should be treated to improve body iron stores.

The U.S. Olympic Committee feels that all elite athletes should have their hemoglobin checked at least once a year.[218] If abnormal, 3–6 months of iron therapy is recommended for menstruating females. If therapy is unsuccessful, or the athlete is male or a nonmenstruating female, a thorough medical evaluation is recommended, including a stool guaiac to check for GI bleeding and lab tests for iron status (serum ferritin, iron-binding capacity, erythrocyte protoporphyrin).[219]

It is very difficult to help a person recover from iron deficiency with diet alone.[195] Oral iron therapy must often be considered, consisting of ferrous sulfate and meat supplements.[184] In addition, ascorbic acid can help enhance absorption.[220] However, for some athletes, effective therapy also involves reducing iron losses by decreasing the amount of exercise to more moderate levels.

Despite the prevalence of iron deficiency among runners, iron supplements should not be given routinely to athletes without medical supervision. In addition to the possibility of inducing deficiencies of other trace minerals, such as copper and zinc, a high iron intake can produce an iron overload in some people.[147] Therefore, athletes should be encouraged to increase iron intake by eating foods high in iron. High-iron foods include fortified breakfast cereals, dried fruit, legumes, molasses, lean meats, and nuts. (See Table 9.16.)

Animal tissue has an average of 40% heme iron and 60% nonheme iron, while plant products are composed of 100% nonheme iron.[221] Nonheme iron absorption is enhanced by consuming vitamin C during the meal, and absorption from plant sources is also increased if meat is eaten at the same time. Vegetarian athletes, who may be at special risk for iron deficiency, should be sure to include vitamin C foods with each meal.[222]

PRINCIPLE 6: VITAMIN AND MINERAL SUPPLEMENTS ARE NOT NEEDED

Most studies show that the intake of major vitamins and minerals by people who exercise is above recommended levels. People who exercise are at an advantage because they tend to eat more than sedentary people, thereby providing their bodies with more vitamins and minerals beyond the extra demands of their exercise. The American Dietetic Association, in their publication "Nutrition for Physical Fitness and Athletic Performance for Adults," has stated that "although physical activity increases the need

TABLE 9.16 Iron in 1-Cup Portions of Foods

Food	Iron per Cup of Food (mg)
Pumpkin seeds	20.7
Raisin bran cereal	16.4
Wheat germ	10.3
Sunflower seeds	9.8
Cashews	8.2
Wheat Chex cereal	7.3
Dried apricots	6.1
Grape-Nuts cereal	4.9
Great Northern beans (cooked)	4.9
Soybeans (cooked)	4.9
Almonds	4.8
Peanut butter	4.6
Red kidney beans (cooked)	4.6
Lentils (cooked)	4.2
Prunes	4.0
Blackeye cowpeas (cooked)	3.6
Lima beans (cooked)	3.5
Raisins	3.0
Fish, bass, broiled	2.9
Turkey	2.5
Ham, extra lean	2.1
Lobster	1.9
Tuna	1.5

Note: Although meats have lower concentrations of iron, their iron (heme iron) is more easily absorbed than iron from plant foods (nonheme iron). Vitamin C, however, greatly improves the availability of iron from plant food.

Source: USDA Handbook No. 8 (revised).

for some vitamins and minerals, this increased requirement typically can be met by consuming a balanced high-carbohydrate, moderate-protein, low-fat diet. The increased energy intake of athletes should provide the additional vitamins and minerals necessary if a wide variety of foods is included in the diet."[93] Although a nutritional deficiency can impair physical performance and can cause several other detrimental effects, there is no conclusive evidence of performance enhancement with intakes in excess of the recommended levels.

There is considerable misinformation and exaggeration regarding the relationship between vitamins and minerals, and exercise.[93,183,184,223–228] Coaches' magazines, popular fitness journals, and training table practices of sports superstars send the message that high levels of vitamins and minerals are needed as an energy boost, to maximize performance, to compensate for less-than-optimal diets, to meet the unusual nutrient demands induced by heavy exercise, and to help alleviate the stress of competition. Advocates of supplementation have exaggerated the needs for all 13 recognized vitamins, and have even created some new ones, such as pangamic acid and vitamin B_{15}. (See Tables 9.2–9.5 for the U.S. Recommended Dietary Allowance guidelines.)

The relationship between vitamins/minerals and exercise can be looked at in two ways:[223]

1. Do vitamin and mineral supplements improve performance?

2. Does exercise impose requirements for vitamins and minerals greater than the amounts obtainable from the diet? (See Figure 9.31.)

As discussed in this chapter previously, most studies that have examined the vitamin and mineral contents of athletic diets have found that athletes exceed 67% of the RDA for all vitamins and minerals measured, except for iron for some females. Figure 9.32 shows that male and female Los Angeles marathon runners met or exceeded 100% of the RDA for all major nutrients except for vitamin B_6, and iron for women.[78]

Despite what appear to be adequate diets for athletes (mainly because of their high caloric intakes), many athletes feel the need to supplement their diets with vitamins and minerals. Research evidence shows that between 50 and 80% of elite athletes use vitamin/mineral supplements on a regular basis.[225,229–231] This compares with about 40% of the American public, as measured in recent government surveys.[232] Approximately 3,400 different vitamin and mineral supplement products are on the market and account for $4 billion annually in gross sales.

The American Medical Association, the American Dietetic Association, the American Institute of Nutrition, the Food and Nutrition Board, and the National Council Against Health Fraud have submitted formal statements to the effect that there are no demonstrated benefits of self-supplementation beyond the Recommended Dietary Allowances except in special cases.[13,14,232–234] According to the American Dietetic Association, "The best nutritional strategy for promoting optimal health and reducing the risk of chronic disease is to obtain adequate nutrients from a wide variety of foods."[232]

There are several reasons for advising against vitamin and mineral supplementation by athletes. For one thing, research does not support the value of vitamin and mineral supplementation. For another, high intake of supplements may be problematic.

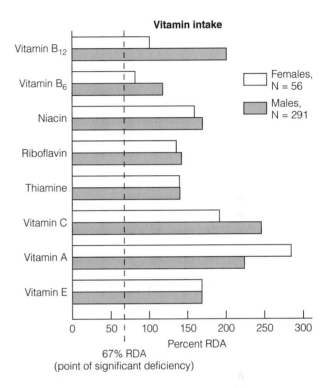

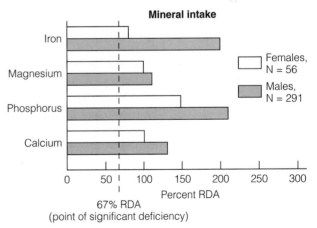

Figure 9.32 In this study of 291 male and 56 female Los Angeles marathon runners, 3-day food records revealed that vitamin (top) and mineral (bottom) intake was adequate except for a slight deficiency of vitamin B_6, and iron for women. *Source:* Nieman DC, Butler JV, Pollett LM, Dietrich SJ, Lutz RD. Nutrient intake of marathon runners. *J Am Diet Assoc* 89:1273–1278, 1989.

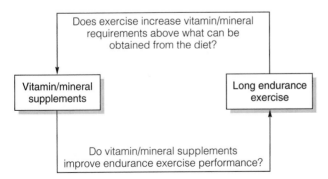

Figure 9.31 Vitamin/mineral–exercise relationship. The relationship between vitamins/minerals and exercise can be looked at in two ways.

Lack of Evidence for Benefits

Extensive reviews of the literature have failed to find any convincing support for the role of supplementation in enhancing performance, hastening recovery, or decreasing the rate of injury in healthy, well-nourished adults undergoing athletic training.[62,223-227] After more than 40 years of research, there is no conclusive evidence to suggest that vitamin supplementation improves the performance of adequately nourished people.[183,184,235-242] For example, in one (double-blind, placebo design) study of 82 athletes from four sports (basketball, gymnastics, rowing, and swimming), 7–8 months of daily supplementation with a high-dose vitamin/mineral tablet failed to affect muscular strength, or aerobic and anaerobic fitness, relative to a control group.[238]

Although heavy endurance exercise is associated with an increased need for many nutrients, including iron, zinc, copper, magnesium, chromium, vitamin B_6, riboflavin, and ascorbic acid, these demands are usually met when the athlete matches energy expenditure through increased consumption of the conventional food supply.[183,184,223-228,242-248]

In general, when the vitamin/mineral biochemical status of athletes and inactive controls are compared, researchers have concluded that sports training has no negative effect and that supplementation in most instances appears unwarranted.[55,59,183,247,248]

This approach is supported in a technical support paper from the American Dietetic Association (ADA).[93] The ADA took the position that extended physical activity may increase the need for some vitamins and minerals, but that these could easily be met by consuming a balanced diet in proportion to the extra caloric requirement. Other reviews of the sports-nutrition literature have also consistently concluded that except in special cases (e.g., iron supplementation for anemic athletes), vitamin and mineral supplementation by athletes is unnecessary.[183-185,223-227]

Many studies have shown clearly that the capacity to exercise is obviously hindered by the development of vitamin-deficiency states, and that performance is returned to normal when the deficiency is corrected.[223-227,249] However, vitamin/mineral deficiencies are rare among athletes.[183,184]

There has been much interest raised recently concerning exercise, generation of oxygen-reactive species or free radicals, and antioxidant nutrients (primarily vitamins E, C, and A, and the mineral selenium).[250-258] During exercise, to meet energy demands, oxygen consumption can increase 10- to 20-fold over consumption at rest. Due to various means (which are still being researched, e.g., increases in catecholamines, lactic acid, hyperthermia, and transient hypoxia), the rise in oxygen consumption results in an "oxidative stress" that leads to the generation of oxygen-reactive species such as the superoxide radical, hydrogen peroxide, and the hydroxyl radical.[250,251] These oxygen-reactive species are defined as molecules or ions containing an unpaired electron, which cause cell and tissue injury. Reactive oxygen species have been implicated in certain diseases and in the aging process.[250-253]

The body is equipped with a sophisticated defense system to scavenge oxygen-reactive species. Antioxidant enzymes (e.g., glutathione peroxidase, superoxide dismutase, catalase) provide the first line of defense, with antioxidant nutrients providing a second line of defense.[250] Because strenuous and prolonged exercise promotes production of oxygen-reactive species, considerable concerns have been raised among experts regarding the ability of the body to cope with the increased oxidative stress.[253] In 1994, Kenneth H. Cooper published his best-selling book, *Dr. Kenneth H. Cooper's Antioxidant Revolution*. In this book, he promoted the concept that high amounts of exercise overwhelm the antioxidant defense systems of the body, and that huge amounts of antioxidant supplements should be ingested to counter the free radicals.

Currently, most researchers in this area disagree with Cooper.[250-252,257] Most studies have shown that chronic physical training augments the physiological antioxidant defenses in several tissues of the body.[250,256,258] The activities of the various antioxidant enzymes are enhanced by physical training, helping to counter the exercise-induced increase in oxygen-reactive species. In general, antioxidant supplementation does not appear necessary and has not been consistently shown to improve performance, minimize exercise-induced muscle cell damage, or maximize recovery.[256,257] However, until more is known, people who exercise regularly and intensely are urged to ingest foods rich in antioxidants (fruits, vegetables, nuts, seeds, and whole grains) to augment the body's defense system against oxygen-reactive species.[257]

Evidence of Possible Problems with High Intake

There are problems associated with very high intakes of vitamins and minerals. Considerable evidence shows that dietary excess of one nutrient may have a detrimental effect on another.[232,259-261] High intakes of specific nutrients, especially fat-soluble vitamins such as A, D, E, and K, can be toxic in themselves and indirectly dangerous because they block the action of other nutrients. Excessive intake of water-soluble vitamins can also cause problems. Too much niacin can in time lead to liver toxicity, too much vitamin C to red blood cell hemolysis and impaired white blood cell activity, and too much vitamin B_6 to peripheral nervous system toxicity and muscle weakness.

A deficiency of one nutrient can be caused by an excess of another.[232] For instance, zinc supplementation can reduce copper status; excessive vitamin C decreases copper absorption; high levels of folic acid decrease zinc absorption and may mask symptoms of vitamin B_{12} deficiency; excess fructose decreases copper absorption; large amounts of calcium, phytates, and fiber in the diet cause the formation of insoluble iron, zinc, or copper complexes, making these minerals unavailable for absorption; high doses of vitamin E can interfere with vitamin K action; excess manganese decreases iron absorption.

In other words, too much of a good thing becomes a definite evil. Water and sunshine are both necessary for life, but excesses of either can kill you. Obviously, it is best to eat a varied diet, for it supplies all of the nutrients in the appropriate amounts.

Some coaches and other leaders still feel that giving supplements is beneficial, even if there is no proven physiological benefit, because the athlete thinks the supplement will help and thus performs better (placebo effect). It would be better to help the athlete believe in something that really works, such as a nutritious, varied diet, high in carbohydrate and liquids, providing both physiological and psychological support.

For the athlete who is poorly nourished (often to "make weight"), the best solution is education to provide a better diet. Supplements can reinforce unhealthy eating habits. Dietary imbalances can get worse in this situation. Thus, every effort must be made to convince athletes that their best nutritional resource for optimum performance is proper eating habits. (See Principle 1 on the "prudent diet.")

PRINCIPLE 7: EXTRA PROTEIN DOES NOT BENEFIT THE ATHLETE

Many people who exercise, especially weight lifters, feel that consumption of high-protein foods and protein supplements is necessary to build muscle mass. The average sedentary person has been advised to consume 0.8 gram of dietary protein per kilogram of body weight. As this section indicates, research is showing that highly active people may need 50–125% more than this because 5–15% of the energy required for long endurance exercise or weight lifting comes from protein, and extra protein is needed for muscle protein synthesis. So, should athletes use protein supplements—or should they concentrate on high-protein foods in their diets? Most experts feel that the traditional food supply provides all of the protein needed, even for athletes during active muscle-building phases.

Changes in Protein Metabolism during Exercise

Interest in the influence of dietary protein intake on athletic performance has been evident since the days of the ancient Greeks and Romans.[262,263] Athletes consumed meat-rich diets, in the belief that they would achieve the strength of the consumed animal.

The importance of protein for athletics has continued to be debated over the years. In 1842, the great German chemist and physiologist, Justus von Liebig, reported that the primary fuel for muscular contraction was derived from muscle protein, and he suggested that large quantities of meat be eaten to replenish the supply.[262,263] A number of studies during the late 1800s, which measured urinary urea excretion failed to confirm his results however, and the concept became established that changes in protein metabolism during exercise are nonexistent or minimal at best.[262]

However, studies using modern technology and improved techniques have concluded that protein is a much more important fuel source during exercise than was previously thought.

Figure 9.33 summarizes protein/amino acid metabolism.[262,263] Amino acids enter the body's free pools from the

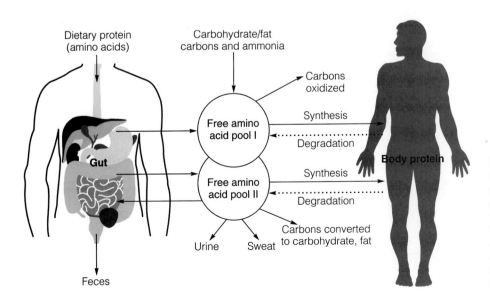

Figure 9.33 Protein/amino acid metabolism. Protein/amino acid metabolism is complex, with amino acids entering and leaving the body's free amino acid pools through several different routes. *Source:* Data from Lemon PWR. Do athletes need more dietary protein nd amino acids? *Int J Sport Nutr* 5: S39–S61, 1995.

diet, from body protein, or from carbons contributed from carbohydrate, fat, and ammonia. Amino nitrogen leaves the free pools to form body protein or exit the body in urine, sweat, and feces. Amino carbons can leave the free pools to form body fat or carbohydrate, or they can exit the body as carbon dioxide.

Exercise has a strong effect on protein/amino acid metabolism.[262–277] Four basic changes in protein metabolism take place with exercise (see Figure 9.34).

1. *Depression of protein synthesis.* During exercise (endurance exercise or heavy weight lifting) normal protein synthesis is depressed by 17–70%, depending on the intensity and duration of the exercise. This depression leaves amino acids available as fuel for the working muscle. Later, during recovery, muscle protein synthesis increases, augmenting incorporation of amino acids into muscle protein (hypertrophy).[262,263,265,274,276]

   The average 70-kg man has 12 kg of protein in his body, nearly half in the actin and myosin myofilaments found in muscle. The body depot of protein is highly labile, with some 200–500 g (50 g nitrogen) of new protein being synthesized every day, and only 10 g nitrogen/day excreted. Five tons of protein are thus synthesized in one's lifetime, while total dietary protein intake is only one ton, indicating the extensive reutilization of body amino acids. For young adults, muscle accounts for 25–30% of total body protein turnover.

The fact that exercise temporarily interrupts this protein turnover and synthesis is very important, making amino acids immediately available for fuel (Figure 9.33). (Following exercise, protein synthesis is accelerated, leading to hypertrophy—temporary unless maintained.)

2. *Increased muscle breakdown.* There is not a clear consensus, but most studies are supporting the concept that exercise leads to a breakdown of the muscle protein.[266,268,269] Hard exercise appears to cause significant muscle cell damage that can be measured when muscle enzymes leak into the plasma. Also, long-term resistance training has been shown to increase 3-methylhistidine excretion, which is a marker for myofibrillar breakdown.[262]

   With the combination of reduced muscle protein synthesis and increased muscle protein breakdown, more amino acids are available in the body for fuel during exercise and the repair and buildup of muscle cells after exercise. For example, endurance-trained individuals at rest have been reported to have 30% higher leucine turnover than sedentary subjects.[264]

3. *Increase in amino acid oxidation.* During rest, 10–20% of ATP regeneration comes from protein. Studies have shown that exercise increases the rate of amino acid oxidation.[264,266,275] During cycling exercise, for example, it has been reported that there is a 240% increase in leucine oxidation, with a 21% decrease in

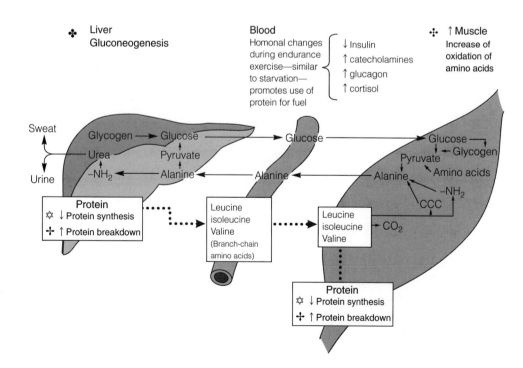

Figure 9.34 Use of protein as fuel during long endurance exercise. This figure summarizes the various pathways by which protein can be used as fuel by the working muscles (see text for an explanation).

leucine synthesis. There is some indication that male endurance athletes may oxidize leucine at a greater rate than female athletes.[266]

4. *Increase in gluconeogenesis.* Sixteen of the amino acids that are in the human body can be changed into glucose by the liver. This gluconeogenic process is extremely important during exercise because it can contribute to the supply of glucose to prevent hypoglycemia during long endurance exercise. During exercise, there is a steady stream of alanine passing from the muscle to the liver, where it is converted into glucose and then enters the blood and feeds the working muscle.[262,263] (See Figure 9.34.) This appears to be most important during prolonged exercise. After 3 hours of exercise, about 60% of glucose used by the working muscle comes from the liver, which is producing glucose from alanine, lactate, glycerol, and other metabolic by-products. Fatty acids are also an important fuel under these conditions.

The increase in liver gluconeogenesis during long endurance exercise and the use of protein for fuel is probably hormonally controlled.[262,263] Exercise causes several changes in blood hormone levels, including a decrease in insulin and increases in catecholamines (epinephrine and norepinephrine), glucagon, and cortisol. These hormonal changes are similar to what happens during starvation (which tends to increase the use of protein for fuel). From the evidence available, it seems likely that endurance exercise and heavy weight lifting cause a transient increase in the use of protein, which is somewhat analogous to the changes caused by starvation.

Practical Implications for Athletes

The practical advice in light of this information is still conjectural. It does appear certain that the contribution of protein as an energy source during endurance training is about 5–15% (instead of next to nothing, as previously thought). The actual amount of protein utilized during such exercise depends on the intensity, duration, and fitness status, with long, hard exercise by trained athletes leading to the greatest protein utilization.[262,263]

Various reviewers have suggested that the current protein RDA is insufficient for both strength and endurance athletes, for whom the actual requirement may be 50–125% higher than the RDA.[262,263] In light of this information, the American Dietetic Association has advised that endurance athletes take in 1–1.5 g/kg daily.[93] For athletes in unusually heavy training, more than 1.5 g/kg may be needed, especially during the initial phases or during unusually heavy periods of exercise.[262,263] The U.S. Olympic Committee has urged that 1–1.5 g/kg body weight a day is usually sufficient for most athletes, provided adequate calories are consumed.[267] For some athletes who restrict calories (e.g., wrestlers, gymnasts, female runners), protein needs may be greater because protein will be used to meet energy needs.[262,263] Adequacy of energy intake is paramount when determining absolute protein need. In general, 1.2–1.4 grams of protein per kilogram of body weight each day is optimal for the majority of endurance athletes[262] (see Table 9.17).

Most endurance athletes are already getting this much protein and do not need to supplement their diets with protein powder or concern themselves with eating high-protein foods. In the study of 347 Los Angeles marathon runners, the average male and female runner consumed 1.4 and

TABLE 9.17 Protein Needs, Intake, and Exercise Requirements

	Protein Intake (grams/day)		Body Weight (kg)	
	Males	Females	Males	Females
Recommended intake level for sedentary Americans (0.8 g/kg)	63	50	79	63
Average sedentary American (actual intake)	96	64	79	63
Average fitness enthusiast (1 g/kg)	75	60	75	60
Recommended level for elite endurance athlete (1.2–1.4 g/kg)	78–91	66–77	65	55
Recommended level for strength athlete (1.4–1.8 g/kg)	126–162	98–126	90	70

Note: Requirements may be higher if caloric intake is low or unusually heavy training is being initiated by novices.

Source: Data from Lemon PWR. Do athletes need more dietary protein and amino acids? *Int J Sport Nutr* 5:S39–S61, 1995.

1.3 g/kg, respectively.[78] Table 9.12 demonstrates that even on a high-carbohydrate diet with relatively little meat and few dairy products, protein intake is still 116 grams, or 13% of total caloric intake. The sedentary public consumes more than 1 gram of protein per kilogram per day, about 16% of total caloric intake.[17] The general public needs to worry more about exercise supplementation than about protein supplementation! (See Table 9.17.)

Several studies have carefully measured the amount of dietary protein needed to keep bodybuilders and weight trainers in positive nitrogen balance.[262,270,271,273] Protein is needed to form increased lean body weight, but more than enough is provided by a normal diet. Most strength and power athletes can enhance muscle development when dietary protein intake ranges between 1.4 and 1.8 g/kg.[262]

There is no good evidence that very high protein intakes (>2 g/kg/day) are either necessary or beneficial.[262,263]

The U.S. Olympic Committee feels that protein supplements are unnecessary, costly, and potentially harmful.[267] There is little scientific evidence that amino acid supplementation enhances the physiological responses to strength training when adequate diets are consumed. As emphasized by the American Dietetic Association, "Even the highest protein requirements can be met easily with a balanced diet that includes a variety of foods. Therefore, excessive protein intake, either through consumption of high-protein foods or protein/amino acid supplements, is unnecessary, does not contribute to athletic performance or increase muscle mass, and actually may be detrimental to health."[93] Box 9.7 reviews recommendations for the vegetarian athlete.

Box 9.7

Special Issues for Vegetarian Athletes

There have been some concerns that the vegetarian athlete is at risk for protein and mineral deficiencies due to lack of meat products in the diet. At an international conference on vegetarian nutrition in 1997 (Loma Linda University, Loma Linda, CA), these and other health issues were addressed. The following conclusions were drawn:

1. *Performance.* The vegetarian diet per se is not associated with improved aerobic endurance performance; however, other benefits make this dietary regimen worthy of consideration by serious athletes.

2. *Carbohydrate intake.* A plant-based diet facilitates a high intake of carbohydrate, which is essential for prolonged exercise.

3. *Potential for suboptimal intake of iron, zinc, and other minerals.* A well-planned vegetarian diet provides the athlete with adequate levels of all known nutrients, although the potential for suboptimal intake of iron, zinc, and trace elements exists if the diet is too restrictive. However, this concern exists for all athletes, vegetarian or nonvegetarian, who have poor dietary habits.

4. *Protein intake.* Although there has been some concern about protein intake for vegetarian athletes, data indicate that all essential and nonessential amino acids can be supplied by plant food sources alone, as long as a variety of foods is consumed

and the caloric intake is adequate to meet energy needs.

5. *Antioxidant nutrients.* Athletes consuming a diet rich in fruits, vegetables, and whole grains receive a high intake of antioxidant nutrients, which help reduce the oxidative stress associated with heavy exertion.

6. *Menstrual irregularity.* There has been some concern that vegetarian female athletes are at increased risk for oligo-amenorrhea, but evidence suggests that low energy intake, not dietary quality, is a major cause.

7. *Health benefits.* While the athlete is most often concerned with performance, long-term health benefits and a reduction in risk of chronic disease have been associated with the vegetarian diet. Studies suggest that a combination of regular physical activity and vegetarian dietary practices provide lower mortality rates than the vegetarian diet or exercise alone.

The vegetarian diet per se is not associated with improved aerobic endurance performance. Although some concerns have been raised about the nutrient status of vegetarian athletes, a varied and well-planned vegetarian diet is compatible with successful athletic endeavor.

Source: Nieman DC. Physical fitness and vegetarian diets: Is there a relationship? *Am J Clin Nutr* (in press).

PRINCIPLE 8: REST AND EAT CARBOHYDRATE BEFORE LONG ENDURANCE EVENTS

The preparation during the last few days and hours before the endurance event can mean the difference between success and failure. In this section, we discuss the concept of "carbohydrate loading" (or "glycogen loading"). The best scheme for endurance athletes preparing for any exercise event lasting longer than 60–90 minutes is to taper off the exercise gradually during the week before the event, while consuming more than 70% carbohydrate during the 3 days before the event. If the exercise event lasts less than 60 minutes, "carbohydrate loading" is unnecessary.

The "pre-event meal" is another important consideration. The meal 3–5 hours before the event should be 500–800 Calories of light, low-fiber starch. There are various pros and cons concerning the use of different sugar solutions.

How to "Carbohydrate Load" before the Big Event

As discussed earlier, the human body has only limited stores of CHO. Exercise training at 60–80% $\dot{V}O_{2max}$ leads to muscle glycogen depletion after 100–120 minutes.[1] Exercise at 80–95% can lead to muscle glycogen depletion even sooner.

Various researchers have therefore tried to manipulate muscle glycogen stores using a combination of the high-CHO diet and varying levels of exercise and rest to increase glycogen levels above normal, in the belief that exercise time to exhaustion could be prolonged.

The original Scandinavian researchers set up a regimen now known as the "classical" method of "muscle glycogen supercompensation." According to this plan, athletes first depleted their muscles of glycogen by eating a low-carbohydrate diet for 3 consecutive days while engaging in intense, prolonged exercise sessions for at least 2 of these days. Next, athletes would "supercompensate" their muscles with glycogen, by resting for 3 days before competition while eating a very high (90%) carbohydrate diet.

This regimen has been found to create muscle glycogen levels as high as 220 mmol/kg wet muscle (with total body CHO stores of more than 1,000 grams).[1,278] Unfortunately, this program causes several undesirable side effects during the depletion phase, including marked physical and mental fatigue, elevation of fat metabolic by-products in the blood (ketosis), low blood sugar levels (hypoglycemia), muscle cell damage, electrocardiographic abnormalities, depression, and irritability.[1,279] In addition, during the high-carbohydrate phase, the athlete often feels heavy and stiff in the legs.

Because of these side effects, researchers have modified the depletion phase.[1,280,281] Instead of 3 days of a low-carbohydrate diet and hard exercise, the modified scheme utilizes a slow tapering of exercise over a 6-day period, without any intensive exercise the day before competition. During the week, the diet should provide more than 8 g CHO/kg (about 70% CHO).[1,282] (See Table 9.12 for a sample menu.) This modified regimen has been found to create muscle glycogen levels of approximately 200 mmol/kg, nearly the same as the old classical method, without the side effects[1] (see Figure 9.35).

With the muscles "loaded" or "supercompensated" with glycogen, endurance athletes are able to maintain their racing pace for longer periods of time. The overall race time is lower, though the pace per mile does not improve. In other words, athletes can maintain speed longer and thus reduce the total time.[1,282–286] In 30-km time trials, for example, carbohydrate-loaded runners are able to run 4–5 minutes faster than when on low-carbohydrate diets.[283,284]

The Pre-Event Meal

The meal before competition can make a difference both physiologically and psychologically. Most sports-nutrition experts advise one or two glasses of water, followed within 20–30 minutes by a light (500–800 kcal) meal of rapidly digestible, low-fiber starch (e.g., cream of wheat hot cereal, white bread, bagels, pasta, refined cereals).[93] The food should be consumed 3–5 hours before the event, so that the stomach will be empty at the time of competition to avoid

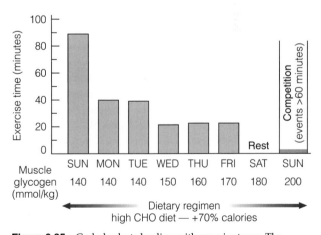

Figure 9.35 Carbohydrate loading with exercise taper. The best scheme for increasing muscle glycogen stores before endurance competition is to consume a high-carbohydrate diet while tapering the exercise to complete rest. *Source:* Sherman WM, Costill DL, Fink WJ, et al. The effect of exercise diet manipulation on muscle glycogen and its subsequent utilization during performance. *Int J Sports Med* 2:114–118, 1981.

uncomfortable feelings of fullness or cramping. The use of proteins, fats, known gas-forming foods, high-fiber foods, and foods known to act as laxatives is not recommended.[1]

Many athletes feel that drinking sports drinks with sugar 30–60 minutes before hard exertion will enhance performance. Earlier studies examining intakes of glucose or sucrose 30–60 minutes before exercise reported that blood glucose rose sharply, causing an increase in blood insulin concentrations, which then stimulated the muscles to utilize blood glucose. This resulted in rebound low blood sugar levels, and later, accelerated muscle glycogen depletion.[287,288]

More recent studies, however, have not been able to confirm these earlier findings.[289–296] The use of 70- to 80-gram glucose solutions (about 280–320 Calories) 30–60 minutes before endurance performance has not been associated with abnormally low blood glucose levels, increased glycogen depletion, or decreased performance. In fact, some researchers report that a carbohydrate meal 30–60 minutes before exercise increases the amount of glucose available to the working muscle, enhancing endurance performance.[289,290]

In one study of 10 well-trained cyclists, researchers found that the best possible pre-event eating schedule was a 200-gram carbohydrate meal (800 Calories) 4 hours before the event, and a 45-gram CHO snack immediately before high-intensity endurance exercise.[297] Figure 9.36 shows the results of an interesting study comparing a large pre-event carbohydrate meal of 1,300 Calories, to 700 Calories of carbohydrate during the exercise, to both schemes used in combination.[298] Cyclers were able to exercise 44% longer when carbohydrates were used both 3 hours before and during exercise.

Some athletes feel that fasting before long endurance exercise will make them feel lighter and more energetic.[299] In one study, a 1-day fast by male marathon runners resulted in a 45% decrease in endurance performance.[104] Fasting caused significant increases in oxygen uptake, heart rate, rating of perceived exertion, ventilation, and psychological fatigue. In general, the metabolic data appeared to suggest that the responses at the start for the runners who had fasted were like those of the runners who had eaten after 90 minutes of exercise (see Figure 9.37). Most other studies have also shown that fasting causes early fatigue and decreased ability to perform.[299]

PRINCIPLE 9: USE OF ERGOGENIC AIDS IS UNETHICAL

Ergogenic aids are defined as substances that increase one's ability to exercise harder. Although there are many worthless ergogenic aids (e.g., bee pollen, B_{15} or pangamic acid, alcohol, wheat germ oil, lecithin, kelp, brewer's yeast, phosphates, L-carnitine, and chromium picolinate), others confer impressive benefits (caffeine, sodium bicarbonate, blood

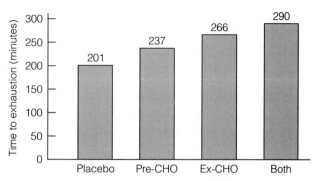

Figure 9.36 Carbohydrate feedings and cycling performance. Three hours prior to exercise, subjects ingested 1,300 Calories as carbohydrate; and during exercise, 700 Calories as carbohydrate. Having carbohydrate in the pre-event meal and during cycling exercise greatly improves endurance time to exhaustion. *Source:* Wright DA, Sherman WM, Dernbach AR. Carbohydrate feedings before, during, or in combination improve cycling endurance performance. *J Appl Physiol* 71:1082–1088, 1991.

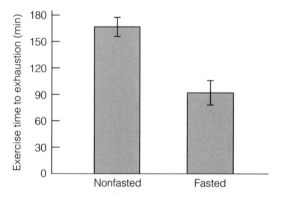

Figure 9.37 The effects of a 1-day fast on running endurance. Fasting for 1 day before long endurance running led to a 45% reduction in exercise time to exhaustion. *Source:* Nieman DC, Carlson KA, Brandstater ME, et al. Running exhaustion in 27-h fasted humans. *J Appl Physiol* 63:2502–2509, 1987.

doping, steroids, etc.). These may enhance performance, but the ethical issues of equitable competition and fair play claim a higher priority.[300–307]

For thousands of years, warriors and athletes have used a wide variety of substances in the attempt to enhance physical performance.[308] The ancient Greek athletes believed in the value of meat and also consumed special herbs and mushrooms; ancient Muslim warriors used hashish; during World War II, some German soldiers experimented with anabolic–androgen steroid hormones to increase their aggressiveness in combat; American soldiers were given the stimulant amphetamine to improve their endurance and attentiveness; amphetamines became popular among bicycle racers in the 1960s, leading to several deaths; strychnine was used by some of the early prizefighters; and many athletes today use everything from anabolic–androgen steroids to caffeine to doses of blood to improve endurance performance.[308]

Why is the use of drugs and ergogenic aids so pervasive today? This is best answered in a statement made in 1972 by the Medical Commission of the International Olympic Committee.[309]

> The merciless rigor of modern competitive sports, especially at the international level, the glory of victory, and the growing social and economical reward of sporting success (in no way any longer related to reality) increasingly forces athletes to improve their performance by any means available.

Categories of Ergogenic Aids

The term *ergogenic* means "tending to increase work." Thus ergogenic aids are any substances or methods that tend to increase performance capacity.[300–307] These aids fall into five categories:

1. *Nutritional aids*—carbohydrates, proteins, vitamins, minerals, iron, water, electrolytes, and miscellaneous substances (e.g., bee pollen, B_{15})
2. *Pharmacological aids*—amphetamines, caffeine, anabolic steroids, alcohol, $NaHCO_3$, recombinant erythropoietin (r-EPO)
3. *Physiological aids*—oxygen, blood doping
4. *Psychological aids*—hypnosis, covert rehearsal strategies, stress management
5. *Mechanical aids*—biomechanical aids, physical warm-up

This section reviews some of the more common nutritional and pharmacological aids.

Miscellaneous Nutritional Aids

Athletes are constantly searching for a "performance edge" through the use of dietary supplements, with some taking large amounts of nutrient preparations, far in excess of recommended levels.[310,311] Most studies show that over half of athletes use supplements, with elite athletes using more than college or high school athletes.[311]

A number of nutritional substances are advocated to improve performance. Included are the various vitamins and minerals, and extracts from various foods. (See Principle 6, on vitamin and mineral supplements.)

Table 9.18 summarizes the ergogenic claims made for a wide variety of natural products and nutritional aids currently available.[309–337] In general, most of the performance claims either are not supported by current research, or research findings have been extrapolated to inappropriate applications. Often, biological functions of some compounds used by the body (e.g., inosine, carnitine, and boron) were

TABLE 9.18   Natural Products and Miscellaneous Nutritional Aids Marketed for Ergogenic Purposes

Product	Claims	Fact
Alcohol	Enhances endurance; alters fatigue; fuel source	Does not enhance endurance; may be ergolytic
Amino acid tablets or capsules	Improves muscle-mass gains, endurance, strength	Most studies show no special benefits
Argentinian bull testes	Potent anabolic agent that increases testosterone	No data to back claims
Arginine/ornithine amino acids	Promotes release of growth hormone	Studies are inconclusive
Bee pollen	Improves metabolism and endurance performance	Best studies show no effect
Boron	Increases testosterone; strengthens muscles	Best studies show no effect
Branch-chain amino acids	Prevents fatigue during long endurance events	Most studies do not support claim
Carnitine	Fat-loss agent ("cutting"); promotes use of fat for fuel	Insufficient data to back claims
Choline	Increases strength and decreases body fat, delays fatigue	No well-designed studies back claims
Chromium picolinate	Increases insulin activity, increases muscle cell uptake of amino acids, decreases body fat	No good data to support claims
Coenzyme Q10	Enhances aerobic performance	Best studies show no improvement
Creatine	Increases anaerobic power; stimulates muscle growth	Well-designed studies both support claims and show no effect
Dibencozide	Potent anabolic agent; increases oxygen transport	No good support for claims

(continued)

TABLE 9.18 Natural Products and Miscellaneous Nutritional Aids Marketed for Ergogenic Purposes *(continued)*

Product	Claims	Fact
Gamma oryzanol / ferulic acid	From rice-bran oil; for metabolic activation; anabolic agent	No data to back claims
Ginseng	Weight loss; energy enhancer; improves mental and physical vigor	Limited data to back claims; best studies show no effect
Inosine	Energy enhancer; improve endurance, strength; weight loss	Insufficient data to back claims; may be ergolytic
Lactate supplement	Regular intake promotes lactate clearance during exercise	Studies do not support claim
Ma-huang	Weight loss; energy enhancer; improves strength and endurance	No data to support performance gains
Pangamic acid / vitamin B_{15}	Improves endurance performance	Best studies show no effect
Phosphate salts	Improves endurance performance	Studies are equivocal
Plant sterols	Anabolic agent; increases growth hormone	No support for claims
Smilax compounds	Increases testosterone; improves muscle mass	No data to support claims
Tryptophan	Increases brain serotonin; delays fatigue, resists pain	Best studies show no effect
Vanadyl sulfate	Builds muscle tissue	Best studies show no effect
Yohimbine	Testosterone enhancer	No data to support claims

Sources: Based on references 309–337.

amplified as performance claims when used in large-dose supplements.

Bodybuilders and strength athletes are the targets of many companies who push various substances as anabolic agents to "naturally" improve body hormone levels, muscle size, and strength.[338] In one study of 309 male and female bodybuilders, 94% took some type of supplement, and 60% spent $25–$100 each month on supplements.[339] The FDA is cracking down on these companies, and misleading claims and false advertising should diminish.[183] It is hoped that most of these ergogenic products will be tested using appropriate scientific methods (double-blind, placebo controlled) so that truth can be separated from error. The Centers for Disease Control, in their review of ergogenic aids marketed to bodybuilders, has emphasized that because of false claims, widespread use, and lack of proper labeling guidelines, "unanticipated effects" may occur.[338] They have urged clinicians to report adverse effects of supplement products to appropriate public health authorities.

Despite such evidence, many athletes are convinced that various nutritional substances do lead to improved performance. If these substances have no value, why do athletes continue to use and believe in them? (See Box 9.8 for guidelines in sorting out hype from the truth.)

The U.S. Food and Drug Administration has concluded that "people are often helped, not by the food or drug being touted, but by a profound belief it will help."[340] In other words, the placebo effect is powerful enough to actually produce a benefit.[341,342] A review of the literature shows that an average of 35% of the members of any group will respond favorably to placebos (with a variation of 0–100%).[341]

The challenge of the health professional working with an athlete is to use this placebo effect to advantage by instilling a "profound belief" in food substances that have proven worth (e.g., carbohydrate, water, and nutritious foods). This can be summarized as follows:

1 (placebo effect) + 0 (substance of no worth) = 1

1 (placebo effect) + 2 (substance of worth) = 3

Use of Caffeine to Improve Performance in Long Endurance Events

Despite the widespread use of caffeinated beverages by Americans, a growing number of studies are providing evidence that this drug is not as benign as once thought.[343–345] Daily caffeine intake has been related to osteoporosis, birth defects, and sleep interference, and this drug exhibits the features of a typical psychoactive substance leading to dependence. One in three Americans consumes approximately 200 mg caffeine (equivalent to 1–2 cups of coffee) per day. Caffeine is an alkaloid present in more than 60 plant species. Peak plasma levels after ingestion occur within 15–45 minutes, with a plasma half-life ranging from 2.5 to 7.5 hours. The metabolism by the liver, storage, and clearance rate of caffeine may vary greatly between acute and chronic users. Table 9.19 summarizes the caffeine content of various beverages, chocolate, and medications.

There is growing evidence that caffeine ingestion (3–9 mg/kg body weight) prior to exercise increases performance during prolonged endurance exercise and short-term intense exercise lasting about 5 minutes.[346–353] Caffeine

---

Box 9.8

Tools for Evaluating Research on Dietary Supplements

The following questions represent some of the key points that may be used to sort out the hype from the truth when evaluating research on dietary supplements.

1. Is there a legitimate rationale for the dietary supplement? Theoretically, the dietary supplement should be able to influence physiological processes involved in exercise, or to improve body composition.

2. Were appropriate subjects studied? If claims are that the dietary supplement augments a certain type of exercise performance, then subjects who are currently engaging in the specific activity should be selected (e.g., weight lifters vs. bodybuilders, runners vs. swimmers, wrestlers vs. gymnasts).

3. How was exercise performance or changes in body composition evaluated? The exercise or body composition test to evaluate the effect of the dietary supplement should be both valid and reliable.

4. Was a placebo used? The dietary supplement should be provided in the appropriate amount and for an appropriate time period to the experimental group of subjects, but a placebo should be used with a control group of subjects. A dietary supplement may work for some individuals, not because of any bona fide physiological effect, but rather because a psychological placebo effect may modify personal behaviors, which are conducive to modifying exercise performance or body mass.

5. Were the subjects randomly assigned to the treatments? Subjects should be randomly assigned to

the dietary supplement or placebo groups. If the study is a crossover design, in which all subjects take both the dietary supplement and the placebo, the order of giving the supplement should be balanced; that is, half of the subjects should take the dietary supplement first, and half take the placebo first. In the second phase of the study, the subjects switch treatments.

6. Was the study double-blind? Neither the subjects nor the investigators interacting with them should know which group receives the dietary supplement or placebo. This is known as a double-blind protocol.

7. Were extraneous factors controlled? Investigators should attempt to control other factors besides the treatment, which may influence exercise performance and body composition. Diet, exercise, and daily physical activities need to be controlled.

8. Were the data analyzed properly? Appropriate statistical techniques should be used to minimize the chance of statistical error.

Well-designed studies published in *peer-reviewed* (reviewed by several other experts) scientific journals serve as the basis for determining the efficacy of dietary supplements. However, a single study does not provide conclusive evidence that a dietary supplement is either effective or ineffective for its stated purpose. The efficacy of dietary supplements must be evaluated by a number of well-designed research studies.

Source: Adapted from Williams M. The gospel truth about dietary supplements. *ACSM's Health & Fitness Journal* 1(1):24–28, 1997.

---

taken 1 hour prior to exercise will enhance endurance performance 10–30%, although individual responses can vary widely.[353]

Caffeine tends to elevate catecholamines and free fatty acids in the blood. When exercising muscles are presented with elevated levels of free fatty acids at the beginning of exercise, the muscles will increase their utilization of fat, sparing the muscle glycogen, resulting in improved endurance. Caffeine also appears to have a "neural" effect, decreasing the perception of effort.[348,351]

The American College of Sports Medicine does not recommend the use of caffeine for enhancement of performance. The International Olympic Committee has banned caffeine present in urine at levels greater than 12 µg/ml urine. It takes about 6 cups of brewed coffee (at 100-mg caffeine per cup) to reach this level.[256] Three tablets of Vivarin® or six tablets of NoDoz® would have the same effect as 6 cups of coffee (see Table 9.19). The ergogenic effects of caffeine are present with urinary caffeine levels that are below the limit of 12 µg/ml, raising serious ethical issues regarding the use of caffeine by athletes.[346,349] Caffeine may have to be added to the list of banned substances. (See Box 9.9.)

TABLE 9.19 Caffeine Sources

Caffeine in drinks and chocolate		Caffeine in medications[c]	
Food Item	Caffeine (mg)	Drug class	Caffeine (mg)
Beverages		**Over-the-counter medications**	
Coffee		*Analgesics*	
Espresso, 2 oz	120	Actamin Super, Aspirin-Free Excedrin, Excedrin Extra Strength	65
Regular, brewed, 6 oz	103	Goody's Headache Powders, Supac, Vanquish	33
Instant, 6 oz	57	Anacin, Anacin Maximum Strength, Buffets II, Cope, Gelpirin, Gensan, P-A-C Revised Formula, Rid-A-Pain Compound	32
Instant, decaf, 6 oz	2		
Tea		*Cold combinations*	
Black, 6 oz[a]	53	Kolephrin, Kolephrin/DM	65
Ooolong, 6 oz[a]	36	Fendol	32
Green, 6 oz[a]	32	Histosal	30
Iced tea, instant, 12 oz	46	*Stimulants*	
Soft drinks, 12 oz[b]		Caffedrine, Keep Alert, NoDoz Maximum Strength, Ultra Pep-Back, Vivarin	200
Jolt Cola	72	Quick Pep	150
Nehi Maxxvm Cola	70	NoDoz, Pep-Back	100
Sundrop	63	Enerjets	75
Kick	58	**Prescription medications**	
Mountain Dew	55	*Analgesics*	
Mello Yello, Surge	53	Cafergot, Ercaf, Ergo-Caff, Gotamine, Wigraine	100
Coca-Cola Classic	47	Amaphen, Femcet, Fioricet, Fiorinal with Codeine No. 3, Idenal with Codeine, Medigesic, Pharmagesic, Two-Dyne	40
Royal Crown Cola	43		
Mr. PiBB, Dr. Pepper, Sunkist Sparkling Lemonade	41	Synalgos-DC	30
Sunkist Orange	40	*Cold combinations*	
Squirt Ruby Red	39	Citra Forte, Hycomine Compound	30
Pepsi	37	*Muscle relaxants*	
A&W Cream Soda	28	Norgesic Forte, Norphadrine Forte, N3 Gesic Forte, Orphenagesic Forte	60
Barq's	23		
Slice Cola	11	Norgesic, Norphadrine, N3 Gesic, Orphenagesic	30
Water, caffeine-enhanced, 12 oz			
Java Water	71		
Krank$_2$O	70		
Water Joe	46		
Aqua Java	43		
Juice drinks, caffeine-enhanced, 12 oz			
Java Juice	90		
XTC	70		
Chocolate			
Baking chocolate, unsweetened, 1 oz	58		
Hershey Special Dark chocolate bar, 1.45 oz	31		
Other milk chocolate candy bars, average, 1.55 oz	11		

[a]Brewed in bag for three minutes.

[b]Diet sodas have roughly the same caffeine content as regular versions.

[c]Table includes only those medications that contain 30 mg of caffeine or more per tablet. All drugs except the stimulants contain active ingredients in addition to caffeine.

Source: Consumer Reports on Health, September, 1997. "Caffeine in Drinks and Chocolate, and in Medications." Copyright © 1997 by Consumers Union of U.S., Inc., Yonkers, NY 10703-1057. Reprinted by permission from Consumer Reports, September 1997.

Box 9.9

Classes of Substances and Methods Prohibited by the International Olympic Committee, Including Substances Subject to Certain Restrictions

Following are various ergogenic aids prohibited for Olympic athletes, during competition.

Prohibited Classes of Substances

1. Stimulants

2. Narcotics

3. Anabolic agents

4. Diuretics

5. Peptide and glycoprotein hormones and analogues (e.g., growth hormone)

Prohibited Methods

1. Blood doping

2. Pharmacological, chemical, and physical manipulation (e.g., use of drugs that alter steroid excretion, or instilling clean urine in the bladder and simulating voiding).

Classes of Drugs Subject to Restrictions

1. Alcohol (restricted in the modern pentathlon)

2. Marijuana

3. Local anesthetics

4. Corticosteroids

5. Beta-blockers

Source: Catlin DH, Murray TH. Performance-enhancing drugs, fair competition, and Olympic sport. *JAMA* 276:231–237, 1996.

"Soda Loading" for Anaerobic Exercise

During high-intensity exercise, the requirement for oxygen exceeds the capacity of the aerobic system, increasing glycolysis and therefore lactic acid levels. The buildup of lactic acid finally inhibits the energy-supplying chemical reactions, resulting in fatigue. Exercise of 1- to 4-minute duration is limited by lactic acid buildup.

Several recent studies have shown that sodium bicarbonate (as found in Alka Seltzer) augments the body's buffer reserve, counteracts the buildup of lactic acid, and improves anaerobic exercise performance.[354–358] The use of sodium bicarbonate in doses of 300 mg/kg (taken all at once or spread out over a 1- to 3-hour period and given

with water) has been shown to improve 400-meter running times by an average of 1.5 seconds and 800-meter running times by 2.9 seconds.[354,355] In general, such doses improve performance during any exercise bout with a large anaerobic component.[356,357] One review of the literature concluded that anaerobic exercise performance is enhanced 27% when using time to exhaustion as the criterion.[356] For the 800-meter, 2.9 seconds translates to a 19-meter advantage, often the difference between first and last place.

The practical implications are that performance can be enhanced in any event demanding hard exercise over a 1- to 4-minute period because the usual limiting factor, lactic acid, is partially controlled and buffered.

As with all ergogenic aids, however, there are some adverse effects. As many as half of those using soda may suffer from "urgent diarrhea" 1 hour after the soda loading is completed. The effects of repeated ingestion are unknown, and caution is advised.

As with caffeine, this use brings up the ethical issue of equitable competition and fair play. Soda loading should be banned because of the unfair advantage it offers. Bicarbonate rises sharply in the urine after sodium bicarbonate is used and can be measured to detect "soda loaders."

Blood Doping for Endurance

Just as Roman gladiators drank the blood of foes to gain strength, modern Olympians have infused the blood of friends, as well as their own, to gain endurance.[359] Increased performance after blood transfusion was first demonstrated in the late 1930s, but the technique did not attract attention until the early 1970s, when it was dubbed "blood doping" by the media. Although earlier studies on blood doping reported mixed results, recent studies have shown that this practice has strong ergogenic value.[359–366]

Blood doping involves removing 900 ml of blood (about 2 units) from an athlete, freeze storing it at 80°C for 6–8 weeks, and then reinfusing the blood back into the athlete 1–7 days before the competition (see Figure 9.38). This increases the hemoglobin about 10%, leading to a 4–11% increase in $\dot{V}O_{2max}$.[365]

Training with a lower amount of red blood cells and blood triggers a physiological response similar to that which occurs when runners train at high altitudes. In general, a runner's performance will drop by 10–20% immediately after the removal of 900 ml of blood, but it will gradually return to normal over the next 6–8 weeks.

Cardiorespiratory endurance performance is improved following the reinfusion because the oxygen-carrying capacity of the blood is greater, cardiac output is increased, lactate levels are reduced and sweating responses are improved.[359–366] Treadmill time to exhaustion is increased, 10-kilometer (6.2-mile) times drop an average of 69 seconds, 5-mile time performances drop an average of 49

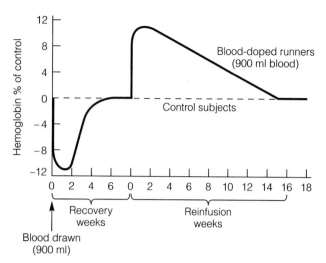

Figure 9.38   Blood-doping scheme. Blood doping usually involves removing 900 ml of one's own blood, storing it for 6–8 weeks as the body builds back to its normal amount, and then, shortly before competition, infusing the 900-ml blood to increase blood volume and hemoglobin to higher than normal levels.   *Source:* Gledhill N. The ergogenic effect of blood doping. *Physician Sportsmed* 11:87–90, 1983.

seconds (10 seconds faster per mile), and 3-mile time performances drop an average of 23.7 seconds.[365]

After blood doping, the hemoglobin level rises about 10% (e.g., to 15–16.5 g/dl). Because the normal range of hemoglobin is 14–18 g/dl, detecting blood doping has proven to be very difficult. Blood doping was forbidden by the International Olympic Committee after the 1984 Olympics, despite the fact that no methods had been devised for unequivocal detection.[364] The American College of Sports Medicine has taken the position that "any blood doping procedure used in an attempt to improve athletic performance is unethical, unfair, and exposes the athlete to unwarranted and potentially serious health risks."[365]

The Food and Drug Administration approved a new drug, erythropoietin (EPO), during the late 1980s. EPO is a hormone produced by the kidney, to stimulate production of red blood cells by the bone marrow. A synthetic form, recombinant EPO (r-EPO) is used to treat kidney patients who have anemia; r-EPO is considered by some athletes to be an easier way to blood dope.[365,367–370] It causes the percentage of red blood cells (hematocrit) in the blood to increase, enhancing oxygen transport capacity. Administering EPO will slowly increase the number of red blood cells over several weeks but the increase will be sustained as long as EPO treatment continues.[365]

Some experts feel that if the hematocrit rises above 55%, the blood gets too thick and may clot more easily, possibly leading to heart attack and stroke.[365] It has been speculated that several cyclists in Europe have died because of r-EPO use, but absolute verification is lacking.[369] Although r-EPO

is available commercially or through the black market, and athletes can administer it by simple injection, they cannot monitor the effects in their circulatory system, and that makes the process risky, not to mention unethical.[370]

Anabolic–Androgenic Steroids for Muscular Strength and Size

Anabolic–androgenic steroids are prescription drugs that have legitimate medical uses, including treatment for anemias, hereditary angioedema, certain gynecological conditions, and protein anabolism.[371] About 3 million prescriptions are given by doctors each year. However, their use in connection with athletic training and muscle building is another matter.

The use of anabolic–androgenic steroids by athletes worldwide has become symbolic of what athletes are willing to go through to achieve excellence and success in competition. The use of steroids by Ben Johnson, which led to his loss of the 1988 Olympic gold medal for the 100-meter dash and of his world record, has been widely reviewed and decried by the media.

Obtaining accurate statistics on steroid use by Americans has proven very difficult. Conservative estimates put the black market cost at $100 million per year, with at least 1 million users.[372–378]

Steroid abuse is particularly common among athletes in strength sports. In one survey of 250 weight lifters, almost half admitted using steroids at some time.[373] In another study of elite power lifters, 33% admitted to having used steroids.[374] Some scientists feel that most steroid abusers are student athletes, bodybuilders, and fitness enthusiasts who are concerned with putting on muscle weight and contouring their bodies.[372,375,376]

Results from nationwide studies of adolescents showed that 4–12% of all male students currently use or have used anabolic steroids.[376,377–379] Over one third of the students initiated use when they were 16 years of age or younger, and users tended to abuse other drugs, as well.

Approximately one in five of these student users reports that a health professional was their primary source. The primary motivation for steroid usage among the high school seniors was strength and appearance. The most common side effects reported were heightened sex drive, acne, and increased body hair. Between 5 and 14% of Division I NCAA athletes use steroids, with incidence of use highest among football athletes.[378]

The problems of anabolic–androgenic steroids can be considered from three different perspectives: pharmacological—the possibility that these substances may provide a real physiological advantage for the athletes; psychological—the importance of winning and the placebo effect of drugs; and ethical—the concept of violation of fair play.[372–391]

Anabolic steroids are synthetic derivatives of testosterone, a male sex hormone, but have greater anabolic activity (building up the body) relative to androgenic activity (masculinization) than testosterone. *Testosterone* is the principal circulating androgen in humans, concentrated 20 times as much in men as in women, and is a powerful agent to increase muscle mass and reduce body fat.[380,387] For example, in one study, subjects were given weekly muscle injections of testosterone for 12 weeks. The average subject gained 16.5 pounds of lean body mass while losing 7.5 pounds of fat, all without changing normal exercise or diet patterns.[380] The average adult male naturally produces 2.5–11.0 milligrams of testosterone daily. The typical steroid abuser often takes more than 100 mg a day, through "stacking" or combining several different brands of steroids.

The esterified steroids are usually given intramuscularly, whereas the alkylated steroids are given orally. The effects of steroids depend on the type used, the size and frequency of the doses, the overall length of treatment, and the route of administration.

A new, alarming trend is the use of other drugs to achieve the "performance-enhancing" effects of steroids. These steroid "alternatives" are sought in order to avoid the stiff penalties now in effect against steroid users. The two most common are gamma hydroxy butyrate (GHB) and clenbuterol. Both drugs are considered potentially dangerous, with serious, immediate side effects.[381] Clenbuterol has been shown to increase skeletal muscle mass 10–20% in 8–14 days.[392]

Anabolic steroids have been used by athletes for decades, in the belief that they increase body mass, muscle tissue, strength, and aggressiveness. More recently, testosterone has been used because it is more difficult to detect in drug screening programs. Although study results have been mixed, an intensive exercise program, coupled with a high-protein diet and anabolic steroids, may increase muscular strength and size for some people.[373,378] One problem in obtaining research data is that athletes use drug combinations and doses that researchers do not replicate in their studies, often for ethical reasons.

Reasons given by athletes for using steroids include decreasing body fat, increasing muscle mass and strength, improving appearance, increasing red blood cell count, and increasing training tolerance (greater intensity, better recovery).[378] Athletes often take doses 10–1,000 times greater than clinical therapeutic doses. (Testimonial evidence suggests that about half of world-class athletes would risk serious or life-threatening adverse drug reactions if they could find a drug that would ensure their winning an Olympic medal.[376]

The side effects are legion[378,381–391] (see Box 9.10). Use of these substances can affect the reproductive system, leading to temporary infertility. Among men, such use may result in atrophy of the testicles, decreased production of

---

Box 9.10

Steroid Side Effects

The side effects of steroid ingestion are legion. These include both established effects and less certain effects.

Established Effects

    Low HDL cholesterol

    Acne

    Genital changes

    Water retention in tissue

    Yellowing of eyes and skin

    Oily, thickened skin

    Stunted growth (when taken before puberty)

    Fetal damage (when taken during pregnancy)

    Coronary artery disease

    Sterility, lowered sperm count in men

    Liver tumors and disease

    Death

Additional effects in women—male-pattern baldness, hairiness, voice deepening, decreased breast size, menstrual irregularities, clitoris hypertrophy

Other Possible Effects

Abdominal pains, hives, chills, euphoria, diarrhea, fatigue, fever, muscle cramps, headache, nausea, vomiting blood, bone pains, depression, impotence, breast development in men, aggressive behavior, urination problems, sexual problems, gallstones, high blood pressure, kidney disease

Sources: See references 381–391.

---

sperm, and reduced levels of several reproductive hormones. Steroids also produce liver abnormalities, decrease HDL cholesterol and increase LDL cholesterol, and increase the incidence of acne. Among women, androgenic hormones produce masculinizing effects (e.g., clitoris enlargement and increased hair growth).

While most of the effects of anabolic steroid use among adults may be reversible, several studies suggest that they may have more serious biophysical consequences for adolescents, particularly with regard to premature skeletal maturation, spermatogenesis, and an elevated risk of injury. However, the long-term health effects of anabolic steroid use are relatively unstudied.[378]

The use of steroids may also expose athletes to a risk of injury to ligaments and tendons, and these injuries may take longer to heal. There is also some evidence of anabolic steroid association with cancer, death, edema, fetal damage, heart disease, prostate enlargement, sterility, swelling of feet or lower legs, and yellowing of the eyes or skin.

It has been known for years that anabolic steroids increase aggressiveness. Athletes using steroids have exhibited increased levels of anger and hostility and overall mood disturbance. Studies also show that in addition to irritability and hostility, steroids increase confusion and forgetfulness, hardly the mental traits coaches desire in their athletes.[386,391]

Creatine Supplementation

Creatine supplementation has been urged as an ergogenic aid for athletes who engage in repeated bouts of short-term, high-intensity exercise.[393–395] Creatine is found in large quantities in skeletal muscle and binds a significant amount of phosphate, providing an immediate source of energy in muscle cells (ATP).[393,394] The reason for consuming supplemental creatine is to increase the skeletal muscle creatine content, in the hope that some of the extra creatine binds phosphate, increasing muscle creatine phosphate content. During repeated bouts of high-intensity exercise (for example, five 30-second bouts of sprinting or cycling exercise, separated by 1–4 minutes of rest), the increased availability of creatine phosphate may improve resynthesis and degradation rates, leading to greater anaerobic ATP turnover and high-power exercise performance.[394]

The estimated daily requirement for creatine is about 2 grams.[394,395] Nonvegetarians typically get about 1 gram of creatine a day from the various meats they ingest, and the body synthesizes another gram in the liver, kidney, and pancreas, using the amino acids arginine and glycine as precursors. Vegetarians have a reduced body creatine pool, suggesting that lack of dietary creatine from avoidance of meat is not adequately compensated by an increase in endogenous creatine production.

Various studies have shown that consuming about 20–25 grams of creatine per day for 5–6 days in a row significantly increases muscle creatine in most people, especially those with low levels to begin with, such as vegetarians.[395] Four to five daily doses of 5 grams each are usually consumed by dissolving creatine in about 250 ml of a beverage throughout the day. Each 5-gram dose of creatine is the equivalent of 1.1 kg of fresh, uncooked steak. There do not appear to be any adverse side effects associated with the oral ingestion of supplemental creatine.

Some[394–397] but not all[398–402] studies have shown that supplemental creatine improves performance during repeated bouts of short-term sprinting, cycling, or swimming. Additional laboratory and field research is needed to help resolve the conflicting findings regarding the ergogenic efficacy of creatine supplementation. Often, when studies differ so widely on the ergogenic effect of a certain supplement, any enhancement in performance will be small at best. While creatine has a variable effect on anaerobic performance, it has no effect on aerobic exercise metabolism and performance.[393]

PRINCIPLE 10: "FAT LOADING" IS NOT RECOMMENDED FOR ENHANCED PERFORMANCE OR HEALTH

Research has shown that athletes have no guarantee of protection from heart disease unless they continue prudent habits of exercise and diet after their days of competition are over. (See Chapter 10.) Even during heavy training, a diet high in saturated fats can raise serum cholesterol to high levels. Regular endurance exercise will not fully negate bad nutritional habits. Fitness enthusiasts and endurance athletes are well advised to consider not only performance, but also general health, in making their dietary choices.

Recently, claims for special diets and nutritional supplements that provide more fat and less carbohydrate for endurance performance have been advanced.[403] It is well known that endurance athletes are capable of sparing body carbohydrate stores through increased fat oxidation during exercise.[404–406] This training-induced effect has led to the premise that a greater availability of fat during exercise, through supplementation or dietary alterations (i.e., "fat loading"), can improve performance by further sparing muscle glycogen.[407]

With endurance training, the muscles become more efficient in using fat for energy, "sparing" the glycogen reserves, allowing the athlete to endure longer before glycogen stores are depleted.[405] One hypothesis is that the increased fat utilization by the endurance athlete at a given work rate increases the intracellular citrate concentration, inhibiting phosphofructokinase (PFK).[407] The inhibition of PFK eventually slows down the rate of glycolysis and glycogenolysis. Because of the ability of the muscle to adapt to aerobic training by increasing fat oxidation, and the well-accepted fact that fatigue is tied to low muscle glycogen levels, it has been speculated that acutely increasing the availability of fatty acids for oxidation through dietary or pharmacological methods might increase the oxidation of fat, sparing muscle glycogen, and therefore improving long-term endurance performance. Before exploring whether this hypothesis is true, the role of fat as a fuel for exercise metabolism is reviewed.

Of the two main fuels stored in the body and used for muscular exercise, fat has several characteristics that would make it a desirable substrate.[408] There is more stored energy (9 Calories/gram) in a gram of fat than in an equal weight of carbohydrate (4 Calories/gram). Typically, about 50,000 to 60,000 Calories of energy are stored as triglycerides in the body of a normal-weight fit individual.[409,410] This large amount of energy is stored in a relatively small amount of adipose tissue (about 13–18 pounds), providing an excellent portable depot of fuel as people move from place to place. In contrast, if all of this energy were stored as glycogen, more than 100 pounds of storage weight would be required, due to binding of heavy water molecules.

Triglyceride is also stored in droplets directly within the muscle fibers, in close proximity to the site of oxidation in the muscle mitochondria. Intramuscular triglyceride accounts for 2,000–3,000 Calories of stored energy, making it a larger source of potential energy than muscle glycogen, which can contribute only about 1,500 Calories.[409,410]

During endurance exercise, lipolysis of triglycerides in both adipose tissue and the muscles is increased after 15–20 minutes by epinephrine stimulation of hormone-sensitive lipase, releasing free fatty acids.[407] Free fatty acids from the blood enter the muscle cell via a carrier-mediated diffusion process. Once inside the muscle cell, the fatty acid is converted to fatty acyl-CoA and then transported across the mitochondrial membrane by an ATP-requiring process via the enzyme complex carnitine palmityl-transferase. In the mitochondria, the acyl-CoA enters the β-oxidation cycle and eventually enters the Krebs cycle, resulting in ATP production.

If the muscle could oxidize fatty acids at a sufficiently high rate during intense exercise, a greater yield of ATP per carbon molecule would occur (1.3-fold) than is possible when relying on carbohydrates. Unfortunately, humans can only slowly convert body fat stores into energy during exercise (less than one third the rate attributed to muscle glycogen).[409,410] About 75% more oxygen is required to completely oxidize fatty acids than glucose, resulting in a much higher stress to the cardiorespiratory system.[1,407] At rest and during low-intensity exercise, fat is the dominant and preferred substrate.[408] However, as the intensity of exercise increases, an increasing proportion of the energy is supplied by carbohydrates. If high-intensity exercise is continued for several hours, muscle glycogen stores slowly become depleted, forcing the muscle cells to use more fatty acids, increasing the sense of effort and strain to the cardiorespiratory system, and ultimately causing a reduction in pace.[1] The primary source of free fatty acids during exercise appear to be intramuscular, rather than adipose tissue triglyceride stores, especially in trained individuals[405,406] (see Figure 9.39).

Dietary and pharmacological methods have been used to increase fatty acid availability and oxidation, in an attempt to spare muscle glycogen and thus enhance long-term endurance performance. Several studies with rats

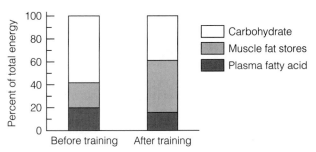

Figure 9.39   Percentage of total energy from carbohydrate and fat during 90–120 minutes cycling at 63% $\dot{V}O_{2max}$ before and after exercise training. Exercise training results in a greater proportion of energy coming from fat, especially fat stored within the muscle.   *Source:* Martin WH, Dalsky GP, Hurly BF, et al. Effect of endurance training on plasma free fatty acid turnover and oxidation during exercise. *Am J Physiol* 265:E708–E714, 1993.

have shown this hypothesis to be true, but the data on humans are at best equivocal.[411]

It is not possible to ingest free fatty acids because they are too acidic and need a protein carrier for intestinal absorption. Thus the only practical way of significantly elevating blood fat levels is by ingesting triglycerides. Normal long-chain dietary triglycerides enter the blood 3–4 hours after ingestion and are bound to chylomicrons. The rate of uptake of triglycerides by muscles during exercise appears to be relatively low. Although medium-chain triglycerides are directly absorbed into the blood and liver and are rapidly broken down to fatty acids and glycerol, only a small amount (about 30 grams) can be ingested without experiencing gastrointestinal discomfort and diarrhea.[412] In general, most studies with medium-chain triglycerides have failed to demonstrate muscle glycogen sparing or enhanced performance.[413]

A technique used in a few research studies to raise plasma levels of free fatty acids is to intravenously infuse a triglyceride emulsion (e.g., Intralipid®), followed by heparin. Thus far, this method has been shown to have minimal, if any, effects on muscle glycogen utilization or performance.[414] Research with normal long-chain dietary triglycerides has centered around the following manipulations:[407]

- High-fat diets for 1–5 days before endurance exercise
- High-fat diets for 2–4 weeks prior to endurance exercise
- High-fat diets immediately before and/or during endurance exercise (after a normal diet)

Nearly all studies have shown that high-fat diets (about 70% of total energy) for several days prior to endurance exercise significantly decrease body carbohydrate stores, reducing endurance time dramatically.[1] Although the relative contribution of fat is increased, performance is impaired because of low muscle glycogen levels. In one study, subjects were fed a high-fat (76% of energy) diet or a high-carbohydrate (76% of energy) diet for 4 days.[415] Subjects then ran to exhaustion on a treadmill at 70% maximal aerobic power. Time to exhaustion following the high-fat diet was decreased by 40%, and all subjects exhibited neurological symptoms of low blood sugar.

A few researchers have studied the effect of 2–4 weeks of a high-fat diet on endurance performance.[416,417] Investigators measured the effect of a 28-day, high-fat diet (with only 20 g carbohydrate per day) on the endurance performance of five well-trained cyclists.[417] Muscle glycogen was decreased by nearly half after the high-fat diet, but the cyclists were able to perform at a moderate intensity (60–65% $\dot{V}O_{2max}$) to the same level as before the diet began. However,

it should be noted that the results may have been quite different, had the intensity been higher.

Researchers have examined the impact of a fatty meal 1–5 hours before exercise after several days of a normal carbohydrate-rich diet, or the use of fat supplements during exercise.[418,419] Potentially, oil supplements just before or during prolonged endurance exercise could cause the muscles to utilize more free fatty acids for fuel, sparing the muscle glycogen that has been built up by a normal carbohydrate-rich diet. Studies thus far, however, have failed to demonstrate improvement in performance.

Taken together, these studies do not support the use of "fat loading" to enhance endurance performance.[407] It should be noted that few studies have explored the issue of "fat loading," and the ones that have been conducted do

SPORTS MEDICINE INSIGHT

A Practical Nutrition Scheme for a Marathon

For the highly active endurance athlete, maximizing muscle glycogen stores for the "big event" is vital. This Sports Medicine Insight deals with the necessary preparation and race-day activities for a marathon-type event (more than 2 hours).

1. Train long and hard to help the muscles adapt. During the months of training for the marathon-type event, train at a hard pace for a minimum of 90–120 minutes several times per month, to train the muscles both to store more glycogen and to utilize fat more efficiently (sparing the glycogen stores). Remember, nutrition is not as important as talent and training. The minimum amount of training for a marathon (26.2 miles) is 50 miles per week for 3 months before the event. The best athletes in the world work up to a schedule of 80–120 miles per week, but this takes many months of gradual training progression.

2. During the months of training, emphasize a high-carbohydrate diet with plenty of rest and water. Adequate recovery from hard training means consuming a high-carbohydrate diet (at least 60–70% of total Calories). The carbohydrate should be primarily starch, not sugar, to ensure adequate vitamin and mineral intake. A wide variety of healthful foods should be used to obtain all nutrients without supplementation. A conscious effort must be made to drink more water than desired.

3. During the week before the event, rest and eat primarily carbohydrate-rich foods. The exercise should gradually taper to total rest the day before the event. During the 3 days just before the event, eat a very high-carbohydrate diet (close to 70–80% of total Calories).

4. In the 3–4 hours before the event, consume a high-carbohydrate meal. About 20–30 minutes before eating the meal, consume two to four glasses of water to ensure that your body is adequately hydrated to provide digestive juices for the meal. The meal should be consumed 3–4 hours before the event, to allow the stomach time to empty all its contents. If the event is early in the day, get up early. The meal should be light (500–800 Calories) and high in carbohydrate, but low in dietary fiber. Refined hot cereal, fruit juices, bagels, white bread and jam, white rice, or pasta (without any fats added) are good choices. Just before the event (5 minutes before), consuming 150–200 Calories of a diluted CHO solution can help maintain blood glucose levels.

5. During the event, drink about 1 liter/hour of a cold sports drink. (Practice during training with various sports drinks until you find one that suits you.)

6. After the event, consume a high-carbohydrate diet to replenish muscle glycogen stores. Recovery from the marathon-type event is hastened by consuming a high-CHO diet soon after the race.

have various methodological flaws. Nonetheless, physiologically, the use of free fatty acids as a major fuel substrate for high-intensity exercise does not seem probable, and even if long-term, high-fat diets lead to some sort of adaptation that allows long-term, moderate-intensity endurance exercise to be performed without impairment, health considerations would forbid an enthusiastic endorsement.[420]

There are data showing that even in athletes training intensively, changes in dietary composition can substantially alter blood lipoprotein levels.[421–423] High-fat diets have also been associated with increased body fat deposition, increasing the difficulty of maintaining an ideal body weight for competition.[411] Although there has been some concern that extremely high carbohydrate diets may lower HDL cholesterol even within athletes training heavily, it is doubtful that this imposes any real impairment in long-term

health because levels still remain above values typical of sedentary subjects.[421,423] Athletes in heavy training should realize, however, that as long as carbohydrate intake is adequate (8–10 g/kg/day), the addition of fat and protein to the diet to meet energy needs does not alter glycogen storage or performance.[424] There is little need for an endurance athlete to be fat-phobic, especially because several studies have shown that total oxidation of fat over the postprandial period is enhanced by long-duration exercise.[425]

There is new evidence that carbohydrate ingestion before, during, and after heavy exertion attenuates the rise in stress hormones, partially abrogating some of the negative immune changes that occur during recovery.[426] Other proven benefits of a high-carbohydrate diet to human health are too important to embrace the unlikely values of a high-fat diet for athletic performance.[427]

SUMMARY

Principle 1: Prudent diet is the cornerstone. The same diet that enhances health (the prudent diet) is the one that also maximizes performance for most athletes. For some athletes in heavy training, however (defined as more than 60–90 minutes a day of aerobic or intermittent anaerobic–aerobic activity), several adaptations beyond the prudent diet are beneficial. Heavy training imposes special nutritional stresses because of the high intensity of effort over a relatively short time period, demanding extra energy, carbohydrate, and water.

Principle 2: Increase total energy intake. Athletes are high energy consumers because of their high working capacities, and high-intensity training levels. Many athletes need more than 50 Calories per kilogram of body weight. Most of this extra energy should come in the form of carbohydrate from grains, dried fruits, breads, and pasta.

Principle 3: Keep the carbohydrate intake high (55–70%) during training. A high-carbohydrate diet is probably the most important nutritional factor for athletes. Body carbohydrate stores (glycogen) are extremely labile because they are the chief fuel source for the working muscle during high-intensity exercise. When muscle glycogen levels drop too low, exercise performance is impaired, and the athlete feels stale and tired and is more prone to injury. Athletes in heavy training need up to 8–10 g CHO/kg in their diet per day (close to 70% of total calories as carbohydrate). The high levels of carbohydrate are usually more than athletes want, so they must be trained to eat high-carbohydrate diets.

Principle 4: Drink large amounts of water during training and the event. Probably the second most important dietary principle for athletes is to drink large quantities of water. As little as a 2% drop in body weight from water loss has been associated with impaired performance. Athletes tend to sweat earlier and more than nonathletes, so they

tend to lose more body water with exercise. The thirst desire of an athlete lags behind actual body needs, so athletes should be encouraged to force fluids beyond what is desired. No electrolytes are needed except in ultramarathon events—they are easily obtained with normal meals after the event. Carbohydrate added to the drink taken during exercise can help maintain blood glucose levels.

Principle 5: Keep a close watch on possible iron deficiency. A number of athletes, especially runners, have Stage 1 iron deficiency, best measured by evaluating serum ferritin levels. All elite athletes are urged to have their iron status checked yearly. To help prevent iron deficiency, runners (especially menstruating females) should consume high-iron foods. Under the supervision of a physician, some runners may benefit from moderate iron supplementation.

Principle 6: Vitamin and mineral supplements are not needed. Most studies show that athletes are above RDA levels for all nutrients (except iron for females). Athletes are at an advantage because their high caloric intakes provide more than adequate quantities of vitamins and minerals. The sedentary are actually at greater risk because of their low caloric intakes. Athletes should not use vitamins or mineral supplements in amounts above the RDA; studies are showing the potential for nutrient imbalances in the body.

Principle 7: Extra protein does not benefit the athlete. Although 5–15% of the energy needed in long endurance exercise or weight lifting come from protein, athletes obtain more than enough protein in their normal diets. There is no need for protein supplements.

Principle 8: Rest and eat carbohydrate before long endurance events. The best scheme for preparing for any exercise event lasting longer than 60–90 minutes is to taper the exercise gradually, while consuming more than 70% carbohydrate during the 7 days before the event. (Depletion of muscle glycogen during the initial phase of "glycogen loading" is no longer recommended.) The pre-event meal should be 500–800 Calories, of light, low-fiber starch, 3–5 hours before the event.

Principle 9: Use of ergogenic aids is unethical. Although there are many worthless ergogenic aids (e.g., bee pollen, B_{15}, alcohol), many provide impressive performance benefits (caffeine, sodium bicarbonate, phosphorus, blood doping). These enhance performance, but the ethical issue of equitable competition and fair play claim a higher priority.

Principle 10: "Fat loading" is not recommended for enhanced performance or health. Research has evaluated the effects of fat in the diet before and during exercise, and performance is not enhanced. Adapting to a high-fat diet for 1 month has been found to aid endurance in some studies, but such adaptation may be harmful to health in the long term. Athletes have no guarantee of protection from heart disease unless they continue prudent habits of exercise and diet after their days of competition are over. Even during heavy training, a diet high in saturated fat can raise serum cholesterol—exercise is not powerful enough to fully negate bad nutritional habits. Athletes can maximize both performance and health through wise dietary choices.

REFERENCES

1. Costill DL. Carbohydrates for exercise: Dietary demands for optimal performance. *Int J Sports Med* 9:1–18, 1988.

2. Mirkin G. *The Sportsmedicine Book.* Boston: Little, Brown, and Co., 1978.

3. Ryan AJ. Anabolic steroids are fool's gold. *Federation Proceedings* 40:2682, 1981.

4. Freeman P. Muscle meals. *California Living,* March 4, 1984.

5. Higdon H. What's diet got to do with it? *Runner's World,* October, 1988.

6. Pritikin N. The brave soldiers in the ironman army travel on their stomachs. *Runner's World,* February, 1984, 127.

7. Sizer FS, Whitney EN. *Nutrition Concepts and Controversies* (7th ed.). Belmont, CA: West / Wadsworth, 1997.

8. Lee RD, Nieman DC. *Nutritional Assessment* (2nd ed.). St. Louis: Mosby, 1996.

9. National Research Council. *Diet and Health: Implications for Reducing Chronic Disease Risk.* Washington, DC: National Academy Press, 1989.

10. U.S. Department of Agriculture. Nutrition and your health: Dietary guidelines for Americans. *Home and Garden Bulletin,* 232. Washington, DC: U.S. Department of Agriculture, 1995.

11. Krauss RM, Deckelbaum RJ, Ernst N, et al. AHA medical / scientific statement: Dietary guidelines for healthy American adults. *Circulation* 94:1795–1800, 1996.

12. American Cancer Society. *Cancer Facts and Figures—1997.* Atlanta: Author, 1997.

13. Food and Nutrition Board, Institute of Medicine. *Recommended Dietary Allowances* (10th ed.). Washington, DC: National Academy Press, 1989.

14. Food and Nutrition Board, Institute of Medicine. *Dietary Reference Intakes for Calcium, Phosphorus, Magnesium, Vitamin D, and Fluoride.* Washington, DC: National Academy Press, 1997.

15. U.S. Department of Agriculture. The food guide pyramid. *Home and Garden Bulletin* 252, 1992.

16. Cleveland LE, Goldman JD, Borrud LG. *Data Tables: Results from USDA's 1994 Continuing Survey of Food Intakes by Individuals and 1994 Diet and Health Knowledge Survey.* Riverdale, MD: Food Surveys Research Group, Beltsville Human Nutrition Research Center, Agricultural Research Service, U.S. Department of Agriculture, 1996.

17. Wilson JW, Enns CW, Goldman JD, et al. *Data Tables: Combined Results from USDA's 1994 and 1995 Continuing Survey of Food Intakes by Individuals and Diet and Health Knowledge Survey.* Riverdale, MD: Food Surveys Research Group, Beltsville Human Nutrition Research Center, Agricultural Research Service, U.S. Department of Agriculture, 1997.

18. Federation of American Societies for Experimental Biology, Life Sciences Research Office. *Third Report on Nutrition Monitoring in the United States: Executive Summary.* Washington, DC: U.S. Government Printing Office, 1995.

19. Cleveland LE, Cook DA, Krebs-Smith SM, Friday J. Method for assessing food intakes in terms of servings based on food guidance. *Am J Clin Nutr* 65(suppl):1254S–1263S, 1997.

20. Krebs-Smith SM, Cook A, Subar AF, Cleveland L, Friday J, Kahle LL. Fruit and vegetable intakes of children and adolescents in the United States. *Arch Pediatr Adolesc Med* 150:81–86, 1996.

21. American Cancer Society. Guidelines on diet, nutrition, and cancer prevention: Reducing the risk of cancer with healthy food choices and physical activity. *CA Cancer J Clin* 46:325–341, 1996.

22. Pietinen P, Rimm EB, Korhonen P, et al. Intake of dietary fiber and risk of coronary heart disease in a cohort of Finnish men: The alpha-tocopherol, beta-carotene cancer prevention study. *Circulation* 94:2720–2727, 1996.

23. Rimm EB, Ascherio A, Giovannucci E, Spiegelman D, Stampfer MJ, Willett WC. Vegetable, fruit, and cereal fiber intake and risk of coronary heart disease among men. *JAMA* 275:447–451, 1996.

24. Van Horn L. Fiber, lipids, and coronary heart disease: A statement for healthcare professionals from the Nutrition Committee, American Heart Association. *Circulation* 95:2701–2704, 1997.

25. American Dietetic Association. Position of the American Dietetic Association: Health implications of dietary fiber. *J Am Diet Assoc* 97:1157–1159, 1997.

26. Marlett JA, Cheung T-F. Database and quick methods of assessing typical dietary fiber intakes using data for 228 commonly consumed foods. *J Am Diet Assoc* 97:1139–1151, 1997.

27. Steinmetz KA, Potter JD. Vegetables, fruit, and cancer prevention: A review. *J Am Diet Assoc* 96:1027–1039, 1996.

28. van Poppel G, Goldbohm RA. Epidemiologic evidence for β-carotene and cancer prevention. *Am J Clin Nutr* 62(suppl):1393S–1402S, 1995.

29. Albanes D, Heinonen OP, Huttunen JK, Taylor PR, et al. Ef-

fects of α-tocopherol and β-carotene supplements on cancer incidence in the alpha-tocopherol beta-carotene cancer prevention study. *Am J Clin Nutr* 62(suppl):1427S–1430S, 1995.

30. Regnstrom J, Nilsson J, Moldeus P, et al. Inverse relation between the concentration of low-density-lipoprotein vitamin E and severity of coronary artery disease. *Am J Clin Nutr* 63:377–385, 1996.

31. Byers T, Guerrero N. Epidemiologic evidence for vitamin C and vitamin E in cancer prevention. *Am J Clin Nutr* 62(suppl):1385S–1392S, 1995.

32. Stampfer MJ, Rimm EB. Epidemiologic evidence for vitamin E in prevention of cardiovascular disease. *Am J Clin Nutr* 62(suppl):1365S–1369S, 1995.

33. Kohlmeier L, Hastings SB. Epidemiologic evidence of a role of carotenoids in cardiovascular disease prevention. *Am J Clin Nutr* 62(suppl):1370S–1376S, 1995.

34. Meyers DG, Maloley PA, Weeks D. Safety of antioxidant vitamins. *Arch Intern Med* 156:925–935, 1996.

35. American Dietetic Association. Position of the American Dietetic Association: Phytochemicals and functional foods. *J Am Diet Assoc* 95:493–496, 1995.

36. Craig WJ. Phytochemicals: Guardians of our health. *J Am Diet Assoc* 97:S199–S204, 1997.

37. Howard BV, Kritchevsky D. Phytochemicals and cardiovascular disease: A statement for healthcare professionals from the American Heart Association. *Circulation* 95:2591–2593, 1997.

38. Clarkson PM. Antioxidants and physical performance. *Crit Rev Food Sci Nutr* 35:131–141, 1995.

39. Sen CK. Oxidants and antioxidants in exercise. *J Appl Physiol* 79:675–686, 1995.

40. Ji LL. Exercise and oxidative stress: Role of the cellular antioxidant systems. *Ex Sport Sci Rev* 23:135–166, 1995.

41. Kanter M. Free radicals and exercise: Effects of nutritional antioxidant supplementation. *Ex Sport Sci Rev* 23:375–397, 1995.

42. Boushey CJ, Beresford SAA, Omenn GS, Motulsky AG. A quantitative assessment of plasma homocysteine as a risk factor for vascular disease. *JAMA* 274:1049–1057, 1995.

43. Lichtenstein AH. Trans fatty acids, plasma lipid levels, and risk of developing cardiovascular disease: A statement for healthcare professionals from the American Heart Association. *Circulation* 95:2588–2590, 1997.

44. Frayn KN, Kingman SM. Dietary sugars and lipid metabolism in humans. *Am J Clin Nutr* 62(suppl):250S–263S, 1995.

45. Wolraich ML, Wilson DB, White W. The effect of sugar on behavior or cognition in children: A meta-analysis. *JAMA* 274:1617–1621, 1995.

46. Peters EM, Goetzsche JM. Dietary practices of South African ultradistance runners. *Int J Sport Nutr* 7:80–103, 1997.

47. Niekamp RA, Baer JT. In-season dietary adequacy of trained male cross-country runners. *Int J Sport Nutr* 5:45–55, 1995.

48. Sjodin AM, Andersson AB, Hogberg JM, Westerterp KR. Energy balance in cross-country skiers: A study using doubly labeled water. *Med Sci Sports Exerc* 26:720–724, 1994.

49. Thompson JL, Manore MM, Skinner JS, Ravussin E, Spraul M. Daily energy expenditure in male endurance athletes with differing energy intakes. *Med Sci Sports Exerc* 27:347–354, 1995.

50. Beidleman BA, Puhl JL, De Souza MJ. Energy balance in female distance runners. *Am J Clin Nutr* 61:303–311, 1995.

51. Horton TJ, Drougas HJ, Sharp TA, Martinez LR, Reed GW, Hill JO. Energy balance in endurance-trained female cyclists and untrained controls. *J Appl Physiol* 76:1937–1945, 1994.

52. Butterworth DE, Nieman DC, Underwood BC, Lindsted KD. The relationship between cardiorespiratory fitness, physical activity, and dietary quality. *Int J Sport Nutr* 4:289–298, 1994.

53. Keith RE, Stone MH, Carson RE, Lefavi RG, Fleck SJ. Nutritional status and lipid profiles of trained steroid-using bodybuilders. *Int J Sport Nutr* 6:247–254, 1996.

54. Nelson Steen S, Mayer K, Brownell KD, Wadden TA. Dietary intake of female collegiate heavyweight rowers. *Int J Sport Nutr* 5:225–231, 1995.

55. Fogelholm GM, Himberg JJ, Alopaeus K, et al. Dietary and biochemical indices of nutritional status in male athletes and controls. *J Am Coll Nutr* 11:181–191, 1992.

56. Butterworth DE, Nieman DC, Butler JV, Herring JL. Feeding patterns of marathon runners. *Int J Sport Nutr* 4:1–7, 1994.

57. Faber M, Spinnler Benadé AJ. Mineral and vitamin intake in field athletes (discus-, hammer-, javelin-throwers and shot-putters). *Int J Sports Med* 12:324–327, 1991.

58. Burke LM, Gollan RA, Read RSD. Dietary intakes and food use of groups of elite Australian male athletes. *Int J Sport Nutr* 1:378–394, 1991.

59. Fogelholm GM, Rehunen S, Gref CG, et al. Dietary intake and thiamin, iron, and zinc status in elite Nordic skiers during different training periods. *Int J Sport Nutr* 2:351–365, 1992.

60. Van Erp-Baart AMJ, Saris WHM, Binkhorst RA, et al. Nationwide survey on nutritional habits in elite athletes: Part I. Energy, carbohydrate, protein, and fat intake. *Int J Sports Med* 10(suppl 1):S3–S10, 1989.

61. Van Erp-Baart AMJ, Saris WHM, Binkhorst RA, et al. Nationwide survey on nutritional habits in elite athletes: Part II. Mineral and vitamin intake. *Int J Sports Med* 10(suppl 1):S11–S16, 1989.

62. Brotherhood JR. Nutrition and sports performance. *Sports Med* 1:350–389, 1984.

63. Burke LM, Diet GD, Read RSD. Diet patterns of elite Australian male triathletes. *Physician Sportsmed* 15(2):140–155, 1987.

64. Ellsworth NM, Hewitt BF, Haskell WL. Nutrient intake of elite male and female Nordic skiers. *Physician Sportsmed* 13(2):78–92, 1985.

65. Hickson JF, Duke MA, Risser WL, et al. Nutritional intake from food sources of high school football athletes. *J Am Diet Assoc* 87:1656–1659, 1988.

66. Nowak RK, Knudsen KS, Schultz LO. Body composition and nutrient intakes of college men and women basketball players. *J Am Diet Assoc* 88:575–578, 1988.

67. Singh A, Evans P, Gallagher KL, Deuster PA. Dietary intakes and biochemical profiles of nutritional status of ultramarathoners. *Med Sci Sports Exerc* 25:328–334, 1993.

68. Sundgot-Borgen J. Risk and trigger factors for the development of eating disorders in female elite athletes. *Med Sci Sports Exerc* 26:414–419, 1994.

69. American Dietetic Association. Timely statement of the American Dietetic Association: Nutrition guidance for adolescent athletes in organized sports. *J Am Diet Assoc* 96:611–612, 1996.

70. Kirchner EM, Lewis RD, O'Connor PJ. Bone mineral density and dietary intake of female college gymnasts. *Med Sci Sports Exerc* 27:543–549, 1995.

71. O'Connor PJ, Lewis RD, Kirchner EM, Cook DB. Eating disorder symptoms in former female college gymnasts: Relations with body composition. *Am J Clin Nutr* 64:840–843, 1996.

72. Walberg-Rankin J, Edmonds CE, Gwazdauskas FC. Diet and weight changes in female bodybuilders before and after competition. *Int J Sport Nutr* 3:87–102, 1993.

73. Thompson J, Manore MM, Skinner JS. Resting metabolic rate and thermic effect of a meal in low- and adequate-energy intake male endurance athletes. *Int J Sport Nutr* 3:194–206, 1993.

74. Faber M, Benadé AJS, van Eck M. Dietary intake, anthropometric measurements, and blood lipid values in weight training athletes (body builders). *Int J Sports Med* 7:342–346, 1986.

75. Sundgot-Borgen J. Nutrient intake of female elite athletes suffering from eating disorders. *Int J Sport Nutr* 3:431–442, 1993.

76. Rosen LW, Hough DO. Pathogenic weight-control behaviors of female college gymnasts. *Physician Sportsmed* 16(9):141–146, 1988.

77. Edwards JE, Lindeman AK, Mikesky AE, Stager JM. Energy balance in highly trained female endurance runners. *Med Sci Sports Exerc* 25:1398–1404, 1993.

78. Nieman DC, Butler JV, Pollett LM, Dietrich SJ, Lutz RD. Nutrient intake of marathon runners. *J Am Diet Assoc* 89:1273–1278, 1989.

79. Horswill CA. Weight loss and weight cycling in amateur wrestlers: Implications for performance and resting metabolic rate. *Int J Sport Nutr* 3:245–260, 1993.

80. Hickner RC, Horswill CA, Welker JM, Scott J, Roemmich JN, Costill DL. Test development for the study of physical performance in wrestlers following weight loss. *Int J Sports Med* 12:557–562, 1991.

81. Walberg Rankin J, Ocel JV, Craft LL. Effect of weight loss and refeeding diet composition on anaerobic performance in wrestlers. *Med Sci Sports Exerc* 28:1292–1299, 1996.

82. American College of Sports Medicine. Weight loss in wrestlers. *Med Sci Sports Exerc* 28:ix–xii, 1996.

83. Butterworth DE, Nieman DC, Perkins R, Warren BJ, Dotson RG. Exercise training and nutrient intake in elderly women. *J Am Diet Assoc* 93:653–657, 1993.

84. Nieman DC, Onasch LM, Lee JW. The effects of moderate exercise training on nutrient intake in mildly obese women. *J Am Diet Assoc* 90:1557–1562, 1990.

85. Blair SN, Jacobs DR, Powell KE. Relationships between exercise or physical activity and other health behaviors. *Public Health Reports* 100:172–179, 1985.

86. Matthews CE, Hebert JR, Ockene IS, Saperia G, Merriam PA. Relationship between leisure-time physical activity and selected dietary variables in the Worcester area trial for counseling in hyperlipidemia. *Med Sci Sports Exerc* 29:1199–1207, 1997.

87. Simoes EJ, Byers T, Coates RJ, Serdula MK, Mokdad AH, Health GW. The association between leisure-time physical activity and dietary fat in American adults. *Am J Public Health* 85:240–244, 1995.

88. Bedgood BL, Tuck MB. Nutrition knowledge of high school athletic coaches in Texas. *J Am Diet Assoc* 83:672–677, 1983. See also *J Am Diet Assoc* 84:1198, 1984.

89. Parr RB, et al. Nutrition knowledge and practice of coaches, trainers, and athletes. *Physician Sportsmed* 12:127, 1984.

90. Barr SI. Nutrition knowledge of female varsity athletes and university students. *J Am Diet Assoc* 87:1660–1664, 1987.

91. Jacobson BH, Gemmell HA. Nutrition information sources of college varsity athletes. *J Appl Sport Res* 5:204–207, 1991.

92. Sossin K, Gizis F, Marquart LF, Sobal J. Nutrition beliefs, attitudes, and resource use of high school wrestling coaches. *Int J Sport Nutr* 7:219–228, 1997.

93. ADA Reports. Position of the American Dietetic Association and the Canadian Dietetic Association: Nutrition for physical fitness and athletic performance for adults. *J Am Diet Assoc* 93:691–696, 1993.

94. McCardle WD, Katch FI, Katch VL. *Exercise Physiology: Energy, Nutrition, and Human Performance* (4th ed.). Baltimore: Williams & Wilkins, 1996.

95. Wilmore JH, Costill DL. *Physiology of Sports and Exercise.* Champaign, IL: Human Kinetics, 1994.

96. Brooks GA, Fahey TD, White TP. *Exercise Physiology: Human Bioenergetics and Its Applications* (2nd ed.). Mountain View, CA: Mayfield Publishing Company, 1996.

97. White JA. Ergogenic demands of a 24 hour cycling event. *Br J Sports Med* 18:165, 1984.

98. Saris WHM, Van Erp-Baart MA, Brouns F, Westerterp KR, Ten Hoor F. Study on food intake and energy expenditure during extreme sustained exercise: The Tour de France. *Int J Sports Med* 10(suppl 1):S26–S31, 1989.

99. Brouns F, Saris WHM, Stroecken J, et al. Eating, drinking, and cycling: A controlled Tour de France simulation study: Part I. *Int J Sports Med* 10(suppl 1):S32–S40, 1989.

100. Brouns F, Saris WHM, Stroecken J, et al. Eating, drinking, and cycling: A controlled Tour de France simulation study: Part II. Effect of diet manipulation. *Int J Sports Med* 10(suppl 1):S41–S48, 1989.

101. Barr SI, Costill DL. Effect of increased training volume on nutrient intake of male collegiate swimmers. *Int J Sports Med* 13:47–51, 1992.

102. Edwards JE, Lindeman AK, Mikesky AE, Stager JM. Energy balance in highly trained female endurance runners. *Med Sci Sports Exerc* 25:1398–1404, 1993.

103. Hagerman FC. Energy metabolism and fuel utilization. *Med Sci Sports Exerc* 24:S309–S314, 1992.

104. Nieman DC, Carlson KA, Brandstater ME, et al. Running exhaustion in 27-h fasted humans. *J Appl Physiol* 63:2502–2509, 1987.

105. Coyle EF, Coggan AR, Hemmert MK, Ivy JL. Muscle glycogen utilization during prolonged strenuous exercise when fed carbohydrate. *J Appl Physiol* 61:165–172, 1986.

106. Bergstrom J, Hermansen L, Hultman E, et al. Diet, muscle glycogen and physical performance. *Acta Physiol Scand* 71:140–150, 1967.

107. Christensen EH, Hansen O. Hypoglykamie, arbeitsfahigkeit und ermudung. *Scand Arch Physiol* 81:172–179, 1939.

108. Christensen EH, Hansen O. Respiratorischer quotient und O_2 aufnahme. *Scand Arch Physiol* 81:180–189, 1939.

109. Fink WJ, Costill DL. Skeletal muscle structure and function. In Maud PJ, Foster C (eds), *Physiological Assessment of Human Fitness.* Champaign, IL: Human Kinetics, 1995.

110. Bergstrom J, Hermansen L, Hultman E, et al. Diet, muscle glycogen and physical performance. *Acta Physiol Scand* 71:140–150, 1967.

111. Bergstrom J, Hultman E. A study of the glycogen metabolism during exercise in man. *Scan J Clin Lab Invest* 19:218–228, 1967.

112. Hargreaves M. Interactions between muscle glycogen and blood glucose during exercise. *Exerc Sport Sci Rev* 25:21–39, 1997.

113. Coyle EF. Substrate utilization during exercise in active people. *Am J Clin Nutr* 61(suppl):968S–979S, 1995.

114. Coggan AR. Plasma glucose metabolism during exercise: Effect of endurance training in humans. *Med Sci Sports Exerc* 29: 620–627, 1997.

115. Walberg-Rankin J. Dietary carbohydrate as an ergogenic aid for prolonged and brief competitions in sport. *Int J Sport Nutr* 5:S13–S28, 1995.

116. Sherman WM. Metabolism of sugars and physical performance. *Am J Clin Nutr* 62(suppl):228S–241S, 1995.

117. O'Brien MJ, Viguie CA, Mazzeo RS, Brooks GA. Carbohydrate dependence during marathon running. *Med Sci Sports Exerc* 25:1009–1017, 1993.

118. Sherman WM, Wimer GS. Insufficient dietary carbohydrate during training: Does it impair athletic performance? *Int J Sport Nutr* 1:28–44, 1991.

119. Ivy JL. Muscle glycogen synthesis before and after exercise. *Sports Med* 11:6–19, 1991.

120. Simonsen JC, Sherman WM, Lamb DR, et al. Dietary carbohydrate, muscle glycogen, and power output during rowing training. *J Appl Physiol* 70:1500–1505, 1991.

121. Kirkendall DT. Effects of nutrition on performance in soccer. *Med Sci Sports Exerc* 25:1370–1374, 1993.

122. Widrick JJ, Costill DL, Fink WJ, et al. Carbohydrate feedings and exercise performance: Effect of initial muscle glycogen concentration. *J Appl Physiol* 74:2998–3005, 1993.

123. Saltin B, Astrand P-O. Free fatty acids and exercise. *Am J Clin Nutr* 57(suppl):752S–758S, 1993.

124. Costill DL, Miller JM. Nutrition for endurance sports: Carbohydrate and fluid balance. *Int J Sports Med* 1:2–14, 1980.

125. Costill DL, Bowers R, Branam G, Sparks K. Muscle glycogen utilization during prolonged exercise on successive days. *J Appl Physiol* 63:2388–2395, 1971.

126. Costill DL, Flynn MG, Kirwan JP, et al. Effects of repeated days of intensified training on muscle glycogen and swimming performance. *Med Sci Sports Exerc* 20:249–254, 1988.

127. Kirwan JP, Costill DL, Mitchell JB, et al. Carbohydrate balance in competitive runners during successive days of intense training. *J Appl Physiol* 65:2601–2606, 1988.

128. Fallowfield JL, Williams C. Carbohydrate intake and recovery from prolonged exercise. *Int J Sport Nutr* 3:150–164, 1993.

129. Sherman WM. Recovery from endurance exercise. *Med Sci Sports Exerc* 24(suppl):S336–S339, 1992.

130. Pascoe DD, Costill DL, Fink WJ, Robergs RA, Zachwieja JJ. Glycogen resynthesis in skeletal muscle following resistive exercise. *Med Sci Sports Exerc* 25:349–354, 1993.

131. Parkin JA, Carey MF, Martin IK, Stojanovska L, Febbraio MA. Muscle glycogen storage following prolonged exercise: Effect of timing of ingestion of high glycemic index food. *Med Sci Sports Exerc* 29:220–224, 1997.

132. Burke LM, Collier GR, Davis PG, Fricker PA, Sanigorski AJ, Hargreaves M. Muscle glycogen storage after prolonged exercise: Effect of the frequency of carbohydrate feedings. *Am J Clin Nutr* 64:115–119, 1996.

133. Hickner RC, Fisher JS, Hansen PA, Racette SB, Mier CM, Turner MJ, Holloszy JO. Muscle glycogen accumulation after endurance exercise in trained and untrained individuals. *J Appl Physiol* 83:897–903, 1997.

134. Van Den Bergh AJ, Houtman S, Heerschap A, et al. Muscle glycogen recovery after exercise during glucose and fructose intake monitored by ^{13}C-NMR. *J Appl Physiol* 81:1495–1500, 1996.

135. Walton P, Rhodes ED. Glycemic index and optimal performance. *Sports Med* 23:164–172, 1997.

136. American College of Sports Medicine. Position stand on exercise and fluid replacement. *Med Sci Sports Exerc* 28:i–vii, 1996.

137. Murray R. Drink more! *ACSM's Health & Fitness Journal* 1(1): 19–50, 1997.

138. Verdaguer-Codina J, Martin DE, Pujol-Amat P, Ruiz A, Prat JA. Climatic heat stress studies at the Barcelona Olympic games, 1992. *Sports Med Train Rehab* 6:167–192, 1995.

139. Sparling PB. Expected environmental conditions for the 1996 summer Olympic games in Atlanta. *Clin J Sport Med* 5:220–222, 1995.

140. Armstrong LE, Maresh CM. The exertional heat illnesses: A risk of athletic participation. *Med Exerc Nutr Health* 2:125–134, 1993.

141. Murray R. Nutrition for the marathon and other endurance sports: Environmental stress and dehydration. *Med Sci Sports Exerc* 24(suppl):S319–S323, 1992.

142. Sawka MN. Physiological consequences of hypohydration: Exercise performance and thermoregulation. *Med Sci Sports Exerc* 24:657–670, 1992.

143. Kenney WL, Johnson JM. Control of skin blood flow during exercise. *Med Sci Sports Exerc* 24:303–312, 1992.

144. Nose H, Mack GW, Shi X, Nadel ER. Shift in body fluid compartments after dehydration in humans. *J Appl Physiol* 65: 318–324, 1988.

145. Gisolfi CV, Wenger CB. Temperature regulation during exercise: Old concepts, new ideas. In Terjung RL (ed), *Exercise and Sport Sciences Reviews*. Lexington: Collamore Press, 1984.

146. Perlmutter EM. The Pittsburgh marathon: 'Playing weather roulette.' *Physician Sportsmed* 14(8):132–138, 1986.

147. Armstrong LE, Hubbard RW, Jones BH, Daniels JT. Preparing Alberto Salazar for the heat of the 1984 Olympic marathon. *Physician Sportsmed* 14(3):73–81, 1986.

148. Gonzalez-Alonso J, Mora-Rodriguez R, Below PR, Coyle EF. Dehydration reduces cardiac output and increases systemic and cutaneous vascular resistance during exercise. *J Appl Physiol* 79:1487–1496, 1995.

149. Murray R. Fluid needs in hot and cold environments. *Int J Sport Nutr* 5:S62–S73, 1995.

150. Greenleaf JE, Harrison MH. Water and electrolytes. In Layman DK (ed), *Nutrition and Aerobic Exercise*. Washington, DC: American Chemical Society, 1986.

151. Coyle EF. Fluid and carbohydrate replacement during exercise: How much and why? *Sports Science Exchange* 7(3):1–6, 1994.

152. Aoyagi Y, McLellan TM, Shephard RJ. Interactions of physical training and heat acclimation: The thermophysiology of exercising in a hot climate. *Sports Med* 23:173–210, 1997.

153. Yamazaki F, Fujii N, Sone R, Ikegami H. Responses of sweating and body temperature to sinusoidal exercise in physically trained men. *J Appl Physiol* 80:491–495, 1996.

154. Barr SI, Costill DL, Fink WJ. Fluid replacement during prolonged exercise: Effects of water, saline, or no fluid. *Med Sci Sports Exerc* 23:811–817, 1991.

155. Noakes TD. Fluid replacement during exercise. *Exerc Sport Sci Rev* 21:297–330, 1993.

156. Hamilton MC, Gonzalez-Alonso J, Montain SJ, Coyle EF. Fluid replacement and glucose infusion during exercise prevent cardiovascular drift. *J Appl Physiol* 71:871–877, 1991.

157. Holtzhausen LM, Noakes TD. The prevalence and significance of post-exercise (postural) hypotension in ultramarathon runners. *Med Sci Sports Exerc* 27:1595–1601, 1995.

158. Rico-Sanz J, Frontera WR, Rivera MA, Rivera-Brown A, Mole PA, Meredith CN. Effects of hyperhydration on total body water, temperature regulation and performance of elite young soccer players in a warm climate. *Int J Sports Med* 17:85–91, 1996.

159. Armstrong LE, Maresh CM, Castellani JW, Bergeron MF, Kenefick RW, LaGasse KE, Riebe D. Urinary indices of hydration status. *Int J Sport Nutr* 4:265–279, 1994.

160. Rehrer NJ. The maintenance of fluid balance during exercise. *Int J Sports Med* 15:122–125, 1994.

161. Wilk B, Bar-Or O. Effect of drink flavor and NaCl on voluntary drinking and hydration in boys exercising in the heat. *J Appl Physiol* 80:1112–1117, 1996.

162. Bassett DR, Nagle FJ, Mookerjee S, et al. Thermoregulatory responses to skin wetting during prolonged treadmill running. *Med Sci Sports Exerc* 19:28–32, 1987.

163. Burke LM, Hawley JA. Fluid balance in team sports: Guidelines for optimal practices. *Sports Med* 24:38–54, 1997.

164. Hawley JA, Dennis SC, Noakes TD. Carbohydrate, fluid, and electrolyte requirements of the soccer player: A review. *Int J Sport Nutr* 4:221–236, 1994.

165. Duchman SM, Ryan AJ, Schedl HP, Summers RW, Bleiler TL, Gisolfi CV. Upper limit for intestinal absorption of a dilute glucose solution in men at rest. *Med Sci Sports Exerc* 29:482–488, 1997.

166. Cunningham JJ. Is potassium needed in sports drinks for fluid replacement during exercise? *Int J Sport Nutr* 7:154–159, 1997.

167. Gisolfi CV, Summers RD, Schedl HP, Bleiler TL. Effect of sodium concentration in a carbohydrate–electrolyte solution on intestinal absorption. *Med Sci Sports Exerc* 10:1414–1420, 1995.

168. Gisolfi CV, Duchman SM. Guidelines for optimal replacement beverages for different athletic events. *Med Sci Sports Exerc* 24:679–687, 1992.

169. Coggan AR, Coyle EF. Carbohydrate ingestion during prolonged exercise: Effects on metabolism and performance. *Exerc Sport Sci Rev* 19:1–40, 1991.

170. Coyle EF. Carbohydrate supplementation during exercise. *J Nutr* 122:788–795, 1992.

171. Coggan AR, Swanson SC. Nutritional manipulations before and during endurance exercise: Effects on performance. *Med Sci Sports Exerc* 24(suppl):S331–S335, 1992.

172. Brouns F, Saris W, Schneider H. Rationale for upper limits of electrolyte replacement during exercise. *Int J Sport Nutr* 2:229–238, 1992.

173. Noakes TD. The hyponatremia of exercise. *Int J Sport Nutr* 2:205–228, 1992.

174. Shirreffs SM, Taylor AJ, Leiper JB, Maughan RJ. Post-exercise rehydration in man: Effects of volume consumed and drink sodium content. *Med Sci Sports Exerc* 28:1260–1271, 1996.

175. Jeukendrup A, Brouns F, Wagenmakers AJM, Saris WHM. Carbohydrate–electrolyte feedings improve 1h time trial cycling performance. *Int J Sports Med* 18:125–129, 1997.

176. Tsintzas OK, Williams C, Singh R, Wilson W, Burrin J. Influence of carbohydrate–electrolyte drinks on marathon running performance. *Eur J Appl Physiol* 70:154–160, 1995.

177. Tsintzas OK, Williams C, Boobis L, Greenhaff P. Carbohydrate ingestion and single muscle fiber glycogen metabolism during prolonged running in men. *J Appl Physiol* 81:801–809, 1996.

178. Millard-Stafford M, Rosskopf LB, Snow TK, Hinson BT. Water versus carbohydrate–electrolyte ingestion before and during a 15-km run in the heat. *Int J Sport Nutr* 7:26–38, 1997.

179. Massicotte D, Peronnet F, Adopo E, Brisson GR, Hillaire-Marcel C. Effect of metabolic rate on the oxidation of ingested glucose and fructose during exercise. *Int J Sports Med* 15:177–180, 1994.

180. Tsintzas K, Liu R, Williams C, Campbell I, Gaitanos G. The effect of carbohydrate ingestion on performance during a 30-km race. *Int J Sport Nutr* 3:127–139, 1993.

181. Yaspelkis BB, Patterson JG, Anderla PA, Ding Z, Ivy JL. Carbohydrate supplementation spares muscle glycogen during variable-intensity exercise. *J Appl Physiol* 75:1477–1485, 1993.

182. Spodaryk K, Czekaj J, Sowa W. Relationship among reduced level of stored iron and dietary iron in trained women. *Physiol Res* 45:393–397, 1996.

183. Fogelholm M. Indicators of vitamin and mineral status in athletes' blood: A review. *Int J Sport Nutr* 5:267–284, 1995.

184. Clarkson PM, Haymes EM. Exercise and mineral status of athletes: Calcium, magnesium, phosphorus, and iron. *Med Sci Sports Exerc* 27:831–843, 1995.

185. Haymes EM, Lamanca JJ. Iron loss in runners during exercise: Implications and recommendations. *Sports Med* 7:277–285, 1989.

186. Pate RR, Miller BJ, Davis JM, Slentz CA, Klingshirn LA. Iron status of female runners. *Int J Sport Nutr* 3:222–231, 1993.

187. Clement DB, Asmundson RC. Nutritional intake and hematological parameters in endurance runners. *Physician Sportsmed* 10:37–43, 1982.

188. Durstine JL, Pate RR, Sparling PB, et al. Lipid, lipoprotein, and iron status of elite women distance runners. *Int J Sports Med* 8(suppl):119–123, 1987.

189. Risser WL, Lee EJ, Poindexter HBW, et al. Iron deficiency in female athletes: Its prevalence and impact on performance. *Med Sci Sports Exerc* 20:116–121, 1988.

190. Magazanik A, Weinstein Y, Dlin RA, et al. Iron deficiency caused by 7 weeks of intensive physical exercise. *Eur J Appl Physiol* 57:198–202, 1988.

191. Eichner ER. Sports anemia, iron supplements, and blood doping. *Med Sci Sports Exerc* (suppl):S315–S318, 1992.

192. Weight LM. Sports anemia: Does it exist? *Sports Med* 16:1–4, 1993.

193. Blum SM, Sherman AR, Boileau RA. The effects of fitness-type exercise on iron status in adult women. *Am J Clin Nutr* 43:456–463, 1986.

194. Bourque SP, Pate RR, Branch D. Twelve weeks of endurance exercise training does not affect iron status measures in women. *J Am Diet Assoc* 97:1116–1121, 1997.

195. Herbert V. Recommended dietary intakes (RDI) of iron in humans. *Am J Clin Nutr* 45:679–686, 1987.

196. Expert Scientific Working Group. Summary of a report on assessment of the iron nutritional status of the United States population. *Am J Clin Nutr* 42:1318–1330, 1985.

197. Looker AC, Dallman PR, Carroll MD, Gunter EW, Johnson CL. Prevalence of iron deficiency in the United States. *JAMA* 277:973–976, 1997.

198. Matter M, Stittfall T, Graves J, et al. The effect of iron and folate therapy on maximal exercise performance in female marathon runners with iron and folate deficiency. *Clinical Science* 72:415–422, 1987.

199. Perkkio MV. Work performance in iron deficiency of increasing severity. *J Appl Physiol* 58:1477–1480, 1985.

200. Li R, Chen X, Yan H, Deurenberg P, Garby L, Hautvast JGAJ. Functional consequences of iron supplementation in iron-deficient female cotton mill workers in Beijing, China. *Am J Clin Nutr* 59:908–913, 1994.

201. Moore RJ, Friedl KE, Tulley RT, Askew EW. Maintenance of iron status in healthy men during an extended period of stress and physical activity. *Am J Clin Nutr* 58:923–927, 1993.

202. Weight LM, Klein M, Noakes TD, Jacobs P. Sports anemia—a real or apparent phenomenon in endurance-trained athletes? *Int J Sports Med* 13:344–347, 1992.

203. Zhu YI, Haas JD. Iron depletion without anemia and physical performance in young women. *Am J Clin Nutr* 66:334–341, 1997.

204. Lamanca JJ, Haymes EM. Effects of low ferritin concentration on endurance performance. *Int J Sport Nutr* 2:376–385, 1992.

205. Klingshirn LA, Pate RR, Bourque SP, Davis JM, Sargent RG. Effect of iron supplementation on endurance capacity in iron-depleted female runners. *Med Sci Sports Exerc* 24:819–824, 1992.

206. Powell PD, Tucker A. Iron supplementation and running performance in female cross-country runners. *Int J Sports Med* 12:462–467, 1991.

207. Telford RD, Bunney CJ, Catchpole EA, et al. Plasma ferritin concentration and physical work capacity in athletes. *Int J Sport Nutr* 2:335–342, 1992.

208. Lamanca JJ, Haymes EM. Effects of iron repletion on $\dot{V}O_{2max}$, endurance, and blood lactate in women. *Med Sci Sports Exerc* 25:1386–1392, 1993.

209. Snyder AC, Dvorak LL, Roepke JB. Influence of dietary iron source on measures of iron status among female runners. *Med Sci Sports Exerc* 21:7–10, 1989.

210. O'Toole ML, Hiller WDB, Roalstad MS, Douglas PS. Hemolysis during triathlon races: Its relation to race distance. *Med Sci Sports Exerc* 20:272–275, 1988.

211. Miller BJ, Pate RR, Burgess W. Foot impact force and intravascular hemolysis during distance running. *Int J Sports Med* 9:56–60, 1988.

212. Waller MF, Haymes EM. The effects of heat and exercise on sweat iron loss. *Med Sci Sports Exerc* 28:197–203, 1996.

213. Stewart JG. Gastrointestinal blood loss and anemia in runners. *Ann Intern Med* 100:843–845, 1984.

214. McMahon LF. Occult gastrointestinal blood loss in marathon runners. *Ann Intern Med* 100:846–847, 1984. See also *Br Med J* 287:1427, 1983.

215. Weight LM, Byrne MJ, Jacobs P. Hemolytic effects of exercise. *Clin Sci* 81:147–152, 1991.

216. Rockey DC, Cello JP. Evaluation of the gastrointestinal tract in patients with iron-deficiency anemia. *N Engl J Med* 329:1691–1695, 1993.

217. Ehn L, Carlmark B, Hoglund S. Iron status in athletes involved in intense physical activity. *Med Sci Sports Exerc* 12:61–64, 1980.

218. International Center for Sports Nutrition, United States Olympic Committee. *Iron and Physical Performance.* Omaha, NE: Author, 1990.

219. Browne RJ. Evaluating and treating active patients for anemia. *Physician Sportsmed* 24(9):79–83, 1996.

220. Schmid A, Jakob E, Berg A, et al. Effect of physical exercise and vitamin C on absorption of ferric sodium citrate. *Med Sci Sports Exerc* 28:1470–1473, 1996.

221. Simmer K, Iles CA, James C, et al. Are iron-folate supplements harmful? *Am J Clin Nutr* 45:122–125, 1987.

222. Nieman DC. Vegetarian dietary practices and endurance performance. *Am J Clin Nutr* 48:754–761, 1988.

223. Belko AZ. Vitamins and exercise—an update. *Med Sci Sports Exerc* 19:S191–S196, 1987.

224. Van der Bek EJ. Vitamins and endurance training: Food for running or faddish claims? *Sports Med* 2:175–197, 1985.

225. Haymes EM. Vitamin and mineral supplementation to athletes. *Int J Sport Nutr* 1:146–169, 1991.

226. Lukaski HC. Micronutrients (magnesium, zinc, and copper): Are mineral supplements needed for athletes? *Int J Sport Nutr* 5:S74–S83, 1995.

227. Clarkson PM, Haymes EM. Trace mineral requirements for athletes. *Int J Sport Nutr* 4:104–119, 1994.

228. Manore MM. Vitamin B6 and exercise. *Int J Sport Nutr* 4:89–103, 1994.

229. Clark N, Nelson M, Evans W. Nutrition education for elite female runners. *Phys Sportsmed* 16(2):124, 1988.

230. Deuster PA, Kyle SB, Moser PB, Vigersky RA, Singh A, Schoomaker EB. Nutritional survey of highly trained women runners. *Am J Clin Nutr* 45:954, 1986.

231. Nieman DC, Gates JR, Butler JV, Pollett LM, Dietrich SJ, and Lutz RD. Supplementation patterns in marathon runners. *J Am Diet Assoc* 89:1615–1619, 1989.

232. American Dietetic Association. Position of the American Dietetic Association: Vitamin and mineral supplementation. *J Am Diet Assoc* 96:73–77, 1996.

233. Council on Scientific Affairs. Vitamin preparations as dietary supplements and as therapeutic agents. *JAMA* 257:1929–1936, 1987.

234. Callaway CW, McNutt K, Rivlin RS. Statement on vitamin and mineral supplements. *Am J Clin Nutr* 46:1075, 1987.

235. Barnett DW, Conlee RK. The effects of a commercial dietary supplement on human performance. *Am J Clin Nutr* 40:586–590, 1984.

236. Keys A. Vitamin supplementation of U.S. Army rations in relation to fatigue and the ability to do muscular work. *J Nutrition* 23:259–269, 1942. See also *Am J Physiol* 144:5, 1945.

237. Weight LM, Noakes TD, Graves J, Jacobs P, Berman PA. Vitamin and mineral status of trained athletes including the effects of supplementation. *Am J Clin Nutr* 47:186, 1988.

238. Telford RD, Catchpole EA, Deakin V, Hahn AG, Plank AW. The effect of 7 to 8 months of vitamin/mineral supplementation on athletic performance. *Int J Sport Nutr* 2:135–153, 1992.

239. Singh A, Moses FM, Deuster PA. Chronic multivitamin–mineral supplementation does not enhance performance. *Med Sci Sports Exerc* 24:726–732, 1992.

240. Read MH, McGuffin SL. The effect of B-complex supplementation on endurance performance. *J Sports Med* 23:178, 1983.

241. Terblanche S, Noakes TD, Dennis SC, Marais DW, Eckert M. Failure of magnesium supplementation to influence marathon running performance or recovery in magnesium-replete subjects. *Int J Sport Nutr* 2:154–164, 1992.

242. Rokitzki L, Sagredos AN, Feub F, Buchner M, Keul J. Acute changes in vitamin B6 status in endurance athletes before and after a marathon. *Int J Sport Nutr* 4:154–165, 1994.

243. Soares MJ, Satvanaravana K, Famii MS, Jacob CM, Ramana YV, Rao SS. The effect of exercise on the riboflavin status of adult men. *Br J Nutr* 69:541–551, 1993.

244. Manore MM, Helleksen JM, Merkel MS, Skinner JS. Longitudinal changes in zinc status in untrained men: Effects of two different 12-week exercise training programs and zinc supplementation. *J Am Diet Assoc* 93:1165–1168, 1993.

245. Anderson RA, Bryden NA, Polansky MM, Deuster PA. Exercise effects on chromium excretion of trained and untrained men consuming a constant diet. *J Appl Physiol* 64:249–252, 1988.

246. Deuster PA, Day BA, Singh A, Douglass L, Moser-Veillon PB. Zinc status of highly trained women runners and untrained women. *Am J Clin Nutr* 49:1295–1301, 1989.

247. Lukaski HC, Hoverson BS, Gallagher SK, Bolonchuk WW. Physical training and copper, iron, and zinc status of swimmers. *Am J Clin Nutr* 51:1093–1099, 1990.

248. Fogelholm M. Micronutrient status in females during a 24-week fitness-type exercise program. *Ann Nutr Metab* 36:209–218, 1992.

249. van der Beck EJ, van Dokkum W, Schrijver J, et al. Thiamin, riboflavin, and vitamins B-6 and C: Impact of combined restricted intake on functional performance in man. *Am J Clin Nutr* 48:1451–1462, 1989.

250. Ji LL. Exercise, oxidative stress, and antioxidants. *Am J Sports Med* 24:S20–S24, 1996.

251. Ji LL. Exercise and oxidative stress: Role of the cellular antioxidant systems. *Exerc Sport Sci Rev* 23:135–166, 1995.

252. Kanter M. Free radicals and exercise: Effects of nutritional antioxidant supplementation. *Exerc Sport Sci* 23:375–397, 1995.

253. Sen CK. Oxidants and antioxidants in exercise. *J Appl Physiol* 79:675–686, 1995.

254. Vasankari TJ, Kujala UM, Vasankari TM, Vuorimaa T, Ahotupa M. Increased serum and low-density-lipoprotein antioxidant potential after antioxidant supplementation in endurance athletes. *Am J Clin Nutr* 65:1052–1066, 1997.

255. Alessio HM, Goldfarb AH, Cao G. Exercise-induced oxidative stress before and after vitamin C supplementation. *Int J Sport Nutr* 7:1–9, 1997.

256. Tiidus PM, Houston ME. Vitamin E status and response to exercise training. *Sports Med* 20:12–23, 1995.

257. Clarkson PM. Antioxidants and physical performance. *Crit Rev Food Sci Nutr* 35:131–141, 1995.

258. Tessier F, Margaritis I, Richard MJ, Moynot C, Marconnet P. Selenium and training effects on the glutathione system and aerobic performance. *Med Sci Sports Exerc* 27:390–396, 1995.

259. Wood RJ, Zheng JJ. High dietary calcium intakes reduce zinc absorption and balance in humans. *Am J Clin Nutr* 65:1803–1809, 1997.

260. Yadrick MK, Kenney MA, Winterfeldt EA. Iron, copper, and zinc status: Response to supplementation with zinc or zinc and iron in adult females. *Am J Clin Nutr* 49:145–150, 1989.

261. Institute of Food Technologists' Expert Panel on Food Safety and Nutrition. Food nutrient interactions. *Food Technology,* October, 1984, 59–63.

262. Lemon PWR. Do athletes need more dietary protein and amino acids? *Int J Sport Nutr* 5:S39–S61, 1995.

263. Lemon PWR. Protein and amino acid needs of the strength athlete. *Int J Sport Nutr* 1:127–145, 1991.

264. Lamont LS, Patel DG, Kalhan PT. Leucine kinetics in endurance-trained humans. *J Appl Physiol* 69:1–6, 1990.

265. Paul GL. Dietary protein requirements of physically active individuals. *Sports Med* 8:154–176, 1989.

266. Phillips SM, Atkinson SA, Tarnopolsky MA, MacDougall JD. Gender differences in leucine kinetics and nitrogen balance in endurance athletes. *J Appl Physiol* 75:2134–2141, 1993.

267. International Center for Sports Nutrition, United States Olympic Committee. *Protein Implications for Athletes.* Omaha, NE: Author, 1990.

268. Hickson JF, Wolinsky I, Rodriguez GP, et al. Failure of weight training to affect urinary indices of protein metabolism in men. *Med Sci Sports Exerc* 18:563–567, 1986.

269. Dohm GL, Tapscott EB, Kasperek GJ. Protein degradation during endurance exercise and recovery. *Med Sci Sports Exerc* 19:S166–S171, 1987.

270. Tarnopolsky MA, Atkinson SA, MacDougall JD, et al. Evaluation of protein requirements for trained strength athletes. *J Appl Physiol* 73:1986–1995, 1992.

271. Lemon PWR, Tarnopolsky MA, MacDougall JD, Atkinson SA. Protein requirements and muscle mass/strength changes during intensive training in novice bodybuilders. *J Appl Physiol* 73:767–775, 1992.

272. Wolfe RR. Does exercise stimulate protein breakdown in humans? Isotopic approaches to the problem. *Med Sci Sports Exerc* 19:S172–S178, 1987.

273. Tarnopolsky MA, MacDougall JD, Atkinson SA. Influence of protein intake and training status on nitrogen balance and lean body mass. *J Appl Physiol* 64:187–193, 1988.

274. Tipton KD, Ferrando AA, Williams BD, Wolfe RR. Muscle protein metabolism in females swimmers after a combination of resistance and endurance exercise. *J Appl Physiol* 81:2034–2038, 1996.

275. El-Khoury AE, Forslund A, Olsson R, et al. Moderate exercise at energy balance does not affect 24-h leucine oxidation or nitrogen retention in healthy men. *Am J Physiol* 273:E394–E407, 1997.

276. Phillips SM, Tipton KD, Aarsland A, Wolf SE, Wolfe RR. Mixed muscle protein synthesis and breakdown after resistance exercise in humans. *Am J Physiol* 273:E99–E107, 1997.

277. Kreider RB, Miriel V, Bertun E. Amino acid supplementation and exercise performance: Analysis of the proposed ergogenic value. *Sports Med* 16:190–209, 1993.

278. Acheson KJ, Schutz Y, Bessard T, et al. Glycogen storage capacity and de novo lipogenesis during massive carbohydrate overfeeding in man. *Am J Clin Nutr* 48:240–247, 1988.

279. Goss FL, Karam C. The effects of glycogen supercompensation on the electrocardiographic response during exercise. *Res Quart Exerc Sport* 58:68–71, 1987.

280. Sherman WM, Costill DL, Fink WJ, et al. The effect of exercise diet manipulation on muscle glycogen and its subsequent utilization during performance. *Int J Sports Med* 2:114–118, 1981.

281. Blom PCS, Costill DL, Vollestad NK. Exhaustive running: Inappropriate as a stimulus of muscle glycogen supercompensation. *Med Sci Sports Exerc* 19:398–403, 1987.

282. Hawley JA, Schabort EJ, Noakes TD, Dennis SC. Carbohydrate-loading and exercise performance: An update. *Sports Med* 24:73–81, 1997.

283. Williams C, Brewer J, Walker M. The effect of a high carbohydrate diet on running performance during a 30-km treadmill time trial. *Eur J Appl Physiol* 65:18–24, 1992.

284. Karlsson J, Saltin B. Diet, muscle glycogen, and endurance performance. *J Appl Physiol* 31:203–206, 1971.

285. Rauch LHG, Rodger I, Wilson GR, Belonje JD, Dennis SC,

Noakes TD, Hawley JA. The effects of carbohydrate loading on muscle glycogen content and cycling performance. *Int J Sport Nutr* 5:25–36, 1995.

286. Maughan RJ, Greenhaff PL, Leiper JB, Ball D, Lambert CP, Gleeson M. Diet composition and the performance of high-intensity exercise. *J Sports Sci* 15:265–275, 1997.

287. Foster C, Costill DL, Fink WJ. Effects of preexercise feedings on endurance performance. *Med Sci Sports Exerc* 11:1–5, 1979.

288. Keller K, Schwarzkopf R. Preexercise snacks may decrease exercise performance. *Physician Sportsmed* 12:89–91, 1984.

289. Gleeson M, Maugham RJ, Greenhaff PL. Comparison of the effects of pre-exercise feeding of glucose, glycerol, and placebo on endurance and fuel homeostasis in man. *Eur J Appl Physiol* 55:645–653, 1986.

290. Sherman WM, Peden MC, Wright DA. Carbohydrate feedings 1 h before exercise improves cycling performance. *Am J Clin Nutr* 54:866–870, 1991.

291. Hargreaves M, Costill DL, Fink WJ, et al. Effect of pre-exercise carbohydrate feedings on endurance cycling performance. *Med Sci Sports Exerc* 19:33–36, 1987.

292. Burelle Y, Peronnet F, Massicotte D, Brisson GR, Hillaire-Marcel C. Oxidation of ^{13}C-glucose and ^{13}C-fructose ingested as a preexercise meal: Effect of carbohydrate ingestion during exercise. *Int J Sport Nutr* 7:117–127, 1997.

293. Short KR, Sheffield-Moore M, Costill DL. Glycemic and insulinemic responses to multiple preexercise carbohydrate feedings. *Int J Sport Nutr* 7:128–137, 1997.

294. Hendelman DL, Ornstein K, Debold EP, Volpe SL, Freedson PS. Preexercise feeding in untrained adolescent boys does not affect responses to endurance exercise or performance. *Int J Sport Nutr* 7:207–218, 1997.

295. Febbraio MA, Stewart KL. CHO feeding before prolonged exercise: Effect of glycemic index on muscle glycogenolysis and exercise performance. *J Appl Physiol* 81:1115–1120, 1996.

296. van Zant RS, Lemon PW. Preexercise sugar feeding does not alter prolonged exercise muscle glycogen or protein catabolism. *Can J Appl Physiol* 22:268–279, 1997.

297. Neufer PD, Costill DL, Flynn MG, et al. Improvements in exercise performance: Effects of carbohydrate feedings and diet. *J Appl Physiol* 62:983–988, 1987.

298. Wright DA, Sherman WM, Dernbach AR. Carbohydrate feedings before, during, or in combination improve cycling endurance performance. *J Appl Physiol* 71:1082–1088, 1991.

299. Aragon-Vargas LF. Effects of fasting on endurance exercise. *Sports Med* 16:255–265, 1993.

300. Williams MH. Ergogenic aids: A means to *Citius, Altius, Fortius,* and Olympic gold? *Res Quart Exerc Sport* 67(suppl): 58–64, 1996.

301. Williams MH. Nutritional supplements for strength trained athletes. *Sports Science Exchange* 6(6):1–6, 1993.

302. Williams MH. The gospel truth about dietary supplements. *ACSM's Health & Fitness Journal* 1(1):24–29, 1997.

303. Catlin DH, Murray TH. Performance-enhancing drugs, fair competition, and Olympic sport. *JAMA* 276:231–237, 1996.

304. Armsey TD, Green GA. Nutrition supplements: Science vs hype. *Physician Sportsmed* 25(6):77–92, 1997.

305. Butterfield G. Ergogenic aids: Evaluating sport nutrition products. *Int J Sport Nutr* 6:191–197, 1996.

306. Knopp WD, Wang TW, Bach BR. Ergogenic drugs in sports. *Clin Sports Med* 16:375–392, 1997.

307. Williams MH. Ergogenic and ergolytic substances. *Med Sci Sports Exerc* 24(suppl):S344–S348, 1992.

308. Strauss RH. *Drugs and Performance in Sports.* Philadelphia: W. B. Saunders Company, 1987.

309. Percy EC. Ergogenic aids in athletics. *Med Sci Sports Exerc* 10: 298–303, 1978.

310. Burke LM, Read RSD. Dietary supplements in sport. *Sports Med* 15:43–65, 1993.

311. Sobal J, Marquart LF. Vitamin/mineral supplement use among athletes: A review of the literature. *Int J Sport Nutr* 4: 320–334, 1994.

312. Kanter MM, Williams MH. Antioxidants, carnitine, and choline as putative ergogenic aids. *Int J Sport Nutr* 5:S120–S131, 1995.

313. Clancy SP, Clarkson PM, DeCheke ME, et al. Effects of chromium picolinate supplementation on body composition, strength, and urinary chromium loss in football players. *Int J Sport Nutr* 4:142–153, 1994.

314. Trappe SW, Costill DL, Goodpaster B, Vukovich MD, Fink WJ. The effects of L-carnitine supplementation on performance during interval swimming. *Int J Sports Med* 15:181–185, 1994.

315. Heinonen OJ. Carnitine and physical exercise. *Sports Med* 22: 109–132, 1996.

316. Brouns F, Fogelholm M, van Hall G, Wagenmakers A, Saris WHM. Chronic oral lactate supplementation does not affect lactate disappearance from blood after exercise. *Int J Sport Nutr* 5:117–124, 1995.

317. Dowling EA, Redondo DR, Branch JD, Jones S, McNabb G, Williams MH. Effect of *Eleutherococcus Senticosus* on submaximal and maximal exercise performance. *Med Sci Sports Exerc* 28:482–489, 1996.

318. Lukaski HC, Bolonchuk WW, Siders WA, Milne DB. Chromium supplementation and resistance training: Effects on body composition, strength, and trace element status of men. *Am J Clin Nutr* 63:954–965, 1996.

319. Fawcett JP, Farquhar SJ, Walker RJ, Thou T, Lowe G, Goulding A. The effect of oral vanadyl sulfate on body composition and performance in weight-training athletes. *Int J Sport Nutr* 6: 382–390, 1996.

320. Weston SB, Zhou S, Weatherby RP, Robson SJ. Does exogenous coenzyme Q10 affect aerobic capacity in endurance athletes? *Int J Sport Nutr* 7:197–206, 1997.

321. Spector SA, Jackman MR, Sabounjian LA, Sakkas C, Landers DM, Willis WT. Effect of choline supplementation on fatigue in trained cyclists. *Med Sci Sports Exerc* 27:668–673, 1995.

322. Starling RD, Trappe TA, Short KR, et al. Effect of inosine supplementation on aerobic and anaerobic cycling performance. *Med Sci Sports Exerc* 28:1193–1198, 1996.

323. Hallmark MA, Reynolds TH, DeSouza CA, Dotson CO, Anderson RA, Rogers MA. Effects of chromium and resistive training on muscle strength and body composition. *Med Sci Sports Exerc* 28:139–144, 1996.

324. Engels HJ, Wirth JC. No ergogenic effects of ginseng (*Panax Ginseng* C.A. Meyer) during graded maximal aerobic exercise. *J Am Diet Assoc* 97:1110–1115, 1997.

325. Porter DA, Costill DL, Zachwieja JJ, et al. The effect of oral coenzyme Q10 on the exercise tolerance of middle-aged, untrained men. *Int J Sports Med* 16:421–427, 1995.

326. Clarkson PM. Effects of exercise on chromium levels: Is supplementation required? *Sports Med* 23:341–349, 1997.

327. Barron RL, Vanscoy GJ. Natural products and the athlete: Facts and folklore. *Ann Pharmacother* 27:607–615, 1993.

328. Grunewald KK, Bailey RS. Commercially marketed supplements for bodybuilding athletes. *Sports Med* 15:90–103, 1993.

329. Woodhouse M, Williams M, Jackson C. The effects of varying doses of orally ingested bee pollen extract upon selected performance variables. *Athletic Training* 22:26–28, 1987.

330. Stensrund T, Ingjer F, Holm H, Stromme SB. L-tryptophan supplementation does not improve running performance. *Int J Sports Med* 6:481–485, 1992.

331. Wheeler KB, Garleb KA. Gamma oryzanol-plant sterol supplementation: Metabolic, endocrine, and physiologic effects. *Int J Sport Nutr* 1:170–177, 1991.

332. Bucci LR, Hickson JF, Wolinsky I, Pivarnik JM. Ornithine supplementation and insulin release in bodybuilders. *Int J Sport Nutr* 2:287–291, 1992.

333. Clarkson PM. Nutritional ergogenic aids: Carnitine. *Int J Sport Nutr* 2:185–190, 1992.

334. Ferrando AA, Green NR. The effect of boron supplementation on lean body mass, plasma testosterone levels, and strength in male bodybuilders. *Int J Sport Nutr* 3:140–149, 1993.

335. Clarkson PM. Nutritional ergogenic aids: Chromium, exercise, and muscle mass. *Int J Sport Nutr* 1:289–293, 1991.

336. Duffy DJ, Conlee RK. Effects of phosphate loading on leg power and high intensity treadmill exercise. *Med Sci Sports Exerc* 18:674–677, 1986.

337. Bredle DL, Stager JM, Brechue WF, Farber MO. Phosphate supplementation, cardiovascular function, and exercise performance in humans. *J Appl Physiol* 65:1821–1826, 1988.

338. Philen RM, Oritz DI, Auerbach SB, Falk H. Survey of advertising for nutritional supplements in health and bodybuilding magazines. *JAMA* 268:1008–1011, 1992.

339. Brill JB, Keane MW. Supplementation patterns of competitive male and female bodybuilders. *Int J Sport Nutr* 4:398–412, 1994.

340. Larkin T. Bee pollen as a health food. *FDA Consumer,* April, 1984, p. 21.

341. Fennema O. The placebo effect of foods. *Food Technology,* December 1984, 57–67.

342. Turner JA, Deyo RA, Loeser JD, Von Korff M, Fordyce WE. The importance of placebo effects in pain treatment and research. *JAMA* 271:1609–1614, 1994.

343. Strain EC, Mumford GK, Silverman K, Griffiths RR. Caffeine dependence syndrome. *JAMA* 272:1043–1048, 1994.

344. Schardt D, Schmidt S. Caffeine: The inside scoop. *Nutrition Action Health Letter* 23(10):1,4–6, 1996.

345. Leonard TK, Watson RR, Mohs ME. The effects of caffeine on various body systems: A review. *J Am Diet Assoc* 87:1048–1053, 1987.

346. Spriet LL. Caffeine and performance. *Int J Sport Nutr* 5: S84–S99, 1995.

347. Nehlig A, Debry G. Caffeine and sports activity: A review. *Int J Sport Med* 15:215–223, 1994.

348. Cole KJ, Costill DL, Starling RD, Goodpaster BH, Trappe SW, Fink WJ. Effect of caffeine ingestion on perception of effort and subsequent work production. *Int J Sport Nutr* 6:14–23, 1996.

349. Pasman WJ, van Baak MA, Jeukendrup AE, de Haan A. The effect of different dosages of caffeine on endurance performance time. *Int J Sports Med* 16:225–230, 1995.

350. Trice I, Haymes EM. Effects of caffeine ingestion on exercise-induced changes during high-intensity, intermittent exercise. *Int J Sport Nutr* 5:37–44, 1995.

351. Jackman M, Wendling P, Friars D, Graham TE. Metabolic, catecholamine, and endurance responses to caffeine during intense exercise. *J Appl Physiol* 81:1658–1663, 1996.

352. Dodd SL, Herb RA, Powers SK. Caffeine and exercise performance: An update. *Sports Med* 15:14–23, 1993.

353. Clarkson PM. Nutritional ergogenic aids: Caffeine. *Int J Sport Nutr* 3:103–111, 1993.

354. Wilkes D, Gledhill N, Smyth R. Effect of acute induced metabolic alkalosis on 800-m racing time. *Med Sci Sports Exerc* 15: 277–280, 1983.

355. Goldfinch J, Naughton LM, Davies P. Induced metabolic alkalosis and its effects on 400-m racing time. *Eur J Appl Physiol* 57:45–48, 1988.

356. Matson LG, Tran ZV. Effects of sodium bicarbonate ingestion on anaerobic performance: A meta-analytic review. *Int J Sport Nutr* 3:2–28, 1993.

357. Linderman JK, Gosselink KL. The effects of sodium bicarbonate ingestion on exercise performance. *Sports Med* 18:75–80, 1994.

358. Horswill CA. Effects of bicarbonate, citrate, and phosphate loading on performance. *Int J Sport Nutr* 5:S111–S119, 1995.

359. Eichner ER. Blood doping: Results and consequences from the laboratory and the field. *Phys Sportsmed* 15(1):121–129, 1987.

360. Gledhill N. The ergogenic effect of blood doping. *Physician Sportsmed* 11:87–90, 1983.

361. Klein HG. Blood transfusion and athletics. *N Engl J Med* 312: 854–856, 1985.

362. Sawka MN, Young AJ. Acute polycythemia and human performance during exercise and exposure to extreme environments. *Ex Sport Sci Rev* 17:265–293, 1989.

363. Jones M, Pedoe DST. Blood doping—a literature review. *Br J Sport Med* 23:84–88, 1989.

364. Berglund B. Development of techniques for the detection of blood doping in sport. *Sports Med* 5:127–135, 1988.

365. American College of Sports Medicine. Position stand on the use of blood doping as an ergogenic aid. *Med Sci Sports Exerc* 28:i–vii, 1996.

366. Young AJ, Sawka MN, Muza SR, et al. Effects of erythrocyte infusion on V̇O2max at high altitude. *J Appl Physiol* 81:252–259, 1996.

367. Porter DL, Goldberg MA. Physiology of erythropoietin production. *Sem Hematol* 31:112–121, 1994.

368. Cowart VS. Erythropoietin: A dangerous new form of blood doping? *Physician Sportsmed* 17(8):115–118, 1989.

369. Ramotar JE. Cyclists' deaths linked to erythropoietin? *Physician Sportsmed* 18(8):48–50, 1990.

370. Wide L, Bengtsson C, Berglund B, Ekblom B. Detection in blood and urine of recombinant erythropoietin administered to healthy men. *Med Sci Sports Exerc* 27:1569–1576, 1995.

371. Council on Scientific Affairs. Medical and nonmedical uses of anabolic–androgenic steroids. *JAMA* 264:2923–2927, 1990.

372. Yesalis CE, Kennedy NJ, Kopstein AN, Bahrke MS. Anabolic–androgenic steroid use in the United States. *JAMA* 270:1217–1221, 1993.

373. American College of Sports Medicine. Position statement on the use of anabolic–androgenic steroids in sports. *Med Sci Sports Exerc* 19:534–539, 1987.

374. Yesalis CE, Herrick RT, Buckley WE, Friedle KE, et al. Self-reported use of anabolic–androgenic steroids by elite power lifters. *Physician Sportsmed* 16(12):91–100, 1988.

375. Council on Scientific Affairs. Drug abuse in athletes: Anabolic steroids and human growth hormone. *JAMA* 259:1703–1705, 1988.

376. Goldberg L, Elliot D, Clarke GN, et al. Effects of a multidimensional anabolic steroid prevention intervention. *JAMA* 276:1555–1562, 1996.

377. Buckley WE, Yesalis CE, Friedl KE, et al. Estimated prevalence of anabolic steroid use among male high school seniors. *JAMA* 260:3441–3445, 1988.

378. Yesalis CE, Bahrke MS. Anabolic–androgenic steroids: Current issues. *Sports Med* 19:326–340, 1995.

379. DuRant RH, Rickert VI, Ashworth CS, Newman C, Slavens G. Use of multiple drugs among adolescents who use anabolic steroids. *N Engl J Med* 328:922–926, 1993.

380. Forbes GB, Porta CR, Herr BE, Griggs RC. Sequence of changes in body composition induced by testosterone and reversal of changes after drug is stopped. *JAMA* 267:397–399, 1992.

381. Ropp KL. Steroid substitutes: No-win situation for athletes. *FDA Consumer*, December, 1992, 8–12.

382. Alen M, Rahkila P. Anabolic–androgenic steroid effects on endocrinology and lipid metabolism in athletes. *Sports Med* 6:327–332, 1988.

383. Glazer G. Atherogenic effects of anabolic steroids on serum lipid levels: A literature review. *Arch Intern Med* 151:1925–1933, 1991.

384. Lubell A. Does steroid abuse cause—or excuse—violence? *Physician Sportsmed* 17(2):176–185, 1989.

385. Pope HG, Katz DL. Affective and psychotic symptoms associated with anabolic steroid use. *Am J Psychiatry* 145:487–490, 1988

386. Su T-P, Pagliaro M, Schmidt PJ, et al. Neuropsychiatric effects of anabolic steroids in male normal volunteers. *JAMA* 269:2760–2764, 1993.

387. Bhasin S, Storer TW, Berman N, et al. The effects of supraphysiologic doses of testosterone on muscle size and strength in normal men. *N Engl J Med* 335:1–7, 1996.

388. Bronson FH, Matherne CM. Exposure to anabolic–androgenic steroids shortens life span of male mice. *Med Sci Sports Exerc* 29:615–619, 1997.

389. Melchert RB, Welder AA. Cardiovascular effects of androgenic–anabolic steroids. *Med Sci Sports Exerc* 27:1252–1262, 1995.

390. Cohen LI, Hartford CG, Rogers GG. Lipoprotein(a) and cholesterol in body builders using anabolic androgenic steroids. *Med Sci Sports Exerc* 28:176–179, 1996.

391. Bahrke MS, Yesalis CE, Wright JE. Psychological and behavioral effects of endogenous testosterone and anabolic–androgenic steroids: An update. *Sports Med* 22:367–390, 1996.

392. Dodd SL, Powers SK, Vrabas IS, Criswell D, Stetson S, Hussain R. Effects of clenbuterol on contractile and biochemical properties of skeletal muscle. *Med Sci Sports Exerc* 28:669–676, 1996.

393. Maughan RJ. Creatine supplementation and exercise performance. *Int J Sport Nutr* 5:94–101, 1995.

394. Greenhaff PL. Creatine and its applications as an ergogenic aid. *Int J Sport Nutr* 5:S100–S110, 1995.

395. Hultman E, Söderlund K, Timmons JA, Cederblad G, Green-haff PL. Muscle creatine loading in men. *J Appl Physiol* 81:232–237, 1996.

396. Volek JS, Kraemer WJ, Bush JA, et al. Creatine supplementation enhances muscular performance during high-intensity resistance exercise. *J Am Diet Assoc* 97:765–770, 1997.

397. Bosco C, Tihanyi J, Pucspk J, et al. Effect of oral creatine supplementation on jumping and running performance. *Int J Sports Med* 18:369–372, 1997.

398. Mujika I, Chatard J-C, Lacoste L, Barale F, Geyssant A. Creatine supplementation does not improve sprint performance in competitive swimmers. *Med Sci Sports Exerc* 28:1435–1441, 1996.

399. Burke LM, Pyne DB, Telford RD. Effect of oral creatine supplementation on single-effort sprint performance in elite swimmers. *Int J Sport Nutr* 6:222–233, 1996.

400. Redondo DR, Dowling EA, Graham BL, Almada AL, Williams MH. The effect of oral creatine monohydrate supplementation on running velocity. *Int J Sport Nutr* 6:213–221, 1996.

401. Terrillion KA, Kolkhorst FW, Dolgener FA, Joslyn SJ. The effect of creatine supplementation on two 700-m maximal running bouts. *Int J Sport Nutr* 7:138–143, 1997.

402. Odland LM, MacDougall JD, Tarnopolsky MA, Elorriaga A, Borgmann A. Effect of oral creatine supplementation on muscle [PCr] and short-term maximum power output. *Med Sci Sports Exerc* 29:216–219, 1997.

403. Pendergast DR, Horvath PJ, Leddy JJ, Venkatraman JT. The role of dietary fat on performance, metabolism, and health. *Am J Sports Med* 24:S53–S58, 1996.

404. Phillips SM, Green HJ, Tarnopolsky MA, Heigenhauser GJF, Hill RE, Grant SM. Effects of training duration on substrate turnover and oxidation during exercise. *J Appl Physiol* 81:2182–2191, 1996.

405. Martin WH. Effect of endurance training on fatty acid metabolism during whole body exercise. *Med Sci Sports Exerc* 29:635–639, 1997.

406. Martin WH, Dalsky GP, Hurley BF, et al. Effect of endurance training on plasma free fatty acid turnover and oxidation during exercise. *Am J Physiol* 265:E708–E714, 1993.

407. Sherman WM, Leenders N. Fat loading: The next magic bullet. *Int J Sport Nutr* 5:S1–S12, 1995.

408. Saltin B, Astrand P-O. Free fatty acids and exercise. *Am J Clin Nutr* 57(suppl):752S–758S, 1993.

409. Coyle EF. Fat metabolism during exercise. *Sports Science Exchange* 8:1–6, 1995.

410. Coyle EF. Substrate utilization during exercise in active people. *Am J Clin Nutr* 61(suppl):968S–979S, 1995.

411. LaPachet RAB, Miller WC, Arnall DA. Body fat and exercise endurance in trained rats adapted to a high-fat and/or high-carbohydrate diet. *J Appl Physiol* 80:1173–1179, 1996.

412. Jeukendrup AE, Saris WH, Schrauwen P, Brouns F, Wagenmakers AJM. Metabolic availability of medium-chain triglycerides coingested with carbohydrates during prolonged exercise. *J Appl Physiol* 79:756–762, 1995.

413. Berning JR. The role of medium-chain triglycerides in exercise. *Int J Sport Nutr* 6:121–133, 1996.

414. Vukovich MD, Costill DL, Hickey MS, Trappe SW, Cole EJ, Fink WJ. Effect of fat emulsion infusion and fat feeding on muscle glycogen utilization during cycle exercise. *J Appl Physiol* 75:1513–1518, 1993.

415. Johannessen A, Hagen C, Galbo H. Prolactin, growth hor-

mone, thyrotropin, 3,5,3'-triiodothyronine, and thyroxine responses to exercise after fat- and carbohydrate-enriched diet. *J Clin Endocrine Metab* 52:56–61, 1981.

416. Lambert EV, Speechly DP, Dennis SC, Noakes TD. Enhanced endurance in trained cyclists during moderate intensity exercise following 2 weeks adaptation to a high fat diet. *Eur J Appl Physiol* 69:287–293, 1994.

417. Phinney SD, Bistrian BR, Evans WJ, Gervina E, Blackburn GL. The human metabolic response to chronic ketosis without caloric restriction: Preservation of submaximal exercise capability with reduced carbohydrate oxidation. *Metabolism* 32: 769–776, 1983.

418. Costill DL, Coyle EF, Dalsky G, Evans W, Fink W, Hoopes D. Effects of elevated plasma free fatty acids and insulin on muscle glycogen usage during exercise. *J Appl Physiol* 43:695–699, 1977.

419. Satabin P, Portero P, Defer G. Metabolic and hormonal responses to lipid and carbohydrate diets during exercise in man. *Med Sci Sports Exerc* 19:218–223, 1987.

420. Nieman DC. Carbohydrates or fats: Which is best for endurance exercise? *Veg Nutr: Int J* 1:17–21, 1997.

421. Leddy J, Horvath P, Rowland J, Pendergast D. Effect of a high or a low fat diet on cardiovascular risk factors in male and female runners. *Med Sci Sports Exerc* 29:17–25, 1997.

422. Lukaski HC, Bolonchuk WW, Klevay LM, Mahalko JR, Milne DB, Sandstead HH. Influence of type and amount of dietary lipid on plasma lipid concentrations in endurance athletes. *Am J Clin Nutr* 39:35–44, 1984.

423. Thompson PD, Cullinane EM, Eshleman R, Kantor MA, Herbert PN. The effects of high-carbohydrate and high-fat diets on the serum lipid and lipoprotein concentrations of endurance athletes. *Metabolism* 33:1003–1010, 1984.

424. Burke LM, Collier GR, Beasley SK, Davis PG, Fricker PA, Heeley P, Walder K, Hargreaves M. Effects of coingestion of fat and protein with carbohydrate feedings on muscle glycogen storage. *J Appl Physiol* 78:2187–2192, 1995.

425. Tsetsonis N, Hardman, AE, Mastana SS. Acute effects of exercise on postprandial lipemia: A comparative study in trained and untrained middle-aged women. *Am J Clin Nutr* 65: 525–533, 1997.

426. Nieman DC. Immune response to heavy exertion. *J Appl Physiol* 82:1385–1394, 1997.

427. White R, Frank E. Health effects and prevalence of vegetarianism. *West J Med* 160:465–471, 1994.

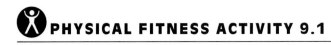

PHYSICAL FITNESS ACTIVITY 9.1

Rating Your Diet by the Food Pyramid

The food pyramid shown early in this chapter is an excellent guide to help you eat healthfully while obtaining all known vitamins and minerals. How close is your diet to the recommendations of the Food Pyramid?

Step 1   Write down *everything* (all fluids and foods) that you ate yesterday.

Food or Beverage	How Much?

Step 2   Referring to Table 9.20, how many servings did you eat from each food group?

Bread, Cereal, Rice, and Pasta Group _____

Vegetable Group _____

Fruit Group _____

Milk, Yogurt, and Cheese Group _____

Meat, Poultry, Fish, Dry Beans, Eggs, and Nuts Group _____

TABLE 9.20 What Counts as a Serving?

Food Groups

Bread, Cereal, Rice, and Pasta

| 1 slice of bread | 1 ounce of ready-to-eat cereal | $^1/_2$ cup of cooked cereal, rice, or pasta |

Vegetable

| 1 cup of raw leafy vegetables | $^1/_2$ cup of other vegetables, cooked or chopped raw | $^3/_4$ cup of vegetable juice |

Fruit

| 1 medium apple, banana, orange | $^1/_2$ cup of chopped, cooked, or canned fruit | $^3/_4$ cup of fruit juice |

Milk, Yogurt, and Cheese

| 1 cup of milk or yogurt | $1^1/_2$ ounces of natural cheese | 2 ounces of processed cheese |

Meat, Poultry, Fish, Dry Beans, Eggs, and Nuts

| 2–3 ounces of cooked lean meat, poultry, or fish | $^1/_2$ cup of cooked dry beans, 1 egg, or 2 tablespoons of peanut butter count as 1 ounce of lean meat |

TABLE 9.21 Sample Diets for a Day at Three Calorie Levels

	Low (about 1,600)	Moderate (about 2,200)	High (about 2,800)
Bread group servings	6	9	11
Vegetable group servings	3	4	5
Fruit group servings	2	3	4
Milk group servings	2–3[a]	2–3[a]	2–3[a]
Meat group[b] (ounces)	5	6	7

[a]Women who are pregnant or breastfeeding, teenagers, and young adults to age 24 need 3 servings.
[b]Meat group amounts are in total ounces.

Step 3 Using the food pyramid at the right and Table 9.21, how do you think your diet compares with the food pyramid? Make sure to adapt servings to your estimated caloric needs.

_____

_____

_____

_____

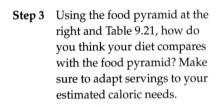

Fats, Oils, and Sweets
USE SPARINGLY

Milk, Yogurt, and Cheese Group
2-3 SERVINGS

Vegetable Group
3-5 SERVINGS

Bread, Cereal, Rice, and Pasta Group
6-11 SERVINGS

Key
These symbols show fat and added sugars in foods
● - Fat (naturally occurring and added)
▼ - Sugars (added)

Meat, Poultry, Fish, Dry Beans, Eggs, and Nuts Group
2-3 SERVINGS

Fruit Group
2-4 SERVINGS

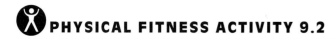

PHYSICAL FITNESS ACTIVITY 9.2

What Is the Carbohydrate Quality of Your Diet?

Starch and most types of dietary fiber are complex carbohydrates. Chemically, they are chains of many sugar molecules. Sugars include table sugar (sucrose), honey, corn syrup, and such, which are simple carbohydrates.

During digestion, starches and sugars are broken down into simple sugar molecules before being absorbed into the body and used for energy. The links between the sugar molecules in dietary fiber cannot be broken by human digestive enzymes. Thus, fiber passes down the intestinal tract and forms bulk for the stool.

Take the following quiz to check your diet for starch and fiber.

	Seldom or never	1–2 times/ week	3–4 times/ week	Almost daily
How often do you eat:				
1. Several servings of breads, cereals, pasta, or rice?	_____	_____	_____	_____
2. Starch vegetables such as potatoes, corn, or peas, or dishes made with dry beans or peas?	_____	_____	_____	_____
3. Whole-grain breads or cereals?	_____	_____	_____	_____
4. Several servings of vegetables?	_____	_____	_____	_____
5. Whole fruit with skins and /or seeds (apples, pears, berries, etc.)?	_____	_____	_____	_____

The best answer to all of the preceding is "Almost daily." Breads, cereals, and other grain products and starch vegetables provide starch. Whole-grain products and fruits and vegetables, especially those with edible skins and seeds, are good sources of fiber.

Note: If you would like a full, computerized analysis of your diet, an excellent computer software program for nutritional analysis can be obtained from

Wellsource Inc.
PO Box 569
15431 SE 82 Dr., Ste. E
Clackamas, OR 97015
503-656-7446

Ask for "Nutrition Profile Plus."

PHYSICAL FITNESS ACTIVITY 9.3

Case Study: Female Vegetarian Fitness Enthusiast with Anemia

Review the data summarized here, which was gathered from a female vegetarian who had been exercising faithfully each day for more than 10 years. Answer the following questions, based on information presented in this chapter, and then discuss your answers with your instructor.

Demographic Data

Age	47 years	Height	66.25 inches
Weight	130 pounds	Percent body fat	16% ("lean")
$\dot{V}O_{2max}$	43.5 ml/kg/min ("good")		
Exercise habits	Daily brisk walking, 30–45 minutes; more than 10 years		

3-Day Food Record Nutrient Intake

Energy intake	2602 Calories/day	Carbohydrate	560 g (86%)
Protein	37 g (6%)	Fat	23 g (8%)
Cholesterol	30.1 mg (<300)	Dietary fiber	29.4 g (20–35)
Iron	17.9 mg (119% RDA)	Zinc	12.2 mg (102%)
Copper	2.3 mg (within RDA range)	Calcium	499 mg (62%)
Vitamin B$_6$	2.62 mg (164%)	Vitamin B$_{12}$	1.2 μg (60%)
Vitamin A	1328 μg RE (166%)	Vitamin C	137 mg (228%)
Vitamin E	4.82 mg α-TE (60%)		

Food exchanges (servings per day)

Meat	1.4 (from legumes)	Milk	0
Bread	6.6	Fruit	12
Vegetable	2.7		

Blood Lipid and Iron Status

Serum cholesterol	178 mg/dl	Serum iron	32 μg/dl (60–180)
HDL cholesterol	51 mg/dl (3:4 ratio)	Hemoglobin	10.2 g/dl (12–16)
Hematocrit	31.4% (37–47)		

1. What would you recommend that this vegetarian woman do to improve her iron status?

_____

_____

2. What changes would you recommend in her diet? (Consider iron, protein, and vegetarian issues.)

_____

_____

PART

IV

Physical Activity and Disease

10

Heart Disease

Regular physical activity or cardiorespiratory fitness decreases the risk of cardiovascular disease mortality in general and of coronary heart disease in particular. The level of decreased risk of coronary heart disease attributable to regular physical activity is similar to that of other lifestyle factors such as keeping free from cigarette smoking.

—Physical Activity and Health: A Report of the Surgeon General, 1996

The circulatory system includes the heart, lungs, arteries, and veins. The normal heart is a strong, muscular pump a little larger then the human fist; within the normal lifetime, it will faithfully beat nearly 3 billion times, pumping 42 million gallons of blood (see Figure 10.1). Unfortunately, many hearts have their work cut short by various diseases related to unhealthy lifestyles.[1,2]

Heart disease is the leading killer of people in the United States and developed countries worldwide (see Figure 10.2)[3]. In this chapter, each of the four major risk factors for heart disease—cigarette smoking, high blood pressure, high blood cholesterol levels, and inactivity—are reviewed, with special attention given to prevention. Each risk factor is also linked to the effects of physical inactivity.

HEART DISEASE

Heart disease, or cardiovascular disease (CVD), comprises diseases of the heart and its blood vessels. CVD is not a single disorder, but a general name for more than 20 different diseases of the heart and its vessels. (See Box 10.1 for a glossary of terms.) The American Heart Association has reminded us that although we have made tremendous progress in fighting CVD, they have been the leading cause of death among Americans in every year but one (1918) since 1900.[1] Every 33 seconds, an American dies of CVD, the underlying cause of just under 1 million deaths annually.

Four of every 10 U.S. coffins contain victims of CVD (see Table 10.1).[1]

Deaths, however, do not tell the whole story, in that of the 260 million Americans alive today, nearly one in four live with some form of CVD. Also, one survey of 90,000 adults in the United States found that only 18% reported having no risk factors for heart disease. In other words, an alarming number of Americans either have CVD or are headed in that direction.[1]

Cancer, according to most surveys, is the disease people fear the most. CVD deserves more respect, however, maintains the National Center for Health Statistics. According to their most recent computations, if all forms of major cardiovascular disease were eliminated, total life expectancy would rise by nearly 10 years. If all forms of cancer were abolished, the gain would be just 3 years.[1]

Atherosclerosis, the build-up of fatty, plaque material in the inner layer of blood vessels, is the underlying factor in 85% of CVD.[4–7] When atherosclerotic plaque blocks one or more of the heart's coronary blood vessels, the diagnosis is coronary heart disease (CHD), the major form of CVD (see Figure 10.3).

Often, a blood clot forms in the narrowed coronary blood artery, blocking the blood flow to the part of the heart muscle supplied by that artery. This causes a heart attack, or what clinicians call a myocardial infarction (MI). Each year, as many as 1,100,000 Americans have a heart attack, and about one third of them die as a result.[1,2]

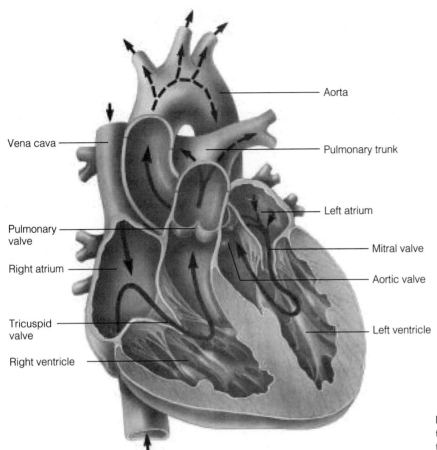

Aorta

Vena cava

Pulmonary trunk

Left atrium

Pulmonary valve

Mitral valve

Right atrium

Aortic valve

Tricuspid valve

Left ventricle

Right ventricle

Figure 10.1 Within the normal lifetime, the average heart will beat nearly 3 billion times, pumping 42 million gallons of blood.

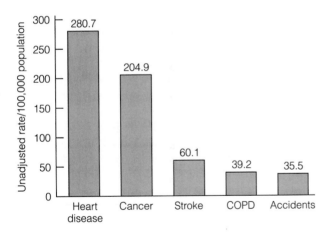

Figure 10.2 Comparison of death rates, 1995. Death rates for the top five leading causes of death in the United States. *Source:* Anderson RN, Kochanek KD, Murphy SL. *Report of Final Mortality Statistics, 1995: Monthly Vital Statistics Report* 45 (11), suppl 2. Hyattsville, MD: National Center for Health Statistics, 1997.

Atherosclerosis can also block blood vessels in the brain (leading to a stroke) or legs (defined as peripheral artery disease).[1] Stroke kills over 150,000 Americans each year and is the third largest cause of death. Peripheral artery disease affects up to 20% of older people and leads to pain in the legs brought on by walking (intermittent claudication). Patients with peripheral artery disease are able to walk only short distances before they must rest to relieve the pain in their legs, brought on by poor circulation due to atherosclerosis. The atherosclerotic plaques range from small yellow streaks to advanced lesions with ulceration, *thrombosis* (formation or existence of a blood clot within the blood vessel system), hemorrhage, and calcification.[4–7]

There are several stages in the development of atherosclerosis[2] (see Figure 10.4). First, the arterial wall is injured by a variety of factors, including high blood pressure

Box 10.1

Glossary of Terms Used in Heart Disease

Following is a list of terms related to heart disease.

aneurysm: A ballooning-out of the wall of a vein, an artery, or the heart, due to weakening of the wall by disease, injury, or an abnormality present at birth.

angina pectoris: Medical term for chest pain due to coronary heart disease; a condition in which the heart muscle does not receive enough blood, resulting in pain in the chest.

angiocardiography: An x-ray examination of the blood vessels or chambers of the heart, by tracing the course of a special fluid (called a contrast medium or dye) visible by x-ray, which has been injected into the bloodstream. The x-ray pictures made are called "angiograms."

angioplasty: A procedure sometimes used to dilate (widen) narrowed arteries; a catheter with a deflated balloon on its tip is passed into the narrowed artery segment, the balloon inflated, and the narrowed segment widened.

arrhythmia (or **dysrhythmia):** An abnormal rhythm of the heart.

arteriosclerosis: Commonly called "hardening of the arteries," this includes a variety of conditions that cause artery walls to thicken and lose elasticity.

atherosclerosis: A form of arteriosclerosis, in which the inner layers of artery walls become thick and irregular due to deposits of fat, cholesterol, and other substances; This buildup is sometimes called "plaque"; as the interior walls of arteries become lined with layers of these deposits, the arteries become narrowed, and the flow of blood through them is reduced.

blood clot: A jellylike mass of blood tissue formed by clotting factors in the blood; this clot can then stop the flow of blood from an injury; blood clots can also form inside an artery with walls damaged by atherosclerotic buildup and can cause a heart attack or stroke.

blood pressure: The force or pressure exerted by the heart in pumping blood; the pressure of blood in the arteries.

bradycardia: Slowness of the heartbeat.

capillaries: Microscopically small blood vessels between arteries and veins, which distribute oxygenated blood to the body's tissues.

cardiac arrest: The stopping of the heartbeat, usually because of interference with the electrical signal (often associated with coronary heart disease).

cardiopulmonary resuscitation (CPR): A technique combining chest compression and mouth-to-mouth breathing; used during cardiac arrest to keep oxygenated blood flowing to the heart muscle and brain until advanced cardiac life support can be started or an adequate heartbeat resumes.

cardiovascular: Pertaining to the heart and blood vessels ("cardio" means heart; "vascular" means blood vessels); the circulatory system of the heart and blood vessels is the cardiovascular system.

carotid artery: A major artery in the neck.

catheterization: The process of examining the heart by introducing a thin tube (catheter) into a vein or artery and passing it into the heart.

cerebral embolism: A blood clot formed in one part of the body and then carried by the bloodstream to the brain, where it blocks an artery.

cerebral hemorrhage: Bleeding within the brain, resulting from a ruptured aneurysm or a head injury.

cerebral thrombosis: Formation of a blood clot in an artery that supplies part of the brain.

cerebrovascular accident: Also called *cerebral vascular accident, apoplexy,* or *stroke;* an impeded blood supply to some part of the brain, resulting in injury to brain tissue.

cholesterol: A fatlike substance found in animal tissue and present only in foods from animal sources, such as whole-milk dairy products, meat, fish, poultry, animal fats, and egg yolks.

circulatory system: Pertaining to the heart, blood vessels, and the circulation of the blood.

collateral circulation: A system of smaller arteries closed under normal circumstances, which may open up and start to carry blood to part of the heart when a coronary artery is blocked; can serve as alternative routes of blood supply.

coronary arteries: Two arteries arising from the aorta, which arch down over the top of the heart, then branch and provide blood to the heart muscle.

coronary artery disease: Conditions that cause narrowing of the coronary arteries, so blood flow to the heart muscle is reduced.

coronary bypass surgery: Surgery to improve blood supply to the heart muscle; most often performed when narrowed coronary arteries reduce the flow of oxygen-containing blood to the heart itself.

coronary heart disease: Disease of the heart caused by atherosclerotic narrowing of the coronary arteries, likely to produce angina pectoris or heart attack; a general term.

(continued)

Glossary of Terms Used in Heart Disease *(continued)*

coronary occlusion: An obstruction of one of the coronary arteries, thereby hindering blood flow to some part of the heart muscle.

coronary thrombosis: Formation of a clot in one of the arteries that conduct blood to the heart muscle; also called coronary occlusion.

echocardiography: A diagnostic method in which pulses of sound are transmitted into the body, and the echoes returning from the surfaces of the heart and other structures are electronically plotted and recorded to produce a "picture" of the heart's size, shape, and movements.

electrocardiogram (ECG or EKG): A graphic record of electrical impulses produced by the heart.

embolus: A blood clot that forms in a blood vessel in one part of the body and then is carried to another part of the body.

endarterectomy: Surgical removal of plaque deposits or blood clots in an artery.

endothelium: The smooth inner lining of many body structures, including the heart (endocardium) and blood vessels.

heart attack: Death of, or damage to, part of the heart muscle, due to an insufficient blood supply.

ischemia: Decreased blood flow to an organ, usually due to constriction or obstruction of an artery.

ischemic heart disease: Also called *coronary artery disease* and *coronary heart disease*; applied to heart ailments (a) caused by narrowing of the coronary arteries, and (b) therefore characterized by a decreased blood supply to the heart.

lipoprotein: The combination of lipid surrounded by a protein, which makes it soluble in blood.

lumen: The opening within a tube, such as a blood vessel.

myocardial infarction: The injury to or death of an area of the heart muscle (*myocardium*), resulting from a blocked blood supply to that area.

myocardium: The muscular wall of the heart; contracts to pump blood out of the heart and then relaxes as the heart refills with returning blood.

nitroglycerin: A drug that causes dilation of blood vessels and is often used in treating angina pectoris.

plaque: Also called atheroma; a deposit of fatty (and other) substances in the inner lining of the artery wall, characteristic of atherosclerosis.

risk factor: An element or condition involving certain hazard or danger; when referring to the heart and blood vessels, a risk factor is associated with an increased chance of developing cardiovascular disease, including stroke.

stroke: Also called *apoplexy, cerebrovascular accident,* or *cerebral vascular accident;* loss of muscle function, vision, sensation, or speech, resulting from brain cell damage, caused by an insufficient supply of blood to part of the brain.

subarachnoid hemorrhage: Bleeding from a blood vessel on the surface of the brain into the space between the brain and the skull.

thrombus: A blood clot that forms inside a blood vessel or cavity of the heart.

transient ischemic attack (TIA): A temporary strokelike event that lasts for only a short time and is caused by a temporarily blocked blood vessel.

ventricular fibrillation: A condition in which the ventricles contract in a rapid, unsynchronized, uncoordinated fashion, so no blood is pumped from the heart.

Source: American Heart Association. *Heart and Stroke Facts.* Dallas: Author, 1997.

(hypertension), high blood cholesterol levels (*hypercholesterolemia*), oxidized low-density lipoproteins (LDL), cigarette smoking, toxins and viruses, and blood flow turbulence.

These injuries lead to a change or impairment in the normal function of the *endothelium* (the lining cells), and a chronic inflammatory response ensues.[4,6] In response to the injury, monocytes and T cells (both are special types of immune cells) penetrate through the endothelium into the underlying *intima* (inner layer of the arterial wall).[2,4] The monocytes are then converted to *macrophages,* scavenger cells that ingest oxidized LDL and other substances. Key to

the entire process is the malign interaction of LDL particles, especially the oxidized form, with the endothelium and the monocytes.[5] As reviewed in Chapter 9, a high intake of saturated fats and cholesterol, combined with a low fruit and vegetable intake, has been implicated in the formation of oxidized LDL. By accumulating large amounts of cholesterol from oxidized LDL, the macrophages are transformed into foam cells. In addition, oxidized LDL causes further injury to the endothelium, attracting even more monocytes, inducing a vicious cycle that leads to the development of a fatty streak, a precursor to plaque.[2]

TABLE 10.1 Statistics on Heart Disease

Prevalence	58,200,000	Cardiovascular disease
	50,000,000	Hypertension (adults)
	13,900,000	Coronary heart disease
	4,000,000	Stroke
Cardiovascular disease deaths	960,592	42% of all deaths; 17% occur before age 65
Heart attack deaths	481,287	number 1 cause of death
	250,000	Per year, die before reaching hospital
	1,100,000	Projected heart attacks of which one third will die
Stroke	157,991	3,890,000 victims alive today; number 3 cause of death
CAB (coronary artery bypass) surgery	573,000	Coronary bypass operations ($44,820 average cost)
PTCA procedures	419,000	Balloon angioplasty ($20,370 average cost)

Source: American Heart Association. *1998 Heart and Stroke Statistical Update.* Dallas: Author, 1997.

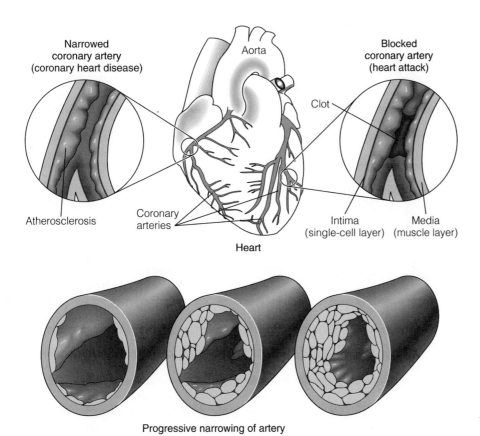

Figure 10.3 Atherosclerosis can form in the coronary arteries, resulting in a progressive narrowing of the lumen (artery passage). If a clot forms, blood flow through the coronary artery can be blocked, resulting in a heart attack.

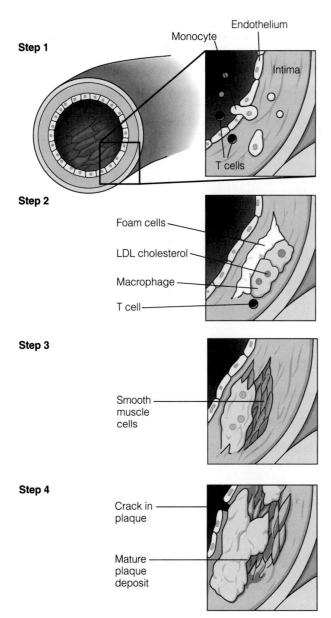

Figure 10.4 How atherosclerosis develops. Step 1—Injury to inner lining of intima. Monocytes and T cells penetrate into intima. *Step 2*—Monocytes are converted to macrophages and scavenge oxidized LDL, turning into foam cells. *Step 3*—Smooth-muscle cells migrate into intima and divide. Macrophages and smooth-muscle cells release collagen and other proteins. *Step 4*—The mature plaque is a complex collection of foam cells, proteins, smooth-muscle cells, and cholesterol debris. The plaque can harden, crack, and then cause blood clots to form. *Source: The Johns Hopkins White Papers.* Baltimore, MD: Johns Hopkins Medical Institutions, 1996.

The injured and impaired endothelial cells attract platelets and begin to release growth factors that stimulate the migration of smooth-muscle cells from the outer layers of the artery wall into the intima, where they proliferate abnormally. The macrophages and smooth-muscle cells begin to release collagen and other proteins, which form the fibrous component of atherosclerosis. The engorged foam cells then die and release cholesterol debris into the artery wall.[2]

The mature plaque is made up of a complex mixture of foam cells, smooth-muscle cells, cholesterol debris, and fibrous proteins. Over time, the plaque may become hardened or calcified and then develop cracks and ulcers, prompting the formation of blood clots that can suddenly close up the narrowed artery lumen, causing a heart attack.[2,4–7] Later in this chapter, important issues such as the treatment and reversal of atherosclerosis are discussed.

There is increasing evidence that atherosclerosis begins in childhood and progresses from fatty streaks to raised lesions in adolescence and young adulthood (see Figure 10.5).[8,9] In one autopsy study of 1,079 men and 364 women who had died from external causes between the ages of 15 and 34, researchers found dramatic differences in the severity of atherosclerosis, depending on blood LDL cholesterol levels and lifestyle habits such as smoking and fat-rich diets.[9] Men and women who smoked and/or had elevated LDL cholesterol experienced the greatest amount of atherosclerosis. The researchers warned that teenagers and young adults place themselves at increased risk of early heart attack unless good lifestyle habits are practiced beginning in childhood. As summarized in Figure 10.6, approximately two thirds of elderly women and three fourths of elderly men have subclinical or clinical atherosclerosis and cardiovascular disease.[10] In other words, the majority of elderly people in the United States have atherosclerosis (whether they know it or not), a process that began when they were children and teenagers.[9,10]

CORONARY HEART DISEASE

Coronary heart disease (CHD) (also referred to as *coronary artery disease* [CAD]) is the major form of heart disease.[1] Nearly one of every five deaths is the result of CHD, making it the single leading cause of death in the United States. About every 20 seconds, an American suffers from a heart attack, and each minute an American dies from one.[1]

The heart muscle, like every other organ of the body, needs its own blood supply. The heart is not nourished by the blood that is being pumped to the lungs and body (Figure 10.1). The heart's blood is supplied through the *coronary arteries* (three major branches) (Figure 10.3). The narrowing, hardening, and blocking of these arteries by atherosclerosis leads to CHD. A blood clot may form in a narrowed coronary artery and block the flow of blood to the part of the heart muscle supplied by that artery. This is referred to as a *myocardial infarction* or *heart attack*.

When part of the heart muscle does not get enough blood (oxygen and nutrients), it begins to die. CHD can cause chest pain, called *angina pectoris,* which can occur

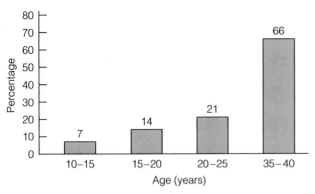

Figure 10.5 Prevalence of atherosclerosis in coronary blood vessels, according to age. Evidence of atherosclerosis is noticeable among children and is almost universal among middle-aged individuals in Western societies. *Source:* Data from Stary HC. The sequence of cell and matrix changes in atherosclerotic lesions of coronary arteries in the first 40 years of life. *Eur Heart J* 11(suppl):3–19, 1990.

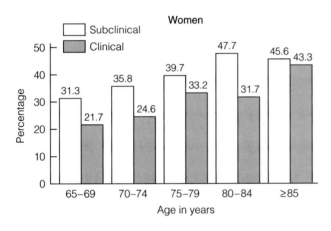

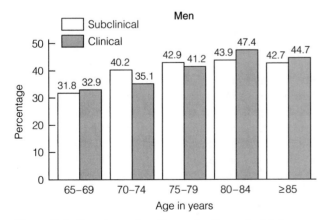

Figure 10.6 Prevalence of cardiovascular disease in elderly Americans. About two thirds of elderly women and three fourths of elderly men have subclinical (i.e., not yet apparent except through special tests) or clinical atherosclerosis and cardiovascular disease. *Source:* Data from Kuller L, et al. Prevalence of subclinical atherosclerosis and cardiovascular disease and association with risk factors in the cardiovascular health study. *Am J Epidemiol* 139:1164–1179, 1994.

---

during emotional excitement or physical exertion. (The treadmill ECG test for victims of angina pectoris can cause a depression of the ST segment. See Chapter 4.) Over 7 million Americans have angina pectoris.[1]

The first indications of a heart attack may be any of several warning signals, including those listed in Box 10.2. Unfortunately, in half of men and two thirds of women who died suddenly of CHD, there were no previous symptoms of this disease.[1]

STROKE

Stroke is a form of cardiovascular disease that affects the blood vessels supplying oxygen and nutrients to the brain[1] (see Figure 10.7).

Most strokes occur because the arteries in the brain become narrow from either a buildup of plaque material or atherosclerosis. Atherosclerosis is the underlying factor for both heart attacks and strokes (sometimes called "brain attacks"). Clots can then totally block the blood flow, causing the stroke. These clots are of two types: a clot that forms in the area of the narrowed brain blood vessel is called a thrombus; a clot that floats in from another area is an embolus. Three fourths of strokes are caused by these clots that plug narrowed brain arteries.[1,11]

Other strokes occur when a blood vessel in the brain or on its surface ruptures and bleeds (hemorrhagic stroke). Of-

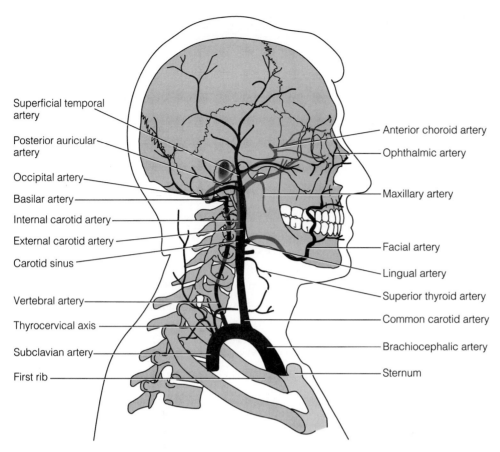

Superficial temporal artery

Posterior auricular artery

Occipital artery

Basilar artery

Internal carotid artery

External carotid artery

Carotid sinus

Vertebral artery

Thyrocervical axis

Subclavian artery

First rib

Anterior choroid artery

Ophthalmic artery

Maxillary artery

Facial artery

Lingual artery

Superior thyroid artery

Common carotid artery

Brachiocephalic artery

Sternum

Figure 10.7 Stroke is a form of CVD that affects the arteries of the central nervous system. A stroke (or "brain attack") occurs when a blood vessel carrying oxygen and nutrients to the brain bursts or is clogged by a blood clot or some other particle. Deprived of oxygen, brain nerve cells cannot function and die within minutes.

ten, the hemorrhage occurs when a spot in a brain artery has been weakened from atherosclerosis or high blood pressure. Hemorrhagic strokes are less common than those caused by clots but are far more lethal.

About 500,000 Americans suffer a new or recurrent stroke each year.[1] About 3 in 10 people who have a stroke die within a year, 6 in 10 within 8 years. Each year, stroke kills over 150,000 Americans, accounting for 1 of every 15 U.S. deaths. It is the third largest cause of death, ranking behind diseases of the heart and cancer. Of those who survive, half suffer long-term disabilities, needing help caring for themselves or when walking.

The good news about stroke is that death rates have fallen dramatically during the latter part of the twentieth century. Between 1950 and 1995 alone, stroke death rates fell an amazing 70%.[1,11] The American Heart Association urges that the best way to prevent a stroke from occurring is to reduce the risk factors for stroke (see Box 10.3). Seventy percent of all strokes occur in people with high blood pressure, making it the most important risk factor for stroke. In

fact, stroke risk varies directly with blood pressure. Additional risk factors that can be treated include cigarette smoking, obesity, excessive alcohol intake, high blood cholesterol levels, diabetes mellitus, and physical inactivity.[1,11] Several other stroke risk factors are categorized by the American Heart Association as unchangeable, including increasing age, being male, being African American, prior stroke, and heredity. Strokes are more common in the southeastern United States, the so-called "Stroke Belt," than in other areas of the United States. Incidence of stroke is strongly related to age, with the highest death rates found among people 85 years of age and over. The incidence of stroke is about 19% higher for men than for women, while African Americans have more than a 60% greater risk of death and disability from stroke than European Americans do. The highest U.S. stroke death rates are found among African American males.[1,11]

Warning signals of stroke include unexplained dizziness; sudden temporary weakness or numbness on one side of the face, arm, leg, or body; temporary loss of speech;

Box 10.3

Risk Factors for Stroke

Various risk factors contribute to the possible occurrence of stroke; most of these can be treated.

Risk Factors That Can Be Treated

1. High blood pressure (number 1 risk factor)
2. Personal history of heart disease
3. Cigarette smoking
4. High red blood cell count (makes clots more likely)
5. Transient ischemic attacks (TIAs)
6. Physical inactivity
7. Excessive alcohol intake
8. Obesity
9. Elevated blood cholesterol
10. Diabetes mellitus
11. Illicit drug use (especially cocaine)
12. Acute triggers (e.g., emotional stress)
13. High homocysteine levels
14. Asymptomatic carotid stenosis

Risk Factors That Cannot Be Changed

1. Age
2. Male—19% higher risk than for females
3. Race—African Americans have 60% elevated risk
4. Personal history of stroke
5. Heredity—family history
6. Geographic location—southeastern U.S.
7. Season—during periods of extreme temperatures
8. Socioeconomic—more likely among the poor

Sources: American Heart Association. *Heart and Stroke Facts.* Dallas: Author, 1997; Helgason CM, Wolf PA. AHA Prevention Conference IV: Prevention and rehabilitation of stroke. *Circulation* 96:701–707, 1997.

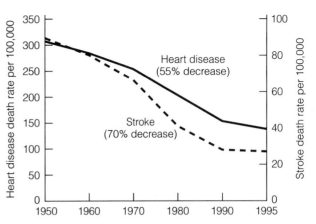

Figure 10.8 Trends in age-adjusted death rates: Heart disease and stroke. Death rates from heart disease and stroke have fallen sharply since 1950. *Source:* National Center for Health Statistics. *Health, United States, 1996–97 and Injury Chartbook.* Hyattsville, MD: 1997.

TRENDS IN CARDIOVASCULAR DISEASE

From 1920 to 1950, there was a sharp rise in deaths from heart disease, primarily from acute myocardial infarction among men.[12] The causes are unknown, but during this time, Americans moved off farms into cities, began driving cars, and increased their consumption of saturated fats and cigarettes. In 1953, awareness of the growing epidemic grew, with the publication of a study of American soldiers killed in action in Korea.[13] Of 300 autopsies on soldiers, whose average age was 22 years, 77.3% of the hearts showed some gross evidence of coronary arteriosclerosis. Of all cases, 12.3% had plaques causing luminal narrowing of more than 50%.

Since the 1950s, the trend has reversed—the sharp rise of the earlier period has been followed by an equally sharp fall in deaths from heart disease.[14–17] From 1950 to 1995, CVD death rates dropped by 55%, which is one of the greatest public health successes of the twentieth century (see Figure 10.8).[14] Men and women of all races shared in the encouraging downward mortality trend. Despite the pronounced overall reduction in heart disease mortality in the United States, Americans still experience higher death rates than their counterparts in many industrialized nations.[1]

The death rate attributable to stroke has been declining for more than 65 years in the United States.[14] Increasing control of hypertension (through lifestyle adjustments and modification) is probably the major cause of this decline. About 70% of people with high blood pressure report taking action to bring it under control, and 29% have achieved success.[18]

Much has been written regarding the causes of this dramatic turnaround.[1,2,15–18] Although estimates vary, about

temporary dimness or loss of vision in one eye; or sudden severe, unexplained headaches.[1] About 10% of strokes are preceded by "little strokes," called *transient ischemic attacks* (TIA). Of those who have had TIAs, about 36% will later have a stroke. Thus, TIAs are extremely important warning signs for stroke.[1,11]

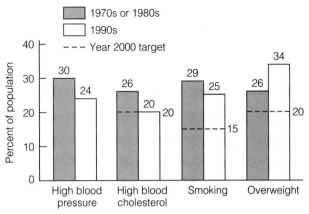

Figure 10.9 Prevalence of modifiable risk factors for heart disease and stroke: United States. Despite the continuing prevalence of overweight, the prevalence of high blood pressure, high blood cholesterol, and smoking has dropped sharply between surveys conducted in the 1970s or 1980s, and those in the 1990s. *Note:* No year 2000 goal was set for high blood pressure prevalence.

TABLE 10.2 Risk Factors for Heart Disease, According to the American Heart Association

Risk Factors	% U.S. Adults with Risk Factor
Major risk factors that *can* be changed	
1. Cigarette / tobacco smoke	25%
2. High blood pressure	24% ($\geq 140/90$ mm Hg)
3. High blood cholesterol	19% (≥ 240 mg/dl)
4. Physical inactivity	60%
5. Obesity	35% (body mass index ≥ 25 kg/m^2)
6. Diabetes	6%
Major risk factors that *cannot* be changed	
1. Heredity	—
2. Being male	—
3. Increasing age	13% (over age 65)
Contributing factor	
1. Individual response to stress	—

Source: American Heart Association. *1998 Heart and Stroke Statistical Update: Heart and Stroke Facts.* Dallas: Author, 1997.

half of the decline in CVD mortality rates has been related to risk-factor improvements, and the other half to improvements in the treatment of CVD.

Americans appear to be heeding the extensive health information about reducing risk factors for heart disease.[1,14,18] Since the early 1970s, Americans have become increasingly health conscious and appreciative of the importance of preventive medicine. Figure 10.9 summarizes the hopeful signs of progress Americans are making in the control of heart disease risk factors.[18]

RISK FACTORS FOR HEART DISEASE

Risk factors are defined as personal habits or characteristics that medical research has shown to be associated with an increased risk of heart disease. Up until 1992, the American Heart Association did not include physical inactivity in its list of "major risk factors that can be changed," which included cigarette smoking, high blood pressure, and high blood cholesterol. Inactivity was listed along with obesity, stress, and diabetes as "contributing factors."[1,19] In 1998, obesity and diabetes were upgraded from "contributing" risk factors to "major" risk factors.

Heredity, sex (being a male), and increasing age have been listed for many years as "risk factors that cannot be changed." Table 10.2 outlines the current list of heart disease risk factors observed by the American Heart Association, along with the prevalence of each factor. Notice that among the risk factors listed, inactivity is by far the most prevalent, followed by obesity, cigarette smoking, and high blood pressure, and then high blood cholesterol.

Why did the American Heart Association wait so long to include physical inactivity as a major risk factor for heart

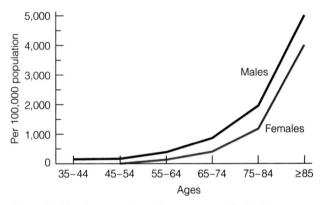

Figure 10.10 Coronary heart disease age-specific death rates by age and sex: United States, 1993 mortality, final data. *Source:* National Center for Health Statistics.

disease? The primary reason was that good research data to support this relationship had been lacking until recently. Most of the earlier studies showed that physically active, compared to inactive, people had a lower risk for heart disease, but critics contended that such findings did not control for other important factors. The importance of physical inactivity as a risk factor for CVD is reviewed later in this chapter.

The American Heart Association has urged that although there is little that can be done about being a male or getting older, those factors do have a strong effect on risk for heart disease, as shown in Figure 10.10.[2]

The risk factors listed in Table 10.2 do not explain all heart disease. In fact, 30–70% of CHD deaths (depending on the group being studied) are not explained by established risk factors.[20] Many other factors are probably important, but not enough is known to include them at this time. For example, blue-collar workers and people with less education have higher CHD death rates than do white-collar workers and those with more education.[1,21,22]

Potential risk factors include stature (short people have higher risk), baldness, low social support, avoidance of postmenopausal hormone therapy, high uric acid levels, high plasma levels of homocysteine, hyperinsulinemia, high levels of blood fibrinogen, emotional distress, a hostile personality, and a host of others.[23–32]

People with a family history of premature CHD are at a risk two to five times that of those with no family CHD history, particularly if first-degree relatives are involved. The role of genetic factors in atherosclerosis is difficult to evaluate precisely, however, because various coronary risk factors tend to cluster within families, as well.[1,33,34]

The danger of heart attack increases with the number of risk factors (see Figure 10.11). Often, people who are stricken with heart disease have several risk factors, each of which is only marginally abnormal. The Centers for Disease Control has calculated the proportions of coronary heart disease deaths attributable to five major risk factors[35] (see Figure 10.12). According to their estimates (which factor in both the strength of each risk factor's association to heart disease and the percentage of the U.S. population that has the risk factor) high serum cholesterol and inactivity rank

first and second, respectively, in their overall impact on heart disease in the United States. The recent increase in obesity prevalence should drive this risk factor upwards in the ranking when this analysis is revised.

The Harvard Medical School has summarized what can be expected in regard to lowering heart disease risk when people quit smoking, decrease their blood cholesterol or blood pressure, become active, or maintain ideal weight.[36] This is summarized in Figure 10.13. These data show that primary prevention of CVD is an effective strategy that should be integrated throughout American society (see Table 10.3).[19,37]

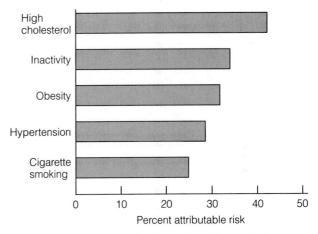

Figure 10.12 Proportion of coronary heart disease deaths attributable to five major risk factors. Rank order of five leading risk factors for heart disease and their overall impact on this disease in America. *Source:* Hahn RA, Teutsch SM, Rothenberg RB, Marks JS. Excess deaths from nine chronic diseases in the United States, 1986. *JAMA* 264:2654–2659, 1990.

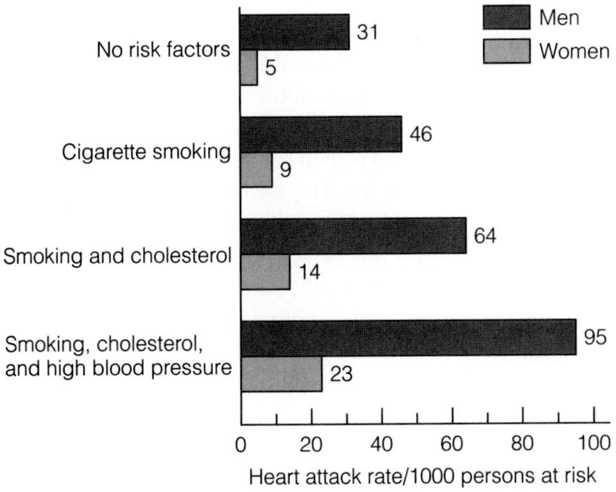

Figure 10.11 Chance of heart attack within 8 years, by risk factors present. This chart shows that a combination of three risk factors can increase the likelihood of heart attack. This chart uses an abnormal blood pressure level of 150 mm Hg (systolic) and a cholesterol level of 260 mg/dl in a 55-year-old male and female. *Source:* American Heart Association, 1997. *Heart and Stroke Statistical Update.* Dallas: Author, 1996.

- ■ Quitting cigarette smoking
  50–70% decrease within 5 years

- ■ Decreasing blood cholesterol
  2–3% decrease for each 1% drop in cholesterol (among people with an elevated level)

- ■ Decreasing high blood pressure
  2–3% decrease for each 1 mm Hg drop in diastolic pressure

- ■ Becoming physically active
  45% decrease for those who maintain active lifestyle

- ■ Maintenance of ideal body weight
  35–55% decrease for maintaining ideal weight vs. obesity (obesity defined as more than 20% above desirable weight)

Figure 10.13 Lifestyle and heart disease risk reduction: Achievable reductions in risk (independent contribution of each risk factor). Improving lifestyle and altering risk factors has a powerful impact on lowering heart disease risk. *Source:* Manson JE, Tosteson H, Ridker PM, et al. The primary prevention of myocardial infarction. *N Engl J Med* 326:1406–1413, 1992.

TABLE 10.3 **Strategies for Primary Prevention of Heart Disease and Stroke**

Risk Factor	Strategies[a]
High blood pressure ($\geq 140/90$ mm Hg)	Weight reduction, promotion of physical activity, reduced salt and alcohol intake
Smoking	Smoking cessation programs, physician counseling, nicotine patches, legislation
High serum cholesterol (≥ 240 mg/dl)	Reduced saturated fat intake, weight reduction, physical activity (to raise HDL cholesterol)
Obesity (>20% desirable weight)	Low-fat, low-energy diet; promotion of long-term physical activity; behavior change
Physical inactivity and irregular exercise habits	Worksite fitness programs, community fitness facilities, physician counseling
Diabetes and impaired glucose tolerance	Weight reduction, promotion of physical activity, dietary improvement
Estrogens	Consider estrogen replacement therapy in postmenopausal women, especially those with multiple CHD risk factors

[a]The first goal of prevention is to prevent the development of risk factors. People should be instructed about adopting healthy life habits to prevent CVD, and this education should be family oriented. Ideally, risk-factor prevention begins in childhood.

Sources: Bronner LL, Kanter DS, Manson JE. Primary prevention of stroke. *N Engl J Med* 333:1392–1400, 1995; Grundy SM, Balady GJ, Criqui MH, et al. Guide to primary prevention of cardiovascular diseases: A statement for healthcare professionals from the task force on risk reduction. *Circulation* 95:2329–2331, 1997.

TREATMENT OF HEART DISEASE

When a person's heart muscle does not get as much blood as it needs, due to blockage of the coronary blood vessels (called myocardial ischemia), the person may experience chest pain, called angina pectoris. Angina pectoris can be treated with drugs that affect either the supply of blood to the heart muscle or the heart's demand for oxygen.[1] Nitroglycerin is the drug most often used, as it relaxes the veins and coronary arteries. Other drugs can be used to reduce blood pressure and thus decrease the heart's workload and need for oxygen.

Invasive techniques may also be used, which improve the blood supply to the heart. In 1959, cardiologists first began to insert thin tubes (catheters) into the coronary arteries of patients with angina, to inject a liquid contrast agent to detect atherosclerotic plaques.[2] This procedure is called *coronary angiography.*

For the next two decades, when this procedure detected severe narrowing of the coronary arteries, there was usu-

ally only one recourse—coronary artery bypass graft surgery (CABGS). In this surgery, surgeons take a blood vessel from another part of the body (usually the leg or from inside the chest wall) and construct a detour around the blocked part of a coronary artery (see Figure 10.14). One end of the vessel is attached above the blockage, and the other to the coronary artery just beyond the blocked area, restoring blood supply to the heart muscle.

In 1977, a Swiss cardiologist revolutionized cardiology by developing a technique to open coronary arteries with special catheters bearing inflatable balloons on the tips (called percutaneous transluminal coronary angioplasty or PTCA).[38] In PTCA, the balloon is positioned using a catheter and wire adjacent to the atherosclerotic plaque, and then inflated. This squashes and cracks the plaque, widening the narrowed coronary artery (see Figure 10.14).

PTCA is performed more than 400,000 times a year in the United States, compared to about 500,000 for CABGS.[1] Although these techniques are common and fairly successful in at least alleviating pain symptoms, various problems and limitations have led many researchers to investigate new techniques.[39] One problem with PTCA is that in 25–50% of patients, the coronary artery renarrows, usually within the first 6 months. Also, in about 5% of cases, physicians cannot open the vessel using PTCA. On the other hand, CABGS is expensive ($44,200 average cost), and long-term studies have not been able to determine that the procedure significantly lengthens the life of the patient.[2,38]

Three new techniques are laser angioplasty (or ablation), directional coronary atherectomy (DCA), and coronary stent (see Figure 10.14).[1,2,38] With *laser angioplasty*, light, heat, and other strategies are used to burn away plaque material. With *DCA*, a special cutting device with a balloon is positioned by the atherosclerotic plaque material. The opening in the cylinder is turned toward the plaque, and the balloon is inflated, to force the plaque into the window of the cylinder. An external motor rotates the cutting blade at approximately 1800 revolutions per minute, grinding up plaque material, which is then sucked into the catheter by a vacuum pressure device. The *coronary stent* is a metallic wire tube that is implanted at the site of a narrowed coronary artery to keep the vessel open. Each of these techniques have various strengths and limitations, and research is ongoing to determine the circumstances in which they apply best.

CAN ATHEROSCLEROSIS BE REVERSED WITHOUT SURGERY?

Obviously, preventing atherosclerosis from forming in the first place is the primary goal for all who value their health. If an individual has had a heart attack, however, or is at high risk for one because of poor lifestyle habits, can the accumulation of atherosclerotic plaque be reversed through

**Percutaneous Transluminal
Coronary Angioplasty (PTCA)**
A catheter is inserted into a groin artery and threaded
up to the blocked coronary artery. The balloon is then
inflated several times, compressing the plaque against
the arterial wall.

Coronary Artery Bypass Surgery
A segment of a blood vessel from another
part of the body (the saphenous vein in the
leg or the preferred choice, the internal
mammary artery in the chest) is used as a
graft. A venous graft is performed by sewing
one end of the vein into the aorta and the
other end into the blocked artery at a point
beyond the blockage. Alternatively, an
internal mammary artery is redirected to a
place beyond the obstructed coronary artery.
Thus, blood is carried around the point of
obstruction, effectively "bypassing" the
blockage. If necessary, multiple coronary
artery blockages can be bypassed in a single
operation.

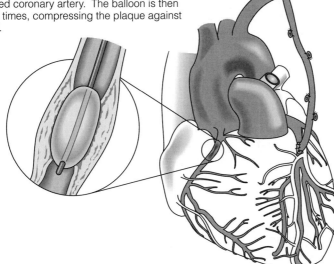

Atherectomy utilizes a mechanical device—either a
rotating blade or a drill—to shave plaque off of the artery
wall. The tiny pieces of plaque debris are then swept or
suctioned into a small compartment in the device and
removed when the catheter is withdrawn.

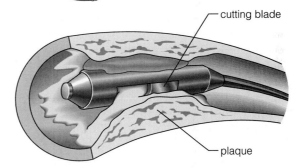

cutting blade

plaque

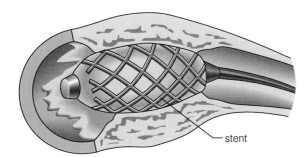

stent

Coronary stents —flexible, stainless steel tubes that are
permanently implanted in a coronary artery to keep it propped
open—are used in conjunction with balloon angioplasty. The stent
is initially collapsed around a deflated balloon and is threaded to
the site of the blockage. When the balloon is inflated, the stent
expands and locks into position.

Laser ablation does not actually use a laser beam to
vaporize plaque. Instead, laser light, emitted from the tip
of the catheter, is used to heat a probe that burns plaque
away from the artery wall, layer by layer.

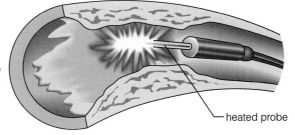

heated probe

Figure 10.14   Treatment of coronary heart disease.   *Source: The Johns Hopkins White Papers.* Baltimore, MD: Johns
Hopkins Medical Institutions, 1996.

improvements in diet, exercise, weight loss, smoking cessation, and stress management, and initiation of drug therapy?[40-50] (This is termed "secondary prevention."[49])

Since early in the twentieth century, regression of atherosclerosis has been demonstrated in many different types of animals, including rabbits, roosters, pigs, and monkeys.[40] In the typical animal experiment, atherosclerosis is promoted by diets high in fat and cholesterol, followed by a vegetarian "regression" diet that leads to a reduction in plaque size within 20 to 40 months.[41] (The earliest human studies were with World War II prisoners who had been subjected to semistarvation diets in prisoner camps and were found at autopsy to have far less atherosclerosis than well-nourished people.)

Since the mid-1970s, controlled trials have convincingly demonstrated that intensive drug and diet therapy to lower LDL cholesterol and raise HDL cholesterol retards the progression of coronary atherosclerosis, promotes regression, and thus decreases the incidence of coronary events.[40-50] In one review of 12 studies, intensive drug, diet, and/or lifestyle interventions with heart disease patients reduced their LDL cholesterol by 33% while increasing HDL cholesterol 15% over an average of 3.3 years.[41] Among control patients not on the intervention regimen, 52% experienced progression, 9% regression, and 39% no change in atherosclerotic disease, in comparison to 24%, 27%, and 49%, respectively, among patients on treatment. More impressively, treatment patients experienced 50% fewer cardiovascular events (heart attacks, deaths, unstable ischemia, etc.). In general, secondary prevention stabilizes progression of atherosclerosis in about half of patients and induces regression in about one fourth of patients.[49]

In several trials, the effect of lifestyle interventions without drug therapy was investigated. In a randomized, controlled 1-year study, a treatment group was placed on an extremely low-fat vegetarian diet (7% calories as fat) and given stress management and moderate exercise.[45] The treatment subjects lost an average of 22 pounds and lowered their average cholesterol from 227 to 172 mg/dl (24% reduction), with 82% experiencing regression, compared to 42% among controls. Patients in the treatment group also reported a 91% reduction in the frequency of angina pain, compared to a 165% rise among controls. A 39-month study of 90 heart disease patients in England has confirmed the value of diet therapy, showing that diet alone can retard the overall progression and increase overall regression of coronary artery disease.[46]

A study from Germany examined the effects of exercise on regression of coronary atherosclerosis.[47] Heart disease patients were randomized either to an intervention group that exercised several hours a week or a control group receiving standard care. After 1 year, among patients exercising, regression of coronary artery disease was measured for 28% of patients, progression for 10%, and no change for 62%, while among controls, the results were 6%, 45%, and 49%, respectively. The researchers concluded that regression of coronary artery disease is likely among patients who expend 2,200 Calories per week in exercise (about 5–6 hours weekly). This same research team has also shown that for patients combining exercise with a low-fat diet, coronary artery disease progresses at a slower pace than for a control group on standard care.[48] The challenge, as these researchers have noted, is getting patients to adhere to the improved lifestyle over long time periods.

Obviously, prevention of atherosclerosis in the first place is the best strategy to follow, and this can be accomplished for most people by avoidance of smoking, eating a diet low in saturated fat and cholesterol, maintaining ideal weight, exercising regularly, managing stress, and keeping blood pressure and cholesterol under control. Interestingly, these are the same strategies that are effective in treating coronary artery disease. The rest of this chapter deals with prevention of heart disease by emphasizing management of the major risk factors.

CIGARETTE SMOKING

Cigarette smoking has been described as the single most preventable cause of premature death in the United States.[51] The Office of the Surgeon General of the United States has been vigilant in warning Americans about the negative consequences of cigarette smoking. On January 11, 1964, the surgeon general released the first report on smoking and health, concluding that "cigarette smoking is causally related to lung cancer." This historic report was widely covered by the media and brought an immediate outcry from the tobacco industry, which continues unabated to the present.

A Leading Cause of Death

The Department of Health and Human Services has ranked tobacco as the leading cause of death in the United States, followed by diet and inactivity, and then alcohol (see Figure 10.15).[52] Nearly one out of every five deaths is the result of cigarette smoking. Over 400,000 Americans die each year from diseases caused by smoking, and (as shown in Figure 10.16) smoking kills more through cardiovascular disease than through cancer.[53] Smoking causes an additional 10 million Americans to suffer increased rates of various debilitating and chronic diseases, including bronchitis, emphysema, peptic ulcer disease, and arteriosclerosis. Attainment of a tobacco-free society would add 15 years of life to each of the more than 400,000 individuals who would have experienced tobacco-related deaths.

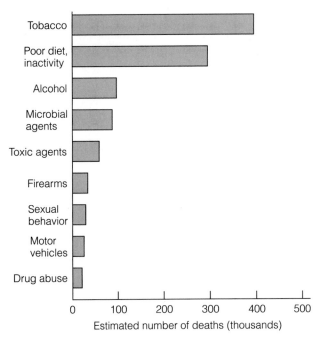

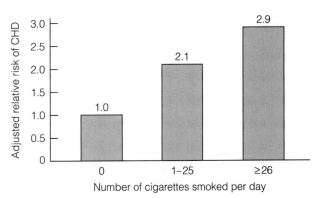

Figure 10.17 Cigarette smoking and coronary heart disease. Risk of coronary heart disease is nearly tripled for heavy smokers. *Source:* Neaton JD, Wentworth D. Serum cholesterol, blood pressure, cigarette smoking, and death from coronary heart disease. *Arch Intern Med* 152:56–64, 1992.

Figure 10.15 Actual causes of death in the United States. The Department of Health and Human Services has ranked tobacco as the leading cause of death in the United States. *Source:* McGinnis JM, Foege WH. Actual causes of death in the United States. *JAMA* 270:2207–2212, 1993.

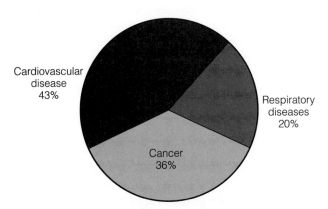

Figure 10.16 Smoking-related deaths: Over 400,000 deaths/year. Smoking is related to more than 400,000 deaths a year, with the largest proportion due to cardiovascular disease. *Source:* Cigarette smoking—Attributable mortality and years of potential life lost—United States, 1990. *MMWR* 42(33):645–647, 1993.

Smoking is a strong and independent risk factor for all forms of CVD, including CHD, stroke, and peripheral artery disease.[54–58] Using data from the multiple risk factor intervention trial (MRFIT), death from coronary heart disease has been shown to be about three times greater among heavy smokers (more than 25 cigarettes a day) than among nonsmokers (see Figure 10.17).[54] Data from the MRFIT study

have also demonstrated that at every level of serum cholesterol or blood pressure, smoking doubles or triples the death rate from coronary heart disease (see Figure 10.18).[54] These three risk factors work closely together, with the result that smokers with high blood cholesterol and blood pressure levels have coronary heart disease death rates approximately 20 times greater than those found among nonsmokers with low blood cholesterol and low blood pressure.

Many underlying mechanisms have been proposed as leading to the hazardous effects of smoking on cardiovascular health. Exposure to tobacco smoke causes abnormalities in endothelial cell function, promotes formation of blood clots, decreases HDL cholesterol levels, and increases the stiffness of both muscular and elastic arteries.[56–58]

Recent Trends

As shown in Figure 10.19, the proportion of U.S. adults who smoke has fallen sharply since the 1960s, so that today only one in four still have the habit.[14,59] If trends continue, the Year 2000 goal of 20% is likely to be met. Table 10.4 shows that cigarette smoking is still a major problem among some segments of the American society, however, particularly blue-collar workers, those with little education, and various minority groups.

Cigarette smoking almost always begins in the adolescent years. It has been estimated that approximately 6,000 young persons try a cigarette each day, with half becoming daily smokers.[60] In other words, more than 1 million young persons start to smoke each year, adding about $10 billion during their lifetimes to the cost of health care in the United States. The prevalence of tobacco use among adolescents is increasing, with one out of three high school students reporting current cigarette use. Cigarette smoking among

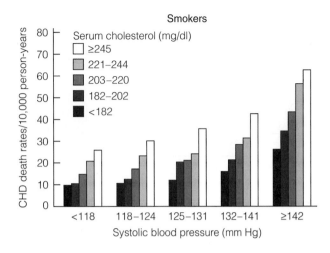

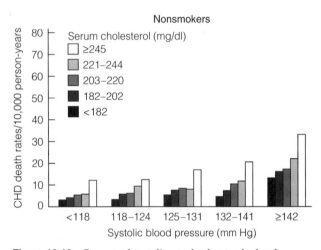

Figure 10.18 Coronary heart disease death rates, by level of serum cholesterol and systolic blood pressure. Compare the coronary heart disease death rates among cigarette smokers (top graph) with those of nonsmokers (bottom graph). In general, death rates at every level of cholesterol or blood pressure is doubled or tripled for smokers. Also notice that the death rate is 20-fold different between individuals with high versus low levels of all risk factors.

Source: Neaton JD, Wentworth D. Serum cholesterol, blood pressure, cigarette smoking, and death from coronary heart disease. *Arch Intern Med* 152:56–64, 1992.

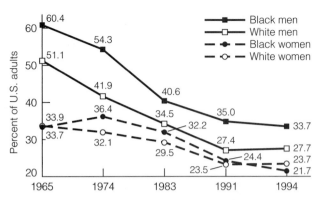

Figure 10.19 Trends in cigarette smoking status: U.S. adults (18 years of age and older). The proportion of U.S. adults who smoke has fallen strongly since the mid-1960s, although the decline has slowed during the 1990s. *Source:* National Center for Health Statistics. *Health, United States, 1996–97 and Injury Chartbook.* Hyattsville, MD: 1997.

adolescents has also been linked to other problems, including marijuana use, binge drinking, and fighting.[61]

The mean number of cigarettes smoked daily per smoker is 20, or one pack a day. Per capita consumption of cigarettes peaked during the 1960s, around the time of the first surgeon general's report, and has since fallen sharply, particularly during the 1980s (see Figure 10.20).[62] Social influences and legislation have had a strong impact on the prevalence of smoking in America. Public attitudes toward smoking have changed, in large part due to the contemporary evidence that many adverse health effects are related to passive smoking (breathing someone else's cigarette smoke).

The National Cancer Institute has concluded that "there is no longer any doubt that exposure to environmental tobacco smoke (ETS) is a cause of death and disease among nonsmokers."[63] A panel of science advisors also told the Environmental Protection Agency (EPA) in October of 1992 that there was enough evidence to classify secondhand tobacco smoke as a cause of cancer for humans and of serious respiratory problems for infants and young children. In January of 1993, after 2 years of revisions and intense debate, the EPA put their stamp of approval on this historic report.[64]

The report estimated that 3,000 lung cancer deaths each year can be attributed to ETS, and that parental smoking causes as many as 300,000 lung infections, including bronchitis and pneumonia, among children each year. Of equal importance, EPA estimates that ETS is causally related to additional episodes and increased severity of preexisting asthma among children and exacerbates symptoms of approximately 20% of the estimated 2–5 million asthmatic children annually. There is increasing evidence that ETS increases the risk for CHD.[65,66] In the United States, 37,000 CHD deaths per year have been linked to ETS.[66] The National Institute for Occupational Safety and Health (NIOSH) recommends eliminating smoking in all workplaces.[67] The only alternative, according to NIOSH, is restricting smoking to completely separated smoking lounges, with independent ventilation systems exhausting secondhand smoke outside.

Smokeless Tobacco

Two types of *smokeless tobacco*—snuff and chewing tobacco—are in current use.[68] *Snuff* is a cured, finely ground tobacco that either can be taken nasally or, more commonly today, placed in small quantities between cheek and gum. *Chewing tobacco* comes in several forms, including loose-leaf, plug,

TABLE 10.4 Percentage of Persons Ages ≥18 Years Who Were Current Cigarette Smokers, by Selected Characteristics—United States, Year 2000 Objectives Supplement of the National Health Interview Survey, 1995

Characteristic	Men (n = 7,423)		Women (n = 9,790)		Total (n = 17,213)	
	%	(95% CI)	%	(95% CI)	%	(95% CI)
Race/Ethnicity						
White, non-Hispanic	27.1	(± 1.5)	24.1	(± 1.3)	25.6	(± 1.0)
Black, non-Hispanic	28.8	(± 3.7)	23.5	(± 3.1)	25.8	(± 2.6)
Hispanic	21.7	(± 2.9)	14.9	(± 2.1)	18.3	(± 1.8)
American Indian / Alaskan Native	37.3	(± 17.2)	35.4	(± 13.9)	36.2	(± 10.6)
Asian / Pacific Islander	29.4	(± 8.6)	4.3	(± 3.1)	16.6	(± 4.6)
Education (yrs)						
≤8	28.4	(± 4.2)	17.8	(± 2.8)	22.6	(± 2.5)
9–11	41.9	(± 4.4)	33.7	(± 3.5)	37.5	(± 2.9)
12	33.7	(± 2.3)	26.2	(± 1.8)	29.5	(± 1.4)
13–15	25.0	(± 2.6)	22.5	(± 2.2)	23.6	(± 1.6)
≥16	14.3	(± 1.8)	13.7	(± 1.8)	14.0	(± 1.4)
Age group (yrs)						
18–24	27.8	(± 3.9)	21.8	(± 3.0)	24.8	(± 2.4)
25–44	30.5	(± 1.8)	26.8	(± 1.6)	28.6	(± 1.2)
45–64	27.1	(± 2.1)	24.0	(± 2.0)	25.5	(± 1.5)
≥65	14.3	(± 2.1)	11.5	(± 1.5)	13.0	(± 1.3)
Poverty Status						
At or above	25.9	(± 1.3)	21.8	(± 1.1)	23.8	(± 0.9)
Below	36.9	(± 4.3)	29.3	(± 2.9)	32.5	(± 2.5)
Unknown	26.9	(± 5.7)	21.0	(± 3.5)	23.5	(± 3.2)
Total	**27.0**	**(± 1.2)**	**22.6**	**(± 1.1)**	**24.7**	**(± 0.8)**

Source: CDC. Cigarette smoking among adults—U.S., 1995. *MMWR* 46:1218–1220, 1997.

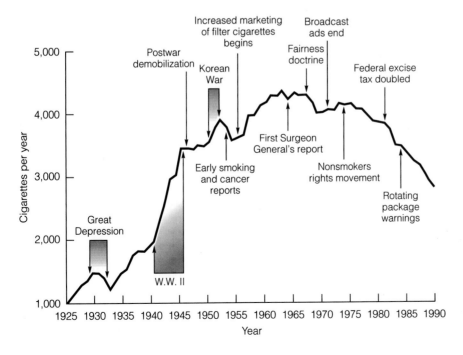

Figure 10.20 Per capita consumption of cigarettes, 1925–1990 (18 years of age and older). Per capita consumption of cigarettes has been strongly influenced by social and political forces. *Source:* U.S. Department of Health and Human Services. *Strategies to Control Tobacco Use in the United States: A Blueprint for Public Health Action in the 1990's.* USDHHS, Public Health Service, National Institutes of Health, National Cancer Institute. NIH Publication No. 92-3316, 1991.

and twist, all of which can be chewed directly and then spit out.

Consumption of moist snuff, now the most popular (and dangerous) form of smokeless tobacco, tripled from the 1970s to the 1990s.[69] An estimated 5.3 million adults (2.9%) are users of smokeless tobacco, with prevalence highest among those 18 to 24 years of age. About one in five male high school students uses smokeless tobacco.[69]

The resurgence in popularity of smokeless tobacco can be linked to advertising campaigns by tobacco companies to promote users as "macho." Adolescent and young adult males are the target of marketing strategies by tobacco companies that link such use with athletic performance and virility. Use of oral snuff is widespread among professional baseball players (about 4 out of 10), encouraging this behavior among adolescent and young adult males.[70]

Snuff and chewing tobacco are associated with a variety of serious adverse effects, especially oral cancer.[68] Holding tobacco in the mouth brings multiple carcinogenic chemicals into contact with the lining of the mouth. This can lead to the formation of white patches called leukoplakia (present in 46% of professional baseball players using smokeless tobacco), some of which then make the final transformation to cancer. Smokeless tobacco may also affect reproduction, longevity, the cardiovascular system, and oral health (bad breath, abrasion of teeth, gum recession, periodontal bone loss, and tooth loss), and it is highly addictive.[68]

Smoking Cessation

The nicotine from tobacco is highly addictive, making smoking cessation one of the most difficult of all health behavior changes.[71] In 1996, the U.S. Agency for Health Care Policy and Research published guidelines for smoking cessation, based on a thorough review of the literature and guidance from a panel of experts.[72] Key points for physicians included these:

- Every person who smokes should be offered smoking cessation treatment at every visit to a physician.
- Clinicians should ask about and record the tobacco-use status of every patient.
- Cessation treatments even as brief as 3 minutes per visit are effective.
- More intense treatment is more effective in producing long-term abstinence from tobacco.
- Nicotine replacement therapy, clinician-delivered social support, and skills training are the three most effective components of smoking cessation treatment. Nicotine nasal spray has been approved for use in the United States by the Food and Drug Administration, joining the nicotine patch and gum as effective available interventions.

- Health-care systems should make institutional changes that result in the systematic identification of, and intervention with, all tobacco users at every visit.

Many different types of smoking cessation providers are effective, including physicians, nurses, dentists, psychologists, pharmacists, and health educators. The following recommendations may be helpful for smoking cessation specialists:[72]

- Assess the smoker who has entered an intervention program to determine motivation and other psychological or medical conditions that may affect success in quitting.
- Use a variety of clinical specialists during the smoking cessation sessions.
- Ensure that the program is sufficiently intensive (sessions should last at least 20–30 minutes, with four to seven sessions spread out over at least 2 weeks).
- Use a variety of program formats (individual and group counseling, and supplementary self-help materials).
- Include effective counseling techniques (e.g., problem solving, social support).
- Target the smoker's motivation to quit (i.e., make the motivation relevant to the person's total situation, review potential risks of smoking, ask the patient to identify the potential benefits of quitting, and repeat these steps, as needed).
- Provide relapse prevention intervention (work to prevent long-term risks of relapse through long-term follow-up contacts, with an emphasis on alleviation of such problems as weight gain, depression, withdrawal symptoms, and lack of social support).
- Offer nicotine replacement therapy.

According to the surgeon general, there are many benefits to the smoker who quits:[51]

- *Reduced overall death rates.* After 15 years off cigarettes, the risk of death from all causes for ex-smokers returns to nearly the level of persons who have never smoked.
- *Reduced heart disease risk.* After just 1 year off cigarettes, the excess risk of heart disease caused by smoking is reduced by half.
- *Reduced lung cancer risk.* The risk of lung cancer for ex-smokers drops to as much as one half that of continuing smokers after 10 years. Risk of many other cancers is also lowered.
- *Improved life quality.* Ex-smokers have fewer days of illness and health complaints, better overall health status, and fewer lung problems. Ex-smokers can ex-

ercise more easily, feel better about themselves, and experience an increased sense of control.

Exercise and Tobacco

Smoking and sports do not mix, and today it is quite rare to find an elite athlete who smokes. When Michael Jordan, who does not smoke, won his first National Basketball Association title, *Sports Illustrated* put him on the cover with a cigar in his mouth, prompting many readers to scold the magazine for portraying their icon in such a misleading fashion.

Cross-sectional studies have shown that the prevalence of smoking among people who exercise is much lower than that of the general population. One study of 2,300 participants in the Los Angeles marathon reported that only 3% were smokers.[73] The 1990 Youth Risk Behavior Survey showed that there was a much lower incidence of smoking among adolescents involved in vigorous physical activity and interscholastic sports than among those exercising little.[74] Other studies have shown that youths who smoke exercise less than those who abstain, and they are prone to other high-risk behaviors, such as drinking, drug use, carrying weapons, failure to wear seat belts, and engaging in physical fights.[75]

Many studies have confirmed that smokers tend to exercise less than nonsmokers.[76-81] Among military personnel, the amount of physical activity has been found to vary inversely with the number of cigarettes smoked.[79,80] With respect to the 3,300 offspring in the Framingham study, increasing levels of physical activity were associated with fewer cigarettes smoked per day.[81] As depicted in Figure 10.21,

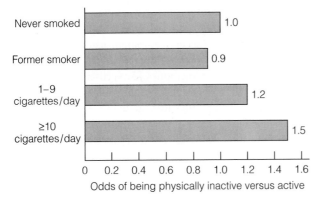

Figure 10.21 Odds of being a physically inactive person by smoking habit: Study of 30,000 Americans, by the Centers for Disease Control and Prevention. The odds of being physically inactive rise with the increasing use of cigarettes. *Source:* Simoes EJ, Byers T, Coates RJ, Serdula MK, Mokdad AH, Heath GW. The association between leisure-time physical activity and dietary fat in American adults. *Am J Public Health* 85:240–244, 1995.

the odds of being physically inactive are highest in those smoking more than 10 cigarettes per day.[76]

The U.S. Surgeon General has speculated that smokers are less likely than nonsmokers to make regular exercise a part of their lives, in part because exercise is more difficult for them.[51] Many studies have documented that smoking is associated with a decrease in the ability to perform vigorous exercise because of decreased lung function, increased blood levels of carboxyhemoglobin, a blunted heart rate response to exercise, and decreased maximal oxygen consumption.[79,80,82–94]

At rest, and to a smaller extent during exercise, nicotine from smoking cigarettes increases the heart rate and blood pressure, decreases the heart's blood output, and increases the oxygen demands of the heart muscle.[83,84] Nicotine also increases lactate levels in the blood during exercise, which can make people feel fatigued or feel like quitting exercise when it rises high enough.[86,90] In animal studies, nicotine has been found to decrease the ability to engage in long endurance exercise such as swimming or running.[87]

The resistance to air flow after smoking is increased in the lung passageways, making it harder to deliver air and oxygen to the lungs during hard exercise.[82,83,85,88,89,92] In some people, cigarette smoke can trigger asthma symptoms, making it nearly impossible to exercise until symptoms subside.[88] A fitness study of more than 3,000 Navy personnel in San Diego concluded that smoking is "a detriment to physical readiness even among these relatively young military personnel."[79]

In one study of 1,000 young recruits in the Air Force, the distance each was able to run in 12 minutes was directly related to the amount of cigarettes smoked, with those smoking more than 30 cigarettes a day in the worst shape.[93] In Switzerland, nearly 7,000 19-year-old military conscripts were studied, and performance in the 12-minute run was found to be inversely related to both the number of cigarettes smoked and the number of years with the habit[80] (see Figure 10.22).

A 7-year study of 1,400 Norwegians showed that physical fitness and lung function declined at a significantly faster rate in those who smoked, compared to nonsmokers.[82] In other words, smokers are less fit to begin with, because of their smoking, and then they lose more fitness and lung function as time passes.

Can the initiation of an exercise program be used to improve success in smoking cessation? Ken Cooper of the Cooper Institute for Aerobics Research in Dallas, Texas, has written that "smokers who get involved in aerobic exercise become more aware of how smoking has decreased their ability to process oxygen. In short, they find they become winded more easily than their fellow exercisers. This helps create a desire to quit smoking."[95]

Proof of this assertion has been hard to come by, however. A cross-sectional study by the Centers for Disease Control and Prevention reported that 81% of men and 75%

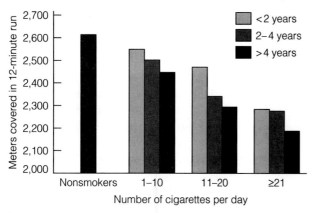

Figure 10.22   Performance in 12-minute run, according to smoking status of 6,592 Swiss 19-year-old military conscripts. The number of meters covered in the 12-minute run was lowest in military conscripts smoking more than a pack a day for more than 4 years.   *Source:* Marti B, Abelin T, Minder CE, Vader JP. Smoking, alcohol consumption, and endurance capacity: An analysis of 6,500 19-year-old conscripts and 4,100 joggers. *Prev Med* 17:79–92, 1988.

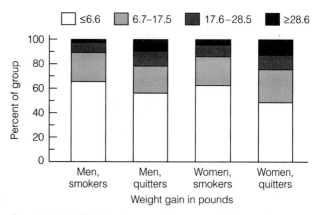

Figure 10.23   Weight gain over a 10-year period by smoking status: Mean adjusted weight gain for quitters was 6.2 pounds for men, 8.4 pounds for women. In this 10-year study of 9,000 Americans, major weight gain (more than 28.6 pounds) occurred in 9.8% of the men and 13.4% of the women who quit smoking.   *Source:* Williamson DF, Madans J, Anda RF, et al. Smoking cessation and severity of weight gain in a national cohort. *N Engl J Med* 324:739–745, 1991.

of women runners who had smoked cigarettes quit after beginning recreational running.[96] Another study of 347 marathon runners, 38% of whom were former smokers, showed that about two thirds of them claimed that running had helped them quit.[97] Two prospective studies, however, have failed to confirm this finding.[98,99] Blair of the Aerobics Research Center was unable to show that individuals voluntarily increasing their physical fitness level were more likely than nonexercisers to reduce smoking.[98] Similarly, a 1-year, randomized, controlled, exercise training study of 160 women and 197 men failed to demonstrate any effect of exercise on smoking cessation.[99]

However, in one study of more than 1,000 men and women who had participated in smoking cessation clinics at Kaiser Permanente medical centers, those who had increased their exercise after trying to quit were more likely to be nonsmokers 1 year later than those who had not.[51] In another study of 2,086 smokers living in New England, those who were successful in quitting smoking were more likely than nonquitters to report efforts to increase exercise.[100]

There is not yet conclusive evidence that exercise helps people stop smoking, but most smoking cessation programs include exercise as a vital component. "Exercise, such as walking, jogging, or bicycling" is included within the *Clinical Practice Guideline on Smoking Cessation* from the U.S. Department of Health and Human Services as a coping skill to handle stress and the urge to smoke.[72]

The Clinical Research Center at the Mayo Clinic includes exercise in the center's 2-week, comprehensive, inpatient, smoking cessation program for hard-core smokers.[101] Also included are group therapy, stress management, daily lectures, supervised recreational activities, and nicotine patches.

The 1-year quit rate is 29%. Although it is not possible to separate out the effects of exercise, these clinicians, along with many others, view exercise as an integral part of smoking cessation efforts.

Although nearly all smokers admit that their habit increases the risk of early death from cancer and heart disease, many are still unwilling to quit, frequently citing their fear of weight gain.[51,102–108] The use of smoking as a weight-control strategy, risky though it may be, appears to be a powerful motivation for continued smoking among a large percentage of smokers. In a nationwide survey in Australia, ex-smokers frequently listed weight gain as the number one disadvantage of quitting.[102] Among continuing smokers, weight gain was a close second to irritability.

Cigarettes have long been associated with slenderness. As early as 1925, Lucky Strike launched its "Reach for a Lucky Instead of a Sweet" campaign, using testimonials from famous women such as Amelia Earhart and Jean Harlow.[102] This campaign continues. Advertisements targeted at women still emphasize ultraslimness, sophistication, beauty, luxury, and popularity with men.

Unfortunately, there is an element of truth to these advertisements—smoking does promote weight loss. Studies have established that the average smoker weighs about 7 pounds less than a comparable nonsmoker.[105] People who start smoking lose weight, while those who quit gain, with women adding on an average of 8 pounds and men 6 pounds. A 10-year study of 9,000 Americans by the Centers for Disease Control and Prevention confirmed that major weight gain (more than 28.6 pounds) can be expected for 10% of men and 13% of women who quit smoking[104] (see Figure 10.23). The relative risk of major weight gain in those who quit smoking (as compared with those who continued to smoke) was 8:1 in men and 5:8 in women. Two thirds of all smokers who quit will gain weight, with the odds increasing for those who smoke more than 15 cigarettes per day. The researchers concluded that major weight gain is strongly related to smoking cessation, but that the average weight gain is rather small, meaning that it is unlikely to negate the health benefits of smoking cessation.

Not only do smokers tend to weigh less than nonsmokers, some studies even suggest they have less body fat, despite eating the same amount and exercising less.[109] It appears that smoking elevates the metabolic rate by 6–10%, and that when people quit, the rate falls back to its original level.[110–113] Then if appetite and food intake are increased, as is commonly reported by those who quit, weight gain is inevitable.

As reviewed by the surgeon general,[51] most studies show that food intake, especially of sweet foods, increases after quitting, resulting in 200–250 extra Calories a day. About one third of the weight gain has been ascribed to the fall in metabolic rate, one third to an increase in caloric consumption, and the other third to unmeasured factors.[111]

For several reasons, then, regular exercise is especially recommended for people quitting smoking.[51] First of all, smokers typically have poor levels of fitness, and initiation of regular exercise can improve their fitness and help improve their general health status. Second, because weight gain is common, burning extra calories through exercise may help to bring the body into better caloric balance. For example, data from the Nurses' Health Study showed that weight gain after smoking cessation was cut in half when subjects simultaneously increased their level of physical activity.[114] Regular exercise can decrease the levels of various risk factors and can reduce the risk for heart disease and some cancers, helping to counter some of the negative disease consequences of smoking.[51] There is also some evidence that exercise enhances long-term maintenance of smoking cessation.[115]

Finally, many individuals use smoking as a method of coping with stress and find the habit to be relaxing. Within 2 hours after quitting, typical feelings of nicotine withdrawal include irritability, frustration, anger, difficulty in concentrating, restlessness, depression, impatience, disrupted sleep, and impaired ability to work.[51] These feelings peak within the first 24 hours, then gradually decline, usually subsiding completely within 1 month.

As emphasized in Chapter 14, exercise is an excellent substitute for smoking in improving psychological mood state and alleviating anxiety and depression, thereby helping the quitter cope with some of the immediate negative mood states.[116] As reported by Ken Cooper, "I have received hundreds of letters from cigarette smokers telling me how they could never break the habit until they started exercising."[95]

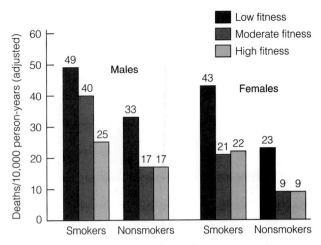

Figure 10.24 Death rates according to fitness status and smoking status. Fit smokers have lower death rates than unfit nonsmokers. *Source:* Blair SN, Kampert JB, Kohl HW, et al. Influences of cardiorespiratory fitness and other precursors on cardiovascular disease and all-cause mortality in men and women. *JAMA* 276:205–210, 1996.

For smokers who cannot or will not quit, exercise is still encouraged, to reduce risk of heart disease and early death. Data from the Cooper Institute for Aerobics Research have shown that smokers who maintain a high level of physical fitness have lower death rates from all causes than do low-fitness nonsmokers.[117] The lowest death rates, however, are found among men and women who avoid smoking while maintaining moderate-to-high physical fitness levels (see Figure 10.24).

HYPERTENSION

As described in Chapter 4, *blood pressure* is the force of the blood pushing against the walls of the arteries. The heart beats about 60–75 times each minute, and the blood pressure is at its greatest when the heart contracts, pumping blood into the arteries. This is called *systolic blood pressure*. When the heart is resting briefly between beats, the blood pressure falls, termed *diastolic blood pressure*. According to the National High Blood Pressure Education Program, *hypertension* is defined as present when diastolic measurements on at least two separate occasions average 90 mm Hg or higher, and/or systolic measurements are 140 mm Hg or higher[118] (see Table 4.1).

In the United States and most other Western societies, the large majority of residents experience a progressive age-related rise in blood pressure (see Figure 4.2). As a result, the incidence and prevalence of hypertension rise steadily with each additional decade of life. Two million new hypertensives are added each year to the pool of patients in the

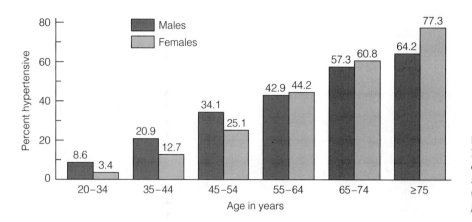

Figure 10.25 Hypertension prevalence by age and sex: 24% (43 million) of U.S. adults have hypertension. *Source:* National Center for Health Statistics. *Health, United States, 1996–97 and Injury Chartbook.* Hyattsville, MD: 1997.

United States, so that by old age, about two thirds of Americans have this disease[119] (see Figure 10.25).

It is important to stress that in unacculturated societies, age-related increases in blood pressure are uncommon. Thus, it does not appear that hypertension is the inevitable consequence of old age. Animal, clinical, and epidemiological research have indicated that in societies where salt and alcohol intakes are high, potassium intake is low, and physical inactivity and obesity are the norm, incidence of hypertension is high.[119–121]

Estimates based on the 1988–1994 National Health and Nutrition Examination Survey indicate that approximately 43 million, or 24%, of all adults in the United States have high blood pressure, while another 30 million have high-normal blood pressures.[119,122,123] One out of three hypertensives are unaware they have the problem, and only half are on appropriate medication.[123] Even of those on medication, 80% still have blood pressures exceeding 140/90 mm Hg.

The good news is that in the United States, between 1960 and 1991, average systolic and diastolic blood pressures fell about 10 and 5 mm Hg, respectively. Prevalence of high blood pressure has decreased for every age–sex–race subgroup, except black men age 50 and older.[122,123]

Health Problems

High blood pressure usually does not give early warning signs; for this reason, it is known as the "silent killer." High blood pressure kills more than 37,000 Americans each year and contributes to the deaths of more than 700,000, reports the National Center for Health Statistics.[124] High blood pressure increases the risk for coronary heart disease and other forms of heart disease, stroke, and kidney failure.[124–127]

According to the National Heart, Lung, and Blood Institute, when blood pressure is not detected and treated, it can cause[124]

- The heart to get larger, which may lead to heart failure

- Small blisters (aneurisms) to form in the brain's blood vessels, which may cause a stroke[126]

- Blood vessels in the kidneys to narrow, which may cause kidney failure

- Arteries throughout the body to harden faster, especially those in the heart, brain, and kidneys, which can cause a heart attack, stroke, or kidney failure[125,127]

High blood pressure also affects the brain. People with elevated blood pressure in middle age are more likely to suffer 25 years later from loss of cognitive abilities—memory, problem solving, concentration, and judgment.[128] This loss further translates into a diminished capacity to function independently in old age.

Using data from the large-scale MRFIT study, researchers have documented that cardiovascular and stroke mortality increases progressively with incremental increases in blood pressure from the optimal level of less than 120/80 mm Hg[119,120] (see Figures 10.26 and 10.27).

Rationale for Primary Prevention of Hypertension

Controlled clinical trials have clearly demonstrated that when hypertensives use drugs to control their condition, risk of cardiovascular mortality decreases.[119,129–131] However, there are several reasons why hypertension experts promote lifestyle therapy in the form of proper diet, exercise, maintenance of ideal weight, and alcohol restriction, as the foundation of hypertension treatment.[119,132–134]

First of all, identifying and then treating all hypertensives in the United States are considered nearly impossible tasks, compounded by the problem that a significant proportion are unaware of their condition. Drug treatment requires a lifelong commitment, because drug therapy does not cure hypertension.

Many hypertensives are not fully compliant in administering their drug therapy, and as a result, only one in five on medication have their blood pressure under 140/90 mm

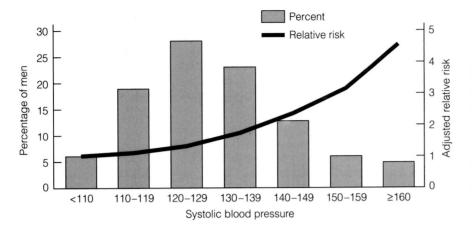

Figure 10.26 Systolic blood pressure and cardiovascular mortality: 12.5-year study of 347,978 men (MRFIT)—prevalence and risk. Data from the MRFIT study have shown that risk of cardiovascular mortality rises sharply with increase in systolic blood pressure. *Source:* Data from Stamler J, Stamler R, Neaton JD. Blood pressure, systolic and diastolic, and cardiovascular risks: US population data. *Arch Intern Med* 153:598–615, 1993.

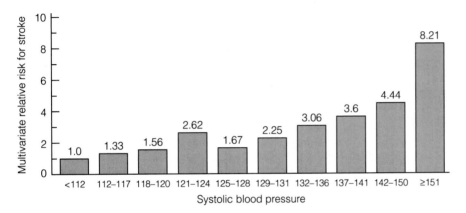

Figure 10.27 Systolic blood pressure and stroke mortality: 12.5-year study of 347,978 men (MRFIT). Data from the MRFIT study have shown that risk of stroke mortality rises sharply with increase in systolic blood pressure. *Source.* Data from Stamler J, Stamler R, Neaton JD. Blood pressure, systolic and diastolic, and cardiovascular risks: US population data. *Arch Intern Med* 153:598–615, 1993.

Hg. Even those who derive optimal benefit from their antihypertensive treatment are likely to have a higher risk of morbidity and mortality than their untreated normotensive counterparts.[119] (See Table 10.5 for a review of drugs used to treat hypertension.)

Many hypertensive treatment regimens are expensive (especially those with new drugs), and almost all carry the potential for some adverse side effects. Some hypertensive drugs (thiazides and loop diuretics, for example) have negative effects on serum lipid and lipoprotein levels.[135] Beta-blockers have a tendency to lower HDL cholesterol and to raise triglycerides. This can pose a problem for many patients, because 40% of hypertensives also have high blood cholesterol levels. A final consideration is that many hypertensives sustain vascular damage to their heart, brain, eyes, or kidneys before they come to the attention of a health-care provider.

For all these reasons, it makes sense to emphasize primary prevention of hypertension in two ways.[119] The first approach, called the "population strategy," is designed to mobilize the population to follow prudent lifestyle practices, utilizing the mass media and educational systems, with support from the food industry and health-care providers. With such an approach, even a small decrease in the population's average blood pressure can lead to a substantial decrease in CVD risk. For example, it has been estimated that a 2 mm Hg shift downward in the overall systolic blood pressure might reduce the annual mortality from stroke by 6% and from coronary heart disease by 4%.[119,133]

The second approach, called the "targeted strategy," attempts to lower blood pressure among those who are most likely to need it. These include those whose blood pressure is in the high normal range, those with a family history of hypertension, members of susceptible minority populations (African Americans and Hispanic Americans), the elderly, and those who are overweight, consume excessive amounts of sodium, are physically inactive, or have a high intake of alcohol. Experience in clinical trials indicates that a targeted intervention that lowers diastolic blood pressure by as little as 1–3 mm Hg may reduce the incidence of hypertension by as much as 20–50%.[119]

The Joint National Committee on Detection, Evaluation, and Treatment of High Blood Pressure of the National Institutes of Health has urged that lifestyle modifications be used as "definitive or adjunctive therapy for hypertension."[94] An attempt should be made with all Stage 1 and Stage 2 (mild and moderate) hypertensive patients to con-

TABLE 10.5 Main Classes of Common Blood Pressure Drugs

The National Institutes of Health recommend that most people start with drugs from either or both of the two oldest, best-studied classes: diuretics and beta-blockers. The newer classes—mainly calcium channel blockers and drugs known as ACE inhibitors—should be reserved for cases where there's a compelling medical reason or where the top choices fail to control blood pressure adequately. Those guidelines notwithstanding, people with hypertension who are already doing well on a particular drug from any one of those classes—except a short-acting calcium channel blocker—should probably stick with that drug rather than switch to another one.

Drug	Monthly Cost[a]	How It Works	Possible Side Effects	Special Considerations
Diuretics				
Chlorothiazide (Diuril) Chlorthalidone (Hygroton) Hydrochlorothiazide (Esidrix, HydroDIURIL)	$5–$25	Prompts kidneys to excrete sodium, which reduces blood volume and thus blood pressure.	Frequent urination, impotence, muscle weakness.[b]	One of the oldest, best-studied classes of blood pressure drugs, proven to prevent deadly complications of hypertension. Recommended, alone or in combination with beta-blockers, as first-line therapy for most people.
Beta-blockers				
Atenolol (Tenormin) Metoprolol (Lopressor, Toprol-XL) Propranolol (Inderal LA)	$10–$30	Slows heartbeat and lessens force of heart's contractions.	Insomnia, slow pulse, weakness, impotence, decreased sex drive.	See above. Also effective against angina, certain heart rhythm disorders, and migraine headaches. Not recommended for people with asthma, chronic bronchitis, or circulatory problems in the hands or legs.
Calcium channel blockers (long-acting)				
Amlodipine (Norvasc) Diltiazem (Cardizem CD Dilacor-XR) Nifedipine (Adalat CC, Procardia XL) Verapamil (Calan SR, Isoptin SR)	$40–$55	Prevents calcium from enabling muscle cells to constrict around the blood vessels, thus dilating the vessels.	Constipation, dizziness, flushing, gum overgrowth, headaches, impotence, palpitations, swollen legs.	Reduces blood pressure, but not proven to prevent complications of hypertension. Often best for hypertensive patients with certain heart rhythm disorders or medical conditions that are worsened by beta-blockers.
ACE inhibitors				
Captopril (Capoten) Enalapril (Vasotec) Lisinopril (Prinivil, Zestril)	$30–$55	Dilates blood vessels by blocking angiotensin-converting enzyme, which can indirectly cause artery walls to constrict.	Cough, rash, weakness, impotence, loss of taste, potassium retention (see right).	Reduces blood pressure, but not proven to prevent complications of hypertension. Often best for people with heart failure or diabetes. However, can also lead to high blood levels of potassium, so periodic blood tests are required.

[a]Price ranges include generic versions, available for diuretics, beta-blockers, and the ACE inhibitor captopril. Cost data provided by Scott-Levin, a subsidiary of PMSI.

[b]Muscle weakness may be remedied by taking prescribed potassium supplements, or switching to a "potassium-sparing" diuretic combination, such as triamterene and hydrochlorothiazide (Dyazide, Maxzide).

Source: Consumer Reports on Health, October, 1996. Common Blood Pressure Drugs. Copyright © 1996 by Consumers Union of U.S., Inc., Yonkers, NY 10703-0157. Reprinted by permission from Consumer Reports, October, 1996.

trol blood pressure with lifestyle changes for at least 3–6 months prior to initiating drug therapy. Even when drug therapy is indicated, weight loss and other lifestyle modifications "should continue to be pursued vigorously."[118]

According to these experts, lifestyle modifications offer "multiple benefits at little cost and with minimal risk. Even when not adequate in themselves to control hypertension, they may reduce the number and doses of antihypertensive medications needed to manage the condition." Also, because so many hypertensive patients have additional risk factors for premature cardiovascular disease, it makes good sense for clinicians to "vigorously encourage their patients to adopt these lifestyle modifications."[118]

Figure 10.28 shows the relative value of lifestyle treatment alone versus lifestyle and drug therapy combined.[136,137] In this 1-year study, mild hypertensives were randomized to

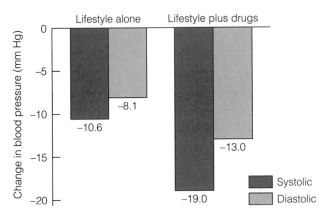

Figure 10.28 Treatment of mild hypertension in 900 people across 1 year: Lifestyle (weight loss, decrease in sodium, and exercise) and drug therapy. Lifestyle modifications have proven to be an effective first-step treatment for persons with mild hypertension. *Source:* Treatment of Mild Hypertension Research Group. The treatment of mild hypertension study: A randomized, placebo-controlled trial of a nutritional–hygienic regimen along with various drug monotherapies. *Arch Intern Med* 151:1413–1423, 1991.

receive lifestyle modifications with either a placebo or one of five different drugs. After 12 months, weight loss averaged 10 pounds, sodium intake had decreased by 23%, and leisure-time physical activity had nearly doubled. Although the additional drug therapy helped to reduce the blood pressure even further, lifestyle alone was found to be an effective first-step treatment for those with mild hypertension.[137]

One of the challenges with lifestyle modification is the poor compliance of most patients in eating less salt, exercising, and maintaining ideal weight. The more compliant the patient, the less likely drug therapy will be required to control hypertension.

Lifestyle Modifications to Lower Blood Pressure

Box 10.4 outlines the lifestyle modifications for preventing and treating hypertension, as recommended by the Joint National Committee on Detection, Evaluation, and Treatment of High Blood Pressure.[118] Of these, weight loss, reduced sodium intake, reduced alcohol consumption, and exercise have the strongest documented efficacy.[119] Table 10.6 shows the suggested treatment for hypertension, for people in various risk groups, in several blood pressure stages.

Weight Control

Studies have identified a strong relationship between body weight and blood pressure.[118,119,134–143] (See discussion in Chapter 13.) Being overweight results in a two- to sixfold increase in the risk of developing hypertension, with the

---

Box 10.4

Lifestyle Modifications for Hypertension Control or Overall Cardiovascular Risk

Following are recommended lifestyle changes for preventing and treating hypertension.

- Lose weight if overweight.
- Limit alcohol intake to no more than 1 oz (30 mL) ethanol (e.g., 24 oz [720 mL] beer, 10 oz [300 mL] wine, or 2 oz [60 mL] 100-proof whiskey) per day or 0.5 oz (15 mL) ethanol per day for women and lighter weight people.
- Increase aerobic physical activity (30–45 minutes most days of the week).
- Reduce sodium intake to no more than 100 mmol per day (2.4 g sodium or 6 g sodium chloride).
- Maintain adequate intake of dietary potassium (approximately 90 mmol per day).
- Maintain adequate intake of dietary calcium and magnesium for general health.
- Stop smoking and reduce intake of dietary saturated fat and cholesterol for overall cardiovascular health.

Source: National High Blood Pressure Education Program. *The Sixth Report of the Joint National Committee on Detection, Evaluation, and Treatment of High Blood Pressure.* National Heart, Lung, and Blood Institute, National Institutes of Health, NIH Publication No. 98-4080. Bethesda, MD: National Institutes of Health, 1997.

---

risk climbing in a stepwise manner with increasing body weight.

Clinical trials with hypertensive and even normotensive subjects have documented that loss of excess weight reduces both systolic and diastolic blood pressure, and has been identified as the most effective of the lifestyle strategies tested.[119,140,143] Figure 10.29 shows the results of one 18-month study of over 500 subjects with high-normal blood pressure.[138] Weight reduction was shown to be an effective lifestyle intervention, with the greatest decreases in blood pressure correlating with those who lost the most weight. Although the goal for subjects randomized to the weight-loss group was to achieve a weight loss of at least 10 pounds through diet and exercise modifications, only 45% of the men and 26% of the women were able to meet this. As discussed in Chapter 13, weight loss is a difficult task for most people, and requires unusual discipline and motivation.

TABLE 10.6   Treatment for Hypertension, Based on Stage and Risk Factors

Blood Pressure Stages (mm Hg)	Risk Group A (no risk factors, no TOD/CCD)[b]	Risk Group B (at least 1 risk factor, not including diabetes; no TOD/CCD)	Risk Group C (TOD/CCD and/or diabetes, with or without other risk factors)
High-normal (130–139 / 85–89)	Lifestyle modification	Lifestyle modification	Drug therapy[c]
Stage 1 (140–159 / 90–99)	Lifestyle modification (up to 12 months)	Lifestyle modification[d] (up to 6 months)	Drug therapy
Stages 2 and 3 (≥160 / ≥100)	Drug therapy	Drug therapy	Drug therapy

For example, a patient with diabetes and a blood pressure of 142/94 mm Hg plus left ventricular hypertrophy should be classified as having Stage 1 hypertension with target organ disease (left ventricular hypertrophy) and with another major risk factor (diabetes). This patient would be categorized as Stage 1, Risk Group C, and recommended for immediate initiation of pharmacological treatment.

[a]Lifestyle modification should be adjunctive therapy for all patients recommended for pharmacological therapy. Major risk factors include smoking, dyslipidemia, diabetes mellitus, age older than 60 years, sex (men and postmenopausal women), and family history of cardiovascular disease—women under age 65 or men under age 55. Target organ damage (TOD) and clinical cardiovascular disease (CCD) include heart diseases (left ventricular hypertrophy, angina/prior myocardial infarction, prior coronary revascularization, and heart failure), stroke or transient ischemic attack, nephropathy, peripheral arterial disease, and retinopathy.
[b]TOD/CCD indicates target organ disease/clinical cardiovascular disease.
[c]For patients with multiple risk factors, clinicians should consider drugs as initial therapy plus lifestyle modifications.
[d]For those with heart failure, renal insufficiency, or diabetes.

Source: National High Blood Pressure Education Program. *The Sixth Report of the Joint National Committee on Detection, Evaluation, and Treatment of High Blood Pressure.* National Heart, Lung, and Blood Institute, National Institutes of Health, NIH Publication No. 98-4080. Bethesda, MD: National Institutes of Health, 1997.

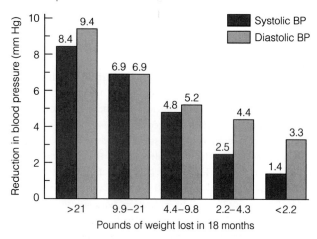

Figure 10.29 Weight loss and effect on blood pressure: 18-month study of more than 500 subjects with high-normal blood pressures. Among subjects with high-normal blood pressure (diastolic blood pressure between 80 and 89 mm Hg), those losing the most weight experienced the greatest reduction in blood pressure. *Source:* Data from Stevens VJ, Corrigan SA, Obarzanek E, et al. Weight loss intervention in Phase I of the trials of hypertension prevention. *Arch Intern Med* 153:849–858, 1993.

Reduced Sodium Chloride Intake

Most people in Western societies consume a diet that contains between 2,500 and 5,000 mg of sodium (about 6–12 g of salt or sodium chloride) per person per day. As discussed in Chapter 9, average daily sodium intake from food alone exceeds 4,000 mg for each U.S. man, and almost 3,000 mg for each woman. These values do not include sodium from salt added to foods at the table. This is far in excess of the physiological need for salt and appears to be substantially more than that eaten by our ancestors or people living in isolated societies. When high salt intake is prolonged throughout the lifetime of a population, the majority will eventually experience a rise in blood pressure.[119]

Sodium is essential for a wide variety of functions in the body. Although needs vary from person to person, a minimum of 500 mg sodium per day is considered necessary to maintain physiological balance for adults, although up to 2,000–3,000 mg per day is considered safe and adequate. As reviewed in Chapter 9, 1 teaspoon of salt (5 g) has 2,000 mg of sodium. The Joint National Committee on Detection, Evaluation, and Treatment of High Blood Pressure recommends less than 2,300 milligrams a day to prevent hypertension.[118]

In the INTERSALT study, a large international epidemiological study of 10,000 people living in 32 countries, a 1-teaspoon difference in salt consumption was associated with a 2.2 mm Hg difference in systolic blood pressure.[144,145] The same study showed that consuming 1 teaspoon less salt a day was associated with a 9 mm Hg attenuation in the rise of systolic blood pressure between the ages of 25 and 55 years.[144,145] In another study of 47,000 individuals, 1 teaspoon of salt was associated with differences in systolic blood pressure that ranged from 5 mm Hg at ages 15–19, to 10 mm Hg at ages 60–69, with the difference even larger for those with higher blood pressures.[146] In general, the risk of hypertension is lower when salt intake is lower.[147]

In clinical trials with hypertensive patients, lowering salt consumption by about ½ teaspoon a day reduces systolic blood pressure by about 5 mm Hg and diastolic blood pressure by 2.5 mm Hg.[118] Adaptation to long-term salt reduction is possible with appropriate counseling. Although the taste for salt is innate, this can be altered, resulting in a decreased intake of 30–50%.[148]

Sauces, dressings, processed meats, cheese, soup, and some breakfast cereals are especially high in sodium. Nutrition experts recommend these steps for keeping sodium intake below recommended levels:[124]

- Learn to read food labels, and avoid foods high in sodium.
- Choose more fresh fruits and vegetables.
- Reduce use of salt during cooking, and use herbs, spices, and low-sodium seasonings.
- Avoid using the salt shaker on prepared foods at the table.

- Limit the use of foods with visible salt on them (snack chips, salted nuts, crackers, etc.).

Potassium appears to help reduce blood pressure by increasing the amount of sodium excreted in the urine and by promoting other favorable physiological changes.[119,149,150] The *sodium-to-potassium ratio* (Na:K) has been explored as a potentially useful indicator of hypertension risk.[150] In the INTERSALT study, changing the Na:K from 3 to 1 equated to a 3.4 mm Hg drop in systolic blood pressure.[144] The average Na:K ratio in the United States is 1.2–1.3, but 0.60 is recommended (which means consuming more potassium than sodium from the diet). Table 10.7 summarizes the categories of foods that are useful (or counterproductive) for improving the Na:K ratio.

Although some studies have indicated that low calcium and magnesium intake may be associated with an increased prevalence of hypertension, the data are inconsistent, and there appears to be no justification for using supplements beyond what is obtained in a varied and balanced diet.[118,119]

Moderation of Alcohol Intake

Studies have identified a positive association between an alcohol intake of 40 grams of ethanol per day (3 drinks or more) and increased blood pressure.[118,119] The prevalence of high blood pressure is four times greater for heavy drinkers than for those who abstain. Also, when hypertensive men who are heavy drinkers discontinue their alcohol intake, their blood pressure falls. For these reasons, hypertensive patients who drink alcohol-containing beverages should be counseled to limit their daily intake to 1 ounce of ethanol a day.[118] As reviewed in Chapter 9, a standard drink contains 0.5 ounce of ethanol (as found in one 12-oz can of beer, one 4-oz glass of wine, or 1.5 oz of 80-proof spirits).

TABLE 10.7   Sodium and Potassium Levels for Various Food Groups

Low-Sodium, High-Potassium Foods	
Fruits and fruit juices	Pineapple, grapefruit, pears, strawberries, watermelon, raisins, bananas, apricots, oranges, etc.
Low-sodium cereals	Oatmeal (unsalted), Roman Meal hot cereal, Shredded Wheat, etc.
Nuts (unsalted)	Hazel nuts, macadamia nuts, almonds, peanuts, cashews, coconut, etc.
Vegetables	Summer squash, zucchini, eggplant, cucumber, onions, lettuce, green beans, broccoli, etc.
Beans (dry, cooked)	Great Northern, lentils, lima beans, red kidney beans, etc.
High-Sodium, Low-Potassium Foods	
Fats	Butter, margarine, salad dressings
Soups	Onion soup, mushroom soup, chicken noodle soup, tomato soup, split pea soup, etc.
Breakfast cereals	Corn flakes, Product 19, Wheaties, Total, Nutri-Grain, etc.
Breads	All varieties except for low-sodium brands
Processed meats	Bacon, canned meats, sausages, etc.
Cheeses	Nearly all varieties, except when specifically labeled as low sodium

(a) Alcohol drinking status of Americans

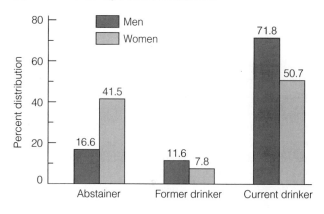

(b) Alcohol consuption by Americans who drink

Level of alcohol consumption in past 2 weeks for current drinkers

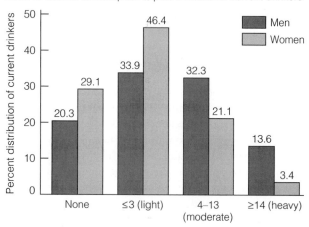

Figure 10.30 Of current drinkers, 13.6% of men and 3.4% of women drink heavily. *Source:* National Center for Health Statistics. *Health, United States, 1996–97 and Injury Chartbook.* Hyattsville, MD: 1997.

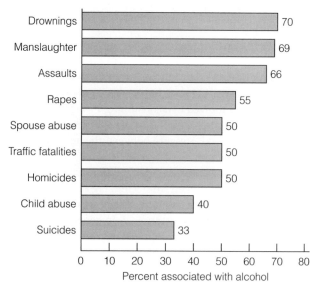

Figure 10.31 Violence and injuries associated with alcohol: National Institute on Alcohol Abuse and Alcoholism. Alcohol is associated with a large proportion of the violence and injuries in America. *Source:* Alcohol, Drug Abuse, and Mental Health Administration, National Institute on Alcohol Abuse and Alcoholism. *Seventh Special Report to the U.S. Congress on Alcohol and Health.* Rockville, MD: U.S. Department of Health and Human Services, 1990.

Alcoholism has been defined as[151]

> a primary, chronic disease with genetic, psychosocial, and environmental factors influencing its development and manifestations. The disease is often progressive and fatal. It is characterized by impaired control over drinking, preoccupation with the drug alcohol, use of alcohol despite adverse consequences, and distortions in thinking, most notably denial. Each of these symptoms may be continuous or periodic.

Several questionnaires have been developed to help people determine whether they have alcoholic tendencies.[152] (See Physical Fitness Activity 10.4 at the end of this chapter.)

The National Institute on Alcohol Abuse and Alcoholism reports that 15.1 million in the United States are either alco-

holics or alcohol abusers.[153] As summarized in Figure 10.30, 72% of men and 51% of women are current drinkers.[14] Of current drinkers, 13.6% of men and 3.4% of women drink heavily (≥14 drinks/week). Alcohol consumption on a per capita basis has been gradually declining since peaking during the late 1970s.[153]

Alcohol affects almost every organ system in the body, either directly or indirectly.[153] The liver (the primary site of alcohol metabolism) is most susceptible. In the gastrointestinal tract, regular alcohol use can precipitate inflammation of the esophagus and pancreas, exacerbate existing peptic ulcers, and cause some cancers (e.g., breast cancer in women). When alcohol accounts for a high percentage of caloric intake, it can lead to significant nutritional deficiencies. Alcohol affects immune, endocrine, and reproductive functions and is a well-documented cause of neurological problems, including dementia, blackouts, seizures, hallucinations, and peripheral neuropathy.

Alcohol is the third leading cause of death in the United States, causing over 100,000 deaths yearly from injuries, certain types of cancer, and liver disease, and it is related to a large percentage of the violence in this country (see Figure 10.31). Nearly half of the trauma beds in the United States are occupied by patients who were injured while under the influence of alcohol.[154] Each year, alcohol-related motor-vehicle crashes result in more than 17,000 deaths, one third of them involving people under the age of 25 years.[155]

TABLE 10.8   Summary of the Relationship between Blood Alcohol Concentration (BAC) and Clinical Symptoms

BAC (g/100 ml of blood or g/210 l of breath)	Stage	Clinical Symptoms
0.01–0.05	Subclinical	Behavior nearly normal by ordinary observation
0.03–0.12	Euphoria	Mild euphoria, sociability, talkativeness Increased self-confidence; decreased inhibitions Diminution of attention, judgment, and control Beginning of sensorimotor impairment Loss of efficiency in finer performance tests
0.09–0.25	Excitement	Emotional instability; loss of critical judgment Impairment of perception, memory, and comprehension Decreased sensory response; increased reaction time Reduced visual acuity, peripheral vision, and glare recovery Sensorimotor incoordination, impaired balance Drowsiness
0.18–0.30	Confusion	Disorientation, mental confusion; dizziness Exaggerated emotional stages Disturbances of vision and of perception of color, form, motion, and dimensions Increased pain threshold Increased muscular incoordination; staggering gait; slurred speech Apathy, lethargy
0.25–0.40	Stupor	General inertia; approaching loss of motor functions Markedly decreased response to stimuli Marked muscular incoordination; inability to stand or walk Vomiting; incontinence Impaired consciousness; sleep or stupor
0.35–0.50	Coma	Complete unconsciousness Depressed or abolished reflexes Subnormal body temperature Incontinence Impairment of circulation and respiration Possible death
0.45+	Death	Death from respiratory arrest

Source: Intoximeters Inc.: http://intox.com/

As a rule of thumb, one standard drink consumed within 1 hour will produce a blood alcohol level (BAL; also BAC, for blood alcohol concentration) of 0.02 in a 150-pound male. Five beers consumed within 1 hour will cause the BAL to rise to 0.10, which violates the drinking and driving laws of most states. (See Table 10.8 for a summary of the relationship between blood alcohol content and clinical symptoms.) About 40% of all Americans will be involved in an alcohol-related crash during their lifetime.[155]

In contrast to these negative effects, alcohol use has been consistently related to lowered risk of coronary heart disease for both men and women, usually on the order of 20–50%.[156–160] Figure 10.32 shows the results of one large study of more than 50,000 health professionals, in which intake of more than two drinks a day was associated with a 47% reduction in risk of coronary heart disease.[156] In a Kaiser Permanente study of more than 120,000 people, coronary heart disease mortality was reduced among drinkers, compared with lifelong nondrinkers.[157]

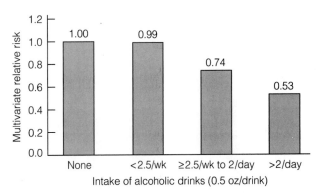

Figure 10.32 Alcohol consumption and risk of coronary heart disease: Health professionals follow-up study of 51,529 middle-aged men. Drinking more than two drinks a day was associated with a 47% reduction in risk of coronary heart disease in this study of more than 50,000 health professionals. *Source:* Data from Rimm EB, Giovannucci EL, Willett WC, et al. Prospective study of alcohol consumption and risk of coronary disease in men. *Lancet* 338:464–468, 1991.

The epidemiological evidence suggests that all alcoholic beverages are similarly protective, and that there is no special effect of red wine over beer or spirits.[158,160,161] The cardioprotective effect of alcohol appears to be due to its effect in raising HDL cholesterol 10–15% and reducing clot formation.[158] Alcoholics, however, have an increased risk of death from heart disease due to ultrastructural changes in the heart tissue resulting from chronic exposure to ethanol.[153] This can lead to sudden death from abnormal heart arrhythmias.

The cardiovascular benefit of light-to-moderate alcohol consumption must be balanced against the risks of cancer and other causes of death.[162,163] When different levels of alcohol consumption are linked to all causes of death, two to six drinks per day are associated with the highest risk of death[162] (see Figure 10.33). In fact, two drinks a day or more increase the risk of mortality by more than 50%. In other words, the benefits on coronary heart disease mortality are more than offset by an increased risk of death from other causes, including cancer.[162,163]

Researchers have been reluctant to advise the public to "drink for your heart." Investigators from the MRFIT research project, for example, found that light-to-moderate drinkers were at lower risk for coronary heart disease but then stated, "alcohol consumption, however, cannot be recommended because of the known adverse effects of excess alcohol use."[159] Researchers from Harvard reported that alcohol consumption reduces risk of coronary heart disease for both men and women, but have written, "our society is so lacking in effective social controls on alcohol abuse and pays such a heavy price for its inadequate response that . . . the thought of a public policy promoting alcohol consumption runs strongly against the grain, however much it might capture at least some hearts."[160] In other words, there are too many problems associated with drinking in our society to recommend this approach for heart disease reduction. The cure would be far worse than the disease.

Physical Activity

As explained in Chapter 4, when a person engages in aerobic exercise, the systolic blood pressure and heart rate will increase, while the diastolic blood pressure changes little. Immediately following the exercise bout, the systolic blood pressure of hypertensive men will fall below pre-exercise values by 20–30 mm Hg, and that of normotensive men by 8–12 mm Hg, an effect that lasts for 20–120 minutes (see Figure 10.34).[164–166] There are many potential mechanisms for this "postexercise hypotensive effect," including relaxa-

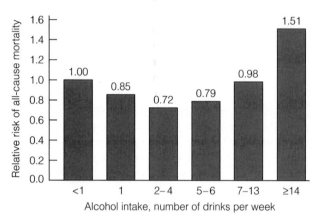

Figure 10.33 Alcohol consumption and all-cause mortality: Physicians' health study, 10.7-year follow-up of 22,071 men. The "J" curve relationship between alcohol consumption and all-cause mortality risk. *Source:* Camargo CA, Hennekens CH, Gaziano JM, Glynn RJ, Manson JE, Stampfer MJ. Prospective study of moderate alcohol consumption and mortality in US male physicians. *Arch Intern Med* 157:79–85, 1997.

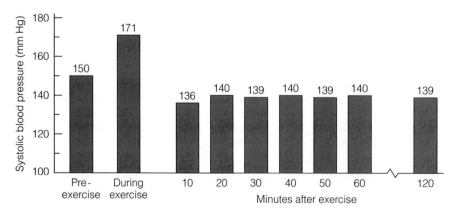

Figure 10.34 The systolic blood pressure response to 45 minutes of exercise: Treadmill walking, 70% of heart rate reserve, in 18 men with high blood pressure. In this study of men with high blood pressure, 45 minutes of brisk treadmill walking lowered the blood pressure below resting levels for at least 2 hours. The decrease was related to a widening and relaxation of the blood vessels. *Source:* Rueckert PA, Slane PR, Lillis DL, Hanson P. Hemodynamic patterns and duration of post-dynamic exercise hypotension in hypertensive humans. *Med Sci Sports Exerc* 28:24–32, 1996.

tion and vasodilation of blood vessels in the legs and visceral organ areas.[164] The blood vessels may relax after each exercise session because of body warming effects, local production of certain chemicals (e.g., lactic acid and nitric oxide), decreases in nerve activity, and changes in certain hormones and their receptors.[164–167] Over time, as the exercise is repeated, there is growing evidence that a long-lasting reduction in resting blood pressure can be measured, which may in part be due to the acute drop in blood pressure that occurs after each bout.

Interestingly, if the blood pressure surges too steeply (i.e., well above 200 mm Hg) during a standardized exercise

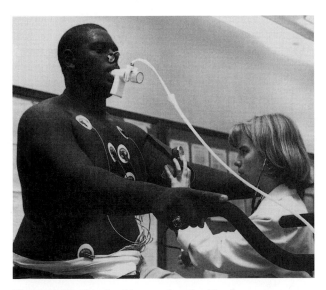

Figure 10.35 People with normal resting blood pressures who experience elevated blood pressure responses during graded exercise testing are at increased risk of developing future resting hypertension.

test, risk of future hypertension or heart disease is unusually high, even in subjects with normal resting blood pressures[168,169] (see Figure 10.35). In one study, for example, the prevalence of hypertension on follow-up among normotensive subjects with a hypertensive response to exercise testing was 2.1 to 3.4 times higher than that among subjects with a normotensive response.[168] In another study, exercise blood pressure was found to be a better predictor of future heart attack than resting blood pressure.[169] The American College of Sports Medicine (ACSM) has urged that if exercise test results are available, patients with an exaggerated blood pressure response should be counseled about their increased risk of developing hypertension at rest in the future, and they should be given appropriate advice regarding health habits that might ameliorate their increased risk.[170]

Exercise has a strong effect in treating high blood pressure. The ACSM and other reviewers have concluded that people with mild hypertension can expect systolic and diastolic blood pressures to fall an average of 8–10 mm Hg and 6–10 mm Hg, respectively, in response to regular aerobic exercise.[170–174] This benefit is independent of changes in body weight or diet (which can result in greater reductions). Even for people with normal resting blood pressures, exercise training can be expected to lower the systolic and diastolic blood pressures by an average of 4 mm Hg and 3 mm Hg, respectively.[171]

The improvement in blood pressure with exercise training may extend to patients with severe hypertension, but few studies exist to confirm this. Figure 10.36 shows the results of one study of African American men with severe hypertension.[173] Subjects exercised for several months, engaging in stationary cycling, three times a week, 20 to 60 minutes a session at 60–80% of maximum heart rate. As a safety precaution, prior to initiating exercise training, dia-

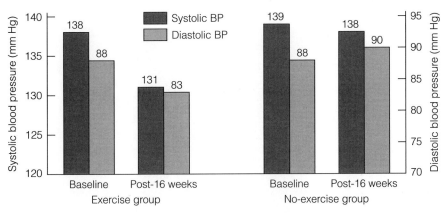

Figure 10.36 Effects of exercise in African American men with severe hypertension: 16 weeks of cycling, three sessions/week, 20–60 minutes/session, at 60–80% maximum heart rate. Moderate exercise training was effective in reducing blood pressure in African Americans with severe hypertension. All subjects were on medication. *Source:* Kokkinos PF, Narayan P, Colleran JA, et al. Effects of regular exercise on blood pressure and left ventricular hypertrophy in African-American men with severe hypertension. *N Engl J Med* 333:1462–1467, 1995.

stolic blood pressures were reduced at least 10 mm Hg with medication. As shown in Figure 10.36, exercise subjects experienced strong decreases in blood pressure after 16 weeks. Exercise training continued for an additional 16 weeks, and doses of medication were reduced in 71% of the exercise subjects, but none of the controls. The results suggest that severe hypertension can be managed effectively with a combination of drug therapy and regular, moderately intense exercise. Most important, medications necessary to control blood pressure without exercise can be curtailed substantially as patients continue exercising.

Most studies show that exercise training acts quickly to improve blood pressure among hypertensives, with most of the effect taking place within the first few weeks. Further reductions in blood pressure may occur if the exercise training is maintained for more than 3 months. Figure 10.37 summarizes results from a study in which hypertensives exercised aerobically three times a week for 10 weeks, while taking a diuretic, a beta-blocker, or a placebo.[174] Exercise alone without drugs resulted in an impressive 8 mm Hg drop in the diastolic blood pressure within the first month, with drug therapy adding a little extra benefit. Interestingly, most of the improvement in blood pressure occurred during the first week, with some additional progress measured as the training continued.

The aerobic exercise program does not have to be too demanding to improve resting blood pressure. In fact, moderate-intensity exercise such as brisk walking may have an even greater blood-pressure-lowering effect than higher intensity training (e.g., running) for some people. The important exercise criterion is frequency—near-daily activity helps the body experience the beneficial blood-pressure-lowering effects of regular exercise.[170]

ACSM does not recommend weight training as the only form of exercise for hypertensives.[170] Weight training does not appear to be as effective in lowering blood pressure as aerobic exercise, although it is an excellent way to increase muscular strength and is recommended for overall physical fitness.[175] Experts recommend, however, that hypertensives avoid maximal lifts and instead emphasize weight lifts that they can repeat for 10–15 repetitions.[170]

Can regular exercise training prevent hypertension from developing? Several major epidemiological studies have been conducted, supporting this idea.[176–178] In general, sedentary and unfit normotensive individuals have a 20–50% increased risk of developing hypertension during follow-up when compared with their more active and fit peers[170] (see Figure 10.38). In a 6- to 10-year study of 15,000 Harvard male alumni, for example, those who did not engage in vigorous sports and activity were at 35% greater risk of hypertension than those who did, and this relationship held at all ages, 35–74 years.[176] In a 4-year study in Dallas, unfit individuals were found to be 52% more likely to develop hypertension than were those who were fit.[177]

Studies on both adults and children have consistently shown that physical activity and fitness are linked to a more favorable blood pressure level, compared to an inactive lifestyle.[170,179–181] In one study of 8,283 male recreational runners, those running more than 50 miles a week, compared to less than 10 miles a week, showed a 50% reduction in prevalence of hypertension and a 50% reduction in the use of medications to lower blood pressure.[179] A study of nearly 5,000 Dutch women showed that blood pressure was lowest in those spending the most time exercising in various sports.[180]

People with high blood pressure have been shown to be less fit (about 30%) than those with normal blood pressures.[182] Thus, regular aerobic exercise is critical for hypertensive patients to improve physical fitness and life quality,

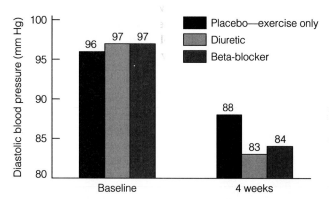

Figure 10.37 Exercise versus drug therapy for hypertension: All subjects exercised three times per week and were randomly assigned to a placebo or a drug group. Exercise training had a strong effect in lowering blood pressure, with drug therapy having only a small additional effect. *Source:* Data from Kelemen MH, Effron MB, Valenti SA, Stewart KJ. Exercise training combined with antihypertensive drug therapy: Effects on lipids, blood pressure, and left ventricular mass. *JAMA* 263:2766–2771, 1990.

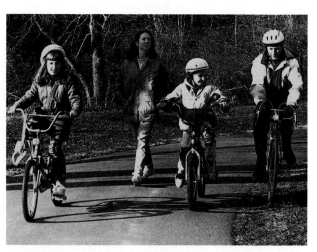

Figure 10.38 Regular exercise is associated with a lower risk of developing high blood pressure.

and to lower risk of heart disease. Data from the Cooper Institute for Aerobics Research have shown that death rates are lower in highly fit people, even when their blood pressures are high, as compared to people with low aerobic fitness and normal blood pressures.[117]

HIGH BLOOD CHOLESTEROL

As reviewed earlier in this chapter, high blood cholesterol is a major risk factor for heart disease.[183–186] Figure 10.39 shows that risk of CHD rises sharply with increase in blood cholesterol levels.[54]

The body makes it own cholesterol and also absorbs cholesterol from certain kinds of foods, specifically all animal products (i.e., meats, dairy products, and eggs). Cholesterol is essential for the formation of bile acids (used in fat digestion) and some hormones, and it is a component of cell membranes and of brain and nerve tissues.[185]

Thus, some cholesterol is necessary to keep the body functioning normally. However, when blood cholesterol levels are too high, some of the excess (especially the oxidized form of LDL cholesterol) is deposited in the artery walls, increasing the risk of heart disease.[4–10, 183] In contrast, according to many studies, when blood cholesterol levels are lowered through lifestyle changes and medication, risk of coronary heart disease decreases.[40–46] As reviewed earlier, for every 1% reduction in blood cholesterol, the occurrence of coronary heart disease is reduced 2% or 3%.[36]

Prevalence of High Blood Cholesterol

Experts urge that everyone know their cholesterol level and have it checked at least once every 5 years (or every year if heart disease risk is high).[186,187] Americans are more "cholesterol conscious" than ever before. A poll by the National Heart, Lung, and Blood Institute showed that 75% of Americans have had their cholesterol checked, and about half can recall their own cholesterol level. Figure 10.40 summarizes the blood cholesterol levels of Americans. Notice the strong increase in serum cholesterol levels with age, especially among women.[14,188–190]

According to the National Cholesterol Education Program, blood cholesterol levels can be categorized as follows:[186]

- Desirable—less than 200 mg/dl
- Borderline-high—200–239 mg/dl
- High—240 mg/dl and above

Despite an impressive (7.7%) drop from the 1960s, 19% of Americans still have high blood cholesterol levels, and 30% have borderline-high levels[14] (see Figures 10.41 and 10.42). The American average for serum cholesterol is 203 mg/dl, and if present trends continue, the Healthy People Year 2000 goal of 200 mg/dl will probably be achieved.[14,188] Some populations around the world with very low risk of heart disease have blood cholesterol levels below 160 mg/dl, a level now regarded by some experts as within the

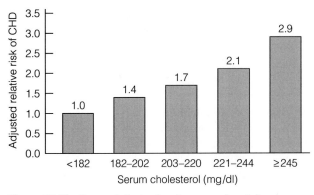

Figure 10.39   Serum cholesterol and coronary heart disease: MRFIT of 316,099 white men, with 12-year follow-up, including 6,327 CHD deaths. In this 12-year study (MRFIT) of more than 300,000 men, risk of coronary heart disease climbed sharply with increase in serum cholesterol.   *Source:* Data from Neaton JD, Wentworth D. Serum cholesterol, blood pressure, cigarette smoking, and death from coronary heart disease. *Arch Intern Med* 152: 56–64, 1992.

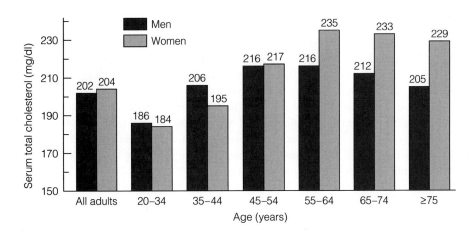

Figure 10.40   Mean serum total cholesterol levels among U.S. adults, 1988–1994. Serum cholesterol levels rise with increase in age.   *Source:* National Center for Health Statistics. *Health, United States, 1996–97 and Injury Chartbook.* Hyattsville, MD: 1997.

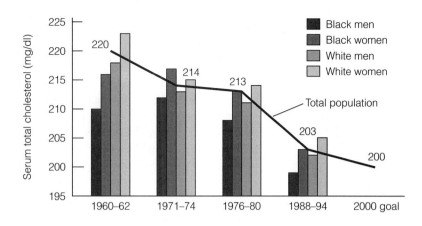

Figure 10.41 Declining serum total cholesterol levels among U.S. adults: Overall mean = 203 mg/dl; 7.7% decrease since 1960; 19% of U.S. population has ≥240 mg/dl cholesterol. Serum total cholesterol levels have fallen consistently since the 1960s for all groups in the United States. *Source:* National Center for Health Statistics. *Health, United States, 1996–97 and Injury Chartbook.* Hyattsville, MD: 1997.

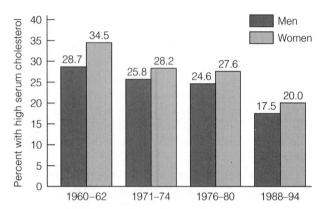

Figure 10.42 Percentage of population with high serum cholesterol (≥240 mg/dl). Prevalence of high blood cholesterol (≥240 mg/dl) has fallen to only 19% in 1988–1994. *Source:* National Center for Health Statistics. *Health, United States, 1996–97 and Injury Chartbook.* Hyattsville, MD: 1997.

"optimal" zone.[184] In the Framingham Heart Study, for example, a study initiated during the 1950s, heart disease has been extremely rare among those with blood cholesterol levels within the optimal zone.[191]

Description of Lipoproteins

To transport the cholesterol and triglycerides, the body utilizes various protein packets, called lipoproteins. There are three major lipoproteins in the fasting blood: *high-density lipoprotein* (HDL), *low-density lipoprotein* (LDL), and *very-low density lipoprotein* (VLDL). Figure 10.43 outlines the protein and lipid composition of each lipoprotein. HDL is the smallest and densest lipoprotein, being nearly half protein. LDL carries the most cholesterol (60–70% of all the serum cholesterol). VLDL is mostly triglyceride.[185,192]

The protein part of the lipoprotein is called *apoprotein*. Apoproteins are important in activating or inhibiting certain enzymes involved in the metabolism of fats. They are identified by letters. HDL, for example, has several differ-

ent apoproteins, the important ones being Apo A-I and Apo A-II. LDL is high in Apo B.

The HDL particle appears to act as a type of shuttle as it takes up cholesterol from the blood and body cells and transfers it to the liver, where it is used to form bile acids.[159,186,193–195] The bile acids are involved in the digestion process, with some of them passing out with the stool, thus providing the body with a major route for excretion of cholesterol. HDLs have for this reason been called the "garbage trucks" of the blood system, collecting cholesterol and dumping it into the liver.

LDL, on the other hand, is formed after VLDL gives up its triglycerides to body cells. LDLs are high in cholesterol and take their cholesterol to various body cells, where it is deposited for cell functions. When LDL cholesterol is too high, it contributes to the buildup of atherosclerosis (see Figure 10.44).[5,186]

LDL cholesterol levels are classified by the National Cholesterol Education Program (NCEP) of the National Heart, Lung, and Blood Institute, National Institutes of Health as follows:[186]

- Desirable—less than 130 mg/dl
- Borderline-high—130–159 mg/dl
- High—160 mg/dl and above

LDL cholesterol levels should be as low as possible, with optimal levels falling below 100 mg/dl.

HDL cholesterol (HDL-C) concentration is emerging as an important measure of heart disease risk, and the National Institutes for Health have urged that HDL-C determinations accompany measurements of total cholesterol when healthy individuals are being assessed for coronary heart disease risk.[186,193] Various studies have shown that a 1% rise in HDL-C reduces coronary heart disease risk 2–3%, and that people with the highest HDL-C have heart disease death rates 2–3 times lower than those with the lowest HDL-C levels.[194,196,197]

Mean HDL-C levels are higher among women (56 mg/dl) than men (46 mg/dl) and change little with increase in

Lipoproteins

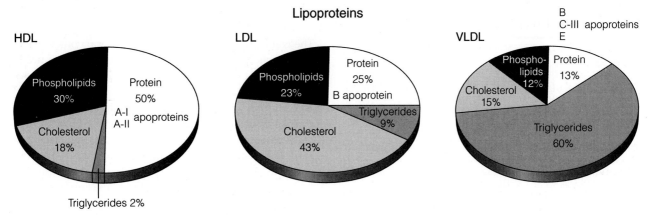

Figure 10.43 Lipoproteins. There are three different kinds of lipoproteins in fasting blood. *Source:* Haskell WL. The influence of exercise on the concentrations of triglyceride and cholesterol in human plasma. *Exerc Sport Sci Rev* 12:205–244, 1984.

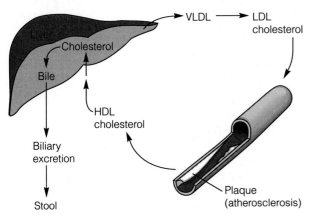

Figure 10.44 Functions of lipoproteins. LDL and HDL have opposing functions. HDL takes cholesterol to the liver, where it is changed to bile and eventually excreted in the stool. This is the body's major method of reducing its cholesterol stores.

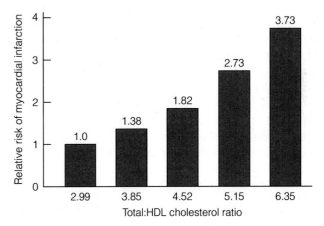

Figure 10.45 Total:HDL cholesterol ratio and myocardial infarction: Physicians' health study, Harvard Medical School; 246 case–control pairs. In this case–control study of heart attack victims, risk climbed sharply with rise in the ratio of total-to-HDL cholesterol. *Source:* Data from Stampfer MJ, Sacks FM, Salvini S, Willett WC, Hennekens CH. A prospective study of cholesterol, apolipoproteins, and the risk of myocardial infarction. *N Engl J Med* 325:373–381, 1991.

age. HDL-C is also higher among blacks than whites.[188] The National Cholesterol Education Program regards HDL-C levels below 35 mg/dl as an important risk factor, with optimal values rising above 60 mg/dl.[186]

Because of the importance of HDL-C, various ratios have been used to improve prediction of heart disease risk. HDL-C can be expressed as a percentage of the total cholesterol, or more commonly, as[195,198,199]

$$\frac{\text{total cholesterol}}{\text{HDL–C}}$$

This ratio has been extremely useful in estimating heart disease risk, as shown in Figure 10.45. In this study of 246 men who had suffered a heart attack versus 246 controls, risk of heart attack climbed sharply with increase in the ratio.[199] A ratio below 3.0 is optimal, while 5.0 and above is considered high risk. For every unit the ratio falls (e.g.,

5.0 to 4.0), risk of coronary heart disease decreases 53%.[199] The average American adult male has a 4.6 ratio, the average female, 4.0.[195] The elderly, the obese, and smokers have higher ratios, while females, alcohol users, blacks, and active people have lower ratios.[195]

The status of serum triglyceride levels as a risk factor for heart disease is less clear. Table 10.9 summarizes NCEP guidelines for classifying serum triglycerides.[186,188] In studies, a high triglyceride level has been found to predict heart disease, but when adjusted for other risk factors, its usefulness as an independent predictor is lost.[193,200,201] However, in cases of people with low HDL-C levels, diabetes, obesity (especially central), and hypertension, and of young adults with multiple risk factors, risk of heart disease increases

TABLE 10.9 Guidelines for Classifying Serum Triglyceride Levels

Serum Triglyceride	mg/dl
Normal triglycerides	<200
Borderline-high triglycerides	200–399
High triglycerides	400–1,000
Very high triglycerides	>1,000

Source: From National Cholesterol Education Program. 1993. *Second Report of the Expert Panel on Detection, Evaluation, and Treatment of High Blood Cholesterol in Adults.* Bethesda, MD: U.S. Department of Health and Human Services, Public Health Service; National Institutes of Health; National Heart, Lung, Blood Institute.

as the triglyceride level increases.[193] Figure 10.46 shows the average serum triglyceride levels for American males and females.[188] Optimal triglyceride values are less than 110 mg/dl, and the levels for athletes are usually below 80 mg/dl.[192] Triglycerides can be lowered by losing weight, exercising aerobically, and reducing alcohol intake. High-sugar diets may increase triglyceride levels for some people.

Most medical laboratories do not measure the LDL-C, but rather calculate it, based on measurements of total cholesterol, HDL-C, and triglycerides. As shown in Figure 10.43, all three lipoproteins carry cholesterol. Thus, the total cholesterol equals the cholesterol in the LDL, HDL, and VLDL. In the indirect procedure, an estimate of the VLDL-C is made by multiplying triglycerides by 20%. The equation is as follows:[202]

$$\text{LDL-C} = \text{total cholesterol} - [\text{HDL-C} + (0.20 \times \text{triglycerides})]$$

For example, if the total cholesterol is 200 mg/dl, HDL-C is 50 mg/dl, and triglycerides are 100 mg/dl:

$$\text{LDL-C} = 200 - [50 + (0.20 \times 100)] = 130 \text{ mg/dl}$$

Treatment of Hypercholesterolemia

The National Cholesterol Education Program offers practical detection and treatment recommendations for health professionals.[186] According to the NCEP guidelines shown in Figure 10.47, all Americans are urged to have their blood cholesterol, HDL-C, and CHD risk factors assessed. If the cholesterol is under 200 mg/dl and the HDL-C over 35 mg/dl, measurements are considered desirable. The intensity of treatment for other people is based on the overall risk status, as shown in Figure 10.47, with more aggressive intervention given to high risk individuals. Final treatment decisions are based on the LDL-C.

For people needing dietary therapy, the NCEP urges that a minimum of 6 months of intensive dietary change, exercise, weight control, and counseling be given.[186] For the first 3 months, the "Step 1" diet should be tried (fat calories <30%, dietary cholesterol <300 mg/day, saturated fat calories 8—10%). If this is unsuccessful, 3 months of the "Step 2" diet is indicated (diet cholesterol <200 mg/day, saturated fat calories <7%) (see Physical Fitness Activity 10.5). If diet and lifestyle therapy do not work, and the LDL-C is high, drug therapy may be initiated. Table 10.10 summarizes dietary and drug treatment decision guidelines.[186]

The NCEP urges that elderly persons in good health not be excluded from therapy, although patients of advanced age or those with severe competing illnesses are not suitable candidates.[186]

Regarding drug therapy, the statins (lovastatin, pravastatin, simvastatin) are highly effective in reducing LDL-C and raising HDL-C and appear to be generally well-tolerated during long-term use. Other major classes of drugs that are recommended include bile acid resin, nicotinic acid, and estrogen replacement for women.[203–206] Table 10.11 summarizes the pros and cons of the various common cholesterol medications.

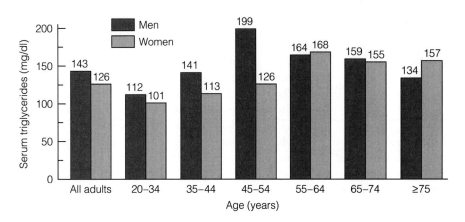

Figure 10.46 Mean serum triglyceride levels among U.S. adults, 1988–1991. Serum triglyceride levels for young male adults are higher than for females; the pattern tends to be reversed in old age. *Source:* Data from Johnson CL, Rifkind BM, Sempos CT, et al. Declining serum total cholesterol levels among US adults. The National Health and Nutrition Examination Surveys. *JAMA* 269:3002–3008, 1993.

(a) Detection, evaluation and treatment of high cholesterol in adults

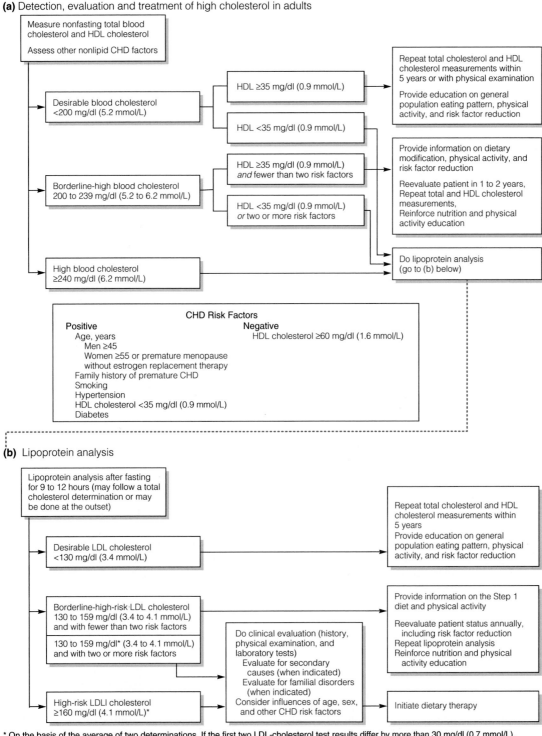

* On the basis of the average of two determinations. If the first two LDL-cholesterol test results differ by more than 30 mg/dl (0.7 mmol/L), a third test result should be obtained within 1 to 8 weeks and the average value of the three tests used.

Figure 10.47 Detection and treatment recommendations of high blood cholesterol from the National Cholesterol Education Program. (a) Detection, evaluation, and treatment of high cholesterol in adults; (b) lipoprotein analysis. *Source:* Expert Panel on Detection, Evaluation, and Treatment of High Blood Cholesterol in Adults. Summary of the second report of the National Cholesterol Education Program (NCEP) expert panel on detection, evaluation, and treatment of high blood cholesterol in adults (adult treatment Panel II). *JAMA* 269:3015–3023, 1993.

TABLE 10.10   Treatment Decisions Based on LDL-C

The initiation level is the LDL-C level at which either dietary or drug therapy should begin, given the various conditions, such as whether CHD and risk factors are present. The goal of therapy is to bring levels of LDL within the LDL goal.

Dietary Therapy	Initiation Level	LDL Goal
Without CHD and with fewer than 2 risk factors	≥160 mg/dl	<160 mg/dl
Without CHD and with 2 or more risk factors	≥130 mg/dl	<130 mg/dl
With CHD	>100 mg/dl	≤100 mg/dl

Drug Treatment	Consideration Level	LDL Goal
Without CHD and with fewer than 2 risk factors	≥190 mg/dl[a]	<160 mg/dl
Without CHD and with 2 or more risk factors	≥160 mg/dl	<130 mg/dl
With CHD	≥130 mg/dl[b]	≤100 mg/dl

[a]In men under 35 years of age and premenopausal women with LDL-C levels 190–219 mg/dl, drug therapy should be delayed except in high-risk patients, such as those with diabetes.
[b]In patients with CHD whose LDL-C levels are 100–129 mg/dl, the physician should exercise clinical judgment in deciding whether to initiate drug treatment.

Source: National Cholesterol Education Program, 1993. *Second Report of the Expert Panel on Detection, Evaluation, and Treatment of High Blood Cholesterol in Adults,* Bethesda, MD: U.S. Department of Health and Human Services, Public Health Service; National Institutes of Health; National Heart, Lung, Blood Institute.

Figure 10.48 summarizes the screening guidelines for children and adolescents.[207] Because the atherosclerotic process begins in childhood and progresses slowly into adulthood, the NCEP urges that all children and youths adopt a low-fat (<30%), low-cholesterol (<300 mg/day), low-saturated-fat (<10%) diet, and that those in high-risk families be screened as shown in Figure 10.48.

Diet and Other Lifestyle Measures

Several organizations have published dietary recommendations for both the prevention and the treatment of hypercholesterolemia.[185,186,208] The NCEP and AHA guidelines are summarized in Box 10.5. In general, the guidelines urge Americans to consume less saturated animal fat and cholesterol and include more carbohydrates and fiber while moderating sodium, energy, and alcohol intake (see Physical Activity 10.5).

Table 10.12 outlines a 3-day menu that both meets the "Step 2" diet guidelines of the NCEP and meets all vitamin and mineral intake recommendations. Notice the wide variety of fruits and vegetables that provide "antioxidant" vitamins, now thought to be crucial in reducing oxidized-LDL. Table 10.13 summarizes information on saturated fat and cholesterol from various food groups.

To have a favorable TC/HDL-C ratio, the total cholesterol (TC) and LDL-C must be lowered and the HDL-C elevated through an application of both dietary and lifestyle factors. A summary of the important factors for elevating HDL-C is given in Box 10.6, and for lowering LDL-C and total cholesterol, in Box 10.7. These factors are listed in order of approximate importance, as summarized from various reviews of the literature.[185,208–214] Aerobic exercise, weight reduction, smoking cessation, and moderate alcohol consumption, each favorable, affects HDL-C, while dietary changes and weight reduction lower LDL-C. As is emphasized in the next section, aerobic exercise has little independent effect on LDL-C and on total cholesterol.

Improvements in lifestyle can have strong, relatively quick effects on total cholesterol, HDL-C, and LDL-C, depending on the initial levels and the degree of change.[208,215,216] The Pritikin Program is a 21-day residential program where high-risk individuals are put on an extremely low-fat (<10% Calories), high-fiber, high-carbohydrate, primarily vegetarian diet, with 1–2 hours of daily moderate exercise.[215]

As shown in Figure 10.49, major improvements are seen in total cholesterol, LDL-C, and triglycerides, with most of the changes occurring within the first 2 weeks. Notice that HDL-C fell 12–19%, which is common during periods where large improvements are being made in the diet. Over time, as the body weight is stabilized and exercise continues, the HDL-C tends to increase a bit. Although the

TABLE 10.11 Common Cholesterol Medications

Drug	Monthly Cost[a]	Therapeutic Effects[b]	Potential Side Effects[b]	Pros and Cons	Good Candidates
Statins (HMG-CoA reductase inhibitors)			**Major:** Elevated liver enzymes, which occasionally signal significant liver problems; rarely, muscle inflammation. **Minor:** *Common:* Headache, indigestion, abdominal pain, flatulence, diarrhea, nausea. *Less common:* Constipation, respiratory infection, fatigue, heartburn, dizziness, rash, insomnia, blurred vision.	**Advantages:** All except fluvastatin reduce "bad" LDL cholesterol more than other cholesterol medications. All less likely to cause uncomfortable side effects. Atorvastatin reduces triglycerides effectively. **Disadvantages:** All increase "good" HDL and (except for atorvastatin) reduce triglycerides much less than some other drugs. Periodic liver tests required. Long-term risks not known.	People who need very large reduction in LDL or who can't tolerate side effects or inconvenience of other cholesterol medications. (Those who need maximum possible reduction in LDL—or any large reduction in LDL plus significant decrease in triglycerides—should consider atorvastatin. Those who need only moderately large LDL reduction should consider fluvastatin, the least expensive statin.)
Atorvastatin: Lipitor	$74	LDL: ↓35–60% HDL: ↑5–15% Triglycerides: ↓15–40%			
Lovastatin: Mevacor	$78	LDL: ↓20–40% HDL: ↑5–15%			
Pravastatin: Pravachol	$65				
Simvastatin: Zocor	$80	Triglycerides: ↓10–20% LDL: ↓20–25% HDL: ↑5–10%			
Fluvastatin: Lescol	$40	Triglycerides: ↓5–10%			
Nicotinic acid (niacin)		LDL: ↓10–30% HDL: ↑15–35% Triglycerides: ↓20–50%	**Major:** Abnormal liver function, increased blood sugar levels, abnormal heart rhythms. **Minor:** *Common:* Facial flushing, itching, rash, abdominal pain, nausea, dry skin. *Less common:* Vomiting, diarrhea.	**Advantages:** Reduces LDL levels fairly effectively and triglycerides very effectively and raises HDL more than any other drug. Cheapest option. **Disadvantages:** More likely (particularly sustained-release form) than other cholesterol drugs to disrupt liver function; periodic liver tests required. Facial flushing often bothersome.[c]	People who need improvement in HDL, improvement in triglycerides, moderately large reduction in LDL, or any combination of those three.
Generic	$9				
Niacor	$22				
Nicolar	$65				
Slo-Niacin	$17				
Bile acid resins		LDL: ↓15–30% HDL: ↑5% Triglycerides: ↑5–20%	**Major:** None. **Minor:** *Common:* Constipation. *Less common:* Abdominal pain, heartburn, belching, flatulence, nausea, vomiting, diarrhea.	**Advantages:** Reduce LDL fairly effectively and pose no major risks. **Disadvantages:** Often cause constipation.[d] Tend to raise triglycerides. Inconvenient and sometimes unpleasant to take. Can interact with several common drugs or nutrients.	People who need moderately large reduction in LDL and are concerned about risks of other cholesterol medications.
Cholestyramine					
Questran (powder)	$58				
Questran Light (powder)	$65				
Colestipol					
Colestid (tablets)	$49				
Colestid (granules)	$68				
Gemfibrozil		LDL: ↓10–15% HDL: ↑10–20% Triglycerides: ↓20–50%	**Major:** Abnormal heart rhythms; muscle disorders, sometimes painful; abnormal liver or kidney function; increased risk of gallstones. **Minor:** *Common:* Indigestion, abdominal pain, diarrhea. *Less common:* Headache, fatigue, dizziness, nausea, vomiting.	**Advantages:** Reduces triglycerides very effectively and increases HDL. Less likely than resins or niacin to cause uncomfortable side effects. **Disadvantages:** Reduces LDL levels less than other cholesterol drugs and has more major risks.	People who need improvements in triglycerides, HDL, or both, and who cannot tolerate niacin, including many type II diabetics.
Generic	$35				
Gemcor	$35				
Lopid	$68				

[a] Cost based on average dosage, derived mostly from data provided by Scott-Levin, a division of PMSI Scott-Levin, Inc.

[b] All major side effects are uncommon, except increased blood sugar levels from niacin (5–10% of patients). Rare side effects are not listed, except muscle inflammation from statin medications. Consult package insert for possibly harmful interactions with other drugs. In particular, cholestyramine and colestipol can each decrease absorption of several drugs, notably certain blood pressure medications, anticoagulants, and vitamins; and gemfibrozil can increase the effects of anticoagulants.

[c] Flushing can be minimized by taking niacin with meals, or by taking aspirin (325 mg) or ibuprofen (200 mg) an hour before taking niacin.

[d] Consuming more fiber or fluids may help relieve constipation.

Source: Consumer Reports on Health, April 1997. "Common Cholesterol Medications." Copyright © 1997 by Consumers Union of U.S., Inc., Yonkers, NY 10703-1057. Reprinted by permission from Consumer Reports, April 1997.

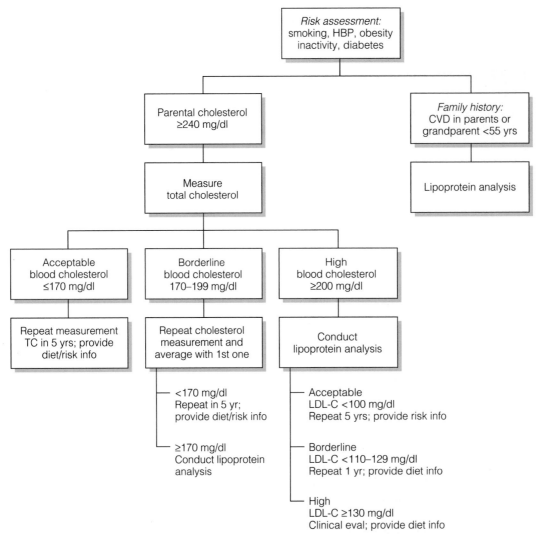

Figure 10.48 Blood cholesterol screening in children and adolescents. Cholesterol screening guidelines for children and youths: HBP, high blood pressure; TC, total cholesterol; and CVD, cardiovascular disease. *Source:* National Cholesterol Education Program. *The Expert Panel on Blood Cholesterol Levels in Children and Adolescents.* U.S. Department of Health and Human Services, National Institutes of Health, publication no. N4LB1. Rockville, MD: Author, 1991.

Pritikin diet is extreme for most people and probably can't be followed for extended periods, it does show what is possible when used therapeutically for several weeks.

Role of Exercise

In the 1970s, several published studies showed that low levels of HDL-C were related to coronary heart disease.[193] About the same time, the first reports that exercise may be related to improved HDL-C levels were published.[192,217] In an early Stanford University study of male and female long-distance runners and sedentary controls, HDL-C was found to be substantially higher in the runners[217,218] (see Fig-

ure 10.50). Total blood cholesterol, LDL-C, and triglycerides were reported to be much lower among the runners. Because of the cross-sectional nature of the research design, however, group disparities in blood fats and lipoproteins could have been due to factors other than exercise, including diet, body fat, and genetic background.[219–221]

In two more recent and larger studies of male and female runners, a dose–response relationship between miles run per week and HDL-C has been reported[179,222] (see Figure 10.51). In both of these studies, runners training the most had the highest HDL-C, and no evidence of a plateau or ceiling effect was seen. In other words, moderate amounts of running were better than little or none, while even more running was related to even higher HDL-C levels.[223] For the

Box 10.5

National Cholesterol Education Program/American Heart Association Guidelines for Dietary Prevention and Treatment of High Serum Cholesterol Levels and Coronary Heart Disease

The NCEP and the AHA recommend the following dietary guidelines for preventing and treating hypercholesterolemia and CHD.

- Total fat intake should be less than 30% of Calories.

- Saturated fat intake should be less than 10% of Calories (for Step 2, less than <7%).

- Polyunsaturated fat intake should not exceed 10% of Calories; monounsaturated fat should not exceed 15%.

- Cholesterol intake should not exceed 300 mg/day (Step 2, 200 mg/day).

- Carbohydrate intake should constitute 55% or more of Calories, with emphasis on complex carbohydrates and high-fiber foods

- Protein intake should provide about 15% of the Calories.

- Sodium intake should not exceed 2,400 mg/day.

- Alcoholic consumption should be moderate (<2 drinks per day for men, <1 drink per day for women).

- Total Calories should be sufficient to maintain the individual's recommended body weight.

- A wide variety of foods should be consumed.

Sources: American Heart Association. Position statement: Dietary guidelines for healthy American adults: A statement for health professionals from the Nutrition Committee. *Circulation* 94:1795–1800, 1996; Expert Panel on Detection, Evaluation, and Treatment of High Blood Cholesterol in Adults. Summary of the second report of the National Cholesterol Education Program (NCEP) expert panel on detection, evaluation, and treatment of high blood cholesterol in adults (adult treatment panel II). *JAMA* 269:3015–3023, 1993.

TABLE 10.12 Three-Day Menu Outline for a Healthy Heart

All vitamins and minerals exceed recommended intake levels.

Nutrient Information

Calories	2,000 per day		Cholesterol	140 milligrams	
Protein	86 grams	(17% of Calories)	Saturated fat	13 grams	(6% of Calories)
Fat	55 grams	(25% of Calories)	Dietary fiber	30 grams	
Carbohydrate	290 grams	(58% of Calories)	Caffeine	170 milligrams	
Sodium	2,800 milligrams				

Day 1 Breakfast

½	Grapefruit: raw, white, all areas
4	Pancakes: plain, and buttermilk, made with eggs and milk, 4-inch diameter
2 tsp.	Margarine: soft, unspecified oils with salt
1 cup	Applesauce: canned, unsweetened, without ascorbic acid
¼ tsp.	Cinnamon, ground
½ cup	Milk, cow's, low-fat, 1% fat
8 fl. oz.	Coffee, brewed, prepared with tap water

Day 1 Lunch

2 oz.	Fish/shellfish; tuna, canned drained solids, light meat, canned in water
2 slices	Bread: whole wheat
1 piece	Lettuce: iceberg, raw, leaf
2 tsp.	Salad dressing: mayonnaise, soybean oil, with salt
1	Carrot, raw
1	Apple, raw, with skin
1 cup	Soup: tomato rice, with water
6	Crackers: saltines
¾ cup	Grape juice: canned/bottled, unsweetened

Day 1 Dinner

3 oz.	Beef: composite of trimmed retailed cuts, all grades, separated lean, cooked, 0-in fat
1	Potato: baked, flesh only, without salt
1 cup	Broccoli: frozen, chopped, boiled, drained, without salt
1 ear	Corn: sweet, yellow, boiled, drained, without salt
3 tsp.	Margarine: soft, unspecified oils, with salt
2	Peaches, raw
1 cup	Milk: cow's, low-fat, 1% fat

Day 2 Breakfast

1 cup	Yogurt: fruit flavored, low-fat
1	English muffin, plain
1	Orange, raw, all varieties
2 tsp.	Margarine: soft, unspecified oils, with salt added
8 fl. oz.	Coffee: brewed, prepared with tap water

(continued)

TABLE 10.12   Three-Day Menu Outline for a Healthy Heart (continued)

Day 2 Lunch

¾ cup	Sauce: spaghetti, canned
1 cup	Spaghetti: enriched, cooked with no salt
1½ cup	Lettuce: iceberg, raw
½	Tomato: red, ripe, raw
¼ cup	Carrots: raw, shredded
¼ cup	Cucumber: not pared, raw, sliced
2 tbs.	Salad dressing: Italian, diet, with salt
1 tbs.	Seeds: sunflower seed kernels, dried
1 slice	Bread: French or Vienna, enriched
1 tsp.	Margarine: soft, unspecified oils, with salt added
⅛ tsp.	Garlic powder
1 serving	Grapes: European type (adherent skin)
1 cup	Tea: brewed

Day 2 Dinner

3 oz.	Chicken: breast, meat only, roasted
¾ cup	Rice: brown, long, cooked, without salt
1 cup	Carrots: boiled, drained, without salt
1	Roll/Bun: brown and serve, enriched
2 tsp.	Margarine: soft, unspecified oils, with salt
1 cup	Milk: cow's, low-fat, 1% fat
1 cup	Strawberries: raw
1 slice	Cake: angel food, baked from mix, enriched, made with water and flavorings

Day 3 Breakfast

2	Cereal: shredded wheat, large biscuits
2 tsp.	Sugar: brown, pressed down
2 slices	Bread: whole wheat, toasted
1	Banana
4 tsp.	Nuts: peanut butter, with salt
1 cup	Milk: cow's, low-fat, 1% fat
8 fl. oz.	Coffee: brewed, prepared with tap water

Day 3 Lunch

2 oz.	Turkey: light, no skin, roasted
1 oz.	Cheese: natural, mozzarella, part skim
2 slices	Bread: whole wheat
2 tsp.	Salad dressing: mayonnaise, soybean oil, with salt
½ cup	Broccoli: raw, chopped
½ cup	Cauliflower: raw, 1-inch pieces
2 tbs.	Salad dressing: Thousand Island, low-calorie, with salt
1	Pear, raw
3	Cookies: oatmeal with raisins
1½ cup	Carbonated beverage low-calorie, cola, with aspartame

Day 3 Dinner

3 oz.	Pork: cured, ham, whole, separated lean only, roasted
1	Sweet potato: baked, flesh only
1 cup	Beans: snap, green, boiled with salt
2 tsp.	Margarine: soft, unspecified oils, with salt added
1 cup	Apple juice: canned/bottled, unsweetened, without added ascorbic acid
1 cup	Melon: cantaloupe, raw, cubed
½ cup	Ice milk: vanilla, soft serve

men, but not the women, runners, LDL-C and triglyceride levels dropped sharply with increase in running distance. However, once again, whether the improved blood lipoprotein profile among the more serious runners was due to genetics, or to a superior diet and body composition, could not be fully determined.

Weight loss, in and of itself, has a powerful effect on blood fats and lipoproteins. With weight loss, the total cholesterol, LDL-C, and triglycerides decrease greatly, while HDL-C increases (but only when weight loss has been maintained and stabilized)[224-226] (see Chapter 13). Some researchers have estimated that the total cholesterol drops about 1 mg/dl for every pound lost (decreases are greatest for those with the highest blood cholesterol levels).[227] In other words, if a subject changes weight from 180 to 160 pounds, blood cholesterol could be expected, on average, to decrease 20 mg/dl (e.g., from 205 to 185 mg/dl).

As discussed in the previous section, improvements in dietary habits also have a favorable effect on blood lipids and lipoproteins.[225-227] Going from the typical American diet to the one recommended by the American Heart Association can decrease the total cholesterol by 5–15% (de-

---

Box 10.6

Lifestyle Factors That Increase High-Density Lipoprotein Cholesterol (HDL-C)

The following factors are listed in approximate order of importance.

1. Aerobic exercise, at least 90 minutes per week
2. Weight reduction and leanness
3. Smoking cessation
4. Moderate alcohol consumption

Sources: Based on references 19, 36, 51, 192, 193, 195.

---

pending on the initial level).[225] Going to more extreme diets, such as the 21-day Pritikin Program diet (<10% total fat), can have very strong effects on the total cholesterol and LDL-C (20–25% decreases), and triglycerides (20–40% decreases)[215] (Figure 10.49).

TABLE 10.13 Fat and Cholesterol in Food

Food	Amount	Percent Calories from Total Fat	Percent Calories from Saturated Fat	Cholesterol (milligrams)
Fruits		Low	Low	0
Vegetables		Low	Low	0
Grains		Low	Low	0
Nuts		High	Moderate	0
Avocado		88	17	0
Coconut, dried		88	76	0
Margarine	1 tbs.	100	18	0
Milk, nonfat	1 cup	—	—	5
Milk, low-fat	1 cup	30	17	22
Cottage cheese, 4% fat	½ cup	35	20	24
Cheese—pasteurized type	1 oz	73	40	25
Cream (half & half)	¼ cup	79	58	26
Ice cream, regular	½ cup	49	27	27
Cheese, cheddar	1 oz	72	40	28
Milk, whole	1 cup	48	27	34
Butter	1 tbs.	100	55	35
Tuna, canned	3 oz	38	10	55
Chicken, cooked	3 oz	19	6	74
Pork, cooked	3 oz	73	26	76
Beef, cooked	3 oz	77	37	80
Lamb, cooked	3 oz	61	34	83
Egg yolk	One	71	43	220
Liver, fried	2 oz	43	13	250

There are three types of fatty acids in foods. Most foods contain all three, with one of them being present in the greatest proportion.

			Effect on Blood Cholesterol
Saturated fatty acids	Coconut oil Palm kernel oil Chocolate Milk, cheese, Butter, cream	Beef, veal Palm oil Lard Pork Chicken	↑
Monounsaturated fatty acids	Avocados Flounder Olive oil, Canola oil Almonds	Haddock Peanut oil, peanuts Cottonseed oil	→
Polyunsaturated fatty acids	Soft margarine (most) Sesame oil Mayonnaise Soybean oil	Corn oil Sunflower oil Safflower oil	↓

Source: Nieman DC, Butterworth DE, Nieman CN. *Nutrition.* Dubuque: W. C. Brown Publishers, 1992. Used with permission.

Box 10.7

Lifestyle Factors That Reduce Low-Density Lipoprotein Cholesterol (LDL-C) and Total Cholesterol

The following factors are listed in approximate order of importance.

1. Reduction of dietary saturated fat intake (especially meat and dairy fats) and of intake of trans fatty acids (mainly from hydrogenated fats)

2. Reduction in body weight

3. Reduction in dietary cholesterol intake (found in all animal foods)

4. Increase in dietary polyunsaturated and monounsaturated fatty acids (mainly from plant foods, fish, and olives)

5. Increase in carbohydrate and dietary water-soluble fibers (especially fruits and vegetables, beans, and oat products)

6. Control of stress (weak evidence)

7. Reduction of dietary caffeine, coffee consumption (weak evidence)

Sources: Based on references 32, 36, 185, 208–214.

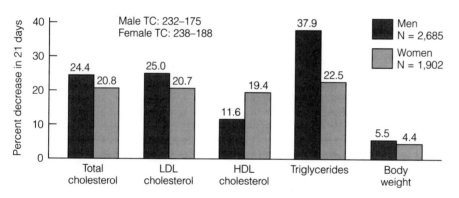

Figure 10.49   Effects of lifestyle modification on serum lipids: Pritikin Program—21 d, <10% fat, high-fiber, carb diet, 1–2 h exercise/d. The Pritikin Program has shown that large blood lipid changes in a short period of time are possible when major lifestyle changes are made.   *Source:* Data from Barnard RJ. Effects of life-style modification on serum lipids. *Arch Intern Med* 151:1389–1394, 1991.

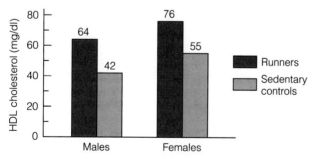

Figure 10.50   High-density lipoprotein cholesterol in male and female runners and sedentary controls. Cross-sectional studies dating back to the 1970s have consistently shown that highly active people have higher HDL cholesterol levels than do inactive people.   *Source:* Wood PD, Haskell WL, Stern MP, Lewis S, Perry C. Serum lipoproteins distributions in male and female runners. *Ann NY Acad Sci* 301: 748–763, 1997.

These studies show that weight loss and dietary changes can have dramatic effects on the blood lipids and lipoproteins. Often, when people begin exercise programs, improvements in dietary habits and body composition occur. Studies using randomized, controlled designs have carefully demonstrated that changes in blood cholesterol and fats with exercise training are very much affected by parallel changes in body weight and diet.[224–229]

A growing consensus among investigators is that when changes in body weight and dietary habits are controlled for, exercise training alone can be expected to increase HDL-C and to decrease triglyceride levels, with little or no effect on LDL-C.[217–237] Figure 10.52 summarizes the results of one study where changes in body weight and diet in both young and old men were minimized and controlled.[229] After 6 months of training intensely 5 days a week, 45 minutes

(a) 2,906 healthy, nonsmoking men

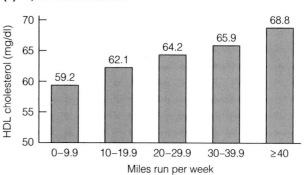

(b) 1,837 female runners

Figure 10.51   Miles run per week and high-density lipoprotein cholesterol. For both men and women, HDL cholesterol levels rise with increase in miles run.   *Sources:* (a) Williams PT. Relationship of distance run per week to coronary heart disease risk factors in 8283 male runners: The national runners' health study. *Arch Intern Med* 157:191–198, 1997. (b) Williams PT. High-density lipoprotein cholesterol and other risk factors for coronary heart disease in female runners. *N Engl J Med* 334:1298–1303, 1996.

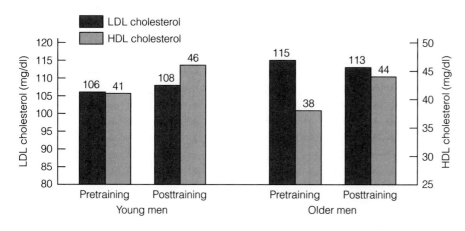

Figure 10.52   Exercise and lipoproteins in young and older men, without change in weight / diet; 6 months exercise, 5 days / week, 45 minutes / session, high intensity. When weight loss and diet are kept constant, exercise training increases HDL cholesterol, but not LDL cholesterol, in both young and older adult men.
Source: Data from Schwartz RS, Cain KC, Shuman WP, et al. Effect of intensive endurance training on lipoprotein profiles in young and older men. *Metabolism* 41: 649–654, 1992.

per session aerobic fitness in the young and older subjects improved 18% and 22%, respectively. No significant changes in LDL cholesterol were found (because diet and body weight were kept near prestudy levels), while HDL cholesterol improved 14%–15%. Triglycerides were low in the young subjects before starting the study, so exercise training had no further effect. For the older subjects, triglycerides fell strongly.

Figure 10.53 shows the results of a 12-week study of 90 overweight women, randomized to one of four groups: controls, walking (five 45-minute sessions per week, 60–75% maximum heart rate), diet (1,200–1,300 kcal per day), and diet and walking.[237] Subjects in the two diet groups lost an average of 17 pounds in 12 weeks, while the control and walking groups stayed within 2 pounds of their starting weight. Notice that serum cholesterol did not change in the control or walking groups but decreased 20–25% in the two

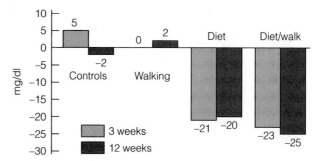

Figure 10.53   Cholesterol changes in response to diet and exercise (12 weeks) in 90 overweight women, randomized to one of four groups. Exercise alone does not improve serum cholesterol levels. Diet-induced weight loss, however, causes a quick and sharp decrease.   *Source:* Butterworth DE, Nieman DC, Henson DA, Utter A. Blood lipid response to exercise and energy restriction in obese women. *Am J Clin Nutr* (in press).

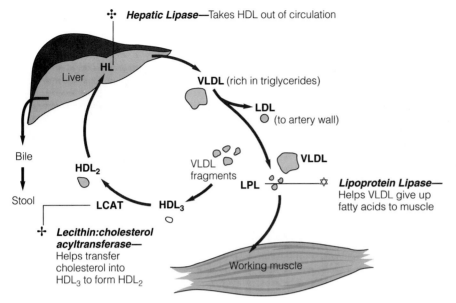

☩ **Hepatic Lipase**—Takes HDL out of circulation

Figure 10.54 Formation and elimination of HDL. HDL is formed within the blood by the action of two key enzymes (lipoprotein lipase [LPL] and lecithin: cholesterol acyltransferase [LCAT]) and then taken out of circulation by hepatic lipase (HL). Active people tend to have higher LPL and LCAT and lower HL enzyme activity levels.

diet groups. Most of the improvement in serum cholesterol occurred within the first 3 weeks.

How much exercise is necessary to improve the lipid profile? Most researchers agree that an exercise program equal to a moderate jog or brisk walk for at least 30 minutes per session, three to five times per week, is necessary before improvements in HDL-C can be measured.[217,231,232,238] In terms of energy expenditure, about 1,000 calories per week of moderate-to-high intensity, aerobic-type exercise is required to produce favorable changes in blood fats and lipoproteins.

At this basic, minimum exercise level, changes in HDL-C and triglyceride levels are sometimes small and variable, depending on the individual. Exercise programs with high duration (e.g., 45 minutes or longer), intensity, and frequency (i.e., near daily) produce the strongest effects on HDL-C and triglycerides. Total cholesterol and LDL-C, however, appear to be little affected by exercise training, even when it is intensive, unless body weight is decreased or dietary saturated fats are lowered at the same time.

Many studies testing the effect of moderate amounts of walking on HDL-C in women have failed to show significant changes.[221,230,231,237] However, when researchers increase the overall exercise volume and intensity, HDL-C does improve.[222,231,234] In other words, women require greater volumes of exercise than men to improve their HDL-C because of their initially higher levels.

Although there is increasing evidence that regular aerobic exercise increases HDL-C and lowers blood triglyceride levels, the exact mechanism explaining these positive changes is still being determined. At present, most researchers have concentrated their efforts on the interplay of important enzymes that regulate the breakdown and for-

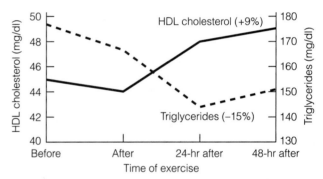

Figure 10.55 Changes in HDL cholesterol and triglyceride levels after exercise in 39 middle-aged men with high cholesterol, who cycled 30–60 minutes, burning 350 calories. A single session of exercise (30–60 min of cycling) lowers triglycerides and elevates HDL cholesterol for at least 2 days. *Source:* Data from Crouse SF, O'Brien BC, Rohack JJ, et al. Changes in serum lipids and apolipoproteins after exercise in men with high cholesterol: Influence of intensity. *J Appl Physiol* 79:279–286, 1995.

mation of HDL-C and triglycerides.[239–244] Regular exercise alters the activity of the regulatory enzymes in a favorable manner. The end result is that aerobically fit, compared to unfit, individuals appear to clear triglycerides from the blood more quickly, produce more HDL-C, and keep HDL-C in circulation longer[242,243] (see Figure 10.54).

Studies have shown that single bouts of aerobic exercise, especially when prolonged and intense, result in immediate and significant increases in HDL-C[245–251] (Figure 10.55). This acute increase in HDL-C has been linked to the breakdown of triglycerides during exercise.[239] Certain enzymes (especially lipoprotein lipase in the walls of the capillaries) break down the triglycerides during exercise, allowing the muscles to take in fat for fuel and energy production.

As the exercise program is maintained on a regular basis, the acute changes in HDL-C and triglycerides, which persist for at least 24–48 hours, result in a chronic improvement. In other words, the favorable lipid profiles of trained individuals may actually be related to short-term changes that occur during or immediately after a single bout of exercise, which over time add up to higher HDL-C and lower triglyceride levels.

The largest acute increase in HDL-C occurs following unusually heavy exertion.[246,250,251] For example, after a marathon race, HDL-C can increase 15–25%.[250,251] Triglycerides drop sharply at the same time, as the muscles use fats for fuel. In one report of 29 triathletes who finished the 1994 Hawaii Ironman World Championship, blood triglyceride levels dropped an average of 39%.[246]

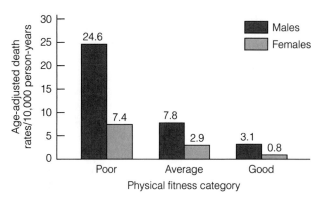

Figure 10.56 Physical fitness and cardiovascular mortality: 8-year study of 10,224 men and 3,120 women. A poor level of physical fitness was associated with much higher death rates for cardiovascular disease than were average or good fitness levels, in this study conducted at the Cooper Institute for Aerobics Research in Dallas. *Source:* Data from Blair SN, Kohl HW, Paffenbarger RS, Clark DG, Cooper KH, Gibbons LW. Physical fitness and all-cause mortality: A prospective study of healthy men and women. *JAMA* 262:2395–2401, 1989.

EXERCISE AND CORONARY HEART DISEASE PREVENTION

Up until 1992, the American Heart Association did not include physical inactivity in their list of "major risk factors that can be changed," which included cigarette smoking, high blood pressure, and high blood cholesterol[252,253] (see Table 10.2). Previously, inactivity was listed along with obesity, stress, and diabetes as "contributing factors." Until recently, good research data to support the relationship between coronary heart disease (CHD) and inactivity had been lacking. Most of the earlier studies showed that physically active, compared to inactive, people had a lower risk for CHD, but critics contended that other important factors (e.g., diet, family history) were not controlled for.

For example, in one of the earliest (1953) published studies, London bus drivers who sat and drove were found to be at higher risk for CHD than the conductors who moved through the double-decker buses collecting tickets.[254] However, critics claimed that the drivers may have been at higher risk for CHD to begin with, and self-selected themselves to an easier, sit-down type of job.

Ralph Paffenbarger of Stanford University has done more than any other researcher to silence the criticism and to advance the cause of exercise as a valuable preventive measure. In 1970, Paffenbarger published data showing that San Francisco longshoremen who engaged in little physical labor on the job were at 60% greater risk for CHD death than colleagues engaging in physically demanding work.[255]

In 1978, the first of several reports on college alumni were released, demonstrating that active alumni were at lower CHD risk than their inactive counterparts.[256] In these studies, Paffenbarger carefully controlled for other CHD risk factors, showing that the sedentary lifestyle in and of itself was related to CHD.[255–259]

Physical activity habits are difficult to measure and are largely based on information provided by the subjects. Cardiorespiratory fitness, however, is an objective measure and can be assessed rather easily. Steven Blair of the Cooper Institute for Aerobics Research has been a leader in evaluating the relationship between fitness and coronary heart and cardiovascular diseases.[117,260] He has used maximal treadmill testing to measure cardiorespiratory fitness in a large group of men and women since 1970. Blair has found that a low level of fitness is a strong risk factor for CVD, in both men and women[260] (see Figure 10.56).

Although more research is needed with women, several studies suggest that physical inactivity affects CHD risk to the same degree in both men and women. In one study of older women in the Seattle area, CHD risk was decreased 50% with moderate amounts of exercise.[261] Another study showed that the odds for CHD for sedentary women are more than doubled when compared to the odds for their more active counterparts.[262] As depicted in Figure 10.57, results from a 7-year study of more than 40,000 Iowa women showed that increasing frequency of both moderate and vigorous physical activity was associated with a reduced risk of death from cardiovascular disease.[263]

In 1987, a landmark review article was published by researchers from the Centers for Disease Control and Prevention (CDC)[264] (see Table 10.14). Forty-three studies were reviewed, and not one reported a greater risk for CHD among active participants. Two thirds of the studies supported the finding that physically active versus inactive people have less CHD, and the studies following the best

TABLE 10.14 Relationship between Physical Activity/Physical Fitness and Coronary Heart Disease

Study Location	Subject Groups Compared	Relative Risk
London postal, civil servants	Active postmen vs. sedentary	2.0
London transport busworkers	Active conductors vs. drivers	2.3
U.S. railroad workers	Active section men vs. clerks	2.0
North Dakota farmers	Active farmers vs. nonfarmers	1.8
Washington D.C. postal workers	Active carriers vs. clerks	2.8
Italy residents	Heavy workers vs. sedentary	3.1
Greek islands residents	Heavy workers vs. sedentary	2.0
San Francisco longshoremen	Heavy workers vs. light tasks	1.6
Harvard alumni	Heavy leisure exercise vs. light	1.6
Framingham, MA, male residents	High vs. low amounts of exercise	1.9
Los Angeles firefighters/police officers	Good vs. low physical fitness	2.4
Gothenberg, Sweden residents	Good vs. low physical fitness	2.3
North Karelia male residents	Heavy workers vs. light	1.6
Seattle residents	High-intensity leisure vs. none	2.5
MRFIT study subjects	High vs. low fitness	1.5
Eastern Finland	Active vs. sedentary, high vs. low fitness	3.3
U.S. railroad workers	Good vs. low physical fitness	1.4
Honolulu heart study	Active vs. inactive elderly	1.5
Lipid Research Clinic	High vs. low physical fitness	2.7
British civil servants	Vigorous exercise vs. none	2.6
Harvard alumni	Initiating exercise vs. remaining sedentary	1.4
Norwegian men	High vs. low fitness	1.6
Iowa women	High vs. low-moderate activity	2.0
U.S. biracial men and women	High vs. low activity	1.7
Alameda County residents	Moderate vs. low activity	1.2
Finnish men	High vs. low activity	3.6
Boston men and women	High vs. low activity	2.5

Sources: See references 254–284. Based primarily on reviews by Powell et al.[264] and Berlin and Golditz.[265]

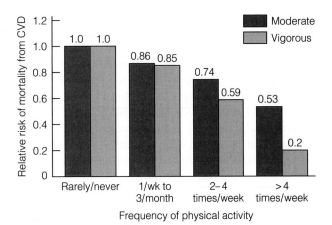

Figure 10.57 Physical activity and CVD mortality in postmenopausal women. Risk of CVD mortality in women decreases as the frequency of both moderate and vigorous physical activity increases. *Source:* Kushi LH, Fee RM, Folsom AR, Mink PJ, Anderson KE, Sellers TA. Physical activity and mortality in postmenopausal women. *JAMA* 277:1287–1292, 1997.

research design were the ones most likely to support this relationship.

In general, the studies summarized in Table 10.14 show that the risk for CHD among physically inactive people is twice that of people who are relatively active.[254–284] This risk is similar to that reported for high blood pressure, high blood cholesterol, and cigarette smoking. According to the CDC, regular physical activity should be as vigorously promoted for CHD prevention as for blood pressure control, dietary improvements to lower serum cholesterol and control weight, and smoking cessation.[264] The CDC feels that given the large proportion of Americans who do not exercise at appropriate levels (nearly 60%), the incidence of CHD that can actually be attributed to lack of regular physical activity is significant (see Figure 10.12).

One of the most important reasons why active people have less CHD is that other risk factors are typically under control, as well[285–288] (see Figure 10.58). For example, relatively few active people smoke cigarettes, are obese or dia-

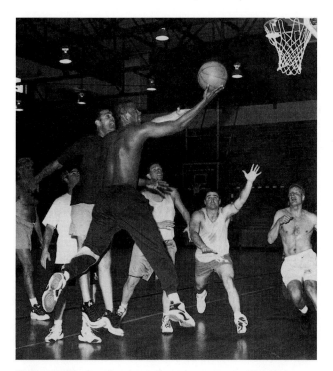

Figure 10.58 Regular physical activity is associated with a lower prevalence for most of the major risk factors of coronary heart disease.

betic, have high blood cholesterol, or experience high blood pressure. Active people have lower blood triglycerides, more HDL-C, and generally report less anxiety and depression. Although there is some controversy as to whether exercise or self-selection is responsible for these reduced risk factors, most experts feel that exercise does have a direct effect in bringing many CHD risk factors under control.[287]

There are other important reasons why regular exercise is identified with lower CHD risk. Coronary arteries of endurance-trained individuals can expand more, are less stiff in older age, and wider than those of unfit subjects.[289,290] Even if some plaque material is present, the coronary arteries of fit people are wide enough to diminish the risk of total closure leading to a heart attack. Although the issue is not yet settled, there is some evidence that exercise may decrease the potential for clot formation.[291–293] In other words, with larger, more compliant coronary arteries, and a diminished likelihood of forming clots, the active individual is at lower risk for a heart attack. The heart muscle itself becomes bigger and stronger with regular exercise. Although still under study, there is some indication that the fit heart develops extra blood vessels, enhancing blood and oxygen delivery.[294]

Exercise must be regular in order for CHD risk to be lowered. In college alumni studies, Paffenbarger noted that current physical activity habits were much more important when considering CHD risk than were those from early adulthood.[259] Former college athletes who dropped their sports-playing habits had higher death rates thereafter than their teammates who continued to exercise moderately vigorously into middle or later age.[257] In contrast, college students who had avoided athletics in college but subsequently took up a more active lifestyle experienced the same low risk of mortality as alumni who had been moderately vigorous all along.

More recent results from the college alumni studies also support this concept. Risk of premature death from CHD was increased if physical activity was reduced below favorable levels, and risk was lowered if physical activity was increased.[258,295] Adopting a regular exercise program was found to be as beneficial in lowering CHD risk as quitting smoking and avoiding obesity and hypertension.

These results are similar to those of Blair, who showed that individuals maintaining or improving fitness over a 5-year span were less likely to die from CVD than those who stayed unfit.[296] Men in the Aerobics Center Longitudinal Study who improved their fitness during the 5-year study had a 64% reduction in risk of death, greater than for any of the other risk factors.

There has been some debate as to the volume and intensity of exercise essential for lowering CHD risk.[253] Some studies have indicated that regular and vigorous exercise is necessary, while others suggest that exercise of moderate duration and intensity is sufficient to reduce CHD risk.[297] There is increasing consensus that while moderate exercise is a sufficient threshold for lowering CHD risk, additional benefit is gained when people are willing to exercise more vigorously for longer periods of time.[297,298] However, the relationship does not appear to be linear. The greatest benefit in lowering CHD risk occurs when sedentary people adopt moderate physical activity habits, with some additional protection gained as the duration and intensity of exercise are raised to a higher level (see Figure 10.59).

Blair has emphasized that as little as 2 miles of brisk walking on most days of the week would result in the moderate level of fitness shown to be protective in the Aerobics Center Longitudinal Study.[260] Other studies suggest a level of activity just a bit higher, the equivalent of 2–3 miles of brisk walking each day of the week.[259,277,281,283]

An expert panel convened by the National Institutes of Health concluded that activity that reduces CVD risk factors does not require a structured or vigorous exercise program.[298] The majority of benefits of physical activity can be gained by performing moderate-intensity activities. The NIH recommends that all children and adults set a long-term goal to accumulate at least 30 minutes or more of moderate-intensity physical activity on most, or preferably all, days of the week.

Some researchers, however, urge that people should not be misled to believe that a casual approach to fitness is sufficient. In one study from Finland, 1,453 middle-aged men who were initially free of CHD for 5 years were followed, classified according to the frequency and intensity of their leisure-time physical activity.[281] Men who engaged

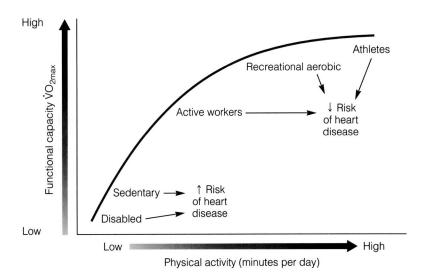

Figure 10.59 The spectrum of physical activity and cardiovascular fitness. Very high $\dot{V}O_{2max}$ values are not necessary to reduce risk of CHD. However, at least moderate physical activity is important and is usually associated with higher than average $\dot{V}O_{2max}$ values.

in moderate-to-strenuous activity for at least 2.2 hours per week had a risk of heart attack that was less than half that of the least active men. Only moderate-to-strenuous aerobic activities such as brisk walking, jogging, bicycling, or cross-country skiing were shown to confer protection. Nonconditioning activities such as slow walking, fishing, easy yard work or gardening, hunting, or picking berries did not lower CHD risk.

EXERCISE AND STROKE PREVENTION

Physical inactivity is still not recognized by the American Heart Association as a primary risk factor for stroke.[1] Instead, physical inactivity is classified as a "secondary risk factor" because it affects the risk of stroke "indirectly by increasing the risk of heart disease (which is a primary risk factor for stroke)."

A growing number of research studies have established a link between physical activity and decrease in stroke, although the link has not been as firmly established as the link to CHD.[37] More than 15 major studies that have been published, and the more recent ones using the best research designs have reported a strong protective effect of regular exercise for both men and women.[299] Although some earlier studies did not report a protective effect, no study has found that regular exercise *increases* the risk for stroke.

It makes sense that if regular physical activity *lowers* CHD risk (a relationship that is well established), stroke risk should also be lowered, given the common underlying cause (atherosclerosis). The first research study providing evidence that physical activity may be related to a decreased risk of stroke was published by Paffenbarger in 1967.[300] Among 50,000 college alumni, those men who were not varsity athletes during their college years had nearly a twofold increased risk of death from stroke, compared to that of the varsity athletes.

In an extended follow-up of 17,000 college alumni, Paffenbarger rated the men according to their leisure-time physical activity. Men in the lowest category of physical activity (those expending less than 500 calories per week) died from stroke at a rate that was 1.7 times higher than that for those who were most active (more than 2,000 calories per week).[257] Another study of Dutch stroke patients and controls also established that men and women exercising the most during their leisure time exhibited the lowest risk of stroke (73%), when compared to those who were sedentary.[301] However, even those reporting regular light activity during their leisure time (walking or cycling each week) experienced a 51% decreased risk of stroke.

Five studies published in the 1990s have provided the best evidence that physically active men and women suffer less from strokes.[302–306] In one study of 105 stroke patients and 161 controls, an increasing protection from stroke was experienced as the duration of exercise in earlier years increased.[302] Risk of stroke fell 56% in those who had engaged in regular and vigorous exercise from ages 15 to 25, with some additional protection afforded those who exercised throughout adulthood.

In a 22-year study of 7,530 men of Japanese ancestry living in Hawaii, physical inactivity was found to be a strong risk factor for stroke caused by clots among nonsmoking middle-aged men (relative risk of 2.8) and for hemorrhagic stroke in older men ages 55–68 (relative risk of 3.7)[303] (see Figure 10.60).

Although the evidence is far from conclusive, data from several studies suggest that while moderate physical activity is sufficient to lower the risk for stroke, further benefit is gained with increasing amounts and intensity of exercise. For example, in one 9.5-year study of 7,735 British middle-aged men, those who were moderately active experienced a 40% decrease in stroke risk, while those who were vigorously active had an even greater decrease (70%)[304] (see Figure 10.61).

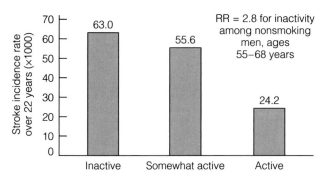

Figure 10.60 Stroke risk and physical activity, in Japanese men living in Hawaii. Incidence rates for stroke among 7,530 Japanese men living in Hawaii were much higher in those who were physically inactive versus active. *Source:* Abbott RD, Rodriguez BL, Burchfiel CM, Curb JD. Physical activity in older middle-aged men and reduced risk of stroke: The Honolulu heart program. *Am J Epidemiol* 139:881–893, 1994.

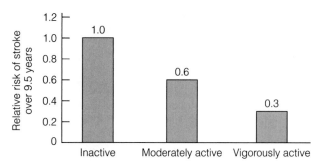

Figure 10.61 Physical activity and stroke risk in British men. Risk of stroke was lowest in British men exercising vigorously. *Source:* Wannamethee G, Shaper AG. Physical activity and stroke in British middle aged men. *BMJ* 304:597–601, 1992.

SPORTS MEDICINE INSIGHT

Cardiac Rehabilitation

As discussed earlier in this chapter, each year, about 1.5 million Americans have a heart attack.[1] Although one third die soon after, the majority live to face an uncertain future. People who survive the acute stage of a heart attack have a chance of illness and death two to nine times higher than the general population. During the first year after having a heart attack, 27% of men and 44% of women will die. More than 11 million Americans alive today have a history of heart attack, angina pectoris (chest pain), or both.

Cardiovascular operations and procedures to treat heart disease are part of a growing industry. Total vascular and cardiac surgeries now number over 4.4 million per year, including diagnostic cardiac catheterizations, coronary artery bypass graft surgery, percutaneous transluminal coronary angioplasty, open-heart surgery, heart transplants, and pacemaker insertions.[1]

Cardiac rehabilitation programs were first developed in the 1950s in response to the growing epidemic of heart disease.[307–312] Participants include people who have CHD, those who have had a heart attack, and surgery patients. Many programs admit people who have multiple CHD risk factors but have not yet been diagnosed with CVD. The goal is to prepare cardiac patients to return to productive, active, and satisfying lives, with a reduced risk of recurring health problems (see Box 10.8).

In cardiac rehabilitation programs, the emphasis is usually on lifestyle change, optimization of drug therapy, vocational counseling, and group and family therapy. Regarding lifestyle change, exercise is considered the cornerstone, but weight control, smoking cessation, and dietary therapy are also essential.[310,311] During the early days of cardiac rehabilitation, it was common practice to have the heart attack patient stay in bed a minimum of 2–3 weeks. As research began to demonstrate the importance of early and progressive physical activity, a four-phase plan was developed, which is now standard in most programs[308] (see Figure 10.62).

Patients with no complications are expected to progress from phase I through phase III within 1 year after an acute cardiac event. Phase IV is designed for lifelong exercise participation. Phase I involves easy walking and bed exercises during the first 5–14 days while the patient is in the coronary care unit of the hospital. Phase II is an outpatient program lasting 1–3 months, with the patient exercising aerobically in the hospital or clinic under careful supervision. Phase III lasts 6–12 months and is a supervised aerobic exercise program in a community setting.

Exercise programs for cardiac patients should be highly individualized and should involve an initial slow, gradual progression of the exercise duration and intensity. Aerobic activities should be emphasized, with a

(continued)

Cardiac Rehabilitation (continued)

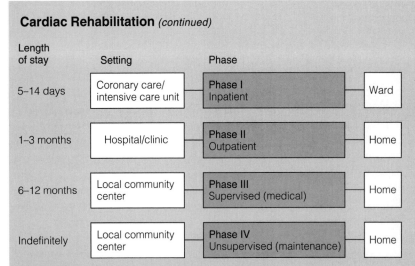

Figure 10.62 Modern cardiac rehabilitation program summary. There are four phases to the modern cardiac rehabilitation program. Participants include people who have CHD, people who have had a myocardial infarction (MI), those with coronary artery disease who have not had an MI, and surgery patients. Patients with no complications are expected to progress from phase I through phase III within 1 year after an acute cardiac event. Phase IV is designed for lifelong participation. Cardiac rehabilitation programs are found at many different sites, including hospitals, YMCAs, universities, community centers, and medical clinics. *Source:* Adapted from Wilson PK. Cardiac rehabilitation: Then and now. *Physician Sportsmed* 16(9):75–84, 1988.

minimum frequency of 3 days per week, 20–40 minutes each session, at a moderate, comfortable intensity. Some resistance exercise, but at a low intensity, is recommended to help build up weakened muscles.[313]

Unfortunately, only 15% of eligible cardiac patients actually participate in cardiac rehabilitation programs.[310] For a variety of reasons, these programs are not feasible or desirable for the vast majority of patients. One problem is that phases II and III involve medical supervision at a designated site (hospital, clinic, or fitness center). This presents time and transportation obstacles for many patients. Home-based programs are an attractive alternative and provide a convenient setting that can also involve the support of family members.

Several pertinent questions have been raised regarding cardiac rehabilitation programs. Do they increase the aerobic fitness of cardiac patients? Do they lengthen life and lower the risk of new cardiac events? Are they safe?

Many studies have clearly shown that cardiac patients who exercise regularly improve their aerobic fitness.[310,312] $\dot{V}O_{2max}$ increases by an average of 20%, according to most studies, and anginal symptoms often disappear or take longer to develop during a certain exercise load.

Researchers have been unable to provide a clear picture as to whether exercise by cardiac patients leads to longer life or fewer subsequent heart attacks.[314] Two re-

view articles have shown that when all studies are gathered together, total and CVD mortality are reduced 20–25% for patients in cardiac rehabilitation programs, compared to those not participating.[310,312] However, the programs involved more than just exercise training, so it is difficult to quantify the role of exercise alone.

Comprehensive cardiac rehabilitation programs that include exercise, diet, and other health behavior changes do help patients keep their CHD risk factors under tighter control.[310] Perhaps more importantly, studies show that patients in cardiac rehabilitation programs report an improved quality of life.

Cardiac rehabilitation programs are safe.[310,312,315] The estimated incidence of heart attack in supervised cardiac rehabilitation programs is only 1 per 294,000 patient-hours, and of death, 1 per 784,000 patient-hours.[310] Over 80% of patients who have been reported to suffer a cardiac arrest have been successfully resuscitated with prompt defibrillation.

The American College of Sports Medicine concludes that "most patients with coronary artery disease should engage in individually designed exercise programs to achieve optimal physical and emotional health. . . . Appropriate exercise programs for patients with coronary artery disease have multiple documented benefits, which can be achieved with a high level of safety."[310]

Box 10.8

Cardiac Rehabilitation Clinical Care Guidelines: Executive Summary from the Agency for Health Care Policy and Research

Cardiovascular disease is the leading cause of morbidity and mortality in the United States, accounting for more than 50% of all deaths. Coronary heart disease (CHD), with its clinical manifestations of stable angina pectoris, unstable angina, acute myocardial infarction, and sudden cardiac death, affects 13.5 million Americans. The almost 1 million survivors of myocardial infarction and the 7 million patients with stable angina pectoris are candidates for cardiac rehabilitation, as are the 309,000 patients who undergo coronary artery bypass graft (CABG) surgery and the 362,000 patients who undergo percutaneous transluminal coronary angioplasty (PTCA) and other transcatheter procedures each year. An estimated 4.7 million patients with heart failure may also be eligible. Although beneficial outcomes from cardiac rehabilitation services can be expected in most of these patients, few such patients currently participate in cardiac rehabilitation programs.

The U.S. Public Health Service definition of *cardiac rehabilitation*, used by the panel, states that "cardiac rehabilitation services are comprehensive, long-term programs involving medical evaluation, prescribed exercise, cardiac risk factor modification, education, and counseling. These programs are designed to limit the physiologic and psychological effects of cardiac illness, reduce the risk for sudden death or reinfarction, control cardiac symptoms, stabilize or reverse the atherosclerotic process, and enhance the psychosocial and vocational status of selected patients." This set of guidelines provides recommendations for cardiac rehabilitation services for patients with CHD and with heart failure, including those awaiting or following cardiac transplantation.

These guidelines are designed for use by health practitioners who provide care to patients with cardiovascular disease. These include physicians (primary care, cardiologists, and cardiovascular surgeons), nurses, exercise physiologists, dietitians, behavioral medicine specialists, psychologists, and physical and occupational therapists. The information can guide clinical decision making regarding referral and follow-up of patients for cardiac rehabilitation services, as well as administrative decisions regarding the availability of and access to cardiac rehabilitation services.

These guidelines detail the outcomes that result from cardiac rehabilitation services. The interventions examined involve two parallel applications: (1) exercise training and (2) education, counseling, and behavioral interventions. The panel emphasizes the added effectiveness of multifactorial cardiac rehabilitation services integrated in a comprehensive approach.

Outcomes of Cardiac Rehabilitation Services

The results of cardiac rehabilitation services, based on reports in the scientific literature, are summarized in these guidelines. The most substantial benefits include

- Improvement in exercise tolerance
- Improvement in symptoms
- Improvement in blood lipid levels
- Reduction in cigarette smoking
- Improvement in psychosocial well-being and reduction of stress
- Reduction in mortality

Improvement in Exercise Tolerance

Cardiac rehabilitation exercise training improves objective measures of exercise tolerance in both men and women, including elderly patients, with CHD and with heart failure. This functional improvement occurs without significant cardiovascular complications or other adverse outcomes. Appropriately prescribed and conducted exercise training should be an integral component of cardiac rehabilitation services and particularly benefits patients with decreased exercise tolerance. Maintenance of exercise training is required to sustain improvement in exercise tolerance.

Improvement in Symptoms

Cardiac rehabilitation exercise training decreases symptoms of angina pectoris in patients with CHD and decreases symptoms of heart failure in patients with left

(continued)

Cardiac Rehabilitation Clinical Care Guidelines: Executive Summary from the Agency for Health Care Policy and Research *(continued)*

ventricular systolic dysfunction. Following exercise rehabilitation, improvement in clinical measures of myocardial ischemia, as identified by electrocardiographic (ECG) and nuclear cardiology techniques, provides objective support for the reported symptomatic improvement. Exercise training of patients with left ventricular systolic dysfunction provides added symptomatic improvement to that achieved by appropriate medication management.

Improvement in Blood Lipid Levels

Multifactorial cardiac rehabilitation in patients with CHD, including exercise training and education, results in improved lipid and lipoprotein levels. Exercise training as a sole intervention has not effected consistent improvement in lipid profiles. Optimal lipid management requires specifically directed dietary and, when medically indicated, pharmacological management as a component of multifactorial cardiac rehabilitation.

Reduction in Cigarette Smoking

Multifactorial cardiac rehabilitation, with well-designed educational and behavioral components, reduces cigarette smoking. Between 16% and 26% of patients can be expected to stop smoking. These smoking cessation rates enhance the spontaneously high smoking cessation rates in most populations following a coronary event. Scientific evidence, consensus reports, and scientific reviews in the nonrehabilitation setting, including the surgeon general's messages since 1965, lend strong support that education, counseling, and behavioral interventions are beneficial for smoking cessation.

Improvement in Psychosocial Well-Being and Stress Reduction

Exercise training enhances measures of psychological and social functioning, particularly as a component of multifactorial cardiac rehabilitation. Improvement in psychological status and functioning, including measures of emotional stress and reduction of the Type-A behavior pattern, is consistent with the improvement in psychosocial outcomes that occurs in nonrehabilitation settings.

Reduction in Mortality

A survival benefit for patients who participate in cardiac rehabilitation exercise training is suggested from the scientific data, but this cannot be attributed solely to exercise training because many studies involved multifactorial interventions. Meta-analysis of the randomized controlled trials of exercise rehabilitation in patients following myocardial infarction establishes a reduction in mortality approximating 25% at 3-year follow-up. This reduction in mortality approaches that resulting from pharmacological management of patients following myocardial infarction with beta-blocking drugs or patients with left ventricular systolic dysfunction with angiotensin-converting enzyme (ACE) inhibitor therapy. The reduction in cardiovascular mortality was 26% in multifactorial randomized trials of cardiac rehabilitation and 15% in trials that involved only an exercise intervention. The panel concludes that multifactorial cardiac rehabilitation services can reduce mortality in patients following myocardial infarction.

Safety

The safety of cardiac rehabilitation exercise training is inferred from aggregate analysis of clinical experience. None of the more than three dozen randomized controlled trials of cardiac rehabilitation exercise training in patients with CHD, involving over 4,500 patients, described an increase in morbidity or mortality in rehabilitation, compared with control patient groups. A survey of 142 cardiac rehabilitation programs in the United States, involving patients participating in exercise rehabilitation from 1980 to 1984, reported, based on aggregate data, a low rate of nonfatal myocardial infarction of 1 per 294,000 patient-hours; the cardiac mortality rate was 1 per 784,000 patient-hours. A total of 21 episodes of cardiac arrest occurred, with successful resuscitation of 17 patients. Thus, the safety of exercise rehabilitation is established by the very low rates of occurrence of myocardial infarction and cardiovascular complications during exercise training.

Source: Agency for Health Care Policy and Research. Full text can be downloaded from http://text.nlm.nih.gov/.

SUMMARY

1. Death from heart disease (also called cardiovascular disease, CVD) is the leading killer among people in developed countries worldwide.

2. Atherosclerosis is the underlying factor in 85% of CVD deaths. Coronary heart disease (CHD) is the major form of heart disease and is caused by atherosclerosis and clotting in the coronary arteries.

3. An estimated 50 million Americans have hypertension (systolic BP ≥140 mm Hg and/or diastolic BP ≥90 mm Hg), making it the most prevalent form of CVD.

4. Nearly 1 million Americans die each year from CVD, representing 42% of all deaths. More than half a million die from heart attacks each year.

5. Since the 1950s, CHD deaths have dropped by 55% and stroke deaths by 70%. Most of the decline in CHD is related to changes in lifestyle.

6. Risk factors for heart disease include being male, family history, cigarette smoking, hypertension, inactivity, high serum cholesterol, low HDL-C, history of stroke or peripheral vascular disease, and severe obesity. The danger of heart attack increases with the number of risk factors.

7. Cigarette smoking is the most important of the known modifiable risk factors for CHD.

8. The relationship between exercise and smoking is complex. Many studies have shown that smoking before exercise adversely affects performance. Very few active people smoke. More study needs to be done to determine the role of physical activity in reducing the desire for cigarette smoking. Weight gain is a likely outcome of smoking cessation and is related to the effect of smoking on energy expenditure.

9. The 1993 Joint National Committee on Detection, Evaluation, and Treatment of High Blood Pressure has organized a treatment scheme emphasizing non-drug approaches (especially weight reduction, salt restriction, exercise, and moderation of alcohol consumption) as a first line of defense, and then a step-care therapy approach with various drugs to treat hypertension.

10. Heavy drinking has been consistently associated with increased risk of death from heart disease. Ethanol use alters lipoprotein metabolism and blood lipid profiles, increasing HDL-C and VLDL-C. There is good evidence that moderate drinking has a protective effect against coronary heart disease, but recommendations to increase alcohol consumption are ill-advised because of other overriding health concerns.

11. Following a bout of aerobic exercise, blood pressures fall for at least 20–120 minutes. Studies have shown that both physical fitness and habitual aerobic activity are associated with a decreased risk of hypertension. Exercise training is associated with lower blood pressures among hypertensive people.

12. Nineteen percent of Americans have blood cholesterol levels above 240 mg/dl. Death rates for CHD climb steadily when serum cholesterol levels rise above 180 mg/dl.

13. There are three major lipoproteins in the fasting blood: HDL, LDL, and VLDL. LDL and HDL have opposing functions. HDL takes cholesterol to the liver, where it is changed to bile and eventually excreted in the stool. LDL takes cholesterol to the artery wall. The level of HDL-C and the ratio of total cholesterol to HDL-C are important measures of heart disease risk.

14. The National Cholesterol Education Program (NCEP) guidelines for classification and treatment of hypercholesterolemia were reviewed. The NCEP dietary recommendations are based on reduction of dietary saturated fat and cholesterol, with increased intake of complex carbohydrate foods.

15. Lifestyle factors that increase HDL-C include aerobic exercise, weight control, smoking cessation, and moderate alcohol consumption. Lifestyle factors that decrease LDL-C center around low intake of saturated fat and cholesterol with weight reduction.

16. A consistent finding is that with weight loss, the total cholesterol, LDL-C, and triglyceride levels decrease, while HDL-C levels increase. The independent effect of aerobic exercise during weight loss, however, is limited to improving the magnitude of change in the triglycerides and HDL-C, but not total cholesterol and LDL-C.

17. HDL is formed within the blood by the action of two key enzymes, LPL and LCAT, and then taken out of circulation by hepatic lipase. Active people tend to have higher LPL and LCAT and lower HL enzyme activity levels.

18. Epidemiological studies have left little doubt as to the existence of a strong inverse relationship between physical exercise and risk of coronary heart disease. These observations suggest that in CHD prevention programs, regular physical activity should be promoted as vigorously as control of blood pressure, dietary modification to lower serum cholesterol, and smoking cessation.

19. The favorable effect of physical activity in decreasing CVD is probably due to several factors. One of the major factors is that regular physical activity is associated with a reduction of the major risk factors of heart disease.

20. Cardiac rehabilitation has been organized to help restore coronary artery bypass surgery patients and other heart disease patients to productive life. The emphasis in cardiac rehabilitation is usually on lifestyle changes, as well as optimization of drug therapy. Exercise is considered the cornerstone of cardiac rehabilitation, but weight control, cessation of cigarette smoking, group therapy and family counseling, vocational counseling, a low-calorie, low-fat diet, systematic follow-up examinations, and careful drug therapy are also important. There are four phases to the modern cardiac rehabilitation program.

REFERENCES

1. American Heart Association. *1998 Heart and Stroke Statistical Update: Heart and Stroke Facts.* Dallas: Author, 1997.

2. *The Johns Hopkins White Papers: Coronary Heart Disease.* Baltimore, MD: Johns Hopkins Medical Institutions, 1996.

3. Anderson RN, Kochanek KD, Murphy SL. Report of final mortality statistics, 1995. *Monthly Vital Statistics Report* 45(11), supplement 2. Hyattsville, MD: National Center for Health Statistics, 1997.

4. Watanabe T, Haraoka S, Shimokama T. Inflammatory and immunological nature of atherosclerosis. *Int J Cardiol* 54(suppl): S51–S60, 1997.

5. Sniderman AD, Pedersen T, Kjekshus J. Putting low-density lipoproteins at center stage in atherogenesis. *Am J Cardiol* 79: 64–67, 1997.

6. Vogel RA. Coronary risk factors, endothelial function, and atherosclerosis: A review. *Clin Cardiol* 20:426–432, 1997.

7. Selwyn AP, Kinlay S, Creager M, Libby P, Ganz P. Cell dysfunction in atherosclerosis and the ischemic manifestations of coronary artery disease. *Am J Cardiol* 79:17–23, 1997.

8. Stary HC. The sequence of cell and matrix changes in atherosclerotic lesions of coronary arteries in the first 40 years of life. *Eur Heart J* 11(suppl):3–19, 1990.

9. McGill HC, McMahan CA, Malcom GT, Oalmann MC, Strong JP. Effects of serum lipoproteins and smoking on atherosclerosis in young men and women: The PDAY research group. Pathobiological determinants of atherosclerosis in youth. *Arterioscler Thromb Vasc Biol* 17:95–106, 1997.

10. Kuller L, Borhani N, Furberg C, et al. Prevalence of subclinical atherosclerosis and cardiovascular disease and association with risk factors in the cardiovascular health study. *Am J Epidemiol* 139:1164–1179, 1994.

11. Helgason CM, Wolf PA. American Heart Association Prevention Conference IV: Prevention and rehabilitation of stroke. *Circulation* 96:701–707, 1997.

12. Eichner ER. Exercise and heart disease: Epidemiology of the "exercise hypothesis." *Amer J Med* 75:1008–1023, 1986.

13. Enos WF, Holmes RH, Beyer J. Coronary disease among United States soldiers killed in action in Korea. *JAMA* 152: 1090–1093, 1953.

14. National Center for Health Statistics. *Health, United States, 1996–97 and Injury Chartbook.* Hyattsville, MD: 1997.

15. Hunink MGM, Goldman L, Tosteson ANA, et al. The recent decline in mortality from coronary heart disease, 1980–1990: The effect of secular trends in risk factors and treatment. *JAMA* 277:535–542, 1997.

16. Sytkowski PA, D'Agostino RB, Belanger A, Kannel WB. Sex and time trends in cardiovascular disease incidence and mortality: The Framingham heart study, 1950–1989. *Am J Epidemiol* 143:338–350, 1996.

17. Traven ND, Kuller LH, Ives DG, Rutan GH, Perper JA. Coronary heart disease mortality and sudden death: Trends and patterns in 35- to 44-year-old white males, 1970–1990. *Am J Epidemiol* 142:45–52, 1995.

18. National Center for Health Statistics. *Healthy People 2000 Review, 1995–96.* Hyattsville, MD: Public Health Service, 1996.

19. Grundy SM, Balady GJ, Criqui MH, et al. Guide to primary prevention of cardiovascular diseases: A statement for healthcare professionals from the task force on risk reduction. *Circulation* 95:2329–2331, 1997.

20. Maher JE, Raz JA, Bielak LF, Sheedy PF, Schwartz RS, Peyser PA. Potential of quantity of coronary artery calcification to identify new risk factors for asymptomatic atherosclerosis. *Am J Epidemiol* 144:943–953, 1996.

21. Lynch JW, Kaplan GA, Cohen RD, Tuomilehto J, Salonen JT. Do cardiovascular risk factors explain the relation between socioeconomic status, risk of all-cause mortality, cardiovascular mortality, and acute myocardial infarction? *Am J Epidemiol* 144:934–942, 1996.

22. Garrison RJ, Gold RS, Wilson PWF, Kannel WB. Educational attainment and coronary heart disease risk: The Framingham offspring study. *Prev Med* 22:54–64, 1993.

23. Kaplan GA, Salonen JT, Cohen RD, et al. Social connections and mortality from all causes and from cardiovascular disease: Prospective evidence from eastern Finland. *Am J Epidemiol* 128:370–380, 1988.

24. Modan M, Or J, Karasik A, et al. Hyperinsulinemia, sex, and risk of atherosclerotic cardiovascular disease. *Circulation* 84: 1165–1175, 1991.

25. Boushey CJ, Beresford SAA, Omenn GS, Motulsky AG. A quantitative assessment of plasma homocysteine as a risk factor for vascular disease: Probable benefits of increasing folic acid intakes. *JAMA* 274:1049–1057, 1995.

26. Hebert PR, Rich-Edwards JW, Manson JE, et al. Height and incidence of cardiovascular disease in male physicians. *Circulation* 88:1437–1443, 1993.

27. Nabulsi AA, Folsom AR, White A, et al. Association of hormone-replacement therapy with various cardiovascular risk factors in postmenopausal women. *N Engl J Med* 328: 1069–1075, 1993.

28. Frohlich ED. Uric acid: A risk factor for coronary heart disease. *JAMA* 270:378–379, 1993.

29. Kannel WB, Wolf PA, Castelli WP, D'Agostino RB. Fibrinogen and risk of cardiovascular disease. *JAMA* 258:1183–118, 1987.

30. Ford ES, Freeman DS, Byers T. Baldness and ischemic heart

disease in a national sample of men. *Am J Epidemiol* 143: 651–657, 1996.

31. Leor J, Poole K, Kloner RA. Sudden cardiac death triggered by an earthquake. *N Engl J Med* 334:413–419, 1996.

32. Deary IJ, Fowkes FGR, Donnan PT, Housley E. Hostile personality and risks of peripheral arterial disease in the general population. *Psychosomatic Med* 56:197–202, 1994.

33. Sorensen TIA, Nielsen GG, Andersen PK, Teasdale TW. Genetic and environmental influences on premature death in adult adoptees. *N Engl J Med* 318:727–732, 1988.

34. Marenberg ME, Risch N, Berkman LF, Floderus B, De Faire U. Genetic susceptibility to death from coronary heart disease in a study of twins. *N Engl J Med* 330:1041–1046, 1994.

35. Hahn RA, Teutsch SM, Rothenberg RB, Marks JS. Excess deaths from nine chronic diseases in the United States, 1986. *JAMA* 264:2654–2659, 1990.

36. Manson JE, Tosteson H, Ridker PM, et al. The primary prevention of myocardial infarction. *N Engl J Med* 326:1406–1413, 1992.

37. Bronner LL, Kanter DS, Manson JE. Primary prevention of stroke. *N Engl J Med* 333:1392–1400, 1995.

38. Opening blocked coronary arteries. *Harvard Heart Letter* 3(9): May, 1993.

39. Writing Group for the Bypass Angioplasty Revascularization Investigation Investigators. Five-year clinical and functional outcome comparing bypass surgery and angioplasty in patients with multivessel coronary disease: A multicenter randomized trial. *JAMA* 277:715–721, 1997.

40. Loscalzo J. Regression of coronary atherosclerosis. *N Engl J Med* 323:1337–1339, 1990.

41. Brown BG, Zhao XQ, Sacco DE, Albers JJ. Lipid lowering and plaque regression: New insights into prevention of plaque disruption and clinical events in coronary disease. *Circulation* 87:1781–1789, 1993.

42. Waters D, Lespérance J. Regression of coronary atherosclerosis: An achievable goal? Review of results from recent clinical trials. *Am J Med* 91 (suppl 1B):10S–17S, 1991.

43. Amsterdam EA, Hyson D, Kappagoda CT. Nonpharmacologic therapy for coronary artery atherosclerosis: Results of primary and secondary trials. *Am Heart J* 128:1344–1352, 1994.

44. Gould KL, Ornish D, Scherwitz L, et al. Changes in myocardial perfusion abnormalities by positron emission tomography after long-term, intense risk factor modification. *JAMA* 274:894–901, 1995.

45. Ornish D, Brown SE, Scherwitz LW, et al. Can lifestyle changes reverse coronary artery heart disease? *Lancet* 336:129–133, 1990.

46. Watts GF, Lewis B, Brunt JNH, et al. Effects on coronary artery disease of lipid-lowering diet, or diet plus cholestyramine, in the St Thomas' atherosclerosis regression study (STARS). *Lancet* 339:563–569, 1992.

47. Hambrecht R, Niebauer J, Marburger C, et al. Various intensities of leisure time physical activity in patients with coronary artery disease: Effects on cardiorespiratory fitness and progression of coronary atherosclerotic lesions. *J Am Coll Cardiol* 22:468–477, 1993.

48. Schuler G, Hambrecht R, Schlierf G, et al. Regular physical exercise and low-fat diet: Effects on progression of coronary artery disease. *Circulation* 86:1–11, 1992.

49. Merz CN, Rozanski A, Forrester JS. The secondary prevention of coronary artery disease. *Am J Med* 102:572–581, 1997.

50. Stark RM. Review of the major intervention trials of lowering coronary artery disease risk through cholesterol reduction. *Am J Cardiol* 78:13–19, 1996.

51. U.S. Department of Health and Human Services. *The Health Benefits of Smoking Cessation.* U.S. Department of Health and Human Services, Public Health Service, Centers for Disease Control, Center for Chronic Disease Prevention and Health Promotion, Office on Smoking and Health. DHHS Publication No. (CDC) 90-8416. Washington, DC: Superintendent of Documents, 1990.

52. McGinnis JM, Foege WH. Actual causes of death in the United States. *JAMA* 270:2207–2212, 1993.

53. Cigarette smoking—attributable mortality and years of potential life lost—United States, 1990. *MMWR* 42(33):645–647, 1993.

54. Neaton JD, Wentworth D. Serum cholesterol, blood pressure, cigarette smoking, and death from coronary heart disease. *Arch Intern Med* 152:56–64, 1992.

55. Wannamethee SG, Shaper AG, Whincup PH, Walker M. Smoking cessation and the risk of stroke in middle-aged men. *JAMA* 274:155–160, 1995.

56. Bartecchi CE, MacKenzie TD, Schrier RW. The human costs of tobacco use. *N Engl J Med* 330:907–911, 975–980, 1994.

57. Waters D, Lesperance J, Gladstone P, et al. Effects of cigarette smoking on the angiographic evolution of coronary atherosclerosis. *Circulation* 94:614–621, 1996.

58. Stefanadis C, Tsiamis E, Vlachopoulos C, et al. Unfavorable effect of smoking on the elastic properties of the human aorta. *Circulation* 95:31–38, 1997.

59. CDC. Cigarette smoking among adults—United States, 1994. *MMWR* 45(27):588–590, 1996.

60. CDC. The great American smokeout. *MMWR* 45(44):961–966, 1996.

61. Escobedo LG, Reddy M, DuRant RH. Relationship between cigarette smoking and health risk and problem behaviors among US adolescents. *Arch Pediatr Adolesc Med* 151:66–71, 1997.

62. U.S. Department of Health and Human Services. *Strategies to Control Tobacco Use in the United States: A Blueprint for Public Health Action in the 1990s.* USDHHS, Public Health Service, National Institutes of Health, National Cancer Institute. NIH Publication No. 92-3316, 1991.

63. U.S. Department of Health and Human Services. *Major Local Tobacco Control Ordinances in the United States.* USDHHS, Public Health Service, National Institutes of Health, National Cancer Institute. NIH Publication No. 93-3532, 1993.

64. U.S. Environmental Protection Agency. *Respiratory Health Effects of Passive Smoking: Lung Cancer and Other Disorders.* U.S. Environmental Protection Agency, Office of Research and Development. Washington, DC: U.S. EPA, 1992.

65. Steenland K, Thun M, Lally C, Heath C. Environmental tobacco smoke and coronary heart disease in the American Cancer Society CPS-II cohort. *Circulation* 94:622–628, 1996.

66. Kritz H, Schmid P, Sinzinger H. Passive smoking and cardiovascular risk. *Arch Intern Med* 155:1942–1948, 1995.

67. National Institute for Occupational Safety and Health. *Current Intelligence Bulletin 54. Environmental Tobacco Smoke in the Workplace: Lung Cancer and Other Health Effects.* U.S. Department of

Health and Human Services, Centers for Disease Control, National Institute for Occupational Safety and Health, June 1991. DHHS Publication No. (NIOSH) 91-108.

68. U.S. Department of Health and Human Services. *Smokeless Tobacco and Health: An International Perspective.* USDHHS, Public Health Service, National Institutes of Health, National Cancer Institute. NIH Publication No. 93-3461, 1992.

69. Use of smokeless tobacco among adults—United States, 1991. *MMWR* 42(14):263–266, 1993. See also *MMWR* 45(20):413–418, 1996.

70. Ernster VL, Grady DG, Greene JC, et al. Smokeless tobacco use and health effects among baseball players. *JAMA* 264: 218–224, 1990.

71. Report of the Surgeon General. *The Health Consequences of Smoking: Nicotine Addiction.* Washington, DC: U.S. Department of Health and Human Services, Publication No. CDC 88-8406, 1988.

72. The Smoking Cessation Clinical Practice Guidelines Panel and Staff. The Agency for Health Care Policy and Research smoking cessation clinical practice guidelines. *JAMA* 275: 1270–1280, 1996.

73. Nieman DC, Johansen LM, Lee JW, Cermak J, Arabatzis K. Infectious episodes in runners before and after the Los Angeles marathon. *J Sports Med Phys Fit* 30:316–328, 1990.

74. Escobedo LG, Marcus SE, Holtzman D, Giovino GA. Sports participation, age at smoking initiation, and the risk of smoking among US high school students. *JAMA* 269:1391–1395, 1993. See also *JAMA* 270:938, 1993.

75. Williard JC, Schoenborn CA. *Relationship between Cigarette Smoking and Other Unhealthy Behaviors among Our Nation's Youth: United States, 1992, Advance Data from Vital and Health Statistics* (no. 263). Hyattsville, MD: National Center for Health Statistics, 1995.

76. Simoes EJ, Byers T, Coates RJ, Serdula MK, Mokdad AH, Heath GW. The association between leisure-time physical activity and dietary fat in American adults. *Am J Public Health* 85:240–244, 1995.

77. Frisk J, Brynhildsen J, Ivarsson T, Persson P, Hammar M. Exercise and smoking habits among Swedish postmenopausal women. *Br J Sports Med* 31:217–223, 1997.

78. Lazarus NB, Kaplan GA, Cohen RD, Leu D-J. Smoking and body mass in the natural history of physical activity: Prospective evidence from the Alameda County study, 1965–1974. *Am J Prev Med* 5:127–135, 1989.

79. Conway TL, Cronan TA. Smoking, exercise, and physical fitness. *Prev Med* 21:723–734, 1992.

80. Marti B, Abelin T, Minder CE, Vader JP. Smoking, alcohol consumption, and endurance capacity: An analysis of 6,500 19-year-old conscripts and 4,100 joggers. *Prev Med* 17:79–92, 1988.

81. Dannenberg AL, Keller JB, Wilson WF, Castelli WP. Leisure time physical activity in the Framingham offspring study. *Am J Epidemiol* 129:76–88, 1989.

82. Erikssen SL, Thaulow E. Smoking habits and long-term decline in physical fitness and lung function in men. *Br Med J* 311:715–718, 1995.

83. Huie MJ. The effects of smoking on exercise performance. *Sports Med* 22:355–359, 1996.

84. Symons JD, Stebbins CL. Hemodynamic and regional blood flow responses to nicotine at rest and during exercise. *Med Sci Sports Exerc* 28:457–467, 1996.

85. Gold DR, Wang X, Wypij D, Speizer FE, Ware JH, Dockery DW. Effects of cigarette smoking on lung function in adolescent boys and girls. *N Engl J Med* 335:931–937, 1996.

86. Colberg SR, Casazza GA, Horning MA, Brooks GA. Metabolite and hormonal response in smokers during rest and sustained exercise. *Med Sci Sports Exerc* 27:1527–1534, 1995.

87. Temocin S, Erenmemisoglu A, Suer C, Beydagi H. Effect of nicotine on swimming exercise in rats. *Jpn J Physiol* 43:567–570, 1993.

88. Agudo A, Bardagi S, Romero PV, Gonzalez CA. Exercise-induced airways narrowing and exposure to environmental tobacco smoke in schoolchildren. *Am J Epidemiol* 140:409–417, 1994.

89. Frette C, Barrett-Connor E, Clausen JL. Effect of active and passive smoking on ventilatory function in elderly men and women. *Am J Epidemiol* 143:757–765, 1996.

90. Huie MJ, Casazza GA, Horning MA, Brooks GA. Smoking increases conversion of lactate to glucose during submaximal exercise. *J Appl Physiol* 80:1554–1559, 1996.

91. Sidney S, Sternfield B, Gidding SS, et al. Cigarette smoking and submaximal exercise test duration in a biracial population of young adults: The CARDIA study. *Med Sci Sports Exerc* 25:911–916, 1993.

92. Higgins MW, Enright PL, Kronmal RA, et al. Smoking and lung function in elderly men and women: The cardiovascular health study. *JAMA* 269:2741–2748, 1993.

93. Cooper KH, Gey GO, Bottenberg RA. Effects of cigarette smoking on endurance performance. *JAMA* 203(3):123–126, 1968.

94. Pederson LL, Poulin M, Lefcoe NM, Donald AW, Hill JS. Does cigarette smoking affect the fitness of young adults? *J Sports Med Phys Fitness* 32:96–105, 1992.

95. Cooper KH. *Aerobics.* New York: Bantam Books, 1968. See also *The New Aerobics.* New York: Bantam Books, 1970.

96. Koplan JP, Powell KE, et al. An epidemiologic study of the benefits and risks of running. *JAMA* 248:3118–3121, 1982.

97. Nieman DC, Butler JV, Pollett LM, Dietrich SJ, Lutz RD. Nutrient intake of marathon runners. *J Am Diet Assoc* 89: 1273–1278,1989.

98. Blair SN, Goodyear NN, Wynne KL, Saunders RP. Comparison of dietary and smoking habit changes in physical fitness improvers and nonimprovers. *Prev Med* 13:411–420, 1984.

99. King AC, Haskell WL, Taylor CB, Kraemer HC, DeBusk RF. Group- versus home-based exercise training in healthy older men and women. *JAMA* 266:1535–1542, 1991.

100. Derby CA, Lasater TM, Vass K, Gonzalez S, Carleton RA. Characteristics of smokers who attempt to quit and of those who recently succeeded. *Am J Prev Med* 10:327–334, 1994.

101. Hurt RD, Dale LC, Offord KP, Bruce BK, McClain FL, Eberman KM. Inpatient treatment of severe nicotine dependence. *Mayo Clin Proc* 67:823–828, 1992.

102. Gritz ER, Klesges RC, Meyers AW. The smoking and body weight relationship: Implications for intervention and post-cessation weight control. *Ann Beh Med* 11(4):144–153, 1989.

103. Grunberg NE. Cigarette smoking and body weight: Current perspective and future directions. *Ann Beh Med* 11(4):154–157, 1989.

104. Williamson DF, Madans J, Anda RF, et al. Smoking cessation and severity of weight gain in a national cohort. *N Engl J Med* 324:739–745, 1991.

105. Klesges RC, Meyers AW, Winders SE, French SN. Determining the reasons for weight gain following smoking cessation: Current findings, methodological issues, and future directions for research. *Ann Beh Med* 11(4):134–143, 1989.

106. Flegal KM, Troiano RP, Pamuk ER, Kuczmarski RJ, Campbell SM. The influence of smoking cessation on the prevalence of overweight in the United States. *N Engl J Med* 333:1165–1170, 1995.

107. Swan GE, Carmelli D. Characteristics associated with excessive weight gain after smoking cessation in men. *Am J Public Health* 85:73–77, 1995.

108. Caan B, Coates A, Schaefer C, Finkler L, Sternfeld B, Corbett K. Women gain weight 1 year after smoking cessation while dietary intake temporarily increases. *J Am Diet Assoc* 96:1150–1155, 1996.

109. Klesges RC, Eck LH, Isbell TR, Fulliton W, Hanson CL. Smoking status: Effects on the dietary intake, physical activity, and body fat of adult men. *Am J Clin Nutr* 51:784–789, 1990.

110. Perkins KA, Epstein LH, Stiller RL, et al. Metabolic effects of nicotine after consumption of a meal in smokers and nonsmokers. *Am J Clin Nutr* 52:228–233, 1990.

111. Moffatt RJ, Owens SG. Cessation from cigarette smoking: Changes in body weight, body composition, resting metabolism, and energy consumption. *Metabolism* 40:465–470, 1991.

112. Collins LC, Cornelius MF, Vogel RL, Walker JF, Stamford BA. Effect of caffeine and/or cigarette smoking on resting energy expenditure. *Int J Obes Relat Metab Disord* 18:551–556, 1994.

113. Hofstetter A, Schutz Y, Jequier E, Wahren J. Increased 24-hour energy expenditure in cigarette smokers. *N Engl J Med* 314:79–82, 1986.

114. Kawachi I, Troisi RJ, Rotnitzky AG, Coakley EH, Colditz GA. Can physical activity minimize weight gain in women after smoking cessation? *Am J Public Health* 86:999–1004, 1996.

115. Marcus B, Albrecht AE, Niaura RS, et al. Exercise enhances the maintenance of smoking cessation in women. *Addict Behav* 20:87–92, 1995.

116. Brown DR, Croft JB, Anda RF, Barrett DH, Escobedo LG. Evaluation of smoking on the physical activity and depressive symptoms relationship. *Med Sci Sports Exerc* 28:233–240, 1996.

117. Blair SN, Kampert JB, Kohl HW, et al. Influences of cardiorespiratory fitness and other precursors on cardiovascular disease and all-cause mortality in men and women. *JAMA* 276:205–210, 1996.

118. National High Blood Pressure Education Program. *The Fifth Report of the Joint National Committee on Detection, Evaluation, and Treatment of High Blood Pressure.* National Heart, Lung, and Blood Institute, National Institutes of Health, NIH Publication No. 93-1088. Bethesda, MD: National Institutes of Health, 1993.

119. National High Blood Pressure Education Program. *Working Group Report on Primary Prevention of Hypertension, National Heart, Lung, and Blood Institute.* Hyattsville, MD: National Institutes of Health, 1992.

120. Stamler J, Stamler R, Neaton JD. Blood pressure, systolic and diastolic, and cardiovascular risks: US population data. *Arch Intern Med* 153:598–615, 1993.

121. Cooper R, Rotimi C, Ataman S, et al. The prevalence of hypertension in seven populations of West African origin. *Am J Public Health* 87:160–168, 1997.

122. Burt VL, Whelton P, Roccella EJ, et al. Prevalence of hypertension in the US adult population. *Hypertension* 25:305–313, 1995.

123. Burt VL, Cutler JA, Higgins M, et al. Trends in the prevalence, awareness, treatment, and control of hypertension in the adult US population: Data from the Health Examination Surveys, 1960–1991. *Hypertension* 26:60–69, 1995.

124. National Heart, Lung, and Blood Institute. *High Blood Pressure: Treat It for Life.* Washington, DC: U.S. Government Printing Office, 1994.

125. Kannel WB. Blood pressure as a cardiovascular risk factor: Prevention and treatment. *JAMA* 275:1571–1576, 1996.

126. Lindenstrom E, Boysen G, Nyboe J. Influence of systolic and diastolic blood pressure on stroke risk: A prospective observational study. *Am J Epidemiol* 142:1279–1290, 1995.

127. Chobanian AV, Alexander RW. Exacerbation of atherosclerosis by hypertension: Potential mechanisms and clinical implications. *Arch Intern Med* 156:1952–1956, 1996.

128. Launer LJ, Masaki K, Petrovitch H, Foley D, Havlik RJ. The association between midlife blood pressure levels and late-life cognitive function: The Honolulu–Asia aging study. *JAMA* 274:1846–1851, 1995.

129. Psaty BM, Smith NL, Siscovick DS, et al. Health outcomes associated with antihypertensive therapies used as first-line agents: A systematic review and meta-analysis. *JAMA* 277:739–745, 1997.

130. Curb JD, Pressel SL, Cutler JA, et al. Effect of diuretic-based antihypertensive treatment on cardiovascular disease risk in older diabetic patients with isolated systolic hypertension. *JAMA* 276:1886–1892, 1996.

131. Kaplan NM, Gifford RW. Choice of initial therapy for hypertension. *JAMA* 275:1577–1580, 1996.

132. Grimm RH, Flack JM, Grandits GA, et al. Long-term effects on plasma lipids of diet and drugs to treat hypertension. *JAMA* 275:1549–1556, 1996.

133. Cook NR, Cohen J, Hebert PR, Taylor JO, Hennekens CH. Implications of small reductions in diastolic blood pressure for primary prevention. *Arch Intern Med* 155:701–709, 1995.

134. Grimm RH, Grandits GA, Cutler JA, et al. Relationships of quality-of-life measures to long-term lifestyle and drug treatment in the treatment of mild hypertension study. *Arch Intern Med* 157:638–648, 1997.

135. Working Group on Management of Patients with Hypertension and High Blood Cholesterol. National Education Programs Working Group report on the management of patients with hypertension and high blood cholesterol. *Ann Int Med* 114:224–237, 1991.

136. Neaton JD, Grimm RH, Prineas RJ, et al. Treatment of mild hypertension study: Final results. *JAMA* 270:713–724, 1993.

137. Treatment of Mild Hypertension Research Group. The treatment of mild hypertension study: A randomized, placebo-controlled trial of a nutritional–hygienic regimen along with various drug monotherapies. *Arch Intern Med* 151:1413–1423, 1991.

138. Stevens VJ, Corrigan SA, Obarzanek E, et al. Weight loss intervention in phase I of the trials of hypertension prevention. *Arch Intern Med* 153:849–858, 1993.

139. Davis BR, Blaufox MD, Oberman A, et al. Reduction in long-term antihypertensive medication requirements: Effects of weight reduction by dietary intervention in overweight persons with mild hypertension. *Arch Intern Med* 153:1773–1782, 1993.

140. Trials of Hypertension Prevention Collaborative Research Group. The effects of nonpharmacologic interventions on blood pressure of persons with high normal levels. *JAMA* 267:1213–1220, 1992.

141. Liu K, Ruth KJ, Flack JM, et al. Blood pressure in young blacks

and whites: Relevance of obesity and lifestyle factors in determining differences. The CARDIA study. *Circulation* 93:60–66, 1996.

142. Curhan GC, Chertow GM, Willett WC, et al. Birth weight and adult hypertension and obesity in women. *Circulation* 94: 1310–1315, 1996.

143. Trials of Hypertension Prevention Collaborative Research Group. Effects of weight loss and sodium reduction intervention on blood pressure and hypertension incidence in overweight people with high-normal blood pressure. *Arch Intern Med* 157:657–667, 1997.

144. Stamler J. The INTERSALT Study: Background, methods, findings, and implications. *Am J Clin Nutr* 65(suppl):626S–642S, 1997.

145. Stamler J, Rose G, Stamler R, Elliott P, Dyer A, Marmot M. INTERSALT study findings: Public health and medical care implications. *Hypertension* 14:570–577, 1989.

146. Law MR, Frost CD, Wald NJ. By how much does dietary salt reduction lower blood pressure? I. Analysis of observational data among populations. *Br J Med* 302:811–815, 1991.

147. Beard TC, Blizzard L, O'Brien DJ, Dip G, Dwyer T. Association between blood pressure and dietary factors in the dietary and nutritional survey of British adults. *Arch Intern Med* 157: 234–238, 1997.

148. National Heart, Lung, and Blood Institute Workshop on Salt and Blood Pressure. *Hypertension* 17(1)(suppl):1–215, 1991.

149. Siani A, Strazzullo P, Giacco A, et al. Increasing the dietary potassium intake reduces the need for antihypertensive medication. *Ann Int Med* 115:753–759, 1991.

150. Tobian L. Dietary sodium chloride and potassium have effects on the pathophysiology of hypertension in humans and animals. *Am J Clin Nutr* 65(suppl):606S–611S, 1997.

151. Morse RM, Flavin DK. The definition of alcoholism. *JAMA* 268:1012–1014, 1992.

152. Kitchens JM. Does this patient have an alcohol problem? *JAMA* 272:1782–1787, 1994.

153. *Seventh Special Report to the U.S. Congress on Alcohol and Health.* Alcohol, Drug Abuse, and Mental Health Administration: National Institute on Alcohol Abuse and Alcoholism. Rockville, MD: U.S. Department of Health and Human Services, 1990.

154. Gentilello LM, Donovan DM, Dunn CW, Rivara FP. Alcohol interventions in trauma centers: Current practice and future directions. *JAMA* 274:1043–1048, 1995.

155. Liu S, Siegel PZ, Brewer RD, Mokdad AH, Sleet DA, Serdula M. Prevalence of alcohol-impaired driving: Results from a national self-reported survey of health behaviors. *JAMA* 277: 122–125, 1997.

156. Rimm EB, Giovannucci EL, Willett WC, et al. Prospective study of alcohol consumption and risk of coronary disease in men. *Lancet* 338:464–468, 1991.

157. Klatsky AL, Armstrong MA, Friedman GD. Risk of cardiovascular mortality in alcohol drinkers, ex-drinkers and nondrinkers. *Am J Cardiol* 66:1237–1242, 1990.

158. Pearson TA. AHA science advisory: Alcohol and heart disease. *Circulation* 94:3023–3025, 1996.

159. Suh I, Shaten J, Cutler JA, Kuller LH. Alcohol use and mortality from coronary heart disease: The role of high-density lipoprotein cholesterol. *Ann Int Med* 116:881–887, 1992.

160. Stampfer MJ, Rimm EB, Walsh DC. Commentary: Alcohol, the heart, and public policy. *Am J Pub Health* 83:801–804, 1993.

161. Marques-Vidal P, Ducimetiere P, Evans A, Cambou JP, Arveiler D. Alcohol consumption and myocardial infarction: A case–control study in France and Northern Ireland. *Am J Epidemiol* 143:1089–1093, 1996.

162. Camargo CA, Hennekens CH, Gaziano JM, Glynn RJ, Manson JE, Stampfer MJ. Prospective study of moderate alcohol consumption and mortality in US male physicians. *Arch Intern Med* 157:79–85, 1997.

163. Fuchs CS, Stampfer MJ, Colditz GA, et al. Alcohol consumption and mortality among women. *N Engl J Med* 332: 1245–1250, 1995.

164. Brown SP, Li H, Chitwood LF, Anderson ER, Boatwright D. Blood pressure, hemodynamic, and thermal responses after cycling exercise. *J Appl Physiol* 75:240–245, 1993.

165. DiCarlo SE, Collins HL, Howard MG, Chen CY, Scislo TJ, Patil RD. Postexertional hypotension: A brief review. *Sports Med Train Rehab* 5:17–27, 1994.

166. Rueckert PA, Slane PR, Lillis DL, Hanson P. Hemodynamic patterns and duration of post-dynamic exercise hypotension in hypertensive humans. *Med Sci Sports Exerc* 28:24–32, 1996.

167. Shen W, Zhang X, Zhao G, Wolin MS, Sessa W, Hintze TH. Nitric oxide production and NO synthase gene expression contribute to vascular regulation during exercise. *Med Sci Sports Exerc* 27:1125–1134, 1995.

168. Benbassat J, Froom P. Blood pressure response to exercise as a predictor of hypertension. *Arch Intern Med* 146:2053–2055, 1986.

169. Mundal R, Kjeldsen SE, Sandvik L, Erikssen G, Thaulow E, Erikssen J. Exercise pressure predicts mortality from myocardial infarction. *Hypertension* 27:324–329, 1996.

170. ACSM Position Stand. Physical activity, physical fitness, and hypertension. *Med Sci Sports Exerc* 25:i–x, 1993.

171. Kelley G, Tran ZV. Aerobic exercise and normotensive adults: A meta-analysis. *Med Sci Sports Exerc* 27:1371–1377, 1995.

172. Kelley G. Effects of aerobic exercise on ambulatory blood pressure: A meta-analysis. *Sports Med Train Rehab* 7:115–131, 1996.

173. Kokkinos PF, Narayan P, Colleran JA, et al. Effects of regular exercise on blood pressure and left ventricular hypertrophy in African-American men with severe hypertension. *N Engl J Med* 333:1462–1467, 1995.

174. Kelemen MH, Effron MB, Valenti SA, Stewart KJ. Exercise training combined with antihypertensive drug therapy: Effects on lipids, blood pressure, and left ventricular mass. *JAMA* 263:2766–2771, 1990.

175. Kelley G. Dynamic resistance exercise and resting blood pressure in adults: A meta-analysis. *J Appl Physiol* 82:1559–1565, 1997.

176. Paffenbarger RS, Wing AL, Hyde RT, Jung DL. Physical activity and incidence of hypertension in college alumni. *Am J Epidemiol* 117:245–256, 1983.

177. Blair SN, Goodyear NN, Gibbons LW, et al. Physical fitness and incidence of hypertension in healthy normotensive men and women. *JAMA* 252:487–490, 1984.

178. Paffenbarger RS, Jung DL, Leung RW, Hyde RT. Physical activity and hypertension: An epidemiological view. *Ann Med* 23:319–327, 1991.

179. Williams PT. Relationship of distance run per week to coronary heart disease risk factors in 8283 male runners: The national runners' health study. *Arch Intern Med* 157:191–198, 1997.

180. Pols MA, Peeters PHM, Twisk JWR, Kemper HCG, Grobbee DE. Physical activity and cardiovascular disease risk profile in women. *Am J Epidemiol* 146:322–328, 1997.

181. Dwyer T, Gibbons LE. The Australian schools health and fitness survey: Physical fitness related to blood pressure but not lipoproteins. *Circulation* 89:1539–1544, 1994.

182. Lim PO, MacFadyen RJ, Clarkson PBM, MacDonald TM. Impaired exercise tolerance in hypertensive patients. *Ann Intern Med* 124:41–55, 1996.

183. Grundy SM. Cholesterol and coronary heart disease: The 21st century. *Arch Intern Med* 157:1177–1184, 1997.

184. Verschuren WMM, Jacobs DR, Bloemberg BPM, et al. Serum total cholesterol and long-term coronary heart disease mortality in different cultures: Twenty-five year follow-up of the seven countries study. *JAMA* 274:131–136, 1995.

185. National Research Council. *Diet and Health: Implications for Reducing Chronic Disease Risk.* Washington, DC: National Academy Press, 1989.

186. Expert Panel on Detection, Evaluation, and Treatment of High Blood Cholesterol In Adults. Summary of the second report of the National Cholesterol Education Program (NCEP) expert panel on detection, evaluation, and treatment of high blood cholesterol in adults (adult treatment panel II). *JAMA* 269:3015–3023, 1993.

187. Task Force on Risk Reduction, American Heart Association. Cholesterol screening in asymptomatic adults: No cause to change. *Circulation* 93:1067–1068, 1996.

188. Johnson CL, Rifkind BM, Sempos CT, et al. Declining serum total cholesterol levels among US adults: The National Health and Nutrition Examination Surveys. *JAMA* 269:3002–3008, 1993.

189. Sempos CT, Cleeman JI, Carroll MD, et al. Prevalence of high blood cholesterol among US adults. *JAMA* 269:3009–3014, 1993.

190. Giles WH, Anda RF, Jones DH, et al. Recent trends in the identification and treatment of high blood cholesterol by physicians: Progress and missed opportunities. *JAMA* 269:1133–1138, 1993.

191. Castelli WP, Garrison RJ, Wilson PWF, et al. Incidence of coronary heart disease and lipoprotein cholesterol levels: The Framingham study. *JAMA* 256:2835–2838, 1986.

192. Haskell WL. The influence of exercise on the concentrations of triglyceride and cholesterol in human plasma. *Exerc Sport Sci Rev* 12:205–244, 1984.

193. NIH Consensus Development Panel on Triglyceride, High-Density Lipoprotein, and Coronary Heart Disease. Triglyceride, high-density lipoprotein, and coronary heart disease. *JAMA* 269:505–510, 1993.

194. Miller M, Seidler A, Kwiterovich PO, Pearson TA. Long-term predictors of subsequent cardiovascular events with coronary artery disease and "desirable" levels of plasma total cholesterol. *Circulation* 86:1165–1170, 1992.

195. Linn S, Fulwood R, Carroll M, et al. Serum total cholesterol: HDL cholesterol ratios in US white and black adults by selected demographic and socioeconomic variables (NHANES II). *Am J Public Health* 81:1038–1043, 1991.

196. Corti MC, Guralnik JM, Salive ME, et al. HDL cholesterol predicts coronary heart disease mortality in older persons. *JAMA* 274:539–544, 1995.

197. Jacobs DR, Mebane IL, Bangdiwala SI, et al. High density lipoprotein cholesterol as a predictor of cardiovascular disease mortality in men and women: The Follow-up Study of the Lipid Research clinics prevalence study. *Am J Epidemiol* 131:32–47, 1990.

198. Grover SA, Coupal L, Hu XP. Identifying adults at increased risk of coronary disease: How well do the current cholesterol guidelines work? *JAMA* 274:801–806, 1995.

199. Stampfer MJ, Sacks FM, Salvini S, Willett WC, Hennekens CH. A prospective study of cholesterol, apolipoproteins, and the risk of myocardial infarction. *N Engl J Med* 325:373–381, 1991.

200. LaRosa JC. Triglycerides and coronary risk in women and the elderly. *Arch Intern Med* 157:961–968, 1997.

201. Criqui MH, Heiss G, Cohn R, et al. Plasma triglyceride level and mortality from coronary heart disease. *N Engl J Med* 328:1220–1225, 1993.

202. DeLong DM, Delong ER, Wood PD, et al. A comparison of methods for the estimation of plasma low- and very low-density lipoprotein cholesterol. *JAMA* 256:2372–2377, 1986.

203. Andrews TC, Raby K, Barry J, et al. Effect of cholesterol reduction on myocardial ischemia in patients with coronary disease. *Circulation* 95:324–328, 1997.

204. Hebert PR, Gaziano JM, Chan KS, Hennekens CH. Cholesterol lowering with statin drugs, risk of stroke, and total mortality. *JAMA* 278:313–321, 1997.

205. Johannesson M, Jonsson B, Kjekshus J, Olsson AG, Pedersen TR, Wedel H. Cost effectiveness of simvastatin treatment to lower cholesterol levels in patients with coronary heart disease. *N Engl J Med* 336:332–336, 1997.

206. Davidson MH, Testolin LM, Maki KC, von Duvillard S, Drennan KB. A comparison of estrogen replacement, pravastatin, and combined treatment for the management of hypercholesterolemia in postmenopausal women. *Arch Intern Med* 157:1186–1192, 1997.

207. National Cholesterol Education Program. *The Expert Panel on Blood Cholesterol Levels in Children and Adolescents.* U.S. Department of Health and Human Services, National Institutes of Health, Publication no. N4LB1. Rockville, MD: Author, 1991.

208. American Heart Association. Position statement: Dietary guidelines for healthy American adults: A statement for health professionals from the nutrition committee. *Circulation* 94:1795–1800, 1996.

209. Hegsted DM, Ausman LM, Johnson JA, Dallal GE. Dietary fat and serum lipids: An evaluation of the experimental data. *Am J Clin Nutr* 57:875–883, 1993.

210. Kris-Etherton PM, Yu S. Individual fatty acid effects on plasma lipids and lipoproteins: Human studies. *Am J Clin Nutr* 65(suppl):1628S–1644S, 1997.

211. Markovitz JH, Smith D, Raczynski JM, et al. Lack of relations of hostility, negative affect, and high-risk behavior with low plasma lipid levels in the coronary artery risk development in young adults study. *Arch Intern Med* 157:1953–1959, 1997.

212. Howell WH, McNamara DJ, Tosca MA, Smith BT, Gaines JA. Plasma lipid and lipoprotein responses to dietary fat and cholesterol: A meta-analysis. *Am J Clin Nutr* 65:1747–1764, 1997.

213. Van Horn L. Fiber, lipids, and coronary heart disease: A statement for healthcare professionals from the nutrition committee, American Heart Association. *Circulation* 95:2701–2704, 1997.

214. Lichtenstein AH. Trans fatty acids, plasma lipid levels, and risk of developing cardiovascular disease: A statement for

healthcare professionals from the nutrition committee, American Heart Association. *Circulation* 95:2588–2590, 1997.

215. Barnard RJ. Effects of life-style modification on serum lipids. *Arch Intern Med* 151:1389–1394, 1991.

216. Walford RL, Harris SB, Gunion MW. The calorically restricted low-fat nutrient-dense diet in Biosphere 2 significantly lowers blood glucose, total leukocyte count, cholesterol, and blood pressure in humans. *Proc Natl Acad Sci* 89:11533–11537, 1992.

217. Wood PD. Physical activity, diet, and health: Independent and interactive effects. *Med Sci Sports Exerc* 26:838–843, 1994.

218. Wood PD, Haskell WL, Stern MP, Lewis S, Perry C. Serum lipoprotein distributions in male and female runners. *Ann NY Acad Sci* 301:748–763, 1977.

219. MacAuley D, McCrum EE, Stott G, et al. Physical fitness, lipids, and apolipoproteins in the Northern Ireland health and activity survey. *Med Sci Sports Exerc* 29:1187–1191, 1997.

220. Toth MJ, Gardner AW, Poehlman ET. Training status, resting metabolic rate, and cardiovascular disease risk in middle-aged men. *Metabolism* 44:340–347, 1995.

221. Nieman DC, Warren BJ, O'Donnell KA, Dotson RG, Butterworth DE, Henson DA. Physical activity and serum lipids and lipoproteins in elderly women. *J Am Geriatr Assoc* 41:1339–1344, 1993.

222. Williams PT. High-density lipoprotein cholesterol and other risk factors for coronary heart disease in female runners. *N Engl J Med* 334:1298–1303, 1996.

223. Kokkinos PF, Holland JC, Narayan P, Colleran JA, Dotson CO, Papademetriou V. Miles run per week and high-density lipoprotein cholesterol levels in healthy, middle-aged men: A dose–response relationship. *Arch Intern Med* 155:415–420, 1995.

224. Katzel LI, Bleecker ER, Colman EG, Rogus EM, Sorkin JD, Goldberg AP. Effects of weight loss vs aerobic exercise training on risk factors for coronary disease in healthy, obese, middle-aged and older men. *JAMA* 274:1915–1921, 1995.

225. Dengel JL, Katzel LI, Goldberg AP. Effect of an American Heart Association diet, with or without weight loss, on lipids in obese middle-aged and older men. *Am J Clin Nutr* 62:715–721, 1995.

226. Andersen RE, Wadden TA, Bartlett SJ, Vogt RA, Weinstock RS. Relation of weight loss to changes in serum lipids and lipoproteins in obese women. *Am J Clin Nutr* 62:350–357, 1995.

227. Nieman DC, Haig JL, Fairchild KS, et al. Reducing-diet and exercise-training effects on serum lipids and lipoproteins in mildly obese women. *Am J Clin Nutr* 52:640–645, 1990.

228. Schwartz RS. The independent effects of dietary weight loss and aerobic training on high density lipoproteins and apolipoprotein A-1 concentrations in obese men. *Metabolism* 36:165–171, 1987.

229. Schwartz RS, Cain KC, Shuman WP, et al. Effect of intensive endurance training on lipoprotein profiles in young and older men. *Metabolism* 41:649–654, 1992.

230. Hinkleman L, Nieman DC. The effects of moderate exercise training on body composition and serum lipids and lipoproteins in mildly obese women. *J Sports Med Phys Fit* 33:49–58, 1993.

231. Lokey EA, Tran ZV. Effects of exercise training on serum lipid and lipoprotein concentrations in women: A meta-analysis. *Int J Sports Med* 10:424–429, 1989.

232. Tran ZV, Weltman A. Differential effects of exercise on serum lipid and lipoprotein levels seen with changes in body weight. *JAMA* 254:919–924, 1985.

233. Wood PD, Stefanick MI, Williams PT, Haskell WL. The effects on plasma lipoproteins of a prudent weight-reducing diet, with or without exercise, in overweight men and women. *N Engl J Med* 325:461–466, 1991.

234. Duncan JJ, Gordon NF, Scott CB. Women walking for health and fitness: How much is enough? *JAMA* 266:3295–3299, 1991.

235. King AC, Haskell WL, Young DR, Oka RK, Stefanick ML. Long-term effects of varying intensities and formats of physical activity on participation rates, fitness, and lipoproteins in men and women aged 50 to 65 years. *Circulation* 91:2596–2604, 1995.

236. Leaf DA, Parker DL, Schaad D. Changes in $\dot{V}O_{2max}$, physical activity, and body fat with chronic exercise: Effects on plasma lipids. *Med Sci Sports Exerc* 29:1152–1159, 1997.

237. Butterworth DE, Nieman DC, Henson DA, Utter A. Blood lipid response to exercise and energy restriction in obese women. *Am J Clin Nutr* (in press).

238. Marrugat J, Elosua R, Covas MI, Molina L, Rubies-Prat T. Amount and intensity of physical activity, physical fitness, and serum lipids in men. *Am J Epidemiol* 143:562–569, 1996.

239. Tsetsonis NV, Hardman AE, Mastana SS. Acute effects of exercise on postprandial lipemia: A comparative study in trained and untrained middle-aged women. *Am J Clin Nutr* 65:525–533, 1997.

240. Aldred HE, Perry IC, Hardman AE. The effect of a single bout of brisk walking on postprandial lipemia in normolipidemic young adults. *Metabolism* 43:836–841, 1994.

241. Ziogas GG, Thomas TR, Harris WS. Exercise training, postprandial hypertriglyceridemia, and LDL subfraction distribution. *Med Sci Sports Exerc* 29:986–991, 1997.

242. Pronk NP. Short term effects of exercise on plasma lipids and lipoproteins in humans. *Sports Med* 16:431–448, 1993.

243. Thompson PD, Cullinane EM, Sady SP, et al. High density lipoprotein metabolism in endurance athletes and sedentary men. *Circulation* 84:140–152, 1991.

244. Tsopanakis C, Kotsarellis D, Tsopanakis A. Plasma lecithin: Cholesterol acyltransferase activity in elite athletes from selected sports. *Eur J Appl Physiol* 58:262–265, 1988.

245. Crouse SF, O'Brien BC, Rohack JJ, et al. Changes in serum lipids and apolipoproteins after exercise in men with high cholesterol: Influence of intensity. *J Appl Physiol* 79:279–286, 1995.

246. Ginsburg GS, Agil A, O'Toole M, Rimm E, Douglas PS, Rifai N. Effects of a single bout of ultraendurance exercise on lipid levels and susceptibility of lipids to peroxidation in triathletes. *JAMA* 276:221–225, 1996.

247. Tsetsonis NV, Hardman AE. The influence of the intensity of treadmill walking upon changes in lipid and lipoprotein variables in healthy adults. *Eur J Appl Physiol* 70:329–336, 1995.

248. Lee R, Nieman DC, Raval R, Blankenship J, Lee J. The effects of acute moderate exercise on serum lipids and lipoproteins in mildly obese women. *Int J Sports Med* 12:537–542, 1991.

249. Angelopoulos TJ, Robertson RJ, Goss FL, Metz KF, LaPorte RE. Effect of repeated exercise bouts on high density lipoprotein-cholesterol and its subfractions HDL2-C and HDL3-C. *Int J Sports Med* 14:196–201, 1993.

250. Skinner ER, Watt C, Maughan RJ. The acute effect of marathon running on plasma lipoproteins in female subjects. *Eur J Appl Physiol* 56:451–456, 1987.

251. Goodyear LJ, van Houten DR, Fronsoe MS, et al. Immediate

and delayed effects of marathon running on lipids and lipoproteins in women. *Med Sci Sports Exerc* 22:588–592, 1990.

252. American Heart Association. Statement on exercise: Benefits and recommendations for physical activity programs for all Americans. *Circulation* 86:340–343, 1992.

253. Fletcher GF, Balady G, Blair SN, et al. Statement on exercise: Benefits and recommendations for physical activity programs for all Americans. *Circulation* 94:857–862, 1996.

254. Morris JN, Heady JA, Raffle PAB, Parks JW. Coronary heart disease and physical activity of work. *Lancet* 2:1053–1057, 1953.

255. Paffenbarger RS, Laughlin ME, Gima AS, et al. Work activity of longshoremen as related to death from coronary heart disease and stroke. *N Engl J Med* 282:1109–1114, 1970.

256. Paffenbarger RS, Wing AL, Hyde RT. Physical activity as an index of heart attack risk in college alumni. *Am J Epidemiol* 108:161–175, 1978.

257. Paffenbarger RS, Hyde RT, Wing AL, Steinmetz CH. A natural history of athleticism and cardiovascular health. *JAMA* 252:491–495, 1984.

258. Paffenbarger RS, Hyde RT, Wing AL, Lee I-M, Jung DL, Kampert JB. The association of changes in physical-activity level and other lifestyle characteristics with mortality among men. *N Engl J Med* 328:538–545, 1993.

259. Paffenbarger RS, Kampert JB, Lee IM. Physical activity and health of college men: Longitudinal observations. *Int J Sports Med* 18(suppl 3):S200–S203, 1997.

260. Blair SN, Kohl HW, Paffenbarger RS, Clark DG, Cooper KH, Gibbons LW. Physical fitness and all-cause mortality: A prospective study of healthy men and women. *JAMA* 262:2395–2401, 1989.

261. Lemaitre RN, Heckbert SR, Psaty BM, Siscovick DS. Leisure-time physical activity and the risk of nonfatal myocardial infarction in postmenopausal women. *Arch Intern Med* 155:2302–2308, 1995.

262. Eaton CB, Lapane KL, Garber CA, Assaf AR, Lasater TM, Carleton RA. Sedentary lifestyle and risk of coronary heart disease in women. *Med Sci Sports Exerc* 27:1535–1539, 1995.

263. Kushi LH, Fee RM, Folsom AR, Mink PJ, Anderson KE, Sellers TA. Physical activity and mortality in postmenopausal women. *JAMA* 277:1287–1292, 1997.

264. Powell KE, Thompson PD, Caspersen CJ, Kendrick JS. Physical activity and the incidence of coronary heart disease. *Ann Rev Public Health* 8:253–287, 1987.

265. Berlin JA, Colditz GA. A meta-analysis of physical activity in the prevention of coronary heart disease. *Am J Epidemiol* 132:612–628, 1990.

266. Sobolski J, Kornitzer M, Backer GD, et al. Protection against ischemic heart disease in the Belgian physical fitness study: Physical fitness rather than physical activity? *Am J Epidemiol* 125:601–610, 1987.

267. Mundal R, Erikssen J, Rodahl K. Assessment of physical activity by questionnaire and personal interview with particular reference to fitness and coronary mortality. *Eur J Appl Physiol* 56:245–252, 1987.

268. Scragg R, Stewart A, Jackson R, Beaglehole R. Alcohol and exercise in myocardial infarction and sudden coronary death in men and women. *Am J Epidemiol* 126:77–85, 1987.

269. Leon AS, Connett J, Jacobs DR, Rauramaa R. Leisure-time physical activity levels and risk of coronary heart disease and death: The multiple risk factor intervention trial. *JAMA* 258:2388–2395, 1987.

270. Salonen JT, Slater JS, Tuomilehto J, Rauramaa R. Leisure time and occupational physical activity: Risk of death from ischemic heart disease. *Am J Epidemiol* 127:87–94, 1988.

271. Slattery ML, Jacobs DR. Physical fitness and cardiovascular disease mortality: The US railroad study. *Am J Epidemiol* 127:571–580, 1988.

272. Donahue RP, Abbott RD, Reed DM, Yano K. Physical activity and coronary heart disease in middle-aged and elderly men: The Honolulu heart program. *Am J Public Health* 78:683–685, 1988.

273. Ekelund LG, Haskell WL, Johnson JL, et al. Physical fitness as a predictor of cardiovascular mortality in asymptomatic North American men: The Lipid Research Clinics Mortality Follow-up Study. *N Engl J Med* 319:1379–1384, 1988.

274. Morris JN, et al. Vigorous exercise in leisure-time: Protection against coronary heart disease. *Lancet* 2:1207, 1980.

275. Siscovick DS, Weiss NS, et al. The incidence of primary cardiac arrest during vigorous exercise. *N Eng J Med* 311:874–877, 1984.

276. Siscovick DS, Weiss NS, et al. Habitual vigorous exercise and primary cardiac arrest: Effect of other risk factors on the relationship. *J Chron Dis* 37:625–631, 1984.

277. Sandvik L, Erikssen J, Thaulow E, et al. Physical fitness as a predictor of mortality among healthy, middle-aged Norwegian men. *N Engl J Med* 328:533–537, 1993.

278. Folsom AR, Arnett DK, Hutchinson RG, Liao F, Clegg LX, Cooper LS. Physical activity and incidence of coronary heart disease in middle-aged women and men. *Med Sci Sports Exerc* 29:901–909, 1997.

279. Goldberg RJ, Burchfiel CM, Benfante R, Chiu D, Reed DM, Yano K. Lifestyle and biologic factors associated with atherosclerotic disease in middle-aged men: 20-year findings from the Honolulu heart program. *Arch Intern Med* 155:686–694, 1995.

280. Leon AS, Myers MJ, Connett J. Leisure time physical activity and the 16-year risks of mortality from coronary heart disease and all-causes in the Multiple Risk Factor Intervention Trial (MRFIT). *Int J Sports Med* 18(suppl 3):S208–S215, 1997.

281. Lakka TA, Venalainen JM, Rauramaa R, Salonen R, Tuomilehto J, Salonen JT. Relation of leisure-time physical activity and cardiorespiratory fitness to the risk of acute myocardial infarction in men. *N Engl J Med* 330:1549–1554, 1994.

282. Kaplan GA, Strawbridge WJ, Cohen RD, Hungerford LR. Natural history of leisure-time physical activity and its correlates: Associations with mortality from all causes and cardiovascular disease over 28 years. *Am J Epidemiol* 144:793–797, 1996.

283. Haapanen N, Miilunpalo S, Vuori I, Oja P, Pasanen M. Characteristics of leisure time physical activity associated with decrease risk of premature all-cause and cardiovascular disease mortality in middle-aged men. *Am J Epidemiol* 143:870–880, 1996.

284. O'Connor GT, Hennekens CH, Willett WC, et al. Physical exercise and reduced risk of nonfatal myocardial infarction. *Am J Epidemiol* 142:1147–1156, 1995.

285. Pols MA, Peeters PHM, Twisk JWR, Kemper HCG, Grobbee DE. Physical activity and cardiovascular disease risk profile in women. *Am J Epidemiol* 146:322–328, 1997.

286. Raitakari OT, Taimela S, Porkka KVK, et al. Associations between physical activity and risk factors for coronary heart disease: The cardiovascular risk in young Finns study. *Med Sci Sports Exerc* 29:1055–1061, 1997.

287. Rauramaa R, Leon AS. Physical activity and risk of cardiovas-

cular disease in middle-aged individuals. *Sports Med* 22:65–69, 1996.

288. Bijnen FCH, Feskens EJM, Caspersen CJ, et al. Physical activity and cardiovascular risk factors among elderly men in Finland, Italy, and the Netherlands. *Am J Epidemiol* 143:553–561, 1996.

289. Haskell WL, Sims C, Myll J, Bortz WM, Goar FG, Alderman EL. Coronary artery size and dilating capacity in ultradistance runners. *Circulation* 87:1076–1082, 1993.

290. Vaitkevicius PV, Fleg JL, Engel JH, et al. Effects of age and aerobic capacity on arterial stiffness in healthy adults. *Circulation* 88(part 1):1456–1462, 1993.

291. Stratton JR, Chandler Wl, Schwartz RS, et al. Effects of physical conditioning of fibrinolytic variables and fibrinogen in young and old healthy adults. *Circulation* 83:1692–1697, 1991.

292. Koenig W, Sund M, Doring A, Ernst E. Leisure-time physical activity but not work-related physical activity is associated with decreased plasma viscosity. *Circulation* 95:335–341, 1997.

293. Chandler WL, Schwartz RS, Stratton JR, Vitiello MV. Effects of endurance training on the circadian rhythm of fibrinolysis in men and women. *Med Sci Sports Exerc* 28:647–655, 1996.

294. Laughlin MH. Effects of exercise training on coronary circulation: Introduction. *Med Sci Sports Exerc* 26:1226–1229, 1994.

295. Paffenbarger RS, Kampert JB, Lee I-M, Hyde RT, Leung RW, Wing AL. Changes in physical activity and other lifeway patterns influencing longevity. *Med Sci Sports Exerc* 26:857–865, 1994.

296. Blair SN, Kohl HW, Barlow CE, Paffenbarger RS, Gibbons LW, Macera CA. Changes in physical fitness and all-cause mortality: A prospective study of healthy and unhealthy men. *JAMA* 273:1093–1098, 1995.

297. U.S. Department of Health and Human Services. *Physical Activity and Health: A Report of the Surgeon General.* Atlanta, GA: U.S. Department of Health and Human Services, Centers for Disease Control and Prevention, National Center for Chronic Disease Prevention and Health Promotion, 1996.

298. NIH Consensus Development Panel on Physical Activity and Cardiovascular Health. Physical activity and cardiovascular health. *JAMA* 276:241–246, 1996.

299. Bouchard C, Shephard RJ, Stephens T. *Physical Activity, Fitness, and Health.* Champaign, IL: Human Kinetics, 1994.

300. Paffenbarger RS, Williams JL. Chronic disease in former college students: XII. Early precursors of fatal stroke. *Am J Public Health* 57:1290–1299, 1967.

301. Herman B, Schmitz B, Leyten ACM, et al. Multivariate logistic analysis of risk factors for stroke in Tilburg, the Netherlands. *Am J Epidemiol* 118:514–525, 1983.

302. Shinton R, Sagar G. Lifelong exercise and stroke. *BMJ* 307:231–234, 1993.

303. Abbott RD, Rodriquez BL, Burchfiel CM, Curb JD. Physical activity in older middle-aged men and reduced risk of stroke: The Honolulu heart program. *Am J Epidemiol* 139:881–893, 1994.

304. Wannamethee G, Shaper AG. Physical activity and stroke in British middle aged men. *BMJ* 304:597–601, 1992.

305. Kiely DK, Wolf PA, Cupples LA, Beiser AS, Kannel WB. Physical activity and stroke risk: The Framingham study. *Am J Epidemiol* 140:608–620, 1994.

306. Gillum RF, Mussolino ME, Ingram DD. Physical activity and stroke incidence in women and men: The NHANES I epidemiologic follow-up study. *Am J Epidemiol* 143:860–869, 1996.

307. Pollock ML, Wilmore JH, Fox SM. *Exercise in Health and Disease.* Philadelphia: W. B. Saunders Co., 1984.

308. Wilson PK. Cardiac rehabilitation: Then and now. *Physician Sportsmed* 16(9):75–84, 1988.

309. American College of Sports Medicine. *ACSM's Exercise Management for Persons with Chronic Diseases and Disabilities.* Champaign, IL: Human Kinetics, 1997.

310. American College of Sports Medicine. Position stand: Exercise for patients with coronary artery disease. *Med Sci Sports Exerc* 26:i–v, 1994.

311. Smith SC, Blair SN, Criqui MH, et al. Preventing heart attack and death in patients with coronary disease. *Circulation* 92:2–4, 1995.

312. Haskell WL. The efficacy and safety of exercise programs in cardiac rehabilitation. *Med Sci Sports Exerc* 26:815–823, 1994.

313. Verrill DE, Ribisl PM. Resistive exercise training in cardiac rehabilitation. *Sports Med* 21:347–383, 1996.

314. O'Conner GT, Buring JE, Yusaf S, et al. An overview of randomized trials of rehabilitation with exercise after myocardial infarction. *Circulation* 80:234, 1989.

315. Van Camp SP, Peterson RA. Cardiovascular complications of outpatient cardiac rehabilitation programs. *JAMA* 256:1160–1163, 1986.

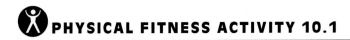 **PHYSICAL FITNESS ACTIVITY 10.1**

Heart Disease Risk

Playing the Odds—What Is Your Heart Disease Risk Score?

Heart disease continues to be the cause of the greatest number of deaths among adult Americans. Using this simple worksheet, you can calculate your heart disease risk score. Following each risk factor, circle the number that applies to you. Total your score, and compare it with the norms. You will need your systolic blood pressure (the higher pressure when the heart beats) and blood cholesterol measurements to take this test. If you have not been measured, we highly recommend you see your doctor or local public health department very soon.

Risk Factor 1—Heredity

Do you have a father or brother who had heart disease before age 55, or a mother or sister with heart disease before age 65?

No	0
Yes but just 1 individual in family	3
Yes, with more than 1 individual	4

Risk Factor 2—Age/gender

Are you a male 45 years of age or older, or a female 55 years of age or older?

No	0
Yes	4

Risk Factor 3—Cigarette smoking

Never have smoked or quit more than 15 years ago	0
Ex-smoker (quit less than 15 years ago)	1
Smoke 1–20 cigarettes/day	2
Smoke 21–40 cigarettes/day	3
Smoke 41 or more cigarettes/day	4

Risk Factor 4—High blood pressure

Your systolic blood pressure is

≤ 120 mm Hg	0
121–129 mm Hg	1
130–139 mm Hg	2
140–149 mm Hg	3
≥ 150 mm Hg	4

Risk Factor 5—High blood cholesterol

Your serum cholesterol is

< 200 mg/dl	0
200–219 mg/dl	1
220–239 mg/dl	2
240–259 mg/dl	3
≥ 260 mg/dl	4

Risk Factor 6—Inactivity

How often do you usually engage in physical exercise that moderately or strongly increases your breathing and heart rate, and makes you sweat, for at least a total of 30 minutes a day, such as in brisk walking, cycling, swimming, jogging, manual labor, etc.?

5 or more times per week	0
3 or 4 times per week	1
2 times per week	2
1 time per week	3
None	4

Risk Factor 7—Obesity

How would you rate your body weight?

Close to ideal	0
About 10–20 pounds overweight	1
About 21–50 pounds overweight	2
About 51–100 pounds overweight	3
More than 100 pounds overweight	4

Risk Factor 8—Stress

How would you describe the stress you experience?

Low or moderate levels of stress	0
High stress but am able to cope with it	1
High stress and often feel unable to cope	2
Very high stress but trying to cope with it	3
Very high stress and unable to cope with it	4

Risk Factor 9—Diabetes

Have you been diagnosed with diabetes by a doctor?

No	0
Yes	4

Your Heart Disease Risk Score

Classification	*Total Points*
Very low risk	Less than 5
Low risk	6–10
Moderately high risk	11–15
High risk	16–20
Very high risk	More than 20

Sources: This is based on information from the Framingham Heart Study (*Circulation* 83:356-362, 1991) and the MRFIT research project (*Arch Intern Med* 152:56-64, 1992).

⊗ PHYSICAL FITNESS ACTIVITY 10.2

Coronary Heart Disease Risk Prediction

Coronary heart disease continues to be the greatest cause of death among adult Americans. Using this simple worksheet, you can calculate your 5- and 10-year CHD risk. Circle the points associated with your personal risk-factor information. (The tables in this worksheet are taken from the Framingham Heart Study, which provides the best available data.)

Age, Female (yr)

Age	Points	Age	Points
30	−12	41	1
31	−11	42–43	2
32	−9	44	3
33	−8	45–46	4
34	−6	47–48	5
35	−5	49–50	6
36	−4	51–52	7
37	−3	53–55	8
38	−2	56–60	9
39	−1	61–67	10
40	0	68–74	11

Age, Male (yr)

Age	Points	Age	Points
30	−2	48–49	9
31	−1	50–51	10
32–33	0	52–54	11
34	1	55–56	12
35–36	2	57–59	13
37–38	3	60–61	14
39	4	62–64	15
40–41	5	65–67	16
42–43	6	68–70	17
44–45	7	71–73	18
46–47	8	74	19

HDL Cholesterol

HDL-C	Points	HDL-C	Points
25–26	7	51–55	−1
27–29	6	56–60	−2
30–32	5	61–66	−3
33–35	4	67–73	−4
36–38	3	74–80	−5
39–42	2	81–87	−6
43–46	1	88–96	−7
47–50	0		

Total Cholesterol (mg/dl)

Cholesterol	Points	Cholesterol	Points
139–151	−3	220–239	2
152–166	−2	240–262	3
167–182	−1	263–288	4
183–199	0	289–315	5
200–219	1	316–330	6

Systolic Blood Pressure (mm Hg)

SBP	Points	SBP	Points
98–104	−2	140–149	3
105–112	−1	150–160	4
113–120	0	161–172	5
121–129	1	173–185	6
130–139	2		

Smoking, Diabetes, and Electrocardiography (ECG-LVH)

	Points	
	Yes	No
Cigarette smoking	4	0
Diabetes		
Male	3	0
Female	6	0
ECG-LVH[a]	9	0

[a]LVH means that the doctor has told you that you have enlargement of the left ventricle of the heart, due to heart disease.

Total Score (add up points from all charts)

$$\underbrace{\qquad}_{\text{(Age)}} + \underbrace{\qquad}_{\text{(Total Chol)}} + \underbrace{\qquad}_{\text{(HDL)}} + \underbrace{\qquad}_{\text{(SBP)}} + \underbrace{\qquad}_{\text{(Smoking)}}$$

$$+ \underbrace{\qquad}_{\text{(Diabetes)}} + \underbrace{\qquad}_{\text{(ECG-LVH)}} = \underbrace{\qquad}_{\text{(Total)}}$$

Based on your total points, this table indicates your probability of dying from coronary heart disease in the next 5 or 10 years. Compare your 10-year probability with that of the average American.

Probability (%)

Points	5 yr	10 yr	Points	5 yr	10 yr
<1	<1	<2	17	6	13
2	1	2	18	7	14
3	1	2	19	8	16
4	1	2	20	8	18
5	1	3	21	9	19
6	1	3	22	11	21
7	1	4	23	12	23
8	2	4	24	13	25
9	2	5	25	14	27
10	2	6	26	16	29
11	3	6	27	17	31
12	3	7	28	19	33
13	3	8	29	20	36
14	4	9	30	22	38
15	5	10	31	24	40
16	5	12	32	25	42

Compare with Average 10-Year Risk

Age (yr)	Probability (%)	
	Women	Men
30–34	<1	3
35–39	<1	5
40–44	2	6
45–49	5	10
50–54	8	14
55–59	12	16
60–64	13	21
65–69	9	30
70–74	12	24

Source: Framingham Heart Study. *Circulation* 83:356–362, 1991.

PHYSICAL FITNESS ACTIVITY 10.3

Women: How Good Are You to Your Heart?

Until recently, heart researchers have concentrated on men, but half of the 500,000 people who die of heart attacks in the United States each year are women. Just like men, women can reduce their risk. They can eat a low-fat diet, exercise, not smoke, and learn to manage stress. Women past menopause can reduce their risk by taking estrogen supplements—but must consider evidence that they may be raising other health risks. Women can also seek treatment for high blood pressure, diabetes, and high cholesterol, all conditions that raise heart disease risks.

Adopting a heart-healthy lifestyle is particularly important for women who have built-in risks, such as a family history of heart disease at an early age.

To assess your risk, take this test, developed especially for women by the Arizona Heart Institute & Foundation in Phoenix.

Points		Fill in your points
	Age	
5	51 and over	_____
2	35–50	_____
0	34 and under	_____
	Family history	
	If you have parents, brothers, or sisters who have had a heart attack, stroke, or heart bypass surgery at	
5	Age 55 or before	_____
3	Age 56 or after	_____
0	None or don't know	_____
	Personal history	
	Have you had	
20	A heart attack	_____
10	Angina, heart bypass surgery, angioplasty, stroke, or blood vessel surgery	_____
0	None of the above	_____
	Smoking	
	Current smoker: How many cigarettes per day?	
20	5 or more	_____
10	4 or fewer	_____
	If you are a smoker currently taking oral contraceptives:	
2[a]	Under 35 years old	_____
5[a]	35 and older	_____
	Or...	
	Previous smoker who quit less than 2 years ago: How many cigarettes did you smoke per day?	

Points		Fill in your points
10	5 or more	_____
5	4 or fewer	_____
	Or...	
0	Never smoked or quit more than 2 years ago	_____
	Blood pressure	
	If you have had your blood pressure taken in the last year, was it	
6	Elevated or high (either or both readings above 160/95)	_____
3	Borderline (between 140/90 and 160/95)	_____
0	Normal (below 140/90) or don't know	_____
	Hormone status	
	If you have undergone natural menopause, what was your age at its start?	
1	41 or older	_____
2	40 or younger	_____
	If you have had a total hysterectomy, what was your age when it was done?	
1	41 or older	_____
3	40 or younger	_____
2[b]	If you take an oral estrogen supplement	_____
1[b]	If you are still menstruating	_____
	Exercise	
	Do you engage in any aerobic activity, such as brisk walking, jogging, bicycling, or swimming for more than 20 minutes?	
6	Less than once a week	_____
3	1 or 2 times a week	_____
0	3 or more times a week	_____

Points		Fill in your points

Blood Fats

If you have had your cholesterol and blood fat levels checked in the past year, score your risk here:

6	Cholesterol over 240	_____
3	From 200 to 240	_____
0	Under 200	_____
1[a]	If your HDLs are lower than 45	

Or . . .

If you know your cholesterol-to-HDL ratio, use this section to score your risk:

6	7.1 and above	_____
3	3.6–7.1	_____
0	3.5 or below	_____

Or . . .

If you do not know your blood fat levels, use this section to score your risk: Which of the following best describes your eating pattern?

6	High fat: Red meat, fast foods or fried foods daily; more than 7 eggs per week; regular consumption of butter, whole milk, and cheese	_____
3	Moderate fat: Red meat, fast foods or fried foods 4–6 times per week; 4–7 eggs weekly; regular use of margarine, vegetable oils, or low-fat dairy products	_____
0	Low fat: Poultry, fish, and little or no red meat, fast foods, fried foods or saturated fats; fewer than 3 eggs per week; minimal margarine and vegetable oils; primarily non-fat dairy products	_____

Points		Fill in your points

Diabetes

If you have diabetes (blood sugar level above 140), your age when you found out:

6	40 or before	_____
4	41 or older	_____
0	Do not have diabetes	_____

Body mass

First calculate your Body Mass Index (BMI) with the following formula:

Weight (pounds) $\times$ 0.45 = (W)

Height (inches) $\times$ .025 = (H)

Divide W by H squared—that is, W divided by (H $\times$ H) = BMI

Example: A woman is 120 pounds and 5 feet 6 inches (66 inches) tall:

$120 \times .45 = 54$ (W)

$66 \times .025 = 1.65$ (H)

$54 \div (1.65 \times 1.65) = 19.8$ BMI

| 2 | If your BMI is 27 or greater | _____ |
| 0 | If your BMI is below 27 | _____ |

Now measure your waist and hips and divide your waist measurement by your hip measurement. For example, if your waist is 26, hips 36: $26 \div 36 = 0.7$.

| 1 | If your waist-to-hip ratio is 0.8 or greater | _____ |
| 0 | If your ratio is 0.79 or less | |

Stress

Are you easily angered and frustrated?

6	Most of the time	_____
3	Some of the time	_____
0	Rarely	_____

Scoring

15 points or below: Low risk. Maintain your heart-healthy status by watching your weight, blood pressure, and blood fat levels; get regular check-ups, and don't smoke.

16-32 points: Medium risk. Personal factors or lifestyle habits may be increasing your vulnerability. See your doctor and take this test with you to get advice on how you can improve your heart-healthy status.

33 points or above: If you are not already being treated for heart disease, see your doctor immediately and take this test with you. You must seek ways to reduce your risk.

---

[a]Add
[b]Subtract
[c]Use score from only one section of Blood Fats.

Source: Arizona Heart Institute & Foundation.

PHYSICAL FITNESS ACTIVITY 10.4

Testing for Alcoholism: The Alcohol Use Disorders Identification Test (AUDIT) from the World Health Organization

Questions	Points					Your tally
	0	1	2	3	4	
1. How often do you have a drink containing alcohol?	Never	Monthly or less	2 to 3 times per month	2 to 3 times per week	4 or more times per week	_____
2. How many drinks do you have on a typical day when you are drinking?	None	1 or 2	3 or 4	5 or 6	7 to 9[a]	_____
3. How often do you have more than 3 drinks (women) or 5 drinks (men) on one occasion?	Never	Less than monthly	Monthly	Weekly	Daily or almost daily	_____
4. How often during the past year have you found that you were unable to stop drinking once you had started?	Never	Less than monthly	Monthly	Weekly	Daily or almost daily	_____
5. How often during the past year have you failed to do what was normally expected from you because of drinking?	Never	Less than monthly	Monthly	Weekly	Daily or almost daily	_____
6. How often during the past year have you needed a first drink in the morning to get yourself going after a heavy drinking session?	Never	Less than monthly	Monthly	Weekly	Daily or almost daily	_____
7. How often during the past year have you had a feeling of guilt or remorse after drinking?	Never	Less than monthly	Monthly	Weekly	Daily or almost daily	_____
8. How often during the past year have you been unable to remember what happened the night before because you had been drinking?	Never	Less than monthly	Monthly	Weekly	Daily or almost daily	_____
9. Have you or someone else ever been injured as a result of your drinking?	Never	Yes, but not in past year (2 points)		Yes, during the past year (4 points)		_____
10. Has a relative, doctor, or other health worker been concerned about your drinking or suggested you cut down?	Never	Yes, but not in past year (2 points)		Yes, during the past year (4 points)		_____

Scoring: A score of 8 points or more indicates a possible drinking problem and the need for a thorough assessment.   TOTAL = _____

[a]Score 5 points if your response is 10 or more drinks on a typical day.

Source: U.S. Preventive Services Task Force. *Guide to Clinical Preventive Services,* 2nd ed. Baltimore: Williams & Wilkins, 1996.

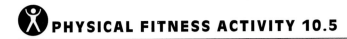

PHYSICAL FITNESS ACTIVITY 10.5

How "Heart Healthy" Is Your Diet?

As discussed in this chapter, all Americans have been advised by the National Cholesterol Education Program to adopt the "Step 1" diet.[140] For those with high-risk blood lipid profiles, the "Step 2" diet is recommended (see Table 10.15). The following questionnaire "MEDFICTS" has been developed by the National Heart, Lung, and Blood Institute to help Americans see how well they are adhering to these dietary recommendations.

TABLE 10.15   Dietary Therapy of High Blood Cholesterol

Nutrient[a]	Recommended Intake	
	Step 1 Diet	**Step 2 Diet**
Total fat	30% or less of total calories	
Saturated fatty acids	8–10% of total calories	Less than 7% of total calories
Polyunsaturated fatty acids	Up to 10% of total calories	
Monounsaturated fatty acids	Up to 15% of total calories	
Carbohydrates	55% or more of total calories	
Protein	Approximately 15% of total calories	
Cholesterol	Less than 300 mg/day	Less than 200 mg/day
Total calories	To achieve and maintain desirable weight	

[a]Calories from alcohol not included.

Source: National Cholesterol Education Program.[140]

MEDFICTS: Dietary Assessment Questionnaire
(**M**eats, **E**ggs, **D**airy, **F**ried foods, **I**n baked goods, **C**onvenience foods, **T**able fats, **S**nacks)

Directions: For each food category for both Group 1 and Group 2 listings: Please check a box in the "Weekly Consumption" column and in the "Serving Size" column. If patient rarely or never eats the food listed, please check only the "Weekly Consumption" box.

FOOD CATEGORY			WEEKLY CONSUMPTION Rarely/Never	3 or less serv/wk	4 or more serv/wk	SERVING SIZE Small	Average	Large	SCORE For office use

M Meats
- Average amount per day: 6 oz (equal in size to 2 decks of playing cards)
- Base your estimation on the food you consume the most

Group 1

Beef	Processed Meats	Pork and Others
Ribs	Regular hamburger	Pork shoulder
Steak	Fast food hamburger	Pork chops, roast
Chuck blade	Bacon	Pork ribs
Brisket	Lunch meat	Ground pork
Ground beef	Sausage	Regular ham
Meat loaf	Hot dogs	Lam steaks, ribs, chops
Corned beef	Knockwurst	Organ meats
		Poultry with skin

Weekly Consumption: □ Rarely/Never, ▨ 3 pts (3 or less serv/wk), ▨ 7 pts (4 or more serv/wk) × Serving Size: ▨ 1 pt (Small), ▨ 2 pts (Average), ▨ 3 pts (Large) = _____

Group 2

Lean Cuts of Beef	Low-Fat Processed Meats	Poultry, Fish, Meat
Sirloin tip	Low-fat lunch meat	Poultry without skin
Flank steak	Low-fat hot dogs	Fish, seafood
Round steak	Canadian bacon	Lamb flank, leg-shank, sirloin, roast
Rump roast		Lean ham cured and fresh
Chuck arm roast		Pork loin chops, tenderloin
		Veal chops, cutlets, roast
		Venison

Weekly Consumption: □, □, □   Serving Size: □, □, ▨ * 6 pts (Large) = _____

E Eggs   • Weekly consumption is expressed as times/week

Group 1

| Whole eggs, Yolks | | | | ▨ 3 pts | ▨ 7 pts | ≤ 1 / 1 pt | 2 / 2 pts | ≥ 3 / 3 pts | = _____ |

Group 2

| Egg whites, Egg substitutes (1/2 cup = 2 eggs) | | | □ | □ | □ | ≤ 1 | 2 | ≥ 3 | |

D Dairy

Milk   • Average serving: 1 cup

Group 1

Whole milk, 2% milk, 2% buttermilk, Yogurt (whole milk)
□ ▨ 3 pts ▨ 7 pts × ▨ 1 pt ▨ 2 pts ▨ 3 pts = _____

Group 2

Skim milk, 1% milk, Skim milk—buttermilk
Yogurt (nonfat & low-fat)
□ □ □ □ □ □

Cheese   • Average serving: 1 oz.

Group 1

Cream cheese, Cheddar, Monterey Jack, Colby, Swiss, American processed, Blue cheese
Regular cottage cheese and Ricotta (1/2 cup)
□ ▨ 3 pts ▨ 7 pts × ▨ 1 pt ▨ 2 pts ▨ 3 pts = _____

Group 2

Low-fat & fat-free cheeses, Skim-milk mozzarella
String cheese
Low-fat & fat-free cottage cheese, and Skim-milk ricotta (1/2 C)
□ □ □ □ □ □

Frozen Desserts   • Average serving: 1/2 cup

Group 1

Ice cream, Milk shakes
□ ▨ 3 pts ▨ 7 pts × ▨ 1 pt ▨ 2 pts ▨ 3 pts = _____

Group 2

Ice milk, Frozen yogurt
□ □ □ □ □ □

*Score 6 points if this box is checked

Comments_____ Total _____

FOOD CATEGORY

	WEEKLY CONSUMPTION			SERVING SIZE			SCORE
	Rarely/ Never	3 or less serv/wk	4 or more serv/wk	Small	Average	Large	For office use

F **Fried Foods**   • Average serving: see below
Group 1
French fries, Fried vegetables: (1/2 cup)
   *Fried chicken, fish, and meat: (3 oz.)
      *Check meat category also

Weekly: □ | ▨ 3 pts | ▨ 7 pts × Serving: ▨ 1 pt | ▨ 2 pts | ▨ 3 pts = _____

Group 2
Vegetables—not deep fried
Meat, poultry, or fish—prepared by baking, broiling,
   grilling, poaching, roasting, stewing

□ | ▨ | ▨   ▨ | ▨ | ▨

I **In Baked Goods**   • Average serving: 1 serving
Group 1
Doughnuts, Biscuits, Butter rolls, Muffins, Croissants,
Sweet rolls, Danish, Cakes, Pies, Coffee cakes, Cookies

□ | ▨ 3 pts | ▨ 7 pts × ▨ 1 pt | ▨ 2 pts | ▨ 3 pts = _____

Group 2
Fruit bars, Low-fat cookies/cakes/pastries, Angel food cake,
Homemade baked goods with vegetable oils

□ | □ | □   □ | □ | □

C **Convenience Foods**   • Average serving: see below
Group 1
Canned, Packaged, or Frozen dinners: e.g., Pizza
(1 slice), Macaroni & cheese (about 1 cup), Pot pie (1),
   Cream soups (1 cup)

□ | ▨ 3 pts | ▨ 7 pts × ▨ 1 pt | ▨ 2 pts | ▨ 3 pts = _____

Group 2
Diet/Reduced calorie or reduced fat dinners (1 dinner)

□ | □ | □   □ | □ | □

T **Table Fats**   • Average serving: see below
Group 1
Butter, Stick margarine: 1 pat
Regular salad dressing or mayonnaise, Sour cream: 1–2 Tbsp.

□ | ▨ 3 pts | ▨ 7 pts × ▨ 1 pt | ▨ 2 pts | ▨ 3 pts = _____

Group 2
Diet and tub margarine, Low-fat & fat-free salad dressings
Low-fat & fat-free mayonnaise

□ | □ | □   □ | □ | □

S **Snacks**   • Average serving: per package
Group 1
Chips (potato, corn, taco), Cheese puffs, Snack mix, Nuts,
Regular crackers, Regular popcorn
Candy (milk chocolate, caramel, coconut)

□ | ▨ 3 pts | ▨ 7 pts × ▨ 1 pt | ▨ 2 pts | ▨ 3 pts = _____

Group 2
Air-popped or low-fat popcorn, Low-fat crackers, Hard candy,
Licorice, Fruit rolls, Bread sticks, Pretzels, Fat-free chips
Fruit

□ | □ | □   □ | □ | □

Directions for scoring:
Multiply Weekly Consumption points (3 or 7) by Serving
Size points (1, 2, 3) for Group 1 foods only except for
a large serving of Group 2 meats

Example: ▨ | ▨ ✓ | ▨ | ▨ | ▨ ✓
            3 pts   7 pts   1 pt   2 pts   3 pts
3 × 7 = 21 points
Add score on page 1 and page 2 to get Final Score

Key
40–70 – Step I Diet
less than 40 – Step II Diet

▨ = Foods high in fat, saturated fat,
      and/or cholesterol

Total   _____
Score from
page 1   + _____
Final Score   _____

Comments: _____
      (Note frequent use of foods high in fat or saturated fat, e.g., coffee creamer, whipped topping)

Source: National Cholesterol Education Program, National Heart, Lung, and Blood Institute, 1993.

CHAPTER
11

Cancer

Physical activity can help protect against some cancers, either by balancing caloric intake with energy expenditure or by other mechanisms.

—American Cancer Society, 1996

There are many types of cancers, but they can all be characterized by uncontrolled growth and spread of abnormal cells.[1,2] If the spread is not controlled, it can result in death, as vital passageways are blocked and the body's oxygen and nutrient supplies are diverted to support the rapidly growing cancer (see Figure 11.1).

Cancer is a general term used to indicate any of the more than 100 types of malignant tumors or neoplasms.[1,2] A *neoplasm* is defined as an abnormal tissue that grows by cellular proliferation more rapidly than normal and continues to grow after the stimuli that initiated the new growth cease. Neoplasms show a lack of structural organization and coordination with the surrounding normal tissue, and they usually form a distinct mass of tissue, which may be either benign (noncancerous tumor) or malignant (cancer). A *malignant cancer* is one that invades surrounding tissues and is usually capable of producing *metastases* (the spread of cancer cells from one part of the body to another). Often, the malignant cancer may recur after attempted removal and is likely to cause death unless adequately treated through radiation, chemotherapy, and surgery.

Two classifications of tumors are carcinoma and sarcoma. A *carcinoma* is any of the various malignant neoplasms derived from epithelial tissue (the lining or covering cells of tissues). Carcinomas occur more frequently in the skin and large intestine, the lung and prostate gland in men, and the lung and breast in women. A *sarcoma* is a connective-tissue neoplasm and is usually highly malignant.

Humans are made up of approximately 60 trillion cells. Each cell contains *DNA*, the blueprint for making enzymes that drive unique chemical reactions. Researchers have estimated that the DNA in each cell receives a "hit" once every 10 seconds from damaging molecules.[3] Most of the DNA injury comes from a class of chemicals known as *oxidants*, by-products of the normal process by which cells turn food into energy. Although much of the damage is repaired, over a lifetime, unrepaired damage accumulates. Both aging and cancer can be attributed in large part to the accumulation of damage to DNA. Alteration of the DNA affects more than the cell in which it occurs; when the affected cell divides, the defective blueprint is passed on to all the descendants of that cell.

Normally, the cells that make up the body reproduce and divide in an orderly manner, so that old cells are replaced and cell injuries repaired. Certain environmental (e.g., oxidants and other chemicals, radiation, and viruses) and internal (e.g., hormones, immune conditions, and inherited mutations) factors contribute to the process by which some cells undergo abnormal changes and begin the process toward becoming cancer cells.[1] These abnormal cells may grow into tumors, some of which are cancerous, but others benign. The formation of cancer (*carcinogenesis*) is a long process (often longer than 10 years) and goes through three stages: initiation, promotion, and progression. The end result is a loss of control over cellular proliferation.

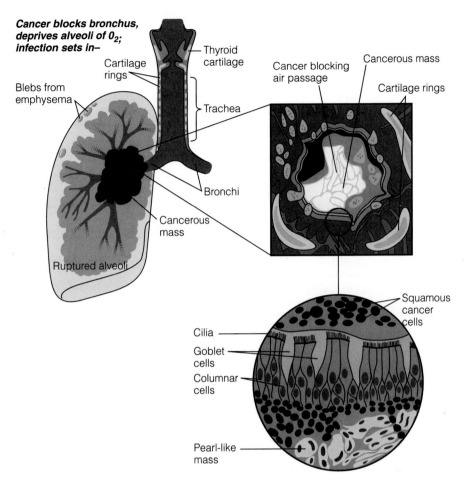

Cancer blocks bronchus, deprives alveoli of O_2; infection sets in–

Figure 11.1 Lung cancer. Squamous cancer cells (O) completely line the bronchial wall. Numerous hard, pearl-like masses (R), made of keratin, have been deposited in the cancerous tissue. With the cancer unchecked and uncontained, the conquest is all but complete. Cancer, blocking the bronchus, also deprives the alveoli of oxygen and makes them ripe for infection by bacteria, which flourish in defenseless tissue.

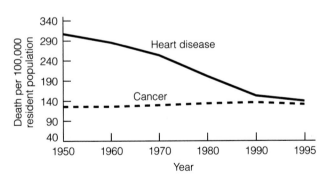

Figure 11.2 Changes in age-adjusted death rates for heart disease and cancer. Death rates for heart disease have fallen sharply since 1950, while those for cancer have risen slightly. *Source:* National Center for Health Statistics. *Health, United States, 1996–97 and Injury Chartbook.* Hyattsville, MD: 1997.

CANCER STATISTICS

Although heart disease has been the leading cause of death in the United States since the 1950s, cancer will probably replace heart disease as the top killer soon after the year 2000.[4–7] (Table 11.1 and Figure 11.2). Since the 1950s, death rates for heart disease have fallen steeply (55%). Meanwhile, the war against cancer has been largely unsuccess-

ful.[5] Between 1950 and 1990, age-adjusted death rates for cancer rose 7.7%, due primarily to the sharp increase in lung cancer.[1,7] As depicted in Figure 11.3, death rates for many other major cancer sites have leveled off or declined since the 1930s. From 1991 to 1995, total cancer deaths fell 3.1%, marking the first decline since cancer statistics were first kept in the 1930s.[7] The decline is expected to continue at about 2% per year and has been attributed to reduced ciga-

TABLE 11.1 Ten Leading Causes of Death, United States, 1995

Rank	Cause of Death	Crude Death Rate per 100,000 Population	Percent of Total Deaths
1	Heart diseases	280.7	31.9
2	Cancer	204.9	23.3
3	Cerebrovascular diseases	60.1	6.8
4	Chronic obstructive pulmonary diseases (COPD)	39.2	4.5
5	Accidents	35.5	4.0
6	Pneumonia and influenza	31.6	3.6
7	Diabetes mellitus	22.6	2.6
8	HIV infection	16.4	1.9
9	Suicide	11.9	1.4
10	Cirrhosis of liver	9.6	1.1

Source: Monthly Vital Statistics Report, 45(11), Supplement 2. Hyattsville, MD: National Center for Health Statistics, June 12, 1997.

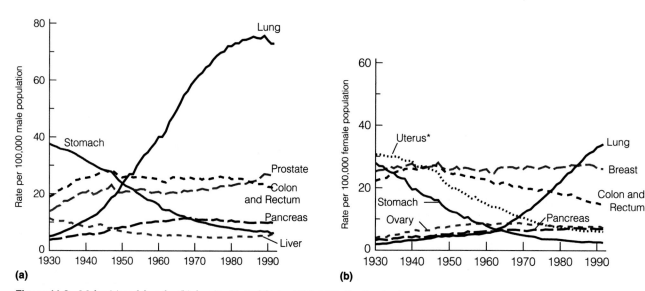

(a)   **(b)**

Figure 11.3 Males (a) and females (b), by site, United States 1930–1993. Death rates for most cancer sites except the lung have leveled off or decreased since 1930.
Note: Due to changes in ICD coding, numerator information has changed over time. Rates for cancers of the liver, lung, uterus, ovary, and colon and rectum are affected by these coding changes. Denominator information for the years 1930–1959 and 1991–1993 is based on intercensal population estimates, while denominator information for the years 1960–1989 is based on postcensal recalculation of estimates. Rate estimates for 1968–1989 are most likely of a better quality.
*Uterine cancer death rates for cervix and corpus combined.
Sources: American Cancer Society. *Cancer Facts & Figures–1997.* Atlanta: Author, 1997. Reprinted by the permission of the American Cancer Society, Inc. Parker SL, Tong T, Bolden S, Wingo PA. Cancer statistics, 1997. *CA Cancer J Clin* 47:5027, 1997. Vital Statistics of the United States, 1993.

TABLE 11.2   Basic Cancer Facts and Figures, United States

New cancer cases per year	1,400,000 (plus 900,000 skin cancers)
Cancer deaths per year	560,000 (1,500 per day)
Rank as cause of death	Second (behind heart disease)
Percentage of total U.S. deaths	23.3%
Cancer death trends	Steady, slight rise from 1950 to 1990; small decrease since 1990
Lifetime risk of developing cancer	48% for males, 38% for females
Survival rate for all cancers, 5 years	40%
Americans alive with a history of cancer	7.4 million
Cost of cancer	$104 billion per year, nationwide
Cancer causes	33% poor nutrition 30% tobacco use

Source: American Cancer Society. *Cancer Facts & Figures, 1997.* Atlanta: Author, 1997. Reprinted by the permission of the American Cancer Society, Inc.

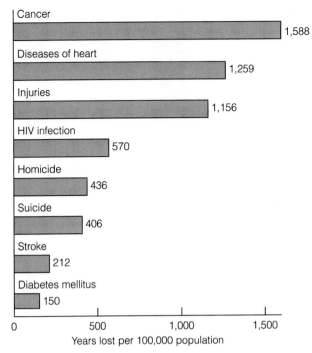

Figure 11.5   Years of potential life lost before age 75. Cancer ranks highest as the cause of years of potential life lost before age 75.   *Source:* National Center for Health Statistics. *Health, United States, 1996–97 and Injury Chartbook.* Hyattsville, MD: 1997.

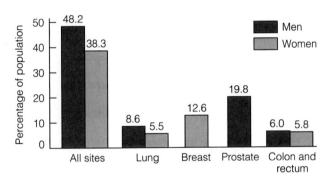

Figure 11.4   Lifetime probability of developing cancer, excluding skin cancer. Nearly one half of men and almost 4 in 10 women will develop cancer within their lifetimes.   *Sources:* American Cancer Society. *Cancer Facts & Figures–1997.* Atlanta: Author, 1997; Parker SL, Tong T, Bolden S, Wingo PA. Cancer statistics, 1997. *CA Cancer J Clin* 47:5027, 1997.

rette smoking (and a concomitant decrease in male lung cancer death rates) and improved screening and treatment.[7]

The American Cancer Society has estimated that the lifetime risk of developing cancer is a staggering 48% for men and 38% for women[1] (see Figure 11.4). About 1.4 million Americans are diagnosed with cancer each year (not including the more than 900,000 cases of skin cancer)[1,2] (see Table 11.2). Each year, over ½ million Americans die of cancer, about 1,500 each day. Just under one in four deaths each

year in the United States are from cancer. Cancer can strike at any age and, as outlined in Figure 11.5, represents the number one cause of years of potential life lost before age 75.[4] The leading cancer killer for both men and women is lung cancer, followed by prostate or breast cancer, and colorectal cancer.[1,2] (see Figures 11.6 and 11.7).

A huge interest in and acceptance of alternative and complementary cancer therapies (see Box 11.1) has arisen because of the high lifetime risk for cancer, the absence of significant gains in treatment for the major cancers (despite decades of research and billions of dollars spent since initiation of the war on cancer), the painful side effects of traditional medical treatment for cancer, and widespread public distrust and dissatisfaction with establishment medicine. Unfortunately, most alternative therapies have no proven worth, may delay conventional care, often cost a great deal, can be directly toxic, and raise false hope.

In the early 1900s, few cancer patients had much hope of long-term survival. In the 1930s, fewer than 1 in 5 patients was alive 5 years after treatment. Now, 4 of 10 patients who get cancer live 5 or more years after diagnosis.[1,2] With regular screening and self-exams, cancer can often be detected early, greatly enhancing the success of treatment.

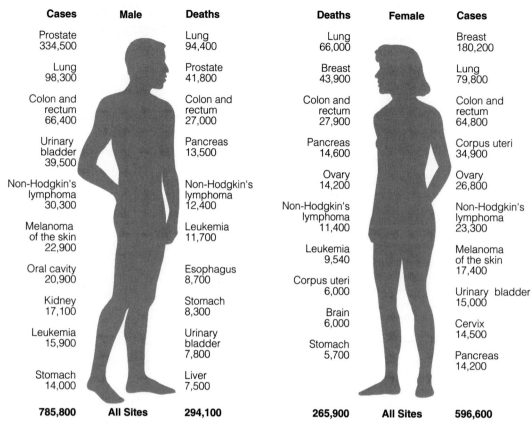

Cases	Male	Deaths		Deaths	Female	Cases

Cases — Male:
Prostate 334,500
Lung 98,300
Colon and rectum 66,400
Urinary bladder 39,500
Non-Hodgkin's lymphoma 30,300
Melanoma of the skin 22,900
Oral cavity 20,900
Kidney 17,100
Leukemia 15,900
Stomach 14,000

Deaths — Male:
Lung 94,400
Prostate 41,800
Colon and rectum 27,000
Pancreas 13,500
Non-Hodgkin's lymphoma 12,400
Leukemia 11,700
Esophagus 8,700
Stomach 8,300
Urinary bladder 7,800
Liver 7,500

Deaths — Female:
Lung 66,000
Breast 43,900
Colon and rectum 27,900
Pancreas 14,600
Ovary 14,200
Non-Hodgkin's lymphoma 11,400
Leukemia 9,540
Corpus uteri 6,000
Brain 6,000
Stomach 5,700

Cases — Female:
Breast 180,200
Lung 79,800
Colon and rectum 64,800
Corpus uteri 34,900
Ovary 26,800
Non-Hodgkin's lymphoma 23,300
Melanoma of the skin 17,400
Urinary bladder 15,000
Cervix 14,500
Pancreas 14,200

| **785,800** | **All Sites** | **294,100** | | **265,900** | **All Sites** | **596,600** |

Figure 11.6 Leading sites of new cancer cases and deaths—1997 estimates, excluding basal and squamous cell skin cancer and in situ carcinomas except bladder. While prostate and breast cancers occur most often, lung cancer is the chief cancer killer among both males and females. *Sources:* American Cancer Society. *Cancer Facts & Figures–1997.* Atlanta: Author, 1997. Reprinted by the permission of the American Cancer Society, Inc. Parker SL, Tong T, Bolden S, Wingo PA. Cancer statistics, 1997. *CA Cancer J Clin* 47:5027, 1997.

Table 11.3 summarizes the American Cancer Society recommendations for the early detection of cancer in the general population.[1] Table 11.4 outlines signs and symptoms for five major cancers. Screening examinations, conducted regularly by a health-care professional can result in the detection of cancers at earlier stages, when treatment is more likely to be successful. More than half of all new cancer cases occur in nine screening-accessible cancer sites (breast, colon, rectum, prostate, tongue, mouth, cervix, testis, and skin). The relative survival rate for these cancers is 80% but could rise to 95% if all Americans participated in regular cancer screenings.[1] As shown in Figure 11.8, 5-year relative survival rates for cancer are much improved when the cancer is diagnosed prior to regional and distant body spread.[1,2]

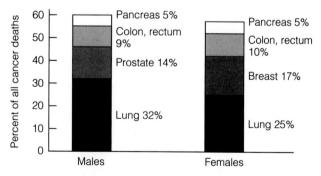

Figure 11.7 Leading cancer death sites for males and females. The top four cancer killers represent about 60% of all cancer deaths. *Sources:* American Cancer Society. *Cancer Facts & Figures–1997.* Atlanta: Author, 1997; Parker SL, Tong T, Bolden S, Wingo PA. Cancer statistics, 1997. *CA Cancer J Clin* 47:5027, 1997.

CANCER PREVENTION

Cancer death rates vary widely throughout the world, as summarized in Figure 11.9.[2] For example, colorectal cancer is rare in southwest Asia and equatorial Africa, but common throughout northwestern Europe, the United States, and Canada. Breast cancer rates are four to seven times higher in the United States than in Asia, and this difference

Box 11.1

Alternative Cancer Therapies Popular Today

To bring structure to the wide and fast-changing universe of alternative therapies, the Office of Alternative Medicine, National Institutes of Health, groups them into seven categories:

1. Diet and nutrition
2. Mind–body techniques
3. Bioelectromagnetics
4. Alternative systems of medical practice (or traditional and folk remedies)
5. Pharmacological and biological treatments
6. Manual healing methods
7. Herbal medicine

Diet and Nutrition

Anticancer diets and nutritional supplements are among the earliest alternative cancer treatments. Many alternative cancer clinics include special diets as part of their overall treatments. Conventional medicine has come to recognize that cancer risk can be reduced through the consumption of fruits, vegetables, and fiber; the avoidance of excessive dietary fat; and the ingestion of antioxidants. However, alternative anticancer diets go further, proponents often claiming that a given diet can cure cancer. Extending claims beyond those that research supports is a hallmark of many alternative treatments.

Mind–Body Techniques

Good documentation exists for the effectiveness of meditation, biofeedback, and yoga in stress reduction and the control of particular physiological reactions. Some proponents argue that patients can use mental attributes and mind–body work to prevent or cure cancer. Attending to the psychological health of cancer patients is a funda-

mental component of good cancer care. Support groups, good doctor–patient relationships, and the emotional and instrumental help of family and friends are vital. However, the idea that patients can influence the course of their disease through mental or emotional work is not substantiated and can evoke feelings of guilt and inadequacy when disease continues to advance despite patients' spiritual or mental efforts.

Bioelectromagnetics

Bioelectromagnetics is the study of living organisms and their interactions with electromagnetic fields. Bioelectromagnetic therapies use the low-frequency portion of the electromagnetic spectrum. Proponents claim that magnetic fields penetrate the body and heal damaged tissues, including cancers, but there are virtually no good data to support this claim.

Traditional and Folk Remedies

This category includes ancient systems of healing that often are based on concepts of human physiology different from those accepted by modern Western science. Two of the most popular healing systems are traditional Chinese medicine and India's Ayurveda, popularized by best-selling author and physician Deepak Chopra. The term "Ayur Veda" comes from the Sanskrit words "ayur" (life) and "veda" (knowledge). Ayurveda's 5,000-year-old healing techniques are based on the classification of people into one of three predominant body types. There are specific remedies for disease and regimens to promote health for each body type. Ayur Veda has a strong mind–body component, stressing the need to keep consciousness in balance. It uses techniques such as yoga and meditation to do so. Traditional Chinese medicine is distinguished by its focus on *chi*, the life force, which flows

(continued)

is not explained by genetics. Prostate cancer is more common in North America and northwestern Europe and is relatively rare in the Near East, Africa, Central America, and South America. For reasons not fully understood, African Americans have the highest rates for prostate cancer in the world. Prostate cancer rates in China and Japan, for example, are one tenth those of U.S. blacks.

Researchers have reported that when migrants move to a nation with high cancer death rates, their mortality from certain types of cancers, especially colon, breast, and prostate, increase.[8,9] The death rate for colorectal cancer in Japa-

nese immigrants to the United States is three to four times greater than that of Japanese residents in Japan. Puerto Ricans in New York City suffer more colon cancer than those remaining in Puerto Rico. When women migrate from geographic areas with low breast cancer risk to nations such as Australia, Canada, and the United States, their breast cancer risk climbs steeply, even within the lifetime of the migrant. Among older first-generation Japanese American women, for example, incidence of breast cancer is almost seven times higher than that of older Japanese women living in Japan. Chinese Americans and Japanese

Alternative Cancer Therapies Popular Today (continued)

through postulated energy channels known as *meridians*. Traditional Chinese medicine relies on exercise techniques such as Qi Gong and Tai Chi to strengthen and balance chi. In addition to Qi Gong and Tai Chi, traditional Chinese medicine uses acupuncture, acupressure, and a full herbal pharmacopeia, with remedies for most ailments, including cancer.

Pharmacological and Biological Treatments

This class of treatments remains highly controversial. Probably the best-known and most popular pharmacological therapy today is the use of antineoplastons, developed by physician Stanislaw Burzynski and available at his clinic in Houston, Texas. Data are lacking to support this therapy.

Immunoaugmentive therapy (IAT) was developed by the late Lawrence Burton and offered in his clinic in the Bahamas. Burton's therapy is based on balancing four protein components in the blood. This injected therapy, as with antineoplastons, relies on strengthening the patient's immune system. Documentation of IAT's efficacy remains anecdotal.

Interest in shark cartilage as a cancer therapy was spurred by a 1992 book written by I. William Lane, *Sharks Don't Get Cancer*, and by a television special that displayed apparent remissions in patients with advanced cancer treated with shark cartilage in Cuba. Despite lack of positive evidence, shark cartilage pills and suppositories are widely publicized and are available in health-food stores throughout the United States.

Another well-known biological remedy, Cancell, is especially popular in the Midwest and in Florida. Proponents claim that it returns cancer cells to a "primitive state" from which they can be digested and rendered inert. The FDA found no basis for proponent claims of Cancell's effectiveness against cancer.

Popular metabolic therapies are banned in the United States but are readily available in Tijuana, Mexico. One of the best-known clinics is the Gerson clinic, where treatment is based on the notion that toxic products of cancer cells accumulate in the liver, leading to liver failure and death. Gerson's treatment aims to counteract liver damage with a low-salt, high-potassium diet and coffee enemas.

Manual Healing Methods

Manual healing includes a variety of touch and manipulation techniques. Osteopathic and chiropractic doctors were among the earliest groups to use manual methods. Hands-on massage is a useful adjunctive technique for cancer patients and others for its stress-reducing benefits. One of the most popular manual healing methods is therapeutic touch, which, despite its name, involves no direct contact. In therapeutic touch, healers move their hands a few inches above a patient's body and remove alleged blockages to the patient's energy field.

Herbal Medicine

Herbal remedies typically are part of traditional and folk healing processes with long histories of use. Herbs come from Asia, Europe, Africa, and North America; some form of herbal medicine is found is most areas of the world. Although many herbal remedies are claimed to have anticancer effects, only a few have gained substantial popularity as alternative cancer therapies. The FDA does not examine herbal remedies for safety and effectiveness, and most have not been formally tested for side effects. There have been recent reports in the literature of severe liver and kidney damage from a limited number of herbal remedies, including chaparral tea. These reports underscore the fact that "natural" products are not necessarily safe or harmless.

Source: Cassileth BR, Chapman CC. Alternative and complementary cancer therapies. *Cancer* 77(6), 1996. Copyright © 1996 American Cancer Society. Reprinted by permission of Wiley-Liss, Inc., a subsidiary of John Wiley & Sons, Inc.

Americans have prostate cancer rates that are higher than those of their counterparts in Asia. It is widely believed that environmental factors, particularly dietary patterns, account for most of these marked variations in colon, breast, and prostate cancer rates.[9]

Table 11.4 lists the important risk factors for the leading cancer sites (locations in the body).[1,10] Notice the importance of dietary factors (33% of all cancers) and of cigarette smoking (30% of all cancers). Other important risk factors include reproductive factors (especially for breast cancer), environmental factors (especially radiation and radon exposure and air pollution), family history, physical inactivity, and obesity.

The most common cancer for women is breast cancer. The risk of breast cancer increases with age. Between 40% and 50% of breast cancer can be explained by four well-established risk factors: never had children, late age at first live birth, high education and socioeconomic status, and family history of breast cancer.[1] Early age at menarche, late age at menopause, and obesity are also important risk fac-

**TABLE 11.3   Summary of American Cancer Society Recommendations
for the Early Detection of Cancer in Asymptomatic People**

Test or Procedure	Sex	Age	Frequency
Sigmoidoscopy, preferably flexible	M & F	50 and over	Every 3–5 years
Fecal occult blood test	M & F	50 and over	Every year
Digital rectal examination	M & F	40 and over	Every year
Prostate exam[a]	M	50 and over	Every year
Pap test	F		All women who are or who have been sexually active, or have reached age 18, should have an annual Pap test and pelvic examination. After a woman has had three or more consecutive satisfactory normal annual examinations, the Pap test may be performed less frequently, at the discretion of her physician.
Breast self-examination	F	20 and over	Every month
Breast clinical examination	F	20–40	Every 3 years
		Over 40	Every year
Mammography[b]	F	40–49	Every 1–2 years
		50 and over	Every year

[a]Annual digital rectal examination and prostate-specific antigen should be performed on men age 50 and older. If either is abnormal, further evaluation should be considered.
[b]Screening mammography should begin by age 40.

Source: American Cancer Society. *Cancer Facts and Figures, 1997.* Atlanta: Author, 1997. Reprinted by permission of the American Cancer Society, Inc.

**TABLE 11.4   Major Risk Factors and Signs and Symptoms
for Major Cancer Sites**

Lung Cancer

Risk factors

Cigarette smoke (causes 87% of all lung cancer)
Exposure to certain industrial substances (e.g., arsenic, asbestos)
Radiation exposure
Residential radon exposure
Air pollution
Tuberculosis
Exposure to environmental tobacco smoke in nonsmokers

Signs and symptoms

Persistent cough
Sputum streaked with blood
Chest pain
Recurring pneumonia or bronchitis

Colorectal Cancer

Risk factors

Personal / family history of colorectal cancer or polyps
Inflammatory bowel disease
Physical inactivity
High-fat and / or low-fiber diet
Inadequate intake of fruits and vegetables

Signs and symptoms

Rectal bleeding or blood in the stool
Change in bowel habits

(continued)

TABLE 11.4 **Major Risk Factors and Signs and Symptoms**
for Major Cancer Sites *(continued)*

Breast Cancer

Risk factors

Increasing age	Personal or family history of breast cancer
Never had children	Some forms of benign breast disease
First childbirth after age 30	BRCA1 and BRCA2 gene mutations
Early menarche	Late menopause
Higher education	Lengthy exposure to postmenopausal estrogen
Alcohol consumption	Higher socioeconomic status
Physical inactivity	High dietary fat intake (international contrast)
Obesity	

Signs and symptoms

Abnormality that shows up on a mammogram before it can be felt

Breast changes that persist (lump, thickening, swelling, dimpling, skin irritation, distortion, retraction, scaliness, pain, nipple tenderness)

Prostate Cancer

Risk factors

Age (over 80% are diagnosed after age 65)

Being African American

High dietary fat intake (international contrast)

Family history (may be genetic or environmental)

Live in North America or northwestern Europe

Signs and symptoms

Weak or interrupted urine flow

Inability to urinate or difficulty starting or stopping the urine flow

Need to urinate frequently, especially at night

Blood in the urine

Pain or burning on urination

Continuing pain in lower back, pelvis, upper thighs

Skin Cancer

Risk factors

Excessive exposure to ultraviolet radiation

Fair complexion

Occupational exposure to coal tar, pitch, creosote, arsenic, radium

Family history

Multiple or atypical *nevi* (malformed, pigmented skin spots)

Signs and symptoms

Any change on the skin, especially size or color of a mole or dark spot

Scaliness, oozing, bleeding, or change in appearance of a bump or nodule

Spread of pigmentation beyond its border

Change in sensation, itchiness, tenderness, or pain

Source: American Cancer Society. *Cancer Facts & Figures, 1997.* Atlanta: Author, 1997. Reprinted by permission of the American Cancer Society, Inc.

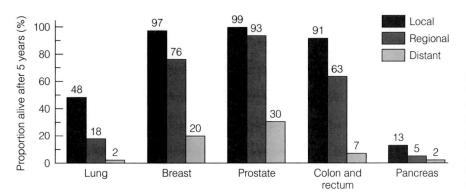

Figure 11.8 Five-year relative survival rates for cancer, by stage at diagnosis. Cancer survival rates are much higher when the cancer is detected early. *Sources:* American Cancer Society. *Cancer Facts & Figures—1997.* Atlanta: Author, 1997; Parker SL, Tong T, Bolden S, Wingo PA. Cancer statistics, 1997. *CA Cancer J Clin* 47:5027, 1997.

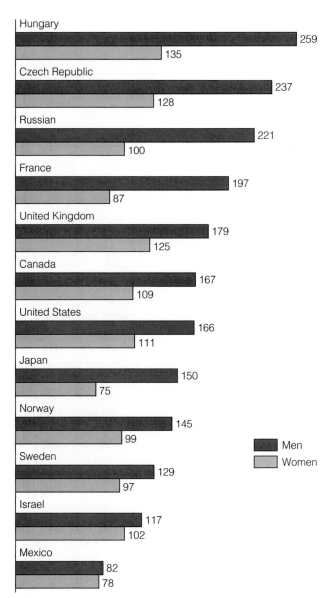

Figure 11.9 Cancer around the world: age-adjusted death rates per 100,000. Cancer death rates vary widely throughout the world. *Source:* Parker SL, Tong T, Bolden S, Wingo PA. Cancer statistics, 1997. *CA Cancer J Clin* 47:5027, 1997.

tors. Certain types of breast cancer are strongly heritable, and studies with identical twins have shown that if one twin has breast cancer, the risk for the other twin is six times greater than normal, and it usually occurs in the same breast (right or left).[1,2] The development of breast cancer is related to female hormones, given that it occurs many times more frequently in women than in men and can be prevented by removal of the ovaries early in life. Any factor that lessens reproductive hormone exposure for a women (e.g., later menarche or early menopause) reduces breast cancer risk.

Prostate cancer is the most common cancer in men. The prostate is a walnut-sized gland tucked away under the bladder and adjacent to the rectum. It provides about a third of the fluid that propels sperm during sex. Prostate cancer rates are about one third higher for black men than for white men. More than 80% of all prostate cancers occur in men over age 65. Studies show that prostate cancer risk is 11 times higher among those who have a brother or a father with prostate cancer.

Lung cancer is the most common cause of cancer death for both men and women. As summarized in Tables 11.4 and 11.5 and Box 11.2, tobacco use is related to lung cancer and many other types of cancers, accounting for about 3 in 10 cancer deaths.[1,2,11–18] Figure 11.10 shows that a strong dose–response relationship exists between lung cancer deaths rates and the number of cigarettes smoked per day.[11] Smoking is responsible for 87% of all lung cancers.[1] Long-term users of smokeless tobacco have a high risk of oral cancer.[1] Each year, about 3,000 nonsmoking adults die of lung cancer as a result of breathing the smoke of other people's cigarettes.[15] New evidence has linked cigarette smoking to prostate, breast, and pancreatic cancers, thus demonstrating that tobacco use is associated with each of the five leading cancer killers.[13–18]

The American Cancer Society has urged that to reduce cancer risk, people should avoid all tobacco use; consume

TABLE 11.5 Lifestyle Habits Are Linked to a Wide Variety of Cancers

Cancer	Estimated Number of Deaths per Year	Smoking	Low Consumption of Fruits & Vegetables	Lack of Exercise	High Consumption of Fat	Use of Smokeless Tobacco	High Consumption of Meat	Obesity	Consumption of Alcohol
Lung	160,000	★★★	★★★	★					
Colon and rectum	55,000	★	★★★	★★★	★★		★	★★	★
Breast	45,000	★	★	★★	★			★★	★★
Prostate	42,000	★	★	★★	★★		★	★★	★
Stomach	14,000	★★	★★						
Kidney	12,000	★★★						★★	
Esophagus	11,200	★★★	★★			★★★			★★
Oral cavity	8,500	★★★	★★			★★★			★★
Endometrium	6,000		★★		★★			★★★	
Larynx	4,000	★★★	★★			★★★			★★

Key: ★★★ A solid body of evidence suggests a link between this habit and cancer.

★★ Numerous studies pointing in the same direction suggest a plausible link.

★ Some research indicates a connection; other studies show no association. The jury is still out.

Source: Tufts University Diet & Nutrition Letter, December, 1996.

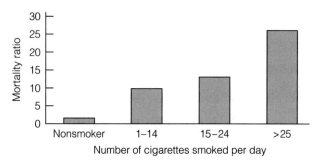

Figure 11.10 Cigarette smoking and lung cancer. A strong dose–response relationship exists between lung cancer death rates and number of cigarettes smoked per day. *Source:* Carbone D. Smoking and cancer. *Am J Med* 93(1A):13S–17S, 1992.

low-fat, high-fiber diets containing plenty of whole grains, fruits, and vegetables; be physically active and maintain a healthy weight; limit consumption of alcoholic beverages; and limit exposure to ultraviolet radiation[1,10] (see Box 11.2). (Visit the American Cancer Society's WWW home page at http://www.cancer.org/.)

Physically active individuals often spend much time outdoors exposed to ultraviolet radiation. Over 900,000 skin cancers are diagnosed each year, most of them highly curable basal cell or squamous cell cancers.[1] The most lethal form of skin cancer is melanoma, which is diagnosed in more than 40,000 persons each year. As outlined in Table 11.4, major risk factors for skin cancer include excessive expo-

sure to ultraviolet radiation, fair complexion, family history, and either multiple or atypical *nevi* (malformed, pigmented skin spots). (See Physical Fitness Activity 11.1 at the end of this chapter.)

Of all lifestyle and environmental factors, dietary habits have been most closely linked to cancer[10] (see Tables 11.4 and 11.5 and Box 11.2). Numerous studies have shown that daily consumption of vegetables and fruits is associated with a reduced risk of lung, colon, pancreas, oral cavity and pharynx, esophagus, endometrium, and stomach cancers.[19–29] The types of vegetables or fruits that most often appear to be protective against cancer are raw vegetables, allium vegetables (e.g., onions, garlic, red pepper), carrots, green vegetables, cruciferous vegetables (e.g., broccoli, cabbage, brussels sprouts), and tomatoes.[19] Vegetables and fruits contain more than 100 beneficial vitamins, minerals, fiber, and other substances. These substances include vitamins (in particular, the antioxidant vitamins A, C, E, and the provitamin beta-carotene), minerals (calcium, selenium), fiber, and nonnutritive constituents (e.g., dithiolthiones, isothiocyanates, isoflavones, protease inhibitors, saponins, phytosterols, lutein, lycopene, and allium compounds).[19,20] These food substances, alone or together, may be responsible for reducing cancer risk. As depicted in Figure 11.11, substances in fruit and vegetables may interrupt the cancer process at several different phases.[19]

Intake of a wide variety of fruits and vegetables is recommended, yet surveys indicate that less than one in four

---

Box 11.2

Cancer Prevention Guidelines from the American Cancer Society

---

The American Cancer Society recommends these steps for preventing cancer.

Practice Good Nutrition and Exercise Habits

1. Choose most of the foods you eat from plant sources. Eat five or more servings of fruits and vegetables each day; eat other foods from plant sources, such as breads, cereals, grain products, rice, pasta, or beans several times each day.

2. Limit your intake of high-fat foods, particularly from animal sources. Choose foods low in fat; limit consumption of meats, especially high-fat meats.

3. Be physically active; achieve and maintain a healthy weight. Physical activity can help protect against some cancers, either by balancing caloric intake with energy expenditure or by other mechanisms.

4. Limit consumption of alcoholic beverages, if you drink at all. Alcoholic beverages, along with cigarette smoking and use of snuff and chewing tobacco, cause cancers of the oral cavity, esophagus, and larynx. Studies have also noted an association between alcohol consumption and an increased risk of breast cancer.

Avoid All Tobacco

Lung cancer mortality rates are 23 times higher for male smokers and 11 times higher for female smokers. In addition to being responsible for 87% of lung cancers, smoking is also associated with cancers of the mouth, pharynx, larynx, esophagus, pancreas, uterine cervix, kidney, and bladder. Smoking accounts for 29% of all cancer deaths. Oral cancer occurs several times more frequently among snuff dippers compared with non–tobacco users. The excess risk of cancer of the cheek and gum may reach nearly 50-fold among long-term snuff users. Cigar smokers have 4–10 times the risk of nonsmokers of dying from laryngeal, oral, or esophageal cancers. Each year, about 3,000 nonsmoking adults die of lung cancer, as a result of breathing the smoke of other people's cigarettes. Secondhand smoke contains at least 14 known or probable human carcinogenic chemicals.

Avoid Environmental Cancer Risks

1. *Chemicals.* Some chemicals show definite evidence of human carcinogenicity (e.g., benzene, asbestos, vinyl chloride, arsenic, aflatoxin).

2. *Radiation.* Only high-frequency radiation, ionizing radiation (e.g., radon and x-rays), and ultraviolet radiation have been proven to cause human cancer.

3. *Unproven risks.* These include pesticides, nonionizing radiation (e.g., radiowaves, microwaves, radar, and electrical and magnetic fields associated with electric currents), toxic wastes, and nuclear power plants.

Source: American Cancer Society. *Cancer Facts & Figures, 1997.* Atlanta: Author, 1997. Reprinted by permission of the American Cancer Society, Inc.

Americans eat five or more servings a day.[10,19] The American Cancer Society does not recommend the use of dietary supplements because "the few studies in human populations that have attempted to determine whether supplements can reduce cancer risk have yielded disappointing results."[10] Although there has been some concern about pesticide residues on plant foods, cancer experts have concluded that there is no good evidence that a high ingestion of fruits and vegetables increases pesticide intake enough to enhance risk of cancer.[30]

The antioxidant vitamins in fruits and vegetables appear to improve immune function, scavenge free radicals and singlet oxygen particles (both of which can damage cell membranes), and play a role in numerous biological sys-

tems and the synthesis of hormones, neurotransmitters, collagen, and many other substances.[19–24] As cells use oxygen to "burn" their fuel, one of the by-products is free radicals. *Free radicals* contain one or more unpaired electrons and can be harmful because they attack the vital components of the cell. Beta-carotene can prevent singlet oxygen from producing free radicals, transforming the singlet oxygen into a stable oxygen species lacking the energy to engage in harmful reactions against cells.[22,23] It has been calculated that one molecule of beta-carotene can quench as many as 1,000 molecules of singlet oxygen. Other carotenoids (there are more than 600 in nature) can also participate in this process.[22] Vitamin C is also an important reducing agent and free-radical scavenger and additionally prevents or reduces

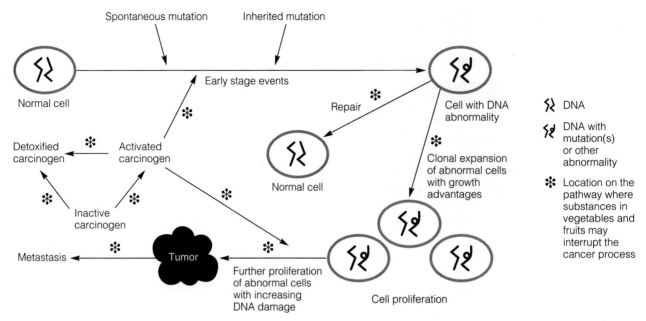

Spontaneous mutation   Inherited mutation

Early stage events

Normal cell

Repair

Cell with DNA abnormality

Detoxified carcinogen   Activated carcinogen

Normal cell

Clonal expansion of abnormal cells with growth advantages

Inactive carcinogen

Metastasis   Tumor

Further proliferation of abnormal cells with increasing DNA damage

Cell proliferation

DNA

DNA with mutation(s) or other abnormality

Location on the pathway where substances in vegetables and fruits may interrupt the cancer process

Figure 11.11 Schematic of cancer process. *Source:* Steinmetz KA, Potter JD. Vegetables, fruit, and cancer prevention: A review. *J Am Diet Assoc* 96:1027–1039, 1996. Copyright © 1996 The American Dietetic Association. Reprinted by permission.

the formation of certain cancer-causing chemicals, such as nitrosamines.[19–21] Vitamin E is a potent antioxidant and has been related to inhibition of tumors in animal studies.[19,20]

Vitamin C is found in most fruits and vegetables. Beta-carotene, which is partially converted to vitamin A in the body, is plentiful in carrots, green leafy vegetables, sweet potatoes, winter squash, cantaloupe, and tomatoes. Carotenoids are a group of pigments that contribute to the yellow, orange, or red coloration of fruits and vegetables. Beta-carotene is the most plentiful carotenoid found in foods consumed by humans. Vitamin E is available in cereal grains, several vegetable oils, sunflower seeds, nuts, and kale.

Dietary fiber is a term used to cover several types of food components (e.g., cellulose, pectins, hemicellulose, lignins, gums) that are not digested in the human intestinal tract. These substances, abundant in whole grains, fruits, and vegetables, consist largely of complex carbohydrates of diverse chemical composition (see Chapter 9). A large number of studies indicate that colon cancer is low in human populations on other continents, who live on diets of largely unrefined food high in dietary fiber.[10,31,32] Researchers have estimated that if people would increase their fiber intake by 13 grams per day, a 31% reduction in colorectal cancer risk would result.[31] Currently, the average American male and female consumes 13.7 and 18.5 grams of dietary fiber a day, respectively, far below the recommended amount of 20–35 grams per day (see Chapter 9).

There are several mechanisms whereby fiber may protect against colon cancer.[10,31,32] Fiber has the ability to bind

to bile acids, which are released into the intestine from the liver, to aid in digestion of fat. High-fat diets increase bile acid production, ultimately increasing the exposure of the bowel to secondary bile acids, which are produced when colon bacteria degrade the primary bile acids from the liver. Fiber, however, binds the bile acids, increases stool bulk, dilutes the concentration of secondary bile acids and other cancer-causing chemicals, and speeds up the transit of the fecal mass through the colon. Additionally, some of the water-soluble fibers (from fruits and vegetables) are fermented by the colonic bacteria into volatile free fatty acids, which may be directly anticarcinogenic.

Whether dietary fiber reduces the risk of other cancers is uncertain. It has been hypothesized that dietary fiber may reduce breast cancer risk because fiber reduces the intestinal reabsorption of estrogens excreted with bile acids from the liver.[33] Although some animal studies suggest that dietary fiber does reduce breast cancer risk, the evidence in humans is inconclusive.

The American Cancer Society recommends reducing total dietary fat intake primarily by decreasing use of animal products.[10] Substantial evidence suggests that excessive fat intake increases the risk of developing cancers of the colon and rectum, prostate, and endometrium.[10,34–38] Several studies have shown a link between consumption of meat, especially red meats, and cancers at several sites, most notably the colon and prostate.[35–37]

There is still controversy regarding the relationship between dietary fat and breast cancer.[39–42] Over 60 years ago, researchers showed that diets high in fat increased the risk of breast tumors in rodents.[33] Around the world, the per capita fat consumption, especially of animal fat, is highly correlated with national breast cancer mortality rates.[42] Breast cancer incidence rates have increased substantially in the United States during the twentieth century, as has per capita fat consumption. However, in various cohort studies where women are followed for 3–20 years, few have found that high fat intake increases the risk of developing breast cancer.[39] Randomized trials of fat reduction have been proposed as a means of resolving the uncertainty about the association between dietary fat and breast cancer.[41] The government is mounting the Women's Health Initiative, a $628 million trial involving 164,000 women. The study will help determine whether low-fat diets that are also high in fruits, vegetables, and grains lead to fewer cases of breast cancer.

For colon cancer, the association with dietary fat is much clearer.[10,25,26,28,31,32,36–38] In Western countries, the rates of colon cancer are up to 10 times those of many Far Eastern and developing nations.[1] Rapid increases in rates of colon cancer occur among offspring of migrants from low-risk to high-risk areas.[9] The per capita consumption of meat or an-imal fat (but not vegetable fat) is highly correlated with national rates of colon cancer worldwide.[9,36–38] As discussed previously, high-fat diets increase the excretion of bile acids, which can then act as tumor promoters in the colon. In one study of 88,751 nurses, intake of animal fat and red meat was positively associated with the risk of colon cancer, with the risk 89% higher for intake of animal fat and 77% higher for red meat intake in women consuming the highest amounts[36] (see Figure 11.12).

A strong correlation between national consumption of fat and national rate of mortality from prostate cancer has been reported.[9,35] As summarized in Figure 11.13, a high intake of animal fat, especially fat from red meat, has been associated with an elevated risk of advanced prostate cancer.[35] These findings support recommendations from the American Cancer Society to lower intake of dietary animal fat and red meat to reduce risk of cancer.[10]

Heavy drinkers of alcohol, especially those who are also cigarette smokers, are at unusually high risk for cancers of the oral cavity, larynx, and esophagus.[10] Cancer risk increases with the amount of alcohol consumed and may start to rise with intake of as few as two drinks per day. Some evidence also suggests that regular alcohol consumption

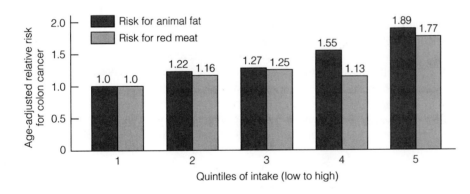

Figure 11.12 Relation of meat and animal fat to risk of colon cancer, 6-year prospective study of women. Colon cancer risk rises with increase in dietary intake of animal fat and red meat. *Source:* Willett WC, Stampfer MJ, Colditz GA, et al. Relation of meat, fat, and fiber intake to the risk of colon cancer in a prospective study among women. *N Engl J Med* 323:1664–1672, 1990.

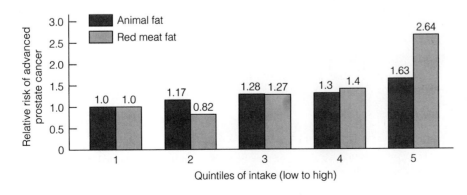

Figure 11.13 Animal fat and risk of prostate cancer, study of 47,855 health professionals. Prostate cancer risk rises with increase in dietary intake of animal fat and red meat. *Source:* Giovannucci E, Rimm EB, Colditz GA, Stampfer MJ, Chute CC, Willett WC. A prospective study of dietary fat and risk of prostate cancer. *J Natl Cancer Inst* 85: 1571–1579, 1993.

increases breast cancer risk in women, perhaps by increasing estrogen levels in the body.[43,44] Heavy alcohol intake can result in liver cirrhosis, which may be associated with liver cancer.[10] There is limited evidence that high alcohol intake also increases the risk for colon and prostate cancers.[45,46] The American Cancer Society advises that people should "limit consumption of alcoholic beverages, if you drink at all."[10]

PHYSICAL ACTIVITY AND CANCER

In 1996, regular physical activity was finally added to the list of cancer prevention measures advocated by the American Cancer Society[1,10] (Figure 11.14). The American Heart Association also took a long time (until the early 1990s) to add physical inactivity as a risk factor for heart disease (Chapter 10). The link between chronic disease and inactivity is a difficult one to establish because the relationship is complex, with many other difficult-to-measure lifestyle factors affecting the process.

Evidence is mounting that inactivity does contribute to the development of cancer.[47-50] In 1997, an international panel of cancer experts concluded that as many as 30–40% of all cancer cases worldwide could be avoided if people ate a healthy diet, avoided obesity, and got enough exercise.[51] The panel proposed a rigorous exercise goal: Take a brisk walk for about an hour daily (or the equivalent) and exercise vigorously at least 1 hour total each week if you have a sedentary job.

Although the epidemic of heart disease during the mid-twentieth century diverted the attention of researchers, the fact that cancer deaths now nearly equal those of heart disease has revitalized the nation's determination to wage war against cancer.

Inactivity As a Risk Factor for Cancer

The idea that increased physical exercise may be of benefit in preventing cancer is not a new one.[48] More than 70 years ago, researchers in Australia observed that primitive tribes who labored continuously for food had lower rates of cancer than people from more civilized societies.[52] Other scientists and physicians observed early in this century that most cancer patients had led relatively sedentary lives, and that men who had worked hard all their lives had less cancer than those who tended to sit during their day of work.[53]

These findings lay dormant until the mid-1970s, when researchers throughout the world took up the question anew. Since then, many studies have bolstered the evidence of an exercise–cancer connection. Active animals, former athletes, people employed in active occupations, and those who exercise during after-work hours have been compared with their sedentary counterparts. In general, depending on the type of cancer site investigated, they have been found to have a lower risk of cancer.[47-50] The Institute for Aerobics Research in Dallas, for example, showed that over an 8-year period, physically unfit men had four times the overall cancer death rate of the most fit men, with an even wider spread found among the women[54] (see Figure 11.15).

Some investigators have injected animals with certain types of cancer-causing chemicals, divided them into exercise and nonexercise groups, and then measured the size and time of cancer appearance. Results show that exercise tends to retard cancer growth at several different sites.[55-60] The activity of certain cells from the immune system—especially natural killer cells, cytotoxic T cells, and macrophages—appears to be enhanced with exercise, with improved cancer-fighting proficiency.[55,60]

Large groups of people have been followed for extended periods of time to see whether those who exercise regularly have less cancer than those who follow an inac-

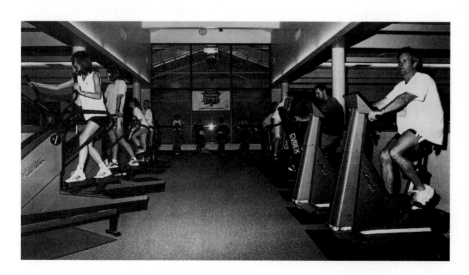

Figure 11.14 In 1996, regular physical activity was finally added to the list of cancer-preventive measures advocated by the American Cancer Society.

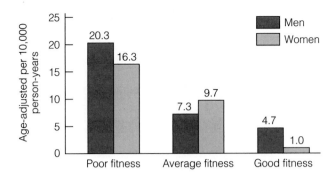

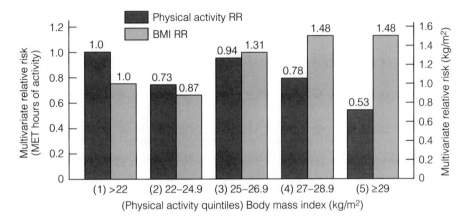

Figure 11.15 Cancer death rates according to fitness status. Cancer death rates were substantially higher in relatively unfit subjects, compared to those with moderate or high levels of fitness. *Source:* Blair SN, Kohl HW, Paffenbarger RS, et al. Physical fitness and all-cause mortality: A prospective study of healthy men and women. *JAMA* 262:2395–2401, 1989.

Figure 11.16 Physical activity and risk for colon cancer, 47,723 health professionals, 40–75 years old, 1986–1992; both low activity and high BMI, RR = 4.9 (extreme tertiles). Men who are most active and leanest experience the lowest risk of colon cancer. *Source:* Giovannucci E, Ascherio A, Rimm EB, Colditz GA, Stampfer MJ, Willett WC. Physical activity, obesity, and risk for colon cancer and adenoma in men. *Ann Intern Med* 122:327–334, 1995.

tive lifestyle. The most impressive results have shown a protective effect of exercise against three common cancer killers: colon, breast, and prostate cancer.[47–50] Although more research is needed, most experts feel that it is unlikely that physical activity has a strong influence on cancers at other sites such as the lung, pancreas, bladder, stomach, or oral cavity.[48,61]

Physical Activity and Colon Cancer

Exercise is most beneficial in preventing cancer of the colon, as compared with other cancer sites.[62] More than 40 studies have been published, looking at both occupational and leisure-time physical activity and the risk of colon cancer.[47,48,63–80] Three fourths of these studies have shown that physically active, compared to inactive, people have less colon cancer, with the best-designed studies showing the strongest relationship.[48] The protective effect of physical activity against colon cancer has been seen in several countries, including China, Sweden, Japan, and the United States.

A frequent finding has been that people who tend to sit the majority of their workday or remain inactive in their leisure time have a 30–100% greater risk of contracting colon cancer.[63–80] For example, researchers at the University of Southern California studied nearly 3,000 men with colon

cancer and compared them with the rest of the male population of Los Angeles County.[77] The men who worked at sedentary jobs were found to have a 60% greater colon cancer risk.

In one study of 163 colon cancer patients and 703 controls, 2 hours or more per week of vigorous leisure-time physical activity (e.g., running, bicycling, swimming laps, racquet sports, calisthenics, and rowing) lowered colon cancer risk by 40%.[65] Researchers at Harvard University studied 48,000 male health professionals and showed that colon cancer risk was decreased 50% in the most physically active men, compared to their sedentary peers[64] (Figure 11.16). The protective effect was most evident in men who exercised on average about 1–2 hours a day. Men who were both physically inactive and obese had a colon cancer risk that was nearly five times higher than that of their active and lean counterparts. A 12-year study of nearly 90,000 nurses has confirmed that the protective effect of regular physical activity against colon cancer also appears in women[63] (Figure 11.17).

One theory explaining the inverse relationship between physical activity and colon cancer risk is that each exercise bout stimulates muscle movement (peristalsis) of the large intestine.[81–83] In one study, subjects who ran or cycled for 1 hour each day for a week experienced significantly faster mean whole-gut transit times[81] (see Figure 11.18). This shortens the time that various cancer-causing chemicals in

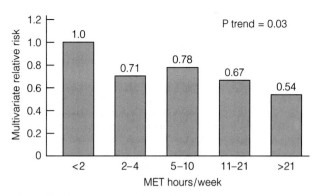

Figure 11.17 Physical activity and risk for colon cancer in women, 12-year study of 89,448 nurses (Nurses Health Study). Colon cancer risk drops by almost half in women who are most active. *Source:* Martinez ME, Giovannucci E, Spiegelman D, Hunter DJ, Willett WC, Colditz GA. Leisure-time physical activity, body size, and colon cancer in women. *J Natl Cancer Inst* 89:948–955, 1997.

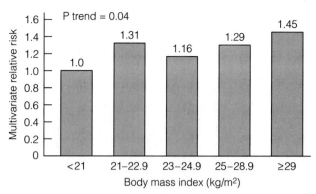

Figure 11.19 Body mass index (BMI) and risk for colon cancer in women, 12-year study of 89,448 nurses (Nurses Health Study). Obesity increases the risk for colon cancer. *Source:* Martinez ME, Giovannucci E, Spiegelman D, Hunter DJ, Willett WC, Colditz GA. Leisure-time physical activity, body size, and colon cancer in women. *J Natl Cancer Inst* 89:948–955, 1997.

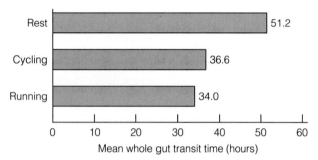

Figure 11.18 Effect of moderate exercise on whole-gut transit time: Subjects either ran, cycled, or rested for 1 hour each day for a week. Exercise intensity = 50% $\dot{V}O_{2max}$; dietary fiber intake the same during each phase. *Source:* Oettlé GJ. Effect of moderate exercise on bowel habit. *Gut* 32:941–944, 1991.

the fecal matter (e.g., secondary bile acids) stay in contact with the cells that line the colon. In other words, exercise has a similar effect on the colon to that of dietary fiber. It is well-known that those who exercise suffer less often from constipation than do the sedentary. In one large national survey, people were asked, "do you have trouble with your bowels that makes you constipated?" Among middle-aged adults, twice as many of those reporting "little exercise" had trouble with constipation, compared to highly active people.[84]

Other theories have been proposed. One of them links exercise, caloric intake, and obesity with colon cancer. In animal studies, when caloric intake is slightly below body needs, cancer risk is lowered.[85] In fact, this is one of the strongest variables controlling cancer incidence in animals. Regular exercise seems to help some people control their diet intakes. As a result, active people tend to be less obese, which is important because obesity in and of itself pro-

motes several different types of cancer, including colon cancer[63,64,66,86] (see Figures 11.16 and 11.19). Overall energy balance appears to be an important factor related to colon cancer. In one study of 2,073 colon cancer patients and 2,466 controls, those at greatest risk of colon cancer had the most unfavorable energy balance, in that they were physically inactive, had high energy intakes, and were obese.[69] Both obesity and physical inactivity promote higher levels of insulin in the blood, a hormone that increases the growth rate of cells lining the colon and hence their likelihood of turning cancerous.

Active people may also eat more dietary fiber, enhancing their protection against colon cancer. For example, in the study from Harvard University reviewed earlier, highly active men ate 29 grams of dietary fiber a day, more than double the intake (12 grams) of the inactive men.[64] It should be noted, however, that even after controlling for dietary fiber intake, physical activity, in and of itself, still lowered colon cancer risk.

Physical Activity and Breast Cancer

There is increasing evidence that women who engage in vigorous exercise from early in life may gain some protection against breast cancer[48,87–96] (Figure 11.20). Relatively few human studies have been conducted, but only one in four have failed to establish a protective effect of physical activity against breast cancer. In animal studies, vigorous physical activity has been associated with an inhibition of chemically induced breast cancer.[55,97,98]

For example, a review of the death records for some 25,000 women in Washington state revealed that those who had worked in physically demanding jobs had a low breast

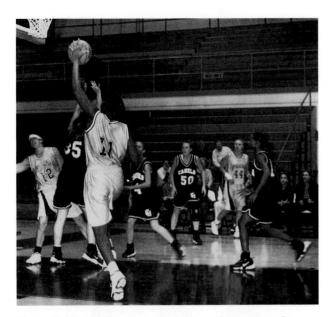

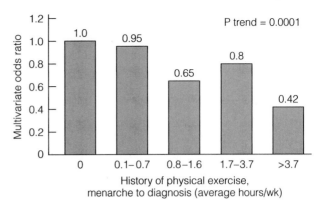

Figure 11.21 Physical exercise and reduced risk of breast cancer, 545 cases (diagnosed under age 40) versus 545 controls. The risk for breast cancer was reduced by more than half in women exercising more than 3.7 hours per week since early in life. *Source:* Bernstein L, Henderson BE, Hanisch R, Sullivan-Halley J, Ross RK. Physical exercise and reduced risk of breast cancer in young women. *J Natl Cancer Inst* 86:1403–1408, 1994.

Figure 11.20 There is increasing evidence that women who engage in vigorous exercise from early in life may gain protection against breast cancer.

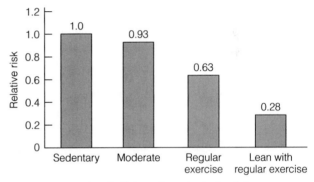

Figure 11.22 Leisure-time physical exercise and reduced risk of breast cancer, 14-year study of 25,624 Norwegian women. Breast cancer risk was lowest in women who were lean and regularly active. *Source:* Thune I, Brenn T, Lund E, Gaard M. Physical activity and the risk of breast cancer. *N Engl J Med* 336:1269–1275, 1997.

cancer risk.[78] Another study of 6,888 women with breast cancer and 9,539 controls showed that women who had exercised vigorously on a near-daily basis between the ages of 14 and 22 had a 50% reduction in breast cancer risk.[95]

The lifetime occurrence rate of breast cancer in women was studied in 2,622 former college athletes and 2,776 non-athletes.[92] The nonathletes had an 86% higher risk for breast cancer than the former athletes throughout their lifetimes. Of interest is that the athletes were leaner and had a later age of menarche and an earlier age of menopause than the nonathletes.

The relationship between breast cancer and physical activity was studied in 545 premenopausal women with breast cancer and 545 controls.[88] As shown in Figure 11.21, the risk for breast cancer was reduced by more than half in women exercising more than 3.7 hours per week starting early in life. In a 14-year study of more than 25,000 Norwegian women, regular physical exercise was associated with a 37% reduction in breast cancer risk.[89] If the women were both lean and regularly active, risk was reduced 72% (Figure 11.22). In a case–control study in Australia, a decrease in risk of breast cancer was found with increasing levels of physical activity and was most evident for women who engaged in vigorous exercise.[96]

Exercise might reduce the risk of breast cancer via several mechanisms.[99–103] As discussed earlier, the cumulative exposure to ovarian hormones is an important factor causing breast cancer.[101,102] Women who exercise vigorously from childhood tend to have a later onset of menarche, may experience some missed menstrual cycles, and are generally leaner, all of which decrease exposure of the breast tissue to estrogen. However, very strenuous exercise is required before the number of ovulatory cycles is reduced.[103]

Obesity, especially the gynoid type, in which fat accumulates around the waist, increases the risk of breast cancer.[99,103] Fat stores provide the substrate for the conversion of androgens to estrogens, increasing the concentration of estrogen in the body.[103] For this reason, some experts feel that reduction of body fat with regular exercise may be one of the chief protective mechanisms against breast cancer. Obesity is also associated with higher blood insulin levels, which promote the growth of breast cancer cells. Thus, active athletic women may be protected from breast cancer because of the indirect effects of exercise on reducing exposure to their own hormones.[103]

The critical role that the female hormone estrogen plays in cancer risk has also been shown for cancer of the uterus.[1] Estrogen stimulates cell division within the lining of the uterus, increasing the risk for cancer cell development. As with breast cancer, uterine cancer risk is increased in women who are obese, who experience a late menopause, or undergo prolonged estrogen therapy. Ovarian cancer risk is elevated in women who have never had children or who have a family history of ovarian cancer. Although more research is needed, there is evidence from several human studies that sedentary women are at substantially greater risk for female reproductive cancers than are those who are moderately to highly physically active.[87,90,92,104–106] In one study, participation in college athletics was related to a reduced lifetime risk of both uterine and ovarian cancer.[90,92] Nonathletes had more than 2.5 times the risk of female reproductive cancers than did former college athletes. Studies in Europe, China, and the United States have each shown that physical inactivity increases the risk for uterine cancer.[104–106] Researchers from the National Cancer Institute have shown that physically inactive women may be at increased risk of endometrial cancer by virtue of their tendency to be obese.[106]

Physical Activity and Prostate Cancer

Prostate cancer is the most frequently diagnosed cancer in men, and physical activity has been studied for its effect on the incidence and mortality due to this cancer.[107–112] Fewer than 20 studies of physical activity and prostate cancer risk have been published, and slightly more than half of these have found inactivity to be a significant risk factor.[48,111]

Recent studies using the best research designs have generally supported a relationship between physical activity and prostate cancer.[76,79,107–112] Researchers in Norway followed 53,242 men for an average of 16 years and found that risk of prostate cancer was reduced by more than half in those who walked during their work hours and also engaged in regular leisure-time exercise.[109] This protective effect, however, was found only among men older than 60 years of age. These results are similar to those of a well-designed study of 17,719 college alumni, in which risk of prostate cancer was reduced 47% in highly active versus sedentary men age 70 years and older.[107]

At the Cooper Clinic in Dallas, nearly 13,000 men were studied during 1970–1989.[108] All the men were given maximal exercise treadmill tests, divided into various fitness groups, and then tracked for development of prostate cancer over time. As shown in Figure 11.23, men in the highest versus the lowest fitness group had a 74% reduced risk of developing prostate cancer. The men were also divided into different physical activity groups, and those exercising

more than 1,000 Calories per week had less than half the risk of prostate cancer of their more sedentary counterparts.

As with breast cancer, there is an attractive explanation for why regular physical activity may lower prostate cancer risk.[111] Research suggests that higher levels of the male hormone testosterone may contribute to the development of prostate cancer.[1] Animal studies have shown that prostate cancer can be provoked by injecting them with testosterone. As explained earlier, African Americans have the highest prostate cancer incidence rates in the world, which are almost entirely attributed to their higher testos-

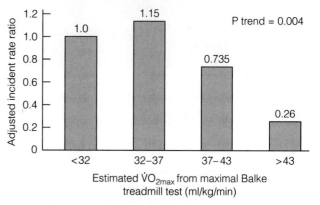

Figure 11.23 Cardiorespiratory fitness and prostate cancer, 12,975 men studied during 1970–1990. Increasing aerobic fitness was related to the lowest risk of prostate cancer. *Source:* Oliveria SA, Kohl HW, Trichopoulos D, Blair SN. The association between cardiorespiratory fitness and prostate cancer. *Med Sci Sports Exerc* 28:97–104, 1996.

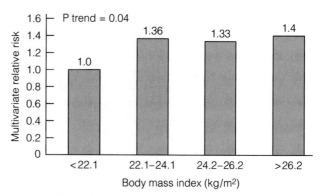

Figure 11.24 Body mass index (BMI) and risk for prostate cancer death, 18-year study of 135,000 male construction workers in Sweden. Obesity was linked to a greater risk of prostate cancer in this large study of men. *Source:* Andersson SO, Wolk A, Bergstrom R, Adami HO, Engholm G, Englund A, Nyren O. Body size and prostate cancer: A 20-year follow-up study among 135,006 Swedish construction workers. *J Natl Cancer Inst* 89: 385–389, 1997.

terone levels (15% higher than those of other American males).[1] Antitestosterone therapy is the treatment of choice for advanced prostate cancer.

Most studies have demonstrated that testosterone concentrations are depressed in trained athletes.[113] In other words, repeated bouts of exercise may lower blood levels of testosterone. The net effect is that highly active men may expose their prostate to less testosterone, reducing their risk of prostate cancer. Obesity promotes prostate cancer risk, as depicted in Figure 11.24.[114,115] Thus, regular and vigorous exercise may lower prostate cancer risk by enhancing leanness.

SPORTS MEDICINE INSIGHT

Exercise and Treatment of Cancer

Fred Lebow, the founder of the New York City marathon and an active marathoner, was diagnosed with brain cancer in 1990. Even as he underwent chemotherapy, he continued to run, first on the roof of the hospital and then back out on the roads and paths of New York's Central Park. In 1992, he and an old friend, nine-time New York City marathon winner Grete Waitz of Norway, ran the entire 26.2 mile course. Just before the 1994 New York City marathon, runners throughout the world were saddened to hear that Fred Lebow had died at age 62 after a second bout with brain cancer.

Lebow's fight against cancer was well known and has raised the question of whether he should have cut back on his training after being diagnosed with cancer. In other words, can too much exercise be harmful to the cancer patient? On the other hand, can moderate amounts be beneficial?

Very few studies have been conducted in this area.[116–121] In one study, researchers followed 451 breast cancer patients for an average of 5–6 years, while the patients reported their weekly levels of light, moderate, and vigorous physical activity.[119] No link between exercise habits and survival from breast cancer could be measured. Animal research has determined that breast cancer risk is decreased by exercise during the earliest stages of cancer formation, but not after the cancer has become established.[55]

Despite the limited research data, many experts still feel that moderate exercise may have several important benefits. According to Roy Shephard, of the University of Toronto in Canada, "Exercise has an immediate mood-elevating effect, and thus can be of particular help to the cancer victim. It also stimulates appetite, and encourages the retention of muscle tissue. These effects should slow the clinical course of the disease, setting back the age at death, while also increasing the quality of the remaining years of life."[49]

The American College of Sports Medicine has made several recommendations regarding exercise for cancer patients:[116]

- Exercise testing and training should be individualized to the patient.
- For survivors of cancer (in remission or after cure), exercise training should have the objective of returning them to their former level of physical and psychological function—or better.
- For persons who are undergoing therapy for cancer, exercise training should have the objective of maintaining endurance, strength, and level of function. Cancer therapy exhausts physical and emotional reserves, so a good use of exercise training is an attempt to maintain these resources.

The Santa Barbara Athletic Club provides an exercise training program for cancer patients who are referred from a local cancer-treatment center.[117] The program has three components—aerobic, strength, and stretching/ relaxation training. Results from the program have shown that cancer patients can experience major gains in upper- and lower-body strength and in aerobic fitness. Patients also reported improvement in ability to engage in household tasks and recreational activities.

In Sweden, 200 cancer patients were assigned by researchers either to the "Starting Again" program or to the control condition.[120] The treatment program emphasized physical training, information, and coping skills. According to the researchers from the Karolinska Hospital in Stockholm, the patients in the program experienced greater physical strength and an improved mood state.

There is some concern that intensive exercise undertaken for extended periods of time may be detrimental. Several studies suggest that in animals, intense, forced, high-volume exercise enhances the spread of certain types of cancer.[55,57,59] Until more is known, it would be prudent to urge that cancer patients undergoing treatment exercise moderately each day, while avoiding intensive exercise.

SUMMARY

1. *Cancer* is defined as the uncontrolled growth and spread of abnormal cells, which can result in death, as vital passageways are blocked and the body's oxygen and nutrient supplies are diverted.

2. Cancer ranks a close second to heart disease as the leading cause of death in the United States. Since 1991, cancer death rates have fallen slightly, due in part to reduced smoking and to improved screening and treatment.

3. Dietary factors are responsible for about one third of all cancers, and cigarette smoking for about 30%. The American Cancer Society has urged that to reduce cancer risk, people should avoid all tobacco use, consume low-fat, high-fiber diets containing plenty of whole grains, fruits, and vegetables, be physically active and maintain a healthy weight, limit consumption of alcoholic beverages, and limit exposure to ultraviolet radiation.

4. In 1996, regular physical activity was finally added to the list of cancer prevention measures advocated by the American Cancer Society. The most impressive research results have shown a protective effect of exercise against three common cancer killers: colon, breast, and prostate cancer.

5. Exercise is most beneficial in preventing cancer of the colon, as compared with other cancer sites. Proposed mechanisms include faster movement of fecal material through the large intestine, decreased body fat stores, and improved overall energy balance.

6. There is increasing evidence that women who engage in vigorous exercise from early in life may gain some protection against breast cancer. Proposed mechanisms include reduced estrogen exposure, decreased body fat stores, and lower blood insulin levels.

7. Recent studies using the best research designs have generally supported a relationship between physical activity and prostate cancer. Proposed mechanisms include lower blood levels of testosterone and reduced body fat stores.

8. Exercise does not appear to improve the process of cancer treatment. Nonetheless, exercise for cancer patients is recommended to improve fitness, life quality, and morale.

REFERENCES

1. American Cancer Society. *Cancer Facts & Figures—1997.* Atlanta: Author, 1997.

2. Parker SL, Tong T, Bolden S, Wingo PA. Cancer statistics, 1997. *CA Cancer J Clin* 47:5027, 1997.

3. Ames BN, Shigenaga MK, Hagen TM. Oxidants, antioxidants, and the degenerative diseases of aging. *Proc Nat Acad Sci* 90: 7915–7922, 1993.

4. National Center for Health Statistics. *Health, United States, 1996–97 and Injury Chartbook.* Hyattsville, MD: 1997.

5. Bailar JC, Gornik HL. Cancer undefeated. *N Engl J Med* 336: 1569–1574, 1997.

6. Chevarley F, White E. Recent trends in breast cancer mortality among white and black US women. *Am J Public Health* 87: 775–781, 1997.

7. Cole P, Rodu B. Declining cancer mortality in the United States. *Cancer* 78:2045–2048, 1996.

8. Doll R, Peto R. The causes of cancer: Quantitative estimates of avoidable risks of cancer in the United States today. *J Natl Cancer Inst* 66:1191–1308, 1981.

9. National Research Council. *Diet and Health: Implications for Reducing Chronic Disease Risk.* Washington, DC: National Academy Press, 1989.

10. American Cancer Society. Guidelines on diet, nutrition, and cancer prevention: Reducing the risk of cancer with healthy food choices and physical activity. *CA Cancer J Clin* 46:325–341, 1996.

11. Carbone D. Smoking and cancer. *Am J Med* 93(1A):13S–17S, 1992.

12. McCusker K. Mechanisms of respiratory tissue injury from cigarette smoking. *Am J Med* 93:1A:18S–21S, 1992.

13. Rodriquez C, Tatham LM, Thun MJ, Calle EE, Heath CW. Smoking and fatal prostate cancer in a large cohort of adult men. *Am J Epidemiol* 145:466–475, 1997.

14. Ambrosone CB, Freudenheim JL, Graham S, et al. Cigarette smoking, N-acetyltransferase 2 genetic polymorphisms, and breast cancer risk. *JAMA* 276:1494–1501, 1996.

15. U.S. Environmental Protection Agency. *Respiratory Health Effects of Passive Smoking: Lung Cancer and Other Disorders.* U.S. Environmental Protection Agency, Office of Research and Development. Washington, DC: U.S. EPA, 1992.

16. Morabia A, Bernstein M, Heritier S, Khatchatrian N. Relation of breast cancer with passive and active exposure to tobacco smoke. *Am J Epidemiol* 143:918–928, 1996.

17. Fuchs CS, Colditz GA, Stampfer MJ, et al. A prospective study of cigarette smoking and the risk of pancreatic cancer. *Arch Intern Med* 156:2255–2260, 1996.

18. Couglin SS, Neaton JD, Sengupta A. Cigarette smoking as a predictor of death from prostate cancer in 348,874 men screened for the Multiple Risk Factor Intervention Trial. *Am J Epidemiol* 143:1002–1006, 1996.

19. Steinmetz KA, Potter JD. Vegetables, fruit, and cancer prevention: A review. *J Am Diet Assoc* 96:1027–1039, 1996.

20. Block G, Patterson B, Subar A. Fruit, vegetable, and cancer prevention: A review of the epidemiological evidence. *Nutr Cancer* 18:1–29, 1992.

21. Block G. Epidemiologic evidence regarding vitamin C and cancer. *Am J Clin Nutr* 54:1310S–1314S, 1991.

22. Bendich A. Clinical importance of beta carotene. *Perspect Appl Nutr* 1(1):14–22, 1993.

23. Pool-Zobel BL, Bub A, Muller H, Wollowski I, Rechkemmer G. Consumption of vegetables reduces genetic damage in humans: First results of a human intervention trial with carotenoid-rich foods. *Carcinogenesis* 18:1847–1850, 1997.

24. Verhoeven DT, Verhagen H, Goldbohm RA, van den Brandt PA, van Poppel G. A review of mechanisms underlying anti-carcinogenicity by brassica vegetables. *Chem Biol Interact* 103:79–129, 1997.

25. Potter JD. Risk factors for colon neoplasia—epidemiology and biology. *Eur J Cancer* 31A:1033–1038, 1995.

26. Giovannucci E, Willett WC. Dietary factors and risk of colon cancer. *Ann Med* 26:443–452, 1994.

27. Yong LC, Brown CC, Schatzkin A, Dresser CM, Slesinski MJ, Cox CS, Taylor PR. Intake of vitamins E, C, and A and risk of lung cancer: The NHANES I epidemiologic follow-up study. *Am J Epidemiol* 146:231–243, 1997.

28. Witte JS, Longnecker MP, Bird CL, Lee ER, Frankl HD, Haile RW. Relation of vegetable, fruit, and grain consumption to colorectal adenomatous polyps. *Am J Epidemiol* 144:1015–1025, 1996.

29. Ocke MC, Bueno-de-Mesquita HB, Feskens EJM, van Staveren WA, Kromhout D. Repeated measurements of vegetables, fruits, beta-carotene, and vitamins C and E in relation to lung cancer. *Am J Epidemiol* 145:358–365, 1997.

30. Ritter L. Report of a panel on the relationship between public exposure to pesticides and cancer. *Cancer* 80:2019–2033, 1997.

31. Howe GR, Benito E, Castelleto R, et al. Dietary intake of fiber and decreased risk of cancers of the colon and rectum: Evidence from the combined analysis of 13 case–control studies. *J Natl Cancer Inst* 84:1887–1896, 1992.

32. Potter JD. Reconciling the epidemiology, physiology, and molecular biology of colon cancer. *JAMA* 268:1573–1577, 1992.

33. Hunter DJ, Willett WC. Diet, body size, and breast cancer. *Epidemiol Rev* 15:110–132, 1993.

34. Kuller LH. Dietary fat and chronic diseases: Epidemiologic overview. *J Am Diet Assoc* 97(suppl):S9–S15, 1997.

35. Giovannucci E, Rimm EB, Colditz GA, Stampfer MJ, Chute CC, Willett WC. A prospective study of dietary fat and risk of prostate cancer. *J Natl Cancer Inst* 85:1571–1579, 1993.

36. Willett WC, Stampfer MJ, Colditz GA, et al. Relation of meat, fat, and fiber intake to the risk of colon cancer in a prospective study among women. *N Engl J Med* 323:1664–1672, 1990.

37. Giovannucci E, Rimm EB, Stampfer MJ, Colditz GA, Ascherio A, Willett WC. Intake of fat, meat, and fiber in relation to risk of colon cancer in men. *Cancer Res* 54:2390–2397, 1994.

38. Van der Meer R, Lapre JA, Govers MJ, Kleibeuker JH. Mechanisms of the intestinal effects of dietary fats and milk products on colon carcinogenesis. *Cancer Lett* 114:75–83, 1997.

39. Hunter DJ, Spiegelman D, Adami HO, et al. Cohort studies of fat intake and the risk of breast cancer—a pooled analysis. *N Engl J Med* 334:356–361, 1996.

40. Boyd NF, Greenberg C, Lockwood G, Little L, Martin L, Byng J, Yaffe M, Tritchler D. Effects at two years of a low-fat, high-carbohydrate diet on radiologic features of the breast: Results from a randomized trial. *J Natl Cancer Inst* 89:488–496, 1997.

41. Greenwald P, Sherwood K, McDonald SS. Fat, caloric intake, and obesity: Lifestyle risk factors for breast cancer. *J Am Diet Assoc* 97(suppl):S24–S30, 1997.

42. Sasaki S, Horacsek M, Kesteloot H. An ecological study of the relationship between dietary fat intake and breast cancer mortality. *Prev Med* 22:187–202, 1993.

43. Friedenreich CM, Howe GR, Miller AB, Jain MG. A cohort study of alcohol consumption and risk of breast cancer. *Am J Epidemiol* 137:512–520, 1993.

44. Longnecker MP, Newcomb PA, Mittendorf R, et al. Risk of breast cancer in relation to lifetime alcohol consumption. *J Natl Cancer Inst* 87:923–929, 1995.

45. Giovannucci E, Rimm EB, Ascherio A, Stampfer MJ, Colditz GA, Willett WC. Alcohol, low-methionine–low-folate diets, and risk of colon cancer in men. *J Natl Cancer Inst* 87:265–273, 1995.

46. Hayes RB, Brown LM, Schoenberg JB, et al. Alcohol use and prostate cancer risk in US blacks and whites. *Am J Epidemiol* 143:692–697, 1996.

47. Lee I-M. Exercise and physical health: Cancer and immune function. *Res Quart Exerc Sport* 66:286–291, 1995.

48. Lee I-M. Physical activity, fitness and cancer. In Bouchard C, Shephard RJ, Stephens T (eds), *Physical Activity, Fitness, and Health: International Proceedings and Consensus Statement*. Champaign, IL: Human Kinetics, 1994.

49. Shephard RJ. Exercise in the prevention and treatment of cancer: An update. *Sports Med* 15:258–280, 1993.

50. Sternfeld B. Cancer and the protective effect of physical activity: The epidemiological evidence. *Med Sci Sports Exerc* 24:1195–1209, 1992.

51. Hellmich N. Fighting cancer: Diet and exercise. *USA Today*, October 1, 1997.

52. Cherry T. A theory of cancer. *Med J Aust* 1:425–438, 1922.

53. Sivertsen I, Dahlstrom AW. The relation of muscular activity to carcinoma: A preliminary report. *J Cancer Res* 6:365–378, 1922.

54. Blair SN, Kohl HW, Paffenbarger RS, et al. Physical fitness and all-cause mortality: A prospective study of healthy men and women. *JAMA* 262:2395–2401, 1989.

55. Hoffman-Goetz L, Husted J. Exercise and breast cancer: Review and critical analysis of the literature. *Can J Appl Physiol* 19:237–252, 1994.

56. Roebuck BD, McCaffrey J, Baumgartner KJ. Protective effects of voluntary exercise during the postinitiation phase of pancreatic carcinogenesis in the rat. *Cancer Res* 50:6811–6816, 1990.

57. Cohen LA, Choi K, Wang CX. Influence of dietary fat, caloric restriction, and voluntary exercise in N-nitrosomethylurea-induced mammary tumorgenesis in rats. *Cancer Res* 48:4276–4283, 1988.

58. MacNeil B, Hoffman-Goetz L. Chronic exercise enhances in vivo and in vitro cytotoxic mechanisms of natural immunity in mice. *J Appl Physiol* 74:388–395, 1993.

59. Cohen LA, Boylan E, Epstein M, Zang E. Voluntary exercise and experimental mammary cancer. *Adv Exp Med Biol* 322:41–59, 1992.

60. Woods JA, Davis JM. Exercise, monocyte / macrophage function, and cancer. *Med Sci Sports Exerc* 26:147–156, 1994.

61. Thune I, Lund E. The influence of physical activity on lung-cancer risk: A prospective study of 81,516 men and women. *Int J Cancer* 70:57–62, 1997.

62. U.S. Department of Health and Human Services. *Physical Activity and Health: A Report of the Surgeon General*. Atlanta, GA: U.S. Department of Health and Human Services, Centers for

Disease Control and Prevention, National Center for Chronic Disease Prevention and Health Promotion, 1996.

63. Martinez ME, Giovannucci E, Spiegelman D, Hunter DJ, Willett WC, Colditz GA. Leisure-time physical activity, body size, and colon cancer in women. *J Natl Cancer Inst* 89: 948–955, 1997.

64. Giovannucci E, Ascherio A, Rimm EB, Colditz GA, Stampfer MJ, Willett WC. Physical activity, obesity, and risk for colon cancer and adenoma in men. *Ann Intern Med* 122:327–334, 1995.

65. Longnecker MP, De Verdier MG, Frumkin H, Carpenter C. A case–control study of physical activity in relation to risk of cancer of the right colon and rectum in men. *Int J Epidemiol* 24: 42–50, 1995.

66. Giovannucci E, Colditz GA, Stampfer MJ, Willett WC. Physical activity, obesity, and risk of colorectal adenoma in women (United States). *Cancer Causes Control* 7:253–263, 1996.

67. Lee I-M, Paffenbarger RS. Physical activity and its relation to cancer risk: A prospective study of college alumni. *Med Sci Sports Exerc* 26:831–837, 1994.

68. White E, Jacobs EJ, Daling JR. Physical activity in relation to colon cancer in middle-aged men and women. *Am J Epidemiol* 144:42–50, 1996.

69. Slattery ML, Potter J, Caan B, Edwards S, Coates A, Ma KN, Berry TD. Energy balance and colon cancer—beyond physical activity. *Cancer Res* 57:75–80, 1997.

70. Brownson RC, Chang JC, Davis JR, Smith CA. Physical activity on the job and cancer in Missouri. *Am J Public Health* 81: 639–642, 1991.

71. Wannamethee G, Shaper AG, Macfarlane PW. Heart rate, physical activity, and mortality from cancer and other noncardiovascular diseases. *Am J Epidemiol* 137:735–748, 1993.

72. Slattery ML, Schumacher MC, Smith KR, West DW, Abd-Elghany N. Physical activity, diet, and risk of colon cancer in Utah. *Am J Epidemiol* 128:989–999, 1988.

73. Ballard-Barbash R, Schatzkin A, Albanes D, et al. Physical activity and risk of large bowel cancer in the Framingham study. *Cancer Res* 50:3610–3613, 1990.

74. Thun MJ, Calle EE, Namboodiri MM, et al. Risk factors for fatal colon cancer in a large prospective study. *J Natl Cancer Inst* 84:1491–1500, 1992.

75. Fraser G, Pearce N. Occupational physical activity and risk of cancer of the colon and rectum in New Zealand males. *Cancer Causes Control* 4(1):45–50, 1993.

76. Brownson RC, Zahm SH, Chang JC, Blair A. Occupational risk of colon cancer: An analysis by anatomic subsite. *Am J Epidemiol* 130:675–687, 1989.

77. Garabrant DH, Peters JM, Mack TM, et al. Job activity and colon cancer risk. *Am J Epidemiol* 119:1005–1014, 1984.

78. Vena JE, Graham S, Zielezny M, et al. Lifetime occupational exercise and colon cancer. *Am J Epidemiol* 122:357–365, 1985.

79. Vena JE, Graham S, Zielezny M, Brasure J, Swanson MK. Occupational exercise and risk of cancer. *Am J Clin Nutr* 45: 318–327, 1987.

80. Gerhardsson M, Norell SE, Kiviranta H, et al. Sedentary job and colon cancer. *Am J Epidemiol* 123:775–780, 1986.

81. Oettlé GJ. Effect of moderate exercise on bowel habit. *Gut* 32: 941–944, 1991.

82. Keeling WF, Martin BJ. Gastrointestinal transit during mild exercise. *J Appl Physiol* 63:978–981, 1987. See also *J Appl Physiol* 68:1350–1353, 1990.

83. Cordain L, Latin RW, Behnke JJ. The effects of an aerobic running program on bowel transit time. *J Sports Med* 26:101–104, 1986.

84. Sandler RS, Jordan MC, Shelton BJ. Demographic and dietary determinants of constipation in the US population. *Am J Public Health* 80:185–189, 1990.

85. Kritchevsky D. Caloric restriction and experimental tumorigenesis. *Nutrition Today,* January/February 1993, 25–27. See also *Ca-A Cancer J Clin* 41(6):328–333, 1991.

86. Garfinkel LE. Overweight and cancer. *Ann Intern Med* 103: 1034–1036, 1985.

87. Kramer MM, Wells CL. Does physical activity reduce risk of estrogen-dependent cancer in women? *Med Sci Sports Exerc* 28:322–334, 1996.

88. Bernstein L, Henderson BE, Hanisch R, Sullivan-Halley J, Ross RK. Physical exercise and reduced risk of breast cancer in young women. *J Natl Cancer Inst* 86:1403–1408, 1994.

89. Thune I, Brenn T, Lund E, Gaard M. Physical activity and the risk of breast cancer. *N Engl J Med* 336:1269–1275, 1997.

90. Frisch RE, Wyshak G, Albright NL, et al. Lower lifetime occurrence of breast cancer and cancers of the reproductive system among former college athletes. *Am J Clin Nutr* 45: 328–325, 1987.

91. Wyshak G, Frisch RE, Albright NL, Albright TE, Schiff I. Lower prevalence of benign diseases of the breast and benign tumors of the reproductive system among former college athletes compared to non-athletes. *Br J Cancer* 54:841–845, 1986.

92. Frisch RE, Wyshak G, Albright NL, et al. Lower prevalence of breast cancer and cancers of the reproductive system among former college athletes compared to non-athletes. *Br J Cancer* 52:885–891, 1985.

93. Fraser GE, Shavlik D. Risk factors, lifetime risk, and age at onset of breast cancer. *Ann Epidemiol* 7:375–382, 1997.

94. Coogan PF, Newcomb PA, Clapp RW, Trentham-Dietz A, Baron JA, Longnecker MP. Physical activity in usual occupation and risk of breast cancer (United States). *Cancer Causes Control* 8:626–631, 1997.

95. Mittendorf R, Longnecker MP, Newcomb PA, et al. Strenuous physical activity in young adulthood and risk of breast cancer (United States). *Cancer Causes Control* 6:347–353, 1995.

96. Friedenreich CM, Rohan TE. Physical activity and risk of breast cancer. *Eur J Cancer Prev* 4:145–151, 1995.

97. Thompson HJ, Westerlind KC, Snedden JR, Briggs S, Singh M. Inhibition of mammary carcinogenesis by treadmill exercise. *J Natl Cancer Inst* 87:453–455, 1995.

98. Thompson HJ. Effect of exercise intensity and duration on the induction of mammary carcinogenesis. *Cancer Res* 54(suppl7): 1960S–1963S, 1994.

99. Shephard RJ. Exercise and cancer: Linkages with obesity? *Int J Obesity* 19(suppl 4):S62–S68, 1995.

100. Trentham-Dietz A, Newcomb PA, Storer BE, Longnecker MP, Baron J, Greenberg ER, Willett WC. Body size and risk of breast cancer. *Am J Epidemiol* 145:1011–1019, 1997.

101. Kelsey JL, Gammon MD, John EM. Reproductive factors and breast cancer. *Epidemiol Rev* 15:36–46, 1993.

102. Pike MC, Spicer DV, Dahmoush L, Press MF. Estrogens, progestogens, normal breast cell proliferation, and breast cancer risk. *Epidemiol Rev* 15:17–34, 1993.

103. McTiernan A. Exercise and breast cancer—time to get moving? *N Engl J Med* 336:1311–1312, 1997.

104. Shu XO, Hatch MC, Zheng W, Gao YT, Brinton LA. Physical activity and risk of endometrial cancer. *Epidemiol* 4(4):342–349, 1993.

105. Levi F, La Vecchia C, Negri E, Franceschi S. Selected physical activities and the risk of endometrial cancer. *Br J Cancer* 67:846–851, 1993.

106. Sturgen SR, Brinton LA, Berman ML, et al. Past and present physical activity and endometrial cancer risk. *Br J Cancer* 68:584–589, 1993.

107. Lee IM, Paffenbarger RS, Hsieh CC. Physical activity and risk of prostatic cancer among college alumni. *Am J Epidemiol* 135:169–179, 1992.

108. Oliveria SA, Kohl HW, Trichopoulos D, Blair SN. The association between cardiorespiratory fitness and prostate cancer. *Med Sci Sports Exerc* 28:97–104, 1996.

109. Thune I, Lund E. Physical activity and the risk of prostate and testicular cancer: A cohort study of 53,000 Norwegian men. *Cancer Causes Control* 5:549–556, 1994.

110. Andersson SO, Baron J, Wolk A, Lindgren C, Bergstrom R, Adami HO. Early life risk factors for prostate cancer: A population-based case–control study in Sweden. *Cancer Epidemiol Biomarkers Prev* 4:187–192, 1995.

111. Oliveria SA, Lee IM. Is exercise beneficial in the prevention of prostate cancer? *Sports Med* 23:271–278, 1997.

112. Albanes D, Blair A, Taylor PR. Physical activity and risk of cancer in the NHANES I Population. *Am J Public Health* 79:744–750, 1989.

113. Hackney AC. The male reproductive system and endurance exercise. *Med Sci Sports Exerc* 28:180–189, 1996.

114. Andersson SO, Wolk A, Bergstrom R, Adami HO, Engholm G, Englund A, Nyren O. Body size and prostate cancer: A 20-year follow-up study among 135,006 Swedish construction workers. *J Natl Cancer Inst* 89:385–389, 1997.

115. Giovannucci E, Rimm EB, Stampfer MJ, Colditz GA, Willett WC. Height, body weight, and risk of prostate cancer. *Cancer Epidemiol Biomarkers Prev* 6:557–563, 1997.

116. American College of Sports Medicine. *ACSM's Exercise Management for Persons with Chronic Diseases and Disabilities.* Champaign, IL: Human Kinetics, 1997.

117. Durak EP, Lilly PC. Cancer rehab in the health club. *Fitness Management,* February 1997, 30–32.

118. Dimeo F, Fetscher S, Lange W, Mertelsmann R, Keul J. Effects of aerobic exercise on the physical performance and incidence of treatment-related complications after high-dose chemotherapy. *Blood* 90:3390–3394, 1997.

119. Rohan TE, Fu W, Hiller JE. Physical activity and survival from breast cancer. *Eur J Cancer Prev* 4:419–424, 1995.

120. Berglund G, Bolund C, Gustafsson UL, Sjoden PO. One-year follow-up of the "Starting Again" group rehabilitation program for cancer patients. *Eur J Cancer* 30A:1744–1751, 1994.

121. Demark-Wahnefried W, Hars V, Conaway MR, et al. Reduced rates of metabolism and decreased physical activity in breast cancer patients receiving adjuvant chemotherapy. *Am J Clin Nutr* 65:1495–1501, 1997.

PHYSICAL FITNESS ACTIVITY 11.1

Test Your Risk from UV Radiation

Your risk of skin cancer is related to your skin type and the amount of time you spend in the sun. How sensitive are you?

	Yes	No
1. I have blond or red hair.	❏	❏
2. I have light-colored eyes (blue, gray, green).	❏	❏
3. I freckle easily.	❏	❏
4. I have many moles.	❏	❏
5. I had two or more blistering sunburns as a child.	❏	❏
6. I spent lots of time in a tropical climate as a child.	❏	❏
7. There is a family history of skin cancer.	❏	❏
8. I work outdoors.	❏	❏
9. I spend a lot of time in outdoor activities.	❏	❏
10. I like to spend as much time in the sun as I can.	❏	❏

Note: Score 10 points for each "Yes." Add another 10 points if you go to tanning parlors or use a sun lamp.

Score

80–110 *High-risk zone*
Limit time in the sun, always wear a sunscreen outdoors, and use protective clothing and a hat.

40–70 *Increased risk*
Use a sunscreen and hat regularly. Avoid exposure at midday, when the sun is most intense.

10–30 *Still at risk*
Use a sunscreen regularly.

Source: FDA Consumer, July / August 1995.

PHYSICAL FITNESS ACTIVITY 11.2

Eating Smart for Cancer Prevention

How Do You Rate?

Following is a quick, simple eating quiz for all ages, which looks at how your diet compares to the American Cancer Society's guidelines. Below each category of food are examples. When rating yourself, think of foods similar to those listed, which are in your diet. Circle the points for the answer you choose, then total your points. Compare your score with the analysis at the end of the quiz. Remember: A poor score does not mean that you will get cancer, nor does a high score guarantee that you will not. Nonetheless, your score will give you a clue to how you eat now and where you need to improve to reduce your cancer risks.

Important: This eating quiz is really for self-information and does not evaluate your intake of essential vitamins, minerals, protein, or calories. If your diet is restricted in some ways (e.g., you are a vegetarian or have allergies) you may want to get professional advice.

Oils and Fats		Points
(butter, margarine, shortening, mayonnaise, sour cream, lard, oil, salad dressing)	I always add these to foods in cooking and/or at the table.	0
	I occasionally add these to foods in cooking and/or at the table.	1
	I rarely add these to foods in cooking and/or at the table	2
	I eat fried foods 3 or more times a week.	0
	I eat fried foods 1 to 2 times a week.	1
	I rarely eat fried foods.	2

Dairy Products		
	I drink whole milk.	0
	I drink 1%, 2% milk.	1
	I drink nonfat milk.	2
	I eat ice cream almost every day.	0
	Instead of ice cream, I eat ice milk, low-fat frozen yogurt, and sherbet.	1
	I eat only fruit ices, seldom eat frozen dairy desserts.	2
	I eat mostly high-fat cheese (jack, Cheddar, Colby, Swiss, cream).	0
	I eat both low- and high-fat cheeses.	1
	I eat mostly low-fat cheese (pot, 2% cottage, skim-milk mozzarella).	2

Snacks		
(potato/corn chips, buttered popcorn, candy bars)	I eat these every day.	0
	I eat some occasionally.	1
	I seldom or never eat these snacks.	2

Baked Goods		Points
(pies, cakes, cookies, sweet rolls, doughnuts)	I eat them 5 or more times a week.	0
	I eat them 2 to 4 times a week.	1
	I seldom eat baked goods or eat only low-fat baked goods.	2

Poultry and Fish*		
	I rarely eat these foods.	0
	I eat them 1 to 2 times a week.	1
	I eat them 3 or more times a week.	2

Low-Fat Meats*		
(extra lean hamburger, round steak, pork loin roast, tenderloin, chuck roast)	I rarely eat these foods.	0
	I eat these foods occasionally.	1
	I eat mostly fat-trimmed red meats.	2

High-Fat Meats*		
(luncheon meats, bacon, hot dogs, sausage, steak, regular and lean ground beef)	I eat these every day.	0
	I eat these foods occasionally.	1
	I rarely eat these foods.	2

Cured and Smoked Meat and Fish*		
(luncheon meats, hot dogs, bacon, ham, and other smoked or pickled meats and fish)	I eat these foods 4 or more times a week.	0
	I eat these foods 1 to 3 times a week.	1
	I seldom eat these foods.	2

Legumes		
(dried beans and peas: kidney, navy, lima, pinto, garbanzo, split pea, lentil)	I eat legumes less than once a week.	0
	I eat these foods 1 to 2 times a week.	1
	I eat them 3 or more times a week.	2

(continued)

Whole Grains and Cereals		Points
(whole-grain breads, brown rice, pasta, whole-grain cereals)	I seldom eat such foods.	0
	I eat them 2 to 3 times a day.	1
	I eat them 4 or more times daily.	2

Vitamin C–Rich Fruits and Vegetables		
(citrus fruits and juices, green peppers, strawberries, tomatoes)	I seldom eat them.	0
	I eat them 3 to 5 times a week.	1
	I eat them 1 to 2 times a day.	2

Dark Green and Deep Yellow Fruits and Vegetables**		
(broccoli, greens, carrots, peaches)	I seldom eat them.	0
	I eat them 1 to 2 times a week.	1
	I eat them 3 to 4 times a week.	2

Vegetables of the Cabbage Family		
(broccoli, cabbage, Brussels sprouts, cauliflower)	I seldom eat them.	0
	I eat them 1 to 2 times a week.	1
	I eat them 3 to 4 times a week.	2

Alcohol		
	I drink more than 2 oz. daily.	0
	I drink alcohol every week but not daily.	1
	I occasionally or never drink alcohol.	2

Personal Weight		Points
	I'm more than 20 lbs. over my ideal weight.	0
	I'm 10 to 20 lbs. over my ideal weight.	1
	I am within 10 lbs. of my ideal weight.	2

TOTAL SCORE		_____

* If you do not eat meat, fish, or poultry, give yourself a 2 for each meat category.

** Dark green and yellow fruits and vegetables contain beta-carotene, which your body can turn into vitamin A, which helps protect you against certain types of cancer-causing substances.

Scoring

0–12   A Warning Signal: Your diet is too high in fat and too low in fiber-rich foods. It would be wise to assess your eating habits to see where you could make improvements.

13–17   Not Bad! You're Partway There: You still have a way to go. Review the Food Guide Pyramid (see Chapter 9). This will help you determine where you can make a few improvements.

18–36   Good for You! You're Eating Smart: You should feel very good about yourself. You have been careful to limit your fats and eat a varied diet. Keep up the good habits and continue to look for ways to improve.

Source: The American Cancer Society.

There is a strong link between type 2 diabetes and sedentary living. The biggest benefits appear to be found among those who incorporate some level of regular physical activity into their daily lives. Physical activity, as recommended by the Surgeon General, would seem to be a prudent strategy for all people, especially those who are at risk or have type 2 diabetes.

—Andrea Kriska, University of Pittsburgh, Graduate School of Public Health

Diabetes mellitus gets it name from the ancient Greek work for *siphon* (a kind of tube) because early physicians noted that diabetics tend to be unusually thirsty and to urinate a lot. The *mellitus* part of the term is from the Latin version of the ancient Greek word for honey, used because doctors in centuries past diagnosed the disease by the sweet taste of the patient's urine.

Diabetes impairs the body's ability to burn the fuel or glucose it gets from food for energy. Glucose is carried to the body's cells by the blood, but the cells need insulin, which is made by the pancreas, to allow glucose to move inside. Without insulin, glucose accumulates in the blood and then is dumped into the urine by the kidneys (see Figure 12.1).

This sometimes happens because the cells of the pancreas that make insulin—the beta cells—are mostly or entirely destroyed by the body's own immune system. The patient then needs insulin injections to survive and is diagnosed with type 1 diabetes. In type 2 diabetes, the person's beta cells do make insulin, but the patient's tissues are not sensitive enough to the hormone and use it inefficiently.

PREVALENCE AND INCIDENCE OF DIABETES MELLITUS

Approximately 15.7 million Americans (5.9%) have diabetes.[1-4] Of these, 10.3 million are diagnosed and 5.4 million undiagnosed. It is estimated that another 13.4 million persons have impaired fasting glucose, placing them at high risk for the development of diabetes.[2,4] Each year, just under 800,000 new cases of diabetes are diagnosed. Forty percent of all diabetics (6.3 million) are age 65 years or older, and among the elderly, nearly one in five has diabetes (see Figure 12.2). About one in twelve American adults 20 years and older has diabetes, with the ratio rising to one in nine among Mexican Americans and African Americans. There are approximately 123,000 cases of diabetes in U.S. children and teenagers. Type 1 diabetes accounts for 5–10% of all diagnosed cases, with type 2 diabetes accounting for 90–95%.[2,4]

DEFINITION AND DESCRIPTION OF DIABETES MELLITUS

Diabetes mellitus is defined as a group of metabolic diseases characterized by high blood glucose (i.e., hyperglycemia) resulting from defects in insulin secretion, insulin action, or both.[2] The chronic hyperglycemia of diabetes is associated with long-term damage, dysfunction, and failure of various organs, especially the eyes, kidneys, nerves, heart, and blood vessels.

Symptoms of hyperglycemia include excessive urination (*polyuria*), excessive and prolonged thirst (*polydipsia*), weight loss, sometimes with excessive eating (*polyphagia*),

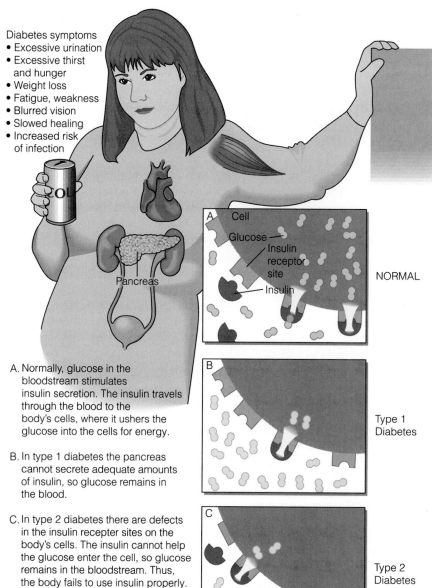

Diabetes symptoms
- Excessive urination
- Excessive thirst and hunger
- Weight loss
- Fatigue, weakness
- Blurred vision
- Slowed healing
- Increased risk of infection

Pancreas

A   Cell
Glucose
Insulin receptor site
Insulin
NORMAL

B
Type 1 Diabetes

C
Type 2 Diabetes

A. Normally, glucose in the bloodstream stimulates insulin secretion. The insulin travels through the blood to the body's cells, where it ushers the glucose into the cells for energy.

B. In type 1 diabetes the pancreas cannot secrete adequate amounts of insulin, so glucose remains in the blood.

C. In type 2 diabetes there are defects in the insulin recepter sites on the body's cells. The insulin cannot help the glucose enter the cell, so glucose remains in the bloodstream. Thus, the body fails to use insulin properly. In some patients, the pancreas makes some insulin, but not enough.

Figure 12.1   Symptoms and effects of diabetes. The cells need insulin to allow glucose to move inside. Diabetes mellitus is a group of diseases characterized by high levels of blood glucose resulting from defects in insulin secretion, insulin action, or both.

and blurred vision[1-4] (see Box 12.1). Impairment of growth and susceptibility to certain infections may also occur. Acute, life-threatening consequences of diabetes include hyperglycemia with *ketoacidosis* (acidosis caused by production of ketone bodies in uncontrolled diabetes).

Complications of Diabetes

Diabetes mellitus is related to many health problems, costing society nearly $100 billion each year in direct and indirect costs.[1,4] Long-term complications of diabetes include[1-4]

- *Heart disease.* Heart disease is the leading cause of diabetes-related deaths. Adults with diabetes have heart disease death rates about two to four times as high as the rates of adults without diabetes (see Figure 12.3).

- *Stroke.* The risk of stroke is two to four times higher in people with diabetes (Figure 12.3).

- *Overall mortality.* Since 1932, diabetes has ranked among the 10 leading causes of death in the United States, and is currently ranked seventh (see Table 11.1).[5] It is the cause of nearly 60,000 deaths annually

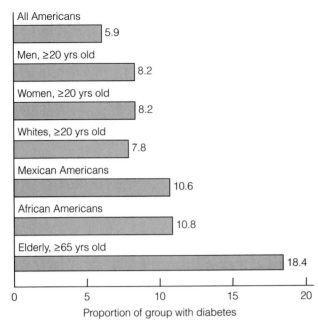

Figure 12.2 Prevalence of diabetes mellitus in the United States—15.7 million Americans have diabetes (10.3 million diagnosed, 5.4 million undiagnosed). One in 12 American men and women have diabetes, with proportions highest among the elderly. *Source:* Centers for Disease Control and Prevention. *National Diabetes Fact Sheet: National Estimates and General Information on Diabetes in the United States.* Atlanta, GA: U.S. Department of Health and Human Services, Centers for Disease Control and Prevention, 1997.

Box 12.1

The Symptoms of Diabetes

The symptoms of type 1 diabetes differ somewhat from those of type 2 diabetes.

Type 1

- Frequent urination
- Unusual thirst
- Extreme hunger
- Unusual weight loss
- Extreme fatigue
- Irritability

Type 2

- Any type 1 symptoms
- Frequent infections
- Blurred vision
- Cuts or bruises that are slow to heal
- Tingling or numbness in the hands or feet
- Recurring skin, gum, or bladder infections

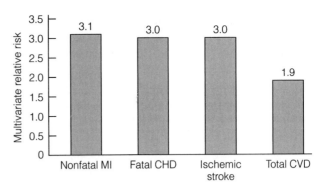

Figure 12.3 Diabetes and risk of cardiovascular disease in women: Relative risk after control for other known risk factors. Risk of nonfatal and fatal heart disease and stroke for diabetics was tripled in this large 8-year study of U.S. nurses. *Source:* Data from Manson JE, Colditz GA, Stampfer, MJ, et al. A prospective study of maturity-onset diabetes mellitus and risk of coronary heart disease and stroke in women. *Arch Intern Med* 151:1141–1147, 1991.

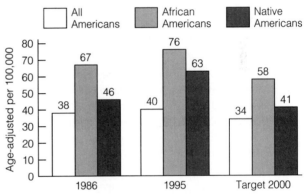

Includes all mentions of diabetes on death certificates

Figure 12.4 Diabetes-related mortality rate. Diabetes-related mortality rates are especially high among African Americans and Native Americans, with no progress made since 1986 in decreasing the rates to year 2000 goals established by the Public Health Service. *Source:* National Center for Health Statistics. *Healthy People 2000 Review, 1997.* Hyattsville, MD: Public Health Service, 1997.

and contributes to at least an additional 130,000 deaths. Studies have found death rates to be twice as high among middle-aged people with diabetes as among middle-aged people without diabetes. Figure 12.4 shows that mortality rates from diabetes mellitus rose between 1986 and 1995.[6]

- *High blood pressure.* An estimated 60–65% of people with diabetes have high blood pressure.

- *Blindness.* Diabetes is the leading cause of new cases of blindness in adults 20–74 years old. Diabetic retinopathy causes 12,000–24,000 new cases of blindness each year.

- *Kidney disease.* Diabetes is the leading cause of end-stage renal disease, accounting for about 40% of new cases. About 30,000 people with diabetes develop end-stage renal disease each year, with about 100,000 receiving dialysis or kidney transplantation.

- *Nervous system disease.* About 60–70% of people with diabetes have mild to severe forms of nervous system damage (which often includes impaired sensation or pain in the feet or hands, slowed digestion of food in the stomach, carpal tunnel syndrome, and other nerve problems). Severe forms of diabetic nerve disease are a major contributing cause of lower-extremity amputations.

- *Amputations.* More than half of lower-limb amputations in the United States occur among people with diabetes. From 1993 to 1995, about 67,000 amputations were performed each year among people with diabetes.

- *Dental disease. Periodontal disease* (a type of gum disease that can lead to tooth loss) occurs with greater frequency and severity among people with diabetes. Periodontal disease has been reported to occur among 30% of people age 19 years or older with type 1 diabetes.

- *Complications of pregnancy.* The rate of major congenital malformations in babies born to women with preexisting diabetes varies from 0% to 5% among women who receive preconception care to 10% among women who do not receive preconception care. Between 3% and 5% of pregnancies among women with diabetes result in death of the newborn; the rate for women who do not have diabetes is 1.5%.

- *Other complications.* Diabetes can directly cause acute life-threatening events, such as diabetic ketoacidosis and hyperosmolar nonketotic coma. People with diabetes are more susceptible to many other illnesses. For example, they are more likely to die of pneumonia or influenza than people who do not have diabetes.

- *Psychosocial dysfunction.* Psychological problems, depression, and anxiety often arise in patients and their families, due to the emotional and social impact of diabetes and to the demands of therapy.[7] Type 2 diabetics have been reported to be at increased risk for the development of dementia such as Alzheimer's disease.[8]

Classification of Diabetes Mellitus

There are four categories of diabetes mellitus:[2]

- Type 1 diabetes
- Type 2 diabetes

- Gestational diabetes (develops during the pregnancy, but disappears afterward)
- Other specific types of diabetes (result from specific genetic syndromes, surgery, drugs, malnutrition, infections, and other illnesses)

Since 1997, diabetes experts have recommended eliminating the old categories of "insulin-dependent diabetes mellitus" (IDDM) and "non–insulin-dependent diabetes mellitus" (NIDDM) because they are based on treatment, which can vary considerably, and does not indicate the underlying problem.[2] Further, in discussing the types of diabetes, the use of Arabic (type 1 and type 2) rather than Roman (type I and type II) numerals is recommended, to prevent confusion (e.g., type II being read as "type eleven"). (Box 12.2 provides a listing of websites where updated information on diabetes is available.)

Type 1 Diabetes Mellitus

Approximately 700,000 Americans have type 1 diabetes, a disease characterized by destruction of the pancreatic beta cells that produce insulin, usually leading to absolute insulin deficiency—that is, a total failure to produce insulin.[1–4] People with type 1 diabetes are prone to ketoacidosis (a life-threatening acidosis of the body due to the production of ketone bodies during fatty acid breakdown). Risk factors are less well defined for type 1 diabetes than for type 2 diabetes, but autoimmune, genetic, and environmental factors are involved. There are two major forms of type 1 diabetes:[2]

1. *Immune-mediated diabetes* results from an autoimmune destruction of the beta cells; it typically starts in children or young adults who are slim but can arise in adults of any age. In this form of diabetes, the rate of beta cell destruction is quite variable, being rapid in some individuals (mainly infants and children) and slow in others (mainly adults). Immune-mediated diabetes commonly occurs in childhood and adolescence, but it can occur at any age, even in the eighth and ninth decades of life. Autoimmune destruction of beta cells has multiple genetic predispositions and is also related to environmental factors that are still poorly defined.

2. *Idiopathic diabetes* refers to rare forms of the disease that have no known cause. This form of diabetes is strongly inherited and lacks immunological evidence for beta cell destruction.

Type 2 Diabetes Mellitus

Type 2 diabetes usually arises because of insulin resistance, in which the body fails to use insulin properly, combined with relative (rather than absolute) insulin deficiency.[2,9] People with type 2 can range from predominantly insulin

Take Charge of Your Diabetes, updated guidelines for persons with diabetes, is available on the World Wide Web site of CDC's Division of Diabetes Translation, National Center for Chronic Disease Prevention and Health Promotion, at http://www.cdc.gov/nccdphp/ddt/tcoyd.htm. This document provides information about the value of teamwork to control glucose, community and family support, and steps to help promote health and prevent complications.

Additional information about diabetes is available from websites of the following organizations:

- CDC's National Center for Chronic Disease Prevention and Health Promotion, Division of Diabetes Translation—http://www.cdc.gov/diabetes
- CDC's National Center for Health Statistics—http://www.cdc.gov/nchswww/nchshome.htm
- Department of Veterans Affairs—http://www.va.gov/health/diabetes
- Health Resources and Services Administration—http://www.hrsa.dhhs.gov
- Indian Health Service—http://www.ihs.gov/IHSmain.html
- National Diabetes Information Clearinghouse, National Institute of Diabetes and Digestive and Kidney Diseases of the National Institutes of Health—http://www.niddk.nih.gov
- Office of Minority Health, US Department of Health and Human Services—http://www.omhrc.gov
- American Association of Diabetes Educators—http://www.diabetesnet.com/aade.html
- American Diabetes Association—http://diabetes.org
- Juvenile Diabetes Foundation International—http://www.jdfcure.com

- *Type 2 diabetes develops gradually.* For a long period of time before type 2 is detected or noticed, blood glucose levels are often high enough to cause pathological changes in various organs and tissues, without clinical symptoms.[9]

- *Most do not need insulin.* At least initially, and often throughout their lifetime, type 2 diabetics do not need insulin treatment to survive.

- *Not ketosis prone.* Ketoacidosis seldom occurs spontaneously in type 2 diabetics.

- *Has multiple risk factors.* Type 2 diabetes typically occurs in people who are over 45 years old, overweight, and sedentary, and who have a family history of diabetes. Most patients with type 2 diabetes are obese, and obesity itself causes some degree of insulin resistance. Type 2 diabetes occurs more frequently in women with prior gestational diabetes mellitus, and in individuals with high blood pressure and high blood LDL cholesterol and triglycerides. African Americans, Hispanic/Latino Americans, Native Americans, and some Asian Americans and Pacific Islanders are at particularly high risk for type 2 diabetes.[1–4,10] (See Physical Fitness Activity 12.1 at the end of this chapter.) Many type 2 diabetics have the "insulin resistance syndrome" (sometimes called the "X" syndrome), which includes obesity, high blood pressure, high blood insulin levels, and dyslipidemia. This syndrome is strongly associated with high morbidity and mortality rates.[10]

- *Has a genetic link.* Type 2 diabetes is often associated with a strong genetic predisposition, but the genetics of this form of diabetes are complex and not clearly defined.

Testing and Diagnosis

In 1997, an international expert committee recommended lowering the number for diagnosis on the most commonly used test for diabetes and has urged that consideration be given to wide-scale screening and testing in order to detect diabetes at an earlier stage and help prevent or delay the onset of serious and costly complications.[2] The expert committee was convened under the auspices of the American Diabetes Association. The expert committee's work is an update of a similar process last undertaken in 1979 by the National Diabetes Data Group, and its recommendations are based on a 2-year review of more than 15 years of research.

The new recommendations are based on data from population-based research showing that serious complications of diabetes begin earlier than previously thought. For

resistant with relative insulin deficiency to predominantly deficient in insulin secretion with some insulin resistance. Approximately 15.3 million Americans have type 2 diabetes, making this the most common type.[4]

Chief characteristics of type 2 diabetes include the following:[2]

the first time, the committee also recommends that the health-care community consider testing for diabetes in all adults starting at age 45, and if normal, repeat testing at 3-year intervals.[2] Testing should be considered at a younger age, or be carried out more frequently, in individuals at high risk for diabetes.

Diabetes can be diagnosed in any one of the following three ways, confirmed on a different day (by any one of the three methods):[2]

- A *fasting plasma glucose* that is equal to or greater than 126 mg/dl (after no caloric intake for at least 8 hours)

- A *casual plasma glucose* (taken at any time of day, without regard to time of last meal) that is equal to or greater than 200 mg/dl, with the classic diabetes symptoms of increased urination, increased thirst, and unexplained weight loss

- An *oral glucose tolerance test* (OGTT) value that is equal to or greater than 200 mg/dl in the 2-hour sample (For the OGTT, the glucose load should contain 75 grams of anhydrous glucose dissolved in water.)

The fasting plasma glucose is the preferred test and is recommended for testing and diagnosis because of its ease of administration, convenience, acceptability to patients, and lower cost (compared to the OGTT).[2] The categories of fasting plasma glucose values are as follows:

- <110 mg/dl = normal fasting glucose
- 110 to 125 mg/dl = impaired fasting glucose
- ≥126 mg/dl = diagnosis of diabetes (after confirmation on a separate day)

The hemoglobin A_{1c} test (also known as HbA1c or glycosylated hemoglobin) is not, at this time, recommended for diagnosis. The hemoglobin A_{1c} test, however, is used to assess the effectiveness of treatment of patients with diabetes because it is a good measure of long-term blood glucose concentrations. Hemoglobin A_{1c} levels of 7% or higher often require pharmacological intervention, while those below 7% can generally be treated with diet, exercise, and weight loss.[11] It should also be noted that the finger-prick test used by people with diabetes to monitor their blood glucose levels, and sometimes used at health fairs and diabetes risk assessments among the general public, is not considered a diagnostic procedure.[2]

Impaired Fasting Glucose

A fasting plasma glucose value of 110 mg/dl is the upper limit of normal blood glucose. There are two categories of impaired glucose metabolism (or impaired glucose homeostasis) that are considered risk factors for future diabetes and cardiovascular disease:[2]

1. *Impaired fasting glucose* (IFG), a new category, when fasting plasma glucose is >110 to 126 mg/dl; about 13.4 million persons, 7.0% of the population, are estimated to have impaired fasting glucose

2. *Impaired glucose tolerance* (IGT), when results of the more complicated oral glucose tolerance test are ≥140 but <200 mg/dl (in the 2-hour sample)

A plasma glucose value of 60–110 mg/dl is normal. Many people feel they are afflicted with hypoglycemia or low blood sugar, a condition popularized in several books devoted to this topic. However, true hypoglycemia is a rare condition seen in less than 1% of the general population.[12] Hypoglycemia is diagnosed when the plasma glucose level drops below 50 mg/dl within a few hours of eating a regular meal, while the patient is experiencing symptoms (weakness, fatigue, stress, headache, trembling, etc.). If the symptoms and low plasma glucose level appear together after the meal, and if the symptoms are relieved soon after eating, hypoglycemia is diagnosed. Hypoglycemia is actually more common among diabetics who use too high a dose of insulin or use it at the wrong time in relationship to dietary and exercise habits.

Risk Factors and Screening for Diabetes

Testing for diabetes should be considered in all adults starting at age 45, and if normal, these tests should be repeated at 3-year intervals[2] (see Figure 12.5). Physicians should consider testing at a younger age, or more frequently, those who are at higher risk of diabetes, including people who have the following characteristics:[2]

- Are obese (more than 20% above their ideal body weight)

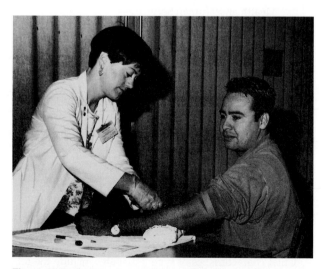

Figure 12.5   Fasting plasma glucose levels should be measured in all adults at age 45 and above, and, if normal, the tests should be reported at 3-year intervals.

- Have a first-degree relative with diabetes
- Are members of a high-risk ethnic group (African American, Hispanic, Native American, Asian)
- Delivered a baby weighing more than 9 pounds or were diagnosed with gestational diabetes mellitus, a condition that can arise during pregnancy and usually disappears thereafter but tends to lead to type 2 in later years
- Are hypertensive (blood pressure at or above 140/90)
- Have an HDL cholesterol level of 35 mg/dl or lower and/or a triglyceride level of 250 mg/dl or higher
- On previous testing, had IFG or IGT

Special Recommendations for Pregnant Women

Gestational diabetes mellitus (GDM) is defined as any degree of glucose intolerance with onset or first recognition during pregnancy.[2] In the majority of cases of GDM, glucose regulation will return to normal after delivery, but it is, nonetheless, a risk factor for the development of diabetes later in life. Although gestational diabetes complicates about 4% of U.S. pregnancies (about 135,000 cases each year), the former recommendation for screening of all pregnant women has been dropped.[2] Pregnant women at low risk who meet *all* of the following criteria do not need to be screened: less than 25 years of age, normal body weight, no family history of diabetes, and not a member of an ethnic group with a high prevalence of diabetes (e.g., Hispanic, Native American, Asian, African American).

Screening for GDM should be performed between 24 and 28 weeks of gestation, and the patient need not be fasting.[2] A plasma glucose value ≥140 mg/dl taken 1 hour after ingesting a 50-gram glucose load indicates the need for a full diagnostic, 100-gram, 3-hour OGTT performed in the fasting state. The diagnosis of GDM requires any two of the four plasma glucose values obtained during the 100-gram OGTT test to meet or exceed these values:[2]

- *Fasting,* 105 mg/dl
- *One hour following ingestion,* 190 mg/dl
- *Two hours,* 165 mg/dl
- *Three hours,* 145 mg/dl

OBESITY AND TYPE 2 DIABETES

Rates for type 2 diabetes rise dramatically as the modernized lifestyle is adopted by people from developing societies. For example, in China, the prevalence of diabetes rose threefold during a recent 10-year period, as changes were made from a traditional to a modernized lifestyle.[13] Among Japanese American men, those retaining a more traditional Japanese lifestyle experienced a reduced prevalence of diabetes.[14]

In the United States, approximately 85% of patients with type 2 diabetes are obese at the time of diagnosis. "Diabesity" has been used to describe this phenomenon. As shown in Figures 12.6 and 12.7, the risk for developing type 2 diabetes rises in direct relationship to the degree of obesity for both men and women.[15-17] In one 5-year study of more than 20,000 U.S. male physicians,[15] risk of type 2 diabetes tripled when the body mass index rose above 26.4 kg/m² (Figure 12.6). In a 14-year study of more than 114,000 female nurses, after adjustment for age, body mass index was the dominant predictor of risk for type 2 diabetes[16] (Figure 12.7). Women who gained weight during the study increased their risk for type 2 diabetes, while those who lost weight decreased their risk. These data indicate that women can minimize the risk for diabetes by achieving a lean body build as a young adult and avoiding even modest weight gain throughout life. Another study showed that for both men and women, gaining just 10 pounds increased the risk for developing diabetes by about 25%.[18]

In severely obese populations, such as the Pima Indians and Nauruans, the prevalence of type 2 diabetes is the highest worldwide.[19] Obesity, especially upper-body or abdominal obesity, is associated with insulin resistance (a decreased ability of the body to respond to the action of insulin, and a reduced number of insulin receptors). A growing number of studies have shown that the risk of type 2 diabetes climbs in direct proportion to the increase in waist circumference or the waist-to-hip ratio (i.e., when the abdominal girth approaches or exceeds the hip girth).[19-21] As shown in Figure 12.8, a 10-inch difference in the waist circumference (e.g., 28 versus 38 inches) increases the risk of type 2 diabetes sixfold.[17] Several other studies have shown that when body weight, especially abdominal fat, is

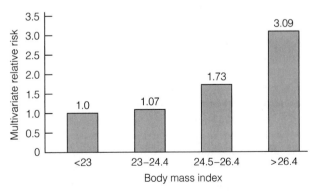

Figure 12.6 Body mass index as a predictor of diabetes: Relative risk of type 2 diabetes. In this 5-year study of 21,271 U.S. male physicians, risk of type 2 diabetes tripled when the body mass index (kg/m²) rose above 26.4. *Source:* Manson JE, Nathan DM, Krolewski AS, et al. A prospective study of exercise and incidence of diabetes among U.S. male physicians. *JAMA* 268: 63–67, 1992.

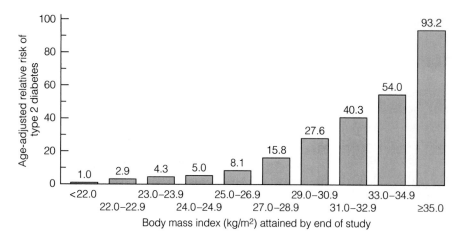

Figure 12.7 Attained body mass index and risk of diabetes, in 114,834 U.S. women age 30–55 years in 1976 and followed 14 years. Risk of type 2 diabetes rises strongly with increase in degree of obesity in women. *Source:* Colditz GA, Willett WC, Rotnitzky A, Manson JE. Weight gain as a risk factor for clinical diabetes mellitus in women. *Ann Intern Med* 122:481–486, 1995.

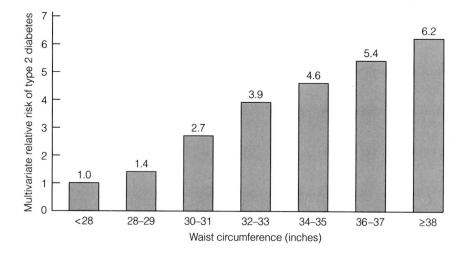

Figure 12.8 Waist circumference and risk of type 2 diabetes, 8-year study of 43,581 nurses. Risk of developing type 2 diabetes rises in direct relationship to waist circumference in women. *Source:* Carey VJ, Walters EE, Colditz GA, et al. Body fat distribution and risk of non-insulin-dependent diabetes mellitus in women: The Nurses' Health Study. *Am J Epidemiol* 145:614–619, 1997.

lost, insulin resistance is reduced, and blood glucose levels either improve or often return to normal.[18–21]

The estimated reduction in the risk of type 2 diabetes associated with maintaining desirable body weight compared with being obese is 50–75%, considerably higher than the 30–50% reduction in risk associated with regular, moderate or vigorous exercise versus a sedentary lifestyle.[19] Thus, avoidance of weight gain with increasing age is the most important prevention measure for type 2 diabetes.[15–23]

Few studies have been conducted on the role of diet in the development of type 2 diabetes. In one 6-year study of more than 65,000 nurses, researchers from the Harvard School of Public Health showed that the risk of developing diabetes was 2.5 times greater in those using refined and processed grain products (low in dietary fiber), compared to those using grains in a minimally refined form (high in fiber)[24] (see Figure 12.9). These same results were confirmed in a cohort of 42,759 men.[25] These studies suggest that grains should be consumed in a minimally refined form to

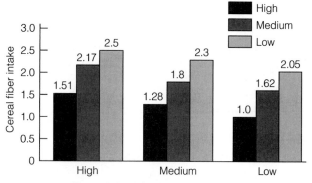

Figure 12.9 Type 2 diabetes risk by cereal fiber intake and glycemic load, 6-year study of 65,173 nurses. The risk of developing diabetes is 2.5 times higher in those using refined and processed grain products that are low in dietary fiber. *Source:* Salmerón J, Manson JE, Stampfer MJ, Colditz GA, Wing AL, Willett WC. Dietary fiber, glycemic load, and risk of non-insulin-dependent diabetes mellitus in women. *JAMA* 277:472–477, 1997.

reduce the risk of type 2 diabetes. It should be noted that while there are few data on dietary habits and risk of developing type 2 diabetes, substantial evidence exists in support of a diet high in carbohydrate and fiber and low in fat in the treatment of types 2 diabetes. (See Sports Medicine Insight at the end of this chapter.) Box 9.3 in Chapter 9 provides more information on the glycemic index.

TREATMENT OF DIABETES

Treatment for either type of diabetes seeks to accomplish what the human body normally does naturally: maintain a proper balance between glucose and insulin. Food makes the blood glucose level rise, while insulin and exercise make it fall. The challenge is to manage these three factors to keep the blood glucose within a narrow range. Training in self-management is integral to the treatment of diabetes. Treatment must be individualized and must address medical, psychosocial, and lifestyle issues.[26–28]

Type 1 Diabetes

Lack of insulin production by the pancreas makes type 1 diabetes particularly difficult to control. Because there is no cure for type 1 diabetes, treatment is lifelong. For the individual with type 1 diabetes, to keep the blood glucose within narrow limits and avoid the medical complications, a regular and consistent lifestyle must be followed.[1,11] Eating times, amounts and types of foods, and physical activity should be consistent from one day to the next. Blood glucose should be measured several times a day, and multiple insulin injections or treatment with an insulin pump is necessary. Periodic measurement of glycosylated hemoglobin is important to monitor long-term glycemic control.[11,29]

Results from a major multicenter study by the Diabetes Control and Complications Trial (DCCT) Research Group have shown that when type 1 diabetes patients keep their blood glucose levels under tight control through intensive care, fewer medical complications develop.[30,31] The study showed that keeping blood glucose levels as close to normal as possible slowed the onset and progression of eye, kidney, and nerve diseases caused by diabetes. In fact, it demonstrated that *any* sustained lowering of blood glucose helps, even if the person has a history of poor control. Elements of intensive management in the DCCT included the following:[30]

- Testing blood glucose levels four or more times a day
- Four daily insulin injections or use of an insulin pump
- Adjustment of insulin doses according to food intake and exercise

- A diet and exercise plan
- Monthly visits to a health-care team composed of a physician, nurse educator, dietitian, and behavioral therapist

One problem with intensive therapy is poor patient compliance and acceptance. In the DCCT, the most significant side effect of intensive treatment was an increase in the risk for low blood glucose episodes severe enough to require assistance from another person (severe hypoglycemia). Because of this risk, DCCT researchers do not recommend intensive therapy for children under age 13, people with heart disease or other advanced complications, older adults, and people with a history of frequent severe hypoglycemia.[30,31] Some patients also gain weight during intensive therapy, suggesting that this plan may not be appropriate for overweight diabetics. DCCT researchers estimated that intensive management doubled the cost of managing diabetes. However, this cost appears to be offset by the reduction in medical expenses related to long-term complications and by the improved quality of life of people with type 1 diabetes.

Implantable, programmable insulin pumps are gaining favor with many diabetes experts.[32,33] Although first considered primarily for type 1 diabetic patients, research data also suggest that type 2 diabetics requiring insulin therapy can also gain benefit.[33] The devices weigh about ½ pound and are surgically implanted just under the skin in the abdomen. A catheter delivers insulin into the abdominal cavity. Insulin refills are performed transcutaneously with a syringe every 4–12 weeks. Long-term studies show that glycemic control is improved with pump therapy.[32,33] Severe hypoglycemia and weight gain are relatively rare, and patients report high satisfaction and improved quality of life.

Type 2 Diabetes

Treatment of type 2 diabetes usually includes diet control, exercise, home blood glucose testing, and in some cases, oral medication and/or insulin.[1,9,26,28] Approximately 30–40% of people with type 2 diabetes require insulin injections. Most experts recommend that a staged approach to diabetic treatment be followed for type 2 diabetes patients.[26] Because the vast majority are obese, weight loss through a healthy diet (i.e., low in fat, with an emphasis on carbohydrates and fiber) and exercise is first recommended. If diet, exercise, and weight loss fail to lower blood glucose levels (most often due to patient noncompliance with the recommended lifestyle changes), the doctor may decide to add an oral sulfonylurea drug, insulin, or both. Sulfonylurea drugs are used only for type 2 diabetes, mainly for patients whose diabetes is judged to be less severe. Insulin is the usual choice for advanced type 2 diabetes cases. Unfortunately, insulin therapy is rarely effective in achieving tight glycemic controls in individuals with type 2 diabetes.[34]

Type 2 diabetes is regarded as largely preventable and treatable through improved lifestyle habits.[19] The single most important objective for the obese individual with type 2 diabetes is to achieve and maintain a desirable body weight.[19,35–39] Weight reduction reduces serum glucose and improves insulin sensitivity, while also favorably influencing several heart disease risk factors. Diabetics who are at high risk for death from heart disease, and who face a future laden with medical complications from high blood glucose levels, have much to gain from losing weight. Unfortunately, various studies have reported that individuals with type 2 diabetes have a poor history of attaining and then maintaining a desirable body weight despite the motivation that comes from having diabetes and seeing improvements in glycemic control with weight loss.[36,38]

Figure 12.10 summarizes how quickly weight loss through a healthy diet and exercise program can influence type 2 diabetes and heart disease risk factors.[35] In this study, 652 type 2 diabetes patients attended the Pritikin Longevity Center 26-day residential program. The group included 212 patients taking insulin and 197 taking oral hypoglycemic agents. The remaining 243 were taking no diabetic medication but had a fasting glucose level above 140 mg/dl. During the 26-day program, the type 2 diabetes patients were involved in daily aerobic exercise, primarily walking (building up to two 1-hour walks each day). Patients were also placed on a high-carbohydrate, high-fiber, low-fat, low-cholesterol, and low-salt diet. Of dietary calories, less than 10% were obtained from fat. The diet contained 35–40 grams of dietary fiber per 1,000 calories, a very high amount according to most standards. During the program, the average patient lost about 10 pounds and experienced great reductions in blood pressure and blood levels of fasting glucose, total cholesterol, and triglycerides. Of patients on insulin, 39% were able to stop therapy, and 71% of patients on oral agents also had their medication discontinued.

Because of the way this study was designed, it is not possible to sort out which lifestyle factor—exercise, weight loss, or improved diet—was most responsible for the impressive results.[35] Although the Pritikin diet has been criticized as being unusually restrictive (and hard to continue once the program stops), the results of this study support a strong emphasis on lifestyle modification consisting of both diet and exercise in the treatment of type 2 diabetes.

Since the 1950s, there has been considerable debate regarding the diet best suited for the diabetic. As is reviewed in the Sports Medicine Insight at the end of this chapter, there has been a progression toward less and less dietary fat and more and more carbohydrate, with an emphasis today on individualizing the diet for each patient.[38] The primary goals of the diabetic diet for type 2 diabetes patients are to lower blood glucose and lipids, blood pressure, and body weight (when necessary). For these reasons, type 2 diabetes patients should follow a healthy and varied diet, with an emphasis on controlling saturated fats.

Impaired Fasting Glucose

As reviewed earlier in this chapter, impaired fasting glucose is a new diagnostic category in which persons have fasting plasma glucose values of 110–125 mg/dl.[2] Scientists are trying to learn how to predict which of these persons will go on to develop diabetes and how to prevent such progression. Several preliminary studies have suggested that improvements in diet and exercise habits can help prevent type 2 diabetes in people with impaired fasting glucose[40] (see Figure 12.11).

EXERCISE AND DIABETES

Researchers have established that type 2 diabetes is less common in physically active, compared to inactive, societies.[15,19,21,23,40–50] Also, as populations have become more sedentary, the incidence of type 2 diabetes has been observed to increase[13,14,42] (Figure 12.12). Type 2 diabetes, for example, is unusually common among some South Pacific

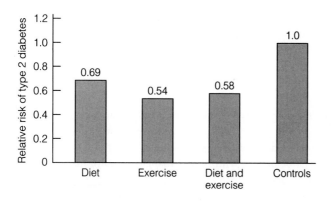

Figure 12.10 Effects of diet and exercise on CHD risk factors in 652 type 2 patients, percentage change after 26-day Pritikin Program (<10% fat, high fiber & carbohydrate diet, 1–2 hours walking/day), in which 71% of subjects taking oral hypoglycemic agents and 39% of those taking insulin discontinued their medication. An intensive diet and exercise program is effective in lowering disease risk factors in type 2 diabetics. *Source:* Barnard RJ, Jung T, Inkeles SB. Diet and exercise in the treatment of NIDDM. *Diabetes Care* 17:1469–1472, 1994.

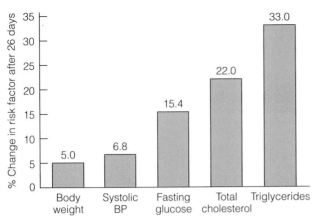

Figure 12.11 Effects of diet and exercise in preventing type 2 diabetes in people with impaired fasting glucose, 6-year study of 530 men and women in China. Diet and exercise were both effective in lowering the risk of developing type 2 diabetes in men and women with impaired fasting glucose. *Source:* Pan XR, Li GW, Hu YH, et al. Effects of diet and exercise in preventing NIDDM in people with impaired glucose tolerance: The Da Qing IGT and diabetes study. *Diabetes Care* 20: 537–544, 1997.

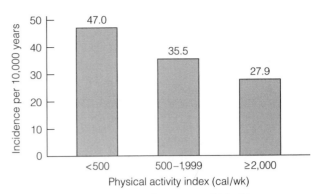

Figure 12.13 Incidence of diabetes among high-risk men, age-adjusted incidence rates of type 2 diabetes. Age-adjusted incidence rates for type 2 diabetes were lowest among the more active "high risk" men (those with obesity, hypertension, or a family history). *Source:* Helmrich SP, Rogland DR, Leung RW, Paffenbarger RS. Physical activity and reduced occurrence of noninsulin-dependent diabetes mellitus. *N Engl J Med* 325: 147–152, 1991.

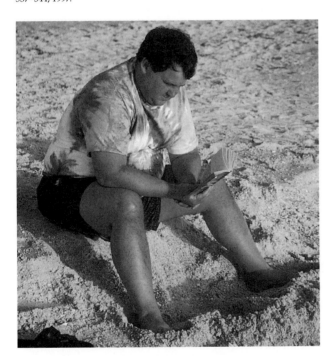

Figure 12.12 Risk of type 2 diabetes is elevated in sedentary societies. (© Myrleen Ferguson / PhotoEdit)

and Native American peoples who have adopted the sedentary habits of the Western world.[19,42] However, experts point out that other environmental and lifestyle factors are probably involved, including changes in body weight and dietary habits.[19]

Physical Activity and Risk of Developing Diabetes

Several major studies have followed large groups of men and women for extended periods of time, measuring the influence of physical activity and inactivity on the risk of developing type 2 diabetes.[15,23,41,44–46,48–50] The studies have provided convincing support for the role of regular physical activity in the prevention of type 2 diabetes.

Data from a 14-year study of nearly 6,000 male alumni of the University of Pennsylvania were published in 1991.[45,51] Leisure-time physical activity was measured and expressed as calories expended per week for walking, stair climbing, and sports. Type 2 diabetes developed in 202 men, and the important finding was that for each 500-Calorie-per-week increase in activity expenditure, the risk of type 2 diabetes was reduced by 6%. For men who were both obese and inactive, the likelihood of developing type 2 diabetes was four times greater than for lean and active men. The protective effect of physical activity was especially strong for men at highest risk for type 2 diabetes, as shown in Figure 12.13. In other words, regular physical activity is an important component of a healthy lifestyle for all adults, but it may be particularly important for those at increased risk for chronic diseases such as type 2 diabetes.

In an 8-year study of 87,253 nurses, women who exercised vigorously at least once a week experienced a 33% reduction in risk of type 2 diabetes.[50] These results are very similar to a 5-year study of 21,271 male physicians[15] (Figure 12.14). Subjects who exercised regularly experienced a 36% reduction in risk of type 2 diabetes, with risk found to

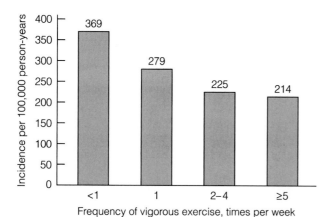

Figure 12.14 Incidence of diabetes among U.S. male physicians, age-adjusted incidence rates of type 2 diabetes. The age-adjusted incidence rate of type 2 diabetes was lower in subjects who exercised vigorously ("enough to work up a sweat") and most frequently in this 5-year study of U.S. physicians. *Source:* Manson JE, Nathan DM, Krolewski AS, et al. A prospective study of exercise and incidence of diabetes among U.S. male physicians. *JAMA* 268:63–67, 1992.

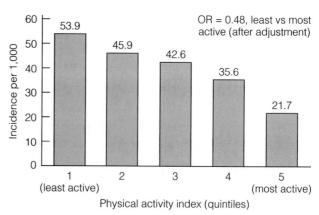

Figure 12.15 Incidence of diabetes among Japanese American men, odds ratio = 0.48, least versus most active (after adjustment). The rate of developing type 2 diabetes was lowest among the most active men. *Source:* Burchfiel CM, Sharp DS, Curb JD, Rodriguez BL, Hwang L-J, Marcus EB, Yano K. Physical activity and incidence of diabetes: The Honolulu heart program. *Am J Epidemiol* 141:360–368, 1995.

be lowest among those exercising most frequently. The benefits of exercise were most pronounced among the obese or those at the highest risk of developing type 2 diabetes.

In Great Britain, 7,735 men were followed for nearly 13 years.[23] The risk of developing type 2 diabetes was found to be reduced by more than 50% among the most physically active when compared to their relatively inactive peers. In Finland, men at high risk for type 2 diabetes who exercised at a moderately intense level for more than 40 minutes per week reduced their risk of developing type 2 diabetes by 64%, compared to men who did not exercise.[41] In Hawaii, a 6-year study of 6,815 Japanese American men came to a similar conclusion.[44] As shown in Figure 12.15, the rate of developing type 2 diabetes was lowest among the most active men, even after adjustment for age, obesity, family history, and other factors known to influence the risk of diabetes. A 10-year study of nearly 3,000 men and women in Finland showed that risk of developing type 2 diabetes was highest among those exercising the least[46] (Figure 12.16).

The Role of Exercise in Treatment of Diabetes

The concept that physical activity is beneficial for the diabetic is not new. It was promoted as a valuable adjunct to diabetic control in 600 A.D. by Chao Yuan-Fang, a prominent Chinese physician of the Sui Dynasty.[52] Even after the isolation of insulin in 1922, exercise was considered one of the three cornerstones of therapy for persons with type 1 diabetes, along with diet and insulin. Although the concept

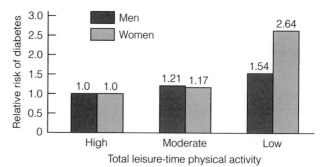

Figure 12.16 Physical activity and risk of type 2 diabetes, 10-year study of 1,340 men and 1,500 women in Finland. Risk of developing type 2 diabetes was highest among men and women exercising the least. *Source:* Haapanen N, Miilunpalo S, Vuori I, Oja P, Pasanen M. Association of leisure time physical activity with the risk of coronary heart disease, hypertension and diabetes in middle-aged men and women. *Int J Epidemiol* 26:739–747, 1997.

that physical activity is beneficial for diabetics is centuries old, there is still considerable controversy regarding its value.

The pancreas secretes two hormones, insulin and glucagon, to help maintain blood glucose levels[53,54] (see Figure 12.17). During rest, when blood glucose levels rise after a meal, insulin is secreted to help move the glucose into the body cells. Receptors on the body cells require that insulin be present before glucose can enter. On the other hand, when blood glucose levels drop, glucagon is secreted to increase blood glucose levels by stimulating the breakdown of liver glycogen.

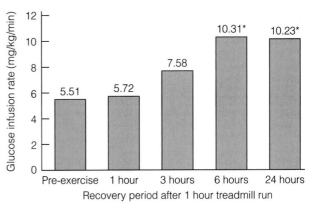

*p < 0.05 vs pre-exercise
Insulin sensitivity defined as glucose infusion rate using the insulin clamp technique

Figure 12.18 Insulin sensitivity after 1 hour of running. Improvements in insulin sensitivity occur within 6 hours of exercise and remain for at least 1 day. *Source:* Oshida Y, Kamanouchi K, Hayamiru S, et al. Effect of training and training cessation on insulin action. *Int J Sports Med* 12:484–486, 1991.

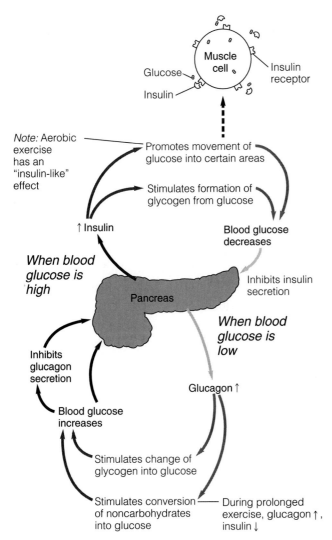

Figure 12.17 Actions of normal pancreas. The pancreas secretes two hormones, insulin and glucagon, to control blood glucose levels. During exercise, glucagon rises while insulin falls to counterbalance the "insulin-like" effect of muscle contraction and the large glucose demands of the working muscle.

During exercise, blood insulin levels drop, while blood glucagon levels increase. These changes take place to counterbalance the insulin-like effect of muscle contraction.[53] As the muscles contract during exercise, they do not require as much insulin to transport glucose into the working cells. The exercising muscle may increase the uptake of glucose 7- to 20-fold during the first 30–40 minutes, depending on the intensity of the exercise. In addition, the insulin receptors become more sensitive to the lower amount of insulin present during exercise.[53–57] This improvement in insulin receptor sensitivity can last for many hours after the exercise bout is over, even for as long as 2 days if the exercise was of long duration and high intensity (see Figure 12.18).

Type 1 Diabetes and Exercise

For nearly 50 years, researchers have known that regular exercise will reduce the insulin requirements of well-controlled type 1 diabetes patients by 30–50%. It appears, however, that each bout of exercise leads to an improvement in insulin sensitivity that lasts for only 1 or 2 days before falling back to pre-exercise levels. In other words, the muscles need regular exercise to maintain an enhanced insulin sensitivity. Bed rest and detraining studies have shown that insulin resistance and impaired glucose tolerance develop quickly, indicating that regular physical activity is required for normal insulin action.[53,54]

A given amount of insulin following exercise is more effective in causing glucose uptake by the cells.[58] The patient with type 1 diabetes who exercises regularly will need smaller than normal insulin doses or will have to increase food intake. Although regular exercise leads to reduced insulin requirements for individuals with type 1 diabetes, studies have failed to show that long-term glucose control is improved, according to the American Diabetic Association (ADA).[59] The ADA still feels that people with type 1 diabetes have much to gain from exercising regularly because of the potential to improve cardiovascular fitness and psychological well-being, and for social interaction and recreation.

Exercise Precautions for Individuals with Type 1 Diabetes

The ADA has urged that safe participation in all forms of exercise, consistent with an individual's lifestyle, should be a primary goal for people with type 1 diabetes.[59] However, physical exercise is not without risks to individuals with type 1 diabetes. While nondiabetic individuals usually experience little change in blood glucose levels during exercise, type 1 diabetes patients may experience an increase (i.e., hyperglycemia) or a decrease (hypoglycemia), depending on their initial levels.[60] Type 1 diabetes patients who have very high blood glucose levels (above 250 mg/dl), with ketones in their urine, can experience a rapid rise in blood glucose upon starting exercise and can develop ketosis. For this reason, individuals with type 1 diabetes should postpone exercise until they have gotten their blood glucose under control through proper diet and insulin therapy.[59]

For most patients with type 1 diabetes who begin exercising, the principal risk is hypoglycemia.[59,60] The ADA cautions that many variables, including fitness, duration and intensity of exercise, and time of exercise regarding insulin administration and meals will affect the metabolic response to exercise.[59] Hypoglycemia is most likely to occur when the exercise is prolonged or intense, when the blood glucose prior to exercise was near normal, and when the exercise takes place shortly after insulin injection into a muscle used during the bout.

To avoid hypoglycemia during or after exercise, a regular pattern of exercise and diet should be adopted, with frequent blood glucose measurements to test the body's response[59,60] (see Box 12.3). Each individual with type 1 diabetes is unique and will need to discover for her- or himself the best schedule to follow to keep the blood glucose under tight control. Exercise should be performed at the same convenient time every day, at approximately the same intensity and for the same amount of time. Morning appears to be preferable to evening for most persons with type 1 diabetes because episodes of delayed hypoglycemia may occur during sleep following late-day exercise.[59,60]

Exercise should not be performed at the time of peak insulin effect (i.e., within 1 hour after an injection of short-acting insulin).[60] Because of the insulin-like effect of exercise, the person with type 1 diabetes initiating an exercise program will have to reduce insulin (by about one third) dosage and/or increase food intake.[59,60] Insulin injections should not be at sites of the body that will be exercised soon thereafter (e.g., thighs that will be used in running or cycling).

During prolonged physical activity, 60–120 calories of carbohydrate (i.e., the amount found in 1–2 cups of most sports drinks) is recommended for each 30 minutes of activity.[60] A meal 1–3 hours before exercise is recommended, and fluids should be taken during and after exercise to avoid dehydration. A carbohydrate snack is recommended soon after unusually strenuous exercise.

Not long ago, the terms *diabetic* and *athlete* seemed mutually exclusive. Today, partly because of the advent of blood glucose self-monitoring and the recognition that ex-

---

Box 12.3

Guidelines for Type 1 Diabetics

The following steps are crucial for type 1 diabetics to avoid hyperglycemia or hypoglycemia during and after exercise.

1. Ingest 40–60 grams of carbohydrate prior to exercise lasting up to 30 minutes. For exercise beyond 30 minutes, consume 15–30 grams carbohydrate for every 30 minutes of moderately intense exercise. A meal 1–3 hours before exercise is recommended.

2. Consume a snack of slowly absorbed carbohydrate (e.g., legumes, fructose, pasta, milk) following prolonged exercise sessions.

3. Reduce the insulin dose before exercise:

   a. *Intermediate-acting insulin.* Reduce by 30–35% on the day of exercise. Inject insulin at least 1 hour before exercise.

   b. *Short-acting insulin.* Omit dose of short-acting insulin that precedes exercise.

   c. *Continuous subcutaneous infusion.* Reduce mealtime increment when exercising just before or after a meal.

4. Avoid exercising the muscle area underlying injections of short-acting insulin for at least 1 hour.

5. Monitor blood glucose before, during, and after exercise.

6. Learn individual glucose responses to different types of exercise.

Source: Young JC. Exercise prescription for individuals with metabolic disorders: Practical considerations. *Sports Med* 19:43–53, 1995.

---

ercise brings multiple benefits, many diabetics have entered the sporting arena with the approval and support of their physicians.[59–63] Nationally known athletes with diabetes have included Ty Cobb, Jackie Robinson, Catfish Hunter, Bobby Clarke, Scott Verplank, and Wade Wilson. Most experts feel that as long as diabetic athletes understand the interactions among diet, exertion, and insulin and are aware of their unique reactions to exercise, they can safely engage in almost any sport or activity.[61–63] Participation in sports during childhood may enhance self-image, provide a sense of accomplishment, and lead to social interactions that are conducive to optimal emotional development. Exercise can also serve as an incentive for children and adolescents to attain tighter control of their blood glucose.[61-63]

No two diabetics respond to exercise in exactly the same way. With the guidance of a physician, athletes with type 1 diabetes, through a process of trial and error, can discover what adjustments in carbohydrate, insulin dosage, or a combination of the two work best. This process requires frequent blood glucose monitoring and correction.[60] The most appropriate exercises for diabetic patients involve predictable levels of physical expenditure. Competitive cyclists, marathon runners, cross-country skiers, and triathletes can all maintain glycemic control by frequent self-testing and adjustment before, during, and after training sessions and events. These sports are compatible with good diabetic control because they involve predetermined distance, duration, and intensity of competition, as well as predictable frequency. Therefore, these activities permit the athlete to anticipate his or her physical needs.

Several of the long-term complications of diabetes may be worsened by exercise[59,60,64,65] (see Box 12.4). Vigorous exercise may precipitate heart attack when there is underlying coronary heart disease, a common medical problem in diabetics. Type 1 diabetes patients over 40 years of age, individuals who have had diabetes for 10 years or more, or those with established complications should first undergo a thorough medical exam that includes a graded exercise stress test. For the majority of type 1 diabetics, however, exercise is safe and improves their quality of life. In one cohort of 548 type 1 diabetics followed for 7 years, regular physical activity was not found to be detrimental with regard to mortality.[64] Disease risk factors are generally under better control in physically active compared to inactive type 1 diabetic patients.[66] A survey of 2,800 U.S. adults with diabetes showed that regular exercise was the only self-management behavior to predict improved quality of life.[67]

There is some concern that large and sustained increase in blood pressure during heavy exertion may accelerate the development of eye or kidney problems in type 1 diabetes patients.[65] Until more is known, diabetics with these complications are cautioned to avoid sustained heavy exercise such as vigorous weight lifting or prolonged, intense aerobic activity. Diabetics with nerve and blood vessel damage in their feet and legs should be particularly careful to avoid cuts, blisters, and pounding exercises of the lower extremities (e.g., running, high-impact aerobic dance).[59,60] Good footwear, careful foot hygiene, and regular inspection is necessary.

Type 2 Diabetes and Exercise

The major aim of therapy for patients with type 2 diabetes is to improve insulin sensitivity through appropriate use of

---

Box 12.4
Benefits and Risks of Exercise for Individuals with Diabetes

Diabetics must be cautious about the possible risks of exercise, but the possible benefits are great, as well.

Possible Benefits

1. Decreased blood glucose
2. Increased insulin sensitivity
3. Improved blood lipoprotein profile and lowered blood pressure
4. Improved cardiorespiratory fitness
5. Usefulness as adjunct to diet for weight reduction
6. Increased sense of well-being and quality of life

Possible Risks

1. Hypoglycemia during or after exercise
2. Increased blood glucose values among poorly controlled patients
3. Complications of atherosclerotic cardiovascular disease
4. Degenerative joint disease
5. Worsening of diabetic complications

Source: Young JC. Exercise prescription for individuals with metabolic disorders: Practical considerations. *Sports Med* 19:43–53, 1995.

---

diet, exercise, and weight reduction. In contrast to results with type 1 diabetes patients, regular exercise by persons with type 2 diabetes does lead to improved long-term diabetic control.[68-77] For obese type 2 diabetes patients on insulin, a combination of exercise and weight reduction can reduce insulin requirements by up to 100%. Improved glucose control has been shown for both middle-aged and elderly type 2 diabetes patients who exercise regularly, due in part to the frequent lowering of the blood glucose level and enhancement of insulin sensitivity with each exercise session.[70,74] Insulin resistance was once thought to be an inevitable part of the aging process, but now there is evidence that age-related declines in physical activity and changes in body composition are largely responsible.[54,70,74]

According to the ADA, patients who are most likely to respond favorably are those with mildly to moderately impaired glucose tolerance and hyperinsulinemia.[59] The ADA cautions that the benefits of exercise typically outweigh the risks if attention is paid to minimizing potential exercise complications. All individuals with type 2 diabetes who are about to start an exercise program should have a thorough medical exam to uncover previously undiagnosed complications due to diabetes.

For most individuals with type 2 diabetes who have been given medical clearance to begin exercising, near daily physical activity, for 20–45 minutes, at a moderate-to-somewhat-high intensity level, is recommended.[60] A high frequency of exercise is essential because the residual effects of an acute exercise bout on glucose tolerance last for only 1 or 2 days. Also, for the obese individual with type 2 diabetes, near-daily activity will help ensure that an adequate number of calories are expended to assist in weight loss.

Exercise sessions of less than 20 minutes duration appear to have little benefit for diabetic control, while sessions lasting more than 45 minutes increase the risk of hypoglycemia.[59,60] Low-intensity exercise (50% of $\dot{V}O_{2max}$) is just as effective as high-intensity exercise (75% of $\dot{V}O_{2max}$) in enhancing insulin sensitivity in diabetics, as long as the caloric expenditure is equated by increasing the duration of the low-intensity exercise bouts.[56]

Because persons with type 2 diabetes are often poorly conditioned, an easy start to the exercise program with gradual progression is advised.[60] Aerobic, endurance-type activities involving large-muscle groups, such as cycling, brisk walking, and swimming, are recommended. Weight training exercises designed to improve muscle endurance through high repetitions with moderate weight will help avoid high blood pressure responses. Each exercise session should begin with an appropriate warm-up and cool-down period.

Several studies have shown that resistance training is feasible and beneficial for type 2 diabetics.[54,71] Data suggest that both an increase in abdominal fat and a loss of muscle mass are highly associated with the development of insulin resistance in type 2 diabetics.[54] Resistance training can help prevent muscle atrophy and stimulate muscle development, improving overall glycemic control. For example, in one 3-month study of type 2 diabetic subjects, a progressive resistance training program (moderate intensity, high volume) twice a week improved muscle size and muscular endurance while lowering glycosylated hemoglobin levels.[71]

Unfortunately, studies have shown that the majority of diabetics do not exercise regularly, and they tend to exercise less than people who do not have diabetes. According to one national survey, only about one in three people with diabetes reported exercising regularly, and less than one in five burned 2,000 calories or more per week in exercise.[78]

With regular exercise, persons with type 2 diabetes respond to a 100-gram oral glucose load with significantly lower blood glucose and insulin levels.[54] Various mechanisms have been proposed for the beneficial role of physical activity in the treatment of insulin resistance, impaired glucose tolerance, and type 2 diabetes:[54]

- Exercise training results in a preferential loss of fat from the central regions of the body. This is important because abdominal fat accumulation is highly related to the development of insulin resistance.

- Skeletal muscle is the largest mass of insulin-sensitive tissue in the body. Therefore, a reduction in muscle mass could reduce the effectiveness of insulin to clear blood glucose. Exercise training can prevent muscle atrophy and build muscle mass, helping to alleviate insulin resistance.

- With deconditioning, insulin loses its ability to vasodilate skeletal muscle and increase muscle blood flow. With regular exercise, this problem is countered, improving the control of insulin over blood glucose.

- A reduced number of insulin receptors has been reported in obese individuals and those with type 2 diabetes. Exercise training appears to increase insulin receptor numbers.

- With regular exercise, skeletal muscle insulin action is improved and is associated with an increase in the insulin-regulatable glucose transporters, GLUT4 (one type of glucose transporter located within the cell), and enzymes responsible for the phosphorylation, storage, and oxidation of glucose.

- Conditioned muscles have a greater density of oxidative fibers and capillaries that favor improved glucose tolerance.

SUMMARY

1. *Diabetes mellitus* is defined as a group of metabolic diseases characterized by high blood glucose resulting from defects in insulin secretion, insulin action, or both. The chronic hyperglycemia of diabetes is associated with long-term damage, dysfunction, and failure of various organs, especially the eyes, kidneys, nerves, heart, and blood vessels.

2. Of the 15.7 million American with diabetes, type 1 accounts for 5–10% and type 2 for 90–95%.

3. There are four categories of diabetes mellitus: type 1, type 2, gestational diabetes, and other specific types. Type 1 diabetes is characterized by destruction of the pancreatic beta cells that produce insulin, usually

SPORTS MEDICINE INSIGHT

Dietary Management for Diabetics

Treatment of diabetes is related to both exercise and nutrition. It is important that the sports medicine specialist understand nutritional principles in order to give professional counseling and referral.

In 1994, the American Diabetes Association submitted their position statement entitled "Nutrition Recommendations and Principles for People with Diabetes Mellitus."[38] A brief summary of these principles follows. Table 12.1 shows that there has been a progression of change throughout the twentieth century regarding the diet best suited for the diabetic. Today, there is an emphasis that the diet should be individualized for each patient.

NUTRITIONAL THERAPY AND TYPE 1 DIABETES

A meal plan based on the individual's usual food intake should be determined and used as a basis for integrating insulin therapy into the usual eating and exercise patterns. It is recommended that individuals using insulin therapy eat at consistent times synchronized with the time-action of the insulin preparation used. Further, individuals need to monitor blood glucose levels and adjust insulin doses for the amount of food usually eaten. Intensified insulin therapy, such as multiple daily injections or use of an insulin pump, allows considerable flexibility in when and what individuals eat.

NUTRITIONAL THERAPY AND TYPE 2 DIABETES

- Emphasis should be placed on achieving glucose, lipid, and blood pressure goals. Although weight loss is desirable, long-term success has not been achieved by many patients.

- Improved food choices are illustrated by *Dietary Guidelines for Americans* and the *Food Guide Pyramid* (see Chapter 9).

- About 10–20% of the daily caloric intake should come from protein.

- Less than 10% of Calories should come from saturated fat. The amount of fat is dependent on desired glucose, lipid, and weight outcomes. If lipids and weight are normal, <30% fat and <10% saturated fat (SAFA) is recommended. If LDL-C is high, NCEP Step 2 guidelines are in order (<30% fat, <7% SAFA, <300 mg cholesterol). Low-fat diets are effective for weight loss.

- The percentage of Calories derived from carbohydrate will vary based on eating habits and glucose and lipid goals. Simple sugars can be a part of the meal plan and do not impair blood glucose control.

- Nonnutritive sweeteners (saccharin, aspartame, acesulfame K) have been approved by the FDA and are safe to consume.

- Dietary fiber recommendations are the same as for the general population (20–35 g/day from a wide variety of food sources).

- Sodium and alcohol intake recommendations are the same as for the general population (<3,000 mg NA/day; <2 alcholic drinks/day).

TABLE 12.1   Changes in the Diabetic Diet

Year	% CHO	% Protein	% Fat
Before 1921	Low calorie	Low calorie	Low calorie
1921	20	10	70
1950	40	20	40
1971	45	20	35
1986	up to 60	12–20	<30
1994	individualized	10–20	individualized; <10% SAFA

(continued)

Dietary Management for Diabetics *(continued)*

DIETARY GOALS FOR DIABETIC MANAGEMENT

- Maintenance of near-normal blood glucose levels by balancing food intake with insulin, medications, and activity levels

- Achievement of optimal serum lipid levels

- Provision of adequate energy for maintaining or attaining reasonable weights for adults and normal growth for children

- Prevention and treatment of acute complications (hypoglycemia, illnesses, exercise-related problems), and long-term complications (renal disease, autonomic neuropathy, hypertension, and cardiovascular disease)

- Improvement of overall health through optimal nutrition (follow the *Dietary Guidelines for Americans* and *Food Guide Pyramid*) (see Chapter 9)

The overall goal of nutrition therapy is to assist people with diabetes in making changes in nutrition and exercise habits leading to improved metabolic control.

The American Diabetes Association and the American Dietetic Association have published the "Exchange Lists for Meal Planning."[79] The six exchange lists make meal planning easier for diabetics, helping the type 1 diabetic to be more consistent and helping the type 2 diabetic to watch Calories more closely. The exchange lists make it easy to identify high-fiber and high-sodium foods.

---

leading to absolute insulin deficiency. Type 2 diabetes usually arises because of insulin resistance, in which the body fails to use insulin properly, combined with relative insulin deficiency. Type 2 diabetes has multiple risk factors, including age, obesity, physical inactivity, family history, ethnicity, previous gestational diabetes, impaired fasting glucose, hypertension, and dyslipidemia.

4. Diabetes can be diagnosed in any one of three ways and must be confirmed on a different day. A fasting plasma glucose that is ≥126 mg/dl is most commonly used.

5. Approximately 85% of patients with type 2 diabetes are obese at the time of diagnosis. The risk for developing type 2 diabetes rises in direct relationship to the degree of obesity.

6. Treatment for either type of diabetes seeks to accomplish what the human body normally does naturally: maintain a proper balance between glucose and insulin. Food makes the blood glucose level rise, while insulin and exercise make it fall. The challenge is to manage these three factors to keep the blood glucose

within a narrow range. Training in self-management is integral to the treatment of diabetes. Treatment must be individualized and must address medical, psychosocial, and lifestyle issues.

7. Type 2 diabetes is less common in physically active, compared to inactive, societies. Several prospective studies have shown that physical activity is protective against type 2 diabetes.

8. Exercise is useful in the treatment of both type 1 and type 2 diabetes. Although regular exercise leads to reduced insulin requirements for individuals with type 1 diabetes, studies have failed to show that long-term glucose control is improved. Regular exercise by persons with type 2 diabetes does lead to improved long-term diabetic control. Several mechanisms were reviewed explaining the beneficial role of physical activity in the treatment of insulin resistance, impaired glucose tolerance, and type 2 diabetes.

9. Physical exercise is not without risk to individuals with type 1 diabetes. These were reviewed in Boxes 12.3 and 12.4.

REFERENCES

1. National Diabetes Data Group, National Institutes of Health. *Diabetes in America* (2nd ed.), NIH Publication No. 95-1468. Bethesda, MD: National Institutes of Health, 1995.

2. Report of the Expert Committee on the Diagnosis and Classification of Diabetes Mellitus. *Diabetes Care* 20:1183–1197, 1997.

3. U.S. Renal Data System. *USRDS 1997 Annual Data Report.* Be-

thesda, MD: National Institutes of Health, National Institute of Diabetes and Digestive and Kidney Disease, 1997.

4. Centers for Disease Control and Prevention. *National Diabetes Fact Sheet: National Estimates and General Information on Diabetes in the United States.* Atlanta, GA: U.S. Department of Health

and Human Services, Centers for Disease Control and Prevention, 1997.

5. National Center for Health Statistics. *Health, United States, 1996–97 and Injury Chartbook.* Hyattsville, MD: Author, 1997.

6. National Center for Health Statistics. *Healthy People 2000 Review, 1997.* Hyattsville, MD: Public Health Service, 1997.

7. Peyrot M, Rubin RR. Levels and risks of depression and anxiety symptomatology among diabetic adults. *Diabetes Care* 20: 585–590, 1997.

8. Leibson CL, Rocca WA, Hanson VA, et al. Risk of dementia among persons with diabetes mellitus: A population-based cohort study. *Am J Epidemiol* 145:301–308, 1997.

9. Dagoga-Jack S, Santiago JV. Pathophysiology of type 2 diabetes and modes of action of therapeutic interventions. *Arch Intern Med* 157:1802–1817, 1997.

10. Horton ES. NIDDM—The devastating disease. *Diab Res Clin Prac* 28(suppl):S3–S11, 1995.

11. Peters AL, Davidson MB, Schriger DL, Hasselblad V. A clinical approach for the diagnosis of diabetes mellitus: An analysis using glycosylated hemoglobin levels. *JAMA* 276:1246–1252, 1996.

12. Anonymous. The lowdown on low blood sugar. *Tufts University Diet and Nutrition Letter,* 13(10), 1995.

13. Pan XR, Yang WY, Li GW, Liu J. Prevalence of diabetes and its risk factors in China, 1994. *Diabetes Care* 20:1664–1670, 1997.

14. Huang B, Rodriquez BL, Burchfiel CM, Chyou PH, Curb JD, Yano K. Acculturation and prevalence of diabetes among Japanese-American men in Hawaii. *Am J Epidemiol* 144:674–681, 1996.

15. Manson JE, Nathan DM, Krolewski AS, et al. A prospective study of exercise and incidence of diabetes among U.S. male physicians. *JAMA* 268:63–67, 1992.

16. Colditz GA, Willett WC, Rotnitzky A, Manson JE. Weight gain as a risk factor for clinical diabetes mellitus in women. *Ann Intern Med* 122:481–486, 1995.

17. Carey VJ, Walters EE, Colditz GA, et al. Body fat distribution and risk of non-insulin-dependent diabetes mellitus in women: The nurses' health study. *Am J Epidemiol* 145:614–619, 1997.

18. Ford ES, Williamson DF, Liu S. Weight change and diabetes incidence: Findings from a national cohort of US adults. *Am J Epidemiol* 146:214–222, 1997.

19. Manson JE, Spelsberg A. Primary prevention of non-insulin-dependent diabetes mellitus. *Am J Prev Med* 10:172–184, 1994.

20. Bosello O, Armellini F, Zamboni M, Fitchet M. The benefits of modest weight loss in type II diabetes. *Int J Obesity* 21(suppl): S10–S13, 1997.

21. Folsom AR, Jacobs DR, Wagenknecht LE, et al. Increase in fasting insulin and glucose over seven years with increasing weight and inactivity of young adults: The CARDIA study. *Am J Epidemiol* 144:235–246, 1996.

22. Torjensen PA, Birkeland KI, Anderssen SA, Hjermann I, Holme I, Urdal P. Lifestyle changes may reverse development of the insulin resistance syndrome: The Oslo diet and exercise study: A randomized trial. *Diabetes Care* 20:26–31, 1997.

23. Perry IJ, Wannamethee AG, Walker MK, Thomson AG, Whincup PH, Shaper AG. Prospective study of risk factors for development of non-insulin dependent diabetes in middle aged British men. *BMJ* 310:560–564, 1995.

24. Salmerón J, Manson JE, Stampfer MJ, Colditz GA, Wing AL, Willett WC. Dietary fiber, glycemic load, and risk of non-insulin-dependent diabetes mellitus in women. *JAMA* 277: 472–477, 1997.

25. Salmerón J, Ascherio A, Rimm EB, et al. Dietary fiber, glycemic load, and risk of NIDDM in men. *Diabetes Care* 20:545–551, 1997.

26. Henry RR, Genuth S. Forum one: Current recommendations about intensification of metabolic control in non-insulin-dependent diabetes mellitus. *Ann Intern Med* 124:175–177, 1996.

27. Glascow RE, Hampson SE, Strycker LA, Ruggiero L. Personal-model beliefs and social-environment barriers related to diabetes self-management. *Diabetes Care* 20:556–561, 1997.

28. U.S. Preventive Services Task Force. *Guide to Clinical Preventive Services* (2nd ed.). Alexandria, VA: International Medical Publishing, 1996.

29. Palta M, Shen G, Allen C, Klein R, D'Alessio D. Longitudinal patterns of glycemic control and diabetes care from diagnosis in a population-based cohort with type 1 diabetes. *Am J Epidemiol* 144:954–961, 1996.

30. The Diabetes Control and Complications Trial Research Group. The effect of intensive treatment of diabetes on the development and progression of long-term complications of insulin-dependent diabetes mellitus. *N Engl J Med* 329:977–986, 1993. See also *Diabetes* 12:1555–1558, 1993.

31. The Diabetes Control and Complications Trial Research Group. Lifetime benefits and costs of intensive therapy as practiced in the diabetes control and complications trial. *JAMA* 276: 1409–1415, 1996.

32. Dunn FL, Nathan DM, Scavini M, Selam JL, Wingrove TG. Long-term therapy of IDDM with an implantable insulin pump. *Diabetes Care* 20:59–64, 1997.

33. Saudek CD, Duckworth WC, Giobbie-Hurder A, et al. Implantable insulin pump vs multiple-dose insulin for non-insulin-dependent diabetes mellitus: A randomized trial. *JAMA* 276: 1322–1327, 1996.

34. Hayward RA, Manning WG, Kaplan SH, Wagner EH, Greenfield S. Starting insulin therapy in patients with type 2 diabetes. *JAMA* 278:1663–1669, 1997.

35. Barnard RJ, Jung T, Inkeles SB. Diet and exercise in the treatment of NIDDM. *Diabetes Care* 17:1469–1472, 1994.

36. Guare JC, Wing RR, Grant A. Comparison of obese NIDDM and nondiabetic women: Short- and long-term weight loss. *Obes Res* 3:329–335, 1995.

37. Beebe CA, Pastors JG, Powers MA, Wylie-Rosett J. Nutrition management for individuals with non-insulin dependent diabetes mellitus in the 1990s: A review by the Diabetes Care and Education Dietetic Practice Group. *J Am Diet Assoc* 91:196–207, 1991.

38. American Diabetes Association. Position statement: Nutritional recommendations and principles for people with diabetes mellitus. *J Am Diet Assoc* 94:504–511, 1994.

39. Anderson JW, Gustafson NJ, Bryant CA, Tietyen-Clark J. Dietary fiber and diabetes: A comprehensive review and practical application. *J Am Diet Assoc* 87:1189–1197, 1987.

40. Pan XR, Li GW, Hu YH, et al. Effects of diet and exercise in preventing NIDDM in people with impaired glucose tolerance: The Da Qing IGT and diabetes study. *Diabetes Care* 20:537–544, 1997.

41. Lynch J, Helmrich SP, Lakka TA, Kaplan GA, Cohen RD, Salo-

nen R, Salonen JT. Moderately intense physical activities and high levels of cardiorespiratory fitness reduce the risk of non-insulin-dependent diabetes mellitus in middle-aged men. *Arch Intern Med* 156:1307–1314, 1996.

42. Monterrosa AE, Haffner SM, Stern MP, Hazuda HP. Sex difference in lifestyle factors predictive of diabetes in Mexican-Americans. *Diabetes Care* 18:448–456, 1995.

43. Pereira MA, Kriska AM, Joswiak ML, et al. Physical inactivity and glucose intolerance in the multiethnic island of Mauritius. *Med Sci Sports Exerc* 27:1626–1634, 1995.

44. Burchfiel CM, Sharp DS, Curb JD, Rodriguez BL, Hwang L-J, Marcus EB, Yano K. Physical activity and incidence of diabetes: The Honolulu heart program. *Am J Epidemiol* 141:360–368, 1995.

45. Helmrich SP, Ragland DR, Leung RW, Paffenbarger RS. Physical activity and reduced occurrence of noninsulin-dependent diabetes mellitus. *N Engl J Med* 325:147–152, 1991.

46. Haapanen N, Miilunpalo S, Vuori I, Oja P, Pasanen M. Association of leisure time physical activity with the risk of coronary heart disease, hypertension and diabetes in middle-aged men and women. *Int J Epidemiol* 26:739–747, 1997.

47. Gudat U, Berger M, Lefèbvre PJ. Physical activity, fitness, and non-insulin-dependent (type II) diabetes mellitus. In Bouchard C, Shephard RJ, Stephens T (eds), *Physical Activity, Fitness, and Health: International Proceedings and Consensus Statement.* Champaign, IL: Human Kinetics, 1994, 669–683.

48. Manson JE, Colditz GA, Stampfer, MJ, et al. A prospective study of maturity-onset diabetes mellitus and risk of coronary heart disease and stroke in women. *Arch Intern Med* 151: 1141–1147, 1991.

49. Frisch RE, Wyshak G, Albright TE, Albright NL, Schiff I. Lower prevalence of diabetes in female former college athletes compared with nonathletes. *Diabetes* 35:1101, 1986.

50. Manson JE, Rimon EB, Stampfer MJ, et al. Physical activity and incidence of noninsulin-dependent diabetes mellitus in women. *Lancet* 338:774–778, 1991.

51. Helmrich SP, Ragland DR, Paffenbarger RS. Prevention of non-insulin-dependent diabetes mellitus with physical activity. *Med Sci Sports Exerc* 26:824–830, 1994.

52. Cantu RC. *Diabetes and Exercise.* Ithaca, New York: Movement Publications, 1982.

53. Ivy JL. The insulin-like effect of muscle contraction. *Exerc Sport Sci Rev* 15:29–54, 1987.

54. Ivy JL. Role of exercise training in the prevention and treatment of insulin resistance and non-insulin-dependent diabetes mellitus. *Sports Med* 24:321–336, 1997.

55. Oshida Y, Kamanouchi K, Hayamiru S, et al. Effect of training and training cessation on insulin action. *Int J Sports Med* 12: 484–486, 1991.

56. Baun B, Zimmerman MB, Kretchmer N. Effects of exercise intensity on insulin sensitivity in women with non-insulin-dependent diabetes mellitus. *J Appl Physiol* 78:300–306, 1995.

57. Dela F, Larsen JJ, Mikines KJ, Ploug T, Petersen LN, Galbo H. Insulin-stimulated muscle glucose clearance in patients with NIDDM: Effects of one-legged physical training. *Diabetes* 44: 1010–1020, 1995.

58. Araujo-Vilar D, Osifo E, Kirk M, Garcia-Estevez DA, Cabezas-Cerrato J, Hockaday TD. Influence of moderate physical exercise on insulin-mediated and non-insulin-mediated glucose uptake in healthy individuals. *Metabolism* 46:203–209, 1997.

59. American Diabetes Association. Diabetes mellitus and exercise. *Diabetes Care* 18(suppl 1):28, 1995. See also *Diabetes Care* 13: 785–789, 1990; *Diabetes Care* 17:924–937, 1994.

60. Young JC. Exercise prescription for individuals with metabolic disorders: Practical considerations. *Sports Med* 19:43–53, 1995.

61. Blackett PR. Child and adolescent athletes with diabetes. *Physician Sportsmed* 16(3):133–149, 1988.

62. Stratton R, Wilson DP, Endres RK. Acute glycemic effects of exercise in adolescents with insulin dependent diabetes mellitus. *Physician Sportsmed* 16(3):150–157, 1988.

63. Robbins DC, Carleton S. Managing the diabetic athlete. *Physician Sportsmed* 17(12):45–54, 1989.

64. Moy CS, Songer TJ, LaPorte RE, Dorman JS, Kriska AM, Orchard TJ, Becker DJ, Drash AL. Insulin-dependent diabetes mellitus, physical activity, and death. *Am J Epidemiol* 137: 74–81, 1993.

65. Albert SG, Bernbaum M. Exercise for patients with diabetic retinopathy. *Diabetes Care* 18:130–132, 1995.

66. Lehmann R, Kaplan V, Bingisser R, Bloch KE, Spinas GA. Impact of physical activity on cardiovascular risk factors in IDDM. *Diabetes Care* 20:1603–1611, 1997.

67. Glasgow RE, Ruggiero L, Eakin EG, Dryfoos J, Chobanian L. Quality of life and associated characteristics in a large national sample of adults with diabetes. *Diabetes Care* 20:562–569, 1997.

68. Estacio RO, Wolfel EE, Regensteiner JG, et al. Effect of risk factors on exercise capacity in NIDDM. *Diabetes* 45:79–85, 1996.

69. Agurs-Collins TD, Kumanyika SK, Have TR, Adams-Campbell LL. A randomized controlled trial of weight reduction and exercise for diabetes management in older African-American subjects. *Diabetes Care* 20:1503–1511, 1997.

70. Yamanouchi K, Shinozaki T, Chikada K, et al. Daily walking combined with diet therapy is a useful means for obese NIDDM patients not only to reduce body weight but also to improve insulin sensitivity. *Diabetes Care* 18:775–778, 1995.

71. Eriksson J, Taimela S, Eriksson K, Parviainen S, Peltonen J, Kujala U. Resistance training in the treatment of non-insulin-dependent diabetes mellitus. *Int J Sports Med* 18:242–246, 1997.

72. Dengel DR, Pratley RE, Hagberg JM, Rogus EM, Goldberg AP. Distinct effects of aerobic exercise training and weight loss on glucose homeostasis in obese sedentary men. *J Appl Physiol* 81: 318–325, 1996.

73. Kang J, Robertson RJ, Hagberg JM, et al. Effect of exercise intensity on glucose and insulin metabolism in obese individuals and obese NIDDM patients. *Diabetes Care* 19:341–349, 1996.

74. Yamanouchi K, Nakajima H, Shinozaki T, et al. Effects of daily physical activity on insulin action in the elderly. *J Appl Physiol* 73:2241–2245, 1992.

75. Lampman RM, Schteingart DE. Effects of exercise training on glucose control, lipid metabolism, and insulin sensitivity in hypertriglyceridemia and non-insulin dependent diabetes mellitus. *Med Sci Sports Exerc* 23:703–712, 1991.

76. Rogers MA, Yamamoto C, King DS, Hagberg JM, Ehsani AA, Holloszy JO. Improvement in glucose tolerance after 1 wk of exercise in patients with mild NIDDM. *Diabetes Care* 11:613–618, 1988.

77. Bayles-Paternostro M, Wing RR, Robertson RJ. Effect of lifestyle activity of varying duration on glycemic control in type II diabetic women. *Diabetes Care* 12:34–37, 1989.

78. Ford ES, Herman WH. Leisure-time physical activity patterns in the U.S. diabetic population. *Diabetes Care* 18:27–33, 1995.

79. American Dietetic Association. *Exchange Lists for Meal Planning.* Chicago: Author, 1995.

PHYSICAL FITNESS ACTIVITY 12.1

Assessing Your Diabetes Risk Score

Are You at Risk?

Write in the points next to each statement that is true for you. If the statement is not true for you, put a zero. Then total your score.

1. I have been experiencing one or more of the following symptoms on a regular basis:

   - excessive thirst — Yes (3) ——
   - frequent urination — Yes (3) ——
   - extreme fatigue — Yes (1) ——
   - unexplained weight loss — Yes (3) ——
   - blurry vision from time to time — Yes (2) ——

2. I am over 30 years old. — Yes (1) ——

3. My weight is equal to or above that listed in Table 12.2. — Yes (2) ——

4. I am a woman who has had more than one baby weighing more than 9 lbs. at birth. — Yes (2) ——

5. I am of Native American descent. — Yes (1) ——

6. I am of Hispanic or African American descent. — Yes (1) ——

7. I have a parent with diabetes. — Yes (1) ——

8. I have a brother or sister with diabetes. — Yes (2) ——

Scoring

- **3–4 points:** You probably are at low risk. But don't just forget about it, especially if you're over 30, overweight, or of African American, Hispanic or Native American descent. Be sure you know the symptoms of diabetes. If you experience any of them, contact your doctor for testing.

- **5 or more points:** You may be at high risk. You even may already have diabetes. See your doctor promptly to find out. Even if you don't have diabetes, know the symptoms. If you experience any of them in the future, you should see your doctor immediately.

TABLE 12.2 Weight Chart (20% over maximum, medium frame)

Height (without shoes)	Weight (pounds, without shoes) Women	Men
4'9"	127	
4'10"	131	
4'11"	134	
5'0"	138	
5'1"	142	146
5'2"	146	151
5'3"	151	155
5'4"	157	158
5'5"	162	163
5'6"	167	168
5'7"	172	174
5'8"	176	179
5'9"	181	184
5'10"	186	190
5'11"		196
6'0"		202
6'1"		208
6'2"		214
6'3"		220

Source: American Diabetes Association.

CHAPTER
13
Obesity

Physical activity might have its most significant effect in preventing, rather than in treating, overweight and obesity.

—Jack Wilmore[1]

In most Western societies today, the overabundance of fat-rich foods and lack of physical activity have created a socioeconomic environment conducive to obesity among a significant proportion of both men and women.[2,3] As we have seen in previous chapters, the prevalence of many other risk factors for chronic disease (e.g., high blood cholesterol and blood pressure) has decreased as of late. As is emphasized in this section, every indication is that the prevalence of obesity has been steadily increasing throughout most of the twentieth century.[2-11]

As defined in Chapter 5, obesity is a condition of excess body fat. This is difficult to measure when conducting national studies, so the National Center for Health Statistics uses various height and weight measures (see Figure 13.1). These studies of Americans since the late 1940s have shown that many are overweight and obese. Obesity affects about

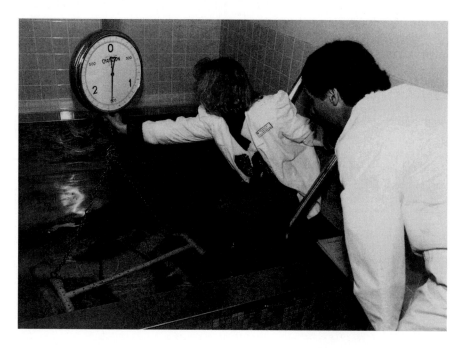

Figure 13.1 Obesity is defined as a condition of excess body fat. This is best measured using underwater weighing techniques, as described in Chapter 5.

97 million adults ages 20 to 74, with the highest rates among the poor and minority groups.[4,5] For both adult men and women, 55% are considered overweight (defined in most national studies as a body mass index ≥ 25 kg/m²).[5] The federal government's year 2000 goal is to reduce the prevalence of overweight in the U.S. adult population to no more than 20%, but trends are in the opposite direction.[12] Figure 13.2 summarizes current estimates of overweight among various groups.[3-8] Comparisons of these figures with data collected during the 1960s demonstrate significant increases in prevalence of overweight for all segments of the American society[4-7] (see Figure 13.3). This is despite increasingly thin ideals in physical appearance for both men and women, a marked departure from ancient standards that held obesity in high esteem.[13] Although the causes of the increase in overweight prevalence are hotly debated, most experts feel that Americans are taking in more calories than in previous decades.[10,11]

Americans are disturbed enough by their body weights to be trying to lose weight in record numbers (33–40% of women and 20–24% of men on any given day are trying to lose weight).[14]

Several international comparisons have shown that Americans are among the heaviest people in the world.[15-17]

For example, the United States has a greater percentage of overweight people than either France or the United Kingdom (Figure 13.4).[15]

National surveys also reveal that a growing proportion of U.S. children and teenagers are overweight.[4,8-10] As depicted in Figure 13.5, overweight prevalence has more than doubled since the 1960s for both children and adolescents. Defining obesity or overweight for children and adolescents is difficult, but experts now recommend that a BMI cutoff point equal to or above the ninety-fifth percentile for age and sex be used to account for growth spurts and other physiological changes.[10,18] Using this conservative method, approximately 14% of children and 12% of adolescents are overweight.[4,10] If the eighty-fifth percentile BMI cutoff point is used, overweight prevalence for American youths rises to 22%.[8]

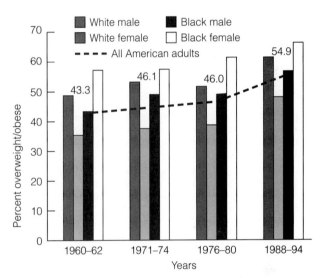

Figure 13.3 Trends in U.S. adult overweight prevalence (BMI ≥ 25 kg/m²). The prevalence of overweight adults has climbed steeply since the 1960s. *Source:* National Center for Health Statistics. *Health, United States, 1996–97 and Injury Chartbook.* Hyattsville, MD: Author, 1997.

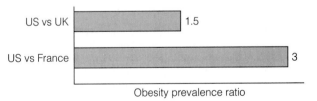

Figure 13.4 Obesity prevalence ratios: U.S. adults compared to adults in France and the United Kingdom (UK). Prevalence ratio = proportion of U.S. adults BMI ≥ 30 kg/m²: France or UK proportion. In the United States, prevalence of obesity is 50% higher than in the United Kingdom, and threefold higher than in France. *Source:* VanItallie TB. Prevalence of obesity. *Endocrinol Metab Clin North Am* 25:887–905, 1996.

Figure 13.2 Overweight adults 20–74 years of age, 1988–1994 (BMI ≥ 25 kg/m²). Obesity prevalence varies widely among different segments of American society, but all are substantially above the federal government's year 2000 goal of no more than 20%. *Source:* National Center for Health Statistics. *Health, United States, 1996–97 and Injury Chartbook.* Hyattsville, MD: Author, 1997.

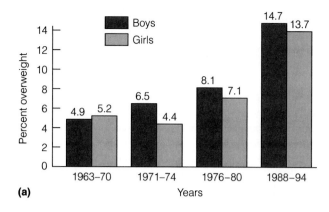

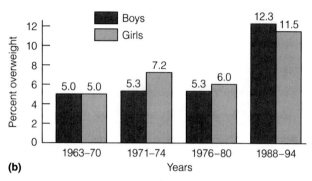

(a)

(b)

Figure 13.5 Trends in U.S. overweight prevalence for (a) children and (b) adolescents, overweight defined as BMI at or above ninety-fifth percentile BMI cutoff based on surveys in the 1960s. Overweight prevalence among children (ages 6–11) and adolescents (ages 12–17) rose sharply since the 1960s. *Source:* National Center for Health Statistics. *Health, United States, 1996–97 and Injury Chartbook.* Hyattsville, MD: Author, 1997.

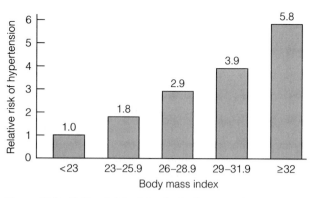

Figure 13.6 BMI and risk of developing hypertension, 8-year study of more than 115,000 nurses. The risk of developing hypertension climbs with the increase in body mass index. *Source:* Witteman JCM, Willett WC, Stampfer MJ, et al. A prospective study of nutritional factors and hypertension among US women. *Circulation* 80:1320–1327, 1989.

HEALTH RISKS OF OBESITY

It has long been suspected that obesity is associated with many health risks, including early death.[19] William Shakespeare has written perhaps the most famous description:

> Make less thy body hence, and more thy grace;
> Leave gormandizing; know the grave doth gape
> For thee thrice wider than for other men.
>
> *King Henry IV, Part II*

However, it was not until 1985 that the health hazards of obesity were first officially recognized by the National Institutes of Health.[20] It is now felt that obesity constitutes one of the more important medical and public health problems of our time.

The National Institutes of Health and several other reviewers have summarized the large number of health problems associated with obesity.[19–24]

- *A psychological burden.* Because of the strong pressures from society to be thin, obese people often suffer feelings of guilt, depression, anxiety, and low self-esteem. In terms of suffering, this may be the greatest burden of obesity, especially among adolescents.[22] Severely obese people are often subjected to prejudice and discrimination.[25] The term "fattism" is used to represent this problem. Social and economic consequences of being obese include reduced income and higher rates of poverty, decreased likelihood of getting married, and poorer academic performance and progress.[26]

- *Increased high blood pressure.* High blood pressure is common among the obese.[27,28] As shown in Figure 13.6 the risk of developing hypertension rises sharply with increase in body mass index.[27] Even among schoolchildren, increases in obesity are associated with corresponding increases in blood pressure.[29] As reviewed in Chapter 10, weight reduction is the single most effective nondrug approach to the control of blood pressure.[28]

- *Increased levels of cholesterol and other lipids in the blood.* The obese, including children, are more likely to have higher blood cholesterol, triglyceride, and LDL-C levels, and lower HDL-C levels.[29–33] Figure 13.7 shows that the ratio of total cholesterol to HDL-C rises with the increase in body mass index.[31] As reviewed in Chapter 10, a high ratio is a strong predictor of heart disease. Weight loss leads to a correction of the negative blood lipid profile, with total cholesterol falling 1 mg/dl for every pound lost.[30]

- *Increased risk of gallstones.* Obesity is a well-recognized risk factor for gallstones, a disease that affects approximately 10–20% of the U.S. population.[34,35] Figure 13.8 shows that the risk for symptomatic gallstones rises sharply with increase in body mass index.[34]

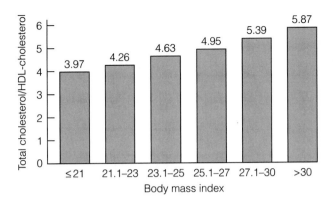

Figure 13.7 Total:HDL-C ratio by body mass index, adult white males, 20–44 years of age, NHANES II. The ratio of total cholesterol to HDL cholesterol rises with an increase in body mass index. *Source:* Denke MA, Sempos CT, Grundy SM. Excess body weight: An underrecognized contributor to high blood cholesterol levels in white American men. *Arch Intern Med* 153: 1093–1103, 1993.

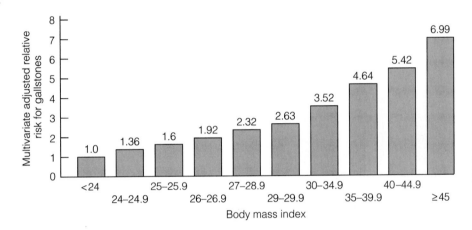

Figure 13.8 Risk of symptomatic gallstones according to obesity status, 8-year study of 90,302 nurses. Risk of gallstones rises sharply with increases in body mass index. *Source:* Stampfer MJ, Maclure KM, Colditz GA, Manson JE, Willett WC. Risk of symptomatic gallstones in women with severe obesity. *Am J Clin Nutr* 55:652–658, 1992.

- *Increased osteoarthritis.* Arthritis and other rheumatic conditions are among the most prevalent diseases in the United States (see Chapter 15).[36,37] Overweight persons are at high risk of osteoarthritis in the knees and hips. Overweight is among the most potent known risk factors for knee osteoarthritis, with persons in the upper 20% of weight having 7–10 times the risk of disease of those in the lowest 20% of weight.[37] In the National Health Interview Survey, the odds of self-reported arthritis and other rheumatic conditions rose with increase in body mass index[36] (see Figure 13.9).

- *Increased diabetes.* The prevalence of diabetes is high among the obese.[38,39] Weight loss by type 2 diabetics often results in dramatic improvements in their blood glucose and insulin levels (see Chapter 12 and Figures 12.6–12.8).

- *Increased cancer.* The American Cancer Society study involving 1 million men and women showed that obese males had a higher mortality rate from cancer of the colon, rectum, and prostate. Obese females had a higher mortality rate from cancer of the gallbladder, bile ducts, breast, uterus, and ovaries[19,40,41] (see Chapter 11, and Figures 11.16, 11.19, and 11.24).

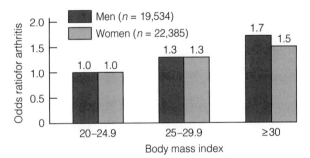

Figure 13.9 Body mass index and odds of arthritis and other rheumatic conditions, National Health Interview Survey, 1989–1991. The odds of self-reported arthritis are highest among those with the highest body mass index. *Source:* CDC. Factors associated with prevalent self-reported arthritis and other rheumatic conditions—United States, 1989–1991. *MMWR* 45: 487–491, 1996.

- *Increased early death.* Hippocrates, the ancient Greek physician, once noted that "sudden death is more common in those who are naturally fat than in the lean." Several modern studies have confirmed the wisdom of Hippocrates. As shown in Figure 13.10, as the body mass increases, mortality from cancer, heart

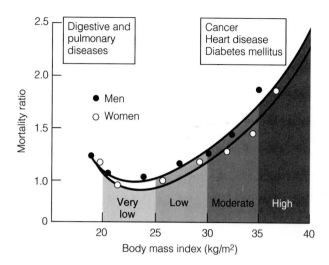

Figure 13.10 Obesity and risk of mortality, J-shaped curve relationship. As the body mass index increases, mortality from heart disease, cancer, and diabetes also increases. Individuals with digestive diseases and pulmonary diseases (mostly due to cigarette smoking) that lead to loss of body weight tend to die early. *Source:* Bray GA, Gray DS. Obesity: Part I. Pathogenesis. *West J Med* 149:429–441, 1988.

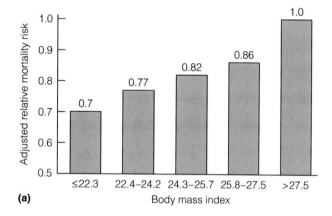

(a)

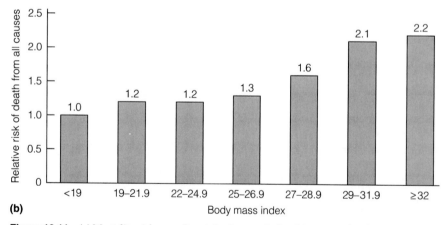

(b)

Figure 13.11 (a) Mortality risk according to body mass index, 26-year study of 8,828 nonsmoking, nondrinking males. In this long-term study of nonsmoking men, no "J" curve was evident, with mortality risk lowest in the leanest men. (b) Mortality risk according to body mass index, 16-year study of 115,195 nonsmoking, weight-stable women; BMI <19.0 vs ≥32.0; risk of cardiovascular disease, 4.1, and cancer, 2.1. As with men, the risk of death from all causes in nonsmoking women is lowest in those with the lowest body mass index. *Sources:* (a) Lindsted K, Tonstad S, Kuzma J. Body mass index and patterns of mortality among Seventh-Day Adventist men. *Int J Obesity* 15:397–406, 1991; (b) Manson JE, Willett WC, Stampfer MJ, Colditz GA, Hunter DJ, Hankinson SE, Hennekens CH, Speizer FE. Body weight and mortality among women. *N Engl J Med* 333: 677–685, 1995.

disease, and diabetes increases.[19,23,40,42] The lower part of the curve, where mortality is increased among the lean, has caused much debate. It appears that this increase is due primarily to the fact that smokers and those with digestive diseases die early and lean. Figure 13.11a shows the results of an interesting 26-year study of nearly 9,000 men who did not drink or smoke.[43] In this study, no "J" curve was evident, suggesting that the lower the body mass index (within reason), the better. This was confirmed in a 16-year study of 115,195 women (see Figure 13.11b).[44] Minimum mortality has been associated with a body weight 10–20% below the average for Americans, after adjustment for cigarette smoking.[44,45] If the American population lost its excess body mass, mortality would be reduced by 15%, corresponding to 3 years of added life expectancy.[42]

In general, the lowest mortality rates from all diseases combined are found among the lean. In one study where men were followed for 55 years, those who had been obese as adolescents were more than twice as likely to die from coronary heart disease.[46] Thus, maintaining leanness from early in life to old age is a primary goal.

- *Increased heart disease.* Obese people have more of the typical risk factors for heart disease (high blood pressure and serum cholesterol levels), and as a result, they die from it at a higher rate.[42–50] As shown in Figure 13.12a, in a large 8-year study of nurses, risk of coronary heart disease more than tripled in those with a body mass index greater than 29 versus those

with an index less than 21.[48] This has been confirmed in a study of U.S. male health professionals (see Figure 13.12b).[50] Risk of stroke also rises with increase in body mass index (see Figure 13.13).[51]

Recent information is showing that it makes a difference where the excess fat is deposited, with respect to medical complications.[50,52–55] The obese people most vulnerable to heart disease, high blood pressure and cholesterol, diabetes, cancers, and early death tend to have more of their fat deposited in abdominal areas rather than the hip and thigh areas.

In other words, health risks are greater for those who have most of their body fat in the upper body, especially the trunk and abdominal areas. This is called *android obesity,* in comparison to *gynoid obesity* (characterized by deposition of body fat in the hips and thighs) (see Figure 13.14). This can be measured by looking at the ratio of waist-to-hip circumferences (WHR) or the waist circumference by itself (see Chapter 5). A high WHR or waist circumference predict more complications from obesity. Figure 13.15 shows the results of a 5-year study of women where risk of both heart disease and cancer rose as the WHR increased.[46] Figure 13.16 shows that risk of stroke rises with increase in the WHR.[52] (Also see Figure 12.8, which depicts the relationship between waist circumference and risk of type 2 diabetes.)

Fat cells in the abdominal area tend to be more active (releasing and taking up fat molecules) than those in the gluteal and femoral areas.[55] When the supply of abdominal fat is too great, the cells release their fat into the blood vessels that go to the liver; the fat that travels to the liver may be linked to negative health consequences. Various re-

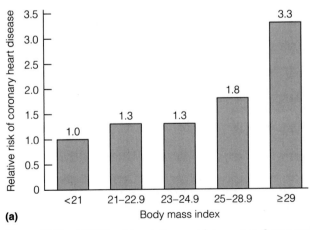

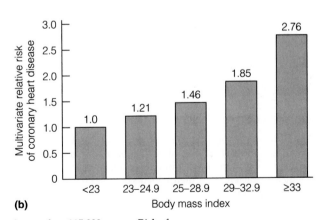

Figure 13.12 (a) BMI and heart disease risk in women, 8-year study of more than 115,000 nurses. Risk of coronary heart disease climbs sharply when the body mass index rises above 29 in women. (b) BMI and risk of coronary heart disease in men, 3-year study of 29,122 U.S. male health professionals. Risk of coronary heart disease rises as the body mass index increases in men. *Sources:* (a) Manson JE, Colditz GA, Stampfer MJ, et al. A prospective study of obesity and risk of coronary heart disease in women. *N Engl J Med* 322:882–889, 1990; (b) Rimm EB, Stampfer MJ, Giovannucci E, Ascherio A, Spiegelman D, Colditz GA, Willett WC. Body size and fat distribution as predictors of coronary heart disease among middle-aged and older US men. *Am J Epidemiol* 141:1117–1127, 1995.

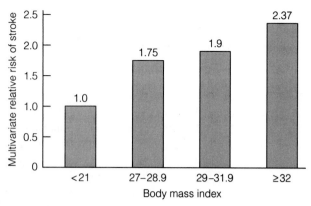

Figure 13.13 Body mass index and risk of ischemic stroke in women, 16-year study of 116,759 women. Risk of ischemic stroke rises with increase in body mass index. *Source:* Rexrode KM, Hennekens CH, Willett WC, Colditz GA, Stampfer MJ, Rich-Edwards JW, Speizer FE, Manson JE. A prospective study of body mass index, weight change, and risk of a stroke in women. *JAMA* 277:1539–1545, 1997.

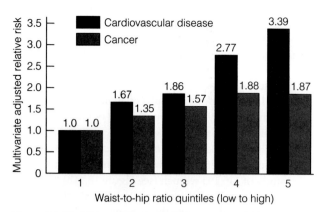

Figure 13.15 Waist-to-hip circumference ratio and disease risk, 5-year-study of 41,837 Iowa women. As the waist-to-hip circumference ratio climbs, risk of both cardiovascular disease and cancer death increases. *Source:* Folsom AR, Kaye SA, Sellers TA, et al. Body fat distribution and 5-year risk of death in older women. *JAMA* 269:483–487, 1993.

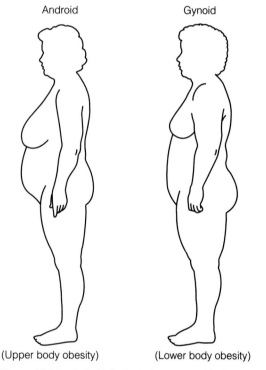

Figure 13.14 *Android obesity* is characterized by high amounts of body fat in the trunk and abdominal areas and is associated with increased medical complications. *Gynoid obesity* is characterized by high amounts of body fat in the hip and thigh areas.

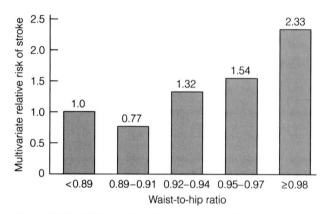

Figure 13.16 Waist-to-hip ratio and risk of stroke, 5-year study of 28,643 U.S. male health professionals. In men, risk of stroke rises with increase in the waist-to-hip ratio. *Source:* Walker SP, Rimm EB, Ascherio A, Kawachi I, Stampfer MJ, Willett WC. Body size and fat distribution as predictors of stroke among US men. *Am J Epidemiol* 144:1143–1150, 1996.

searchers have found that magnetic resonance imaging or computed tomography can image the abdominal fat depot (especially the visceral depot) quite precisely, improving prediction of health risks much better than the WHR (see Chapter 5).

It appears that lifestyle habits have much to do with abdominal fat.[56,57] For example, smoking, alcohol use, and weight cycling appear to preferentially increase abdominal fat stores, whereas exercise decreases them. Weight cycling, or weight fluctuation (i.e., repeated gaining and losing of body weight), has been shown to increase risk of heart disease and death, compared to maintaining a relatively stable weight.[58–60] In general, remaining lean throughout one's lifetime is the safest course to follow to avoid the health risks associated with abdominal obesity, weight cycling, and a high body mass index.[54] For overweight individuals, intentional weight loss, as opposed to unintentional loss of body mass, has been associated with increased longevity and improved quality of life.[61]

THEORIES OF OBESITY

Explaining why so many Americans weigh more than they should has been a source of confusion to researchers and the public alike. Currently, most theories of obesity fall into three categories: genetic and parental influences, high energy intake, and low energy expenditure[62,63] (see Figure 13.17).

Although we know that the development of obesity must involve a prolonged period in which energy intake exceeds energy expenditure, the relative importance of persistent overeating, abnormally low energy expenditure, or the influence of heredity for any particular individual remains controversial.[62]

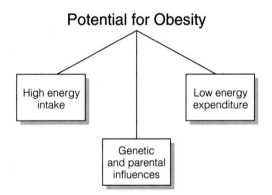

Figure 13.17 The theories of obesity fall into three categories.

Genetic and Parental Influences

Genetic and parental factors are important in explaining why some find it difficult to avoid obesity.[62–65] Jean Mayer reported in 1965 that 80% of the offspring of two obese parents eventually become obese, compared to 40% when one parent is obese and 14% when neither parent is obese.[66] Subsequent research has confirmed the importance of parental obesity in predicting obesity in their offspring, especially when present during the first 10 years of life (see Figure 13.18).

These results, however, gave little indication as to the relative importance of genetics versus the effects of family lifestyle patterns. Researchers have found the study of identical and fraternal twins to be more useful.[67–72] A study comparing adult fraternal and identical twins found that the body weights of the identical twins were much closer together than the body weights of the fraternal twins.[67] When monozygotic twins were reared apart, their body mass indexes were nearly as close as those of monozygotic twins reared together.[69]

A study of adults who had been adopted before the age of 1 year revealed that despite being brought up by their adoptive parents, their body weights were still very similar to those of their biological parents.[68] These studies suggest that shared genes are important in obesity.[71] Animal studies support this conclusion. When animals with inherited forms of obesity are paired with lean littermates and fed exactly the same, they gain more weight and fat.[67]

Other factors related to obesity may have a genetic component, including the resting metabolic rate, energy cost of exercise, level of habitual physical activity, tendency to store fat in the abdominal area, response to overfeeding, and relative rate of carbohydrate to lipid oxidation.[64,70,73–75] In one overfeeding experiment, 12 pairs of monozygotic twins were fed 1,000 extra Calories per day for 84 days.[74] Some subjects gained only 9 pounds, while others gained

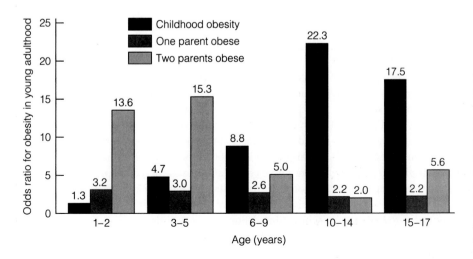

Figure 13.18 Odds for obesity in young adulthood: Parents' versus children's obesity status, retrospective study of 854 U.S. males and females. The odds of obesity in young adulthood are influenced by parental obesity (before the age of 10) and childhood–teenage obesity (especially after the age of 10). *Source:* Whitaker RC, Wright JA, Pepe MS, Seidel KD, Dietz WH. Predicting obesity in young adulthood from childhood and parental obesity. *N Engl J Med* 337:869–873, 1997.

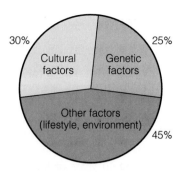

Figure 13.19 Genetic influence of human variation in body fat. Genetic influences on obesity are considered less important than nongenetic influences such as cultural, environmental, and lifestyle factors. *Source:* Bouchard C, Pérusse L, Leblanc C, et al. Inheritance of the amount and distribution of human body fat. *Int J Obesity* 12:205–215, 1988.

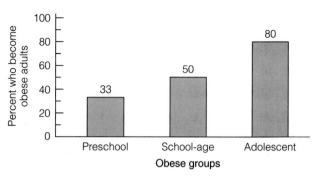

Figure 13.20 Obese children and youths: Percentage of those who become obese adults. The risk of adult obesity is greater for children and youths who are obese at older ages. *Source:* Serdula MK, Ivery D, Coates RJ, Freedman DS, Williamson DF, Byers T. Do obese children become obese adults? A review of the literature. *Prev Med* 22:167–177, 1993.

up to 29 pounds (average was 18). Of interest was the finding that there was at least three times more variance in response between twin pairs than within pairs for weight gains, showing that the amount of weight gain has some genetic basis.

In one research project, 1,698 members of 409 families were studied, including spouses, foster parents–adopted children, siblings by adoption, first-degree cousins, uncles/aunts–nephews/nieces, parents–natural children, full siblings, dizygotic twins, and monozygotic twins.[73] Biological inheritance was found to account for 25% of the variance in fat mass (see Figure 13.19). Nongenetic influences such as lifestyle and environmental and cultural factors were shown to be more important. Subsequent research has confirmed that 25–40% of the variability in human obesity has a genetic basis.[62,76]

These studies demonstrate that some people are more prone to obesity than others because of genetic factors. Such people have to be unusually careful with their dietary and exercise habits to counteract these inherited tendencies and may have to accept a body shape and size that is different than the American ideal portrayed in the media. There is a growing consensus that numerous genes interact with each other and with the environment to express the obesity phenotype.[62–64,76] It is likely that genes that affect both energy intake and energy expenditure are involved. Genes are involved in the regulation of body weight, which is a complex operation involving many different chemical signals, some of which arise from adipose tissue stores and then act in the central nervous system.[62] Leptin, for example, is produced by adipose tissue and acts in the central nervous system through a specific receptor and multiple neuropeptide pathways (under genetic control) to decrease appetite and increase energy expenditure.[62,77]

Most obesity experts feel that obesity is due to both genetic predisposition and environmental circumstances.[62,67,76,78]

In other words, a certain genetic makeup can give an individual a predisposition to obesity, and the appropriate environment can cause the expression of it. For example, the Pima Indians in Arizona were once of normal weight, living as farmers near the Gila River.[62] Their lifestyles favored physical activity and a diet high in complex carbohydrates and low in fat. Today, the Pima Indians have high prevalence rates for obesity and diabetes mellitus, live a sedentary existence, and consume a high-fat and high-alcohol diet. Although modern Pima Indians have the same genetic makeup of their predecessors, their environment has been greatly altered, and their biological disposition to obesity is now well expressed.

Although it is widely believed that fat children become fat adults, only about one third of obese preschool children become obese as adults.[65,79,80] However, about half of obese schoolage children become obese adults, and more than 80% of obese adolescents remain obese into adulthood.[79] The risk of adult obesity is greater for the fattest children and youths and for those with obese parents and grandparents.[65,79,80] (see Figures 13.18 and 13.20).

High Energy Intake

Do obese people eat more? This has been a controversial issue, with researchers on both sides of the issue.[81–85] In studies indicating that obese people do not eat more than normal-weight people do, subjects were asked to record food intake for 1–14 days using food diaries or memory-recall methods. There is now evidence that these methods do not give valid data because obese people tend to underreport their food intake as much as 20–50%.[82,84] Figure 13.21 depicts the result of one study of "diet resistant" subjects who claimed they ate very little, exercised appropriately, yet were obese.[84] When carefully examined by Columbia

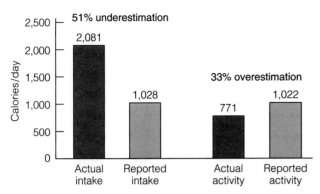

Figure 13.21 bars: 51% underestimation; Actual intake 2,081; Reported intake 1,028; 33% overestimation; Actual activity 771; Reported activity 1,022

Figure 13.21 Actual versus reported energy intake and expenditure, 14-day study of "diet resistant" subjects. In this study, subjects who claimed they are little and had a difficult time losing weight were found to underreport caloric intake and to overestimate energy expenditure. *Source:* Lichtman SW, Pisarska K, Berman ER, et al. Discrepancy between self-reported and actual caloric intake and exercise in obese subjects. *N Engl J Med* 327: 1893–1898, 1992.

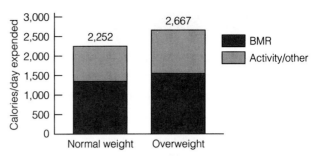

Figure 13.22 bars: BMR, Activity/other; Normal weight 2,252; Overweight 2,667

Figure 13.22 Energy expenditure in normal-weight and overweight women, 2-week study using doubly labeled water; body weight, 131 (26% fat) vs 187 (41%) pounds. Obese people expend more energy than normal-weight people and therefore must be eating more to maintain their excess weight. *Source:* Welle S, Forbes GB, Statt M, Barnard RR, Amatruda JM. Energy expenditure under free-living conditions in normal-weight and overweight women. *Am J Clin Nutr* 55:14–21, 1992.

University researchers during a 2-week period, these subjects were found to be underestimating food intake by about 50% and overestimating physical activity by 33%.

Several researchers have measured energy expenditure using respiratory chambers or doubly labeled water techniques in obese and normal-weight individuals. In these studies, obese people tend to expend and therefore eat about 400–500 Calories more on average each day.[82,86] Figure 13.22 gives the results of a 2-week study of obese and normal-weight women using doubly labeled water, which allowed the subjects to go about their normal duties.[86] Daily energy expenditure was more than 400 Calories higher among the obese women, with half of this due to their higher resting metabolic rates. The investigators concluded that most "overweight subjects must consume more energy than lean subjects to maintain their excess weight."[86] This outcome has also been established in animal studies. For example, fat versus lean rats of the same genetic line have been found to consume significantly more Calories.[87]

There is good reason to believe that the abundance of tasty, calorically rich foods, especially those high in fat, is a major factor in the high prevalence of obesity in Western societies.[88] A consistent finding among many recent studies is that when the intake of dietary fat is high, most adults and children tend to gain weight rather easily and quickly. However, when the intake of dietary fat is low and the intake of carbohydrate and fiber is high, desirable body weight is more readily achieved.[88-96] Cross-cultural studies show that obesity tends to be more prevalent in societies that consume a greater proportion of energy from dietary fat. For example, Americans eat 40% and the Chinese eat 15% of their total energy from fat, yet the Chinese consume 20% more Calories and there is little obesity in China.[97]

There are indications that obese versus lean people tend to choose high-fat and energy-rich foods more often in their day-to-day diets and have different eating behaviors.[85,91,92,98] In one study, obese inpatients at a hospital metabolic ward maintained a high caloric intake by consuming foods of greater caloric density, with occasional binge eating, as compared to leaner subjects.[85] When the eating behavior of 23 normal-weight and 20 obese children was compared, the obese children were found to eat faster and did not slow down their eating rate toward the end of the meal.[98] One fourth to one half of obese patients who seek weight-loss treatment suffer from problems with binge eating.[83] (See Box 13.1 for diagnostic criteria for binge eating.)

There are several reasons why high-fat diets promote obesity more than those high in carbohydrates.[99-108] Higher-fat foods are often perceived as more palatable, leading to a much greater caloric intake. For example, when eating from a range of either high-fat or high-carbohydrate foods, obese subjects have been found to voluntarily consume twice as much energy from the fat items.[96,101] This finding has led to the theory that the appetite-control system may have only weak inhibitory signals to prevent overconsumption of dietary fat. Researchers believe that while glycogen and protein stores in the body are tightly controlled, fat stores are not, allowing a high degree of expansion.[100,101] This may have served a useful purpose eons ago but now means that obesity can be avoided only if dietary fat intake is low.

Dietary fat also has less of a thermogenic effect than does carbohydrate or protein and can thus be stored as adipose tissue rather easily (see Figure 13.23). Dietary carbohydrate, on the other hand, is not readily converted to body fat, even during periods of high intake.[100,102,104-108] In one study, obese and lean men ingested 50% more energy than normal for 2 weeks.[99] In random order, the additional energy was given as either all fat or all carbohydrate. A whole-room calorimeter determined that carbohydrate over-

Box 13.1

Diagnostic Criteria for Binge Eating

Following are key diagnostic criteria for diagnosing binge eating.

1. *Characteristics of binge-eating episodes.* The binge-eating episodes are associated with at least three of the following:

   a. Eating much more rapidly than normal

   b. Eating until feeling uncomfortably full

   c. Eating large amounts of food when not feeling physically hungry

   d. Eating alone because of being embarrassed by how much one is eating

2. *Distress.* The person experiences marked distress regarding binge eating. Feelings include disgust, depression, and extreme guilt after overeating.

3. *Recurrent episodes of binge eating.* An episode of binge eating is characterized by both of the following:

   a. Eating, in a discrete period of time (e.g., within any 2-hour period), an amount of food that is definitely larger than most people would eat in a similar period of time under similar circumstances; and

   b. A sense of lack of control over eating during the episode (e.g., a feeling that one cannot stop eating or control what or how much one is eating).

4. *Frequency.* The binge eating occurs, on average, at least 2 days a week for 6 months.

5. *No connection to other eating disorders.* The binge eating is not associated with the regular use of inappropriate compensatory behaviors (e.g., purging, fasting, excessive exercise) and does not occur exclusively during the course of anorexia nervosa or bulimia nervosa.

Source: American Psychiatric Association. *Diagnostic and Statistical Manual of Mental Disorders* (4th ed.). Washington, DC: American Psychiatric Association, 1994. Copyright © 1994 American Psychiatric Association. Reprinted with permission.

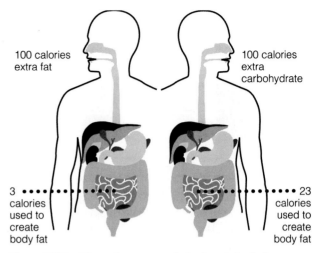

100 calories extra fat

100 calories extra carbohydrate

3 calories used to create body fat

23 calories used to create body fat

Figure 13.23   Dietary fat versus carbohydrate in body fat formation. The body converts dietary fat into body fat more efficiently than it converts dietary carbohydrate into body fat. *Source:* Acheson KJ, Schutz Y, Bessard T, Flatt JP, Jequier E. Carbohydrate metabolism and de novo lipogenesis in human obesity. *Am J Clin Nutr* 45:78–85, 1987.

feeding increased carbohydrate oxidation and total energy expenditure, resulting in 75–85% of the excess energy being stored. Fat overfeeding, however, had minimal effects on fat oxidation and total energy expenditure, leading to storage of 90–95% of excess energy. In other words, excess dietary fat leads to greater fat accumulation in the body than an equal caloric amount of dietary carbohydrate.

A randomized, 11-week crossover study of 16 female subjects by researchers at Cornell University illustrates the importance of keeping dietary fat intake low[93] (see Figure 13.24). Subjects were randomly assigned to either a low-fat diet (22% of calories as fat) or a control diet (37% fat) for 11 weeks, with conditions reversed for another 11 weeks. During the study, subjects were allowed to eat as much food as desired, but they could consume only foods provided by the investigators. The same 41 menu items were offered to the subjects in both groups, but the researchers reduced the quantity of oil, margarine, cream, and so on, used in the preparation of the menu items for subjects on the low-fat diet.

While on the low-fat diet, subjects tended to eat less (237 fewer Calories per day) than when on the control diet, and they lost more weight (5.5 pounds). The results of this study clearly demonstrate that when the fat content of the diet is reduced from 37% to 22% of total Calories, people tend to ingest fewer Calories. Also, it seems that some degree of weight loss can be achieved by simply lowering the amount of fat used during food preparation without the necessity of dieting or voluntarily limiting the amount of food consumed.

In another study, 24 women each consumed a sequence of three 2-week dietary treatments in which 15–20%, 30–35%,

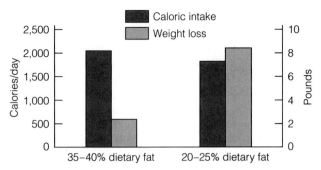

Figure 13.24 Weight loss on a low-fat diet (ad libitum), randomized to low- or high-fat diets for 11 weeks, using same 41 menu items. Low-fat diets promote more weight loss than high-fat diets. *Source:* Kendall A, Levitsky DA, Strupp BJ, Lissner L. Weight loss on a low-fat diet: Consequence of the imprecision of the control of food intake in humans. *Am J Clin Nutr* 53:1124–1129, 1991.

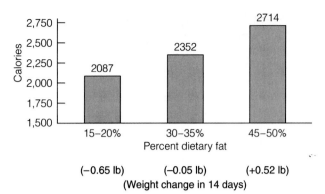

Figure 13.25 Energy intake during 14-day diet, treatments varying in fat content. Reduction in dietary fat is associated with a lower caloric intake and greater weight loss. *Source:* Lissner L, Levitsky DA, Strupp BJ, et al. Dietary fat and the regulation of energy intake in human subjects. *Am J Clin Nutr* 46:886–892, 1987.

or 45–50% of the total Calories was derived from fat.[95] The diets consisted of foods that were similar in appearance and taste, but differed in the amount of high-fat ingredients used. The subjects spontaneously consumed 27% fewer Calories when on the low-fat diet versus the high-fat diet, resulting in significant changes in body weight (see Figure 13.25). Once again, reduction of habitual fat intake was seen by these researchers as a key element for both the prevention and the treatment of obesity "in that it imposes no strict limitations on the quantity of food consumed, but rather emphasizes the selection of low-fat foods."[95]

Of all the current theories attempting to explain the epidemic of obesity in most Western societies, the "high dietary fat intake" hypothesis is most widely accepted by experts. As emphasized in the medical journal *Lancet* by one team of obesity experts:

> Fat calories represent the only candidate for a sufficient chronic energy imbalance to cause obesity, implying that in addition to an increase in exercise and a restriction of total calories . . . a simple reduction in fat intake will lead to weight loss. This approach . . . could serve as the central strategy for the prevention and treatment of obesity at the individual and population levels. . . . Encouraging the food industry to produce and promote low fat products, and educating consumers to choose these products, are probably the best options for population-wide dietary changes.[107]

Low Energy Expenditure

So far we have seen that some people are more prone to obesity because of genetic tendencies and habitual consumption of high-fat diets. Can obesity also develop because total energy expenditure is lower than normal? Is there some type of metabolic defect that predicts increased

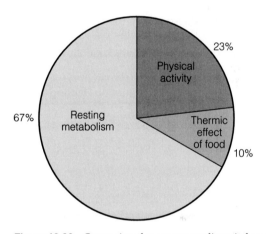

Figure 13.26 Categories of energy expenditure in humans. Approximately 67% of human energy expenditure is from the resting metabolism rate. Sedentary people expend about 23% of their energy in miscellaneous physical activity, and another 10% metabolizing and digesting food. *Source:* Ravussin E, Bogardus C. A brief overview of human energy metabolism and its relationship to essential obesity. *Am J Clin Nutr* 55:242S–245S, 1992.

obesity because the body is burning fewer Calories than it should? Do obese people burn fewer Calories in physical activity?

All humans expend energy in three ways: through the *resting metabolic rate*, physical activity, and digesting and metabolizing food (*thermic effect of food*)[109,110] (see Figure 13.26).

Resting Metabolic Rate

The largest number of Calories expended by most people (except for athletes who train several hours a day) is from the *resting metabolic rate* (RMR). This represents the energy expended by the body to maintain life and normal body functions, such as respiration and circulation. The resting metabolic rate of the average 154-pound male amounts to approximately 1,700 Calories per day, or 60–75% of total daily energy expenditure. This is a considerable amount of energy, equivalent to jogging 17 miles. The RMR varies up to 20–30% among people of the same age, sex, and body weight, but about 65–80% of this variation is due to differences in body composition, with the RMR higher in those with the greatest fat-free mass (muscle, bone, water, etc.).[109-112] RMR falls about 1–2% per decade of adult life, even after adjusting for fat-free mass.[109]

The RMR is best measured by collecting and analyzing expired air (*indirect calorimetry*) several hours after eating. RMR can also be estimated through the use of equations. Table 13.1 summarizes some of the more commonly used equations.[111-115] Because of the tight relationship between RMR and fat-free mass, estimation of RMR is improved especially for obese individuals by using equations 4 and 5 in Table 13.1.[111,112]

As would be expected from these equations, an obese person actually has a higher RMR than a normal-weight person.[111] Obese people, because of the extra weight they carry, have a high fat-free mass—resulting in a higher RMR.

Although obese individuals have elevated RMRs, those levels will fall to normal following achievement of desirable weight.[116,117] The excess weight of mildly and moderately obese people is approximately 25% lean body tissue and 75% fat. With each kilogram of body weight loss, the RMR drops between 10 and 20 Calories per day. A loss of 20 kilograms will reduce RMR by approximately 200–400 Calories per day. As summarized in Figure 13.27, body energy expenditure decreases or increases in parallel with body weight changes.[116]

Although the RMR is closely related to the lean body weight, resting metabolic rate still may vary substantially among people of similar body composition, age, sex, and body weight.[110,111] Heredity may account for as much as 40% of this variation, perhaps by affecting sympathetic nervous activity, which is related to all three major components of energy expenditure.[118] Some researchers have determined that a low RMR is a risk factor for future obesity.[118,119] However, others disagree and have not been able to associate low RMR with future weight gain.[120,121] It makes sense, however, that if for a given body weight and fat-free mass the RMR is lower than found in others, that particular

TABLE 13.1 Equations for Estimating Resting Metabolic Rate

1. Equations by Owens[113]

Males

Resting metabolic rate (Calories/day) = 879 + 10.2 (kg)

Females

Resting metabolic rate (Calories/day) = 795 + 7.18 (kg)

2. Revised Harris–Benedict Equations[114]

Males

Resting metabolic rate (Calories/day)
= 88.362 + (4.799 × ht) + (13.397 × kg) − (5.677 × age)

Females

Resting metabolic rate (Calories/day)
= 447.593 + (3.098 × ht) + (9.247 × kg) − (4.330 × age)

3. World Health Organization Equations[115]

Age Range (years)	Equation for Calories Resting Metabolic Rate	Standard Deviation (actual vs predicted)
Males		
18–30	15.3 (kg) + 679	151
30–60	11.6 (kg) + 879	164
>60	13.5 (kg) + 487	148
Females		
18–30	14.7 (kg) + 496	121
30–60	8.7 (kg) + 829	108
>60	10.5 (kg) + 596	108

4. National Institutes of Health, Phoenix, Arizona, Lab[111]

Resting metabolic rate (Calories/day) = 638 + 15.9 (FFM)

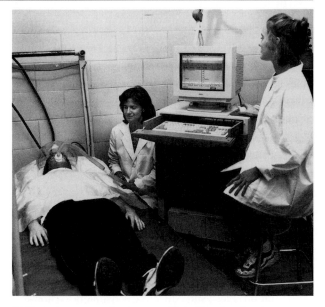

RMR can be measured using a ventilated hood and metabolic cart.

5. University of Vermont[112]

Resting metabolic rate (Calories/day) = 418 + 20.3 (FFM)

Note: kg = body weight in kilograms; ht = height in centimeters; FFM = fat-free mass in kilograms

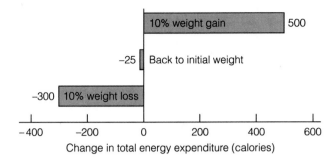

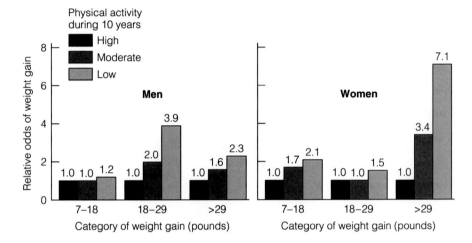

Figure 13.27 Adjustments in body energy expenditure after weight gain or loss, 41 obese and nonobese men and women. Body energy expenditure parallels changes in body weight. *Source:* Leibel RL, Rosenbaum M, Hirsch J. Changes in energy expenditure resulting from altered body weight. *N Eng J Med* 332:621–628, 1995.

Figure 13.28 Recreational physical activity and 10-year weight change: NHANES I epidemiologic follow-up study of 3,515 men and 5,810 women. For both men and women who engaged in low amounts of physical activity, weight gain over a 10-year period was much more likely than for those who engaged in high levels of activity. *Source:* Williamson DF, Madans J, Anda RF, et al. Recreational physical activity and ten-year weight change in a US national cohort. *Int J Obesity* 17:279–286, 1993.

individual will have to compensate by exercising more or eating less in order to avoid obesity.

Physical Activity

All physical activity, all muscular movement, expends energy. The average sedentary person usually expends only 300–800 Calories a day in physical activity, most of this from informal, unplanned types of movement. On the other hand, top athletes usually match their RMR energy expenditure through hard, intense exercise. For optimal health, most physical fitness experts recommend burning at least 200–400 Calories per day through planned exercise (see Chapter 8).

The National Research Council has recommended that the average male and female adult ingest enough Calories each day to match 1.6 and 1.55 times their RMR.[122] This meets the energy needs of those engaging in light-to-moderate activity. For a 72-pound male with an RMR of 1,780, the total energy needed for 1 day would be 1,780 × 1.6 = 2,848 Calories. As physical activity increases, the RMR multiplication factor may rise to between 2 and 3 for many athletes.

It is commonly believed by most obesity experts that the epidemic of obesity in the modern era is in part due to the technological transformations that have made human energy expenditure nigh obsolete during both work and leisure-time pursuits.[123–130] Even when people do exercise during their leisure time, the total daily energy expenditure still falls far short of what was typical during the nineteenth century.[123]

There is some indication that long-term physical activity is related to a lower risk of gaining weight.[124–130] Researchers from the American Cancer Institute followed over 79,000 people for 10 years and found that those engaging in vigorous exercise 1–3 hours a week, or walking for more than 4 hours a week, were better able to ward off weight gain than their more sedentary counterparts.[128] When a group of more than 9,000 men and women were followed for 10 years, major weight gain was much more likely among people with low versus high amounts of physical activity[125] (see Figure 13.28). Among male health professionals, just 30 minutes a day of moderate physical activity was sufficient to reduce the risk of becoming overweight during a 2-year period.[127] In a 10-year study of more than 5,000 Finnish men and women, the odds of significant weight gain were 2.6-fold greater in those reporting no regular exercise, compared to their peers who engaged in regular vigorous exercise[124] (see Figure 13.29). Prospective studies of young children have demonstrated that those with low, compared to high, levels of physical activity gain more body fat.[129,130] Together, these studies indicate that reg-

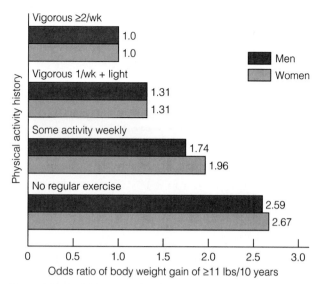

Figure 13.29 Odds for weight gain over 10 years according to physical activity, 10-year study of 5,259 Finnish men and women. The odds of significant weight gain are highest in men and women reporting no regular exercise during a 10-year period. *Source:* Haapanen N, Miilunpalo S, Pasanen M, Oja P, Vuori I. Association between leisure time physical activity and 10-year body mass change among working-aged men and women. *Int J Obesity* 21:288–296, 1997.

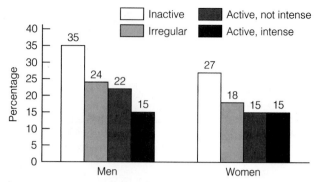

Figure 13.30 Prevalence of overweight by physical activity pattern, CDC BRFSS, 6,125 men, 12,557 women. In cross-sectional studies, the prevalence of obesity has consistently been found to be highest in those reporting no regular physical activity. *Source:* DiPietro L, Williamson DF, Caspersen CJ, Eaker E. The descriptive epidemiology of selected physical activities and body weight among adults trying to lose weight: The behavioral risk factor surveillance system survey, 1989. *Int J Obesity* 17:69–76, 1993.

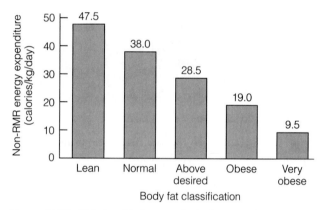

Figure 13.31 Relationship between body fatness and non-RMR energy expenditure, 300 obese and non-obese males and females, measured with the doubly labeled water method. Energy expenditure (non-RMR) is lowest (weight adjusted) in the very obese. *Source:* Schulz LO, Schoeller DA. A compilation of total daily energy expenditures and body weights in healthy adults. *Am J Clin Nutr* 60:676–681, 1994.

ular physical activity is associated with a reduced risk of body weight gain over the long term.

Do the obese exercise more or less than normal-weight people? Although measurement of physical activity is extremely difficult and has hampered our understanding of this issue, most studies show that both obese children and obese adults are less active than normal-weight people.[129–143] Overweight girls have been found to be less active than lean ones while playing sports.[131] For example, obese adolescent girls, when swimming, spend less time actually moving their arms and legs and more time standing and floating than normal-weight girls. While playing tennis, obese girls have been found to be inactive 77% of the time, compared with 56% of the time for normal-weight girls. In general, obese children spend up to 40% less time in physical activity than lean children.[131]

Obese men informally walk an average of 3.7 miles per day, compared to 6 miles per day for men of normal weight; obese women walk 2 miles per day, compared to 4.9 miles per day for normal-weight women.[133] The obese stay in bed longer and spend 17% less time on their feet than normal-weight people do.[134] When given a choice of an escalator or stairs, the obese are more likely than the lean to take the escalator.[42]

In general, there are good data to indicate that physical activity decreases in direct relationship to the degree of obesity.[135,139,140] In cross-sectional studies, the prevalence of obesity is consistently highest in those reporting the least amount of physical activity[140] (see Figure 13.30). As depicted in Figure 13.31, energy expended in activity (Calories/kg/day) falls in direct relationship to the degree of obesity.[139] It has been difficult to know, however, whether inactivity causes obesity or if obesity leads to inactivity.[126] Some researchers feel that because aerobic fitness levels are lower among the obese, exercise is more difficult, and inactivity is then a result of the increase in body fat stores.[137,138]

Although there appears to be a tendency for obese people to be less physically active than normal-weight people, this does not necessarily mean that the total energy expenditure from physical activity is less. Because they weigh more, the obese expend more Calories when they do engage in physical activity. In other words, even though obese people tend to engage in less physical activity than lean

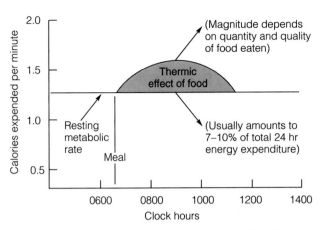

Figure 13.32 Thermic effect of food. The thermic effect of food (TEF) is the energy expended for the digestion, absorption, transport, metabolism, and storage of food.[102] *Source:* Reed GW, Hill JO. Measuring the thermic effect of food. *Am J Clin Nutr* 63:164–169, 1996.

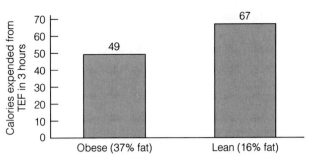

Figure 13.33 Thermic effect of a 720-calorie meal in lean and obese men, thermic effect of food (TEF) = postprandial − postabsorptive RMR. The thermic effect of food is slightly lower among obese, compared to lean, men.[148] *Source:* Segal KR, Edano A, Tomas MB. Thermic effect of a meal over 3 and 6 hours in lean and obese men. *Metabolism* 39:985–992, 1990.

people, they expend more energy in the course of that activity. The end result is that daily energy expenditure from physical activity has been found in most studies to be little different between the obese and the nonobese[119,144] (see Figure 13.22). For this reason, most experts feel that overeating is a more important factor than inactivity in accounting for the large number of obese people in developed countries.[42,107] Nonetheless, most experts agree that increased physical activity is necessary for long-term prevention of weight gain.[140]

Thermic Effect of Food

The *thermic effect of food* (TEF) is the increase in energy expenditure above the RMR that can be measured for several hours after a meal[145–150] (see Figure 13.32). Energy is expended as the body digests, absorbs, transports, metabolizes, and stores the food eaten. The average person's TEF is about 10% of total ingested Calories, or about 200–250

Calories per day for women and about 250–300 Calories per day for men.[145,146] For example, after a meal containing 800 Calories, the body uses about 80 Calories just to process the meal.

The TEF has been found to be higher with larger meals.[147] For normal-weight people, the TEF raises the energy expenditure of the body 40–45% over the RMR 1 hour after a 1,500-Calorie meal; after a 1,000-Calorie meal, there is a 25% increase over the RMR. As depicted in Figure 13.32, the TEF peaks about 60–120 minutes following a meal and lasts up to 4–6 hours.

Do the obese expend fewer Calories in digesting and metabolizing their food than normal-weight people? Most researchers have concluded that obese adults and children have a slightly lower TEF, especially if they are diabetic[145–150] (see Figure 13.33). However, the difference is too small in terms of actual Calories to be important. In addition, most obese people have higher RMRs, due to their increased fat-free mass, more than making up for the small decrease in TEF.[146]

Table 13.2 summarizes information on energy expenditure, comparing obese and nonobese people. The 177 people

TABLE 13.2 Energy Expenditure in 177 Humans (Obese and Nonobese) Studied in a Respiratory Chamber

Variable	Average (Calories/day)	Range (Calories/day)	Obese vs Lean
24-hour energy expenditure	2,292	1,371–3,615	Increased[a]
All types of physical activity	348	138–685	Decreased
Resting metabolic rate	1,813	1,102–2,935	Increased[a]
Thermic effect of food	165	50–476	Little difference

Note: Average weight = 97 kg; range = 47–178 kg.
[a]Increased in an obese person, in comparison to a lean person.

Source: Ravussin E, Lillioja S, Anderson TE, Christin L, Bogardus C. Determinants of 24-hour energy expenditure in man. *J Clin Invest* 78:1568–1578, 1986.

in this study varied widely in weight and degree of obesity. In general, obese people were found to expend more energy each day than nonobese people, despite lower levels of physical activity. This was due primarily to higher RMRs.[119]

TREATMENT OF OBESITY

As we have seen thus far in this chapter, over one half of adults in the United States are classified as overweight and obese. The prevalence of overweight has increased during the twentieth century and is disproportionately high in many subpopulations, including the poor and members of some ethnic groups.[151] Being overweight can seriously affect health and longevity and is a contributing factor to the two leading causes of death in the United States: heart disease and cancer. Although experts still debate the underlying causes, all agree that the basic mechanism is an imbalance between caloric intake and energy expenditure. Evidence suggests that obesity is multifactorial in origin, reflecting genetic, lifestyle, cultural, socioeconomic, and psychological conditions.

Americans appear to be preoccupied with plans and aspirations to lose body weight and spend over $30 billion a year to this end.[151] Using information from four federal surveys, the National Institutes of Health Technology Assessment Conference Panel on Methods for Voluntary Weight Loss and Control has estimated that 33–40% of adult women and 20–24% of men are, during any given time, trying to lose weight, with an additional 28% of both sexes trying to maintain weight.[151] Fifty-seven percent of men and 72% of women report having attempted to lose weight within the previous year. The number of attempts to lose weight in the past 2 years averaged 2.5 for women and 2.0 for men. Figure 13.34 shows the various weight-control practices being used by U.S. adults trying to lose weight, which range from simply measuring body weight on a regular basis to using commercial weight-loss programs.[152] Among high school students, 44% of females and 15% of males report they also are trying to lose weight.[153] Although about one third of Americans see themselves as overweight, less than two thirds of those are actually trying to lose weight.[154] Among those who think their weight is about right, 11% are still trying to lose weight, as are 4% of self-perceived underweight Americans.[154] Concerns about future and current health, fitness, and appearance are cited most frequently by Americans as the most important reasons for trying to lose weight.

Treatment Is Challenging

Treatment of obesity has proven to be one of the greatest challenges facing health professionals. Many obese people

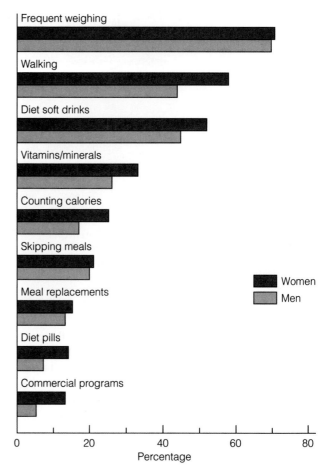

Figure 13.34 Weight-control practices of U.S. adults trying to lose weight: 33–44% of adult women, 20–24% of men trying to lose weight currently; 28% trying to maintain weight. U.S. adults use a wide variety of methods to try to lose weight. These data are from the 1992 Weight Loss Practices Survey sponsored jointly by the U.S. Food and Drug Administration and the National Heart, Lung, and Blood Institute. *Source:* Levy AS, Heaton AW. Weight control practices of U.S. adults trying to lose weight. *Ann Intern Med* 119(7 pt 2):661–666, 1993.

will not stay in treatment. Of those who do, most will not achieve ideal body weight, and of those who lose weight, most will regain it. For most weight-loss methods, there are few scientific studies evaluating their effectiveness and safety.[151] Studies that are available indicate that people can be quite successful losing weight in the short term, but after completing the program or weight-loss scheme, they tend to regain the weight over time.

For example, in a 4-year study of 152 men and women who had participated in a 15-week behaviorally oriented weight-loss program including diet, exercise, and behavior modification, less than 3% of subjects were able to maintain posttreatment weights throughout the 4 years of follow-up observation.[155] Data from a 5-year study of 76 obese women (mean weight 233 pounds) are given in Figure 13.35.[156] At

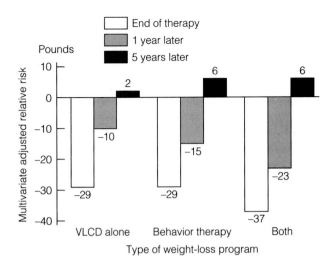

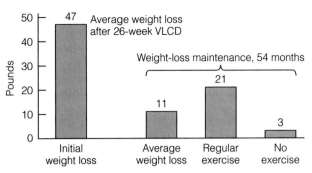

Figure 13.36 Weight-loss maintenance following a very-low-calorie diet program, 54 months of follow-up. Regular exercise over a 4.5-year period following a 26-week VLCD program significantly improved weight-loss maintenance. *Source:* Walsh MF, Flynn TJ. A 54-month evaluation of a popular very low calorie diet program. *J Fam Pract* 41:231–236, 1995.

Figure 13.35 Maintenance of weight loss over 5 years, 76 obese women (mean weight 233 lb) treated for 4–6 months and followed 5 years. Long-term success in maintaining the body weight lost during treatment for obesity has been found in this study and others to be poor. *Source:* Wadden TA, Sternberg JA, Letizia KA, Stunkard AJ, Foster GD. Treatment of obesity by very low calorie diet, behavior therapy, and their combination: A five-year perspective. *Int J Obesity* 13 (suppl 2):39–49, 1989.

baseline, subjects were randomly assigned to one of three weight-loss programs:

1. A very-low-calorie diet (VLCD) of 400–500 Calories per day for 2 months followed by a 1,000- to 1,200-Calorie-per-day diet for 2 more months (designated as "VLCD alone" in Figure 13.35).

2. A 1,200-Calorie-per-day diet plus behavior modification training for 6 months (behavior therapy).

3. Same as group 1, but behavior modification training was included for 6 months ("Both" in the figure).

The data in Figure 13.35 show that although the end-of-treatment and 1-year data are quite impressive, especially for groups receiving behavior therapy, 5 years after treatment, nearly all subjects in each group had returned to their pretreatment weight, with group means actually above starting body weights. Overall, only 5% of subjects maintained all of their weight loss after 5 years, and only 18% maintained a loss greater than 11 pounds, with 64% of subjects regaining all of, or more than, what they had once lost.

Weight-Loss Maintenance

These researchers and others have urged that more vigorous efforts should be put forth to help patients maintain the weight they do lose.[156–162] They recommend that patients participate in at least a 6- to 12-month program of weight-loss maintenance immediately after losing weight (no matter what the method) and that they be prepared to reenter

therapy whenever they show a gain of 10 pounds or more that they cannot lose on their own. During the maintenance program, group and individual counseling with health professionals (especially physicians, who appear to have the most influence with obese patients) and an emphasis on a low-fat diet and regular exercise should be integrated. Behavior treatment should continue after the weight-loss program, by which patients are made aware of their current lifestyle habits through various techniques, including record keeping, problem solving, change in thinking processes, social support, and self-reinforcement.

Several studies have attempted to measure factors that predict long-term maintenance of weight-loss after participation in a weight-loss program or process.[162–165] In one study of 509 obese subjects, predictors of success after 2 years were feeling in control of eating habits, success during actual treatment, frequency of weight measurement, and increase in physical activity.[164] Another study of 118 obese patients followed for more than 3 years showed that weight loss was maintained best in those who reported eating fewer high-fat foods, using the behavioral techniques taught in the program, and exercising more.[165] In the National Weight Control Registry study, a low-fat diet and high levels of physical activity were reported by the majority of subjects who had been successful at long-term maintenance of weight loss.[162]

Several other studies have found that exercise is one of the best markers for long-term success.[166–170] In one study, 90% of women who had lost weight and maintained their losses for more than 2 years reported regular exercise, compared with only 34% of the women who had regained their weight losses.[169] Figure 13.36 shows that weight-loss maintenance was significantly enhanced in subjects who exercised regularly for 4.5 years after a VLCD program, compared to those who avoided exercise.[166]

Weight regain is probably related to several powerful factors, including genetic influences to retain high fat stores, an innate propensity of the human body in general to defend body fat reserves, and failure on the part of the individual to apply new behavioral skills (especially exercise and eating a low-fat diet) because of barriers imposed by family and societal forces. A tremendous amount of support from several sources is necessary for a prolonged time following treatment of obesity to ensure any type of reasonable success.

There are many health benefits associated with weight loss.[151,171,172] Weight loss reduces many of the health hazards associated with obesity, including insulin resistance, diabetes mellitus, hypertension, dyslipidemia (e.g., high cholesterol, low HDL, and high triglycerides), sleep apnea, and osteoarthritis. Among very obese individuals, weight loss has been followed by greater functional status, reduced work absenteeism, less pain, and greater social interaction.[151] However, there are adverse effects of weight loss when it is too rapid (e.g., during fasting or VLCDs), including a greater risk for gallstone formation and cholecystitis, excessive loss of lean body mass, water and electrolyte problems, mild liver dysfunction, and elevated uric acid levels.

Conservative Treatment Guidelines

Obesity has typically been treated as if it is an acute illness, when it is more appropriately viewed as a chronic condition much like heart disease or diabetes.[151,173] Obesity treatment should include efforts not only at the individual but also at community and national levels. Community interventions could include educational and media programs to lower dietary fat consumption and increase physical activity. National policies to improve food-label information or to provide economic support for local community efforts are examples of what could be done to enhance environmental support for individuals struggling to maintain ideal body weight.

Because the ultimate goal of a weight-reduction program is to lose weight and maintain the loss, a nutritionally balanced, low-calorie diet that is applicable to the patient's lifestyle is most appropriate.[158] A comprehensive weight-reduction program that incorporates diet, exercise, and behavior modification is more likely to lead to long-term weight control.[174] (Shape Up America!, a nonprofit organization dedicated to helping people lose weight, has some excellent obesity treatment guidelines that can be downloaded at this website: http://www.shapeup.org.)

For most obese individuals, a weight loss of about 1% total body weight per week is optimal. For example, someone who weighs 200 pounds and wants to weigh 165 pounds should lose no more than an average of 1.5–2 pounds a week. Because each pound of body fat represents about 3,500 Calories, this would require a daily caloric deficit of 750–1,000 Calories, which could be accomplished by increasing energy expenditure through physical activity by 300 Calories a day and reducing dietary fat intake by 450–700 Calories. Each tablespoon of fat represents about 100 Calories, so an emphasis on low-fat dairy products and lean meats, and reduced intake of visible fats (oils, butter, margarine, salad dressings, sour cream, etc.), would be the easiest way to reduce caloric intake without reducing the volume of food eaten.

In summary, conservative treatment for obesity involves three elements:[174,175]

1. *Diet.* The caloric intake should be reduced, preferably by reducing the fat content of the diet, while increasing the complex carbohydrates. In 1998, the National Heart, Lung, and Blood Institute (NHLBI) advised that for most overweight/obese clients, a decrease of 300–1,000 kcal/day will lead to weight losses of ½–2 pounds per week, and a 10% weight loss in six months (the initial goal).[5] The low-calorie diet should be consistent with the NCEP's Step 1 or 2 diet (see Chapter 10).[5]

2. *Exercise.* Energy expenditure should be increased at least 200–400 Calories per day by increasing all forms of physical activity.

3. *Behavior modification.* Several techniques should be employed, including

   • *Self-monitoring*—such as keeping diet diaries, emphasizing the recording of food amounts consumed and circumstances surrounding the eating episode

   • *Control of the events that precede eating*—identification of the circumstances that elicit eating and overeating

   • *Development of techniques to control the act of eating*—typical behavioral modification techniques

   • *Reinforcement through use of rewards*—involving a system of formal rewards that facilitate progress

Although the majority of obese patients will benefit from these guidelines, there are some who carry substantial amounts of body fat, who may need additional forms of therapy to be successful, including the VLCD under medical supervision, drug therapy, and/or gastric-reduction surgery. Figure 13.37 summarizes a treatment scheme for obese patients based on their body mass index or severity of obesity.[176] Box 13.2 summarizes the treatment scheme advocated by Shape Up America! Notice that gastric-reduction surgery is reserved for the most severely obese, while the VLCD and drug therapy are recommended as a consideration for moderately obese patients. These methods

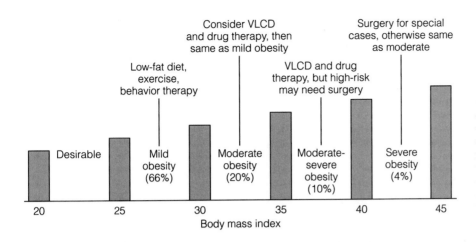

Figure 13.37 Treatment scheme for obesity. Treatment varies according to the severity of obesity. The presence of comorbid conditions and disease risk factors increases the urgency for treatment. The percentages in parentheses represent the proportion of obese people in each category. *Source:* Bray GA. Pathophysiology of obesity. *Am J Clin Nutr* 55:488S–494S, 1992.

Box 13.2

Summary of the Shape Up America! Treatment Model

The treatment model has three fundamental components:

I. Assessment of the patient's health risk

II. Decision: Is the patient eligible for and interested in weight-reduction treatment?

III. Prescription of appropriate treatment strategy and follow-up

Part I. Assessment of Patient's Health Risk

1. *Determine body mass index (BMI).*

2. *Assess comorbid conditions.* Does your patient have any of the following conditions? Hypertension, cardiovascular disease, dyslipidemia, type 2 diabetes, sleep apnea, osteoarthritis, infertility, other conditions.

3. *Identify other risk factors.* Does your patient have any of the following additional risk factors? Waist-to-hip ratio >1.0 in males or >0.8 in females, waist circumference ≥40 inches in males or ≥35 inches in females. Factors requiring clinical judgment: progressive weight gain since adolescence, individual history of obesity, family history of obesity, bulimia nervosa, or binge-eating disorder; depression, anxiety, or stress; and relevant medical or physical conditions, including hyperinsulinemia, breast, colon, or endometrial cancer, menopause, overall disease burden, physical inactivity, and smoking cessation.

4. *Determine patient's BMI-related health risk.* What is your patient's BMI-related health risk? How is

that risk modified by the presence of comorbid conditions and / or other risk factors?

BMI Category	Health Risk Based on BMI	Risk Adjusted for Comorbidity/ Risk Factors
< 25	Minimal	Low
25–26.9	Low	Moderate
27–29.9	Moderate	High
30–34.9	High	Very high
35–39.9	Very high	Extremely high
≥ 40	Extremely high	Extremely high

5. *Determine weight-reduction exclusions.* Does your patient have any conditions that warrant a temporary or permanent exclusion from weight-reduction treatment? *Temporary exclusions* include pregnancy, lactation, unstable mental illness, unstable medical conditions. *Possible exclusions* (require clinical judgment) include cholelithiasis, osteoporosis. *Permanent exclusions* include anorexia nervosa, terminal illness. Weight-reduction treatment is not recommended for pregnant women or for patients with unstable mental or medical conditions.

6. *Assess patient readiness: Is your patient ready to lose weight?* Lack of patient interest or readiness is an indication that weight-reduction treatment is not appropriate—even if such treatment is warranted based on the patient's health risk. For these patients, prevention of weight gain should be the

(continued)

Summary of the Shape Up America! Treatment Model *(continued)*

treatment goal. If the patient denies treatment, it is important to ensure an "informed refusal."

Part II. Decision: Is Patient Eligible for and Interested in Weight-Reduction Treatment?

- If yes, proceed to section on weight reduction (III, 1).

- If no, proceed to section on prevention of weight gain (III, 2).

Part III. Prescription of Appropriate Treatment Strategy and Follow-up

1. *Weight reduction.* If weight-reduction treatment is appropriate, the process is as follows:

   a. Prescribe weight reduction through energy deficit.

      - Select an appropriate target BMI.

      - Create an energy deficit.

      - Establish permanent changes in lifestyle.

      For most patients—especially those with a BMI ≥ 30—a target BMI that is 2 BMI units below their current one is realistic and practical. An energy deficit can only be achieved by consistently expending more energy than consumed in food. Treatment options that support such a strategy include attention to diet, increased physical activity, pharmacological intervention, and surgery. Lifestyle-change strategies should be routinely used in combination with any other treatment option.

   b. Select weight-reduction treatment option. The treatment options available to each patient are based on health risk (see Part I).

Health Risk	Treatment Options Available
Minimal and low	Healthful eating and/or moderate-deficit diet, increased physical activity, lifestyle-change strategies
Moderate	All the above plus low-calorie diet
High and very high	All the above plus pharmacotherapy and very-low-calorie diet
Extremely high	All the above plus surgical intervention

   c. Identify treatment provider and location. What weight-reduction treatment programs or services meet your patient's treatment needs? Consider with your patient which treatment programs and services available within your community would be appropriate for the patient's treatment plan *and* best meets the patient's individual weight-reduction needs.

   d. Monitor progress. Is your patient losing weight? Encourage and recognize success. Reassess patient readiness if necessary.

2. *Prevention of weight gain.* If BMI-related health risk does not warrant weight-reduction treatment, or it does but the patient is not ready for or interested in treatment, a strategy to prevent weight gain is appropriate.

Source: Shape Up America! *Guidance for Treatment of Adult Obesity.* Bethesda, MD: Author, 1996. (http://www.shapeup.org/sua)

---

have evoked considerable discussion, and a brief review of each is given in the next three sections.

Gastric-Reduction Surgery

As noted in Figure 13.37, *severe obesity* is defined as having a body mass index greater than 40 kg/m². Severe obesity is associated with serious medical complications and has proven extremely difficult to treat.

Until recently, severely obese people were rarely able to lose weight and keep it off using traditional methods. The advent of surgical treatments for obesity in the 1940s dramatically changed this picture. Large amounts of weight (up to 200 pounds) can be lost, with up to half of the loss maintained over the long term.[177]

One type of surgery involves radically reducing the volume of the stomach to less than 50 ml by constructing a pouch with a restricted outlet along the lesser curvature of the stomach (called vertical banded gastroplasty)[178] (see Figure 13.38). Another type of surgery is gastric bypass, which involves stapling shut a small portion of the stomach and then connecting it to the small intestine, bypassing the stomach, duodenum, and first portion of the jejunum.

These surgical procedures are major operations, and a decision to use surgery requires assessing the risk–benefit ratio in each case. Only certain people are qualified to un-

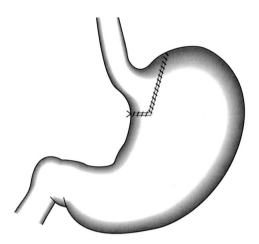

Figure 13.38 Gastric-reduction surgery. Gastric-reduction surgery reduces the volume of the stomach, resulting in dramatic changes in eating habits. *Source:* Kolanowski J. Surgical treatment for morbid obesity. *Br Med Bull* 43:433–444, 1997.

dertake this type of surgery.[177,178] To be cleared for surgery, the patient must show a history of repeated failures to lose weight by acceptable nonsurgical methods, be severely obese (body mass index of over 40 kg/m² for at least 3–5 years or 35–39.9 kg/m² with high-risk comorbid conditions), be experiencing some medical complications from the obesity, and be highly motivated and well informed about the procedure. There must be a commitment by the patient, surgeon, and hospital for a comprehensive lifelong follow-up.[5]

Weight reduction is dramatic and long term. At 5 years postsurgery, half of patients lose more than half of their excess weight, 30% lose 25–50%, while 20% fail to lose significant amounts of weight.[178] Patients go through drastic forced changes in eating habits. The 50-ml stomach resulting from the surgery requires people to eat less during each meal, eat more often, and not have any liquids at mealtime.

The loss in weight and the improvement in eating habits lead to an improvement in blood lipids, glucose, psychological mood state, and overall health in the most morbidly obese subjects who have gastric-reduction surgery.[177–182] However, a subgroup of patients respond poorly to the surgery in terms of failure to lose substantial weight, moderate to life-threatening medical complications, and emotional trauma.[183] Complications occur in 5–10% of cases, but mortality is very rare (0.1%). The most common complications are respiratory problems, severe vomiting, nutritional deficiencies, and wound infections, with the most severe complications being deep venous thrombosis and gastrointestinal leakage.[177,178]

Although severely obese subjects tend to lose more weight with gastric-reduction surgery, some research teams using comprehensive programs have been able to achieve long-term success with the VLCD.[184] Fewer complications are experienced on the VLCD.[185] In general, gastric-reduction surgery should be resorted to only after non-surgical techniques have failed to reduce weight in the obese subject.

Drug Therapy

Appetite-suppressant drugs (also called anorectic or anorexiant medications) have been available for several decades, and although there has been some stigma in their use, recent studies are showing that they may have a role in the treatment of some patients.[186–190] The majority of weight-loss medications prescribed in the 1950s and 1960s were amphetamines and had widespread and indiscriminate use. Between 1970 and 1990, medication usage for the treatment of obesity decreased, and no new medication was approved by the Food and Drug Administration (FDA) for the treatment of obesity until 1996.

In the late 1980s and early 1990s, a series of reports showing sustained weight loss with the use of a combination of fenfluramine hydrochloride and phentermine resin (nicknamed fen-phen) fueled widespread interest from patients, health professionals, and the media.[187] The number of prescriptions written for fenfluramine increased from about 60,000 in 1992 to over 1 million in 1995. In 1996, the FDA approved dexfenfluramine (a more potent form of fenfluramine, with the trade name of Redux) for use up to 1 year in the treatment of obesity.

The explosion of interest led to the development of clinics devoted to the prescription of weight-loss medications. Despite little training or expertise in obesity, many physicians established overnight fen-phen treatment programs with the promise of long-term cure.[190] In the fall of 1997, all this came crashing down when fenfluramine and dexfenfluramine were withdrawn from the market because a high incidence of heart valve defects was found in patients who used them.[189] Redux was also linked to an increased risk of primary pulmonary hypertension, a rare but potentially deadly lung disorder.[187]

Many lessons were learned during the 1990s about the role of medications in the management of obesity. Before listing these, a review of the major medications used in the treatment of obesity is given. Pharmacological treatments include anorexigenic agents (i.e., drugs that decrease appetite), which fall into the following broad categories:[187,188]

- *Catecholaminergic agents* decrease appetite and food intake primarily by increasing the availability of norepinephrine in the brain. Examples include phentermine hydrochloride (trade names include Fastin, Oby-Trim), amphetamines (Biphetamine), benzphetamine (Didrex), phendimetrazine (Bontril, Prelu-2,

X-Trozine), mazindol (Mazanor, Sanorex), and phenyl-propanolamine (Dexatrim, Acutrim).

- *Serotoninergic agonists* decrease appetite by increasing serotonin levels in the brain. Examples include fenfluramine hydrochloride (trade name, Pondimin), dexfenfluramine hydrochloride (Redux), and other antidepressant selective serotonin reuptake inhibitors (SSRIs). Dexfenfluramine both stimulates the release and inhibits the reuptake of central serotonin, thereby increasing brain serotonin and decreasing appetite.

- *Mixed serotoninergic and catecholaminergic reuptake inhibitors,* such as sibutramine (Meridia), acts on both the brain catecholamine and serotonin pathways, blocking the reuptake of norepinephrine and serotonin, and thus increasing the levels of these neurotransmitters in the brain.

Based on the events that took place in the 1990s, several guidelines were developed for practitioners regarding the use of obesity medications:[187]

- Pharmacological agents are a useful adjunct to, but not a substitute for, the necessary changes in dietary and exercise habits.

- Drug therapy for treatment of obesity should be reserved for patients with a body mass index greater than 30 kg/m², or 27 kg/m² in the presence of associated comorbidities (e.g., hypertension, type 2 diabetes, dyslipidemia, osteoarthritis, and cardiovascular disease).[5]

- Moderately obese patients lose about 5–10% of their body weight (about 10–20 pounds) within 4–6 months of using appetite-suppressant drugs such as sibutramine. Most of the weight loss with drug therapy occurs within 6 months. Weight then tends to be maintained or to increase slightly for the duration of treatment. When the weight-loss medications are discontinued, most patients tend to regain the weight that was lost, and several months after discontinuation, there is generally no difference between drug and placebo groups. In other words, these drugs produce a modest weight loss, and the achievement of desirable body weight requires a healthy lifestyle of proper dietary and exercise habits.

- Anorexiant agents should be used with caution and careful monitoring in patients with cardiac arrhythmias, symptomatic cardiovascular disease, diabetes, hypertension, depression, psychiatric illness, and severe systemic disease, such as liver or kidney failure. Anorexiant agents are contraindicated in patients taking monoamine oxidase inhibitors, in patients

with glaucoma, and in pregnant and lactating women.

- There are several potential adverse effects of long-term pharmacotherapy for treatment of obesity:

  Potential for abuse or dependence. This occurs primarily with amphetamines.

  Development of tolerance. Most studies of anorexiant drugs show a plateau in weight loss after 4–6 months of treatment, which probably represents the limits of efficacy, rather than tolerance.

  Avoidance of responsibility. Patients may not take responsibility for their condition.

  Adverse effects. Numerous minor adverse effects include diarrhea, polyuria, dry mouth, sleep disturbance, nausea, sweating, tremor, nervousness, depression, and short-term memory loss, depending on the drug.

Based on a thorough review of the literature, the American Medical Association has taken the stance that "until more data are available, pharmacotherapy cannot be recommended for routine use in obese individuals, although it may be helpful in carefully selected patients. If physicians choose to use medications in the long-term management of obesity, patients should be fully informed about the nonstandard use of some drugs, their potential adverse effects, and the scarcity of long-term studies available.... Ultimately, physician and patient need to balance carefully the potential risks of therapy against the potential benefits of sustained reduction in body weight in the responsive patient."[187]

Very-Low-Calorie Diets

Moderate obesity, defined as a body mass index between 30 and 40 kg/m², is present in about 30% of the obese population (see Figure 13.37). The development of very-low-calorie diets (VLCD) in the 1920s arose out of a need to attain a larger and more rapid weight loss for moderately obese individuals than was possible with conventional diets, while avoiding the dangers of starvation. Deficit diets fall into one of four categories:

- Moderate deficit diet
  = 1,200+ Calories/day for women
  1,400+ Calories/day for men
- Low-calorie diet
  = 800–1,200 Calories/day for women
  800–1,400 Calories/day for men
- Very-low-calorie diet = <800 calories/day
- Fasting = <100 calories/day

Moderately obese people have a high volume of excess fat tissue, which demands the fastest weight loss that can be tolerated with safety and comfort. Fasting is attractive to some patients, but this method raises problems of safety, comfort, and effectiveness. With fasting, 40–50% of the weight loss comes from the lean body weight, compromising health and personal appearance. Conventional reducing diets of 1,200–1,500 Calories produce too slow a weight loss to be practical because of the long time period involved. A compromise between the two, the VLCD, became widespread during the 1970s and has proven very effective (at least in the short term) and safe.[164–170,191–202]

Formerly called the protein-sparing modified fast, the VLCD provides 400–800 Calories per day, or fewer than 12 Calories per kilogram of ideal body weight.[195] Protein is emphasized, to help avoid loss of muscle tissue, with an intake of at least 1 gram protein per kilogram of body weight recommended. Patients can use either special-formula beverages or natural foods such as fish, fowl, or lean meat (along with mineral and vitamin supplements). All subjects should receive 1.5 L water per day and supplementation of minerals, vitamins, and trace elements according to RDA. Carbohydrates are added to diminish ketosis.

In the 1970s, some very-low-calorie commercial preparations were made largely from collagen, a protein of low biological value.[195,196] Reports of sudden deaths and fatal heart arrhythmias led to a formal Public Health Service investigation. Fifty-eight cases of sudden, unexpected death were attributed to the low quantity and quality of the protein in the liquid preparations and to inadequate medical supervision. This report led to a more conservative use and attempts to improve the quality and balance of the nutrients. Most VLCDs now provide 45–100 grams of high-quality protein, carbohydrates, essential fatty acids, vitamins, minerals, and more Calories than initially used (420–800 Calories per day in most preparations). The amount of weight lost over 12–16 weeks with VLCDs providing 800 Calories a day is little different from those providing 420–600, probably the result of improved compliance on the part of the patient.[195] Serious complications of modern VLCDs are unusual.

The primary benefit of VLCDs is that they can produce large weight losses in a large proportion of patients.[194–195] Patients tend to lose 3–5 pounds a week on the VLCD, with the total loss after 12–16 weeks averaging 40–45 pounds. In contrast to fasting, for every 20 pounds lost on the VLCD, 5 of them (25%) are from the lean body mass and 15 (75%) from the fat tissue.[195] In that excess body weight is about one fourth lean body mass, this loss during the VLCD is to be expected. During the first 3–4 days, weight loss is rapid, with weight change due primarily to loss of body water and glycogen. After this, weight loss is slower and is related more to changes in the fat stores, with some loss of pro-

tein.[198] The resting metabolic rate falls 15–20% after just 2 weeks on the VLCD, partially negating the expected weight loss.[199] Upon refeeding, the metabolic rate when adjusted for the loss of fat-free mass is usually reported to be normal.

As with severe obesity, weight loss during the VLCD for moderately obese patients leads to improvement in blood lipids, blood pressure, glycemic control for diabetics, and psychological mood state.[195] Minor side effects during VLCD include fatigue, weakness, dizziness, constipation, hair loss, dry skin, brittle nails, nausea, diarrhea, changes in menses, edema, and cold intolerance. More significant side effects are gout and gallstones. Serum levels of uric acid may rise during VLCDs and lead to a gallbladder attack, especially in patients with a history of gout. Dieting with rapid weight loss appears to increase the risk of gallstone disease. Cardiac complications are considered extremely rare on modern VLCDs when appropriate screening and surveillance procedures are followed. A disadvantage of VLCD programs, as currently conducted, is their high cost (about $3,000 per program).[195] Over the long term, VLCD programs have been estimated to cost $630 per pound lost and maintained.[166]

Unfortunately, about half of patients do not complete VLCD programs, and for those who do, losses are poorly maintained unless unusual effort is expended by a team of dietitians, psychologists, exercise physiologists, and medical personnel for years following the initial program[197] (see Figures 13.35, 13.36, 13.39). In one study of 400 patients, half of the patients who started the VLCD program did not complete the treatment.[200] Patients who completed the treatment lost a mean of 84% of their excess weight but regained an average of 59–82% of their initial excess weight by 30 months follow-up. In another study of 4,026 obese patients in the Optifast (420 Calories protein supplement) treatment program, 25% of patients dropped out within the first 3 weeks.[201] Of the patients remaining in the program, 68% lost weight but did not reach their goal. Of this group, recidivism was extremely high, with only 5–10% maintaining weight loss after 18 months. Thirty-two percent of the patients successfully attained their goal weight. Of this group, 30% of women and 58% of men maintained weight loss to within 10 pounds of posttreatment weight for at least 18 months. Figure 13.39 shows that 3 years after a VLCD program, the average weight of the group differed little from the initial weight, and only 12% were able to maintain more than three fourths of the weight loss.[170]

VLCDs are not appropriate for everyone.[191,195] Selection criteria for VLCD candidates include failure at more conservative approaches to weight loss; a body mass index greater than 30 kg/m² (or indexes of 27–30 kg/m² who have medical conditions that might respond to rapid weight loss); no serious medical conditions (recent heart attack, stroke, his-

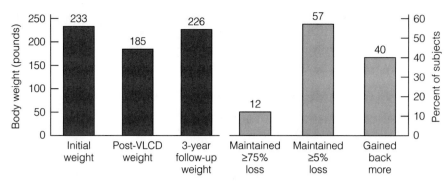

Figure 13.39 Three-year follow-up of 192 participants in a VLCD program. Three years after a VLCD program, average weight differed little from the initial weight, and only 12% were able to maintain more than three fourths of the weight loss. *Source:* Grodstein F, Levine R, Troy L, Spencer T, Colditz GA, Stampfer MJ. Three-year follow-up of participants in a commercial weight loss program: Can you keep it off? *Arch Intern Med* 156:1302–1306, 1996.

tory of heart conduction problems, kidney or liver problems, cancer, type 1 diabetes, or significant psychiatric problems); high motivation; and willingness to commit to establishing new eating behaviors after therapy. The VLCD should be preceded by 2–4 weeks of a well-balanced 1,200 Calorie diet, should last 12–16 weeks, and should then be followed by a gradual refeeding period of 2–4 weeks with foods slowly introduced. During the VLCD, weekly medical exams, with serum electrolytes checked every 2 weeks, are recommended. All VLCD clients should continue in some type of maintenance program to avoid relapse. Behavior modification and aerobic exercise should be included during and after the VLCD.[202]

In 1998, the NHLBI recommended that VLCDs not be used for weight-loss therapy for several reasons:[5]

1. Energy deficits are too great

2. Nutritional inadequacies will occur unless nutrient supplements are used

3. Moderate energy restriction is just as effective as the VLCD in producing long-term weight loss

4. Rapid weight reduction does not allow for gradual acquisition of changes in eating behavior

5. Clients using VLCDs are at increased risk for gallstones.

Weight-Loss Programs and Methods

In their attempts to lose weight, American adults use many methods, including low-calorie foods and beverages, exercise, weight-loss classes, medication, meal substitution, and self-imposed fasting.[203] Although many people attempt to lose weight on their own, a significant proportion use commercial products or join commercial weight-loss programs.

A Consumer Reports survey of 95,000 people showed that although most had tried to lose weight on their own, 24% had used meal-replacement products such as Slim-Fast and DynaTrim, 20% had joined a commercial weight-loss program, and 6% had tried over-the-counter appetite suppressants such as Acutrim and Dexatrim.[204]

To address the efficacy and safety of weight-loss programs, the National Institutes of Health (NIH) and the Food and Drug Administration (FDA) requested data from industry on the success of programs targeted for use by persons with various degrees of obesity.[203] The NIH and FDA concluded that good scientific data are lacking and that "given the importance to public health of reducing obesity, rigorous studies on current weight control practices should be pursued aggressively."

The NIH has recommended that people not be distracted by anecdotal "success" stories or by advertising claims.[151] The Federal Trade Commission has looked into advertising practices by commercial diet companies and has directed them to be more factual in their claims. People seeking help from commercial programs are urged to ask for valid and reliable data backing up claims and for additional information on program characteristics. Box 13.3 provides a listing of reputable organizations that offer good information and programs for the treatment of obesity.[20]

There are several characteristics of desirable weight-loss programs for obese individuals:[204–208]

- Provide or encourage food intake no lower than 1,200 Calories per day, which meets all nutrient needs. The diet plan should be varied, balanced, and conducive to improvement of overall health, with an emphasis on selection of low-fat foods. Diets lower than 1,200 Calories per day are not recommended for most obese individuals because they often are low in essential vitamins and minerals, can lead to excess

Box 13.3

Referral Organizations for Information on Treatment of Obesity

Following are various organizations that offer reliable information on the treatment of obesity.

Professional Organizations and Information Resource Centers

Shape Up America!
6707 Democracy
Boulevard, Suite 107
Bethesda, MD 20817
http://www.shapeup.org

American Obesity
Association
401 N. Michigan Avenue
Chicago, IL 60611-4267
800-98-OBESE

LEARN Program: Lifestyle,
Exercise, Attitudes,
Relationships, Nutrition
The LEARN Education
Center
1555 W. Mockingbird
Lane, Suite 203
Dallas, TX 75235
214-637-7700; 800-736-7323

PACE: Physician-Based
Physical Activity
Assessment Counseling
http://shs.sdsu.edu/pace/
619-594-5949

Weight-Control Information
Network (WIN)
http://www.niddk.nih.gov
800-WIN-8098

Centers for Disease Control
http://www.cdc.gov
888-232-4674

The Walking Magazine
9–11 Harcourt Street
Boston, MA 02116
walking@cowles.com
800-829-3340

American Dietetic
Association
216 W. Jackson Blvd.
Chicago, IL 60606-6995
http://www.eatright.org
312-899-0040; 800-877-1600
(consumer nutrition
hotline)

International Association
Eating Disorder
Professionals (IAEDP)
123 NW 13th St., #206
Boca Raton, FL 33432
407-338-6494

American Society for
Bariatric Surgeons (ASBS)
6717 NW 11th Place
Suite C
Gainesville, FL 32605
352-331-4900

Noncommercial Weight-Loss and Support Organizations

TOPS Club, Inc. (Taking Off
Pounds Sensibly)
Milwaukee, WI
800-932-8677

Overeaters Anonymous (OA)
Rio Rancho, NM
505-891-2664

Commercial Weight-Loss Programs

Weight Watchers
International, Inc.
175 Crossways Park West
Woodbury, NY 11797-2055
800-651-6000

Shapedown Pediatric
Obesity Program
Balboa Publishing
11 Library Place
San Anselmo, CA 94960
shapedown@aol.com
888-724-5245

Richard Simmons Slimmons
9306 Civic Center Dr.
Beverly Hills, CA 90210
310-275-4663

Jenny Craig, Inc.
11355 N. Torrey Rd.
La Jolla, CA 92038-7910
800-775-JENNY

Diet Workshop
50 Cummings Parkway
Woburn, MA 01801
800-488-3438

Clinical Weight-Loss Programs

Health Management
Resources (HMR)
Boston, MA
800-467-6467

Medifast
Healthrite, Inc.
Owings Mills, MD
800-638-7867

Optifast
Sandoz Nutrition
Minneapolis, MN
800-222-9201

---

loss of muscle mass, and lower the resting metabolic rate.

- Do not attempt to make the individual dependent on special products (that the program sells for a profit) rather than teaching them how to make good choices from the conventional food supply. The foods should be acceptable to the dieter in terms of sociocultural background, taste, and cost, and they should be easy to acquire and prepare. Good programs have supermarket and restaurant tours and cooking schools to teach people how to make practical choices and learn new techniques of eating within their day-to-day environments.

- Do not promise or imply dramatic, rapid weight loss (i.e., substantially beyond 1% of body weight per week).

- Include an exercise program that provides a daily caloric expenditure of 300 or more Calories.

- Include the use of behavior modification techniques to identify and eliminate lifestyle habits that contribute to obesity.

- Emphasize that lifestyle changes be lifelong, not just for the duration of the program.

- Do not promote or sell products that are unproven or spurious, such as starch blockers, spirulina, benzocaine, growth hormone releasers, grapefruit pills, fiber diet capsules, sauna belts, body wraps, passive exercise, ear stapling, acupuncture, electric muscle-stimulating devices, human chorionic gonadotrophin injections, or special "cellulite" cures.

Consumer Reports has recommended what many obesity experts now support, which is that "if you want or need to lose weight, you would probably do well to try to reduce on your own, or through a free hospital-based program, before spending money on a commercial weight-loss center. . . . The majority of dieters would probably do better to forget about cutting calories, focus on exercising and eating a healthful diet, and let the pounds fall where they may."[204]

As has been emphasized thus far in this chapter, a fundamental principle of weight loss and control is that for almost all people, a lifelong commitment to a change in lifestyle, behavioral responses, and dietary practices is necessary.[151] For most mildly obese people, modest goals and a slow course will maximize the probability of both losing the weight and keeping it off.

The whole concept of dieting can be criticized on psychological grounds, for going on a diet implies going off it and the resumption of old eating habits. For this reason, one can argue that the most effective diet is not a diet at all but rather a gradual change in eating patterns and a shift to foods that the person can continue to eat indefinitely. This means increasing the intake of complex carbohydrates, particularly in fruits, vegetables, legumes, and cereals, and decreasing the intake of fats and refined sugars. This course of action probably gives the best chance of maintaining the weight that is lost, and it is an eminently safe one. One should not lose weight by any method that cannot be included permanently within a healthy lifestyle.

In other words, the same diet that is being recommended for the treatment and prevention of heart disease, cancer, and diabetes is the same diet that should be used in preventing and treating obesity. This diet is high in carbohydrate, but low in fat. Complex carbohydrates as found in whole grains, vegetables, and fruits are emphasized, and only low-fat meats and dairy products are used. Table 13.3 shows that when comparing the amount of Calories per cup of food, vegetables and fruits have the lowest number of Calories, while sugar and high-fat, low-dietary-fiber foods contain the most.

The Role of Exercise during Weight Loss

Thus far, this chapter has emphasized that regular exercise has proven to be a consistent indicator of the ability to maintain weight loss over the long term following periods of caloric restriction. Also, many studies have shown that obese people tend to exercise less than normal-weight individuals and that active people are leaner.

Although it is often accepted that physical activity is a powerful tool in the treatment of obesity, the best-designed research studies have failed to support this belief. In fact, most researchers in this area now regard exercise as a relatively weak weapon in the "battle of the bulge," with control of caloric intake representing the real power behind weight-loss efforts.[208–214]

There are several misconceptions regarding the role of exercise in weight loss. These are summarized in Box 13.4. Each of these is explained in turn, with the true benefits reviewed later in this chapter.

Misconception 1: Aerobic Exercise Accelerates Weight Loss Significantly, When Combined with a Reducing Diet

Some obese people have been led to believe that if they start brisk walking 2–3 miles a day, significant amounts of body weight will be lost quickly. Most research does not support this idea, even when the exercise program lasts several months. For example, in a randomized, controlled, 1-year study of 160 females and 197 males, three or five 30- to 40-minute exercise sessions per week had no significant effect on body weight despite a 5–8% improvement in cardiorespiratory endurance.[215] Many other studies have come to the same conclusion that when young and old alike exercise moderately in a free-living condition (with no diet control), this amount of exercise ends up being an insufficient stimulus to affect body weight significantly.[208–214,216–220]

Box 13.4

Misconceptions Regarding the Role of Exercise in Weight Loss

Following are some of the most common misconceptions about the role of exercise in weight loss.

1. Accelerates weight loss significantly when combined with a reducing diet.

2. Causes the resting metabolic rate to stay elevated for a long time after the bout, burning extra Calories.

3. Counters the diet-induced decrease in resting metabolic rate.

4. Counters the diet-induced decrease in fat-free mass.

TABLE 13.3   Calories Found in One-Cup Portions of Food

Food	Calories Per Cup	Ranking	Food	Calories Per Cup	Ranking
Vegetable oils	1927		Grape juice	155	
Shortening	1812		Whole milk	150	
Margarine	1616		Oatmeal (cooked)	145	
Butter	1600	Very High	Plain yogurt	144	
Mayonnaise	1582	in Calories	Pineapple juice	139	Moderately
Peanut butter	1520	(fats)	Crabmeat	135	Low
Salad dressing, blue cheese	1234		Corn (cooked)	134	(juices,
Honey	1040		Peas (cooked)	126	soups,
Cake icing	1035		Low-fat milk	121	cereals,
Nuts, macadamia	940		White bread	120	milk)
Jams/preserves	880		Apple juice	116	
Chocolate candy	860		Orange juice	112	
Peanuts, oil roasted	840	High	Rice Krispies	112	
Sunflower seeds	821	(nuts, seeds	Corn Chex	111	
Cashews	787	and sugar)	Nonfat milk	86	
Almonds	766		Oranges	85	
White sugar	720		Pumpkin	83	
Granola	595		Winter squash	79	
Sour cream	492		Pineapple	77	
Dates	489		Blackberries	74	Low
Walnuts	486		Apples	64	(nonfat milk,
Dried pears	472	Moderately	Grapes	58	fruits)
Coconut	466	High	Onions	58	
Cheddar cheese	455	(dried fruit,	Cantaloupe	57	
Raisins	434	cheese, flour)	Beets (cooked)	52	
Flour (wheat, enriched)	420		V-8 Juice	51	
Grape-Nuts	407		Watermelon	50	
Corned beef hash	400		Carrots	48	
Prunes	385		Broccoli (cooked)	46	
Ice cream (16% fat)	349		Strawberries	45	
Sweet potato	344		Green beans	44	
Pork (lean, roasted)	341		Kale (cooked)	41	
Ricotta cheese (skim milk)	340		Kohlrabi (raw)	38	
Ice Cream (10% fat)	269		Summer squash (cooked)	44	
Turkey	262	Moderate	Sprouted mung beans	32	
Ham (roasted)	249	(legumes,	Zucchini (cooked)	28	
Soybeans (cooked)	234	some dairy	Collards (cooked)	27	Very Low
Brown rice (cooked)	232	products, rice)	Cauliflower (raw)	24	(vegetables)
Yogurt (fruit flavored)	231		Cabbage (raw)	22	
Red kidney beans (cooked)	230		Celery	18	
Spanish rice	213		Mushrooms (raw)	18	
Lentils (cooked)	210		Cucumber	14	
Macaroni (cooked)	190	Moderately	Spinach (raw)	12	
Whole-wheat cereal (cooked)	180	Low	Romaine lettuce	8	
Wheat Chex	169	(juices, soups,	Iceberg lettuce	7	
Tomato soup (with milk)	160	cereals, milk)	Swiss chard (raw)	6	

Source: USDA Food Composition Tables (Handbook No. 8 series).

It has been argued that when people begin exercising, they may start eating more, negating the increased energy expenditure from initiation of regular exercise. Instead, perhaps they may alter other areas of their lifestyle (e.g., resting more than normal during the remainder of the day after exercise), diluting the effect of added exercise. For these reasons, researchers have tested the effects of exercise under controlled dietary conditions, where all subjects are fed the same amount of food, while some exercise and others remain sedentary. Even under these conditions, exercise has been found to add little to the weight loss.[221–230]

Figures 13.40 and 13.41 portray the typical findings of researchers who have tested the effect of moderate exercise in accelerating weight loss during a reducing diet.[224,229] In the study summarized in Figure 13.40, 91 obese women were randomized into one of four groups for the 12-week study: control (no exercise or special diet), walking (five 45-minute walking sessions per week at 75% maximum heart rate), diet (1,300 Calories/day), and both diet and walking. In this well-controlled study, walking alone was an insufficient stimulus to decrease body weight compared to the control group. Subjects in the two diet groups lost between 17 and 18 pounds on average (about 1.5 pounds of weight loss per week), with walking providing no added benefit. For the two diet groups, 80–90% of the weight loss was body fat, and walking did not affect this proportion.

Results shown in Figure 13.41 are from a 90-day study of 69 moderately obese females who each were put on a VLCD of 520 Calories a day.[229] Subjects were randomized into four groups: diet only, diet plus aerobic training, diet plus weight training, and diet plus aerobic and weight training. Aerobic training consisted of four sessions a week, with duration increasing from 20 minutes up to 60 minutes per session by the end of the study, at 70% of the heart rate reserve. The weight trainers exercised four times a week, engaging in two to three sets, 6–8 repetitions of several exercises at 70–80% of their one-repetition maximum. As shown in Figure 13.41, exercise had no significant effect on weight loss, with each group losing about 46 pounds, with three fourths of the loss being fat mass and the other fourth, lean body weight (LBW). Exercise also had no effect on the fall in resting metabolic rate (RMR), which averaged about 10% for all groups.

These and other studies demonstrate that in obesity treatment programs lasting 12–20 weeks, only a few extra pounds, at best, will be lost when moderate amounts of aerobic exercise (2–7 hours per week) are combined with a reducing diet.[208–234] Figure 13.42 shows a summary graph of a meta-analysis of 493 studies conducted over a 25-year period. During a typical 15-week program, the combination of diet and exercise can be expected to cause a 24.2 pound weight loss, little different than the 23.5 pounds from diet alone. It appears that in order for aerobic exercise to have a major effect on reduction of body weight, daily exercise

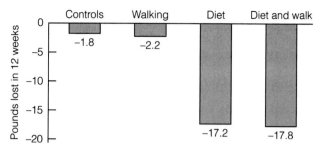

Figure 13.40 Body weight changes in response to diet and/or exercise, 12-week study of 91 obese women; diet = 1,300 Calories/day; exercise = five 45-minute walk sessions/week, 75% MHR. Exercise alone had little effect on weight loss and did not accelerate weight loss significantly beyond the effects due to the reducing diet. *Source:* Utter AC, Nieman DC, Butterworth DE, Henson DA. Body composition and cardiorespiratory fitness responses to energy restriction and moderate exercise training in obese women. *Int J Sport Nutr* (in press).

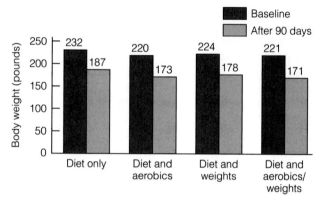

Figure 13.41 Moderate exercise does not enhance weight loss during dieting; 90-day study of 69 obese females, all on 520-Calorie/day formula: Exercise had no effect on RMR (10% decrease) or LBW (¼ of 46-pound loss). *Source:* Donnelly JE, Pronk NP, Jacobsen DJ, Pronk SJ, Jakicic JM. Effects of a very-low-calorie diet and physical training regimens on body composition and resting metabolic rate in obese females. *Am J Clin Nutr* 54:56–61, 1991.

sessions need to be unusually long in duration (more than 1 hour) and high in intensity, something that most obese people cannot do.[228,234,235]

There are several reasons for the weak effect of moderate exercise on weight loss, the primary one being that the net energy expenditure of such exercise sessions is small. From a quantitative point of view, the energy cost of formal exercise is much less than most people believe.[210] The net energy cost of exercise equals the Calories expended during the exercise session minus the Calories expended for the resting metabolic rate and other activities that the individual would have been doing had they not been formally exercising.[231]

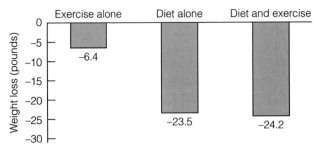

Figure 13.42 Average weight loss during 15-week interventions with diet and/or exercise, meta-analysis of 493 studies over a 25-year period. Exercise alone has a relatively minor effect on weight loss and does not add much to the weight-loss effects of a reducing diet. *Source:* Miller WC, Koceja DM, Hamilton EJ. A meta-analysis of the past 25 years of weight loss research using diet, exercise or diet plus exercise intervention. *Int J Obes Relat Metab Disord* 21:941–947, 1997.

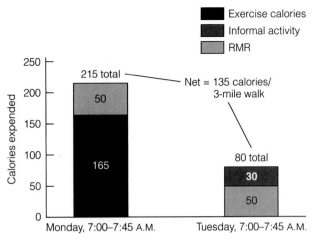

Figures are for a 3-mile walk in 45 minutes by a 154-lb, mildly obese individual

Figure 13.43 The concept of net energy expenditure: Net energy expenditure = gross energy expended − RMR − informal exercise Calories. The net caloric expenditure of moderate exercise is much smaller than many people realize—in this example, only 135 Calories.

For example, the net energy cost of a 3-mile, 45-minute walk for a 70-kg obese woman is only about 130 to 140 Calories (215 total Calories minus 50 Calories for the RMR and 25 to 35 for incidental activity) (see Figure 13.43). One pound of human fat contains approximately 3,500 calories, which means that if all else stayed exactly the same, it would take nearly one month of daily brisk walking (3 miles each session) to lose 1 pound of fat. Many obese people find walking 2–3 miles a day to be the most they can handle without injury, yet much more than this is necessary if significant weight loss is to be achieved.[234,235]

As emphasized by University of Vermont obesity researchers, "The types and intensities of exercise that carry a high energy expenditure for a single bout are basically confined to those that can be undertaken by elite athletes or subjects with an excellent level of physical fitness. On a clinical basis, and especially for the obese patient, it would be unrealistic (even dangerous) to expect [such] a level of exercise performance."[210]

Also, some people may "reward" themselves with extra food (in free-living conditions) or by resting and sitting more after exercising, negating the energy expenditure of the entire exercise bout. A team of researchers from Loughborough University in England had women walk 2.5 hours a week for a whole year and were unable to measure any decrease in body fat, even though the women did not change their diets. The researchers concluded that the walkers may have rested more throughout the day after their walk, thereby erasing the effects of the walking session.[220] More research is needed to test this hypothesis.[232]

The practical advice from these studies is that exercise alone must not be seen as a major weapon in the treatment of obesity. Instead, improvements in the quality and quantity of the diet should take the lead, with exercise relegated to an important supporting role. At the 1992 National Institutes of Health Technology Assessment Conference Panel on Methods for Voluntary Weight Loss and Control, it was concluded, "Weight loss that can be achieved by exercise programs alone is more limited than that which can be obtained by caloric restriction. However, exercise has beneficial effects independent of weight loss . . . and can be an important adjunct to other strategies."[151,233]

Misconception 2: Exercise Causes the Resting Metabolic Rate to Stay Elevated for a Long Time after the Bout, Burning Extra Calories

Another common misconception is that aerobic exercise causes the resting metabolic rate (RMR) to stay elevated for a long time after the bout, burning extra Calories. In general, most researchers have found that the energy expended after aerobic exercise is small unless a great amount of high-intensity exercise is engaged in.[236–241] For example, jogging (12 minutes per mile), walking, or cycling at moderate intensities (40–60% aerobic capacity) for about one half hour causes the RMR to stay elevated for 20–30 minutes, burning 10–12 extra Calories.[236,240] When the intensity is increased to about 75%, RMR is increased for about 35–45 minutes, with 15–30 extra Calories expended. Obviously, this amount of caloric expenditure following exercise is too little to have any significant effect on body weight loss. Even when the duration is quite long (e.g., 80 minutes), the amount of Calories expended afterward through elevation of the RMR is low unless the intensity is high during the entire exercise bout[237–239] (see Figures 13.44 and 13.45). For the obese individual who takes a 20- to 30-minute walk, at most, about 10

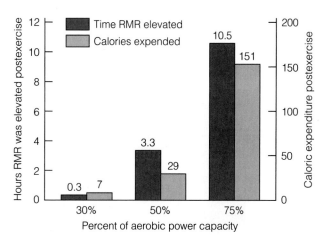

Figure 13.44 Calories burned after 80 minutes of cycling at different intensities, subjects rested in bed for 14 hours postexercise. This study shows the importance of intensity for postexercise RMR elevation. Eighty minutes of high-intensity cycling resulted in 151 extra Calories being burned after exercise. However, most obese individuals are incapable of this amount of exercise. *Source: Bahr R, Sejersted OM. Effect of intensity of exercise on excess postexercise oxygen consumption. Metabolism 40:836–841, 1991.*

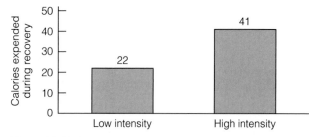

Figure 13.45 Postexercise energy expenditure in women, low-intensity cycling (80 minutes, 50% $\dot{V}O_{2max}$) versus high-intensity (50 minutes, 70% $\dot{V}O_{2max}$). High-intensity exercise for 50 minutes results in a higher postexercise energy expenditure than low-intensity exercise for 80 minutes. *Source: Phelain JF, Reinke E, Harris MA, Melby CL. Postexercise energy expenditure and substrate oxidation in young women resulting from exercise bouts of different intensity. J Am College Nutr 16: 140–146, 1997.*

extra Calories will be burned afterward, hardly enough to be meaningful when balanced against other diet and energy expenditure factors.[210,239]

Is there a chronic effect of exercise training on the RMR beyond that expected with increase in fat-free mass? Potentially, any effect of exercise on the RMR could be important because it represents such a large percentage of the total energy expenditure.[210] There has been some disagreement among researchers on this issue, with some concluding that trained individuals (especially elite athletes) have higher RMRs than sedentary people (when adjusted for differences in lean body weight,[242–244] while others have been unable to establish significant differences.[245–247] However,

there is a growing consensus that when differences in RMR between active and inactive individuals have been found, this has been due more to the acute effect of the previous day's exercise bout (in athletes) than to any real chronic adaptation.[248–250] When athletes have been tested 2 days after hard exercise, no difference in RMR has been found.[248,250] These researchers have suggested that when athletes don't exercise, they also don't eat as much, which means they have a lower caloric turnover and therefore normal RMRs. When training is heavy and food intake is higher, caloric turnover is elevated, along with the RMR. Although these findings are interesting to academicians and researchers, for obese individuals, they have no practical significance because the amount of exercise they can engage in will be too little to have any true chronic effect on RMR beyond that achieved by their higher fat-free mass.

Misconception 3: Exercise Counters the Diet-Induced Decrease in Resting Metabolic Rate

During caloric restriction, the resting metabolic rate drops substantially and is related to the rate of weight loss, averaging 10–20% for VLCDs and up to 20–30% for long-term fasting (see Figure 13.46). Can exercise during caloric restriction counter this diet-induced decrease in the RMR?

Most studies do not support this idea, and when a protective effect of exercise training on RMR is found, it is rather small.[210,211,226–229,251–255] For example, in one study, 12 mildly obese women were put onto 530-Calorie/day diets for 28 days and an exercise program (three sessions per week, 30–45 minutes at 60% $\dot{V}O_{2max}$). RMR dropped 16% despite the exercise program.[252] In another study, half of 13 mildly obese subjects on a 4-week VLCD (720 Calories/day) exercised a total of 27 hours at 50% $\dot{V}O_{2max}$.[223] RMR dropped more in the exercise group than in the sedentary group (10% for both groups in the first week, but then a further 17% drop in the exercise group). Apparently, the exercise session prompted energy conservation in the dieting obese subjects, decreasing the RMR.[254] Figure 13.47 suggests that even when obese subjects are on a mild energy-deficit diet (1,200 Calories/day), aerobic or weight training is an insufficient stimulus to counter the drop in RMR.[226]

Figure 13.48 shows the results of a study reviewed previously[213] (Figure 13.41). Notice that neither aerobic nor resistive training had any effect on the drop in RMR induced by the 520-Calorie/day diet. This may have been because the fat-free mass dropped equally in all groups, important because the RMR is so tightly connected to it.

Misconception 4: Exercise Counters the Diet-Induced Decrease in Fat-Free Mass

During weight loss, the percentage lost as fat-free mass (FFM) increases in proportion to the severity of the Caloric deficit. With total fasting, the body weight loss is close to

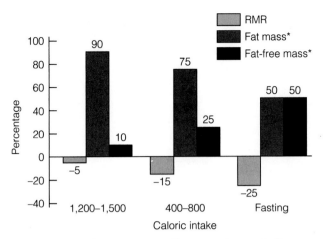

Figure 13.46 Caloric restriction, effect on resting metabolic rate, fat mass, and fat-free mass. Both the resting metabolic rate and the fat-free mass are decreased in parallel with the degree of caloric restriction.

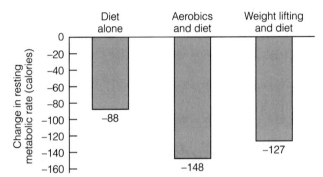

Figure 13.47 Change in resting metabolic rate with diet and / or exercise, 65 moderately obese subjects, 8-week intervention; all on formula diet, 70% RMR (1,200 Calories / day), with exercise three times / week; weight training = three sets, 6 reps, eight stations; aerobics = leg and arm cycling, 70% MHR. Aerobic and weight training were not sufficient to counter diet-induced decrements in RMR.
Source: Geliebter A, Maher MM, Gerace L, Gutin B, Heymsfield SB, Hashim SA. Effects of strength or aerobic training on body composition, resting metabolic rate, and peak oxygen consumption in obese dieting subjects. *Am J Clin Nutr* 66:557–563, 1997.

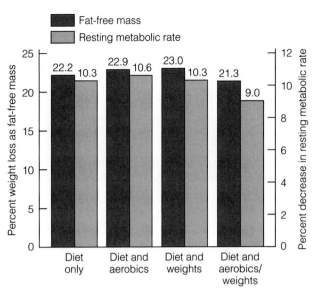

Figure 13.48 Exercise does not counter diet-induced decreases in RMR and FFM; 90-day study of 69 obese females, all on 520-Calorie / day formula, aerobic exercise = 4 days / week, 20 minutes, progressing to 60 minutes / session; weights = 4 days / week, two to three sets, 6–8 repetitions.
Source: Donnelly JE, Pronk NP, Jacobsen DJ, Pronk SJ, Jakicic JM. Effects of a very-low-calorie diet and physical training regimens on body composition and resting metabolic rate in obese females. *Am J Clin Nutr* 54:56–61, 1991.

50% fat and 50% FFM.[256] During a VLCD (with appropriate protein intake), the proportions improve to 75% fat and 25% FFM.[213,229] While on a 1,200–1,500-Calorie diet, the proportions improve even more to 90% fat and 10% fat-free mass[221] (see Figure 13.46). Thus the degree of caloric deprivation appears to be the major controlling factor in determining the magnitude of loss from FFM. As explained earlier in this chapter, excess weight in obese individuals is about 75% fat, 25% FFM. Thus, during weight reduction, some loss of FFM is expected and probably desirable.[257]

Can exercise counter the diet-induced decrease in FFM (if this is the desire of the patient)? In general, both moderate aerobic and strength training programs have been found to have little effect (see reviews[211,213,214,257]). As depicted in Figure 13.48, despite fairly rigorous aerobic and resistive training programs by moderately obese females, FFM still represented about 22% of the 46 pounds that were lost by each group. In another 90-day study, FFM represented one fourth the weight loss in moderately obese females who were on an 800-Calorie diet, despite engaging in strength training three times a week and showing significant improvements in strength (see Figure 13.49).[258]

In general, it appears that the caloric deficit is dominant in its effects on the FFM, with moderate amounts of exercise representing an insufficient stimulus to alter the decrease.

Some individuals trying to lose body fat have been led to believe that the optimal exercise intensity for fat burning is low intensity (e.g., moderate walking). Figure 13.50 shows that when the same individuals exercise moderately (50% $\dot{V}O_{2max}$) or very intensely (80% $\dot{V}O_{2max}$) for 45 minutes, the proportion of fat calories expended is three times greater with moderate exercise (49% versus 16%).[259] However, the moderate exercise bout burns about 40% fewer total Calories. Because 1 pound of body fat is about 3,500 Calories, and any type of food Calorie can be turned into body fat (carbohydrate, protein, or fat), what really matters is energy balance—expending more energy than what is consumed.

Several studies have now confirmed that vigorous and intense, compared to moderate, exercise is associated with

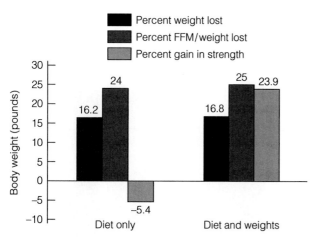

Figure 13.49 Effect of resistance training during weight loss, 14 obese females on 800-VLCD formula for 90 days, three sessions/week, eight exercises, three to four sets, 70–80% 1-RM. During 800-Calorie diets, obese women who lift weights increase their strength but do not experience greater weight loss or protection of their fat-free mass. *Source:* Donnelly JE, Sharp T, Houmard J, et al. Muscle hypertrophy with large-scale weight loss and resistance training. *Am J Clin Nutr* 58:561–565, 1993.

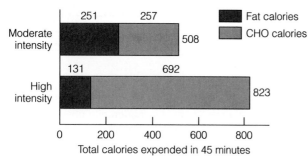

Figure 13.50 Calories from fat and carbohydrate during exercise, 45 minutes of high- (80% $\dot{V}O_{2max}$) versus moderate- (50% $\dot{V}O_{2max}$) intensity exercise. Although moderate exercise may burn more fat Calories than high-intensity exercise, the total Calories expended per unit of time is far less. *Source:* Nieman DC, Miller AR, Henson DA, Warren BJ, Gusewitch G, Johnson RL, Davis JM, Butterworth DE, Herring JL, Nehlsen-Cannarella SL. The effects of high- versus moderate-intensity exercise on lymphocyte subpopulations and proliferative response. *Int J Sports Med* 15:199–206, 1994.

a greater reduction in body fat, especially from the abdominal area.[260-264] For example, in a large study of more than 2,000 middle-aged and elderly men and women in the Netherlands, intensive physical activity such as playing sports was negatively associated with abdominal fat.[262] Another study of more than 2,500 men and women in Canada showed that higher-intensity exercise was associated with a preferential reduction in abdominal fat.[263] There is some evidence that fat in the abdominal, compared to the gluteal, area is more responsive to lipolysis or breakdown from epinephrine (which is elevated during vigorous but not

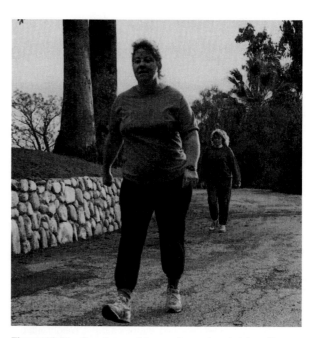

Figure 13.51 Regular aerobic exercise such as brisk walking is associated with several important health benefits for the obese.

moderate exercise).[264] Thus, brisk activity is recommended for overweight individuals when possible because physical training is viewed as an important nonpharmacological tool in the treatment of abdominal obesity and associated metabolic disorders.[261] However, moderately and severely obese subjects should first bring their body mass index below 30 kg/m² before concerning themselves with exercise intensity, due to the injury potential (see section on precautions).

Benefits of Exercise for Weight Loss

If exercise training has relatively little effect during weight-loss programs in accelerating weight loss, or in protecting diet-induced decreases in the RMR and the FFM, then why should obese patients exercise? The main reason is to improve their health. Moderate exercise may be a weak weapon in promoting a great deal of weight loss, but it has much greater power in enhancing health (see Figure 13.51). As outlined in Box 13.5, there are at least five health-related benefits of exercise for obese patients.

Each of these benefits is reviewed in detail elsewhere in this textbook and is perhaps even more important for obese individuals. The improvement in $\dot{V}O_{2max}$ by obese individuals following moderate aerobic exercise programs has been found to vary from 10% to 25% after 5–15 weeks of exercise.[224] (see Figures 13.52 and 13.53).

As reviewed in Chapter 10, weight loss is associated with a dramatic improvement in the blood lipid profile. A consistent finding is that with weight loss, total choles-

Box 13.5

Benefits of Moderate Aerobic Exercise for the Obese Individual

Regular exercise by the obese individual is associated with

1. Improved cardiorespiratory endurance ($\dot{V}O_{2max}$)

2. Improved blood lipid profile, in particular decreased triglycerides and increased HDL-C, with weight loss more responsible for decreases in total cholesterol and LDL-C

3. Improved psychological state, especially increased general well-being and vigor, and decreased anxiety and depression

4. Enhanced group social support, which may improve long-term maintenance of weight loss

5. Decreased risk of obesity-related diseases (e.g., diabetes, heart disease, cancer, hypertension)

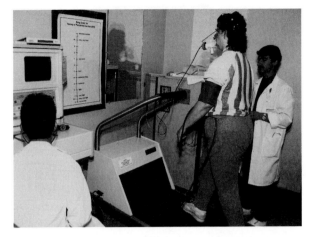

Figure 13.52 Most studies show that a brisk walking program increases $\dot{V}O_{2max}$ in obese subjects.

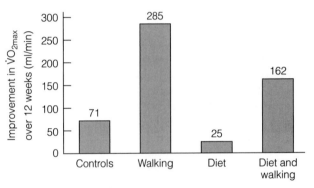

Figure 13.53 $\dot{V}O_{2max}$ changes in response to diet and/or exercise, 12-week study of 91 obese women; diet = 1,300 Calories/day; exercise = five 45-minute walk sessions/week, 75% MHR. Regular brisk walking significantly improves $\dot{V}O_{2max}$ in obese women, whether they are on or off of a reducing diet. *Source:* Utter AC, Nieman DC, Butterworth DE, Henson DA. Body composition and cardiorespiratory fitness responses to energy restriction and moderate exercise training in obese women. *Int J Sport Nutr* (in press).

terol, LDL-C, and triglycerides decrease, while HDL-C increases.[265] The independent effect of aerobic exercise, however, is limited to improving the magnitude of change in the triglycerides and HDL-C, but not total cholesterol and LDL-C.

In addition to the physiological benefits, exercise is associated with feelings of well-being, a reduction in anxiety and depression, and a positive self-concept and elevated mood (see Chapter 14). The strong evidence in this area provides additional support for including exercise within weight-loss programs.[226,227] During weight loss, many individuals experience feelings of depression and irritability, which exercise can help counter. Figure 13.54 shows that exercise and diet together improved depression scores more than diet alone did.[226]

In most obesity studies, subjects exercise together. The social interaction during the weeks of exercising may enhance long-term maintenance of the weight loss. As reviewed earlier in this chapter, exercise has emerged as one of the best predictors of weight-loss maintenance. Exercise may also provide ancillary benefits such as increased group cohesiveness, communication, and opportunities for information passage that persist for months after the program is over.

As discussed at the beginning of this chapter, obesity is associated with many complications, such as heart disease, diabetes, high blood pressure, and high blood cholesterol levels. There is strong evidence that exercise can help to counter each of these complications (see Chapters 10 through 15). As reviewed earlier, there is some evidence

that people who exercise regularly accumulate less fat in the abdominal area than inactive people, promoting a more favorable fat distribution.[266,267] This may be one reason why active people tend to be protected against various chronic diseases and have fewer risk factors for them.

In summary, then, moderate aerobic exercise during weight reduction helps to improve the health status of the individual, while the real power behind weight loss comes from a reduction in the amount of Calories (in particular, the dietary fat) consumed. A moderate reduction in Calories (to about 1,200–1,500/day for mildly obese individuals) promotes loss of fat weight while sparing the lean body weight, whereas aerobic exercise improves the fitness and health status of the dieting individual.

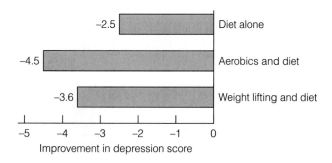

Figure 13.54 Improvement in depression score with diet and/or exercise, in 65 moderately obese subjects, 8-week intervention; all on formula diet, 70% RMR (1,200 Calories/day), with exercise three times/week: weight training = three sets, 6 reps, eight stations; aerobics = leg and arm cycling, 70% MHR. *Source:* Geliebter A, Maher MM, Gerace L, Gutin B, Heymsfield SB, Hashim SA. Effects of strength or aerobic training on body composition, resting metabolic rate, and peak oxygen consumption in obese dieting subjects. *Am J Clin Nutr* 66: 557–563, 1997.

Exercise Precautions for the Obese

There are several exercise precautions for the obese, and their importance increases with the increasing degree of obesity.[268] These include providing for heat intolerance, difficulty breathing, movement restriction, musculoskeletal pain and injury, local muscular weakness, and balance-anxiety.

In addition, the obese are at higher risk for cardiovascular disease, diabetes, and hypertension. However, if the exercise leader is careful to follow appropriate American College of Sports Medicine screening procedures (Chapter 3), has adequately prepared for emergencies, and emphasizes low-to-moderate intensity *non-weight-bearing activities* (such as bicycling, swimming, water exercises, and brisk walking), exercise programs for the severely obese can be conducted safely.

Social reinforcement and compliance are enhanced through group participation in activities that are recreational, fun, and varied, and which offer the participant a feeling of personal success.[269,270] Regimented calisthenics are not generally advisable. On the other hand, music, games, and social interaction will improve compliance.

Another key principle is that exercise need not be formal to be beneficial. It can take place at different times of the day, as a part of regular daily activities (like climbing stairs or walking to a neighbor's house), and as such is often more attractive to the obese, who may want to avoid being noticed during exercise.

SPORTS MEDICINE INSIGHT

Eating Disorders: Bulimia and Anorexia Nervosa

It is an ongoing paradox that our food-laden, sedentary society equates thin with beautiful. On the one hand, our magazine covers, movie stars, and athletic heroes advance the concept that thin is in. On the other hand, we are led (often through advertising) to believe that technological labor-saving devices and sumptuous foods rich in fats and sugars are desirable rewards of a successful society.

It is perhaps not surprising that one sector of our population finds itself extremely disordered in its eating habits—the bulimics and the anorexics. The characteristics of bulimia and anorexia nervosa have been summarized by the American Psychiatric Association[271] (see Box 13.6). People with bulimia, known as bulimics, indulge in *binge eating* (episodes of eating large quantities of food) and *purging* (getting rid of food by vomiting or using laxatives). People with anorexia, known as anorexics or anorectics, severely limit their food intake. Some bulimics may consume up to 20,000 Calories in 8 hours,

sometimes resorting to stealing food or money to support their obsession. The average bulimic binge is 1,200–4,500 Calories, and total daily energy intake averages over 10,000 Calories.[272–274]

Among women 15–40 years of age nationwide, 2–3% are classified as bulimic and 0.2–1.1% are anorexic.[275–285] The National Center for Health Statistics estimates that 10,000 bulimia cases and 11,000 anorexia cases are diagnosed each year, with males accounting for only 5–10%.[272] However, symptoms of bulimia and anorexia, such as binge eating, induced vomiting, and an extreme fear of gaining weight are present in alarming numbers of college students and obese individuals. For example, in one study, 23% of college women and 14% of college men reported episodes of binge eating at least once a week. In addition, 28% of the women and 7% of the men stated that they were "often" to "always" terrified of gaining weight.[279] Among the obese, 20–40% report significant problems with binge eating. There are indications

(continued)

Eating Disorders: Bulimia and Anorexia Nervosa *(continued)*

that the incidence and prevalence of eating disorders are rising.[277]

A startling number of adolescents are practicing unhealthful behaviors to regulate body weight.[283,284] In one study of tenth-grade students, 13% reported the use of vomiting, laxatives, or diuretics to control their weight. These students expressed an abnormal concern with their weight, frequently dieted, and experienced guilt following periods of excessive eating.[284]

There are published reports of abnormal weight-control behaviors in athletes, especially ballet dancers, gymnasts, runners, and swimmers.[278,285] At one competitive-swimming camp, researchers found that of the 900 swimmers ages 9 to 18, 15.4% of the girls and 3.6% of the boys used a variety of abnormal weight-loss techniques to meet the demands of their sport. Girls in particular were likely to misperceive themselves as overweight.[285] Among 93 elite women runners, 13% reported a history of anorexia nervosa, 25% binge eating, 9% bingeing and purging, and 34% abnormal eating practices.[286] In general, athletes are considered to be at increased risk for eating disorders[287-289] (see Chapter 16).

Weight patterns of athletes can be grouped into three categories.[290] First, there are sports such as baseball, where maintenance of low weight is not important. The second category involves sports with specific weight divisions, such as wrestling or boxing. Weight fluctuations can be rapid, frequent (15 times per season), and large (one survey found that the weight of 41% fluctuated 11–20 pounds every week of the season, with an average end-of-season weight gain of from 4 to 5 pounds.) The third category involves sports in which low weights are the norm, such as distance running, gymnastics, figure skating, and ballet. Low weights in this category are necessary for optimal performance and appearance, and participants are often willing to utilize bizarre and unhealthy weight-control measures to attain the necessary weight for competition.

Signs to watch for if someone is suspected of being bulimic and/or anorexic include[287,291]

1. Change in personal weight goal to a much lower standard
2. Dieting accompanied by an increased criticism of own body weight and shape
3. Social isolation, depressive moods
4. Cessation of menstrual periods in women

5. Episodes of hiding food, vomiting, and misusing laxatives, diuretics, and diet pills
6. Relentless, excessive exercise
7. Wearing baggy or layered clothing
8. Bathroom visits immediately after meals

Risk factors for anorexia and bulimia are listed in Table 13.4.[292-294] Eating disorders are associated with multiple risk factors that represent a complex interplay among genetic, psychological, and social processes.[292] Eating disorders are commonly understood to reflect a failed adaptation to the developmental challenges associated with female adolescence. Physical Fitness Activity 13.2 can be used to help detect people with an eating disorder.

Binge eating and the various forms of purging (vomiting, laxative and diuretic use) can cause serious medi-

TABLE 13.4 Risk Factors for Anorexia Nervosa and Bulimia Nervosa

Anorexia Nervosa	Bulimia Nervosa
High parental education and income	Childhood obesity
Early feeding problems	Early onset of menarche
Low self-esteem	Weight concern
High neuroticism	Perfectionism
Maternal over-protectiveness	Low self-esteem
Eating disorders among family members	Social pressure about weight/eating
	Family dieting
	Eating disorders among family members
	Inadequate parenting
	Parental discord
	Parental psychopathology
	Childhood sexual abuse
	Chronic illness (diabetes, asthma, physical disabilities, etc.)

Sources: Neumark-Sztainer D, Story M, Resnick MD, Garwick A, Blum RW. Body dissatisfaction and unhealthy weight-control practices among adolescents with and without chronic illness: A population-based study. *Arch Pediatr Adolesc Med* 149:1330–1335, 1995; Striegel-Moore RH. Risk factors for eating disorders. *Ann N Y Acad Sci* 817:98–109, 1997; Wonderlich SA, Wilsnack RW, Wilsnack SC, Harris RH. Childhood sexual abuse and bulimic behavior in a nationally representative sample. *Am J Public Health* 86:1082–1086, 1996. See also *J Am Acad Child Adolesc Psychiatry* 36:1107–1115, 1997.

(continued)

Eating Disorders: Bulimia and Anorexia Nervosa *(continued)*

cal problems, including stomach dilation and rupture, infection of the lung from vomitus, low body levels of chloride and potassium ions, infection and rupture of the esophagus, enlargement of the salivary glands, and tooth erosion and loss.[295–297] Gastrointestinal complaints are the most common medical complaint of eating-disordered patients and include slow gastric emptying, bloating, constipation, and abdominal discomfort.[296] Death is possible among anorexics—who can literally starve themselves to death. Karen Carpenter, a famous pop singer of the 1970s, died from complications related to her battles with anorexia. She used syrup of ipecac to induce vomiting and died after buildup of the drug irreversibly damaged her heart.[272] Each year, in the United States, approximately 70 people die from anorexia. The resting metabolic rate can fall substantially in anorexics, as noted in Figure 13.55.[298]

What can be done to help the anorexic or bulimic?[299] Generally, they find it difficult to stop on their own, and most experts feel they need specialized professional help—generally in eating disorder clinics. These clinics usually have a staff of professionals, including physicians, psychologists, dietitians, and nurses to meet the varied needs of people with eating disorders. Often, bulimics and anorexics have deep-seated emotional problems at the foundation of their eating problems. Long-term professional care is necessary but can have mixed results. One study of teenagers with anorexia and/or bulimia showed that 5–8 years after treatment, 86% had returned to normal weight and menstrual function.[300] However, a 12-year study of 84 anorexia nervosa patients showed that 11% died, 11% remained anorexic, whereas the rest varied between moderate and good improvement[301] (see Figure 13.56).

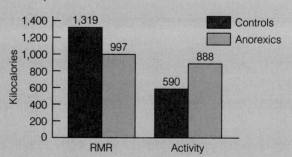

Figure 13.55 Energy expenditure in anorexics versus controls: Anorexics = 94 lb, 11% fat; controls = 124 lb, 25% fat. In this study, females with anorexia nervosa experienced a 25% reduction in their resting metabolic rates due to their low body weights (94 pounds). They partially compensate for this by exercising more. *Source:* Casper RC, Schoeller DA, Kushner R, Hnilicka J, Gold ST. Total daily energy expenditure and activity level in anorexia nervosa. *Am J Clin Nutr* 3:1143–1150, 1991.

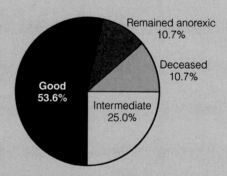

Figure 13.56 12-year follow-up of 84 anorexia nervosa patients: Purging, physical symptoms, older age, and high social status predicted unfavorable course. In this follow-up study, nearly one out of four patients had an unfavorable outcome, while only about one in two had "good" progress.[284] *Source:* Deter HC, Herzog W. Anorexia nervosa in a long-term perspective: Results of the Heidelberg–Mannheim study. *Psychosom Med* 56:20–27, 1994.

Box 13.6

Defining Anorexia Nervosa, Bulimia, and Binge Eating

Eating Disorders

This category of disorders is characterized by severe disturbances in eating behavior. It includes anorexia nervosa and bulimia nervosa, which are symptomatically related. The salient feature of *anorexia nervosa* is a refusal to maintain a minimally normal body weight. *Bulimia nervosa* is characterized by repeated episodes of binge eating followed by inappropriate compensatory behaviors such as self-induced vomiting; misuse of laxatives, diuretics, or other medications; fasting; or excessive exercise. A distorted perception of body shape and weight is an essential feature of both anorexia nervosa and bulimia nervosa. An "eating disorder not otherwise specified" category is also provided for coding disorders that do not meet any specific criteria.

Simple obesity is included in the International Classification of Diseases as a general medical condition but does not appear in the DSM-IV because it has not been established that it is consistently associated with a psychological or behavioral syndrome. However, when there is evidence that psychological factors are of importance in the etiology or course of a particular case of obesity, this can be indicated by noting the presence of psychological factors affecting medical condition.

Disorders of feeding and eating that are usually first diagnosed in infancy or early childhood (i.e., pica, rumination disorder, and feeding disorder of infancy or early childhood).

Anorexia Nervosa

Diagnostic criteria for anorexia nervosa:

1. Refusal to maintain body weight at or above a minimally normal weight for age and height (e.g., weight loss leading to maintenance of body weight less than 85% of that expected; or failure to make expected weight gain during period of growth, leading to body weight less than 85% of that expected).

2. Intense fear of gaining weight or becoming fat, even though underweight.

3. Disturbance in the way in which one's body weight or shape is experienced, undue influence of body weight or shape on self-evaluation, or denial of the seriousness of the current low body weight.

4. Amenorrhea in postmenarchal women, that is, the absence of at least three consecutive menstrual cycles. (A woman is considered to have amenorrhea if her menstrual periods occur only after administration of hormones such as estrogen.)

Restricting type: During the episode of anorexia nervosa, the person does not regularly engage in binge eating or purging behavior (i.e., self-induced vomiting or the misuse of laxatives, diuretics, or enemas).

Bulimia Nervosa

Diagnostic criteria for bulimia nervosa:

1. Recurrent episodes of binge eating. An episode of binge eating is characterized by both of the following:

a. Eating, in a discrete period of time (e.g., within any 2-hour period), an amount of food that is definitely larger than most people would eat during a similar period of time and under similar circumstances, and

b. A sense of lack of control over eating during the episode (e.g., a feeling that one cannot stop eating or control what or how much one eats).

2. Recurrent inappropriate compensatory behavior in order to prevent weight gain, such as self-induced vomiting; misuse of laxatives, diuretics, enemas, or other medications; fasting; or excessive exercise.

3. The binge eating and inappropriate compensatory behaviors both occur, on average, at least twice a week for 3 months.

4. Self-evaluation is unduly influenced by body shape and weight.

5. The disturbance does not occur exclusively during episodes of anorexia nervosa.

Purging type: the person regularly engages in self-induced vomiting or the misuse of laxatives, diuretics, or enemas.

Nonpurging type: The person uses other inappropriate compensatory behaviors, such as fasting or excessive exercise.

Eating Disorder Not Otherwise Specified

This category is for disorders of eating that do not meet the criteria for any specific eating disorder. Examples include

1. All of the criteria for bulimia nervosa are met except binges occur at a frequency of less than twice a week or for a duration of less than 3 months.

2. All of the criteria for anorexia nervosa are met except that, despite substantial weight loss, the individual's current weight is in the normal range.

3. An individual of normal body weight who regularly engages in inappropriate compensatory behavior after eating small amounts of food (e.g., self-induced vomiting after the consumption of two cookies).

4. An individual who repeatedly chews and spits out, but does not swallow, large amounts of food.

5. Binge-eating disorder; recurrent episodes of binge eating in the absence of the regular use of inappropriate compensatory behaviors characteristic of bulimia nervosa.

(continued)

Defining Bulimia, Binge Eating, and Anorexia Nervosa *(continued)*

Binge-Eating Disorder

Diagnostic criteria for binge-eating disorder:

1. Recurrent episodes of binge eating. An episode of binge eating is characterized as specified in regard to bulimia nervosa.[a]

2. The binge-eating episodes are associated with at least three of the following:

    a. Eating much more rapidly than normal.

    b. Eating until feeling uncomfortably full.

    c. Eating large amounts of food when not feeling physically hungry.

    d. Eating alone because of being embarrassed by how much one is eating.

    e. Feeling disgusted with oneself, depressed, or very guilty after overeating.

3. Marked distress regarding binge eating.

4. The binge eating occurs, on average, at least 2 days[a] a week for 6 months.

5. The binge eating is not associated with the regular use of inappropriate compensatory behaviors (e.g., purging, fasting, excessive exercise) and does not occur exclusively during the course of anorexia nervosa or bulimia nervosa.

[a]Method of determining frequency differs from that used for bulimia nervosa; future research should address whether counting the number of days on which binges occur or the number of episodes of binge eating is the preferred method of setting a frequency threshold.

Source: Diagnostic criteria for eating disorders. Reprinted with permission. American Psychiatric Association: *Diagnostic and Statistical Manual of Mental Disorders,* 4th ed. Washington, DC: American Psychiatric Association, 1994. Copyright © 1994 American Psychiatric Association.

SUMMARY

1. This chapter placed emphasis on describing the various theories of obesity and how this major health problem can be treated.

2. The majority of American adults weigh more than they should. Fourteen percent of children and 12% of adolescents are obese.

3. There are many disadvantages associated with obesity, including several diseases such as cancer, diabetes, and heart disease. Obesity is associated with early death.

4. Three major theories of obesity were discussed, with emphasis placed on the importance of genetic and parental influences, dietary factors (especially excess dietary fat), and insufficient energy expenditure.

5. Some people are more prone to obesity due to genetic influences than are others, and they need to be unusually careful in their dietary and exercise habits.

6. When humans eat diets high in fat, excess body fat is formed more easily than it is with a high-carbohydrate, high-fiber diet. Including more fruits, vegetables, legumes, and whole grains in the diet while moderating high-fat, low-fiber foods such as oils, margarine, butter, cheese, and fatty meats is probably the most important measure for controlling obesity.

7. Although obese people have higher resting metabolic rates than normal-weight people because of their greater lean body weight, they tend to exercise less than lean people. However, most studies have found that overeating is more prominent than underexercising in explaining obesity.

8. Following a meal, energy is expended by the body to process the food. This is the *thermic effect of food.* Some obese people may have a slightly lower than average thermic effect of food, but this does not appear to be a major factor explaining why people gain excess weight.

9. Obesity is very difficult to treat. There are three classifications of obesity, and each requires different approaches.

10. *Severe obesity* (BMI ≥ 40 kg/m²) is defined as weighing more than double the ideal weight. In certain cases, gastric-reduction surgery is recommended.

11. *Moderate obesity* is defined as having a BMI of 30–39.9 kg/m². Because of the high amounts of excess body fat, the very-low-calorie diet can be effective but should be administered only under medical supervision. Drug therapy should also be considered.

12. The majority of obese people are *mildly obese* (BMI 25–29.9 kg/m²). For them, a weight loss of about

1% total body weight per week is optimal—utilizing a combination of improved diet, increased exercise, and appropriate behavioral modification.

13. To lose 1 pound of fat, an excess of 3,500 Calories must be expended over caloric intake.

14. The caloric intake should be reduced, generally by reducing the fat content of the diet and increasing the complex carbohydrate content. Weight watchers must beware of the many "quick and easy" weight-loss methods.

15. Four misconceptions regarding the role of physical activity in weight reduction were reviewed, including the theories that aerobic exercise accelerates weight loss significantly when combined with a reducing diet; causes the resting metabolic rate to stay elevated for a long time after the exercise bout, burning extra Calories; counters the diet-induced decrease in resting metabolic rate; and counters the diet-induced decrease in fat-free mass.

16. There are several important benefits of exercise for the obese, including these effects of moderate aerobic activity: improved cardiorespiratory endurance; improved blood lipid profile; improved psychological state; group social support, which may enhance long-term maintenance of weight loss; and decreased risk of obesity-related diseases.

17. Moderate aerobic exercise during weight reduction helps to improve one's general health status, but the real power behind weight loss comes from a reduction in dietary Calories. The success of a weight-loss program should be measured not only by the total amount of weight lost but also by the quality of the weight loss and final health status.

18. Bulimia and anorexia nervosa are two unhealthy and sometimes life-threatening eating disorders. Bulimics consume large amounts of food within short periods of time and then engage in various purging techniques. People with anorexia nervosa have disturbed perceptions of their body images, which tend to prompt excessive weight loss. Long-term professional care is necessary for both disorders.

REFERENCES

1. Wilmore JH. Increasing physical activity: Alterations in body mass and composition. *Am J Clin Nutr* 63(suppl):456S–460S, 1996.

2. Stamler J. Endemic obesity in the United States. *Arch Intern Med* 153:1040–1044, 1993.

3. U.S. Department of Health and Human Services. *Physical Activity and Health: A Report of the Surgeon General*. Atlanta, GA: U.S. Department of Health and Human Services, Centers for Disease Control and Prevention, National Center for Chronic Disease Prevention and Health Promotion, 1996.

4. National Center for Health Statistics. *Health, United States, 1996–97 and Injury Chartbook*. Hyattsville, MD: Author, 1997.

5. NHLBI Obesity Education Initiative Expert Panel. Clinical Guidelines on the Identification, Evaluation, and Treatment of Overweight and Obesity in Adults. National Heart, Lung, and Blood Institute: www.nhlbi.nih.gov/nhlbi/, 1998.

6. Flegal KM. Trends in body weight and overweight in the U.S. population. *Nutr Rev* 54:S97–S100, 1996.

7. Galuska DA, Serdula M, Pamuk E, Siegel PZ, Byers T. Trends in overweight among US adults from 1987 to 1993: A multi-state telephone survey. *Am J Public Health* 86:1729–1735, 1996.

8. Troiano RP, Flegal KM, Kuczmarski RJ, Campbell SM, Johnson CL. Overweight prevalence and trends for children and adolescents: The National Health and Nutrition Examination Surveys, 1963–1991. *Arch Pediatr Adolesc Med* 149:1085–1091, 1995.

9. Ogden CL, Troiano RP, Briefel RR, Kuczmarski RJ, Flegal KM, Johnson CL. Prevalence of overweight among preschool children in the United States, 1971–1994. *Pediatrics* 99:E1, 1997.

10. National Center for Health Statistics. Update: Prevalence of overweight among children, adolescents, and adults—United States, 1988–1994. *MMWR* 46(9):199–202, 1997.

11. Heini AF, Weinsier RL. Divergent trends in obesity and fat intake patterns: The American paradox. *Am J Med* 102:259–264, 1997.

12. National Center for Health Statistics. *Healthy People 2000 Review, 1997*. Hyattsville, MD: Public Health Service, 1997.

13. Rodin J. Cultural and psychosocial determinants of weight concerns. *Ann Intern Med* 119:643–645, 1993.

14. Piani AL, Schoenborn CA. *Health Promotion and Disease Prevention: United States, 1990*. National Center for Health Statistics Series 10(1185). Hyattsville, MD: National Center for Health Statistics, 1993.

15. VanItallie TB. Prevalence of obesity. *Endocrinol Metab Clin North Am* 25:887–905, 1996.

16. Millar WJ, Stephens T. The prevalence of overweight and obesity in Britain, Canada, and United States. *Am J Public Health* 77:38–41, 1987.

17. Laurier D, Guiguet M, Chau NP, Wells JA, Valleron A-J. Prevalence of obesity: A comparative survey in France, the United Kingdom and the United States. *Int J Obesity* 16:565–572, 1992.

18. Himes JH, Dietz WH. Guidelines for overweight in adolescent preventive services: Recommendations from an expert committee. *Am J Clin Nutr* 59:307–316, 1994.

19. Bray GA. Obesity: Historical development of scientific and cultural ideas. *Int J Obesity* 14:909–926, 1990.

20. National Institutes of Health. Consensus development conference statement: Health implications of obesity. *Ann Intern Med* 103:981–1077, 1985.

21. Wolf AM, Colditz GA. Social and economic effects of body weight in the United States. *Am J Clin Nutr* 63(suppl): 466S–469S, 1996.

22. Cassell JA. Social anthropology and nutrition: A different look at obesity in America. *J Am Diet Assoc* 95:424–427, 1995.

23. Pi-Synyer FX. Medical hazards of obesity. *Ann Intern Med* 119(7 pt 2):655–660, 1993.

24. Gorsky RD, Pamuk E, Williamson DF, Shaffer PA, Koplan JP. The 25-year health care costs of women who remain overweight after 40 years of age. *Am J Prev Med* 12:388–394, 1996.

25. Stunkard AJ, Wadden TA. Psychological aspects of severe obesity. *Am J Clin Nutr* 55:524S–532S, 1992.

26. Gortmaker SL, Must A, Perrin JM, Sobol AM, Dietz WH. Social and economic consequences of overweight in adolescence and young adulthood. *N Engl J Med* 329:1008–1012, 1993.

27. Witteman JCM, Willett WC, Stampfer MJ, et al. A prospective study of nutritional factors and hypertension among US women. *Circulation* 80:1320–1327, 1989.

28. McCarron DA, Reusser ME. Body weight and blood pressure regulation. *Am J Clin Nutr* 63(suppl):423S–425S, 1996.

29. McMurray RG, Harrell JS, Levine AA, Gansky SA. Childhood obesity elevates blood pressure and total cholesterol independent of physical activity. *Int J Obesity Relat Metab Disord* 19:881–886, 1995.

30. Dattilo AM, Kris-Etherton PM. Effects of weight reduction on blood lipids and lipoproteins: A meta-analysis. *Am J Clin Nutr* 56:320–328, 1992.

31. Denke MA, Sempos CT, Grundy SM. Excess body weight: An underrecognized contributor to high blood cholesterol levels in white American men. *Arch Intern Med* 153:1093–1103, 1993.

32. Andersen RE, Wadden TA, Bartlett SJ, Vogt RA, Weinstock RS. Relation of weight loss to changes in serum lipids and lipoproteins in obese women. *Am J Clin Nutr* 62:350–357, 1995.

33. Couillard C, Lemieux S, Moorjani S, et al. Associations between 12 year changes in body fatness and lipoprotein–lipid levels in men and women of the Quebec family study. *Int J Obes Relat Metab Disord* 20:1081–1088, 1996.

34. Stampfer MJ, Maclure KM, Colditz GA, Manson JE, Willett WC. Risk of symptomatic gallstones in women with severe obesity. *Am J Clin Nutr* 55:652–658, 1992.

35. Utter A, Goss F. Exercise and gall bladder function. *Sports Med* 23:218–227, 1997.

36. CDC. Factors associated with prevalent self-reported arthritis and other rheumatic conditions—United States, 1989–1991. *MMWR* 45:487–491, 1996.

37. Felson DT. Weight and osteoarthritis. *Am J Clin Nutr* 63(suppl): 430S–432S, 1996.

38. Colditz GA, Willett WC, Rotnitzky A, Manson JE. Weight gain as a risk factor for clinical diabetes mellitus in women. *Ann Intern Med* 122:481–486, 1995.

39. Carey VJ, Walters EE, Colditz GA, et al. Body fat distribution and risk of non-insulin-dependent diabetes mellitus in women: The Nurses' Health Study. *Am J Epidemiol* 145:614–619, 1997.

40. Lew EA. Mortality and weight: Insured lives and the American Cancer Society studies. *Ann Intern Med* 103:1024–1029, 1985.

41. Ballard-Barbash R, Swanson CA. Body weight: Estimation of risk for breast and endometrial cancers. *Am J Clin Nutr* 63 (suppl):437S–441S, 1996.

42. Bray GA, Gray DS. Obesity: Part I. Pathogenesis. *West J Med* 149:429–441, 1988.

43. Lindsted K, Tonstad S, Kuzma J. Body mass index and patterns of mortality among Seventh-Day Adventist men. *Int J Obesity* 15:397–406, 1991.

44. Manson JE, Willett WC, Stampfer MJ, Colditz GA, Hunter DJ, Hankinson SE, Hennekens CH, Speizer FE. Body weight and mortality among women. *N Engl J Med* 333:677–685, 1995.

45. Must A, Jacques PF, Dallal GE, Bajema CJ, Dietz WH. Long-term morbidity and mortality of overweight adolescents: A follow-up of the Harvard growth study of 1922 to 1935. *N Engl J Med* 327:1350–1355, 1992.

46. Lee IM, Manson JE, Hennekens CH, Paffenbarger RS. Body weight and mortality: A 27-year follow-up of middle-aged men. *JAMA* 270:2823–2828, 1993.

47. Kannel WB, D'Agostino RB, Cobb JL. Effect of weight on cardiovascular disease. *Am J Clin Nutr* 63(suppl):419S–422S, 1996.

48. Manson JE, Colditz GA, Stampfer MJ, et al. A prospective study of obesity and risk of coronary heart disease in women. *N Engl J Med* 322:882–889, 1990.

49. Jousilahti P, Tuomilehto J, Vartiainen E, Pekkanen J, Puska P. Body weight, cardiovascular risk factors, and coronary mortality. *Circulation* 93:1372–1379, 1996.

50. Rimm EB, Stampfer MJ, Giovannucci E, Ascherio A, Spiegelman D, Colditz GA, Willett WC. Body size and fat distribution as predictors of coronary heart disease among middle-aged and older US men. *Am J Epidemiol* 141:1117–1127, 1995.

51. Rexrode KM, Hennekens CH, Willett WC, Colditz GA, Stampfer MJ, Rich-Edwards JW, Speizer FE, Manson JE. A prospective study of body mass index, weight change, and risk of stroke in women. *JAMA* 277:1539–1545, 1997.

52. Walker SP, Rimm EB, Ascherio A, Kawachi I, Stampfer MJ, Willett WC. Body size and fat distribution as predictors of stroke among US men. *Am J Epidemiol* 144:1143–1150, 1996.

53. Folsom AR, Kaye SA, Sellers TA, et al. Body fat distribution and 5-year risk of death in older women. *JAMA* 269:483–487, 1993.

54. Young TK, Gelskey DE. Is noncentral obesity metabolically benign? *JAMA* 274:1939–1941, 1995.

55. Rebuffé-Scrive M, Anderson B, Olbe L, Björntorp P. Metabolism of adipose tissue in intraabdominal depots in severely obese men and women. *Metabolism* 39:1021–1025, 1990.

56. Trosis RJ, Heinold JW, Vokonas PS, Weiss ST. Cigarette smoking, dietary intake, and physical activity: Effects on body fat distribution—the normative aging study. *Am J Clin Nutr* 53: 1104–1111, 1991.

57. Rodin J. Determinants of body fat localization and its implications for health. *Ann Behav Med* 14:275–281, 1992.

58. French SA, Folsom AR, Jeffery RW, Zheng W, Mink PJ, Baxter JE. Weight variability and incident disease in older women: The Iowa women's health study. *Int J Obesity* 21:217–223, 1997.

59. Lee I-M, Paffenbarger RS. Change in body weight and longevity. *JAMA* 268:2045–2049, 1992.

60. Harris TB, Ballard-Barbasch R, Madans J, Makuc DM, Feldman JJ. Overweight, weight loss, and risk of coronary heart

disease in older women: The NHANES I epidemiologic follow-up study. *Am J Epidemiol* 137:1318–1327, 1993.

61. Williamson DF. Intentional weight loss: Patterns in the general population and its association with morbidity and mortality. *Int J Obesity* 21(suppl 1):S14–S19, 1997.

62. Pi-Sunyer FX. Energy balance: Role of genetics and activity. *Ann N Y Acad Sci* 819:29–36, 1997.

63. Bray G, Bouchard C. Genetics of human obesity: Research directions. *FASEB J* 11:937–945, 1997.

64. Bouchard C, Tremblay A. Genetic influences on the response of body fat and fat distribution to positive and negative energy balances in human identical twins. *J Nutr* 127(suppl 5): 943S–947S, 1997.

65. Whitaker RC, Wright JA, Pepe MS, Seidel KD, Dietz WH. Predicting obesity in young adulthood from childhood and parental obesity. *N Engl J Med* 337:869–873, 1997.

66. Mayer J. Genetic factors in human obesity. *Ann NY Acad Sci* 131:412–421, 1965.

67. Stunkard AJ, Foch TT, Hrubec Z. A twin study of human obesity. *JAMA* 256:51–54, 1986.

68. Stunkard AJ, Sorensen TIA, Hanis C, et al. An adoption study of human obesity. *N Engl J Med* 314:193–198, 1986.

69. Stunkard AJ, Harris JR, Pedersen NL, McClearn GE. The body-mass index of twins who have been reared apart. *N Engl J Med* 322:1483–1487, 1990.

70. Bouchard C. Heredity and the path to overweight and obesity. *Med Sci Sports Exerc* 23:285–291, 1991.

71. Sorensen TIA, Holst C, Stunkard AJ. Childhood body mass index—genetic and familial environment influences assessed in a longitudinal adoption study. *Int J Obesity* 16:705–714, 1992.

72. Sorensen TIA, Holst C, Stunkard AJ, Skovgaard LT. Correlations of body mass index of adult adoptees and their biological and adoptive relatives. *Int J Obesity* 16:227–236, 1992.

73. Bouchard C, Pérusse L, Leblanc C, et al. Inheritance of the amount and distribution of human body fat. *Int J Obesity* 12: 205–215, 1988.

74. Bouchard C, Tremblay A, Després JP, et al. The response to long-term overfeeding in identical twins. *N Engl J Med* 322: 1477–1482, 1990.

75. Rice T, Despres JP, Daw EW, et al. Familial resemblance for abdominal visceral fat: The HERITAGE family study. *Int J Obesity* 21:1024–1031, 1997.

76. Bouchard C. Genetics of human obesity: Recent results from linkage studies. *J Nutr* 127:1887S–1890S, 1997.

77. Mistry AM, Swick AG, Romsos DR. Leptin rapidly lowers food intake and elevates metabolic rates in lean and Ob/Ob mice. *J Nutr* 127:2065–2072, 1997.

78. Korkeila M, Kaprio J, Rissanen A, Koskenvuo M. Consistency and change of body mass index and weight: A study on 5967 adult Finnish twin pairs. *Int J Obesity* 19:310–317, 1995.

79. Serdula MK, Ivery D, Coates RJ, Freedman DS, Williamson DF, Byers T. Do obese children become obese adults? A review of the literature. *Prev Med* 22:167–177, 1993.

80. Power C, Lake JK, Cole TJ. Body mass index and height from childhood to adulthood in the 1958 British birth cohort. *Am J Clin Nutr* 66:1094–1101, 1997.

81. Briefel RR, Sempos CT, McDowell MA, Chien SCY, Alaimo K. Dietary methods research in the Third National Health and Nutrition Examination Survey: Underreporting of energy intake. *Am J Clin Nutr* 65(suppl):1203S–1209S, 1997.

82. Heymsfield SB, Darby PC, Muhlheim LS, Gallagher D, Wolper C, Allison DB. The calorie: Myth, measurement, and reality. *Am J Clin Nutr* 62(suppl):1034S–1041S, 1995.

83. Bruce B, Wilfley D. Binge eating among the overweight population: A serious and prevalent problem. *J Am Diet Assoc* 96: 58–61, 1996.

84. Lichtman SW, Pisarska K, Berman ER, et al. Discrepancy between self-reported and actual caloric intake and exercise in obese subjects. *N Engl J Med* 327:1893–1898, 1992.

85. Strain GW, Hershcopf RJ, Zumoff B. Food intake of very obese persons: Quantitative and qualitative aspects. *J Am Diet Assoc* 92:199–203, 1992.

86. Welle S, Forbes GB, Statt M, Barnard RR, Amatruda JM. Energy expenditure under free-living conditions in normal-weight and overweight women. *Am J Clin Nutr* 55:14–21, 1992.

87. Scotellaro PA, Gorski LLJ, Oscai LB. Body fat accretion: A rat model. *Med Sci Sports Exerc* 23:275–279, 1991.

88. Golay A, Bobbioni E. The role of dietary fat in obesity. *Int J Obes Relat Metab Disord* 21(suppl 3):S2–S11, 1997.

89. Ravussin E, Tataranni A. Dietary fat and human obesity. *J Am Diet Assoc* 97(suppl):S42–S46, 1997.

90. Shah M, McGovern P, French S, Baxter J. Comparison of a low-fat, ad libitum complex-carbohydrate diet with a low-energy diet in moderately obese women. *Am J Clin Nutr* 59: 980–984, 1994.

91. Miller WC, Niederpruem MG, Wallace JP, Lindeman AK. Dietary fat, sugar, and fiber predict body fat content. *J Am Diet Assoc* 94:612–615, 1994.

92. Heitmann BL, Lissner L, Sorensen TIA, Bengtsson C. Dietary fat intake and weight gain in women genetically predisposed for obesity. *Am J Clin Nutr* 61:1213–1217, 1995.

93. Kendall A, Levitsky DA, Strupp BJ, Lissner L. Weight loss on a low-fat diet: Consequence of the imprecision of the control of food intake in humans. *Am J Clin Nutr* 53:1124–1129, 1991.

94. Lissner L, Habicht JP, Strupp BJ, et al. Body composition and energy intake: Do overweight women overeat and underreport? *Am J Clin Nutr* 49:320–325, 1989.

95. Lissner L, Levitsky DA, Strupp BJ, et al. Dietary fat and the regulation of energy intake in human subjects. *Am J Clin Nutr* 46:886–892, 1987.

96. Lawton CL, Burley VJ, Wales JK, Blundell JE. Dietary fat and appetite control in obese subjects: Weak effects on satiation and satiety. *Int J Obesity* 17:337–342, 1993.

97. Peoples Republic of China—United States Cardiovascular and Cardiopulmonary Epidemiology Research Group. An epidemiological study of cardiovascular and cardiopulmonary disease risk factors in four populations in the People's Republic of China. *Circulation* 85:1083–1096, 1992.

98. Barkeling B, Ekman S, Rössner S. Eating behavior in obese and normal weight 11-year-old children. *Int J Obesity* 16: 355–360, 1992.

99. Horton TJ, Drougas H, Brachey A, Reed GW, Peters JC, Hill JO. Fat and carbohydrate overfeeding in humans: Different effects on energy storage. *Am J Clin Nutr* 62:19–29, 1995.

100. Swinburn B, Ravussin E. Energy balance or fat balance. *Am J Clin Nutr* 57(suppl):766S–771S, 1993.

101. Blundell JE, Burley VJ, Cotton JR, Lawton CL. Dietary fat and the control of energy intake: Evaluating the effects of fat on meal size and postmeal satiety. *Am J Clin Nutr* 57(suppl): 772S–778S, 1993.

102. Rising R, Alger S, Boyce V, et al. Food intake measured by an automated food-selection system: Relationship to energy expenditure. *Am J Clin Nutr* 55:343–349, 1992.

103. Proserpi C, Sparti A, Schutz Y, Vetta VD, Milon H, Jéquier E. Ad libitum intake of a high-carbohydrate or high-fat diet in young men: Effects on nutrient balances. *Am J Clin Nutr* 66: 539–545, 1997.

104. Sims EAH, Danforth E. Expenditure and storage of energy in man. *J Clin Invest* 79:1019–1025, 1987.

105. Acheson KJ, Schutz Y, Bessard T, Flatt JP, Jéquier E. Carbohydrate metabolism and de novo lipogenesis in human obesity. *Am J Clin Nutr* 45:78–85, 1987.

106. Marin P, Rebuffé-Scrive DM, Björntorp DP. Glucose uptake in human adipose tissue. *Metabolism* 36:1154–1160, 1987.

107. Ravussin E, Swinburn BA. Pathophysiology of obesity. *Lancet* 340:404–408, 1992.

108. Schutz Y, Flatt JP, Jéquier E. Failure of dietary fat intake to promote fat oxidation: A factor favoring the development of obesity. *Am J Clin Nutr* 50:307–314, 1989.

109. Klausen B, Toubro S, Astrup A. Age and sex effects on energy expenditure. *Am J Clin Nutr* 65:895–907, 1997.

110. Ravussin E, Bogardus C. A brief overview of human energy metabolism and its relationship to essential obesity. *Am J Clin Nutr* 55:242S–245S, 1992.

111. Tataranmi PA, Ravussin E. Variability in metabolic rate: Biological sites of regulation. *Int J Obesity* 19(suppl 4):S102–S106, 1995.

112. Arciero PJ, Goran MI, Poehlman ET. Resting metabolic rate is lower in women than in men. *J Appl Physiol* 75:2514–2520, 1993.

113. Owen OE, Holup ML, D'Alessio DA, et al. A reappraisal of the caloric requirements of men. *Am J Clin Nutr* 46:875–885, 1987.

114. Roza AM, Shizgal HM. The Harris Benedict equation reevaluated: Resting energy requirements and the body cell mass. *Am J Clin Nutr* 40:168–182, 1984.

115. Report of a Joint FAO/WHO/UNU Expert Consultation. *Energy and Protein Requirements.* Geneva, Switzerland: World Health Organization, 1985.

116. Leibel RL, Rosenbaum M, Hirsch J. Changes in energy expenditure resulting from altered body weight. *N Engl J Med* 332: 621–628, 1995.

117. Froidevaux F, Schutz Y, Christin L, Jéquier E. Energy expenditure in obese women before and during weight loss, after refeeding, and in the weight-relapse period. *Am J Clin Nutr* 57:35–42, 1993.

118. Ravussin E. Low resting metabolic rate as a risk factor for weight gain: Role of the sympathetic nervous system. *Int J Obesity* 19(suppl 7):S8–S9, 1995).

119. Ravussin E, Lillioja S, Knowler WC, et al. Reduced rate of energy expenditure as a risk factor for body-weight gain. *N Engl J Med* 318:467–472, 1988.

120. Davies PSW, Day JME, Lucas A. Energy expenditure in early infancy and later body fatness. *Int J Obesity* 15:727–731, 1991.

121. Seidell JC, Muller DC, Sorkin JD, Andres R. Fasting respiratory exchange ratio and resting metabolic rate as predictors of weight gain: The Baltimore longitudinal study on aging. *Int J Obesity* 16:667–674, 1992.

122. Food and Nutrition Board, National Research Council. *Recommended Dietary Allowances* (10th ed.). Washington, DC: National Academy Press, 1989.

123. Park RJ. Human energy expenditure from *Australopithecus afarensis* to the 4-minute mile: Exemplars and case studies. *Exerc Sport Sci Rev* 20:185–220, 1992.

124. Haapanen N, Miilunpalo S, Pasanen M, Oja P, Vuori I. Association between leisure time physical activity and 10-year body mass change among working-aged men and women. *Int J Obesity* 21:288–296, 1997.

125. Williamson DF, Madans J, Anda RF, et al. Recreational physical activity and ten-year weight change in a US national cohort. *Int J Obesity* 17:279–286, 1993.

126. DiPietro L. Physical activity, body weight, and adiposity: An epidemiologic perspective. *Exerc Sport Sci Rev* 23:275–303, 1995.

127. Ching PLYH, Willett WC, Rimm EB, Colditz GA, Gortmaker SL, Stampfer MJ. Activity level and risk of overweight in male health professionals. *Am J Public Health* 86:25–30, 1996.

128. Kahn HS, Tatham LM, Rodriguez C, Calle EE, Thun MJ, Heath CW. Stable behaviors associated with adults' 10-year change in body mass index and likelihood of gain at the waist. *Am J Public Health* 87:747–754, 1997.

129. Moore LL, Nguyen USDT, Rothman KJ, Cupples LA, Ellison RC. Preschool physical activity level and change in body fatness in young children. *Am J Epidemiol* 142:982–988, 1995.

130. Klesges RC, Klesges LM, Eck LH, Shelton ML. A longitudinal analysis of accelerated weight gain in preschool children. *Pediatrics* 95:126–130, 1995.

131. Bullen BA, Reed RB, Mayer J. Physical activity of obese and nonobese adolescent girls appraised by motion picture sampling. *Am J Clin Nutr* 14:211–223, 1964.

132. Stefanick ML. Exercise and weight control. *Exerc Sport Sci Rev* 21:363–396, 1993.

133. Chirico AM, Stunkard AJ. Physical activity and human obesity. *N Engl J Med* 263:935–940, 1960.

134. Bloom WL, Eidex MF. Inactivity as a major factor in adult obesity. *Metabolism* 16:679–684, 1967.

135. Tryon WW, Goldberg JL, Morrison DF. Activity decreases as percentage overweight increases. *Int J Obesity* 16:591–595, 1992.

136. Ferraro R, Boyce VL, Swinburn B, De Gregorio M, Ravussin E. Energy cost of physical activity on a metabolic ward in relationship to obesity. *Am J Clin Nutr* 53:1368–1371, 1991.

137. Rowland TW. Effects of obesity on aerobic fitness in adolescent females. *AJDC* 145:764–768, 1991.

138. Voorrips LE, Meijers JHH, Sol P, Seidell JC, van Staveren WA. History of body weight and physical activity of elderly women differing in current physical activity. *Int J Obesity* 16: 199–205, 1992.

139. Schulz LO, Schoeller DA. A compilation of total daily energy expenditures and body weights in healthy adults. *Am J Clin Nutr* 60:676–681, 1994.

140. DiPietro L, Williamson DF, Caspersen CJ, Eaker E. The descriptive epidemiology of selected physical activities and body weight among adults trying to lose weight: The behav-

ioral risk factor surveillance system survey, 1989. *Int J Obesity* 17:69–76, 1993.

141. CDC. Prevalence of physical inactivity during leisure time among overweight persons: Behavioral risk factor surveillance system, 1994. *MMWR* 45(9):185–188, 1996.

142. Davies PSW, Gregory J, White A. Physical activity and body fatness in pre-school children. *Int J Obesity* 19:6–10, 1995.

143. Rising M, Harper IT, Fontvielle AM, Ferraro RT, Spraul M, Ravussin E. Determinants of total daily energy expenditure: Variability in physical activity. *Am J Clin Nutr* 59:800–804, 1994.

144. Maffeis C, Zaffanello M, Pinelli L, Schutz Y. Total energy expenditure and patterns of activity in 8–10-year-old obese and nonobese children. *J Pediatr Gastroenterol Nutr* 23:256–261, 1996.

145. Reed GW, Hill JO. Measuring the thermic effect of food. *Am J Clin Nutr* 63:164–169, 1996.

146. Tataranni PA, Larson DE, Snitker S, Ravussin E. Thermic effect of food in humans: Methods and results from use of a respiratory chamber. *Am J Clin Nutr* 61:1013–1019, 1995.

147. Tai MM, Castillo P, Pi-Sunyer FX. Meal size and frequency: Effect on the thermic effect of food. *Am J Clin Nutr* 54:783–787, 1991.

148. Segal KR, Edano A, Tomas MB. Thermic effect of a meal over 3 and 6 hours in lean and obese men. *Metabolism* 39:985–992, 1990.

149. Maffeis C, Schutz Y, Zoccante L, Micciolo R, Pinelli L. Meal-induced thermogenesis in lean and obese prepubertal children. *Am J Clin Nutr* 57:481–485, 1993.

150. Nelson KM, Weinsier RL, James LD, Darnell B, Hunter G, Long CL. Effect of weight reduction on resting energy expenditure, substrate utilization, and the thermic effect of food in moderately obese women. *Am J Clin Nutr* 55:924–933, 1992.

151. NIH Technology Assessment Conference Panel. Methods for voluntary weight loss and control. *Ann Intern Med* 119(7 pt 2): 764–770, 1993.

152. Levy AS, Heaton AW. Weight control practices of U.S. adults trying to lose weight. *Ann Intern Med* 119(7 pt 2):661–666, 1993.

153. Serdula MK, Collins E, Williamson DF, et al. Weight control practices of U.S. adolescents and adults. *Ann Intern Med* 119 (7 pt 2):667–671, 1993.

154. Horm J, Anderson K. Who in America is trying to lose weight? *Ann Intern Med* 119(7 pt 2):672–676, 1993.

155. Kramer FM, Jeffery RW, Forster JL, Snell MK. Long-term follow-up of behavioral treatment for obesity: Patterns of weight regain among men and women. *Int J Obesity* 13: 123–136, 1989.

156. Wadden TA, Sternberg JA, Letizia KA, Stunkard AJ, Foster GD. Treatment of obesity by very low calorie diet, behavior therapy, and their combination: A five-year perspective. *Int J Obesity* 13(suppl 2):39–46, 1989.

157. Foreyt JP, Goodrick GK. Evidence for success of behavior modification in weight loss and control. *Ann Intern Med* 119 (7 pt 2):698–701, 1993.

158. Hill JO, Drougas H, Peters JC. Obesity treatment: Can diet composition play a role? *Ann Intern Med* 119(7 pt 2):694–697, 1993.

159. Hakala P, Karvetti R-L, Rönnemaa T. Group vs. individual weight reduction programmes in the treatment of severe obesity—A five year follow-up study. *Int J Obesity* 17:97–102, 1993.

160. Williams CL, Campanaro LA, Squillace M, Bollella M. Management of childhood obesity in pediatric practice. *Ann N Y Acad Sci* 817:225–240, 1997.

161. Goodrick GK, Poston WS, Foreyt JP. Methods for voluntary weight loss and control: Update 1996. *Nutrition* 12:672–676, 1996.

162. Klem ML, Wing RR, McGuire MT, Seagle HM, Hill JO. A descriptive study of individuals successful at long-term maintenance of substantial weight loss. *Am J Clin Nutr* 66:239–246, 1997.

163. Foreyt JP, Goodrick GK. Factors common to successful therapy for the obese patient. *Med Sci Sports Exerc* 23:292–297, 1991.

164. Lavery MA, Loewy JW. Identifying predictive variables for long-term weight change after participation in a weight loss program. *J Am Diet Assoc* 93:1017–1024, 1993.

165. Holden JH, Darga LL, Olson SM, et al. Long-term follow-up of patients attending a combination very-low calorie diet and behavior therapy weight loss program. *Int J Obesity* 16: 605–613, 1992.

166. Walsh MF, Flynn TJ. A 54-month evaluation of a popular very low calorie diet program. *J Fam Pract* 41:231–236, 1995.

167. Saris WHM, Koenders MC, Pannemans DLE, van Baak MA. Outcome of a multicenter outpatient weight-management program including very-low-calorie diet and exercise. *Am J Clin Nutr* 56:294S–296S, 1992.

168. Phinney SD. Exercise during and after very-low-calorie dieting. *Am J Clin Nutr* 56:190S–194S, 1992.

169. Kayman S, Bruvold W, Stern JS. Maintenance and relapse after weight loss in women: Behavioral aspects. *Am J Clin Nutr* 52: 800–807, 1990.

170. Grodstein F, Levine R, Troy L, Spencer T, Colditz GA, Stampfer MJ. Three-year follow-up of participants in a commercial weight loss program: Can you keep it off? *Arch Intern Med* 156:1302–1306, 1996.

171. Pi-Sunyer FX. Short-term medical benefits and adverse effects of weight loss. *Ann Intern Med* 119(7 pt 2):722–726, 1993.

172. Higgins M, D'Agostino R, Kannel W, Cobb J. Benefits and adverse effects of weight loss: Observations from the Framingham study. *Ann Intern Med* 119(7 pt 2):758–763, 1993.

173. Atkinson RL. Proposed standards for judging the success of the treatment of obesity. *Ann Intern Med* 119(7 pt 2):677–680, 1993.

174. Brownell KD, Cohen LR. Adherence to dietary regimens 2: Components of effective interventions. *Beh Med* 20:155–163, 1995.

175. Stunkard AJ. Conservative treatments for obesity. *Am J Clin Nutr* 45:1142–1154, 1987.

176. Bray GA. Pathophysiology of obesity. *Am J Clin Nutr* 55: 488S–494S, 1992.

177. National Institutes of Health Consensus Development Conference Panel. Gastrointestinal surgery for severe obesity. *Ann Int Med* 115:956–961, 1991.

178. Kolanowski J. Surgical treatment for morbid obesity. *Br Med Bull* 43:433–444, 1997.

179. Fried M, Peskova M. Gastric banding in the treatment of morbid obesity. *Hepato-Gastroenterology* 44:582–587, 1997.

180. Brolin RE. Critical analysis of results: Weight loss and quality of data. *Am J Clin Nutr* 55:577S–581S, 1992.

181. Kral JG, Sjöström LV, Sullivan MBE. Assessment of quality of life before and after surgery for severe obesity. *Am J Clin Nutr* 55:611S–614S, 1992.

182. Gleysteen JJ. Results of surgery: Long-term effects on hyperlipidemia. *Am J Clin Nutr* 55:591S–593S, 1992.

183. Mason EE, Renquist KE, Jiang D. Perioperative risks and safety of surgery for severe obesity. *Am J Clin Nutr* 55:573S–576S, 1992.

184. Anderson JW, Brinkman VL, Hamilton CC. Weight loss and 2-y follow-up for 80 morbidly obese patients treated with intensive very-low-calorie diet and an education program. *Am J Clin Nutr* 56:244S–246S, 1992.

185. Andersen T, Stokholm KH, Backer OG, Quaade F. Long-term (5-year) results after either horizontal gastroplasty or very-low-calorie diet for morbid obesity. *Int J Obesity* 12:277–284, 1988.

186. Bray GA. Use and abuse of appetite-suppressant drugs in the treatment of obesity. *Ann Intern Med* 119(7 pt 2):707–713, 1993.

187. National Task Force on the Prevention and Treatment of Obesity. Long-term pharmacotherapy in the management of obesity. *JAMA* 276:1907–1915, 1996.

188. Weiser M, Frishman WH, Michaelson MD, Abdeen MA. The pharmacologic approach to the treatment of obesity. *J Clin Pharmacol* 37:453–473, 1997.

189. Connolly HM, Crary JL, McGoon MD, et al. Valvular heart disease associated with fenfluramine–phentermine. *N Engl J Med* 337:581–588, 1997.

190. Kushner R. The treatment of obesity: A call for prudence and professionalism. *Arch Intern Med* 157:602–604, 1997.

191. Wadden TA, Van Itallie TB, Blackburn GL. Responsible and irresponsible use of very-low-calorie diets in the treatment of obesity. *JAMA* 263:83–85, 1990.

192. ADA Reports. Position of the American Dietetic Association: Very-low-calorie weight loss diets. *J Am Diet Assoc* 90:722–726, 1990.

193. Pi-Sunyer FX. The role of very-low-calorie diets in obesity. *Am J Clin Nutr* 56:240S–243S, 1992.

194. Wadden TA. Treatment of obesity by moderate and severe caloric restriction: Results of clinical research trials. *Ann Intern Med* 119(7 pt 2):688–693, 1993.

195. National Task Force on the Prevention and Treatment of Obesity. Very low-calorie diets. *JAMA* 270:967–974, 1993.

196. Howard AN. The historical development of very low calorie diets. *Int J Obesity* 13(suppl 2):1–9, 1989.

197. Wadden TA, Foster GD, Letizia KA, Stunkard AJ. A multicenter evaluation of a proprietary weight reduction program for the treatment of marked obesity. *Arch Intern Med* 152:961–966, 1992.

198. Casper K, Matthews DE, Heymsfield SB. Overfeeding: Cardiovascular and metabolic response during continuous formula infusion in adult humans. *Am J Clin Nutr* 52:602–609, 1990.

199. Foster GD, Wadden TA, Feurer ID, et al. Controlled trial of the metabolic effects of a very-low-calorie diet: Short- and long-term effects. *Am J Clin Nutr* 51:167–172, 1990.

200. Hovell MF, Koch A, Hofstetter R, et al. Long-term weight loss maintenance: Assessment of a behavioral and supplemented fasting regimen. *Am J Public Health* 78:663–666, 1988.

201. Kirschner MA, Schneider G, Ertel NH, Gorman J. An eight-year experience with a very-low-calorie formula diet for control of major obesity. *Int J Obesity* 12:69–80, 1988.

202. Torgerson JS, Lissner L, Lindroos AK, Kruijer H, Sjostrom IL. VLCD plus dietary and behavioral support versus support alone in the treatment of severe obesity: A randomized two-year clinical trial. *Int J Obes Relat Metab Disord* 21:987–994, 1997.

203. Hyman FN, Sempos E, Saltsman J, Glinsmann WH. Evidence for success of caloric restriction in weight loss and control: Summary of data from industry. *Ann Intern Med* 119(7 pt 2):681–687, 1993.

204. Losing weight: What works, what doesn't. *Consumer Reports,* June 1993, 347–357.

205. Shape Up America! *Guidance for Treatment of Adult Obesity.* Bethesda, MD: Author, 1996.

206. National Council Against Health Fraud. NCAHF guidelines for evaluating commercial weight-loss promotions. *NCAHF Newsletter,* March/April, 1987.

207. ADA Reports. Position of the American Dietetic Association: Food and nutrition misinformation. *J Am Diet Assoc* 95:705–707, 1995.

208. Garrow JS. Exercise in the treatment of obesity: A marginal contribution. *Int J Obesity* 19(suppl 4):S126–S129, 1995.

209. Wilmore JH. Variations in physical activity habits and body composition. *Int J Obesity* 19(suppl 4):S107–S112, 1995.

210. Calles-Escandón, Horton ES. The thermogenic role of exercise in the treatment of morbid obesity: A critical evaluation. *Am J Clin Nutr* 55:533S–537S, 1992.

211. Saris WHM. The role of exercise in the dietary treatment of obesity. *Int J Obesity* 17(suppl 1):S17–S21, 1993.

212. Miller WC, Koceja DM, Hamilton EJ. A meta-analysis of the past 25 years of weight loss research using diet, exercise or diet plus exercise intervention. *Int J Obes Relat Metab Disord* 21:941–947, 1997.

213. Donnelly JE, Jakicic J, Gunderson S. Diet and body composition: Effect of very low calorie diets and exercise. *Sports Med* 12:237–249, 1991.

214. Garrow JS, Summerbell CD. Meta-analysis: Effect of exercise, with or without dieting, on the body composition of overweight subjects. *Eur J Clin Nutr* 49:1–10, 1995.

215. King AC, Haskell WL, Taylor B, Kraemer HC, DeBusk RF. Group- vs home-based exercise training in healthy older men and women: A community-based clinical trial. *JAMA* 266:1535–1542, 1991.

216. Warren BJ, Nieman DC, Dotson RG, Adkins CH, O'Donnell KA, Haddock BL, Butterworth DE. Cardiorespiratory responses to exercise training in septuagenarian women. *Int J Sports Med* 14:60–65, 1993.

217. Hinkleman L, Nieman DC. The effects of a walking program on body composition and serum lipids and lipoproteins in overweight women. *J Sports Med Phys Fit* 33:49–58, 1993.

218. Lemarche B, Després J-P, Pouliot M-C, et al. Is body fat loss a determinant factor in the improvement of carbohydrate and lipid metabolism following aerobic exercise training in obese women? *Metabolism* 41:1249–1256, 1992.

219. Blaak EE, Westerterp KR, Bar-Or O, Wouters LJM, Saris WHM. Total energy expenditure and spontaneous activity in relation to training in obese boys. *Am J Clin Nutr* 55:777–782, 1992.

220. Hardman AE, Jones PRM, Norgan NG, Hudson A. Brisk walking improves endurance fitness without changing body fatness in previously sedentary women. *Eur J Appl Physiol* 65:354–359, 1992.

221. Nieman DC, Haig JL, De Guia ED, et al. Reducing diet and exercise training effects on resting metabolic rates in mildly obese women. *J Sports Med* 28:9–88, 1988.

222. Hagan RD, Upton SJ, Wong L, Whittam J. The effects of aerobic conditioning and/or caloric restriction in overweight men and women. *Med Sci Sports Exerc* 18:87–94, 1986.

223. Phinney SD, LaGrange BM, O'Connell M, Danforth E. Effects of aerobic exercise on energy expenditure and nitrogen balance during very low calorie dieting. *Metabolism* 37:758–765, 1988.

224. Utter AC, Nieman DC, Butterworth DE, Henson DA. Body composition and cardiorespiratory fitness responses to energy restriction and moderate exercise training in obese women. *Int J Sports Nutr* (in press).

225. Van Dale D, Saris WHM. Repetitive weight loss and weight regain: Effects on weight reduction, resting metabolic rate, and lipolytic activity before and after exercise and/or diet treatment. *Am J Clin Nutr* 49:409–416, 1989.

226. Geliebter A, Maher MM, Gerace L, Gutin B, Heymsfield SB, Hashim SA. Effects of strength or aerobic training on body composition, resting metabolic rate, and peak oxygen consumption in obese dieting subjects. *Am J Clin Nutr* 66:557–563, 1997.

227. Wadden TA, Vogt RA, Anderson RE, et al. Exercise in the treatment of obesity: Effects of four interventions on body composition, resting energy expenditure, appetite, and mood. *J Consult Clin Psyc* 65:269–277, 1997.

228. Whatley JE, Gillespie WJ, Honig J, Walsh MJ, Blackburn AL, Blackburn GL. Does the amount of endurance exercise in combination with weight training and a very-low-energy diet affect resting metabolic rate and body composition? *Am J Clin Nutr* 59:1088–1092, 1994.

229. Donnelly JE, Pronk NP, Jacobsen DJ, Pronk SJ, Jakicic JM. Effects of a very-low-calorie diet and physical training regimens on body composition and resting metabolic rate in obese females. *Am J Clin Nutr* 54:56–61, 1991.

230. Sweeney ME, Hill JO, Heller PA, Baney R, DiGirolamo M. Severe vs moderate energy restriction with and without exercise in the treatment of obesity: Efficiency of weight loss. *Am J Clin Nutr* 57:127–134, 1993.

231. Hill JO, Melby C, Johnson SL, Peters JC. Physical activity and energy requirements. *Am J Clin Nutr* 62(suppl):1059S–1066S, 1995.

232. Poehlman ET, Melby CL, Goran MI. The impact of exercise and diet restriction on daily energy expenditure. *Sports Med* 11:78–101, 1991.

233. Blair SN. Evidence for success of exercise in weight loss and control. *Ann Intern Med* 119(7 pt 2):702–706, 1993.

234. Schoeller DA, Shay K, Kushner RF. How much physical activity is needed to minimize weight gain in previously obese women? *Am J Clin Nutr* 66:551–556, 1997.

235. Mattsson E, Larsson UE, Rossner S. Is walking for exercise too exhausting for obese women? *Int J Obes Relat Metab Disord* 21:380–386, 1997.

236. Sedlock DA, Fissinger JA, Melby CL. Effect of exercise intensity and duration on postexercise energy expenditure. *Med Sci Sports Exerc* 21:662–666, 1989.

237. Bahr R, Sejersted OM. Effect of intensity of exercise on excess postexercise oxygen consumption. *Metabolism* 40:836–841, 1991.

238. Phelain JF, Reinke E, Harris MA, Melby CL. Postexercise energy expenditure and substrate oxidation in young women resulting from exercise bouts of different intensity. *J Am College Nutr* 16:140–146, 1997.

239. Withers RT, Gore CJ, Mackay MH, Berry MN. Some aspects of metabolism following a 35 km road race. *Eur J Appl Physiol* 63:436–443, 1991.

240. Short KR, Sedlock DA. Excess postexercise oxygen consumption and recovery rate in trained and untrained subjects. *J Appl Physiol* 83:153–159, 1997.

241. Seale JL, VanZant RS, Conway JM. Free-living, 24-hour, and sleeping energy expenditure in sedentary, strength-trained, and endurance-trained men. *Int J Sport Nutr* 6:370–381, 1996.

242. Sjodin AM, Forslund AH, Westerterp KR, Andersson AB, Forslund JM, Hambraeus LM. The influence of physical activity on BMR. *Med Sci Sports Exerc* 28:85–91, 1996.

243. Poehlman ET, Gardner AW, Ades PA, et al. Resting energy metabolism and cardiovascular disease risk in resistance-trained and aerobically trained males. *Metabolism* 41:1351–1360, 1992.

244. Toth MJ, Poehlman ET. Resting metabolic rate and cardiovascular disease risk in resistance- and aerobic-trained middle-aged women. *Int J Obesity* 19:691–698, 1995.

245. Meijer GAL, Westerterp KR, Seyts GHP, Janssen GME, Saris WHM, ten Hoor F. Body composition and sleeping metabolic rate in response to a 5-month endurance-training program in adults. *Eur J Appl Physiol* 62:18–21, 1991.

246. Broeder CE, Burrhus KA, Svanevik LS, Wilmore JH. The effects of aerobic fitness on resting metabolic rate. *Am J Clin Nutr* 55:795–801, 1992.

247. Gilbert JA, Misner JE, Boileau RA, Ji L, Slaughter MH. Lower thermic effect of a meal post-exercise in aerobically trained and resistance-trained subjects. *Med Sci Sports Exerc* 23:825–830, 1991.

248. Schultz LO, Nyomba BL, Alger S, Anderson TE, Ravussin E. Effect of endurance training on sedentary energy expenditure measured in a respiratory chamber. *Am J Physiol* 260:E257–261, 1991.

249. Herring JL, Molé PA, Meredith CN, Stern JS. Effect of suspending exercise training on resting metabolic rate in women. *Med Sci Sports Exerc* 24:59–65, 1992.

250. Bullough RC, Gillette CA, Harris MA, Melby CL. Interaction of acute changes in exercise energy expenditure and energy intake on resting metabolic rate. *Am J Clin Nutr* 61:473–481, 1995.

251. Thompson JL, Manore MM, Thomas JR. Effects of diet and diet-plus-exercise programs on resting metabolic rate: A meta-analysis. *Int J Sport Nutr* 6:41–61, 1996.

252. Mathieson RA, Walberg JL, Gwazdauskas FC, et al. The effect of varying carbohydrate content of a very-low-calorie diet on resting metabolic rate and thyroid hormones. *Metabolism* 35:394–398, 1986.

253. Gornall J, Villani RG. Short-term changes in body composition and metabolism with severe dieting and resistance exercise. *Int J Sport Nutr* 6:285–294, 1996.

254. Westerterp KR, Meijer GAL, Schoffelen P, Janssen EME. Body mass, body composition and sleeping metabolic rate before,

during and after endurance training. *Eur J Appl Physiol* 69: 203–208, 1994.

255. Kempen KPG, Saris WHM, Westerterp KR. Energy balance during an 8-wk energy-restricted diet with and without exercise in obese women. *Am J Clin Nutr* 62:722–729, 1995.

256. Garrow JS. Energy balance in man—an overview. *Am J Clin Nutr* 45:1114–1119, 1987.

257. Marks BL, Rippe JM. The importance of fat free mass maintenance in weight loss programs. *Sports Med* 22:273–281, 1996.

258. Donnelly JE, Sharp T, Houmard J, et al. Muscle hypertrophy with large-scale weight loss and resistance training. *Am J Clin Nutr* 58:561–565, 1993.

259. Nieman DC, Miller AR, Henson DA, Warren BJ, Gusewitch G, Johnson RL, Davis JM, Butterworth DE, Herring JL, Nehlsen-Cannarella SL. The effects of high- versus moderate-intensity exercise on lymphocyte subpopulations and proliferative response. *Int J Sports Med* 15:199–206, 1994.

260. Tremblay A, Simoneau JA, Bouchard C. Impact of exercise intensity on body fatness and skeletal muscle metabolism. *Metabolism* 43:814–818, 1994.

261. Buemann B, Tremblay A. Effects of exercise training on abdominal obesity and related metabolic complications. *Sports Med* 21:191–212, 1996.

262. Visser M, Launer LJ, Deurenberg P, Deeg DJH. Total and sports activity in older men and women: Relation with body fat distribution. *Am J Epidemiol* 145:752–761, 1997.

263. Tremblay A, Després JP, Leblanc C, et al. Effect of intensity of physical activity on body fatness and fat distribution. *Am J Clin Nutr* 51:153–157, 1990.

264. Wahrenberg H, Bolinder J, Arner P. Adrenergic regulation of lipolysis in human fat cells during exercise. *Eur J Clin Invest* 21:534–541, 1991.

265. Stevenson DW, Darga LL, Spafford TR, et al. Variable effects of weight loss on serum lipids and lipoproteins in obese patients. *Int J Obesity* 12:495–502, 1987.

266. Schwartz RS, Shuman WP, Larson V, et al. The effect of intensive endurance exercise training on body fat distribution in young and older men. *Metabolism* 40:545–551, 1991.

267. Kohrt WM, Malley MT, Dalsky GP, Holloszy JO. Body composition of healthy sedentary and trained, young and older men and women. *Med Sci Sports Exerc* 24:832–837, 1992.

268. Foss ML. Exercise concerns and precautions for the obese. In Storlie J, Jordan HA (eds), *Nutrition and Exercise in Obesity Management.* New York: Spectrum Publications, 1984.

269. Franklin BA. Myths and misconceptions in exercise for weight control. In Storlie J, Jordan HA (eds), *Nutrition and Exercise in Obesity Management.* New York: Spectrum Publications, 1984.

270. Zachwieja JJ. Exercise as treatment for obesity. *Endocrinol Metab Clin North Am* 25:965–988, 1996.

271. American Psychiatric Association. *Diagnostic and Statistical Manual of Mental Disorders* (4th ed.). Washington, DC: Author, 1994.

272. Farley D. Eating disorders require medical attention. *FDA Consumer,* March 1992, 27–29.

273. Yanovski SZ, Leet M, Yanovski JA, et al. Food selection and intake of obese women with binge-eating disorder. *Am J Clin Nutr* 56:975–980, 1992.

274. Heterington MM, Altemus M, Nelson ML, Bernat AS, Gold PW. Eating behavior in bulimia nervosa: Multiple meal analyses. *Am J Clin Nutr* 60:864–873, 1994.

275. Pemberton AR, Vernon SW, Lee ES. Prevalence and correlates of bulimia nervosa and bulimic behaviors in a racially diverse sample of undergraduate students in two universities in southeast Texas. *Am J Epidemiol* 144:450–455, 1996.

276. Fredenberg JP, Berglund PT, Dieken HA. Incidence of eating disorders among selected female university students. *J Am Diet Assoc* 96:64–65, 1996.

277. Wakeling A. Epidemiology of anorexia nervosa. *Psychiatry Res* 62:3–9, 1996.

278. Leon GR. Eating disorders in female athletes. *Sports Med* 12: 219–227, 1991.

279. Zuckerman DM, Colby A, Ware NC, Lazerson JS. The prevalence of bulimia among college students. *Am J Public Health* 76:1135–1137, 1986.

280. Schotte DE, Stunkard AJ. Bulimia vs bulimic behaviors on a college campus. *JAMA* 258:1213–1215, 1987.

281. Drewnowski A, Hopkins SA, Kessler RC. The prevalence of bulimia nervosa in the US college student population. *Am J Public Health* 78:1322–1325, 1988.

282. Kurtzman FD, Yager J, Landsverk J, Wiesmeier E, Bodurka DC. Eating disorders among selected female student populations at UCLA. *J Am Diet Assoc* 89:45–53, 1989.

283. Killen JD, Taylor CB, Telch MJ, et al. Depressive symptoms and substance use among adolescent binge eaters and purgers: A defined population study. *Am J Public Health* 77:1539–1541, 1987.

284. Killen JD, Taylor CB, Telch MJ, et al. Self-induced vomiting and laxative and diuretic use among teenagers. *JAMA* 255: 1447–1449, 1986.

285. Dummer GM, Rosen LW, Heusner WW, et al. Pathogenic weight-control behaviors of young competitive swimmers. *Physician Sportsmed* 15(5):75–86, 1987.

286. Clark N, Nelson M, Evans W. Nutrition education for elite female runners. *Physician Sportsmed* 15:75–84, 1987.

287. Wilmore JH. Eating and weight disorders in the female athlete. *Int J Sport Nutr* 1:104–117, 1991.

288. Sundgot-Borgen J. Prevalence of eating disorders in elite female athletes. *Int J Sport Nutr* 3:29–40, 1993.

289. ACSM position stand on the female athlete triad. *Med Sci Sports Exerc* 29:i–ix, 1997.

290. Brownell KD, Steen SN, Wilmore JH. Weight regulation practices in athletes: Analysis of metabolic and health effects. *Med Sci Sports Exerc* 19:546–556, 1987.

291. National Institute of Nutrition. An overview of the eating disorders anorexia nervosa and bulimia nervosa. *Nutrition Today,* May/June 1989, 27–29.

292. Striegel-Moore RH. Risk factors for eating disorders. *Ann N Y Acad Sci* 817:98–109, 1997.

293. Wonderlich SA, Wilsnack RW, Wilsnack SC, Harris RH. Childhood sexual abuse and bulimic behavior in a nationally representative sample. *Am J Public Health* 86:1082–1086, 1996. See also *J Am Acad Child Adolesc Psychiatry* 36:1107–1115, 1997.

294. Neumark-Sztainer D, Story M, Resnick MD, Garwick A, Blum RW. Body dissatisfaction and unhealthy weight-control practices among adolescents with and without chronic illness: A population-based study. *Arch Pediatr Adolesc Med* 149: 1330–1335, 1995.

295. Mehler PS. Eating disorders: 2. Bulimia nervosa. *Hospital Practice*, February 15, 1996.

296. Carney CP, Andersen AE. Eating disorders: Guide to medical evaluation and complications. *Psychiatr Clin North Am* 19: 657–679, 1996.

297. Casper RC. The pathophysiology of anorexia nervosa and bulimia nervosa. *Ann Rev Nutr* 6:299–316, 1986.

298. Casper RC, Schoeller DA, Kushner R, Hnilicka J, Gold ST. Total daily energy expenditure and activity level in anorexia nervosa. *Am J Clin Nutr* 53:1143–1150, 1991.

299. Position of the American Dietetic Association: Nutrition intervention in the treatment of anorexia nervosa and bulimia nervosa. *J Am Diet Assoc* 88:68–71, 1988.

300. Churchill BH, Strauss J. Long-term outcome of adolescents with anorexia nervosa. *Am J Dis Children* 143:1322–1327, 1989.

301. Deter HC, Herzog W. Anorexia nervosa in a long-term perspective: Results of the Heidelberg–Mannheim study. *Psychosom Med* 56:20–27, 1994.

PHYSICAL FITNESS ACTIVITY 13.1

Calculating Your Energy Expenditure

In this physical fitness activity, you will be calculating your average daily Calorie expenditure. As you may remember from your study of this chapter, during any given 24-hour period, the majority of your energy expenditure (if you are no more than moderately active) comes from your resting metabolic rate, with smaller amounts from physical activity and the energy used in digesting and metabolizing your food.

Table 13.5 outlines a method for determining the number of Calories burned each day, combining RMR and physical activity. Notice that Category 1 represents the energy you expend during sleeping or resting in bed, or in other words, your resting metabolic rate. Categories 2 through 9 represent different forms of physical activity, with category 9 being the most intense.

The average female in the United States burns only 1,500–2,000 total Calories per day, and the average male, 2,300–3,000 Calories per day. Those spending more time in categories 6 through 9 will burn more than these amounts.

Estimate the number of Calories you burn in a given day by averaging the number of hours you spend in each activity category. Make sure that your hour total equals 24.

Multiply the number of hours by the Calorie/kg factor and then your weight (in kilograms). The final step is to total the Calories you have estimated in the final column. Your final result should be close to the estimated amount of Calories you consume each day.

TABLE 13.5   Calculating Energy Expenditure

Directions: Estimate the average number of hours you spend in each category. Multiply the Calorie/kg factor times the hours/day and then by your body weight. Put the total number of Calories calculated for each category in the Calorie/Category blank.

Category	Average Hours/Day		Calorie/kg Per Hour		Body Wt (kg)		Calorie/ Category
1	_____	×	1.00	×	_____	=	_____
2	_____	×	1.35	×	_____	=	_____
3	_____	×	2.00	×	_____	=	_____
4	_____	×	2.50	×	_____	=	_____
5	_____	×	3.00	×	_____	=	_____
6	_____	×	4.25	×	_____	=	_____
7	_____	×	5.00	×	_____	=	_____
8	_____	×	6.00	×	_____	=	_____
9	_____	×	8.00	×	_____	=	_____
Total	24					=	_____

Total (24-hour energy expenditure)

Category 1   Sleeping; resting in bed

Category 2   Sitting; eating; listening; writing; etc.

Category 3   Light activity while standing; washing, shaving, combing hair, cooking

Category 4   Slow walking; driving; dressing; showering

Category 5   Light manual work (floor sweeping, window washing, driving a truck, painting, waiting on tables, nursing chores, house chores, electrical work, walking at moderate pace)

Category 6   Leisure activities and sports in a recreational environment (baseball, golf, volleyball, canoeing or rowing, archery, bowling, slow cycling, table tennis, etc.)

Category 7   Manual work at moderate pace (mining, carpentry, house building, snow shoveling, loading and unloading goods)

Category 8   Leisure and sport activities of higher intensity, but not competitive (canoeing, bicycling at less than 10 mph, dancing, skiing, badminton, gymnastics, moderately paced swimming, tennis, brisk walking, etc.)

Category 9   Intense manual work, high-intensity sport activities or sport competition (tree cutting, carrying heavy loads, jogging and running faster than 12 minutes a mile, racquetball, swimming, cross-country skiing, mountain biking, etc.)

Source: Bouchard C, et al. A method to assess energy expenditure in children and adults. *Am J Clin Nutr* 37:461–467, 1983.

PHYSICAL FITNESS ACTIVITY 13.2

Eating Disorder Checksheet

As discussed in the Sports Medicine Insight, a significant number of college-age students have eating disorders. This activity will help determine whether you have an eating disorder.

Place an (X) under the column that applies best to each of the numbered statements.

Section One

Always 0	Very Often 0	Often 0	Some-times 1	Rarely 2	Never 3	
						1. I like eating with other people.
						2. I like my clothes to fit tightly.
						3. I enjoy eating meat.
						4. I have regular menstrual periods.
						5. I enjoy eating at restaurants.
						6. I enjoy trying new rich foods.

Section Two

Always 3	Very Often 2	Often 1	Some-times 0	Rarely 0	Never 0	
						7. I prepare foods for others but do not eat what I cook.
						8. I become anxious prior to eating.
						9. I am terrified about being overweight.
						10. I avoid eating when I am hungry.
						11. I find myself preoccupied with food.
						12. I have gone on eating binges where I feel that I may not be able to stop.
						13. I cut my food into small pieces.
						14. I am aware of the Calorie content of foods that I eat.
						15. I particularly avoid foods with a high carbohydrate content (bread, potatoes, rice, etc.)
						16. I feel bloated after meals.
						17. I feel others would prefer if I ate more.
						18. I vomit after I have eaten.
						19. I feel extremely guilty after eating.
						20. I am preoccupied with a desire to be thinner.

Always 3	Very Often 2	Often 1	Some-times 0	Rarely 0	Never 0	
						21. I exercise strenuously to burn off Calories.
						22. I weigh myself several times a day.
						23. I wake up early in the morning.
						24. I eat the same foods day after day.
						25. I think about burning up Calories when I exercise.
						26. Other people think I am too thin.
						27. I am preoccupied with the thought of having fat on my body.
						28. I take longer than others to eat my meals.
						29. I take laxatives.
						30. I avoid foods with sugar in them.
						31. I eat diet foods.
						32. I feel that food controls my life.
						33. I display self-control around foods.
						34. I feel that others pressure me to eat.
						35. I give too much time and thought to food.
						36. I suffer from constipation.
						37. I feel uncomfortable after eating sweets.
						38. I engage in dieting behavior.
						39. I like my stomach to be empty.
						40. I have the impulse to vomit after meals.

Total your points (use the numbers given at the top of each column for the two sections.)

Norms	Range (0–120 points)
Eating disorder	>50 points
Borderline eating disorder	30–50 points
Normal[a]	<30 points

[a]Average score among those with normal eating habits = 15.4.

Source: Garner DM, Omstead M, Polivy J. Development and validation of a multidimensional eating disorder inventory for anorexia nervosa and bulimia. *Int J Eating Disorders* 2:15–33, 1983. Reprinted by permission of John Wiley & Sons, Inc.

CHAPTER
14

Psychological Health

Mens sana in corpore sano. [A sound mind in a sound body.]

—Homer

As discussed in Chapter 1, the promotion of physical activity is public policy in both the United States and Canada. While directed primarily at the reduction of cardiovascular diseases, obesity, and other chronic diseases, this policy could also have some beneficial effects on the population's mental health. Even a small effect could be significant because mental health problems and stress are so widespread in most Western countries.[1] *Mental health* is a general term used to refer not only to the absence of mental disorders such as schizophrenia, depression, panic attacks, and phobias, but also to the ability of a person to negotiate successfully the daily challenges and social interactions of life.[2]

During any 1-year period, an estimated 52 million American adults (nearly 3 of 10) suffer some form of mental disorder, imposing a $148 billion cost burden. As shown in Table 14.1, anxiety and depressive disorders are most common. The National Institute of Mental Health estimates that there are between 4 and 5 million adults with what are defined as serious mental health disorders.[2–4]

Signs and symptoms of anxiety are widespread throughout the world and are associated with significant disability.[5,6] In the United States, nearly three quarters of the population have one or more unreasonable fears, spells of sudden panic, or general nervousness.[5] Anxiety disorders are two times as prevalent in females as in males, and these include phobias (e.g., social phobia and agoraphobia, with a lifetime prevalence of 14%), generalized anxiety disorder

TABLE 14.1 Mental Illness in the United States

	In Millions
Anxiety: phobia, panic, obsessive–compulsive	23.3
Depression: manic (bipolar disorder), major depression	17.6
Substance-abuse disorders	17.5
Severe cognitive impairment	5.0
Antisocial personality	2.8
Schizophrenia	2.0

Source: National Institute of Mental Health.

(lifetime prevalence of 5%), and panic disorder (lifetime prevalence of 3.5%).[5]

Depression is a pernicious illness associated with episodes of long duration, relapse, and significant social and physical impairment.[7–10] The majority of patients with chronic major depression are misdiagnosed, receive inappropriate or inadequate treatment, or are given no treatment at all.[10] The lifetime estimate for major depression is 17% and is most common among females, the elderly, young adults, and people with less education than a bachelor's degree.[7–10] Box 14.1 lists seven criteria for the diagnosis of depression, and Physical Fitness Activity 14.3 provides a tool for measuring depression.

Box 14.1

Criteria for Diagnosing Depression

Depression may range from mild symptoms to more severe forms. Seven criteria for the diagnosis of depression are

1. Changes in appetite and weight
2. Disturbed sleep
3. Fatigue and loss of energy
4. Loss of interest or pleasure in usual activities
5. Feelings of worthlessness, self-reproach, and excessive guilt
6. Suicidal thinking or attempts
7. Difficulty with thinking or concentration

Source: NIH Consensus Development Panel on Depression in Late Life. Diagnosis and treatment of depression in late life. *JAMA* 268: 1018–1022, 1992.

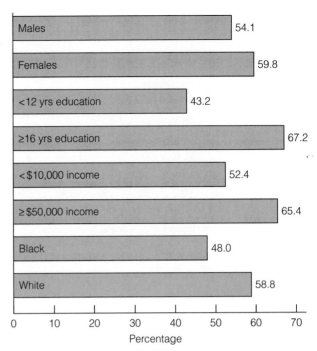

Figure 14.1 Percentage of U.S. adults reporting stress in previous 2 weeks, National Health Interview Survey. More than one half of U.S. adults reported experiencing at least a moderate amount of stress in the 2 weeks preceding the National Health Interview Survey. This prevalence varied according to race, income level, and education.   *Source:* Piani A, Schoenborn C. Health promotion and disease prevention: United States, 1990, National Center for Health Statistics. *Vital Health Stat* 10(185), 1993.

In 1990, the U.S. Public Health Service conducted the National Health Interview Survey, which included questions on the amount of stress experienced in the past 2 weeks and the effect of stress on health.[11] More than one half (57.1%) of U.S. adults reported experiencing at least a moderate amount of stress during the previous 2 weeks, up from 51.4% in 1985 (see Figure 14.1). Individuals with higher education and income reported they were more likely to experience stress. According to a 1995 survey by *Prevention Magazine,* 65% of Americans reported that they were under a great deal of stress one or more times a week, an increase of 10% from 1983.[12] Despite this relatively high prevalence of stress, only 14% of adults had sought help in the previous year for a personal or emotional problem.[4]

As shown in Figure 14.2, negative moods such as depression, loneliness, restlessness, boredom, and feeling upset are experienced by a substantial proportion of Americans.[13] Depression is a major risk factor for suicide, a cause of death that is especially prevalent among elderly men[2] (see Figure 14.3).

THE MEANING OF STRESS

Stress has been defined as any action or situation (stressor) that places special physical or psychological demands on a person—in other words, anything that unbalances one's equilibrium.[14–16] Hans Selye, one of the great pioneers of

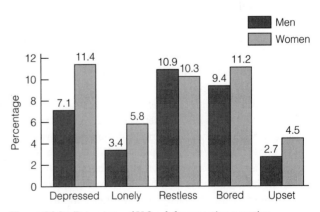

Figure 14.2 Percentage of U.S. adults reporting negative moods in previous 2 weeks, National Health Interview Survey. Of the five negative moods reported in a national government survey, the most prevalent among women was depression and among men restlessness.   *Source:* Schoenborn CA, Norm J. Negative moods as correlates of smoking and heavier drinking: Implications for health promotion. *Advance Data* 236: November 4, 1993.

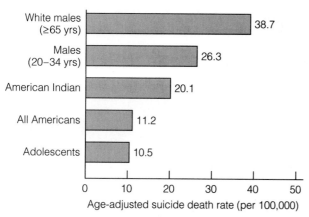

Figure 14.3 Suicide death rates in Americans. Suicide rates are highest in elderly white males. *Source:* National Center for Health Statistics. *Healthy People 2000 Review, 1997.* Hyattsville, MD: Public Health Service, 1997.

medicine and the originator of the concept of stress, wrote in his famous 1956 classic, *The Stress of Life,* "In its medical sense, stress is essentially the rate of wear and tear in the body . . . the nonspecific response of the body to any demand.[17]

There are two types of stress: eustress and distress.[14-18] *Eustress* is good stress and appears to motivate and inspire (e.g., falling in love or exercising moderately). *Distress* is considered bad stress and can be *acute* (quite intense, but then disappears quickly) or *chronic* (not so intense, but lingers for prolonged periods of time). (See Physical Fitness Activities 14.1 and 14.2 for two questionnaires used in measuring stress.) Selye observed that whether a situation was perceived as very good (e.g., getting married) or very bad (e.g., getting divorced), demands were placed on the body and mind, forcing them to adapt. According to Selye, the physiological response or arousal was very similar during both good and bad situations, producing a similar physiological response.[17,18]

Medical research on the effects of stress dates back to the early part of the 1900s, when Walter Cannon of Harvard University first coined the term "fight-or-flight response," now known as the stress response.[19] In this response, the muscles tense and tighten, breathing becomes deep and fast, the heart rate rises and blood vessels constrict, blood pressure rises, the stomach and intestines temporarily halt digestion, perspiration increases, the thyroid gland is stimulated, secretion of saliva slows, blood sugar and fats rise, and sensory perception becomes sharper. These responses are regulated by the nervous system and various hormones, redirecting energy, oxygen, and fuel to allow the body to cope with the physical or emotional stress (see Figure 14.4).

In the 1940s and 1950s, Selye extended Cannon's work, laying the foundation for today's understanding of stress and its medical consequences.[17,18] Experimenting with rats while using various physical stressors such as cold temperature or random electrical shock, Selye discovered that if the stressor was maintained long enough, the body would go through three stages (termed the "general adaptation syndrome"):[18]

1. *Alarm* reaction (essentially the fight-or-flight response)
2. *Resistance* stage (body functions return to normal as the body adjusts)
3. *Exhaustion* stage (alarm symptoms return, leading to disease and death)

Selye and other stress researchers, however, urged recognizing that not all stress is harmful.[14-19] In fact, it appears that humans need some degree of stress to stay healthy. While the human body needs some sort of balance (*homeostasis,* or physiological calm), it also requires occasional arousal to ensure that the heart, muscles, lungs, nerves, brain, and other tissues stay in good shape.

III Effects of High Stress

Chronic stressors (e.g., economic difficulties, intolerable relationships, bodily pain) are thought to be the real villains and have been associated with a growing list of health and disease problems: chronic anxiety and depression, an overabundance of life-change events, repressed feelings of loss, bereavement, emotional distress, lack of social ties, and hostility have been linked to increased risk of hypertension, heart disease, cancer, early death, infection, suppressed immunity, asthma attacks, back pain, chronic fatigue, gastrointestinal distress, headaches, and insomnia.[20-47] For example, a study of 740 men and women in Denmark found that chronic depression was related to a 70% increased risk of heart attack over a 20-year period.[20] Among 1,500 people living in Baltimore, the odds for a heart attack over a 13-year period were doubled in those with a history of *dysphoria* (2 weeks or more of sadness).[21] A cohort of men and women followed for 7–16 years showed that risk of developing hypertension was increased about 80% in those with high anxiety or depression.[22]

A 30-year study of some 1,000 men determined that those who had the highest anger scores on a psychological test taken in their 20s were about three times more likely to have a heart attack and nearly six times more likely to have a stroke during midlife.[23] Anger and mental stress have been described as triggers for heart attacks, especially in those with little education or with preexisting coronary artery disease.[24-29]

Swedish researchers asked some 7,000 men how often they had trouble sleeping or felt tense, irritable, or anxious. Over the next 12 years, the men who said they constantly experienced those symptoms were about 70% more likely

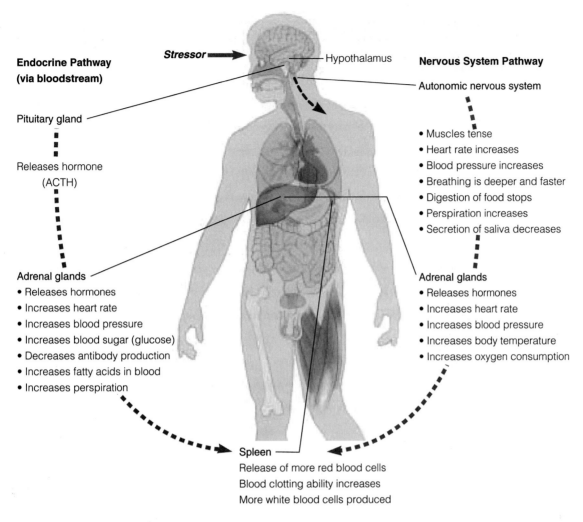

Endocrine Pathway (via bloodstream)

Stressor ⟶

Hypothalamus

Nervous System Pathway

Autonomic nervous system

Pituitary gland

Releases hormone (ACTH)

- Muscles tense
- Heart rate increases
- Blood pressure increases
- Breathing is deeper and faster
- Digestion of food stops
- Perspiration increases
- Secretion of saliva decreases

Adrenal glands
- Releases hormones
- Increases heart rate
- Increases blood pressure
- Increases blood sugar (glucose)
- Decreases antibody production
- Increases fatty acids in blood
- Increases perspiration

Adrenal glands
- Releases hormones
- Increases heart rate
- Increases blood pressure
- Increases body temperature
- Increases oxygen consumption

Spleen
Release of more red blood cells
Blood clotting ability increases
More white blood cells produced

Figure 14.4 The stress response affects the entire body through both hormonal and nerve pathways (RBCs = red blood cells; ACTH = adrenocorticotropic hormone).

to die of a heart attack or stroke than the other men were.[30] Another Swedish study, involving nearly a million people, linked stressful jobs—high pressure or little power to make decisions—with a 60% increase in heart attack risk.[31]

Researchers at Carnegie Mellon University injected cold viruses into the noses of some 400 volunteers and reported that the risk of coming down with a cold was directly related to the stress levels of the subjects.[32] Those experiencing the most stress and tension were almost twice as likely to catch cold as those who reported the least. A study in Australia found that highly stressed people had twice as many days with flu and cold symptoms, compared to those reporting little stress, during a 6-month period.[33] Marital disruption has been linked to depressed immunity and physical illness, with separated partners having about 30% more acute illnesses and physician visits than those who remain married.[34] A lack of social ties has also been linked to a decreased resistance to infection from the common cold.[35]

About 7–12 months following the loss of a spouse, mortality risk is doubled for both men and women.[36,37] Among

women 75 years of age and older with no contact from children, friends, and group organizations, mortality risk is increased two- to threefold.[38] A review of published studies has determined that people who are socially isolated are at increased mortality risk from a number of causes.[39] Among heart disease patients, lack of social support is a risk factor for an additional heart attack.[40,41]

Stress Management Principles

Much has been written about controlling stress. Box 14.2 summarizes the basic formats of stress management often used at work settings.[16] There are five basic stress management principles.[14–19]

Control Stressors

Stressors are everywhere. They cannot all be avoided, but much can be done to reduce, modify, or avoid many of them

Box 14.2

Basic Formats of Stress Management Programs Used at Work Settings

Since the late 1970s, a consistent finding among investigators is that the psychosocial factors of high psychological job demands and low control over the work process (i.e., job strain) are associated with excess cardiovascular disease. About one third of employed workers report that exposure to mental stress is the work condition that most endangers their health. About half of workers report that their job is very stressful, with one fourth characterizing their job as the single greatest cause of stress in their lives. Emerging changes in the work environment (e.g., downsizing and reorganization, flexiplace arrangements, total quality management) and changes in workforce demographics (e.g., cultural diversity) indicate that job stress will continue to be a problem for the foreseeable future.

Stress management interventions are defined as techniques designed to help employees modify their appraisal of stressful situations or deal more effectively with the symptoms of stress. There is great variability in the strategies used to manage stress, but in general, a combination of techniques (e.g., muscle relaxation plus cognitive-behavioral skills training) is more effective than a single technique. Stress management interventions can be grouped into four categories:

1. *Progressive muscle relaxation.* This technique involves focusing attention on muscle activity, learning to identify even small amounts of tension in a muscle group, and practicing the release of tension from the muscles. The underlying theory is that because relaxation and muscle tension are incompatible states, reducing muscle tension levels indirectly reduces autonomic nervous activity and, consequently, anxiety and stress levels.

2. *Biofeedback.* In biofeedback training, a person is provided with information or feedback about the status of a physiological function and, over time, learns to control the activity of that function. For example, the electrical activity produced when muscles tense can be recorded and transformed into a tone, the pitch of which rises as muscle activity increases and falls as muscle activity decreases.

3. *Meditation.* There are several types of meditation techniques. Most of them involve finding a quiet place and sitting comfortably for 20 minutes twice a day. While maintaining a passive attitude toward intruding thoughts, the person repeats some neutral word with each exhalation. Meditation is thought to invoke a "relaxation response," which is the opposite of the stress response.

4. *Cognitive-behavioral skills.* Cognitive methods help people restructure their thinking patterns and are often referred to as cognitive restructuring techniques. *Stress inoculation* (a common form of cognitive-behavioral skills training) involves three stages: (1) education (learning about how one has responded to past stressful experiences), (2) rehearsal (learning various coping techniques such as problem solving, relaxation, and cognitive coping), and (3) application (practicing the skills under simulated conditions).

Sources: Johnson JV, Stewart W, Hall EM, Fredlund P, Theorell T. Long-term psychosocial work environment and cardiovascular mortality among Swedish men. *Am J Public Health* 86:324–331, 1996; Murphy LR. Stress management in work settings: A critical review of the health effects. *Am J Health Promot* 11:112–135, 1996.

in a way that will allow one to accomplish goals. For example, in climbing a tall mountain, one can make the trip miserable by hiking too fast with a heavy backpack, or satisfying and pleasurable by walking at a moderate pace with a lighter load. Same goal, same path, but a completely different experience.

Suppose that a college student is taking a heavy academic load in a subject area (e.g., biochemistry) that is too difficult for him at present, working 15 hours a week to help pay for expenses, living in a crowded and noisy apartment with an unbearable roommate, experiencing constant trans-

portation problems because of a car that keeps breaking down, and dealing with crushing family problems due to the divorce of his parents. The first step would be for the student to sit down, make a list of all his major goals, in order of importance, and then catalog each of the stressors, along with plans to either eliminate or modify them. (See Physical Fitness Activity 14.4 at the end of this chapter.)

For example, finishing biochemistry has a high priority because he must do so to have a chance to achieve his major life goal of becoming a physician. He should give it his first attention (he could increase his study time by quitting work and taking out a loan). He could move closer to campus, find more desirable living accommodations, and walk or bicycle for transportation until finances improve.

Just as in climbing a mountain, stressors often can be managed by controlling the pace of life and the load carried. A key is to avoid crowding too much into the schedule, and learning to control circumstances to allow the pace of life to flow with one's psychological makeup. The important objective is to control your circumstances—don't let them control you.

Let the Mind Choose the Reaction

This strategy is also called "stress reaction management." As mentioned, a stress reaction (the fight-or-flight response) stimulates production of various stress hormones, depressing immune function, increasing blood pressure, and so on. Over time, the response has negative health effects, so the goal is to head off stress reactions before they become chronic.

To understand how to do this, one needs to remember that events only cause stress when they are seen, heard, felt, or sensed by the brain. The mind interprets the event, and the type of interpretation governs the reaction. When a stressor presents itself, one can decide what kind of reaction to have. Usually we have "knee-jerk" reactions to potentially stressful events, without taking the opportunity to calmly reason them out. In other words, we are largely responsible for creating our emotional reactions, and we miss our opportunities to control them.

Once again, the strategy is not new. Marcus Aurelius said long ago, "If you are distressed by anything external, the pain is not due to the thing itself but to your estimate of it. This you have the power to revoke at any time."

So when an event takes place (e.g., a flat tire on your way to work or school), one can choose how to react. One can react with the stress response of anger (e.g., cussing and kicking the tire), or one can choose a calm response by considering practical options (I'll call at the first opportunity and work it out with the boss or professor).

Seek the Social Support of Others

Surveys have shown that as much as one fourth of the American population feels extremely lonely at some time during any given month—especially divorced parents, single mothers, people who have never married, and housewives.[13]

As reviewed in this chapter, when people are socially isolated (few social contacts with family and friends, neighbors, or the "society at large"), they are more vulnerable to sickness, mental stress, and even early death. One 9-year study (of 7,000 residents of Alameda County, California)

found that people with few ties to other people had death rates from various diseases two to five times higher than those with more ties. The researchers measured social ties by looking at whether people were married, the number of close friends and relatives they had and how often they were in contact with them, church attendance, and involvement in informal and formal group associations.[46]

Social support means reaching out to other people, sharing emotional, social, physical, financial, and other types of comfort and assistance. The principle was summarized by the Institute of Medicine (Division of Health Promotion and Disease Prevention): "a lack of family and community supports plays an important role in the development of disease. An absence of social support weakens the body's defenses through psychological stress. Isolated individuals must be identified, and strategies for increasing social contact and diminishing feelings of loneliness must be developed. Clinicians, family, friends, and social institutions bear a responsibility for diminishing social isolation."[48]

Find Satisfaction in Work and Service

Albert Schweitzer once wrote, "I don't know what your destiny will be. But I do know that the only ones among you who will find true happiness are those who find a place to serve." Selye echoed this thought in his book, *Stress without Distress:*[18] "My own code is based on the view that to achieve peace of mind and fulfillment through self-expression, most men need a commitment to work in the service of some cause that they can respect."

Keep Physically Healthy

It is far easier to handle stressors when the body is healthy from adequate exercise, sleep, good food and water, clean air and sunshine, and relaxation.

Problems with sleep have become a modern epidemic that is taking an enormous toll on our bodies and minds. Desperately trying to fit more into the hours of the day, many people are stealing extra hours from the night. The result, say sleep researchers, is a sleep deficit that undermines health, sabotages productivity, blackens mood, clouds judgment, and increases the risk of accidents. Sadly, even those who want to sleep more often cannot. In recent surveys, half of the men and women surveyed said they have had trouble sleeping.

The Better Sleep Council gives several guidelines for improving sleep, including these:

1. Keep regular sleeping hours.

2. Exercise regularly.

3. Cut down on stimulants (coffee, tea, cola drinks, chocolate).

4. Sleep on a good bed.

5. Do not smoke (nicotine is a stronger stimulant than caffeine).

6. Go for quality, not just quantity.

7. Set aside a worry or planning time early in the evening.

8. Do not go to bed stuffed or starved.

9. Develop a sleep ritual.

(See the Sports Medicine Insight at the end of this chapter for more information on sleep.)

PHYSICAL ACTIVITY AND STRESS

One of the most important habits a person can acquire to improve mood state and manage stress is the habit of regular exercise. The rest of this chapter describes how regular physical activity can reduce depression, anxiety, and mental stress, while enhancing psychological well-being and a vigorous attitude toward life.

We have seen that poor psychological health is associated with poor physical health. Is there proof for the converse association? Is a healthy and fit body positively associated with psychological health? Were the ancient Greeks right in their assertion that a physically fit and strong body would lead to a sound mind? Surveys and cross-sectional studies of active, compared to inactive, people strongly support this concept.

The part of the brain that enables us to exercise, the motor cortex, lies only a few millimeters away from the part of the brain that deals with thought and feeling. Might this proximity mean that when exercise stimulates the motor cortex, it has a parallel effect on cognition and emotion?

Since the beginning of time, many have believed in the "cerebral satisfaction" of exercise. The Greeks maintained that exercise made the mind more lucid. Aristotle started his "Peripatetic School" in 335 B.C.—so named because of Aristotle's habit of walking up and down (*peripaton*) the paths of the Lyceum in Athens while thinking or lecturing to his students walking with him. Plato and Socrates had also practiced the art of peripatetics, as did the Roman *Ordo Vagorum* or walking scholars. Centuries later, Oliver Wendell Holmes explained that "in walking the will and the muscles are so accustomed to working together and perform their task with so little expenditure of force that the intellect is left comparatively free."

John F. Kennedy echoed the Greek ideal when he said,

> Physical fitness is not only one of the most important keys to a healthy body, it is the basis of dynamic and creative intellectual activity. Intelligence and skill can only function at the peak of their ca-

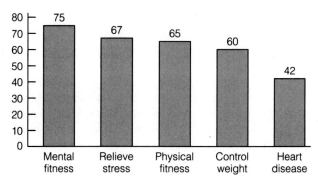

Figure 14.5   Why runners run, *Runner's World* subscriber research. When 700 runners were asked why they ran, the two most important reasons were to "increase mental fitness" and to "relieve stress."   *Source:* Johnsgard KW. Peace of mind. *Runner's World*, April 1990, 73–81.

pacity when the body is strong. Hardy spirits and tough minds usually inhabit sound bodies.

The highly acclaimed 1978 "Perrier Survey of Fitness in America," conducted by Louis Harris and Associates, showed that those who had a deep commitment to exercise reported feeling more relaxed, less tired, more disciplined, more attractive, more self-confident, more productive in work, and in general, more at one with themselves.[49]

The 1988 Campbell's Survey on Well-Being in Canada revealed that physically active people reported less depression and a higher sense of positive well-being than inactive people.[50] A survey by *Runner's World* magazine discovered that although most people start running to "improve physical fitness," most continue to run to "improve mental fitness" and to "relieve stress"[51] (see Figure 14.5).

There have been several national surveys in the United States and in Canada to study the relationship between physical activity and feelings of mental well-being.[49] One of the questionnaires used in national studies was the general well-being schedule (GWBS) (see Physical Fitness Activity 14.1). The GWBS is highly regarded as one of the best measures of stress and mental health. It consists of 18 questions, covering such areas as energy level, satisfaction, freedom from worry, and self-control. A high score on the GWBS reflects an absence of bad feelings, an expression of positive mood state, and low stress.[52]

Figure 14.6 summarizes the findings from the national studies. "The inescapable conclusion from these four national studies," says Stephens, "is that physical activity is positively associated with good mental health, especially positive mood, general well-being, and less anxiety and depression."[49] This relationship was found to be stronger for the older age group (+40 years of age) than for the younger, and for women than for men. Many other cross-sectional studies of aerobically fit individuals of all ages have found them to have more favorable psychological profiles than

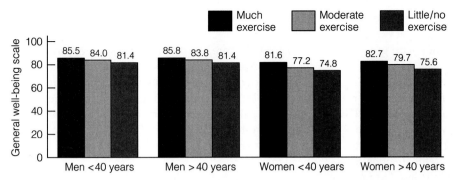

Figure 14.6   General well-being in the general population, by gender, age, and amount of exercise. With increased exercise, scores from the general well-being schedule were higher for all age and gender subgroups measured. (See Physical Fitness Activity 14.1 at the end of this chapter to see how you score.)   *Source:* Stephens T. Secular trends in adult physical activity: Exercise boom or bust? *Res Quart Exerc Sport* 58:94–105, 1987.

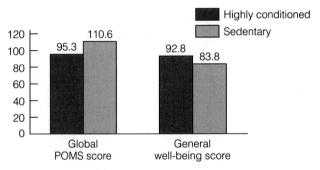

Figure 14.7   Highly conditioned versus sedentary elderly women, mood state and psychological well-being. A comparison of highly conditioned versus sedentary elderly women (mean age = 73 years) revealed superior psychological test scores among the fit subjects. A lower profile of mood states (POMS) score and a higher general well-being score are considered "superior."   *Source:* Nieman DC, Warren BJ, Dotson RG, et al. Physical activity, psychological well-being, and mood state in elderly women. *J Aging Phys Act* 1:22–33, 1993.

their sedentary counterparts.[53–55] In one study of 32 sedentary and 12 highly conditioned elderly women (mean age 73 years), the fit subjects received superior scores on the profile of mood states and the general well-being schedule (see Figure 14.7). (The highly conditioned elderly women were active an average of 1.5 hours a day, and had been exercising for an average of 11 years.[54]) A large study of 5,000 adolescents concluded that emotional well-being was positively associated with the extent of participation in sports and vigorous recreational activity.[55]

There are several problems with cross-sectional studies, however, when evaluating the effect of regular exercise on mental health. Often, the physically active subjects are different from sedentary individuals in many other lifestyle areas (e.g., diet, body weight, genetic endowment), making it difficult to measure the independent role of exercise. The

best study design starts with a group of sedentary subjects who are then randomly assigned to exercise and nonexercise groups and followed for several months to study the effects of exercise on depression, anxiety, mood state, self-concept, and so on.

CONTROLLED STUDIES ON EXERCISE AND STRESS

Randomized, controlled studies on exercise training and stress are difficult and expensive to conduct, and few have followed large enough groups of people for long enough periods of time to draw sound conclusions.[56–59] Nonetheless, as is emphasized in the rest of this chapter, growing evidence supports the survey and cross-sectional reports of superior mental health by physically active people, especially when the studies are long term. According to the 1996 surgeon general's report on physical activity and health, a major conclusion of experts in this area was that "physical activity improves mental health."[57] The report goes on to summarize that "the literature reported here supports a beneficial effect of physical activity on relieving symptoms of depression and anxiety and on improving mood."[57]

Cardiovascular Reactivity to Mental Stress

When individuals are subjected to stressful physical or psychological conditions, they experience an increase in heart rate, blood pressure, plasma catecholamine (stress hormones), and other measures of sympathetic nervous system activation.[60] Typical experiments are designed to measure these variables before and after, exposing subjects to behaviorally challenging procedures such as matching geometric shapes and colors, playing color-word games, or solving arithmetic problems with performance-dependent monetary awards. Studies have compared highly fit versus unfit subjects, or followed exercise and nonexercise groups for several weeks.[56,60–64]

Although not all researchers agree, exercise training is usually associated with a reduction in cardiovascular reactivity to mental stress. In one review of 34 studies with 1,449 subjects, aerobically fit individuals were found to have a significantly reduced stress reactivity to various stressors.[62] If experiments are conducted with careful attention to extraneous factors, exercise training usually leads to a reduction in stress reactivity to behavioral challenges.[60]

This reduction in stress reactivity is felt to be important in day-to-day coping with work and social stressors. Exercise appears to be useful in this regard because as the individual adapts to the increase in heart rate, blood pressure, stress hormones, and other biochemical measures during exercise, the body is strengthened and conditioned to react more calmly when the same responses are elicited during mental stress.

Depression, Anxiety, and Mood Elevation

National surveys have suggested that sedentary adults are at much higher risk for feeling fatigue and depression than those who are physically active.[1,65] In one study of 1,536 Germans, the odds of being depressed were more than three times higher for sedentary versus physically active adults.[66]

Since 1980, numerous reviews of the literature have concluded that exercise is associated with reduced depression, which was also the consensus of the Workshop on Exercise and Mental Health sponsored by the National Institute of Mental Health in 1984.[1,56,57,67–75] Both acute and chronic exercise have been associated with reduced depression, with the greatest improvements seen in clinically depressed subjects who exercise frequently for several months.[70] Two meta-analyses of the literature have shown that all age groups, both men and women, across persons differing in health status gain strong antidepressant effects from regular, long-term aerobic exercise.[70,74]

In general, depressed patients have been found to be physically sedentary and to experience a reduction in their depressive feelings when they initiate regular exercise. It has been proposed that exercise is as effective as group or individual psychotherapy, or meditative relaxation, in alleviating mild-to-moderate depression.[70–73] However, exercise plus psychotherapy have been shown to be better than exercise alone in reducing depression.[72]

As Table 14.1 shows, anxiety disorders, including various phobias, panic attacks, and obsessive–compulsive behavior, are the most prevalent of all mental health problems in the United States. One of the most common measures

of anxiety is the Spielberger State–Trait Anxiety Inventory (STAI).[76]

STAI scores are based on responses to a variety of questions on tension, nervousness, self-confidence, indecisiveness, security, confusion, worry, and so on. Other measures of anxiety include blood pressure, heart rate, skin responses (galvanic, palmar sweating, and skin temperature), central nervous system measures (EEG, electroencephalogram), and electromyography (e.g., muscular tension of the forehead muscles).

Researchers have studied the effects of *acute* (before and after one bout) and *chronic* (before and after several weeks of training) exercise on anxiety. One of the most frequently reported psychological benefits of acute exercise has been a reduction in state anxiety (anxiety the subject feels "right now") following vigorous exercise, an effect that may last up to several hours.[77–84]

Figure 14.8 shows the results of one study of 60 untrained college males who engaged in one of the following activities for 50 minutes: (a) resistance exercise, (b) cycling at 70% of maximum, (c) autogenic relaxation, or (d) resting quietly in a sound chamber.[82] Notice that 1 hour following these sessions, state anxiety was reduced most strongly in the cycling group. In another study, 15 adults completed 20-minute sessions of cycle ergometer exercise on separate days at intensities equal to 40%, 60%, or 70% $\dot{V}O_{2max}$.[81] State anxiety was reduced for 2 hours following all exercise sessions, demonstrating that light-to-heavy intensities are equally effective. The reduction in state anxiety is a consistent finding following aerobic, but not resistance, exercise[84] and occurs during any time of the day.[83]

Exercise training has been linked to a reduction in trait anxiety (anxiety the subject "generally feels"). The reduction in anxiety is most noticeable when exercise is regular,

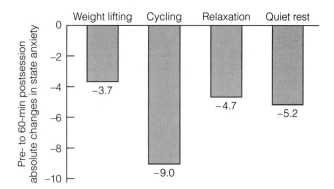

Figure 14.8 Sessions (50 minutes) of cycling, weight lifting, relaxation, and rest, comparative acute effects on state anxiety. State anxiety is decreased most strongly 1 hour following cycling. *Source:* Garvin AW, Koltyn KF, Morgan WP. Influence of acute physical activity and relaxation on state anxiety and blood lactate in untrained college males. *Int J Sports Med* 18:470–476, 1997.

sessions last longer than 30 minutes, and the training programs last several months.[56,77] Figure 14.9 summarizes the results of one study involving 35 sedentary, mildly obese women (mean age 34 years) who were randomly assigned to exercise or nonexercise groups.[85] Women in the exercise group walked briskly five times a week, 45 minutes per session, for 15 weeks, and they experienced a significant reduction in anxiety relative to the nonexercise group. This study supports the idea that moderate aerobic exercise such as brisk walking is a sufficient stimulus to reduce anxiety and tension.[86]

One meta-analysis of 104 studies of 3,048 subjects on the anxiety-reducing effects of exercise came to several conclusions, including the following:[77]

1. Training programs usually need to exceed 10 weeks before there are significant changes in trait anxiety (the anxiety one generally feels).

2. Exercise of at least 20 minutes duration seems necessary to achieve reductions in both state and trait anxiety.

3. Reductions in both state and trait anxiety occur after aerobic, but not anaerobic, exercise training programs.

Psychological mood state is often measured using the profile of mood states (POMS)[87] or the general well-being schedule (GWBS).[52] The POMS consists of 65 adjectives rated on a 5-point scale designed to assess mood during the previous week. The six scales of the POMS are tension/anxiety, depression/dejection, anger/hostility, vigor/activity, fatigue/inertia, and confusion/bewilderment. A POMS global score can be calculated, with a lower score indicating a more favorable mood state.

The GWBS consists of 18 items that generate a total score from six subscale scores that include health concern, energy level, life satisfaction, cheerfulness/depression, ten-sion/relaxation, and emotional stability. A high score on the GWBS represents an expression of positive well-being and the absence of bad feelings (see Physical Fitness Activity 14.1 at the end of this chapter for norms).

Most studies have shown that psychological mood state as measured by the POMS or GWBS is more favorable for active people and can be improved with regular exercise, especially when mood state is unfavorable prior to initiating training.[1,54,85,88–91] Figure 14.10 shows the results from the same study described in Figure 14.9.[85] In this study, 15 weeks of moderate exercise training was associated with improved GWBS total scores, with contributions made from each of the six subscales, especially higher energy levels. Figure 14.11 summarizes results from a randomized study of 91 obese women. Notice that GWBS scores improved

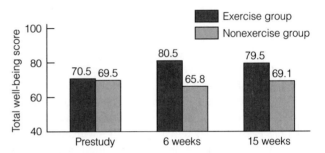

Figure 14.10 Moderate exercise training: Effect on general psychological well-being. General well-being was significantly improved for women who walked briskly for 15 weeks, relative to sedentary controls. *Source:* Cramer SR, Nieman DC, Lee JW. The effects of moderate exercise training on psychological well-being and mood state in women. *J Psychosom Res* 35:437–449, 1991.

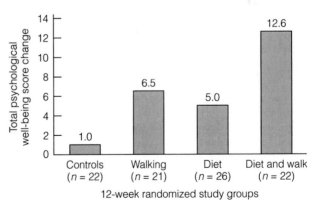

Figure 14.11 Psychological well-being response to diet and/or exercise; controls = mild calisthenics four sessions/week, walking = five 45-minute sessions/week, diet = 1,300 Calories/day. A combination of walking and weight-loss diet was most effective in improving psychological well-being in overweight women. *Source:* Nieman DC, Custer WF, Butterworth DE, Utter AC, Henson DA. Psychological response to exercise training and/or energy restriction in obese women. *J Psychosom Res* (in press).

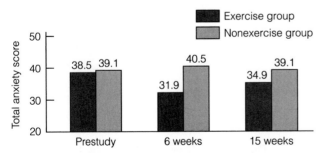

Figure 14.9 Moderate exercise training: Effect on state anxiety. Anxiety scores were significantly reduced in women who walked briskly 5 days a week, 45 minutes per session, for 15 weeks compared to a randomized, nonexercise control group. *Source:* Cramer SR, Nieman DC, Lee JW. The effects of moderate exercise training on psychological well-being and mood state in women. *J Psychosom Res* 35:437–449, 1991.

most in women who both dieted (losing about 17 pounds) and walked regularly.[90]

Self-Esteem

Self-esteem or self-concept is defined as the degree to which individuals feel positive about themselves, and it can be measured by various instruments, including the Rosenberg Self-Esteem Scale.[92] Various reviewers have identified self-esteem as the psychological variable with the greatest potential to be improved with exercise training, especially for those with initially low self-esteem.[53,56,74,93–99] A meta-analysis of the literature has shown a strong link between aerobic fitness training and self-concept in adults.[74]

In one study of young men in a juvenile detention center, 2 hours per week of running and hard basketball led to significant improvements in self-esteem and general psychological mood state.[94] The researchers concluded that vigorous aerobic exercise can provide substantial psychological help for delinquent adolescents. A meta-analysis demonstrated a positive effect for physical activity on the self-esteem of children.[99]

Weight training leads to measurable improvements in muscular strength and size, providing positive feedback that has been associated in many studies with an improvement in self-esteem. In one 12-week study of 60 women randomly assigned to weight training or brisk walking, body image improved for both groups, but more so for the weight lifters.[95] In cardiac patients, strength training has been associated with enhanced self-efficacy.[98]

Mental Cognition

Many people report that they feel "mentally alert" shortly after a bout of exercise and can study with greater attentiveness. A large number of studies have evaluated the effect of both acute and chronic exercise on cognition, using various tests involving word recall, memory searches, name retrieval, and so on.[100–111] Although much more research is needed, exercise does appear to have a positive effect on cognitive performance, especially when complex memory tasks are tested.[103,105,108,111] Results indicate that memory and intellectual function may be improved during or shortly after an exercise session, and following long-term training.[104] Several studies also suggest that exercise is effective in reversing or at least slowing certain age-related declines in cognitive performance.[100–103,107,108,111] Overall, there appears to be some possible influence of exercise on selected measures of cognitive functioning (especially in the elderly), but better-designed studies are needed to confirm this.[56,100,106]

MECHANISMS: HOW PHYSICAL ACTIVITY HELPS PSYCHOLOGICAL HEALTH

Figure 14.12 summarizes the information reviewed in the previous section. In general, most research is supportive of the Greek ideal of a "strong mind in a strong body." Explaining how and why exercise improves psychological health is a topic of active debate at present. Some of the more tenable hypotheses can be grouped as[70,112,113]

1. Cognitive-behavioral
2. Social interaction
3. Time-out/distraction
4. Cardiovascular fitness
5. Monoamine neurotransmitters
6. Endogenous opioids

Cognitive-Behavioral Hypothesis

As a sedentary individual initiates and then maintains a regular exercise program, which most perceive as a difficult

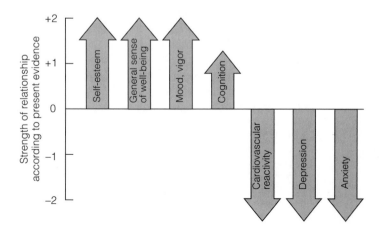

Figure 14.12 Summary of relationship between physical activity and psychological health. This figure summarizes the relationship between physical activity and psychological health, using present evidence. The strength of the relationship is represented on the vertical axis, with "2" representing strong evidence in support and "1" representing preliminary supporting evidence, with more research needed to confirm the association.

task, this accomplishment can result in an increased sense of mastery and self-confidence.[70] In other words, individuals who master something that they perceive as difficult (exercising regularly) may experience a positive change in their psychological health manifested by increased self-confidence, improved self-efficacy (an "I can do it" attitude), ability to cope with personal problems, uplifted vigor and general well-being, and lessening of anxiety and depression. On the other hand, some people may simply report feeling better following exercise because they expect such a change.[77] In the best-designed studies, however, researchers have tried to control for this by using random assignment, the use of mild calisthenic control groups, and concealing the intention of the study from the subjects.[85,112]

Social Interaction Hypothesis

Exercise is often performed with others, leading to improved opportunities for social interaction, pleasure, and personal attention. It has been hypothesized that this could account for the antidepressant and mood elevation effects of exercise. However, in one meta-analysis, exercise was shown to be a significantly better antidepressant than enjoyable group activities alone.[70] In studies that have attempted to control for social interaction, most have concluded that favorable psychological responses to aerobic training were not due to this factor.[85,86,88]

Time-Out/Distraction Hypothesis

This hypothesis maintains that being distracted from stressful stimuli, or taking "time-out" from the daily routine, is responsible for the mood elevation seen with exercise.[70,77] However, the evidence suggests that the mood elevation experienced after exercise is due to more than simply taking time out from one's daily routine. For example, exercise has been found to reduce depression and anxiety more than relaxation (time-out) or enjoyable activities (distraction).[70] Thus, regular exercise may be a more effective long-term mood elevator than habitual relaxation.

Cardiovascular Fitness Hypothesis

According to this theory, mood elevation and a reduction in anxiety and depression are directly related to the level of aerobic fitness ($\dot{V}O_{2max}$). However, several studies have reported that the psychological improvements seen with exercise take place within the first few weeks of treatment before significant increases in aerobic fitness have occurred.[70,85] Also, in some studies, depending on the psychological variable tested, improvement in anaerobic fitness

from weight training was just as effective as gains in aerobic fitness.[70,95]

There is some thinking that aerobic exercise may increase oxygen transport to the brain and elevate deep body temperature, inducing an elevation in mood state.[106] However, the research linking these changes to improved mental health is tenuous at best, and further research is needed before conclusions can be made.

Monoamine Neurotransmitter Hypothesis

Disturbances in the brain secretions of three monoamine neurotransmitters—serotonin, dopamine, and norepinephrine—have been implicated in depression and other psychological disorders.[68,113] There is some evidence that depressed individuals have decreased secretions of these neurotransmitters, and various medications are used to increase their transmission.

There are some indications from animal studies that an acute bout of exercise increases both dopamine and norepinephrine synthesis and metabolism in various parts of the brain, including the midbrain, cortex, and hypothalamus.[114,115] Various reviewers have conjectured that exercise could play a role in the treatment and prevention of depression and other mental disorders by promoting optimal neurotransmitter secretions, but this remains uncertain on the basis of available data.[70,113]

Endogenous Opioid Hypothesis

Opiates have been used for centuries to relieve pain and induce euphoria. In 1975, researchers were successful in isolating chemicals from the body that were found to have morphinelike qualities. Since then, many more endogenous opioids have been identified and can roughly be divided into three groups: endorphins, enkephalins, and dynorphins. These endogenous opioids are widely distributed throughout areas of the central nervous system and influence many important systems of the body, including the cardiovascular, respiratory, and immune systems, and metabolism of fuels.[116–122]

Of special interest has been the β-*endorphin system*, which contributes to the regulation of blood pressure, pain perception, and the control of body temperature. β-endorphin has receptors in the hypothalamus and limbic systems of the brain, areas associated with emotion and behavior.

During vigorous exercise, the pituitary increases its production of β-endorphin, leading to an increase in its concentration in the blood. As Figure 14.13 shows, β-endorphin is a late-acting hormone, rising sharply only during and immediately following intense exercise. In this study, the increase in β-endorphin did not differ significantly between athletes and nonathletes when compared on a percent

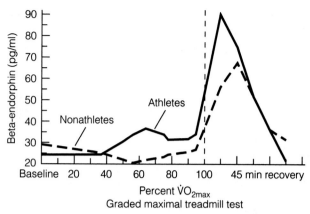

Figure 14.13 Beta-endorphin in athletes versus nonathletes. In this study, sedentary nonathletes and marathon athletes were exercised to exhaustion during a Balke treadmill, graded exercise test. The concentration of β-endorphin in the blood rose sharply during early recovery, in response to near-maximal-intensity exercise. *Source:* Author (unpublished data).

$\dot{V}O_{2max}$ basis. β-endorphin concentrations peaked during recovery at 3–3.5 times resting levels and fell to near-resting levels after 45 minutes of recovery.

Most researchers have found that β-endorphin does not increase unless the exercise intensity exceeds 75% $\dot{V}O_{2max}$ or the duration exceeds 1 hour and the exercise is performed at a steady state between lactate production and elimination.[121]

Although it is widely accepted by the exercising public that endorphins are responsible for exercise-induced euphoria, researchers disagree on the interpretation of the available data. At the center of the debate is whether blood concentrations of β-endorphin actually reflect what is happening in the brain's limbic system, where β-endorphin must activate the central nervous system to produce euphoria.

After the β-endorphin is secreted into the blood by the pituitary gland, it apparently is unable to be able to penetrate the blood–brain barrier to get into the brain. As a result, most researchers have been unable to correlate changes in blood β-endorphin concentrations with reduced tension or pain. Studies show, for example, that although subjects can tolerate more pain than normal during and for 15 minutes after intense exercise, plasma β-endorphin levels do not appear to be related.[122]

However, there is some evidence from animal studies that brain concentrations of β-endorphin increase during exercise.[120] Prolonged, submaximal exercise has been found to increase brain β-endorphin levels and to improve the pain tolerance of rats.

Other animal research suggests that prolonged rhythmic, large-muscle exercise can activate brain opioid systems by triggering certain sensory nerves that go from the muscle to the brain.[120] It is uncertain, however, whether the brain is making its own β-endorphin or whether exercise-induced changes enable β-endorphin to cross the blood–brain barrier and pass into the brain.[121]

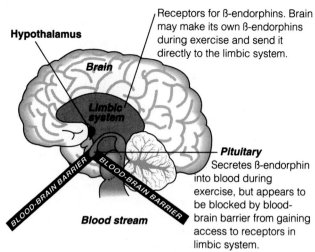

Figure 14.14 Beta-endorphin and the blood–brain barrier. Although it is true that vigorous exercise increases the concentration of β-endorphin in the blood, this complex protein molecule is unable to cross the blood–brain barrier to gain access to the receptors located in the limbic system. However, the brain may be able to make its own β-endorphin during exercise, or this hormone may project into areas of the brain through nerve fibers.

Further research is needed to resolve these issues, but there is evidence that intense exercise may activate brain opioid systems, increasing the pain threshold and improving mood state[120] (see Figure 14.14).

It is more than likely that both the physiological and the psychological mechanisms reviewed in this section play a role in explaining the improvements in psychological mood state seen after exercise.

PRECAUTIONS: EXERCISE ADDICTION, MOOD DISTURBANCE, AND SLEEP DISRUPTION

Morgan from the University of Wisconsin has described individuals with "exercise addiction."[67] They are "addicted" to exercise and have such a commitment that obligations to work, family, and interpersonal relationships, and their ability to utilize medical advice suffer. Such people are also compulsive, use exercise for an escape, are overcompetitive, live in a state of chronic fatigue, are self-centered, and are preoccupied with fitness, diet, and body image. If for any reason exercise has to be discontinued, these individuals experience withdrawal symptoms. Figure 14.15 shows that mood disturbance rises sharply within the first 48 hours of exercise deprivation in habitual exercisers.[123]

Researchers have also reported that mood disturbance can increase when training loads are increased too greatly.[124–127] When swimmers increased their daily training distance from 4,000 to 9,000 meters per day during a 10-day

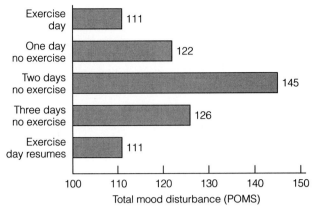

Figure 14.15 Mood disturbance during exercise deprivation in habitual exercisers. Mood disturbance rises sharply within the first 2 days of exercise deprivation in habitual exercisers. *Source:* Mondin GW, Morgan WP, Piering PN, et al. Psychological consequences of exercise deprivation in habitual exercisers. *Med Sci Sports Exerc* 28:1199–1203, 1996.

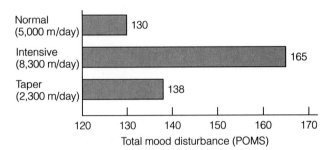

Figure 14.16 Mood disturbance in swimmers during training. Intensive training increases mood disturbance in swim athletes. *Source:* Raglin JS, Koceja DM, Stager JM, Harms CA. Mood, neuromuscular function, and performance during training in female swimmers. *Med Sci Sports Exerc* 28:372–377, 1996.

period, there were significant increases in muscle soreness, depression, anger, fatigue, and overall mood disturbance, along with a reduced general sense of well-being.[125] Figure 14.16 shows that intensive training periods are associated with mood disturbance in athletes.[126] Intense physical exercise such as a competitive marathon (26.2 miles) has been shown to disrupt both rapid eye movement (REM) sleep and total sleep time[128] (see Sports Medicine Insight).

PRACTICAL IMPLICATIONS

Although we are not sure why, the research presented in this chapter has shown that the same amount of exercise that helps the heart also helps the brain. The American College of Sports Medicine has established that three to five, 20–30 minute aerobic exercise sessions per week of moderate-intensity activities such as jogging, swimming, bicycling, or brisk walking are necessary to fully develop the cardiovas-

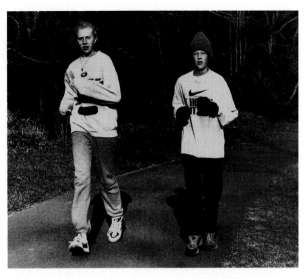

Figure 14.17 If exercise is to be effective in inducing relaxation, it should be noncompetitive, moderate in intensity, and pursued in pleasant surroundings.

cular and respiratory systems. Most of the studies quoted by the ACSM used these same exercise criteria and thus showed that as the heart is strengthened, so is the brain. Shephard of Toronto has advised that if exercise is to be effective in alleviating stress, it should be noncompetitive, moderate in intensity, and pursued in pleasant surroundings[58] (see Figure 14.17).

We can have confidence that in exercise we have a strong weapon to help counter the never-ending onslaught of stress, anxiety, and depression associated with our modern era. Exercise does help, acting as a buffer, reducing the strain of stressful events. Exercise can help to fortify the brain, alleviating anxiety and depression while elevating mood. Stress levels can be reduced by various drugs, but an appropriate program of physical activity is preferred because it has many other positive health effects.[58]

Preliminary research is also indicating that the brain may function better cognitively during exercise. Though we need more research to evaluate the effect of regular exercise on overall mental function, there is evidence that exercise does more than just make people feel better physically.

What this means for busy students and workers everywhere is that time spent in exercise may not be lost in terms of getting the job done. The half-hour exercise session may actually enhance mental functioning to the point of increasing overall time efficiency.

Therefore, the allocation of curricular time to physical education may not hamper academic achievement, as some school boards have thought. Also, exercise breaks for normally sedentary office workers may actually enhance the productivity of a business. Future research should help to resolve some of these questions.

SPORTS MEDICINE INSIGHT

Exercise and Sleep

Sleep disorders are common among humans worldwide. According to a report issued by the National Commission on Sleep Disorders Research, as many as 80 million Americans have serious, incapacitating sleep problems, 20–40% have insomnia, and nearly half of older adults say they cannot get a solid night's rest.[129,130] The vast majority of Americans fail to understand what to do about poor sleep and the consequences.[131]

Sleep loss and sleep disturbances are thought to play a major role in 200,000–400,000 automobile accidents each year, with as many as 13% of accident-related fatalities caused by falling asleep at the wheel.[130] The loss of 1 hour's sleep when most Americans "spring forward" in April to daylight saving time causes an average increase of 7–8% in traffic accidents. Conversely, the switch back to standard time in the fall causes a 7–8% decrease.

Insomnia is defined by the National Institutes of Health as "the perception or complaint of inadequate or poor-quality sleep."[132] Characteristics of insomnia include[132,133]

- Difficulty falling asleep
- Waking up frequently during the night, with difficulty returning to sleep
- Waking up too early in the morning
- Unrefreshing sleep

Advanced age, being female, marital disruption, lower socioeconomic status, and a history of depression have each been linked to insomnia.[132,133] People with chronic insomnia have a diminished ability to concentrate, memory problems, trouble in carrying out daily tasks, and difficulty in working with and getting along with other people. Poor sleep can result in fatigue, increasing the opportunity for human error and accidents. Shift workers account for 20% of the U.S. workforce, and are two to five times more likely to fall asleep on the job than day workers, while exhibiting more stress and irritability, and experiencing more heart disease and stomach/intestinal ailments.

Sleep duration is related to length of life. In one study of a million Americans, those age 45 years or older who reported sleeping more than 10 hours or fewer than 5 hours per night had higher death rates during follow-up than those sleeping about 7 hours a night.[134] Insomnia early in adult life is a risk factor for the development of clinical depression and psychiatric distress.[135]

SLEEP CYCLES

A night's sleep consists of four or five cycles, each of which progresses through several stages.[136,137] Each stage produces specific brain patterns that can be documented by an electroencephalogram (EEG), a record of the electrical impulses generated in the brain. During each night, a person alternates between non–rapid eye movement (NREM) sleep and rapid eye movement (REM) sleep. The entire cycle of NREM and REM sleep takes about 90 minutes. The average adult sleeps 7.5 hours (five full cycles), with 20% of that in REM. By age 70, total nighttime sleep decreases to about 6 hours (four sleep cycles), but the proportion of REM stays at about 20%. Sleep efficiency is reduced in the elderly, with an increased number of awakenings during the night.

In NREM sleep, brain activity, heart rate, respiration, blood pressure, and metabolism (vital signs) slow down, and body temperature falls, as a deep, restful state is reached. Sleep begins with NREM, during which brain waves gradually lengthen through four distinct stages:[136,137]

1. *Stage 1*—characterized by lighter sleep, a slowing down of brain activity and vital signs, and dream-like thoughts
2. *Stage 2*—characterized by slightly deeper sleep and slower vital signs
3. *Stages 3 and 4 (slow-wave sleep)*—characterized by deep sleep, depressed vital signs, and slow, low-frequency, high-amplitude brain activity known as delta waves

Slow-wave sleep usually terminates with the sleeper changing position. The brain waves now reverse their course as the sleeper heads for the active REM stage. The central nervous system puts on a display of physiology so intense that some have described it as a third stage of earthly existence. In REM sleep, the eyes dart about under closed eyelids, and vivid dreams transpire, which can often be remembered. The even breathing of NREM gives way to halting uncertainty, and the heart rhythm speeds or slows unaccountably. The brain is highly active during REM sleep, and overall brain metabolism may be increased above the level experienced when awake.

BETTER SLEEP

Getting a good night's sleep has proven to be a difficult goal for many people in this modern era. The Better Sleep Council has published several guidelines for better sleep. Here are eight guidelines for better sleep.[131]

1. *Keep regular hours.* According to the Better Sleep Council, sleeping late one morning and rising early the next can lead to a "home-bound version of jet lag." To keep the body's biological clock in order, a regular schedule is "the best way to ensure perfect nights."

2. *Cut down on stimulants.* Caffeine from any source (coffee, soft drinks, medications) when taken within 6–8 hours of bedtime can make it harder to sleep, diminish deep sleep, and increase nighttime awakenings.

3. *Sleep on a good bed.* One is less likely to get deep, solid, restful sleep on a bed that is too small, too soft, too hard, or too old.

4. *Don't smoke.* Nicotine is an even stronger stimulant than caffeine. Heavy smokers take longer to fall asleep, awaken more often, and spend less time in REM and deep NREM sleep.

5. *Drink only in moderation.* Alcohol late in the evening can suppress REM and deep NREM sleep and accelerate shifts between sleep stages.

6. *Set aside a worry or planning time early in the evening.* Sleep is better when anxieties, worries, and possible solutions are dealt with before bedtime.

7. *Don't go to bed stuffed or starved.* A big meal late at night forces the digestive system to work overtime, leading to tossing and turning through the night. Going to bed hungry also interferes with sleep.

8. *Exercise regularly.* According to the Better Sleep Council, "exercise enhances sleep by burning off the tensions that accumulate during the day, allowing both body and mind to unwind. While the fit seem to sleep better and deeper . . . you don't have to push to utter exhaustion. A 20- to 30-minute walk, jog, swim or bicycle ride at least three days a week . . . should be your goal. But don't wait too late in the day to exercise. In the evening, you should be concentrating on winding down rather than working up a sweat. . . . The ideal exercise time is late afternoon or early evening, when your workout can help you shift gears from daytime pressures to evening pleasures."

PHYSICAL ACTIVITY AND SLEEP

The Better Sleep Council statements on the value of exercise in improving the quality and quantity of sleep are based on relatively few well-designed studies. There is considerable debate on the value of exercise in improving sleep, due in large part to the difficulty researchers have in measuring sleep quality.[137–141]

Compared to those who avoid exercise, physically fit people claim that they fall asleep more rapidly, sleep better, and feel less tired during the day.[137,140] Scientists have confirmed that people who exercise regularly and intensely do indeed spend more time in slow-wave sleep, a measure of sleep quality, than the inactive.[142–146] In one study, researchers compared the total amount of time spent in slow-wave sleep between very fit runners (training an average of 45 miles a week) and sedentary controls.[146] The runners spent 18% more time in slow-wave sleep than the controls (see Figure 14.18). In another study, sleep quality was compared in sedentary and physically active elderly men and women.[145] The exercise group had greater sleep quality in the form of longer sleep duration, shorter time to fall asleep, and better alertness throughout the day.

Some sleep researchers feel that slow-wave sleep helps restore and revitalize people for the next day.[137–141] When people initiate and maintain vigorous exercise

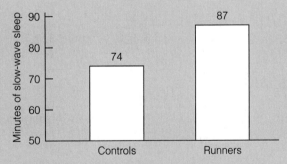

Figure 14.18 Slow-wave sleep in runners and controls. In this study of runners (45 miles/week) and sedentary controls, runners spent 18% more time in slow-wave sleep. *Source:* Trinder J, Paxton S, Montgomery I, Fraser G. Endurance as opposed to power training: Their effect on sleep. *Psychophysiol* 22: 668–673, 1985.

(continued)

Exercise and Sleep (continued)

programs, it would make sense that during sleep, they would have to increase the amount of slow-wave sleep to compensate. In other words, if there is an increase in energy expenditure through exercise, this requires more restoration time in the form of more sleep overall, especially at the deepest level.

Most studies agree with this "theory of restoration."[140,147] In one comprehensive review of the literature on the effects of exercise on sleep quality, it was concluded that individuals who exercise not only fall asleep faster, but also sleep somewhat longer and deeper than individuals who avoid exercise.[139] An exercise bout has the greatest positive impact on sleep quality for those who are elderly or of low fitness. In other words, those who need it the most gain the greatest sleep benefit from exercise.

The longer the duration of the exercise bout (e.g., beyond 1 hour), the better the sleep quality that night, except for unusually severe and prolonged exercise such as ultramarathon running races, which can actually disrupt sleep.[140,141] For example, wakefulness in runners has been reported to be increased on the night following a marathon race.[128]

There is some evidence that high-intensity exercise leading to sweating has a better effect on sleep quality than does low-intensity exercise.[137,140] However, researchers do caution that exercising and sweating close to bedtime can have an adverse effect on sleep quality for both fit and sedentary subjects. This is why the Better Sleep Council recommends avoiding heavy exercise late in the day.[131] During slow-wave sleep, the body temperature falls. If physical activities that raise body temperature and cause sweating are conducted too close to bedtime, sleep quality is disturbed because the body and brain are not able to reach the cooler temperatures needed for deep sleep. However, recent evidence challenges this assumption.[148] In aerobically fit subjects, sleep was not adversely affected by a 1-hour bout of exercise at 60% $\dot{V}O_{2max}$ or by 3 hours of exercise at 70% $\dot{V}O_{2max}$ completed 30 minutes before bedtime.

Most of the studies on exercise and sleep quality have compared fit and unfit individuals, or analyzed the effect of one exercise bout on that night's sleep. There have been very few exercise training studies to determine whether initiating and maintaining an exercise program improves sleep quality.[137–140] In one study of new army recruits, 18 weeks of basic training were found to improve sleep quality by several measures.[143] Most of the sleep quality improvements occurred within the first 9 weeks of training, when the recruits were adapting to the increased exercise.

In a study conducted at Stanford University, physically inactive older adults were assigned to exercise or nonexercise groups for 16 weeks.[149] Subjects in the exercise group engaged in low-impact aerobics and brisk walking for 30–40 minutes, 4 days per week. Exercise training led to improved sleep quality, longer sleep, and a shorter time to fall asleep. The researchers concluded that older adults who often complain of sleep problems can benefit from initiating a regular moderate-intensity endurance exercise program (see Figure 14.19).

SUMMARY

1. Nearly one out of five Americans is affected by one or more mental disorders, and 57% of U.S. adults experience at least a moderate amount of stress on a regular basis.

2. *Stress* was defined as any action or situation that places special demands on a person. Five stress management principles were reviewed.

3. Many studies have shown that being chronically anxious, depressed, or emotionally distressed is associated with deterioration of health.

4. Studies of active people show them to have a better psychological profile than inactive people. However, a strong self-selection bias may be present when comparing active people with the general population. Controlled intervention studies are preferred when looking at the relationship between physical activity and psychological health.

5. A review of national surveys has concluded that physical activity is positively associated with good mental health, defined as positive mood, general sense of well-being, and relatively infrequent symptoms of anxiety and depression.

6. A considerable amount of research has indicated that less aerobically fit people show greater cardio-

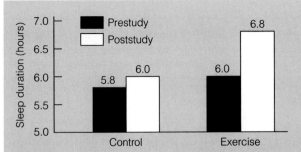

Figure 14.19 Influence of 16 weeks of exercise training on sleep duration in 43 older adults with moderate sleep complaints. Sleep duration increased in older adults exercising four times per week, 30–40 minutes per session, over a 16-week period. *Source:* King AC, Oman RF, Brassington GS, Bliwise DL, Haskell WL. Moderate-intensity exercise and self-rated quality of sleep in older adults. *JAMA* 277:32–37, 1997.

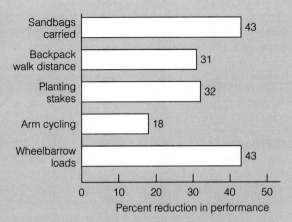

Figure 14.20 Decrease in work/exercise performance after 2 days of sleep deprivation. Sleep deprivation is associated with a decrease in work performance. *Source:* Rodgers CD, Paterson DH, Cunningham DA, et al. Sleep deprivation: Effects on work capacity, self-paced walking, contractile properties and perceived exertion. *Sleep* 18:30–38, 1995.

SLEEP LOSS AND ABILITY TO EXERCISE

It is well documented that lack of sleep negatively affects mood, vigilance, and ability to accomplish complex mental tasks. In regard to the body, most studies have shown that sleep loss of 4–60 hours does not significantly impair the ability to exercise.[150–156] However, sleep-deprived subjects still report that the exercise feels harder to accomplish than normal. In other words, following sleep loss of one or two nights, physical performance does not appear to be significantly impaired, provided that participants are sufficiently motivated.

A group of researchers from Canada studied the effects of 2 days of sleep deprivation on 33 male volunteers.[155] Although the lack of sleep had no effect on muscle strength, work performance decreased significantly (Figure 14.20). The subjects had a difficult time motivating themselves to do such things as carrying sandbags, walking briskly for 30 minutes, or carrying loads with a wheelbarrow. The researchers concluded that although sleep-deprived individuals may have the physiological capacity to do the work, the interference of mood, perception of effort, or even the repetitive nature of the tasks decreases the ability of individuals to maintain a constant level of work output.

vascular and subjective responses to psychological stressors than do those at high levels of aerobic fitness.

7. Most studies support the proposition that depression, anxiety, and mood state in general are favorably affected by regular aerobic exercise.

8. Both aerobic and nonaerobic exercise have been shown to be helpful in improving self-esteem.

9. Preliminary research suggests that short-term memory and intellectual function may be improved during or shortly after an exercise session. More research is needed to study the long-term effects.

10. β-endorphin rises in the blood during intense exercise, but not during low-intensity exercise. Most researchers have found that despite significant decreases in tension during exercise, the increase in β-endorphin is unrelated to the improvement in mood. It appears that the complex β-endorphin protein molecule is unable to cross the blood–brain barrier to gain access to the receptors located in the limbic system. Nonetheless, the brain may be activated by muscular movement to make its own β-endorphin.

11. Exercise may enhance neurotransmitter activity in the brain, increasing the concentrations of brain norepinephrine and serotonin.

12. In the Sports Medicine Insight, sleep and its relationship to exercise were reviewed.

REFERENCES

1. Stephens T. Physical activity and mental health in the United States and Canada: Evidence from four population surveys. *Prev Med* 17:35–47, 1988.

2. National Center for Health Statistics. *Healthy People 2000 Review, 1997.* Hyattsville, MD: Public Health Service, 1997.

3. The Office of Disease Prevention and Health Promotion, U.S. Public Health Service, U.S. Department of Health and Human Services. *Disease Prevention/Health Promotion: The Facts.* Palo Alto: Bull Publishing Company, 1988.

4. Barker PR, Manderscherd RW, Hendershot GE, et al. Serious mental illness and disability in the adult household population: United States, 1989. *Advance Data* 218: September 16, 1992.

5. Eaton WW. Progress in the epidemiology of anxiety disorders. *Epidemiologic Reviews* 17:32–38, 1995.

6. Ormel J, VonKorff M, Ustun B, Pini S, Korten A, Oldehinkel T. Common mental disorders and disability across cultures. *JAMA* 272:1741–1748, 1994.

7. Lebowitz BD, Pearson JL, Schneider LS, et al. Diagnosis and treatment of depression in late life: Consensus statement update. *JAMA* 278:1186–1190, 1997.

8. Blazer DG. The prevalence and distribution of major depression in a national community sample: The national comorbidity survey. *Am J Psychiatry* 151:979–986, 1994.

9. Burvill PW. Recent progress in the epidemiology of major depression. *Epidemiologic Reviews* 17:21–30, 1995.

10. Hirschfeld RMA, Keller MB, Panico S, et al. The national depressive and manic–depressive association consensus statement on the undertreatment of depression. *JAMA* 277:333–340, 1997.

11. Piani A, Schoenborn C. Health promotion and disease prevention: United States, 1990, National Center for Health Statistics. *Vital Health Stat* 10(185), 1993.

12. Prevention Magazine. *The Prevention Index.* Emmaus PA: Rodale Press, 1996.

13. Schoenborn CA, Norm J. Negative moods as correlates of smoking and heavier drinking: Implications for health promotion. *Advance Data* 236: November 4, 1993.

14. Seward BL. *Managing Stress: Principles and Strategies for Health and Wellbeing.* Boston: Jones and Bartlett Publishers, 1994.

15. Chrousos GP, Gold PW. The concepts of stress and stress system disorders: Overview of physical and behavioral homeostasis. *JAMA* 267:1244–1252, 1992.

16. Murphy LR. Stress management in work settings: A critical review of the health effects. *Am J Health Promot* 11:112–135, 1996.

17. Selye H. *The Stress of Life.* New York: McGraw-Hill Book Co., Inc., 1956.

18. Selye H. *Stress without Distress.* New York: New American Library Inc., 1974.

19. Cannon WB. *Bodily Changes in Pain, Hunger, Fear and Rage.* Boston: Charles T. Branford Co., 1953.

20. Barefoot JC, Schroll M. Symptoms of depression, acute myocardial infarction, and total mortality in a community sample. *Circulation* 93:1976–1980, 1996.

21. Pratt LA, Ford DE, Crum RM, Armenian HK, Gallo JJ, Eaton WW. Depression, psychotropic medication, and risk of myocardial infarction: Prospective data from the Baltimore ECA follow-up. *Circulation* 94:3123–3129, 1996.

22. Jonas BS, Franks P, Ingram DD. Are symptoms of anxiety and depression risk factors for hypertension? Longitudinal evidence from the National Health and Nutrition Examination Survey I epidemiologic follow-up study. *Arch Fam Med* 6:43–49, 1997.

23. Thomas CB, Greenstreet RL. Psychobiological characteristics in youth as predictors of five disease states: Suicide, mental illness, hypertension, coronary heart disease and tumor. *Johns Hopkins Med J* 132:16–43, 1973.

24. Everson SA, Kauhanen J, Kaplan GA, Goldberg DE, Julkunen J, Tuomilehto J, Salonen JT. Hostility and increased risk of mortality and acute myocardial infarction: The mediating role of behavioral risk factors. *Am J Epidemiol* 146:142–152, 1997.

25. Mittleman MA, Maclure M, Nachnani M, Sherwood JB, Muller JE. Educational attainment, anger, and the risk of triggering myocardial infarction onset. *Arch Intern Med* 157:769–775, 1997.

26. Kawachi I, Sparrow D, Spiro A, Vokonas P, Weiss ST. A prospective study of anger and coronary heart disease. *Circulation* 94:2090–2095, 1996.

27. Krantz DS, Kop WJ, Santiago HT, Gottdiener JS. Mental stress as a trigger of myocardial ischemia and infarction. *Cardiol Clin* 14:271–287, 1996.

28. Jiang W, Babyak M, Krantz DS, et al. Mental stress-induced myocardial ischemia and cardiac events. *JAMA* 275:1651–1656, 1996.

29. Barefoot JC, Larsen S, von der Lieth L, Schroll M. Hostility, incidence of acute myocardial infarction, and mortality in a sample of older Danish men and women. *Am J Epidemiol* 142:477–484, 1995.

30. Consumers Union. Does stress kill? *Consumer Reports on Health* 7(7):1–3, 1995.

31. Johnson JV, Stewart W, Hall EM, Fredlund P, Theorell T. Long-term psychosocial work environment and cardiovascular mortality among Swedish men. *Am J Public Health* 86:324–331, 1996.

32. Cohen S, Tyrrell DA, Smith AP. Psychological stress and susceptibility to the common cold. *N Engl J Med* 325:606–612, 1991.

33. Graham HMH, Douglas RM, Ryan P. Stress and acute respiratory infection. *Am J Epidemiol* 124:389–395, 1986.

34. Kiecolt-Glaser JK, Glaser R, Cacioppo JT, MacCallum RC, Snydersmith M, Kim C, Malarkey WB. Marital conflict in older adults: Endocrinological and immunological correlates. *Psychosom Med* 59:339–349, 1997.

35. Cohen S, Doyle WJ, Skoner DP, Rabin BS, Gwaltney JM. Social ties and susceptibility to the common cold. *JAMA* 277:1940–1944, 1997.

36. Schaefer C, Quesenberry CP, Wi S. Mortality following conjugal bereavement and the effects of a shared environment. *Am J Epidemiol* 141:1142–1152, 1995.

37. Martikainen P, Valkonen T. Mortality after the death of a spouse: Rates and causes of death in a large Finnish cohort. *Am J Public Health* 86:1087–1093, 1996.

38. Yasuda N, Zimmerman SI, Hawkes W, Fredman L, Hebel JR, Magaziner J. Relation of social network characteristics to 5-year mortality among young-old versus old-old white women in an urban community. *Am J Epidemiol* 145:516–523, 1997.

39. Berkman LF. The role of social relations in health promotion. *Psychosom Med* 57:245–254, 1995.

40. Ruberman W. Psychosocial influences on mortality after myocardial infarction. *N Engl J Med* 311:552–559, 1984.

41. Case RB, Moss AJ, Case N, et al. Living alone after myocardial infarction: Impact on prognosis. *JAMA* 267:515–519, 1992.

42. Wassertheil-Smoller S, Applegate WB, Berge K, et al. Change in depression as a precursor of cardiovascular events. *Arch Intern Med* 156:553–561, 1996.

43. Shekelle RB, Raynor WJ, Ostfeld AM, et al. Psychological depression and 17-year risk of death from cancer. *Psychosom Med* 43:117–1225, 1981.

44. Girard DE. Psychosocial events and subsequent illness—a review. *West J Med* 142:358–363, 1985.

45. Kaplan GA, Salonen JT, Cohen RD, et al. Social connections and mortality from all causes and from cardiovascular disease: Prospective evidence from eastern Finland. *Am J Epidemiol* 128:370–380, 1988.

46. Seeman TE, Kaplan GA, Knudsen L, et al. Social network ties and mortality among the elderly in the Alameda County study. *Am J Epidemiol* 126:714–723, 1987.

47. Orth-Gomer K, Rosengren A, Wilhelmsen L. Lack of social support and incidence of coronary heart disease in middle-aged Swedish men. *Psychosom Med* 55:3743, 1993.

48. Institute of Medicine. *The Second Fifty Years: Promoting Health and Preventing Disability.* Washington, DC: National Academy Press, 1990.

49. Stephens T. Secular trends in adult physical activity: Exercise boom or bust? *Res Quart Exerc Sport* 58:94–105, 1987.

50. Stephens T, Craig CL. *The Well-Being of Canadians: Highlights of the 1988 Campbell's Survey.* Ottawa: Canadian Fitness and Lifestyle Research Institute, 1990.

51. Johnsgard KW. Peace of mind. *Runner's World,* April 1990, 73–81.

52. Fazio AF. *A Concurrent Validation Study of the NCHS General Well-Being Schedule.* Vital and Health Statistics Series Vol. 2, No. 73. (DHEW Pub. No. [HRA] 781347, National Center of Health Statistics. Hyattsville, MD: U.S. Public Health Service.

53. Hughes JR. Psychological effects of habitual aerobic exercise: A critical review. *Prev Med* 13:66–78, 1984.

54. Nieman DC, Warren BJ, Dotson RG, et al. Physical activity, psychological well-being, and mood state in elderly women. *J Aging Phys Act* 1:22–33, 1993.

55. Steptoe A, Butler N. Sports participation and emotional well-being in adolescents. *Lancet* 347:1789–1792, 1996.

56. Biddle S. Exercise and psychosocial health. *Res Quart Exerc Sport* 66:292–297, 1995.

57. U.S. Department of Health and Human Services. *Physical Activity and Health: A Report of the Surgeon General.* Atlanta, GA: U.S. Department of Health and Human Services, Centers for Disease Control and Prevention, National Center for Chronic Disease Prevention and Health Promotion, 1996.

58. Shephard RJ. Exercise and relaxation in health promotion. *Sports Med* 23:211–217, 1997.

59. Glenister D. Exercise and mental health: A review. *J R Soc Health* 116:7–13, 1996.

60. Claytor RP. Stress reactivity: Hemodynamic adjustments in trained and untrained humans. *Med Sci Sports Exerc* 23:873–881, 1991.

61. Holmes DS, McGilley BM. Influence of a brief aerobic training program on heart rate and subjective response to a psychologic stressor. *Psychosom Med* 49:366–374, 1987.

62. Crews DJ, Landers DM. A meta-analytic review of aerobic fitness and reactivity to psychosocial stressors. *Med Sci Sports Exerc* 19:S114–S120, 1987.

63. Sinyor D, Seraganian P. Aerobic fitness level and reactivity to psychosocial stress: Physiological, biochemical, and subjective measures. *Psychosom Med* 45:205–216, 1983.

64. Siconolfi SF. Exercise training attenuated the blood pressure response to mental stress. *Med Sci Sports Exerc* 17:281, 1985.

65. Chen MK. The epidemiology of self-perceived fatigue among adults. *Prev Med* 15:74–81, 1986.

66. Weyerer S. Physical inactivity and depression in the community: Evidence from the upper Bavarian field study. *Int J Sports Med* 13:492–496, 1992.

67. Morgan WP. Affective beneficence of vigorous physical activity. *Med Sci Sports Exerc* 17:94–100, 1985.

68. Dunn AL, Dishman RK. Exercise and the neurobiology of depression. *Exerc Sport Sci Rev* 19:41–98, 1991.

69. O'Connor PJ, Aenchbacher LE, Dishman RK. Physical activity and depression in the elderly. *J Aging Phys Act* 1:34–58, 1993.

70. North TC, McCullagh P, Tran ZV. Effect of exercise on depression. *Exerc Sport Sci Review* 18:379–415, 1990.

71. Martinsen EW. Benefits of exercise for the treatment of depression. *Sports Med* 9:380–389, 1990.

72. Martinsen EW. Exercise and mental health in clinical populations. In Biddle SJH (ed), *European Perspectives on Exercise and Sport Psychology.* Champaign, IL: Human Kinetics, 1995.

73. Martinsen EW, Stephens T. Exercise and mental health in clinical and free-living populations. In Dishman RK (ed), *Advances in Exercise Adherence.* Champaign, IL: Human Kinetics, 1994.

74. McDonald DG, Hodgdon JA. *Psychological Effects of Aerobic Fitness Training.* New York: Springer-Verlag, 1991.

75. Morgan WP. Physical activity, fitness, and depression. In Bouchard C, Shephard RJ, Stephens T (eds), *Physical Activity, Fitness, and Health.* Champaign, IL: Human Kinetics, 1994.

76. Spielberger CD, Gorsuch RL, Lushene RE. *Manual for the State–Trait Anxiety Inventory.* Palo Alto, CA: Consulting Psychology Press, 1970.

77. Petruzzello SJ, Landers DM, Hatfield BD, Kubitz RA, Salazar W. A meta-analysis on the anxiety-reducing effects of acute and chronic exercise: Outcomes and mechanisms. *Sports Med* 11:143–182, 1991.

78. Raglin JS, Turner PE, Eksten F. State anxiety and blood pressure following 30 minutes of leg ergometry or weight training. *Med Sci Sports Exerc* 25:1044–1048, 1993.

79. O'Connor PJ, Carda RD, Graf BK. Anxiety and intense running exercise in the presence and absence of interpersonal competition. *Int J Sports Med* 12:423–426, 1991.

80. O'Connor PJ, Bryant CX, Veltri JP, Gebhardt SM. State anxiety and ambulatory blood pressure following resistance exercise in females. *Med Sci Sports Exerc* 25:516–521, 1993.

81. Raglin JS, Wilson M. State anxiety following 20 minutes of bicycle ergometer exercise at selected intensities. *Int J Sports Med* 17:467–471, 1996.

82. Garvin AW, Koltyn KF, Morgan WP. Influence of acute physical activity and relaxation on state anxiety and blood lactate in untrained college males. *Int J Sports Med* 18:470–476, 1997.

83. Trine MR, Morgan WP. Influence of time of day on the anxiolytic effects of exercise. *Int J Sports Med* 18:161–168, 1997.

84. Koltyn KF, Raglin JS, O'Connor PJ, Morgan WP. Influence of weight training on state anxiety, body awareness and blood pressure. *Int J Sports Med* 16:266–269, 1995.

85. Cramer SR, Nieman DC, Lee JW. The effects of moderate exercise training on psychological well-being and mood state in women. *J Psychosom Res* 35:437–449, 1991.

86. Moses J, Steptoe A, Mathews A, Edwards S. The effects of exercise training on mental well-being in the normal population: A controlled trial. *J Psychosom Res* 33:47–61, 1989.

87. McNair DM, Lorr M, Droppleman LF. *EDITS Manual: Profile of Mood States.* San Diego: Educational and Industrial Testing Service, 1981.

88. Steptoe A, Edwards S, Moses J, Mathews A. The effects of exercise training on mood and perceiving coping ability in anxious adults from the general population. *J Psychosom Res* 33:537–547, 1989.

89. Simons CW, Birkimer JC. An exploration of factors predicting the effects of aerobic conditioning on mood state. *J Psychosom Res* 32:63–75, 1988.

90. Nieman DC, Custer WF, Butterworth DE, Utter AC, Henson DA. Psychological response to exercise training and/or energy restriction in obese women. *J Psychosom Res* (in press).

91. McAuley E, Rudolph D. Physical activity, aging, and psychological well-being. *J Aging Phys Act* 3:67–96, 1995.

92. Wylie RC. *The Self-concept: A Review of Methodological Considerations and Measuring Instruments.* Lincoln: University of Nebraska Press, 1977.

93. Sonstroem RJ. Exercise and self-esteem. *Exerc Sport Sci Rev* 12: 123–155, 1984.

94. MacMahon J, Gross RT. Physical and psychological effects of aerobic exercise in delinquent adolescent males. *Am J Dis Child* 142:1361–1366, 1988.

95. Tucker LA, Mortell R. Comparison of the effects of walking and weight training programs on body image in middle-aged women: An experimental study. *Am J Health Promot* 8(1): 34–42, 1993.

96. DeGeus EJC, Van Doornen LIP, Orlebeke IF. Regular exercise and aerobic fitness in relation to psychological make-up and physiological stress reactivity. *Psychosom Med* 55:347–363, 1991.

97. McAuley E. Physical activity and psychosocial outcomes. In Bouchard C, Shephard RJ, Stephens T (eds), *Physical Activity, Fitness, and Health.* Champaign, IL: Human Kinetics, 1994.

98. Beniamini Y, Rubenstein JJ, Zaichkowsky LD, Crim MC. Effects of high-intensity strength training on quality-of-life parameters in cardiac rehabilitation patients. *Am J Cardiol* 80: 841–846, 1997.

99. Gruber JJ. Physical activity and self-esteem development in children: A meta-analysis. In Stull G, Eckert H (eds), *Effects of Physical Activity on Children: The Academy Papers No. 19.* Champaign, IL: Human Kinetics, 1986.

100. Dustman RE, Emmerson R, Shearer D. Physical activity, age, and cognitive-neuropsychological function. *J Aging Phys Act* 2:143–181, 1994.

101. Williams P, Lord SR. Effects of group exercise on cognitive functioning and mood in older women. *Aust N Z J Public Health* 21:45–52, 1997.

102. Hassmen P, Koivula N. Mood, physical working capacity and cognitive performance in the elderly as related to physical activity. *Aging* (Milano) 9(1–2):136–142, 1997.

103. Chodzko-Zajko WJ, Moore KA. Physical fitness and cognitive functioning in aging. *Exerc Sport Sci Rev* 22:195–220, 1994.

104. Hogervorst E, Riedel W, Jeukendrup A, Jolles J. Cognitive performance after strenuous physical exercise. *Percept Mot Skills* 83:479–488, 1996.

105. Tomporowski PD, Eillis NR. Effects of exercise on cognitive processes: A review. *Psychol But* 99:338–346, 1986.

106. Etnier JL, Landers DM. Brain function and exercise: Current perspectives. *Sports Med* 19:81–85, 1995.

107. Rogers RL, Meyer IS, Mortel KF. After reaching retirement age, physical activity sustains cerebral perfusion and cognition. *J Am Geriat Soc* 38:123–128, 1991.

108. Chodzko-Zajko WJ. Physical fitness, cognitive performance, and aging. *Med Sci Sports Exerc* 23:868–872, 1991.

109. Blomquist K, Danner F. Effects of physical conditioning on information-processing efficiency. *Percept Motor Skills* 65: 175–186, 1987.

110. Blumenthal JA, Madden DJ. Effects of aerobic exercise training, age, and physical fitness on memory-search performance. *Psyc Aging* 3(3):280–285, 1988.

111. Van Boxtel MPJ, Paas FGW, Houx PJ, Adam JJ, Teeken JC, Jolles J. Aerobic capacity and cognitive performance in a cross-sectional aging study. *Med Sci Sports Exerc* 29:1357–1365, 1997.

112. Yeung RR. The acute effects of exercise on mood state. *J Psychosom Res* 40:123–141, 1996.

113. Forge RL. Exercise-associated mood alterations: A review of interactive neurobiologic mechanisms. *Med Exerc Nutr Health* 4:17–32, 1995.

114. Mazzeo RS. Catecholamine responses to acute and chronic exercise. *Med Sci Sports Exerc* 23:839–845, 1991.

115. Dishman RK. Brain monoamines, exercise, and behavioral stress: Animal models. *Med Sci Sports Exerc* 29:63–74, 1997.

116. Goldfarb AH, Jamurtas AZ. Beta-endorphin response to exercise. An update. *Sports Med* 24:8–16, 1997.

117. Sforzo GA, Seeger TF, Pert CB, Pert A, Dotson CO. In vivo opioid receptor occupation in the rat brain following exercise. *Med Sci Sports Exerc* 18:380–384, 1986.

118. Goldfarb AH, Hatfield BD, Sforzo GA, et al. Serum beta-endorphin levels during a graded exercise test to exhaustion. *Med Sci Sports Exerc* 19:78–82, 1987.

119. Farrell PA, Gustafson AB, Morgan WP, et al. Enkephalins, catecholamines, and psychological mood alterations: Effects of prolonged exercise. *Med Sci Sports Exerc* 19:347–353, 1987.

120. Thoren P, Floras IS, Hoffmann P, Seals DR. Endorphins and exercise: Physiological mechanisms and clinical implications. *Med Sci Sports Exerc* 22:417–428, 1990.

121. Schwarz L, Kindermann W. Changes in beta-endorphin levels in response to aerobic and anaerobic exercise. *Sports Med* 13: 25–36, 1992.

122. Droste C, Greenlee MW, Schreck M, Roskamm H. Experimental pain thresholds and plasma beta-endorphin levels during exercise. *Med Sci Sports Exerc* 23:334–342, 1991.

123. Mondin GW, Morgan WP, Piering PN, et al. Psychological consequences of exercise deprivation in habitual exercisers. *Med Sci Sports Exerc* 28:1199–1203, 1996.

124. O'Connor PJ, Morgan WP, Raglin JS. Psychobiologic effects of 3d of increased training in female and male swimmers. *Med Sci Sports Exerc* 23:1055–1061, 1991.

125. Morgan WP, Costill DL, Flynn MG, Raglin JS, O'Connor PJ. Mood disturbance following increased training in swimmers. *Med Sci Sports Exerc* 20:408–414, 1988.

126. Raglin JS, Koceja DM, Stager JM, Harms CA. Mood, neuromuscular function, and performance during training in female swimmers. *Med Sci Sports Exerc* 28:372–377, 1996.

127. Berglund B, Safstrom H. Psychological monitoring and modulation of training load of world-class canoeists. *Med Sci Sports Exerc* 26:1036–1040, 1994.

128. Montgomery I, Trinder J, Paxton S, Fraser G. Sleep disruption following a marathon. *J Sports Med* 25:69–74, 1985.

129. National Center on Sleep Disorders Research and Office of Prevention, Education, and Control, National Heart, Lung, and Blood Institute, National Institutes of Health. *Strategy Development Workshop on Sleep Education.* Bethesda, MD: National Institutes of Health, 1994.

130. Dement WC, Mitler MM. It's time to wake up to the importance of sleep disorders. *JAMA* 269:1548–1550, 1993.

131. Better Sleep Council. *The Sleep Better, Live Better Guide.* Washington, DC: Better Sleep Council, 1990.

132. NHLBI Information Center. *Insomnia,* NIH Publication No. 95-3801. Bethesda, MD: 1995.

133. Kupfer DJ, Reynolds CF. Management of insomnia. *N Engl J Med* 336:341–345, 1997.

134. Hammond EC. Some preliminary findings on physical complaints from a prospective study of 1,064,000 men and women. *Am J Public Health* 54:11–23, 1964.

135. Chang PP, Ford DE, Mead LA, Cooper-Patrick L, Klag MJ. Insomnia in young men and subsequent depression: The Johns Hopkins precursors study. *Am J Epidemiol* 146:105–114, 1997.

136. Long ME. What is this thing called sleep? *National Geographic,* December 1987, 787–821.

137. O'Connor PJ, Youngstedt SD. Influence of exercise on human sleep. *Exerc Sport Sci Rev* 23:105–134, 1995.

138. Driver HS, Taylor SR. Sleep disturbances and exercise. *Sports Med* 21:1–6, 1996.

139. Kubitz KA, Landers DM, Petruzzello SJ, Han M. The effects of acute and chronic exercise on sleep: A meta-analytic review. *Sports Med* 21:277–291, 1996.

140. Youngstedt SD. Does exercise truly enhance sleep? *Physician Sportsmed* 25(10):72–82, 1997.

141. Youngstedt SD, O'Connor PJ, Dishman RK. The effects of acute exercise on sleep: A quantitative synthesis. *Sleep* 20:203–214, 1997.

142. Montgomery I, Trinder J, Paxton SJ. Energy expenditure and total sleep time: Effect of physical exercise. *Sleep* 5:159–168, 1982.

143. Shapiro CM, Warren PM, Trinder J, et al. Fitness facilitates sleep. *Eur J Appl Physiol* 53:1–4, 1984.

144. Edinger ID, Morey MC, Sullivan RJ, et al. Aerobic fitness, acute exercise, and sleep in older men. *Sleep* 16:351–359, 1993.

145. Brassington GS, Hicks RA. Aerobic exercise and self-reported sleep quality in elderly individuals. *J Aging Phys Act* 3:120–134, 1995.

146. Trinder J, Paxton S, Montgomery I, Fraser G. Endurance as opposed to power training: Their effect on sleep. *Psychophysiol* 22:668–673, 1985.

147. Taylor SR, Rogers GG, Driver HS. Effects of training volume on sleep, psychological, and selected physiological profiles of elite female swimmers. *Med Sci Sports Exerc* 29:688–693, 1997.

148. Youngstedt SD, Kripke DF. Late night exercise does not disrupt sleep in physically active individuals. *Sleep Res* 26:222, 1997.

149. King AC, Oman RF, Brassington GS, Bliwise DL, Haskell WL. Moderate-intensity exercise and self-rated quality of sleep in older adults. *JAMA* 277:32–37, 1997.

150. Pilcher JJ, Huffcutt AI. Effects of sleep deprivation on performance: A meta-analysis. *Sleep* 19:318–326, 1996.

151. VanHelder T, Radomski MW. Sleep deprivation and the effect on exercise performance. *Sports Med* 7:235–247, 1989.

152. Mougin F, Simon-Rigaud ML, Davenne D, et al. Effects on sleep disturbances on subsequent physical performance. *Eur J Appl Physiol* 63:77–82, 1991.

153. Chen HI. Effects of 30-h sleep loss on cardiorespiratory functions at rest and in exercise. *Med Sci Sports Exerc* 23:193–198, 1991.

154. Mougin F, Bourdin H, Simon-Rigaud ML, Didier JM, Toubin G, Kantelip JP. Effects of a selective sleep deprivation on subsequent anaerobic performance. *Int J Sports Med* 17:115–119, 1996.

155. Rodgers CD, Paterson DH, Cunningham DA, et al. Sleep deprivation: Effects on work capacity, self-paced walking, contractile properties and perceived exertion. *Sleep* 18:30–38, 1995.

156. Symons JD, VanHelder T, Myles WS. Physical performance and physiological responses following 60 hours of sleep deprivation. *Med Sci Sports Exerc* 20:374–380, 1988.

PHYSICAL FITNESS ACTIVITY 14.1

The General Well-Being Schedule

As described earlier in this chapter, one measure of psychological status that has been used with good success in national surveys is the general well-being schedule (GWBS). The GWBS was designed by the National Center for Health Statistics and consists of 18 items in six subscales covering such constructs as energy level, satisfaction, freedom from worry, and self-control. A high score on the GWBS represents an absence of bad feelings and an expression of positive feelings. Results from national surveys have shown that higher scores for the GWBS are significantly associated with increased amounts of physical activity for all age groups and for both men and women. (See Stephens T. Physical activity and mental health in the United States and Canada: Evidence from four population surveys. *Prev Med* 17:35–47, 1988.)

In this physical fitness activity, the 18 questions of the GWBS are listed, with an interpretation of results.

The General Well-Being Schedule

Instructions: The following questions ask how you feel and how things have been going for you *during the past month.* For each question, mark an "x" for the answer that most nearly applies to you. Since there are no right or wrong answers, it's best to answer each question quickly without pausing too long on any one of them.

1. How have you been feeling in general?
   - 5 ❑ In excellent spirits
   - 4 ❑ In very good spirits
   - 3 ❑ In good spirits mostly
   - 2 ❑ I've been up and down in spirits a lot
   - 1 ❑ In low spirits mostly
   - 0 ❑ In very low spirits

2. Have you been bothered by nervousness or your "nerves"?
   - 0 ❑ Extremely so—to the point where I could not work or take care of things
   - 1 ❑ Very much so
   - 2 ❑ Quite a bit
   - 3 ❑ Some—enough to bother me
   - 4 ❑ A little
   - 5 ❑ Not at all

3. Have you been in firm control of your behavior, thoughts, emotions or feelings?
   - 5 ❑ Yes, definitely so
   - 4 ❑ Yes, for the most part
   - 3 ❑ Generally so
   - 2 ❑ Not too well
   - 1 ❑ No, and I am somewhat disturbed
   - 0 ❑ No, and I am very disturbed

4. Have you felt so sad, discouraged, hopeless, or had so many problems that you wondered if anything was worthwhile?

    0 ❑ Extremely so—to the point I have just about given up

    1 ❑ Very much so

    2 ❑ Quite a bit

    3 ❑ Some—enough to bother me

    4 ❑ A little bit

    5 ❑ Not at all

5. Have you been under or felt you were under any strain, stress, or pressure?

    0 ❑ Yes—almost more than I could bear

    1 ❑ Yes—quite a bit of pressure

    2 ❑ Yes—some, more than usual

    3 ❑ Yes—some, but about usual

    4 ❑ Yes—a little

    5 ❑ Not at all

6. How happy, satisfied, or pleased have you been with your personal life?

    5 ❑ Extremely happy—couldn't have been more satisfied or pleased

    4 ❑ Very happy

    3 ❑ Fairly happy

    2 ❑ Satisfied—pleased

    1 ❑ Somewhat dissatisfied

    0 ❑ Very dissatisfied

7. Have you had reason to wonder if you were losing your mind, or losing control over the way you act, talk, think, feel, or of your memory?

    5 ❑ Not at all

    4 ❑ Only a little

    3 ❑ Some, but not enough to be concerned

    2 ❑ Some, and I've been a little concerned

    1 ❑ Some, and I am quite concerned

    0 ❑ Much, and I'm very concerned

8. Have you been anxious, worried, or upset?

    0 ❑ Extremely so—to the point of being sick, or almost sick

    1 ❑ Very much so

    2 ❑ Quite a bit

    3 ❑ Some—enough to bother me

    4 ❑ A little bit

    5 ❑ Not at all

9. Have you been waking up fresh and rested?

    5 ❑ Every day

    4 ❑ Most every day

    3 ❑ Fairly often

    2 ❑ Less than half the time

    1 ❑ Rarely

    0 ❑ None of the time

10. Have you been bothered by any illness, bodily disorder, pain, or fears about your health?

    0 ❏ All the time

    1 ❏ Most of the time

    2 ❏ A good bit of the time

    3 ❏ Some of the time

    4 ❏ A little of the time

    5 ❏ None of the time

11. Has your daily life been full of things that are interesting to you?

    5 ❏ All the time

    4 ❏ Most of the time

    3 ❏ A good bit of the time

    2 ❏ Some of the time

    1 ❏ A little of the time

    0 ❏ None of the time

12. Have you felt downhearted and blue?

    0 ❏ All of the time

    1 ❏ Most of the time

    2 ❏ A good bit of the time

    3 ❏ Some of the time

    4 ❏ A little of the time

    5 ❏ None of the time

13. Have you been feeling emotionally stable and sure of yourself?

    5 ❏ All of the time

    4 ❏ Most of the time

    3 ❏ A good bit of the time

    2 ❏ Some of the time

    1 ❏ A little of the time

    0 ❏ None of the time

14. Have you felt tired, worn out, used-up, or exhausted?

    0 ❏ All of the time

    1 ❏ Most of the time

    2 ❏ A good bit of the time

    3 ❏ Some of the time

    4 ❏ A little of the time

    5 ❏ None of the time

Note: For each of the following four scales, the words at each end describe opposite feelings. Circle any number along the bar that seems closest to how you have felt generally *during the past month.*

15. How concerned or worried about your health have you been?

Not concerned at all	10	8	6	4	2	0	**Very concerned**

16. How relaxed or tense have you been?

Very relaxed	10	8	6	4	2	0	**Very tense**

17. How much energy, pep, and vitality have you felt?

No energy at all, listless	0	2	4	6	8	10	**Very energetic, dynamic**

18. How depressed or cheerful have you been?

Very depressed	0	2	4	6	8	10	**Very cheerful**

Directions: Add up all the points from the boxes you have checked for each question. Compare your total score with the norms listed in the following table.

National Norms for the General Well-Being Schedule

Stress State	Total Stress Score	% Distribution U.S. Population
Positive well-being	81–110	55%
Low positive	76–80	10%
Marginal	71–75	9%
Indicates stress problem	56–70	16%
Indicates distress	41–55	7%
Serious	26–40	2%
Severe	0–25	<1%

Notes: Figure 14.6 gives the scores for the U.S. population by age, gender, and amount of exercise. Notice that all subgroups reporting "much exercise" fell within the "positive well-being" range of 81–110.

Software for analyzing the General Well-Being Schedule is available from: Wellsource, 15431 S.E. 82nd Dr., Suite F, Clackamas, OR 97015.

PHYSICAL FITNESS ACTIVITY 14.2

Life Hassles and Stress

Survey of Recent Life Experiences

Following is a list of experiences that many people have at some time or other. Please indicate for each experience how much it has been a part of your life *over the past month.*

Intensity of Experience over Past Month

1 = not at all part of my life
2 = only slightly part of my life
3 = distinctly part of my life
4 = very much part of my life

_____ 1. Disliking your daily activities

_____ 2. Lack of privacy

_____ 3. Disliking your work

_____ 4. Ethnic or racial conflict

_____ 5. Conflicts with in-laws or boyfriend's / girlfriend's family

_____ 6. Being let down or disappointed by friends

_____ 7. Conflict with supervisor(s) at work

_____ 8. Social rejection

_____ 9. Too many things to do at once

_____ 10. Being taken for granted

_____ 11. Financial conflicts with family members

_____ 12. Having your trust betrayed by a friend

_____ 13. Separation from people you care about

_____ 14. Having your contributions overlooked

_____ 15. Struggling to meet your own standards of performance and accomplishment

_____ 16. Being taken advantage of

_____ 17. Not enough leisure time

_____ 18. Financial conflicts with friends or fellow workers

_____ 19. Struggling to meet other people's standards of performance and accomplishment

_____ 20. Having your actions misunderstood by others

_____ 21. Cash-flow difficulties

_____ 22. A lot of responsibilities

_____ 23. Dissatisfaction with work

_____ 24. Decisions about intimate relationship(s)

_____ 25. Not enough time to meet your obligations

_____ 26. Dissatisfaction with your mathematical ability

_____ 27. Financial burdens

_____ 28. Lower evaluation of your work than you think you deserve

_____ 29. Experiencing high levels of noise

_____ 30. Adjustments to living with unrelated person(s) (e.g., roommate)

_____ 31. Lower evaluation of your work than you hoped for

_____ 32. Conflicts with family member(s)

_____ 33. Finding your work too demanding

_____ 34. Conflicts with friend(s)

_____ 35. Hard effort to get ahead

_____ 36. Trying to secure loan(s)

_____ 37. Getting "ripped off" or cheated in the purchase of goods

_____ 38. Dissatisfaction with your ability at written expression

_____ 39. Unwanted interruptions of your work

_____ 40. Social isolation

_____ 41. Being ignored

_____ 42. Dissatisfaction with your physical appearance

_____ 43. Unsatisfactory housing conditions

_____ 44. Finding work uninteresting

_____ 45. Failing to get money you expected

_____ 46. Gossip about someone you care about

_____ 47. Dissatisfaction with your physical fitness

_____ 48. Gossip about yourself

_____ 49. Difficulty dealing with modern technology (e.g., computers)

_____ 50. Car problems

_____ 51. Hard work to look after and maintain home

Norms

Add up your points, and compare with the following "life hassle and stress score" norms.

Total "Life Hassle and Stress Score"

Very high stress .... ≥136
High stress 116–135
Average stress 76–115
Low stress 56–75
Very low stress 51–55

Source: Used with permission from Kohn PM, Macdonald JE. The survey of recent life experiences: A decontaminated hassles scale for adults. _J Beh Med_ 15:221–236, 1992.

PHYSICAL FITNESS ACTIVITY 14.3

Depression

The National Institute of Mental Health has estimated that 17.6 million Americans suffer from depression. Only a minority of cases are diagnosed and treated, in part because many of the usual symptoms—feelings of hopelessness, despair, lethargy, self-loathing—tend to discourage the depressed individual from reaching out for help. The majority of cases of depression can be successfully treated, usually with medication, psychotherapy, or both. Nonetheless, the condition must first be identified. The Center for Epidemiologic Studies (CES) has developed a tool for measuring depression, known as the CES-D Scale. Take this test to see how you are feeling.

During the past week	< 1 day	1–2 days	3–4 days	5–7 days
I was bothered by things that don't usually bother me	0	1	2	3
I did not feel like eating; my appetite was poor	0	1	2	3
I felt that I could not shake off the blues even with the help of my family or friends	0	1	2	3
I felt that I was just as good as other people	3	2	1	0
I had trouble keeping my mind on what I was doing	0	1	2	3
I felt depressed	0	1	2	3
I felt everything I did was an effort	0	1	2	3
I felt hopeful about the future	3	2	1	0
I thought my life had been a failure	0	1	2	3
I felt fearful	0	1	2	3
My sleep was restless	0	1	2	3
I was happy	3	2	1	0
I talked less than usual	0	1	2	3
I felt lonely	0	1	2	3
People were unfriendly	0	1	2	3
I enjoyed life	3	2	1	0
I had crying spells	0	1	2	3
I felt sad	0	1	2	3
I felt that people disliked me	0	1	2	3
I could not get "going"	0	1	2	3

Scoring: A score of 22 or higher indicates possible depression. In general, the higher the score, the greater the mood disturbance—even below that threshold.

Source: Radloff LS. The CES-D Scale: A self-report depression scale for research in the general population. *Appl Psychol Meas* 1:385–401, 1977.

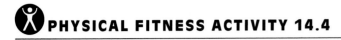 **PHYSICAL FITNESS ACTIVITY 14.4**

Controlling Stressors

Stressors are everywhere. They cannot all be avoided, but much can be done to reduce, modify, or eliminate them in a way that will allow you to accomplish your goals. Follow these three steps:

Step 1   List top five major life goals, in order of importance.
Step 2   List stressors associated with each goal.
Step 3   Summarize plans to modify or eliminate stressors so that goals can be achieved.

Step 1   Top five goals   **Step 2**   Major stressors associated with goal

Goal 1

Goal 2

Goal 3

Goal 4

Goal 5

Step 3   Summarize plans to modify or eliminate stressors so that goals can be achieved.

1. _____

2. _____

3. _____

4. _____

5. _____

6. _____

7. _____

8. _____

9. _____

10. _____

CHAPTER
15

Aging, Osteoporosis, and Arthritis

All parts of the body which have a function, if used in moderation and exercised in labors in which each is accustomed, become thereby healthy, well-developed and age more slowly, but if unused and left idle they become liable to disease, defective in growth, and age quickly.

—Hippocrates

How old would you be if you didn't know how old you were?

—Satchel Paige

The United States has long thought of itself as a nation of youth, and at least in the mind of Ponce deLeon, the "fountain of youth." Americans idolize youth, yearn for it, and spare no expense to regain it (or at least look the part). Yet scientists now regard this nation as an "aging society." In colonial times, for instance, the average age of the population was 16 years. Today it is 33 years, and it will be 42 years in 2030.[1]

The fastest-growing minority in the United States today is the *elderly*—those who reach or pass the age of 65[2] (see Figure 15.1). Figure 15.2 shows that there are now nearly 36 million elderly people in the United States, a figure that will climb to 70 million, or 22% of the population, by the year 2030. The 65 and over group is growing twice as fast as the rest of the population. Most of this growth is due to the fact that the baby-boom generation (people born be-

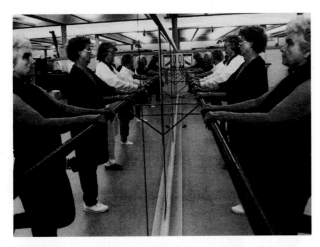

Figure 15.1   The ranks of the elderly are multiplying faster than any other segment of our society.

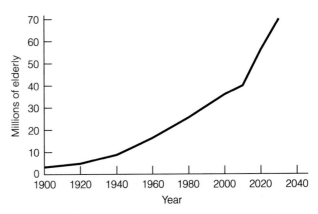

Figure 15.2   Number of elderly, 1900–2030. About 13% of Americans—or one in seven— is now 65 years of age or older. By the year 2030, one in five Americans will be elderly. *Source:* Geographic profile of the aged. *Stat Bull* 74(1):2–9, 1993.

tween 1945 and 1965), which constitutes one third of the U.S. population, is advancing inevitably toward old age.[2] Consider these statistics:[1–6]

- It is difficult to comprehend that in 1900, only 40% of American individuals lived beyond age 65, while in 1995, approximately 80% survived age 65, and 50% lived to be age 79 (see Figure 15.3). Since the mid-1980s, intense interest has been focused on the 85-and-older population (termed the "very old"). This is projected to be the fastest-growing population segment over the next several decades, swelling from 3.1 million in 1990 to approximately 17.7 million by the year 2050.

- Length of life has increased remarkably during the twentieth century (see Figure 15.4). *Life expectancy* at birth (the number of years a newborn baby can expect to live) is now 76 years on average and is

expected to exceed 82 years by the year 2050. Increases in life expectancy at birth during the first half of the twentieth century occurred mainly because of reductions in infant and childhood mortality and control of infectious disease. These reductions meant that more Americans survived to middle age. By contrast, increases in longevity in recent years have largely resulted from decreasing mortality from chronic diseases (primarily heart disease and stroke) among the middle-aged (45–64) and elderly (65–84) populations.

- Life expectancy at age 65 has increased dramatically since mid-century. From 1900 to 1960, life expectancy at age 65 improved only 2.4 years, as compared with 3.1 years from 1960 to 1995. People who are 65 years of age can now expect to live an extra 17–18 years (see Figure 15.5).

Although these trends are generally welcome, public health officials have expressed concern about several issues.[7–10]

- The central issue raised by increasing longevity is that of net gain in active functional years versus total years of disability and dysfunction.[1] As depicted in Figure 15.6, the National Center for Health Statistics estimates that 15% of the average American's life is spent in an "unhealthy" state (impaired by disabilities, injuries, and / or disease).[5] Among the elderly, 5 of their remaining 17 or 18 years, on average, will be unhealthy ones. As summarized in Figure 15.7, the prevalence of risk factors and disease is high among the elderly.[5–8] Nearly nine in ten elderly individuals have one or more chronic health conditions.[7,8]

- Cardiovascular diseases (diseases of the heart and stroke combined) and cancers account for about two thirds of all deaths among the elderly. While the good news is that death rates for heart disease and

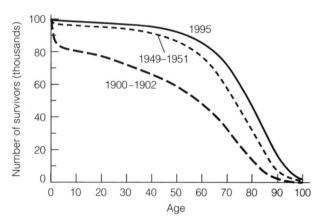

Figure 15.3 Number of survivors from birth to successive ages, total population, United States, 1900–1902, 1949–1951, and 1995. A larger proportion of Americans are now surviving into old age than was the case in 1900. *Source:* Bureau of the Census and National Center for Health Statistics. *U.S. Life Tables.*

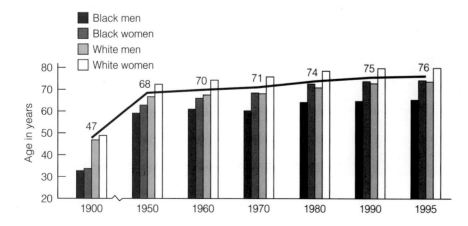

Figure 15.4 Life expectancy at birth by race and gender, average life expectancy = 76 years. Life expectancy has increased 62% since 1900. *Source:* National Center for Health Statistics. *Health, United States, 1996–97 and Injury Chartbook.* Hyattsville, MD: Author, 1997.

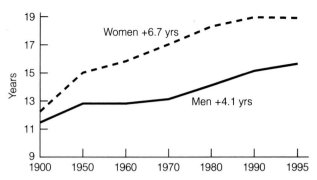

Figure 15.5 Life expectancy at age 65 by gender. People who are 65 years of age can now expect to live to 82.4 years. *Source:* National Center for Health Statistics. *Health, United States, 1996–97 and Injury Chartbook.* Hyattsville, MD: 1997.

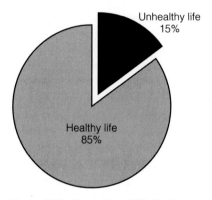

Figure 15.6 Proportion of life that is spent in an "unhealthy" state (impaired by disabilities, disease, injuries), total life expectancy = 76 years. Fifteen percent of life is spent in an "unhealthy" state, a proportion that health officials have targeted as a priority issue for the year 2000. *Source:* National Center for Health Statistics. *Healthy People 2000 Review, 1997.* Hyattsville, MD: Public Health Service, 1997.

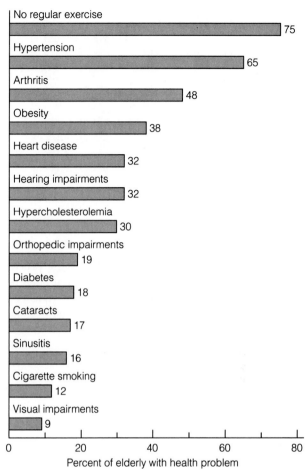

Figure 15.7 Prevalence of risk factors and disease among the elderly. The prevalence of risk factors and disease is high among the elderly. *Sources:* National Center for Health Statistics. *Healthy People 2000 Review, 1997;* Hyattsville, MD: Public Health Service, 1997; National Center for Health Statistics. *Health, United States, 1996–97 and Injury Chartbook.* Hyattsville, MD: Author, 1997.

stroke are declining among the elderly, those for cancer are rising, mainly because of lung cancer.[6]

- Osteoporosis, defined as decrease in bone density, is widespread among the elderly. One third of women over age 65 develop fractures of their spinal bones, and by extreme old age, one of every three women and one of every six men will have had a hip fracture. (This is discussed in more detail later in this chapter.)

- There are several types of senile dementia, the most common form being Alzheimer's disease.[10] Memory loss, especially for recent events, is usually the first sign, followed by more profound and debilitating mental, behavioral, and bodily control impairments. Alzheimer's disease strikes about 10% of people over age 65 and nearly half of those 85 and older. About 4 million Americans have Alzheimer's, and 100,000 die each year because of it. The Centers for Disease Control and Prevention have reported a pronounced increase in the rate of Alzheimer's deaths. The cost of care for these patients is now $100 billion per year.[10]

- The elderly account for over one third of health-care spending and prescription drug use.[10,11] The forecasted increase in people 85 years of age and older may lead to a large increase in use of nursing homes in the future. Financing the health care of the elderly in the future is a serious concern.[9]

THE AGING PROCESS

Aging refers to the normal yet irreversible biological changes that occur throughout a person's lifetime.[12–14] It is a very complex phenomenon and is influenced by genetic,

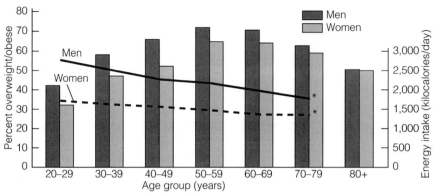

Figure 15.8 Energy intake and overweight adults by age group, 1988–1994. The prevalence of obesity rises until ages 55–64 but then falls in old age. Energy intake is lowest among the elderly. *Sources:* Morley JE. Anorexia of aging: Physiologic and pathologic. *Am J Clin Nutr* 66:760–773, 1997; National Center for Health Statistics. *Health, United States, 1996–97 and Injury Chartbook.* Hyattsville, MD: Author, 1997.

* Energy intake data not available for age 80+

environmental, and lifestyle factors. The aging process takes place at all ages, but for those over 65, it often becomes more manifest, with significant changes in quality of life. There are two major kinds of theories of aging:[12] damage theories and program theories.

Damage theories speculate that with advancing age, we become less able to repair damage caused by internal malfunctions or external assault from oxygen-free radicals to the body. Various biochemical and hormonal changes with aging may finally lead to death. The immune system is less effective in the elderly, and free radicals are less effectively mopped up by scavengers. The body may be less able to combat infection or destroy abnormal body cells.

Program theories of aging suggest that an internal clock starts ticking at conception and is programmed to run just so long. Some researchers feel that human cells can only divide a certain number of times and then stop, leading to death. DNA transcription occurs at lower rates and in significantly altered patterns as cells age.

As a person ages, many changes take place in the body:[7–19]

- *Loss of taste and smell.* The elderly often complain of a decreased ability to taste and enjoy food. Taste buds decrease in number and size, affecting sweet and salty tastes in particular. About 40% of people 80 years or older appear to have difficulty identifying common substances by smell.

- *Periodontal (bone area around the teeth) bone loss.* The majority of the elderly suffer bone loss and disease in the tissues around the teeth as they grow older. As a result, one third of the population over 65 have lost all of their teeth, and about 65% have lost teeth in at least one arch. The end result of this is obvious: Older people tend to choose foods that are easy to chew, leading to a reduced consumption of fresh fruit and vegetables high in dietary fiber.

- *Decrease in gastrointestinal function.* With an increase in age, the stomach cells are less able to secrete digestive juices, interfering with the digestion of protein

and vitamin B_{12}. The small intestine becomes less capable of absorbing some nutrients, and there may also be a reduced ability of the intestine to move its contents through the digestive tract, resulting in constipation. Constipation is further exacerbated by lack of dietary fiber.

- *Loss in visual and auditory function.* Visual function starts to decline around age 45 and worsens gradually thereafter. After age 80, less than 15% of the population has 20/20 vision. Gradual hearing loss generally begins at about age 20 and has been estimated to affect as many as 66% of people reaching 80.

- *Decrease in lean body weight.* The prevalence of obesity is highest in the 55–64 age group, but then falls thereafter. As a person ages, body fat increases, while muscle and bone (or lean body weight) decreases. This leads to a decrease in energy expended during rest, partially explaining why the elderly consume fewer Calories than younger people. The resting metabolic rate decreases by 1–2% per decade starting at about age 20 (see Figure 15.8).

- *Loss of bone mineral mass.* As discussed previously, loss of bone (osteoporosis) is an almost universal phenomenon with increasing age. The resulting fractures often mend with difficulty, resulting in long periods of decreased physical activity and social interaction.

- *Mental impairment.* Senility, also called senile dementia or organic brain syndrome, affects about 60% of the elderly. Some of the problems associated with senile dementia include impairment of memory, judgment, feelings, personality, and ability to speak. Senile dementia of the Alzheimer's type accounts for at least half of all dementia in old age.

- *Decreased ability to metabolize drugs.* The elderly account for about one third of all prescription drug consumption, yet they have a decreased ability to absorb, distribute, metabolize, and excrete both pre-

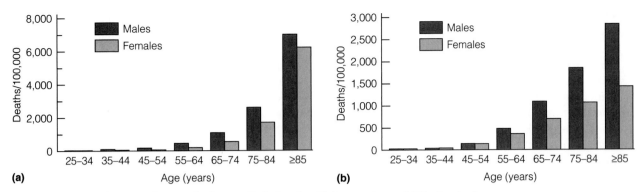

Figure 15.9 Heart disease and cancer death rates climb sharply with increase in age. (a) Death rates for diseases of the heart according to age. (b) Death rates for cancer, according to age. *Source:* National Center for Health Statistics. *Health, United States, 1996–97 and Injury Chartbook.* Hyattsville, MD: Author, 1997.

scription and nonprescription drugs. The majority of the elderly are on more than one prescription drug, and these can interact with each other, affecting nutritional status.

- *High prevalence of chronic disease.* As discussed earlier, up to 88% of the elderly suffer from at least one chronic disease. A variety of diseases are more common among the elderly, including diabetes, cancer, heart disease, high blood pressure, stroke, and arthritis (see Figure 15.9).

- *Neuromuscular changes.* Reaction time, ability to balance, and strength of muscles, tendons, and ligaments decrease with aging, limiting normal activity for many. Accidents increase, and the ability to shop for and prepare food may be hampered.

- *Urinary incontinence.* Up to 20% of the elderly living at home and 75% of those in long-term-care facilities cannot control the muscle that controls urination. This can lead to social isolation, embarrassment, and the decision to live in a nursing home environment.

- *Decrease in liver and kidney function.* The size and function of the liver and kidneys decrease steadily with age, making the removal of metabolic waste products more difficult.

- *Decrease in heart and lung fitness.* With aging, there is a decrease on the order of 8–10% per decade in the ability of the heart and lungs to supply oxygen to the muscles. Most of this is due to the decreasing physical activity of the elderly.

HEALTH HABITS AND AGING

While *life expectancy* is defined as the average number of years of life expected for a population of a given age, *life span* refers to the maximum age obtainable by a particular species. Figure 15.10 shows that the maximum life span var-

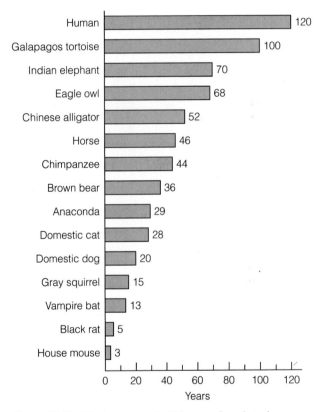

Figure 15.10 Maximum recorded life spans for selected species. The maximum life span varies widely among species. *Source:* Kirkwood TBL. Comparative life spans of species: Why do species have the life spans they do? *Am J Clin Nutr* 55: 1191S–1195S, 1992.

ies widely among species and is thought to be 120 for humans (about 44 years higher than the current average American life expectancy).[14] Several humans have lived to 120 years or more. Arthur Reed of Oakland, California, lived to be 124 years of age. Born the year Lincoln was elected president (1860), he rode his bike on his 100th birthday and held a job until age 116. Shigechigo Isumi of Japan died in 1986 and was reported to be 121 years old. Mary Thompson of Orlando, Florida, died in 1996 at the age of 120. In 1997, Jeanne Calment of France died at age 122.[12]

Currently, accidental deaths, cancer, suicide/homicide, heart disease, congenital anomalies (the number one cause of infant mortality), and the human immunodeficiency virus infection, which causes AIDS, are the leading causes of "years of potential life lost" before age 65.[6] To move life expectancy toward the maximum life span of the human species, these will have to be largely eliminated as major causes of early death. This will require a strong commitment to improved health habits and lifestyles on the part of Americans.

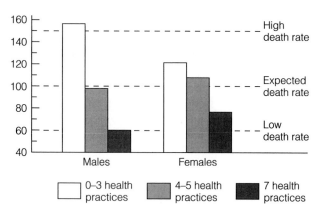

Figure 15.11 Relationship between number of good health habits and mortality. Males and females who follow seven simple health practices have approximately half the mortality of people with three or fewer of these health habits. *Source:* Enstrom JE, Kanim LE, Breslow L. The relationship between vitamin C intake, general health practices, and mortality in Alameda county, California. *Am J Public Health* 76:1124–1130, 1986.

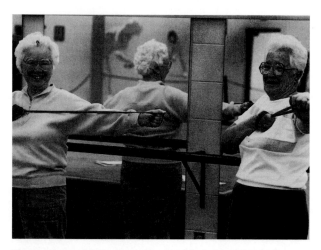

Figure 15.12 Of all age groups, the elderly have the most to gain by being active.

There is much current interest in life-extension strategies including energy restriction (which has been shown to lengthen the life of rodents), hormone supplements, various drugs, antioxidants, and gene manipulation. Much more research is needed to assess effectiveness, safety, and socioeconomic impact.[20,21] Health habits are clearly identified as having a major influence on life expectancy and quality of life during old age[22–28] (see Physical Fitness Activity 15.1). Lester Breslow of UCLA, for example, in his famous study of more than 6,000 people in the San Francisco Bay Area, showed a dramatic difference in death rate between those who followed seven simple health habits (never smoked, moderate alcohol consumption, daily breakfast, no snacking, 7–8 hours of sleep per night, regular exercise, ideal weight) and those who did not[25–28] (see Figure 15.11). Those following all seven health habits were estimated to live 9 years longer than those who did not practice any of them. In addition, the healthful lifestyle followers were only half as likely to have suffered disabilities that kept them from work or limited their day-to-day activities.[25] In other words, habitual healthful living appears not only to promote longevity but also to increase the chance of having the physical ability to enjoy life to its fullest in later years.[22]

EXERCISE AND AGING

As is reviewed in this section, a key ingredient to healthy aging is regular physical activity.[1] Of all age groups, the elderly have the most to gain by being active, including the potential for decreased risk of cardiovascular disease, cancer, high blood pressure, depression, osteoporosis, bone fractures, and diabetes, with improved body composition, fitness, longevity, ability to perform personal-care activities, and management of arthritis or other conditions leading to activity limitations[29–33] (see Figure 15.12). Yet national surveys indicate that only about one fourth of the elderly exercise regularly, which is less than any other age group[31] (see Chapter 1).

Figure 15.13 summarizes the physiological changes that take place in the human body with aging. Interestingly, many of the changes that accompany aging are the same types of changes that can be expected with inactivity and weightlessness.[34–37] The identifying characteristics of both aging and the "disuse syndrome" are a decrease in cardiorespiratory function, obesity, musculoskeletal fragility, and premature aging. However, as is emphasized in this section, older individuals adapt to both resistive and endurance exercise training in a fashion similar to young people.[30] In other words, it makes sense that a significant proportion of the deterioration attributed to aging can be explained by the tendency of people to exercise less as they age.

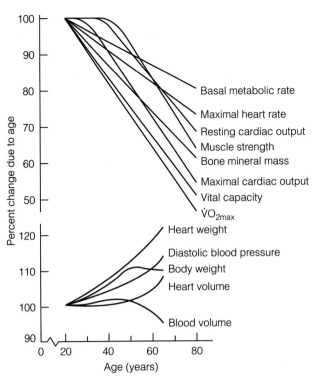

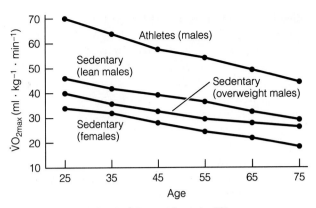

Figure 15.14 Decline in $\dot{V}O_{2max}$ with age in different groups of males and females. $\dot{V}O_{2max}$ decreases by about 8–10% per decade for both males and females, athletes and nonathletes.
Sources: Heath GW, Hagberg JM, Ehsani AA, Holloszy JO. A physiological comparison of young and older endurance athletes. *J Appl Physiol* 51:634–640, 1981; Nieman DC, Pover NK, Segebartt KS, Arabatzis K, Johnson M, Dietrich SJ. Hematological, anthropometric, and metabolic comparisons between active and inactive healthy old old to very old women. *Ann Sports Med* 5:2–8, 1990.

Figure 15.13 Physiological changes with increase in age. Aging is accompanied by a decrease in cardiorespiratory and musculoskeletal functions. Many of these changes also occur during the transition from a trained to an untrained state.

$\dot{V}O_{2max}$ and the Aging Process

Researchers who have evaluated the effects of aging on the cardiorespiratory system have focused on work capacity, or $\dot{V}O_{2max}$. The ability of the body to take in oxygen, transport it, and use it for oxidation of fuel is viewed as the single best variable to define the overall functional changes that occur with aging.[30]

$\dot{V}O_{2max}$ normally declines 8–10% per decade for both males and females after 25 years of age[38–43] (see Figure 15.14). From cross-sectional data, the rate of decline in $\dot{V}O_{2max}$ for men and women is about 0.35–0.50 ml · kg^{-1} · min^{-1} per year, starting at age 25 years.

Why does $\dot{V}O_{2max}$ tend to be low among the elderly? Declining physical activity appears to be a major factor, along with the loss in fat-free mass and increase in fat mass.[44] Two studies of 1,499 men and 409 women have determined that nearly half of the age-related decline in aerobic power is due to changes in body composition and exercise habits.[41,42] Notice in Figure 15.14 that athletic males who are 65–75 years of age have the $\dot{V}O_{2max}$ of young adult sedentary males. Figure 15.15 shows the results of one study that compared highly conditioned and sedentary septuagenarian women.[45] The highly conditioned elderly women (who competed in state and national senior games endur-

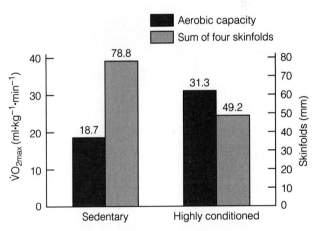

Figure 15.15 Fitness and leanness in highly active elderly women. Septuagenarian women (mean age 73 years) who were highly active, competing in state and national senior games endurance competitions were much leaner and fitter ($\dot{V}O_{2max}$ 67% higher) than their sedentary counterparts.
Source: Warren BJ, Nieman DC, Dotson RG, Adkins CH, O'Donnell KA, Haddock BL, Butterworth DE. Cardiorespiratory responses to exercise training in septuagenarian women. *Int J Sports Med* 14:60–65, 1993.

ance competitions and had been training intensively for an average of 11 years) were much leaner and had a $\dot{V}O_{2max}$ 67% higher than their sedentary counterparts and similar to that of sedentary women 35 years of age (Figure 15.16).

Many other studies have shown that elderly people who are vigorous in their exercise possess high aerobic power (similar to that of sedentary young adults) and are capable of performing at levels once thought unattainable.[33,40,45–50] For example, in 1991, 70-year-old Warren Utes of Illinois set

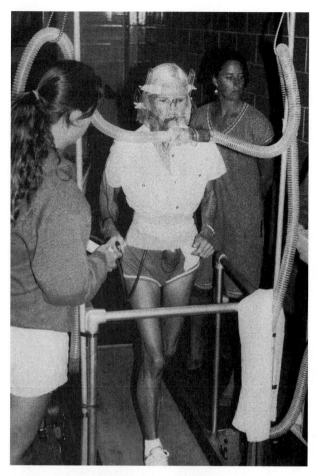

Figure 15.16 This highly conditioned elderly woman (age 67) has a $\dot{V}O_{2max}$ of 35 ml · kg^{-1} · min^{-1}, equal to that of a woman 40 years younger than herself (a subject in study from Figure 15.15).

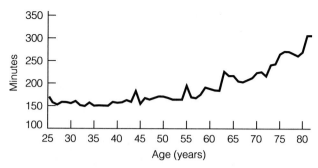

Figure 15.17 John Kelley's Boston marathon times, ages 25 to 82 years. John Kelley raced the Boston marathon every year between the ages of 25 and 82. Despite intensive training, his race time was about twice as slow in old age, compared to when he was a young adult.

an age-group world record of 38:24 for the 10-kilometer race. Sixty-year-old Luciano Acquarone of Italy ran a 2:38 marathon, a pace of 6 minutes a mile, while Derek Turnbull of New Zealand ran 5 kilometers in 16:39 at age 65. At age 49, Evy Palm ran a half-marathon in 1:12:36 in Holland, a time regarded as one of the top-rated, age-graded performances of all time. In 1996, 71-year-old John Keston of England ran a world-best marathon time of 3:01 for those over the age of 70. His goal is to break 3 hours for the marathon, a threshold once thought impossible for septuagenarians. (See the Sports Medicine Insight at the end of the chapter for a discussion of Mavis Lindgren, who has performed well in extreme old age.)

However, even among athletes who exercise vigorously throughout their lifetimes, $\dot{V}O_{2max}$ still declines at a similar rate to that of sedentary individuals (albeit at a much higher absolute level). Some studies have demonstrated that the rate of decline may be reduced for several years during which vigorous exercise is engaged in (with no decrease in

exercise frequency, intensity, or duration), but ultimately, $\dot{V}O_{2max}$ will start falling at normal or accelerated rates later.[45-53] Most scientists now believe that endurance exercise may be effective in reducing the rate for a certain time period, but that the age-related decrease in aerobic power and cardiovascular function cannot be prevented.[30,47-57] A lower stroke volume, heart rate, and arteriovenous oxygen difference all appear to contribute to the age-related decline in $\dot{V}O_{2max}$, even when the individual tries to keep physically active.[55-57]

The bottom line is that at any given age, athletes who exercise vigorously can be fitter than their sedentary counterparts, but because of the aging process, less fit than younger athletes. Studies have confirmed that men achieve peak performance in their 20s for all running and swimming events (e.g., 23 years for sprinting and 28 for marathon running).[58]

A case in point is the 57-year history of John Kelley, the famous runner who competed in the Boston marathon every year between the ages of 25 and 82. As shown in Figure 15.17, despite intensive training and unusual motivation and tenacity, his race time at age 82 was about twice as slow as it was during his 20s and 30s. Running the marathon at age 82 was a tremendous feat in and of itself (something the vast majority of people worldwide cannot do at any age), but the aging process was strong enough to slow him down considerably.

Physical Training by the Elderly

The studies from the previous section were primarily cross-sectional in nature, with researchers comparing older and younger athletes and nonathletes. A more difficult research design is to randomly divide sedentary subjects into exercise and nonexercise groups and then to compare them before and after several months of training. The question of

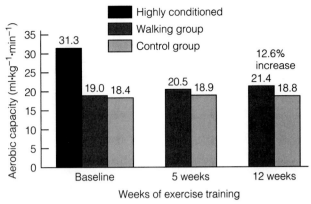

Mean age of women = 73 years

Figure 15.18 Exercise and aerobic capacity in elderly women; highly conditioned subjects had exercised vigorously for an average of 11 years; 12-week training program = 5 days/week, brisk walking, 37 minutes/session at 60% aerobic capacity. Twelve weeks of brisk walking by elderly women led to a 12.6% improvement in $\dot{V}O_{2max}$. The dark bar shows the $\dot{V}O_{2max}$ of a highly conditioned group of elderly women who had been training vigorously for 11 years, competing in state and national senior games competitions. *Source:* Warren BJ, Nieman DC, Dotson RG, Adkins CH, O'Donnell KA, Haddock BL, Butterworth DE. Cardiorespiratory responses to exercise training in septuagenarian women. *Int J Sports Med* 14:60–65, 1993.

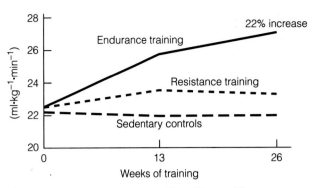

Figure 15.19 Exercise training in 70- to 79-year-olds, endurance training = 3 days/week, 40 minutes/session, 50% increasing to 75–85% $\dot{V}O_{2max}$. After 26 weeks of vigorous endurance training, $\dot{V}O_{2max}$ improved 22% in elderly men and women. *Source:* Hagberg JM, Graves JE, Limacher M, et al. Cardiovascular responses of 70- to 79-yr-old men and women to exercise training. *J Appl Physiol* 66:2589–2594, 1989.

interest has been whether elderly individuals are capable of improving cardiorespiratory and musculoskeletal fitness, and body composition in a fashion similar to that of younger adults. The answer is "yes," but the absolute level attained after training is lower than can be attained when younger.[30]

Cardiorespiratory Training

Although earlier studies suggested that older individuals are not as responsive to aerobic training as their younger counterparts, there is now a growing consensus that the relative increase in $\dot{V}O_{2max}$ over an 8–26 week period is similar between young and old adults.[30,45,55,59–65]

Figure 15.18 shows the result of a randomized controlled study involving women in their 70s.[45] Twelve weeks of brisk walking led to a 12.6% improvement in $\dot{V}O_{2max}$, an increase similar to that reported for younger adults. Notice, however, that $\dot{V}O_{2max}$ was still far below that of younger females (Figure 15.14) or a group of elderly female athletes who had been training intensely for an average of 11 years (Figures 15.15 and 15.18).

In another study of septuagenarian subjects, 26 weeks of high-intensity exercise led to even greater gains (22% increase overall) in aerobic power (see Figure 15.19).[62] Men and women between the ages of 70 and 79 were randomly assigned to endurance training, resistance training, or a control group. Subjects in the endurance group trained

on treadmills, gradually increasing the intensity of exercise from 50% (walking) to 75–85% (walking/jogging) of $\dot{V}O_{2max}$ for 40 minutes per session, 3 days a week. The researchers concluded that "healthy men and women in their 70s increased their $\dot{V}O_{2max}$ to the same relative degree as would be expected in younger individuals in response to a prolonged and vigorous program of endurance exercise training" and that people in their eighth decade of life "have not lost the ability to adapt to endurance exercise training."[62]

There is some concern about exercise-induced injury rates among the elderly. While walking has been associated with low injury rates among the elderly, jogging may induce an unusually high injury rate.[66] Some researchers feel that the elderly, as compared to younger adults, are more fragile and susceptible to musculoskeletal injury during high-impact aerobic activities (such as jogging or aerobic dance) and that such activities as walking, low-impact aerobic dance, or swimming may be preferable (see Figure 15.20).

In general, the same basic exercise prescription principles used for young adults can be applied to the elderly, but with an emphasis on greater caution and slower progression. The elderly are frequently divided into three approximate groupings: the young old, 65–74 years of age; the old old, 74–84 years of age; and the very old, greater than 84 years of age.[67] The question of whether regular cardiorespiratory exercise can improve aerobic power in very old individuals has received little attention, and more research is needed to determine their trainability. At this extreme age, the aging process may dominate so powerfully that little improvement in cardiorespiratory fitness may be experienced.[51] In addition, for many people over age 75, health problems and a lack of motivation may prevent

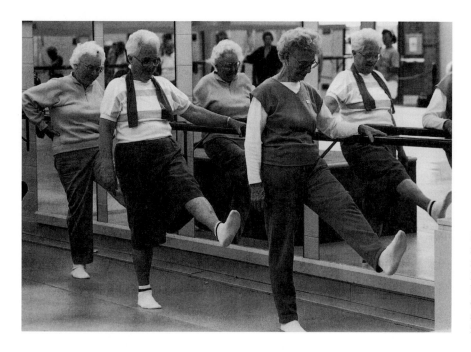

Figure 15.20 The elderly are more fragile and susceptible to musculoskeletal injury during high-impact aerobic activities. Low-impact aerobic dance or other activities such as walking or swimming are preferable to high-impact aerobic dance or jogging.

them from being able to engage in appropriate amounts of exercise.

Muscular Strength and Resistance Training

Muscle strength in most individuals is well preserved to about 45 years of age but then deteriorates by about 5–10% per decade thereafter (see Chapter 6).[30,35,68] The average individual will lose about 30% of muscle strength and 40% of muscle size between the second and seventh decades of life.[30,35] The loss in muscle mass appears to be the major reason strength is decreased among the elderly, with the aging process leading to only minor changes in the muscle's ability to generate tension.[69] Muscle atrophy appears to be the result of loss of both the size and number of muscle fibers.[68]

In older individuals, muscle weakness may compromise common activities of daily living, leading to dependency on others. Also, reduced leg strength may increase the risk of injury through falling. In fact, the capacity of the elderly to remain functionally independent appears to depend less on cardiorespiratory fitness than on muscular fitness.

At issue has been whether the elderly can improve muscular strength by engaging in regular resistance training. Several studies have now shown that the elderly respond to progressive resistance training with relative (but not absolute) improvements in muscular strength and size that compare favorably to responses seen in younger adults.[30,35,68–78] In one study, knee-extension weight training by frail, institutionalized men and women (mean age 90 years) led to dramatic improvements in strength.[76]

Overall, studies suggest that the rate of decline in strength and muscle mass with increase in age can be reduced or even largely reversed by appropriate resistance training. In the words of one reviewer:

> Since older individuals adapt to resistive and endurance exercise training in a similar fashion to young people, the decline in the muscle's metabolic and force-producing capacity can no longer be considered as an inevitable consequence of the aging process. Rather, the adaptations in aging skeletal muscle to exercise training may prevent sarcopenia, enhance the ease of carrying out the activities of daily living, and exert a beneficial effect on such age-associated diseases as Type II diabetes, coronary artery disease, hypertension, osteoporosis, and obesity.[35]

Body Composition Changes

With aging, there is an accumulation of fat and a substantial loss of muscle mass.[79] Comparisons between average young and elderly adults suggest a decrease in the fat-free mass of 15–30% by age 80, with the rate and degree of loss varying widely depending on both genetic and lifestyle influences.[35,79] During middle age, there is typically a gain in body fat, and in some individuals, centralization of body fat with its attendant health risks may also occur.[79] In very old age, both fat-free and fat mass are lost as body weight declines. All the various components of the fat-free mass—muscle and bone mineral mass, and total body water—are decreased in older men and women, relative to young adults. The decline in resting metabolic rate with advancing age is primarily due to this decline in fat-free mass.[69,79]

As reviewed in the previous section, resistance exercise can increase muscle mass and strength in the elderly.[35,79] Elderly individuals can also demonstrate a level of body fat somewhat similar to that of younger persons if they have a consistent physical activity history and control their food intake throughout life.[45] (see Figure 15.15). Although short-term reductions in body fat and gains in muscle mass have been reported in studies with the elderly, the usual age-related changes in body composition may not be completely countered unless aerobic and resistance training are combined. In a study of master athletes, for example, fat weight increased about 2.5 pounds during a 10-year period, while fat-free weight dropped 3–6 pounds, despite heavy endurance training (about 30 miles per week of running).[80]

Physical Activity and Life Expectancy

With an increasingly aged population, there is an urgent need for health practices that can prolong adult vigor and delay the onset and progression of chronic diseases. In other words, prolonging active life expectancy, not just disabled existence, is an important goal. "Medicated survival" by the elderly is a state to be avoided, and exercise is one factor, along with other lifestyle habits, that can improve the quality of life of the elderly.

Can regular exercise lengthen life expectancy? Do active people live longer? This has been an active area of research, and in general, most studies using both cross-sectional and longitudinal research designs suggest the answer is "yes," for both men and women.[81–89] In general, the combined studies indicate that the most active or fit individuals experience death rates that are 25–50% lower than the rates among those least active or fit.[85]

Figure 15.21 shows the results of one interesting cross-sectional study of 2,613 Finnish male world-class athletes who competed during 1920–1965, and 1,712 nonathletes.[81] Using death certificates and other medical records dating up to 1989, the life expectancy of endurance sport athletes (long-distance running and cross-country skiing) was shown to be nearly 6 years greater than that of the nonathletes and 4 years greater than that of power-sport athletes (boxing, wrestling, weight lifting, and throwers in field athletics), with team-sport athletes in an intermediate position (soccer, ice hockey, basketball, jumpers, and sprinters). Many of the athletes (especially the runners and skiers) continued their regular exercise programs throughout life, and both this and genetic selection may have explained their increased life expectancy.

Ralph Paffenbarger of Stanford University showed that Harvard alumni whose weekly energy output in walking, stair climbing, and playing sports totaled 2,000 to 3,500 Cal-

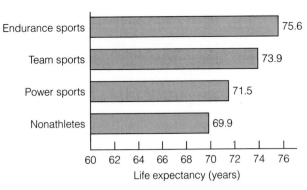

Figure 15.21   Mean life expectancy among athletes versus nonathletes. These cross-sectional data of Finnish male world-class athletes and nonathletes suggest that endurance-sport athletes have a greater life expectancy than athletes from other sports or nonathletes.   *Source:* Sarna S, Sahi T, Koskenvuo M, Kaprio J. Increased life expectancy of world class male athletes. *Med Sci Sports Exerc* 25:237–244, 1993.

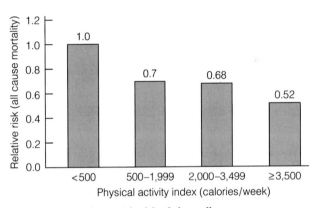

Figure 15.22   Relative risk of death from all causes, among 10,269 Harvard alumni, according to patterns of physical activity. In the Harvard alumni study, the risk of death from all causes was reduced among the physically active. For those exercising at least 2,000 Calories a week, life expectancy was estimated to be about 2 years greater than for the sedentary. *Source:* Paffenbarger PS, Hyde RT, Wing AL, et al. Physical activity, all-cause mortality, and longevity of college alumni. *N Engl J Med* 314: 605–613, 1986.

ories a week experienced a 32% reduction in all-cause death rates[87,88] (see Figure 15.22). For subjects exercising at least 3,500 Calories a week, death rates were about half those of sedentary alumni. In general, life expectancy was found to be about 2 years greater in those exercising at least 2,000 Calories a week. Although this may not seem like much, this is the same impact in epidemiological terms of completely removing cancer from the United States. In practical terms, this improvement in life expectancy can be gained by walking or jogging 8–10 miles a week.

Data from the Cooper Institute for Aerobics Research have shown that the least fit of men and women are about

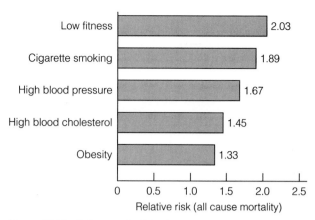

Figure 15.23 Relative risk of death from all causes among 25,341 men, Cooper Institute for Aerobics Research. Low fitness ranks highest as a predictor of early mortality among men. *Source:* Blair SN, Kampert JB, Kohl HW, et al. Influences of cardiorespiratory fitness and other precursors on cardiovascular disease and all-cause mortality in men and women. *JAMA* 276: 205–210, 1996.

twice as likely to die as their fit counterparts.[82] As shown in Figure 15.23, low fitness is one of the strongest risk factors for death from all causes in males and is at least as risky as cigarette smoking.

OSTEOPOROSIS

Osteoporosis is an age-related disorder characterized by decreased bone mass and increased susceptibility to fractures[90-94] (see Figure 15.24). Osteoporosis is defined as a drop in bone density 30% or more below the average bone density of healthy people in their thirties and is classified into primary and secondary forms. *Primary osteoporosis* may occur in two types: Type I osteoporosis (postmenopausal), which is the accelerated decrease in bone mass that occurs when estrogen levels fall after menopause; and Type II osteoporosis (age related), which is the inevitable loss of bone mass with age and occurs in both men and women. *Secondary osteoporosis* may develop at any age as a consequence of hormonal, digestive, and metabolic disorders, as well as prolonged bed rest and weightlessness (space flight) that result in loss of bone mineral mass.

Osteoporosis is a common condition afflicting 25 million Americans and causing each year an estimated 1.5 million fractures of the spinal bones (500,000), hips (300,000), forearms (200,000), and other bones in those 45 years of age and older. Loss of bone mineral content (BMC) is an almost universal phenomenon with increasing age among white men and women in the United States. Overall, almost a third of elderly women will have one or more vertebral fractures. Among those who live to be 90, 33% of women and 17% of men will suffer hip fractures. Of the elderly experiencing a hip fracture, 18–33% will die within 1 year, and most have a significant reduction in quality of life.[93,95]

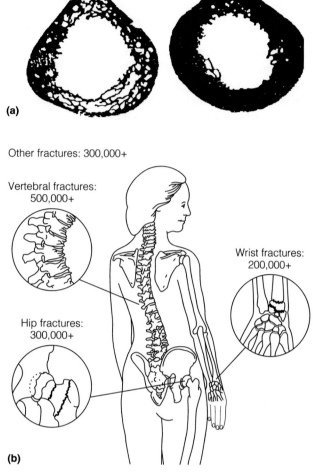

Figure 15.24 *Osteoporosis* is characterized by a decrease in the amount of bone, often so severe that it leads to fractures after even minimal trauma. (a) Cross-sections of normal and osteoporotic bone; (b) the three most common sites of osteoporosis.

The annual cost of osteoporosis in the United States will exceed $60 billion by the year 2000.[91] Obviously, osteoporosis is an important public health problem, exacting on the elderly an enormous economic and medical burden. The problem is likely to increase as the number of elderly people grows.

Several tests can safely and accurately measure bone density. The newest, most accurate version uses a technology called DEXA—dual-energy x-ray absorptiometry. During the painless 15-minute scan, a low-dose, focused beam of radiation creates images of the hip and spine. A computer then calculates how dense the bones are, compared with those of healthy young adults and those of average people the same age. The cost is between $150 and $250. Most experts recommend against routine screening and suggest that DEXA measurements be reserved for high-risk individuals because of the high cost and limited testing resources.[96]

Risk Factors

Bone is a spongy protein matrix in which crystals of calcium and phosphorus salts are embedded.[94] In many bones, there are two distinct regions: an outer, dense shell of compact bone (cortical) and an inner, open, spongelike region of cancellous bone (trabecular). Once produced, bone does not remain as a fixed structure. From birth until death, bone tissue is continually being formed, broken down, and reformed in a process called *remodeling.* The cells that break down bone are called *osteoclasts,* and those that build bone are called *osteoblasts.*

During puberty, rapid increases in bone growth and density occur, with peak bone density achieved between the ages of 20 and 30.[94,97] About 90% of the adult bone mineral content is deposited by the end of adolescence, and this process is affected by both genetic and lifestyle factors.[94] The period between ages 9 and 20 is critical in building up an optimal bone density as a safeguard against losses later in life. Osteoporosis is now viewed as a pediatric health problem.[94] Bone mass is approximately 30% higher in men than in women and about 10% higher in blacks than in whites. Once peak bone mass is reached, osteoclast and osteoblast activity remain in balance until about age 45–50, when osteoclast activity becomes greater than that of the osteoblasts, and adults begin to slowly lose bone mass. At menopause, women normally have an accelerated loss of bone mineral mass (2.5–5% per year) for several years[90,98] (see Figure 15.25). During the course of their lifetimes, women lose about 50% of their trabecular bone and 30% of their cortical bone, while men lose about 30% and 20%, respectively.[92] Although peak bone mass is an important factor explaining why some individuals develop osteoporosis and bone fractures and others do not, differences in bone architecture and structure also appear to be important.[90]

The best strategies for preventing osteoporosis are to build strong bones early in life, and then reduce bone loss in later years (see Physical Fitness Activity 15.2). Several risk factors predict those who should be most concerned about prevention of osteoporosis (see Table 15.1):[92–112]

- *Age.* The older an individual, the greater the risk of osteoporosis, with most experiencing loss of bone mass starting in the fifth decade.

- *Gender.* Women are at greater risk for developing osteoporosis than men (four to one) and generally start with a lower peak bone mass and experience an accelerated loss following menopause.

- *Race.* Caucasian and Asian women are more likely to develop osteoporosis than women of African descent.

- *Bone structure and body weight.* Small-boned and thin women are at greater risk. Elderly individuals who involuntarily lose weight are also at high risk.[103]

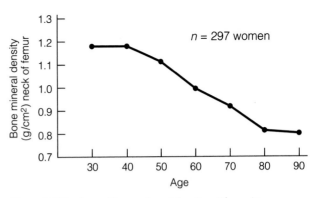

Figure 15.25 Loss of bone mineral density with age in women. Age-related bone loss among U.S. women. *Source:* Melton LJ, Kan SH, Wahner HW, Riggs BL. Lifetime fracture risk: An approach to hip fracture risk assessment based on bone mineral density and age. *J Clin Epidemiol* 41:985–994, 1988.

TABLE 15.1 Scientific Validity of the Risk Factors of Osteoporosis[a]

Well Established	Moderate Evidence
Female (+)	Alcohol (+)
Obesity (−)	Moderate exercise (−)
Black ethnicity (−)	Cigarette smoking (+)
Heavy exercise (−)	Thiazide diuretic use (+)
Age (+)	Using water fluoride (−)
Early menopause (+)	Caffeine use (+)
Removal of ovaries (premenopausal) (+)	High protein intake (+)
Caucasian / Asian (+)	
Use of steroids (+)	
Low calcium intake (+)	
Estrogen use (−)	
Bed rest (+)	
Menstrual irregularity (+)	
Anorexia nervosa (+)	
Family history (+)	
Involuntary weight loss (+)	
Low vitamin D intake (+)	
Use of thyroid hormones (+)	
Use of long-acting sedatives (+)	
Rheumatoid arthritis (+)	
Chronic liver disease (+)	

[a](+) = increased risk; (−) = decreased risk. See text for discussion of risk factors.

- *Menopause/menstrual history.* Normal or early menopause (brought about naturally or because of surgery) increases osteoporosis risk. In addition, women who stop menstruating before menopause because of conditions such as anorexia or bulimia, or because of excessive physical exercise, may also lose bone tissue and develop osteoporosis.

- *Lifestyle.* Smoking, drinking too much alcohol, drinking more than two cups of coffee a day (when combined with a low calcium intake), consuming an inadequate amount of calcium, or getting little or no weight-bearing exercise, increases the chances of developing osteoporosis.[106-110] A high caffeine intake (from any source, including coffee, tea, and other beverages), a high protein intake from meat, fish, and eggs, and a high salt intake accelerate the loss of calcium in the urine, thereby increasing the risk of bone fracture.

- *Medications and disease.* Osteoporosis is associated with certain medications (e.g., cortisone-like drugs, steroids, thyroid hormone, long-acting sedatives) and is a recognized complication of a number of medical conditions, including endocrine disorders (having an overactive thyroid), rheumatoid arthritis, chronic liver disease, and immobilization (e.g., prolonged bed rest).

- *Family history.* Susceptibility to fracture may be, in part, hereditary. Young women whose mothers have histories of vertebral fractures also seem to have reduced bone mass. Some researchers have estimated that 60–80% of bone mass is genetically determined.

There is no cure for osteoporosis, but the National Osteoporosis Foundation does recommend several steps for slowing its progress:

- Diet

- Estrogen and other medications

- Exercise

Estrogens are vitally important for preventing and treating osteoporosis.[105] Estrogens act directly on the bone, increasing its density. Because estrogen is so important for maintaining bone in women, physicians often prescribe estrogen replacement therapy for women at menopause. Estrogen replacement therapy is the predominant way to protect bone during the years of rapid bone loss immediately following menopause. If begun soon after the menopause, estrogen therapy prevents the early phase of bone loss and decreases the incidence of fractures by about 50%.[100] When started later in life, estrogen is also effective in preventing hip fractures. There are other health benefits in using estrogen-replacement therapy, including decreased risk of coronary heart disease (risk drops in half), relief from hot flashes and other unpleasant symptoms of menopause, and decreased risk of colon cancer.[105] (Postmenopausal estrogen use has not been associated with weight gain (a fear that has caused many women to avoid its use).

Taking estrogen alone does increase the risk of uterine cancer, but when combined with synthetic progesterone, the risk is greatly reduced.[105] Although evidence is conflicting, there may be a small increase in risk of breast cancer after 15 years of hormone therapy. New evidence suggests that a high bone mineral density predicts the risk of breast cancer in older women, implying that long-term exposure to estrogen is an important risk factor for breast cancer.[113] These concerns over estrogen have increased interest in the use of other medications for preventing and treating osteoporosis.[112] (see Box 15.1 for a review of drug therapy for osteoporosis).

According to an expert panel convened by the Institutes of Medicine (IOM) in 1997, the optimal calcium intake to facilitate peak bone mass is 1,300 mg/day for children (ages 9–18), 1,000 mg/day for adult men and women (ages 19–50), and 1,200 mg/day for those over the age of 50. This is a significant increase from the previous benchmark, 800–1,200 mg/day, set in 1989 by the National Academy of Sciences (see Chapter 9).

The average male and female teenager takes in 1,151 and 793 mg of calcium per day, respectively. Elderly males and females ingest only 775 and 600 mg per day, respectively, far below the new recommended intake guidelines. The IOM panel urges that the preferred source of calcium is through calcium-rich foods such as dairy products. Calcium-fortified foods and calcium supplements are other means by which optimal calcium intake can be reached in those who cannot meet this need by ingesting conventional foods. Table 15.2 summarizes recommended sources of calcium. Notice that teenagers need to take in the equivalent of more than 4 cups of milk per day to get 1,300 mg of calcium.

There is growing evidence that when calcium intake is appropriate throughout life, a greater bone mass is developed in early adulthood, decreasing the risk of age-related bone loss.[94] When calcium intake is too low (probably below 400–500 mg a day), peak bone mass may be below optimal levels. Too much caffeine, protein, and salt increase calcium loss in the urine.

Can calcium supplementation decrease bone loss after menopause? Several studies suggest "yes," especially when combined with vitamin D and given to postmenopausal women with low calcium intakes from food.[108-111]

The Role of Physical Activity

Can exercise maximize peak bone mass and minimize age-related losses? The use of exercise in the prevention and treatment of osteoporosis has been an active area of re-

Box 15.1

Osteoporosis and Drug Therapy

Although there is no cure for osteoporosis, steps can be taken to slow down its progress. Drug therapy for postmenopausal women may be indicated, upon advice of a physician.

- *Estrogen replacement therapy.* Estrogen has a direct and positive influence on bone cells. Following the loss of estrogen with menopause, bone loss is accelerated. A third to half of all bone loss in women is related to menopause. Because estrogen is so important for maintaining bone in women, physicians often prescribe estrogen replacement therapy for women at menopause. Estrogen replacement therapy is the only way to protect bone during the years of rapid bone loss immediately following menopause.

- *Calcitonin.* For women already suffering osteoporosis, doctors will often prescribe the hormone calcitonin. It is also a treatment for women who cannot or choose not to take estrogen. Calcitonin is a naturally occurring hormone involved in calcium regulation and bone metabolism. Calcitonin safely prevents further bone loss by slowing bone removal and has been reported to provide relief from the pain associated with osteoporosis. An injectable form has been available for several years,

but in 1995, the Food and Drug Association approved a more user-friendly nasal spray (marketed as Miacalcin by Sandoz Pharmaceuticals Corp.).

- *Bisphosphonates.* These are compounds that inhibit bone breakdown and slow bone removal. They have been shown to increase bone density and decrease the risk of fractures. Alendronate sodium, marketed as Fosamax by Merck & Co. Inc., was approved by the Food and Drug Administration in 1995 for treating osteoporosis in postmenopausal women. Research shows that Fosamax decreases the number of hip fractures by half over a 3-year period among women with osteoporosis. This drug has few side effects when used properly. Some reports of serious irritations to the esophagus (the portion of the digestive tract between the throat and stomach) have been linked to taking Fosamax with very little water (6–8 ounces of water should be used to help wash the drug down to the stomach). Experts recommend taking Fosamax first thing in the morning with a full glass of water, and avoiding lying down or consuming anything except water for at least 30 minutes afterward.

Source: National Osteoporosis Foundation.

TABLE 15.2   Calcium in 1-Cup Portions of Food[a]

Food	Calcium in 1-Cup Portions (mg)	Food	Calcium in 1-Cup Portions (mg)
Sesame seeds	1,404	Filbert nuts	216
Mozzarella cheese, skim milk	980	Macaroni and cheese	199
Cheddar cheese	815	Broccoli, cooked	178
Ricotta cheese, skim milk	669	Sunflower seeds	168
Plain yogurt, low-fat	415	Soup—cream of potato with milk	166
Fish, mackerel (canned)	388	Cottage cheese, low-fat	155
Almonds	346	Soybeans, cooked	131
Fish, brook trout	338	Peanuts, roasted	125
Low-fat milk	297		
Lobster	286		
Dried figs	286		
Brazil nuts	246		
Oysters	226		

[a]Recommended intake is 1,000–1,300 mg/day for people 9 years of age and older.

Source: United States Department of Agriculture.

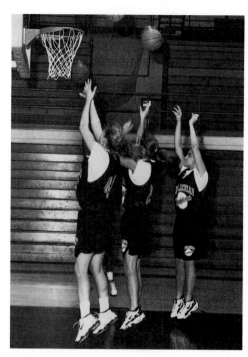

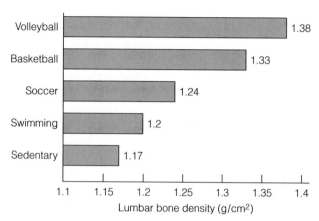

Figure 15.26 Lumbar bone mineral density in female athletes. Sports that require jumping and short bursts of powerful leg movements are associated with the highest bone density in female athletes. *Source:* Lee EJ, Long KA, Risser WL, Poindexter HBW, Gibbons WE, Goldzieher J. Variations in bone status of contralateral and regional sites in young athletic women. *Med Sci Sports Exerc* 27:1354–1361, 1995.

search, and although it is now well accepted that physical activity is essential for the maintenance of bone health, further research is needed to understand the role exercise can play in preventing osteoporosis.[114–119]

It is well known that humans lose bone mass rapidly when gravitational or muscle forces on the legs are decreased or become absent, as in weightlessness, bed rest, or spinal cord injury.[120,121] Healthy individuals who undergo complete bed rest for 4–36 weeks can lose an average of 1% bone mineral content per week, while astronauts in a gravity-free environment can lose bone mass at a monthly rate as high as 4% for trabecular bone and 1% for cortical bone.[122] The bone adapts to imposed stress or lack of stress by forming or losing mass.[119] The bone becomes bigger and denser when stress is applied in excess of normal levels because of stimulation or remodeling. The bone will continue to grow and adapt until it is restructured to handle the new imposed stress. This is one reason why total body weight has been found to be directly related to bone mineral density, with the heaviest people having the greatest bone density.[123]

There are also substantial data showing that athletes have a greater bone density than sedentary controls.[124–130] Weight-bearing activities such as walking, running, and racket sports are more effective in maintaining density of the leg and spinal bones than non-weight-bearing activities

such as bicycling and swimming (see Figure 15.26). The athletes with the greatest bone mineral masses are weight lifters, followed by athletes throwing the shotput and discus, then runners, soccer players, and finally swimmers.

A significant relationship exists between lifetime physical activity, bone mineral mass, and lowered risk of hip fracture in postmenopausal women.[124,127,131–133] Children who engage in sports that produce significant impact loading on their skeletons (e.g., running, gymnastics, and dance) have greater femoral neck bone density than children in sports producing low-impact loads to the bones (e.g., swimming).[126,128,134] This is considered important because a higher peak bone mass may be experienced in these individuals if exercise is maintained, decreasing the risk of osteoporosis later in life.

Some researchers feel that these differences between athletes and nonathletes may be due to factors of heredity and self-selection. In other words, people who tend to do well in sports competition tend to have strong, dense bones to begin with. Although this may be true to a certain extent, studies comparing the active and inactive arms of tennis players, for example, show differences in bone density.[135] This suggests that bones adapt to the exercise stresses imposed directly on them.

Among female athletes (especially runners and other endurance athletes) who lose their menstrual periods, bone mineral density typically decreases.[114,115] The loss in bone density occurs even though they engage in vigorous endurance exercise.[136] However, research with amenorrheic female gymnasts has shown that the extremely high stress on their skeletons from tumbling and dismount landings can actually override the negative effects of low reproductive hormones.[117,137] Thus it appears that in some cases, if the exercise stress is high enough, the bone will strengthen, regardless of the poor hormonal environment.[137] Nonetheless, female endurance athletes who are amenorrheic should attempt to regain their menstrual period or use estrogen therapy to avoid early osteoporosis.[115,117] Running is an insufficient stimulus to counteract the loss of estrogen that occurs with amenorrhea, and few women are willing to undergo the intense gymnastic-like exercise that is necessary to protect bone mass under these conditions.

As emphasized earlier in this section, the foundation for bone health begins early in life. Thus, physical activity that places a load on the bones is essential throughout childhood and the adolescent years. Several studies have demonstrated that adolescents who have stronger muscles through regular exercise also have denser bones, which should translate to a reduced risk of osteoporosis later in life.[115,117,138]

Among older women, researchers have found that a history of lifelong physical activity relates to a greater bone mineral mass and, very importantly, a lowered risk of hip fracture.[131-133] Typically, as people age, both bone density and muscular strength decrease, as shown in Figure 15.27.[117,139] Thus, muscular strength has an important influence on bone mineral density at all sites among women. In other words, if women maintain good muscle strength through intensive exercise, bone density should be better preserved even into old age.[117]

Exercise alone cannot prevent or cure osteoporosis. The American College of Sports Medicine has taken the stance that although "weight-bearing physical activity is essential for the normal development and maintenance of a healthy skeleton . . . exercise cannot be recommended as a substitute for hormone replacement therapy at the time of menopause."[115] In other words, osteoporosis prevention and treatment demand a multifaceted approach.

Exercise has not received enthusiastic support by some authorities as an effective way to treat osteoporosis. Part of the problem has been inadequate research design. The American College of Sports Medicine recommends that five principles be considered when evaluating the success of an exercise program for preventing or treating osteoporosis.[115] These are summarized in Box 15.2. In general, density in a specific bone cannot be expected to increase unless that bone is stressed above normal limits on a long-term, regular basis.

Several studies have shown the value of intensive resistance and weight-bearing training in protecting the skeletons of postmenopausal women.[140-149] In a 1-year study of 39 postmenopausal women, subjects engaged in intensive weight training for 45 minutes, two times a week. The weight trainers improved their strength and muscle mass, and also their bone mineral density when compared to the control subjects[141] (see Figure 15.28). In another 1-year study of postmenopausal women (32 women, 60–72 years of age), subjects walked and jogged and climbed stairs vigorously for 50 minutes a session, three to four times a week. Exercise and estrogen therapy together had the greatest effect on lumbar bone density, with about one third of the improvement due to exercise[140] (see Figure 15.29). These results suggest that the efficacy of estrogen therapy is enhanced by combining it with weight-bearing exercise.

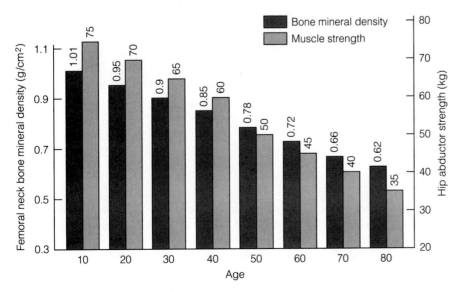

Figure 15.27 Age and bone mineral density and strength in the hip. Typically, as people age, bone density and muscular strength decrease in parallel. *Source:* Snow CM. Exercise and bone mass in young and premenopausal women. *Bone* 18(suppl):51S–55S, 1996.

Box 15.2

ACSM Guidelines on the Prevention and Treatment of Osteoporosis

The ACSM has recommended several guidelines for evaluating the success of an exercise program in preventing or treating osteoporosis.

1. *Principle of specificity.* If the leg bones are stressed by running and jumping, the arm bones will not benefit unless they, too, are stressed with specific exercises (e.g., weight lifting).

2. *Principle of overload.* For a bone to improve its density and strength, the exercise stress must exceed normal levels.

3. *Principle of reversibility.* The positive effect of an exercise program on the skeleton will be lost if the program is stopped.

4. *Principle of initial values.* People with the lowest levels of bone density and strength will experience more improvement from an exercise program than those with normal or above-normal bone density.

5. *Principle of diminishing returns.* Each person has an individual genetic ceiling that limits her or his gains in bone mass. As this ceiling is approached, gains in bone mass will slow and plateau.

Source: American College of Sports Medicine. ACSM position stand on osteoporosis and exercise. *Med Sci Sports Exerc* 27: i–vii, 1995.

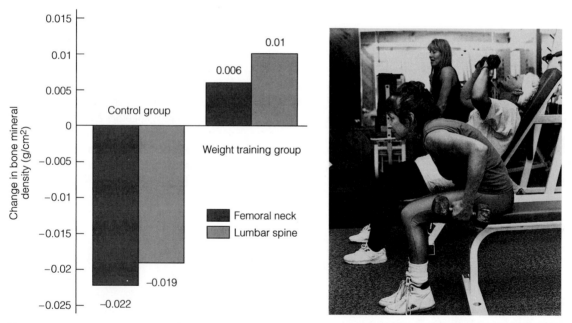

Figure 15.28   Changes in bone mineral density with intensive strength training, 1-year study: two weight-training sessions/week, 45 minutes, high intensity. High-intensity weight training improved bone density in postmenopausal women.   *Source:* Nelson ME, Fiatarone MA, Morganti CM, Trice I, Greenberg RA, Evans WJ. Effects of high-intensity strength training on multiple risk factors for osteoporotic fractures: A randomized controlled trial. *JAMA* 272: 1909–1914, 1994.

One of the chief benefits of regular exercise by the elderly is a decrease in the risk of falling. Falls and the resulting injuries are among the most serious and common medical problems suffered by the elderly. Each year, about 3 in 10 elderly individuals sustain a fall, with 10–15% of falls resulting in serious injuries such as hip fractures.

In its position statement on osteoporosis and exercise, the American College of Sports Medicine has urged that "the optimal program for older women would include activities that improve strength, flexibility, and coordination that may indirectly, but effectively, decrease the incidence of osteoporotic fractures by lessening the likelihood of fall-

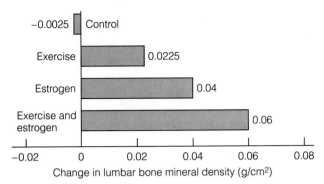

Figure 15.29 Changes in bone with weight-bearing exercise and estrogen, 1-year study: three to four walk/jog/stairclimb sessions/week, 50 minutes/session, high intensity; 32 women, 60–72 years of age. Weight-bearing exercise with estrogen can build lumbar bone density in postmenopausal women. *Source:* Kohrt WM, Snead DB, Slatopolsky E, Birge SJ. Additive effects of weight-bearing exercise and estrogen on bone mineral density in older women. *J Bone Min Res* 10:1303–1311, 1995.

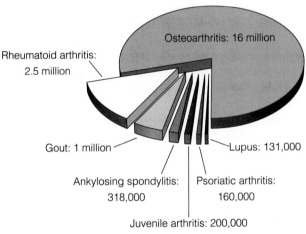

Figure 15.30 Some of the more common of the 100 forms of arthritis and their approximate number of cases in the United States. *Sources:* CDC. Prevalence and impact of arthritis by race and ethnicity—United States, 1989–1991. *MMWR* 45:373–367, 1996; Strange CJ. Coping with arthritis in its many forms. *FDA Consumer*, March 1996, 17–21.

ing."[115] In one large-scale study, researchers studied about 2,300 elderly individuals in six different states and showed that treatments including exercise reduced the risk of falls.[150] In other words, regular weight-bearing and resistance exercise has a twofold benefit for the elderly—an improvement in bone mineral density and a reduced likelihood of falling.

ARTHRITIS

Arthritis and other rheumatic conditions are among the most prevalent chronic conditions in the United States, af-

fecting an estimated 40 million persons in 1995 (one in seven) and a projected 60 million by 2020, according to the Centers for Disease Control and Prevention.[151–153] Women are affected by arthritis more than men—nearly two thirds of people with arthritis are women. Arthritis is the number one cause of disability in America, and it limits everyday activities such as dressing, climbing stairs, getting in and out of bed, or walking, for about 7 million Americans.

Common Types of Arthritis

Arthritis means joint inflammation, a general term that includes over 100 kinds of rheumatic diseases.[152,154,155] Rheumatic diseases are those affecting joints, muscles, and connective tissue, which make up or support various structures of the body. Arthritis is usually chronic and lasts a lifetime. The early warning signs of arthritis include pain, swelling, and limited movement that lasts for more than 2 weeks.

The most common type of arthritis is *osteoarthritis*, affecting more than 16 million Americans and about half of those 65 years of age and older[151–155] (see Figure 15.30). Although this degenerative joint disease is common among the elderly, it may appear decades earlier. Osteoarthritis begins when joint cartilage breaks down, sometimes eroding entirely to leave a bone-on-bone joint. The joint then loses shape, bone ends thicken, and spurs (bony growths) develop. Any joint can be affected, but the feet, knees, hips, and fingers are most common (see Figure 15.31). Osteoarthritis is not fatal, but it is incurable, with few effective treatments. Symptoms of pain and stiffness can persist for long periods of time, leading to difficulty in walking, stair climbing, rising from a chair, transferring in and out of a car, and lifting and carrying.

The second most common form of arthritis is *rheumatoid arthritis*, an autoimmune disease that affects 2.5 million Americans, three times more women than men.[151–154,156] It can strike at any age, but usually appears between ages 20 and 50. Rheumatoid arthritis starts slowly over several weeks to months. The small joints of the hands and the knee joint are most commonly affected, but it can affect most joints of the body. Rheumatoid arthritis is frequently related to severe complications and decline in ability to function, with most patients dying 10–15 years earlier than those who are nonafflicted.

Many joints of the body have a tough capsule lined with a synovial membrane that seals the joint and provides a lubricating fluid. In rheumatoid arthritis, inflammation begins in the synovial lining of the joint and can spread to the entire joint. The inflamed joint lining leads to damage of the bone and cartilage. The space between joints diminishes, and the joint loses shape and alignment (see Figure 15.31). The disease is highly variable (some patients become bed-

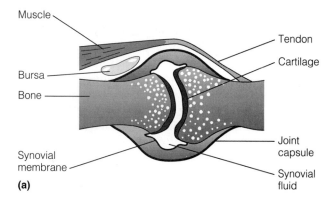

(a)

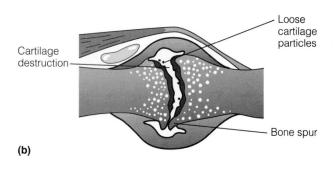

(b)

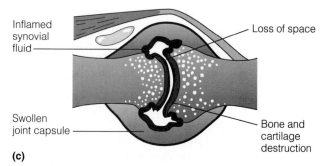

(c)

Figure 15.31 A comparison between a normal joint and joints with arthritis. (a) *Normal joint:* In a normal joint (where two bones come together), the muscle, bursa, and tendon support the bone and aid movement. The synovial membrane (an inner lining) releases a slippery fluid into the joint space. Cartilage covers the bone ends, absorbing shocks and keeping the bones from rubbing together when the joint moves. (b) *Osteoarthritis:* In osteoarthritis, cartilage breaks down and the bones rub together. The joint then loses shape and alignment. Bone ends thicken, forming spurs (bony growths). Bits of cartilage or bone float in the joint space. (c) *Rheumatoid arthritis:* In rheumatoid arthritis, inflammation accompanies thickening of the synovial membrane or joint lining, causing the whole joint to look swollen due to swelling in the joint capsule. The inflamed joint lining enters and damages bone and cartilage, and inflammatory cells release an enzyme that gradually digests bone and cartilage. Space between bones diminishes, and the joint loses shape and alignment. *Source:* Strange CJ. Coping with arthritis in its many forms. *FDA Consumer,* March 1996, 17–21.

ridden, others can run marathons) and difficult to control, and it can severely deform joints.

Other common types of arthritis include *gout* (a metabolic disorder leading to high uric acid and crystal formation in joints), *ankylosing spondylitis* (inflammatory disease of the spine that can result in fused vertebrae and rigid spine), *juvenile arthritis* (involving 200,000 American children), *psoriatic arthritis* (affects about 5% of people with psoriasis, a chronic skin disease), and *systemic lupus erythematosus* (symptoms usually appear in women of childbearing age).[152,154]

Treatment

The key to treatment of arthritis is early diagnosis and a plan individualized to the needs of each patient.[152,154–156] Therapeutic treatment of arthritis has four major goals: easing of pain, decrease of painful inflammation, improvement in function, and lessening of joint damage. Most treatment programs include a combination of patient education, medication, exercise, rest, use of heat and cold, joint protection techniques, and sometimes surgery (for example, total hip replacement surgery). Total hip arthroplasty (THA) is commonly used to treat severe osteoarthritis of the hip, with more than 120,000 such operations performed each year in the United States.[157]

The American College of Rheumatology guidelines advise that treatment include[154]

- *Lifestyle changes*—exercise to strengthen muscles, weight loss to reduce stress on joints, and assistive devices such as canes and wall bars when needed

- *Pain management*—physical therapy, acetaminophen as first-line therapy, and prescription drugs or surgery for more severe pain

- *Patient education*—to inform patients about the disease, provide tools to help overcome pain and help them adjust to their situation

Arthritis symptoms come and go, with a worsening or reappearance of the disease called a *flare*. This can be followed by a remission period that brings welcome relief. The normal up-and-down nature of this painful, incurable disease has led to widespread fraud and quackery.[154] People with arthritis spend nearly a billion dollars a year on unproven remedies, largely diets and supplements. Arthritis patients have been lured by an astounding array of quack devices, including copper or magnetic bracelets, "electronic" mechanisms, vibrating chairs, pressurized enema devices, snake venom, and countless nutritional supplements, including cod liver oil, alfalfa, pokeberries, vinegar, iodine, and kelp. While some of these remedies seem harmless, they can become hurtful if they cause people to abandon conventional therapy.

The FDA also cautions that diet has little to do with arthritis.[152] Gout is the only rheumatic disease known to be helped by avoiding certain foods. Regarding diet, the American College of Rheumatology advises that until more data are available, patients should continue to follow balanced and healthy diets, be skeptical of miraculous claims, and avoid elimination diets and fad nutritional practices.

Overweight persons are at high risk of osteoarthritis in the knees, hips, and hands.[158] For example, the heaviest Americans (those in the upper 20% of body weight) have 7–10 times greater risk of developing osteoarthritis of the knee than those of normal weight. Weight control is an important concern for people with arthritis to help decrease the pressure on the knees and hips.

There are many different kinds of drugs used to treat arthritis.[152,154,159] Anti-inflammatory agents generally work by slowing the body's production of prostaglandins, substances that play a role in inflammation. The most familiar anti-inflammatory agent is aspirin, often a good arthritis treatment. Acetaminophen is recommended as a first-line therapy, at doses up to 4,000 milligrams a day. More than a dozen nonsteroidal anti-inflammatory drugs (NSAIDs) are available, most by prescription only, which fight pain and inflammation. The FDA has approved three NSAIDs for over-the-counter marketing: ibuprofen (marketed as Advil, Nuprin, Motrin, and others), naproxen sodium (sold as Aleve), and ketoprofen (marketed as Actron and Orudis). The most potent anti-inflammatories are corticosteroids.

Disease-modifying drugs are also prescribed by doctors to slow rheumatoid arthritis.[152] These drugs are now used early in the course of the illness to slow down disease advancement. Gold salts, penicillamine, methotrexate, hydroxychloroquine, sulfasalazine, and other powerful drugs, often used in combination, are used to help suppress the immune system.

The Role of Exercise

In the past, doctors often advised arthritis patients to rest and avoid exercise.[160–163] Rest remains important, especially during flares, but inactivity can lead to weak muscles, stiff joints, reduced joint range of motion, and decreased energy and vitality. Rheumatologists today routinely advise a balance of physical activity and rest, individualized to meet special patient needs.

Studies have consistently shown that people with arthritis have weaker muscles, less joint flexibility and range of motion, and lower aerobic capacity, compared to those without arthritis.[160] In addition, individuals with arthritis have been found to be at higher risk for several other chronic diseases, including coronary heart disease, diabetes mellitus, and osteoporosis. Thus, it makes sense that a well-rounded physical fitness program may be of benefit to

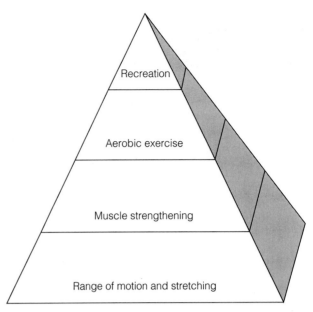

Figure 15.32 Exercise pyramid for patients with arthritis. Exercise treatment for patients with arthritis should be based on the exercise pyramid. *Source:* Hoffman DF. Arthritis and exercise. *Primary Care* 20:895–910, 1993.

those suffering from arthritis. Prior to initiating an exercise program, however, each patient should have an extensive evaluation to assess the severity and extent of joint involvement, presence of systemic involvement, overall functional capacity, and presence of other medical conditions that may interfere with exercise.[161]

Individuals with arthritis will often respond to their pain by limiting their physical activity.[164] Over time, this leads to loss of muscle strength and endurance, which further weakens the joints and sets up a vicious cycle that accelerates arthritis. There are three objectives of exercise for patients with arthritis:[162]

- Preserve or restore range of motion and flexibility around each affected joint
- Increase muscle strength and endurance to enhance joint stability
- Increase aerobic conditioning to improve psychological mood state and decrease risk of disease

As depicted in Figure 15.32, the exercise program should be organized according to the "exercise pyramid," with exercises to develop joint range of motion and flexibility providing the foundation.[160]

- *Range of motion and stretching exercises.* Maintaining joint mobility is very important for all patients with arthritis. Loss of joint range of motion results in a tightening of surrounding tendons, muscles, and other tissues. Acutely inflamed joints should be put through gentle range-of-motion exercises several times per day, with the assistance of a therapist or trained family member. Overzealous stretching or improper technique can have harmful effects on a joint, especially if it is inflamed or is unstable. Utilizing a trained therapist to initially monitor and teach the patient proper technique is recommended. Once the joints become less inflamed, the patient can gradually build up to several sets of 10 repetitions daily of stretching and range-of-motion exercises.

- *Muscle strengthening.* Both isometric and isotonic strengthening exercises are recommended. Isometric exercises can build muscle strength without adverse effects on an acutely inflamed joint. Isotonic exercises (e.g., weight lifting, calisthenics) allow the joints to move through a limited or full range of motion while the muscles are contracting. This type of exercise is recommended when pain and joint inflammation have been controlled and sufficient strength has been achieved through isometric exercise.

- *Aerobic exercise.* In the past, the treatment of arthritis has often excluded aerobic exercise, for fear of increasing joint inflammation and accelerating the disease process. Aerobic exercise, however, has been demonstrated to be a safe and effective treatment for patients who are not in acute flares. Low-impact activities such as swimming, water aerobics, walking, bicycling, low-impact dance aerobics, and rowing can improve aerobic fitness without negatively affecting arthritis. Patients should start with 10–15 minutes of aerobic activity every other day, gradually progressing toward near-daily activity of 30–45 minutes duration at a moderate-to-somewhat-hard intensity. Each aerobic session should begin and end with range-of-motion exercises.

- *Recreational exercise.* Patients with arthritis commonly find golfing, gardening, hiking on gentle terrain, and other hobbies requiring physical activity enjoyable. Many organizations, including the Arthritis Foundation and PACE (People with Arthritis Can Exercise), offer aquatic exercise classes or other group activities. Patients may experience improvements in both fitness and psychological mood state as they engage in group recreational activities.

There are many potential benefits of exercise for the individual with arthritis:[160-163]

- Improvement in joint function and range of motion
- Increase in muscular strength and aerobic fitness to enhance daily activities of living
- Elevation of psychological mood state
- Decrease in loss of bone mass

- Decrease in risk of heart disease, diabetes, hypertension, and other chronic diseases

Can regular exercise improve, retard the progression of, or even cure arthritis? Most researchers who have studied this question now answer, "No."[165-175] While exercise for people with arthritis is important for all the aforementioned reasons, investigators have typically found that exercise training does not improve arthritis, but neither does it worsen the disease process. In other words, exercise does not affect the underlying disease state in people with arthritis one way or the other, but it does improve many other areas of importance to life quality.

In one study, researchers randomly divided 102 patients with osteoarthritis of the knee into walking and control groups.[169] Those in the walking group walked up to 30 minutes, three times a week, for 8 weeks. As shown in Figure 15.33, the walkers experienced a strong increase in their performance during a 6-minute walking test, an effect that was achieved without exacerbating pain or triggering flares. In other words, those with osteoarthritis became fitter with the exercise program, but their disease was neither reversed nor progressed.

In another study, elderly subjects with a history of mild-to-moderate arthritis were divided into four groups: (1) strength training (two sets and 10 reps of eight different weight-machine exercises, 3 days a week), (2) stationary cycle training (35 minutes at 60–75% intensity, 3 days a week), (3) both strength and cycle training, and (4) controls.[165] After 6 months of training, strength improved significantly in all exercise groups, but especially in those who worked out on the weight machines. Joint pain symptoms did not improve or worsen in any group.

In the 18-month FAST (Fitness Arthritis and Seniors Trial) study, 439 adults age 60 years or older, with osteo-

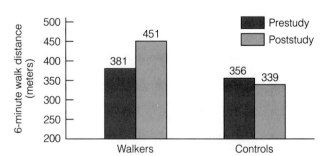

Figure 15.33 Supervised fitness walking in patients with osteoarthritis of the knee, 47 walkers compared to 45 controls after 8 weeks of training (three sessions/week, 90 minutes/session). Exercise training improves walking performance in patients with knee osteoarthritis. *Source:* Kovar PA, Allegrante JP, MacKenzie R, Peterson MGE, Gutin B, Charlson ME. Supervised fitness walking in patients with osteoarthritis of the knee. *Ann Intern Med* 116:529–534, 1992.

arthritis, were randomly divided into one of three groups: (1) health education (no exercise), (2) aerobic exercise (three 40-minute sessions per week), or (3) resistance exercise (three 40-minute sessions per week, with two sets of 12 repetitions of nine exercises).[167] As shown in Figure 15.34, the mean score on the physical disability questionnaire was significantly improved for both exercise groups. Other tests revealed lower pain scores and improved measures of performance with exercise. The researchers concluded that older disabled persons with osteoarthritis of the knee can experience modest improvements in measures of disability, physical performance, and pain as a result of participating in a regular exercise program.

Other researchers have come to the same conclusion: Patients with arthritis are trainable (i.e., they can get stronger and more aerobically fit), and the exercise can be done safely without detrimental effects on the joints.[165–175] However, the results show no effect of training on the disease activity or on the progression of the disease.

Osteoarthritis and Wear and Tear

Some clinicians have defined osteoarthritis as a "wear-and-tear" disease, and fear that high amounts of weight-bearing exercise may increase the risk for osteoarthritis.[176–179] Several important risk factors for osteoarthritis include[160]

- *Increasing age.* By age 75, 85% of people have evidence of osteoarthritis.
- *Joint malalignment.* If the joint is not aligned correctly, a smaller contact area may create stresses that exceed the shock-absorbing capabilities of the joint.

- *Obesity.* Several studies have suggested that obesity increases the risk for osteoarthritis.
- *Repetitive impact to the joint.*

Together, these risk factors and animal studies appear to suggest that osteoarthritis is a wear-and-tear disease. Some animal studies have suggested that animals trained intensely for long time periods have more osteoarthritis.[160] For example, the Husky breed of dogs has increased hip and shoulder arthritis from pulling sleds, while racehorses and workhorses can develop arthritis in their forelegs and hind legs, respectively. Good evidence to confirm these findings in humans is lacking. Earlier studies had suggested that repetitive trauma to joints during work may lead to arthritis. For example, some studies reported increased osteoarthritis in the elbows and knees of miners, the shoulders and elbows of pneumatic drill operators, the hands of cotton workers and diamond cutters, and the spines of dock workers. However, not all of these studies were carried out to contemporary standards, nor have they been confirmed through replication.[160]

Many athletic endeavors place tremendous stress on joints. Baseball, football, basketball, gymnastics, soccer, wrestling, and ballet dancing have each been studied for their effect on osteoarthritis.[176–179] There are many anecdotal reports of famous athletes developing arthritis. Los Angeles Dodger Sandy Koufax, for example, was forced to retire from pitching in 1966 because of an arthritic elbow. However, most experts now feel that participation in vigorous exercise and sports does not increase the risk of osteoarthritis unless the involved joint has some sort of abnormality or previous major injury.[179] Normal joints are well designed to withstand the repetitive stress that comes with physical

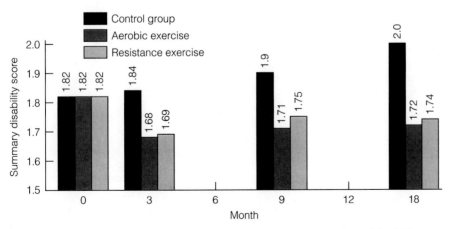

Figure 15.34 Influence of aerobic exercise and resistance exercise on physical disability, 18-month study of 365 older adults with knee osteoarthritis. Physical disability symptoms are reduced in adults with knee osteoporosis who exercise regularly. *Source:* Ettinger WH, Burns R, Messier SP, et al. A randomized trial comparing aerobic exercise and resistance exercise with a health education program in older adults with knee osteoarthritis: The fitness arthritis and seniors trial (FAST). *JAMA* 277: 25–31, 1997.

SPORTS MEDICINE INSIGHT

A Case Study of Mavis Lindgren

The author has been gathering data on Mavis Lindgren, an elderly marathon runner, since 1985. Mavis was sedentary most of her life until age 63, when she began walking for her health. After a few months of slow progression, she started jogging 25–30 miles a week, a routine she faithfully kept for 7 years.

At the age of 70, in response to a challenge laid down by her physician son, she increased her training to 40–50 miles per week and ran her first marathon. Mavis found that she enjoyed the challenge of marathon running and the attention it brought her. Between the ages of 70 and 90, she ran 76 marathons and maintained a training distance of 40–50 miles a week. During this time, she became the oldest woman ever to race to the top of Pike's Peak in Colorado and to finish the New York City marathon.

Figure 15.35 plots the race times for these marathons, as well as the results of 11 treadmill $\dot{V}O_{2max}$ tests that were conducted on Mavis between the ages of 77 and 90. There are several interesting points to be made, especially considering the information in this chapter.

- Between the ages of 80 and 83, Mavis's $\dot{V}O_{2max}$ fell rapidly and then plateaued, despite maintaining a training schedule of 40–50 miles a week. $\dot{V}O_{2max}$ decreased 44% between the ages of 77 and 90, which occurred during a period when her marathon race times increased by about 80%. There are

probably several reasons explaining this loss of aerobic fitness and racing ability, including effects due to the aging process itself and a decline in ability to sustain a high training intensity despite unusually high motivation.

- Between the ages of 77 and 80, her $\dot{V}O_{2max}$ averaged about 38 ml . kg^{-1} . min^{-1}, an aerobic fitness level equal to that of untrained women in their 20s. Despite significant decreases in her aerobic power since age 77, Mavis still has the $\dot{V}O_{2max}$ of a woman about 25 years younger than herself.

Mavis has demonstrated that it is never too late to start exercising, and that an unusually high $\dot{V}O_{2max}$ is possible even in old age when there is a motivation to engage in large amounts of exercise.

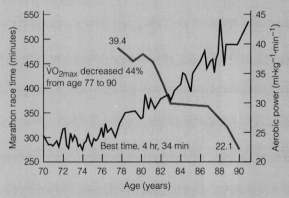

Figure 15.35   Mavis Lindgren's marathon times and aerobic power, 76 marathons from age 70 to 90; first treadmill test age 77, trained 40–50 miles/week each year since age 70. Mavis Lindgren ran 76 marathons between the ages of 70 and 90. Her race times slowed about 80% during a period in which her measured aerobic power fell 44%.

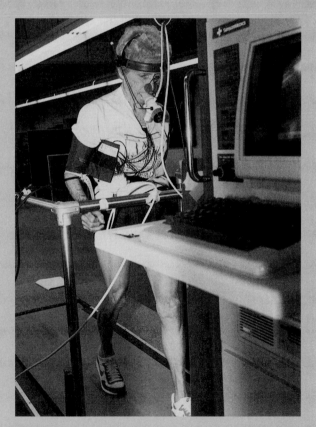

At the age of 80, Mavis Lindgren had the $\dot{V}O_{2max}$ capacity of a woman nearly 60 years younger than herself.

activity. Nonetheless, an injury to the joint alters its ability to handle exercise stress. Several studies of athletes with major knee injuries, for example, have shown that they are at increased risk of premature osteoarthritis.[179]

Long-distance runners have been studied more than any other type of athlete because of the long-term and repetitive stress they experience to joints of their legs. During running, two and one-half to three times the body weight is transmitted to the lower limbs at heel strike. The stresses that the feet and ankles do not absorb are shifted to the knees, hips, and spine. Despite the repetitive stress to their feet and legs, long-distance runners who train for many years do not appear to be at increased risk of osteoarthritis unless they have abnormal biomechanical problems or prior injuries in the hips, knees, or ankles.[177,178]

The injury rate among participants in many sports is quite high. Fortunately, most injuries appear to be limited, with no long-term consequences. If the injury leads to long-term joint instability, however, the risk for osteoarthritis climbs sharply.[179]

SUMMARY

1. The ranks of the aged are increasing rapidly, as heart disease and stroke continue to decrease. The fastest-growing minority in the United States today is the elderly.

2. The average baby born today can expect to live to 76 years of age. Increases in life expectancy at birth during the first half of the twentieth century occurred mainly because of reductions in infant mortality, and recently because of decreasing mortality from chronic diseases.

3. Prominent aging-related concerns include the quality of life in old age, the high prevalence of chronic diseases, osteoporosis, and senile dementia among the elderly, and the financial impact of those problems.

4. *Aging* refers to the normal yet irreversible biological changes that occur during the total years that a person lives. The maximum life span of the human species is thought to be about 120 years. There are several theories of aging, including the damage and the program theories. As a person ages, many changes take place in the body (summarized in the text). Health habits have a major influence on life expectancy.

5. There is great similarity between the physiological changes that accompany aging and those that accompany inactivity. The identifying characteristics of both aging and the disuse syndrome are a decrease in cardiorespiratory function, obesity, musculoskeletal fragility, and (among the inactive) premature aging.

6. Most researchers who have evaluated the effects of aging on the cardiorespiratory system have focused on work capacity, or $\dot{V}O_{2max}$. $\dot{V}O_{2max}$ normally declines 8–10% per decade for both males and females after 25 years of age.

7. Declining physical activity and changes in body composition are responsible in part for the low $\dot{V}O_{2max}$ in old age.

8. The elderly can recapture decades worth of $\dot{V}O_{2max}$ with appropriate (gradual) training.

9. The data suggest that the overall rate of loss of cardiorespiratory function is similar for active and inactive people, but that at any given age, the active conserve more function.

10. Several studies suggest that the elderly can respond to physical training over an 8- to 26-week period in a manner expected of younger people.

11. In general, the same basic exercise prescription principles used for younger adults can be applied for the elderly, but with greater caution and slower progression.

12. Regular physical activity can have a beneficial impact on life expectancy by reducing the life-shortening effects of the various chronic diseases.

13. Osteoporosis is characterized by decreased bone mass and increased susceptibility to fractures. The mainstays of treatment include estrogen replacement, adequate lifelong calcium intake, and appropriate exercise.

14. Weightlessness and bed rest can cause a dramatic loss in bone mass. Cross-sectional studies show that athletes have denser bones than sedentary people. Some studies show that postmenopausal women can retard bone mineral mass loss, or even increase bone density, with appropriate exercise, especially resistance training.

15. Arthritis (joint inflammation) includes over 100 kinds of rheumatic diseases. The two most common are osteoarthritis and rheumatoid arthritis.

16. Based on existing research, professionals recommend a comprehensive physical fitness program designed to improve joint range of motion and flexibility, muscular strength and endurance, and aerobic endurance, all of which are individualized to the patient's special needs and goals. This program is safe and effective and improves quality of life but does not cure arthritis.

REFERENCES

1. Institute of Medicine, Division of Health Promotion and Disease Prevention. *The Second Fifty Years: Promoting Health and Preventing Disability.* Washington, DC: National Academy Press, 1990.

2. Geographic profile of the aged. *Stat Bull* 74(1):2–9, 1993.

3. National Center for Health Statistics. *Vital Statistics of the United States, 1993, Life Tables.* Hyattsville, MD: Author, 1997.

4. Van Nostrand JF, Furner SE, Suzman R, eds. Health data on older Americans: United States, 1992, National Center for Health Statistics. *Vital Health Stat* 3(27), 1993.

5. National Center for Health Statistics. *Healthy People 2000 Review, 1997.* Hyattsville, MD: Public Health Service, 1997.

6. National Center for Health Statistics. *Health, United States, 1996–97 and Injury Chartbook.* Hyattsville, MD: Author, 1997.

7. Hoffman C, Rice D, Sung HY. Persons with chronic conditions: Their prevalence and costs. *JAMA* 276:1473–1479, 1996.

8. Manton KG, Corder L, Stallard E. Chronic disability trends in elderly United States populations: 1982–1994. *Proc Natl Acad Sci USA* 94:2593–2598, 1997.

9. Lubitz J, Beebe J, Baker C. Longevity and medicare expenditures. *N Engl J Med* 332:999–1003, 1995.

10. Small GW, Rabins PV, Barry PP, et al. Diagnosis and treatment of Alzheimer disease and related disorders. *JAMA* 278:1363–1371, 1997.

11. Willcox SM, Himmelstein DU, Woolhandler S. Inappropriate drug prescribing for the community-dwelling elderly. *JAMA* 272:292–296, 1994.

12. Banks DA, Fossel M. Telomeres, cancer, and aging: Altering the human life span. *JAMA* 278:1345–1348, 1997.

13. Baker GT, Martin GR. Biological aging and longevity: Underlying mechanisms and potential intervention strategies. *J Aging Phys Act* 2:304–328, 1994.

14. Kirkwood TBL. Comparative life spans of species: Why do species have the life spans they do? *Am J Clin Nutr* 55:1191S–1195S, 1992.

15. Schiffman SS. Taste and smell losses in normal aging and disease. *JAMA* 278:1357–1362, 1997.

16. Morley JE. Anorexia of aging: Physiologic and pathologic. *Am J Clin Nutr* 66:760–773, 1997.

17. Shephard RJ. Nutrition and the physiology of aging. In Young EA (ed), *Nutrition, Aging, and Health.* New York: Alan R. Liss, Inc., 1986.

18. Russell RM. Changes in gastrointestinal function attributed to aging. *Am J Clin Nutr* 55:1203S–1207S, 1992.

19. Vaughan L, Zurlo F, Ravussin E. Aging and energy expenditure. *Am J Clin Nutr* 53:821–825, 1991.

20. Bernarducci MP, Owens NJ. Is there a fountain of youth? A review of current life extension strategies. *Pharmacotherapy* 16:183–200, 1996.

21. Cefalu WT, Wagner JD, Wang ZQ, et al. A study of caloric restriction and cardiovascular aging in cynomolgus monkeys: A potential model for aging research. *J Gerontol Biol Sci* 52A:B10–B19, 1997.

22. LaCroix AZ, Guralnik JM, Berkman LF, Wallace RB, Satterfield S. Maintaining mobility in late life: II. Smoking, alcohol consumption, physical activity, and body mass index. *Am J Epidemiol* 137:858–869, 1993.

23. Campbell AJ, Busby WJ, Robertson MC. Over 80 years and no evidence of coronary heart disease: Characteristics of a survivor group. *J Am Geriatr Soc* 41:1333–1338, 1993.

24. Black JS, Kapoor W. Health promotion and disease prevention in older people: Our current state of ignorance. *JAGS* 38:168–172, 1990.

25. Breslow L, Breslow N. Health practices and disability: Some evidence from Alameda county. *Prev Med* 22:86–95, 1993.

26. Kaplan GA, Seeman TE, Cohen RD, Knudsen LP, Guralnik J. Mortality among the elderly in the Alameda county study: Behavioral and demographic risk factors. *Am J Public Health* 77(3):307–312, 1987.

27. Belloc NB, Breslow L. Relationship of physical health status and health practices. *Prev Med* 1:409, 1972. See also *Prev Med* 9:469, 1980.

28. Enstrom JE, Kanim LE, Breslow L. The relationship between vitamin C intake, general health practices, and mortality in Alameda county, California. *Am J Public Health* 76:1124–1130, 1986.

29. Paffenbarger RS, Lee IM. Physical activity and fitness for health and longevity. *Res Quart Exerc Sport* 67(suppl):11–28, 1996.

30. Mazzeo RS, Cavanagh P, Evans WJ, Fiatarone M, Hagberg J, McAuely E, Startzell J. Position stand from the American College of Sports Medicine: Exercise and physical activity for older adults. *Med Sci Sports Exerc* (in press).

31. Yusuf HR, Croft JB, Giles WH, Anda RF, Casper ML, Caspersen CJ, Jones DA. Leisure-time physical activity among older adults: United States, 1990. *Arch Intern Med* 156:1321–1326, 1996.

32. DiPetro L. The epidemiology of physical activity and physical function in older people. *Med Sci Sports Exerc* 28:596–600, 1996.

33. Shephard RJ, Kavanagh T, Mertens DJ, Qureshi S, Clark M. Personal health benefits of masters athletics competition. *Br J Sports Med* 29:35–40, 1995.

34. Convertino VA, Bloomfield SA, Greenleaf JE. An overview of the issues: Physiological effects of bed rest and restricted physical activity. *Med Sci Sports Exerc* 29:187–190, 1997.

35. Rogers MA, Evans WJ. Changes in skeletal muscle with aging: Effects of exercise training. *Exerc Sports Sci Rev* 21:65–102, 1993.

36. Lane HW, LeBlanc AD, Putcha L, Whitson PA. Nutrition and human physiological adaptations to space flight. *Am J Clin Nutr* 58:583–588, 1993.

37. Bortz WM. The disuse syndrome. *West J Med* 141:691–694, 1984.

38. Heath GW, Hagberg JM, Ehsani AA, Holloszy JO. A physiological comparison of young and older endurance athletes. *J Appl Physiol* 51:634–640, 1981.

39. Nieman DC, Pover NK, Segebartt KS, Arabatzis K, Johnson M, Dietrich SJ. Hematological, anthropometric, and metabolic comparisons between active and inactive healthy old old to very old women. *Ann Sports Med* 5:2–8, 1990.

40. Smith EL, Gilligan C. Health-related fitness of the older adult. In Drury TF (ed), *National Center for Health Statistics: Assessing Physical Fitness and Physical Activity in Population-Based Surveys,* DHHS Pub. No. (PHS) 89-1253. Public Health Service. Washington, DC: U.S. Government Printing Office, 1989.

41. Jackson AS, Beard EF, Wier LT, Ross RM, Stuteville JE, Blair SN. Changes in aerobic power of men, ages 25–70 yr. *Med Sci Sports Exerc* 27:113–120, 1995.

42. Jackson AS, Wier LT, Ayers GW, Beard EF, Stuteville JE, Blair SN. Changes in aerobic power of women, ages 20–64 yr. *Med Sci Sports Exerc* 28:884–891, 1996.

43. Fitzgerald MD, Tanaka H, Tran ZV, Seals DR. Age-related declines in maximal aerobic capacity in regularly exercising vs. sedentary women: A meta-analysis. *J Appl Physiol* 83:160–165, 1997.

44. Joth MJ, Gardner AW, Ades PA, Poehlman ET. Contribution of body composition and physical activity to age related decline in peak $\dot{V}O_{2max}$ in men and women. *J Appl Physiol* 77:647–652, 1994.

45. Warren BJ, Nieman DC, Dotson RG, Adkins CH, O'Donnell KA, Haddock BL, Butterworth DE. Cardiorespiratory responses to exercise training in septuagenarian women. *Int J Sports Med* 14:60–65, 1993.

46. Wells CL, Boorman MA, Riggs DM. Effect of age and menopausal status on cardiorespiratory fitness in masters women runners. *Med Sci Sports Exerc* 24:1147–1154, 1992.

47. Kasch FW, Boyer JL, Van Camp SP, Verity LS, Wallace JP. The effect of physical activity and inactivity on aerobic power in older men (a longitudinal study). *Physician Sportsmed* 18(4): 73–83, 1990.

48. Trappe SW, Costill DL, Vukovich MD, Jones J, Melham T. Aging among elite distance runners: A 22-yr longitudinal study. *J Appl Physiol* 80:285–290, 1996.

49. Pollock ML, Mengelkoch LJ, Graves JE, Lowenthal DT, Limacher MC, Foster C, Wilmore JH. Twenty-year follow-up of aerobic power and body composition of older track athletes. *J Appl Physiol* 82:1508–1516, 1997.

50. Hagerman FC, Fielding RA, Fiatarone MA, Gault JA, Kirkendall DT, Ragg KE, Evans WJ. A 20-yr longitudinal study of Olympic oarsmen. *Med Sci Sports Exerc* 28:1150–1156, 1996.

51. Stevenson ET, Davy KP, Seals DR. Maximal aerobic capacity and total blood volume in highly trained middle-aged and older female endurance athletes. *J Appl Physiol* 77:1691–1696, 1994.

52. Tanaka H, Seals DR. Age and gender interactions in physiological functional capacity: Insight from swimming performance. *J Appl Physiol* 82:846–851, 1997.

53. Green JS, Crouse SF. The effects of endurance training on functional capacity in the elderly: A meta-analysis. *Med Sci Sports Exerc* 27:920–926, 1995.

54. Coggan AR, Abduljalil AM, Swanson SC, et al. Muscle metabolism during exercise in young and older untrained and endurance-trained men. *J Appl Physiol* 75:2125–2133, 1993.

55. Green JS, Crouse SF. Endurance training, cardiovascular function and the aged. *Sports Med* 16:331–341, 1993.

56. Ogawa T, Spina RJ, Martin WH, et al. Effects of aging, sex, and physical training on cardiovascular responses to exercise. *Circulation* 86:494–503, 1992.

57. Rogers MA, Hagberg JM, Martin WH, Ehsani AA, Holloszy JO. Decline in $\dot{V}O_{2max}$ with aging in master athletes and sedentary men. *J Appl Physiol* 68:2195–2199, 1990.

58. Schultz R, Curnow C. Peak performance and age among superathletes: Track and field, swimming, baseball, tennis, and golf. *J Gerontol* 43:P113–120, 1988.

59. Vitiello MV, Wilkinson CW, Merriam GR, et al. Successful 6-month endurance training does not alter insulin-like growth factor-I in healthy older men and women. *J Gerontol Med Sci* 52A:M149–M154, 1997.

60. Carroll JF, Convertino VA, Wood CE, Graves JE, Lowenthal DT, Pollock ML. Effect of training on blood volume and plasma hormone concentrations in the elderly. *Med Sci Sports Exerc* 27:79–84, 1995.

61. MaKrides L, Heigenhauser GJF, Jones NL. High-intensity endurance training in 20- to 30- and 60- to 70-year-old healthy men. *J Appl Physiol* 69:1792–1798, 1990.

62. Hagberg JM, Graves JE, Limacher M, et al. Cardiovascular responses of 70- to 79-yr-old men and women to exercise training. *J Appl Physiol* 66:2589–2594, 1989.

63. Kohrt WM, Malley MT, Coggan AR, et al. Effects of gender, age, and fitness level on response of $\dot{V}O_{2max}$ to training in 60–71 yr olds. *J Appl Physiol* 71:2004–2011, 1991.

64. Poulin MJ, Paterson DH, Govindasamy D, Cunningham DA. Endurance training of older men: Responses to submaximal exercise. *J Appl Physiol* 73:452–457, 1992.

65. Spina RJ, Ogawa T, Kohrt WM, Martin WH, Holloszy JO, Ehsani AA. Differences in cardiovascular adaptations to endurance exercise training between older men and women. *J Appl Physiol* 75:849–855, 1993.

66. Pollock ML, Carroll JF, Graves JE, et al. Injuries and adherence to walk/jog and resistance training programs in the elderly. *Med Sci Sports Exerc* 23:1194–1200, 1991.

67. Zauber N, Zauber A. Hematologic data of healthy very old people. *JAMA* 257:2181–2184, 1987.

68. Aoyagi Y, Shephard RJ. Aging and muscle function. *Sports Med* 14:376–396, 1992.

69. Frontera WR, Hughes VA, Lutz KJ, Evans WJ. A cross-sectional study of muscle strength and mass in 45- to 78-yr-old men and women. *J Appl Physiol* 71:644–650, 1991.

70. Going S, Williams D, Lohman T. Aging and body composition: Biological changes and methodological issues. *Exerc Sport Sci Rev* 23:411–455, 1995.

71. Phillips WT, Haskell WL. "Muscular fitness"—easing the burden of disability for elderly adults. *J Aging Phys Act* 3: 261–289, 1995.

72. Guralnik JM, Ferrucci L, Simonsick EM, Salive ME, Wallace RB. Lower-extremity function in persons over the age of 70 years as a predictor of subsequent disability. *N Engl J Med* 332: 556–561, 1995.

73. Morganti CM, Nelson ME, Fiatarone MA, Dallal GE, Economos CD, Crawford BM, Evans WJ. Strength improvements with 1 yr of progressive resistance training in older women. *Med Sci Sports Exerc* 27:906–912, 1995.

74. Hurley BF, Redmond RA, Pratley RE, Treuth MS, Rogers MA, Goldberg AP. Effects of strength training on muscle hypertrophy and muscle cell disruption in older men. *Int J Sports Med* 16:378–384, 1995.

75. Brown AB, McCartney N, Sale DG. Positive adaptations to weight-lifting training in the elderly. *J Appl Physiol* 69: 1725–1733, 1990.

76. Fiatarone MA, Marks EC, Ryan ND, Meredith CN, Lipsitz LA, Evans WJ. High-intensity strength training in nonagenarians. *JAMA* 263:3029–3034, 1990.

77. Grimby G, Aniansson A, Hedberg M, et al. Training can improve muscle strength and endurance in 78- to 84-yr-old men. *J Appl Physiol* 73:2517–2523, 1992.

78. Frontera WR, Meredith CN, O'Reilly KP, et al. Strength con-

ditioning in older men: Skeletal muscle hypertrophy and improved function. *J Appl Physiol* 64:1038–1044, 1988.

79. Going SB, Williams DP, Lohman TG, Hewitt MJ. Aging, body composition, and physical activity: A review. *J Aging Phys Act* 2:38–66, 1994.

80. Pollock ML, Foster C, Knapp D, Rod JL, Schmidt DH. Effect of age and training on aerobic capacity and body composition of master athletes. *J Appl Physiol* 62:725–731, 1987

81. Sarna S, Sahi T, Koskenvuo M, Kaprio J. Increased life expectancy of world class male athletes. *Med Sci Sports Exerc* 25: 237–244, 1993.

82. Blair SN, Kampert JB, Kohl HW, et al. Influences of cardiorespiratory fitness and other precursors on cardiovascular disease and all-cause mortality in men and women. *JAMA* 276: 205–210, 1996.

83. Blair SN, Kohl HW, Barlow CE, et al. Changes in physical fitness and all-cause mortality: A prospective study of healthy and unhealthy men. *JAMA* 273:1093–1098, 1995.

84. Lee IM, Hsieh CC, Paffenbarger RS. Exercise intensity and longevity in men: The Harvard alumni health study. *JAMA* 273:1179–1184, 1995.

85. Lee IM, Paffenbarger RS. Do physical activity and physical fitness avert premature mortality? *Exerc Sports Sci Rev* 24: 135–169, 1996.

86. Lissner L, Bengtsson C, Björkelung C, Wedel H. Physical activity levels and changes in relation to longevity: A prospective study of Swedish women. *Am J Epidemiol* 143:54–62, 1996.

87. Paffenbarger PS, Hyde RT, Wing AL, et al. Physical activity, all-cause mortality, and longevity of college alumni. *N Engl J Med* 314:605–613, 1986.

88. Paffenbarger RS, Hyde RT, Wing AL, Lee I-M, Jung DL, Kampert JB. The association of changes in physical-activity level and other lifestyle characteristics with mortality among men. *N Engl J Med* 328:538–545, 1993.

89. Kushi LH, Fee RM, Folsom AR, Mink PJ, Anderson KE, Sellers TA. Physical activity and mortality in postmenopausal women. *JAMA* 277:1287–1292, 1997.

90. Johnston CC, Slemenda CW. Pathogenesis of osteoporosis. *Bone* 17:19S–22S, 1995.

91. National Institutes of Health, Consensus Conference. Osteoporosis. *JAMA* 252:799–802, 1984.

92. Riggs BL, Melton LJ. The prevention and treatment of osteoporosis. *N Engl J Med* 327:620–627, 1992.

93. Ross PD. Osteoporosis: Frequency, consequences, and risk factors. *Arch Intern Med* 156:1399–1411, 1996.

94. Fässler AL, Bonjour JP. Osteoporosis as a pediatric problem. *Pediatr Clin N Am* 42:811–824, 1995.

95. Wolinsky FD, Fitzgerald JF, Stump TE. The effect of hip fracture on mortality, hospitalization, and functional status: A prospective study. *Am J Public Health* 87:398–403, 1997.

96. Scientific Advisory Board, Osteoporosis Society of Canada. Clinical practice guidelines for the diagnosis and management of osteoporosis. *Can Med Assoc J* 155:1113–1133, 1996.

97. Recker RR, Davies M, Hinders SM, et al. Bone gain in young adult women. *JAMA* 268:2403–2408, 1992

98. Melton LJ, Kan SH, Wahner HW, Riggs BL. Lifetime fracture risk: An approach to hip fracture risk assessment based on bone mineral density and age. *J Clin Epidemiol* 41:985–994, 1988.

99. Cauley JA, Lucas LL, Kuller LH, Vogt MT, Browner WS, Cum- mings SR. Bone mineral density and risk of breast cancer in older women: The study of osteoporotic fractures. *JAMA* 276: 1404–1408, 1996.

100. Schneider DL, Barrett-Connor EL, Morton DJ. Timing of postmenopausal estrogen for optimal bone mineral density: The Rancho Bernardo study. *JAMA* 277:543–547, 1997.

101. Meyer HE, Pedersen JI, Løken EB, Tverdal A. Dietary factors and the incidence of hip fracture in middle-aged Norwegians. *Am J Epidemiol* 145:117–123, 1997.

102. Cummings SR, Nevitt MC, Browner WS, et al. Risk factors for hip fracture in white women. *N Engl J Med* 332:767–773, 1995.

103. Ensrud KE, Cauley J, Lipschutz R, Cummings SR. Weight change and fractures in older women. *Arch Intern Med* 157: 857–863, 1997.

104. Kritz-Silverstein D, Barrett-Connor E. Early menopause, number of reproductive years, and bone mineral density in postmenopausal women. *Am J Public Health* 83:983–988, 1993.

105. Col NF, Eckman MH, Karas RH, et al. Patient-specific decisions about hormone replacement therapy in postmenopausal women. *JAMA* 277:1140–1147, 1997.

106. Hollenbach KA, Barrett-Connor E, Edelstein SL, Holbrook T. Cigarette smoking and bone mineral density in older men and women. *Am J Public Health* 83:1265–1270, 1993.

107. Hernandez-Avila M, Colditz GA, Stampfer MJ, et al. Caffeine, moderate alcohol intake, and risk of fractures of the hip and forearm in middle-aged women. *Am J Clin Nutr* 54:157–163, 1991.

108. Lloyd T, Andon MB, Rollings N, et al. Calcium supplementation and bone mineral density in adolescent girls. *JAMA* 270: 841–844, 1993.

109. Reid IR, Ames RW, Evans MC, Gamble GD, Sharpe SJ. Effect of calcium supplementation on bone loss in postmenopausal women. *N Engl J Med* 328:460–464, 1993.

110. Chapuy MC, Arlot ME, Duboeuf F, et al. Vitamin D3 and calcium to prevent hip fractures in elderly women. *N Engl J Med* 327:1637–1642, 1992.

111. Dawson-Hughes B, Harris SS, Krall EA, Dallal GE. Effect of calcium and vitamin D supplementation on bone density in men and women 65 years of age and older. *N Engl J Med* 337: 670–676, 1997.

112. Karpf DB, Shapiro DR, Seeman E, et al. Prevention of nonvertebral fractures by alendronate: A meta-analysis. *JAMA* 277:1159–1164, 1997.

113. Cauley JA, Lucas LL, Kuller LH, Vogt MT, Browner WS, Cum- mings SR. Bone mineral density and risk of breast cancer in older women: The study of osteoporotic fractures. *JAMA* 276: 1404–1408, 1996.

114. Drinkwater BL. Physical fitness, activity and osteoporosis. In Bouchard C, Shephard RJ (eds), *Exercise, Fitness, and Health: A Consensus of Current Knowledge*. Champaign, IL: Human Kinetics, 1994.

115. American College of Sports Medicine. ACSM position stand on osteoporosis and exercise. *Med Sci Sports Exerc* 27:i–vii, 1995.

116. Bailey DA, Faulkner RA, McKay HA. Growth, physical activity, and bone mineral acquisition. *Exerc Sports Sci Rev* 24: 233–263, 1996.

117. Snow CM. Exercise and bone mass in young and premenopausal women. *Bone* 18(suppl):51S–55S, 1996.

118. Snow-Harter C, Marcus R. Exercise, bone mineral density, and osteoporosis. *Exerc Sport Sci Rev* 19:351–388, 1991.

119. Chilibeck PD, Sale DG, Webber CE. Exercise and bone mineral density. *Sports Med* 19:103–122, 1995.

120. Zernicke RF, Vailas AC, Salem GJ. Biomechanical response of bone to weightlessness. *Exerc Sports Sci Rev* 18:167–192, 1990.

121. Bloomfield SA. Changes in musculoskeletal structure and function with prolonged bed rest. *Med Sci Sports Exerc* 29:197–206, 1997.

122. Bailey DA, McCulloch RG. Bone tissue and physical activity. *Can J Sport Sci* 15:229–239, 1990.

123. Edelstein SL, Barrett-Connor E. Relation between body size and bone mineral density in elderly men and women. *Am J Epidemiol* 138:160–169, 1993.

124. Dook JE, James C, Henderson NK, Price RI. Exercise and bone mineral density in mature female athletes. *Med Sci Sports Exerc* 29:291–296, 1997.

125. Lee EJ, Long KA, Risser WL, Poindexter HBW, Gibbons WE, Goldzieher J. Variations in bone status of contralateral and regional sites in young athletic women. *Med Sci Sports Exerc* 27:1354–1361, 1995.

126. Dyson K, Blimkie CJR, Davison KS, Webber CE, Adachi JD. Gymnastic training and bone density in pre-adolescent females. *Med Sci Sports Exerc* 29:443–450, 1997.

127. Hutchinson TM, Whalen RT, Cleek TM, Vogel JM, Arnaud SB. Factors in daily physical activity related to calcaneal mineral density in men. *Med Sci Sports Exerc* 27:745–750, 1995.

128. Nichols DL, Sanborn CF, Bonnick SL, Ben-Ezra V, Gench B, DiMarco NM. The effects of gymnastics training on bone mineral density. *Med Sci Sports Exerc* 26:1220–1226, 1994.

129. Suominen H. Bone mineral density and long term exercise: An overview of cross-sectional athlete studies. *Sports Med* 16:316–330, 1993.

130. Conroy BP, Kraemer WJ, Maresh CM, et al. Bone mineral density in elite junior olympic weightlifters. *Med Sci Sports Exerc* 25:1103–1109, 1993.

131. Greendale GA, Barrett-Connor E, Edelstein S, Ingles S, Haile R. Lifetime leisure exercise and osteoporosis. *Am J Epidemiol* 141:951–959, 1995.

132. Pocock NA, Eisman JA, Yeates MG, et al. Physical fitness is a major determinant of femoral neck and lumbar spine bone mineral density. *J Clin Invest* 78:618–621, 1986.

133. Jaglal SB, Kreiger N, Darlington G. Past and recent physical activity and risk of hip fracture. *Am J Epidemiol* 138:107–118, 1993.

134. Grimston SK, Willows ND, Hanley DA. Mechanical loading regime and its relationship to bone mineral density in children. *Med Sci Sports Exerc* 25:1203–1210, 1993.

135. Pirnay F, Bodeux M, Crielaard JM, Franchimont P. Bone mineral content and physical activity. *Int J Sports Med* 8:331–335, 1987.

136. Micklesfield LK, Lambert EV, Fataar AB, Noakes TD, Myburgh KH. Bone mineral density in mature, premenopausal ultramarathon runners. *Med Sci Sports Exerc* 27:688–696, 1995.

137. Keay N, Fogelman I, Blake G. Bone mineral density in professional female dancers. *Br J Sports Med* 31:143–147, 1997.

138. Nordstrom P, Thorsen K, Nordstrom G, Bergstrom E, Lorentzon R. Bone mass, muscle strength, and different body constitutional parameters in adolescent boys with a low or moderate exercise level. *Bone* 17:351–356, 1995.

139. Aloia JF, Vaswani A, Ma R, Flaster E. To what extent is bone mass determined by fat-free or fat mass? *Am J Clin Nutr* 61:1110–1114, 1995.

140. Kohrt WM, Snead DB, Slatopolsky E, Birge SJ. Additive effects of weight-bearing exercise and estrogen on bone mineral density in older women. *J Bone Min Res* 10:1303–1311, 1995.

141. Nelson ME, Fiatarone MA, Morganti CM, Trice I, Greenberg RA, Evans WJ. Effects of high-intensity strength training on multiple risk factors for osteoporotic fractures: A randomized controlled trial. *JAMA* 272:1909–1914, 1994.

142. Lohman T, Going S, Pamenter R, et al. Effects of resistance training on regional and total bone mineral density in premenopausal women: A randomized prospective study. *J Bone Min Res* 10:1015–1024, 1995.

143. Prince R, Devine A, Dick I, et al. The effects of calcium supplementation (milk powder or tablets) and exercise on bone density in postmenopausal women. *J Bone Min Res* 10:1068–1075, 1995.

144. Kohrt WM, Ehsani AA, Birge SJ. Effects of exercise involving predominantly either joint-reaction or ground-reaction forces on bone mineral density in older women. *J Bone Miner Res* 12:1253–1261, 1997.

145. Sinaki M, Wahner HW, Bergstralh EJ, Hodgson SF, Offord KP, Squires RW, Swee RG, Kao PC. Three-year controlled, randomized trial of the effect of dose-specified loading and strengthening exercises on bone mineral density of spine and femur in nonathletic, physically active women. *Bone* 19:233–244, 1996.

146. Dalsky GP, Stocke KS, Ehsani AA, et al. Weight-bearing exercise training and lumbar bone mineral content in postmenopausal women. *Ann Intern Med* 108:824–828, 1988.

147. Snow-Harter C, Bouxsein ML, Lewis BT, Carter DR, Marcus R. Effects of resistance and endurance exercise on bone mineral status of young women: A randomized exercise intervention trial. *J Bone Miner Res* 7(7):761–769, 1992.

148. Pruitt LA, Jackson RD, Bartels RL, Lehnhard HJ. Weight-training effects on bone mineral density in early postmenopausal women. *J Bone Miner Res* 7(2):179–185, 1992.

149. Prince RL, Smith M, Dick IM, et al. Prevention of postmenopausal osteoporosis: A comparative study of exercise, calcium supplementation, and hormone-replacement therapy. *N Engl J Med* 325:1189–1195, 1991.

150. Province MA, Hadley EC, Hornbrook MC, et al. The effects of exercise on falls in elderly patients: A preplanned meta-analysis of the FICSIT trials. *JAMA* 273:1341–1347, 1995.

151. CDC. Factors associated with prevalent self-reported arthritis and other rheumatic conditions—United States, 1989–1991. *MMWR* 45:487–491, 1996.

152. Strange CJ. Coping with arthritis in its many forms. *FDA Consumer,* March 1996, 17–21.

153. CDC. Prevalence and impact of arthritis by race and ethnicity—United States, 1989–1991. *MMWR* 45:373–376, 1996.

154. Arthritis Foundation. *Arthritis Fact Sheet.* Author, http://www.arthritis.org, 1996.

155. Harris C. Osteoarthritis: How to diagnose and treat the painful joint. *Geriatrics* 48:39–46, 1993.

156. Semble EL. Rheumatoid arthritis: New approaches for its evaluation and management. *Arch Phys Med Rehabil* 76:190–201, 1995.

157. Chang RW, Pellissier JM, Hazen GB. A cost-effectiveness analysis of total hip arthroplasty for osteoarthritis of the hip. *JAMA* 275:858–865, 1996.

158. Felson DT. Weight and osteoarthritis. *Am J Clin Nutr* 63(suppl):430S–432S, 1996.

159. O'Dell JR, Haire CE, Erikson N, et al. Treatment of rheumatoid arthritis with methotrexate alone, sulfasalazine and hydroxychloroquine, or a combination of all three medications. *N Engl J Med* 334:1287–1291, 1996.

160. Hoffman DF. Arthritis and exercise. *Primary Care* 20:895–910, 1993.

161. DiNubile NA. Osteoarthritis: How to make exercise part of your treatment plan. *Physician Sportsmed* 25(7):47–56, 1997.

162. Ytterberg SR, Mahowald ML, Krug HE. Exercise for arthritis. *Baillière's Clin Rheumatol* 8:161–189, 1994.

163. Panush RS. Physical activity, fitness, and osteoarthritis. In Bouchard C, Shephard RJ, Stephens T (eds), *Physical Activity, Fitness, and Health: International Proceedings and Consensus Statement.* Champaign, IL: Human Kinetics, 1994.

164. CDC. Prevalence of leisure-time physical activity among persons with arthritis and other rheumatic conditions—United States, 1990–1991. *MMWR* 46:389–393, 1997.

165. Coleman EA, Buchner DM, Cress ME, Chan BKS, De Lateur BJ. The relationship of joint symptoms with exercise performance in older adults. *J Am Geriatr Soc* 44:14–21, 1996.

166. Ettinger WH, Afable RF. Physical disability from knee osteoarthritis: The role of exercise as an intervention. *Med Sci Sports Exerc* 26:1435–1440, 1994.

167. Ettinger WH, Burns R, Messier SP, et al. A randomized trial comparing aerobic exercise and resistance exercise with a health education program in older adults with knee osteoarthritis: The fitness arthritis and seniors trial (FAST). *JAMA* 277:25–31, 1997.

168. Hochberg MC, Altman RD, Brandt KD. Guidelines for the medical management of knee osteoarthritis. *Arthritis Rheumatology* 38:1541–1546, 1995.

169. Kovar PA, Allegrante JP, MacKenzie R, Peterson MGE, Gutin B, Charlson ME. Supervised fitness walking in patients with osteoarthritis of the knee. *Ann Intern Med* 116:529–534, 1992.

170. Häkkinen A, Häkkinen K, Hannonen P. Effects of strength training on neuromuscular function and disease activity in patients with recent-onset inflammatory arthritis. *Scan J Rheumatol* 23:237–242, 1994.

171. Hanson TM, Hansen G, Langgaard AM, Rasmussen JO. Long-term physical training in rheumatoid arthritis: A randomized trial with different training programs and blinded observers. *Scan J Rheumatol* 22:107–112, 1993.

172. Lyngberg KK, Harreby M, Bentzen H, Frost B, Danneskiold-Samsøe E. Elderly rheumatoid arthritis patients on steroid treatment tolerate physical training without an increase in disease activity. *Arch Phys Med Rehabil* 75:1189–1195, 1994.

173. Noreau L, Moffet H, Drolet M, Parent E. Dance-based exercise program in rheumatoid arthritis: feasibility in individuals with American College of Rheumatology functional class III disease. *Am J Phys Med Rehabil* 76:109–113, 1997.

174. Rall LC, Meydani SN, Kehayias JJ, Dawson-Hughes B, Roubenoff R. The effect of progressive resistance training in rheumatoid arthritis: Increased strength without changes in energy balance or body composition. *Arthritis Rheumatol* 39:415–426, 1996.

175. Rintala P, Kettunen H, McCubbin JA. Effects of a water exercise program for individuals with rheumatoid arthritis. *Sports Med Train Rehab* 7:31–38, 1996.

176. Hannan MT, Felson DT, Anderson JJ, Naimark A. Habitual physical activity is not associated with knee osteoarthritis: The Framingham study. *J Rheumatol* 20:704–709, 1993.

177. Lane NE, Michel B, Bjorkengren A, Oehlert J, Shi H, Bloch DA, Fries JF. The risk of osteoarthritis with running and aging: A 5-year longitudinal study. *J Rheumatol* 20:461–468, 1993.

178. Lane NE, Buckwalter JA. Exercise: A cause of osteoarthritis? *Rheumatic Dis Clin N Am* 19:617–633, 1993.

179. Rangger C, Kathrein A, Klestil T, Glotzer W. Partial meniscectomy and osteoarthritis: Implications for treatment of athletes. *Sports Med* 23:61–68, 1997.

PHYSICAL FITNESS ACTIVITY 15.1

Health Check

As reviewed in this chapter, health habits have a significant impact on life expectancy. In this activity, you can conduct a comprehensive review of your health habits to determine your overall risk for mortality. Note the points given by each of your answers, total them, and then apply them to the norms listed at the end of this activity.

Name: _____   Today's Date: _____

Your age? _____ years   Sex: ❑ Male ❑ Female   How tall are you (without shoes)? _____ feet _____ inches

If male ⩾50 yrs or female ⩾55 yrs = 4 points; all others, 0

How much do you weigh (minimal clothing and without shoes)? _____ pounds

Calculate BMI (kg/m²):   *Points*

Points	BMI	Category
2	<16	**Too lean, may have eating disorder**
0	16–19.9	**Lean, underweight**
0	20–24.9	**Desirable**
2	25–29.9	**Mild obesity (may be due to extra muscle mass)**
3	30–40	**Moderate obesity**
4	>40	**Severe obesity**

What is the most you have ever weighed? _____ pounds

If ±20% or more from present weight = 2 points; if within ±20% = 0 points.

Are you NOW trying to: ❑ Lose weight ❑ Gain weight ❑ Stay about the same ❑ Not trying to do anything

If BMI ⩾ 27, and not trying to do anything = 2 points
If BMI ⩾ 27, and trying to stay the same or gain weight = 1 point
If BMI ⩾ 27 and trying to lose = 0 points

Please check the appropriate box for each question.
Yes No

4   0   Points
❑   ❑   1. Has your father or brother had a heart attack or died suddenly of heart disease before age 55 years; has your mother or sister experienced these heart problems before age 65 years?

4   0
❑   ❑   2. Has a doctor told you that you have high blood pressure (more than 140/90 mm Hg), or are you on medication to control your blood pressure?

    OR   2a. If you know your blood pressure, please check the appropriate category:

        0 ❑ Less than 120/80 mm Hg   3 ❑ 140/90 to 159/99   0 ❑ Do not know

        1 ❑ 120/80 to 129/84   4 ❑ 160/100 to 180/110

        2 ❑ 130/85 to 139/89   5 ❑ More than 180/110

Yes No

4   0

☐   ☐   3. Is your total blood cholesterol greater than 240 mg/dl, or has a doctor told you that your cholesterol is at a high risk level?

   OR   3a. If you know your blood cholesterol, please check the appropriate category:

   0 ☐ Less than 160 mg/dl   2 ☐ 200–219   5 ☐ More than 260

   0 ☐ 160–179   3 ☐ 200–239   0 ☐ Do not know

   1 ☐ 180–199   4 ☐ 240–260

4   0

☐   ☐   4. Do you have diabetes?

3   0

☐   ☐   5. During the past year, would you say that you experienced enough stress, strain, and pressure to have a significant effect on your health?

4   0

☐   ☐   6. Do you eat foods nearly every day that are high in fat and cholesterol such as fatty meats, cheese, fried foods, butter, whole milk, ice cream, or eggs?

---

7. In general, compared to other persons your age, rate how healthy you are:

   1 ☐   2 ☐   3 ☐   3 ☐   4 ☐   5 ☐   6 ☐   7 ☐   8 ☐   9 ☐   10 ☐

   Not at all   Somewhat   Extremely
   healthy   healthy   healthy

1,2 = 3 points; 3,4 = 2 points; 5,6,7 = 1 point; 8,9,10 = 0 points

8. Outside of your normal work or daily responsibilities, how often do you engage in exercise that at least moderately increases your breathing and heart rate, and makes you sweat, for at least 20 minutes (such as brisk walking, cycling, swimming, jogging, aerobic dance, stair climbing, rowing, basketball, racquetball, vigorous yard work, etc.)

0 ☐ 5 or more times per week   1 ☐ 3 to 4 times per week   2 ☐ 1 to 2 times per week

3 ☐ Less than 1 time per week   4 ☐ Seldom or never

9. On average, how many servings of fruit and vegetables do you eat per day? (one serving = 1 medium fruit, ½ cup of chopped, cooked, or canned fruit/vegetable, ¾ cup of fruit or vegetable juice).

4 ☐ none   3 ☐ 1–2   2 ☐ 3–4   1 ☐ 5–6   0 ☐ 7–8   0 ☐ 9 or more

10. On average, how many servings of bread, cereal, rice, or pasta do you eat per day? (one serving = 1 slice of bread, 1 ounce of ready-to-eat cereal, ½ cup of cooked cereal, rice, or pasta).

3 ☐ none   3 ☐ 1–2   2 ☐ 3–5   1 ☐ 6–8   0 ☐ 9–11   0 ☐ 12 or more

11. How have you been feeling in general during the past month?

0 ☐ In excellent spirits   1 ☐ In good spirits mostly   2 ☐ In low spirits mostly

0 ☐ In very good spirits   1 ☐ I've been up and down in spirits a lot   3 ☐ In very low spirits

12. On average, how many hours of sleep do you get in a 24-hour period?

2 ☐ Less than 5   1 ☐ 5 to 6.9   0 ☐ 7 to 9   0 ☐ More than 9

13. How would you describe your cigarette smoking habits?

0 ☐ Never smoked

☐ Used to smoke

   How many years has it been since you smoked? (Check appropriate box)

   3 ☐ Less than 1 year   1 ☐ 6–15

   2 ☐ 1–5   0 ☐ More than 15

❏ Still smoke

How many cigarettes a day do you smoke on average?

3 ❏ 1–10   4 ❏ 21–30   5 ❏ More than 40

3 ❏ 11–20   4 ❏ 31–40

14. How many alcoholic drinks do you consume? (A "drink" is a glass of wine, a wine cooler, a bottle/can of beer, a shot glass of liquor, or a mixed drink.)

0 ❏ Never use alcohol   0 ❏ Less than 1 per week   0 ❏ 1 to 6 per week

0 ❏ 1 per day   3 ❏ 2 to 3 per day   4 ❏ More than 3 per day

15. When driving or riding in a car, do you wear a seat belt:

0 ❏ All or most of the time   1 ❏ Some of the time   2 ❏ Once in awhile   3 ❏ Rarely or never

---

Norms

Total Points	Classification
0–7	Excellent health habits
8–15	Good, but some improvement needed
16–24	Fair, improvement needed
25 or more	Poor, at high risk for disease

PHYSICAL FITNESS ACTIVITY 15.2

Osteoporosis—Can It Happen to You?

Learn more about this bone-thinning disease that causes debilitating fractures of the hip, spine, and wrist. Complete the following questionnaire to determine your risk for developing osteoporosis.

Question	Yes	No
1. Do you have a small thin frame, or are you Caucasian or Asian?	_____	_____
2. Do you have a family history of osteoporosis?	_____	_____
3. Are you a postmenopausal woman?	_____	_____
4. Have you had an early or surgically induced menopause?	_____	_____
5. Have you been taking excessive thyroid medication or high doses of cortisone-like drugs for asthma, arthritis, or cancer?	_____	_____
6. Is your diet low in dairy products and other sources of calcium?	_____	_____
7. Are you physically inactive?	_____	_____
8. Do you smoke cigarettes or drink alcohol in excess?	_____	_____

The more times you answer "yes," the greater your risk for developing osteoporosis. See your physician, and contact the National Osteoporosis Foundation for more information.

Source: National Osteoporosis Foundation, 2100 M Street, N.W., Suite 602, Washington, D.C. 20037.

CHAPTER

16

Exercise Risks

The athlete's habit of body neither produces a good condition for the general purposes of civic life, nor does it encourage ordinary health and the procreation of children. Some amount of exertion is essential for the best habit, but it must be neither violent nor specialized, as is the case with the athlete. It should rather be a general exertion, directed to all the activities of a free man.

—Aristotle

The modern-day fitness movement is not yet 30 years old. It was given its first great impetus in 1968, when Kenneth Cooper, a physician for the Air Force, published his book *Aerobics* (see Chapter 1). In this book, Cooper challenged Americans to take personal charge of their lifestyles and counter the "epidemics" of heart disease, obesity, and rising health-care costs. Millions took up the "aerobic challenge" and began jogging, cycling, walking, and swimming their way to better health—thus starting the new fitness revolution.

Americans are now exercising more than at any other time in our modern era. Exercise is suddenly prestigious. With the prestige, however, have come some real problems.

One product of the added prestige is "overzealousness." Excessive exercise appears to be America's newest elixir in that endless search for the "fountain of youth." Some people, allured by the media reports, and perhaps overreacting to health problems, job dissatisfaction, boredom, marital difficulties, and a fear of growing old, have seized on exercise as a panacea. As many recent articles in the medical literature have shown, excessive training has brought a host of problems.[1] This chapter reviews the major risks of carrying exercise too far.

MUSCULOSKELETAL INJURIES

This section places emphasis on running, aerobic dance, bicycling, and swimming, activities that are popular among

Americans, yet have been associated with significant risk for injury when certain conditions are exceeded. Although walking and gardening are the two most prevalent forms of physical activity (see Chapter 1), there are no published reports indicating that these pose a problem as far as injuries are concerned.

Running Injuries

The muscles, joints, and supporting ligaments and tendons of the legs and feet respond very poorly to excessive exercise, especially activities that require running and jumping (see Figure 16.1).

Many studies have explored the relationship between running and musculoskeletal injuries, and several excellent literature reviews are available. More injury information has been gathered on runners than on any other mode of exercise, due in large part to the rate of injury.[2-16]

The Extent of the Problem

Depending on the study, the 1-year injury incidence rate for runners in the general population varies from 24 to 77% or 2.5–12 injuries per 1,000 hours of running.[2,4] One of the earliest studies conducted by the Centers for Disease Control and Prevention evaluated the injury rates for 2,500 male and female runners for 1 year.[6-9] Thirty-seven percent developed orthopedic injuries serious enough to reduce

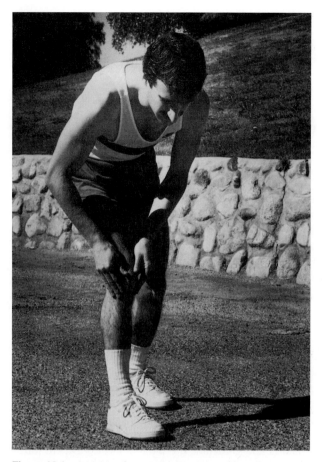

Figure 16.1 Activities that require running and jumping often cause trauma to the muscles, joints, and supporting ligaments and tendons of the legs and feet, especially when done to excess.

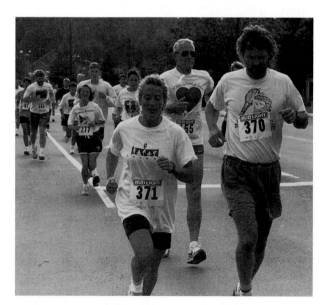

Figure 16.2 According to the Centers for Disease Control and Prevention, the average recreational runner has a one-in-three chance of being injured within any given year.

weekly running mileage. Of these, 38% sought medical consultation for their injuries. The risk of injury increased with weekly running mileage, with 53% injured when running 30–39 miles per week, and 65% injured when running more than 50 miles per week.

Sixty percent of the injuries involved the knee and foot areas. The researchers concluded that the average runner has a one-in-three chance of being injured within any given year, and a one-in-ten likelihood of incurring an injury that will require medical attention (see Figure 16.2). A person running 15 miles a week can count on one injury every 2 years. In a 10-year follow-up study of this cohort of runners, the CDC reported that 53% had at least one injury.[9] As shown in Figures 16.3 and 16.4, injury rates increased with running distance (except for the ≥50 mile/week category), with the knee and foot identified as the most common sites. Almost half of the cohort of runners had quit running, with injury cited as a common cause.[9]

In one of the largest studies ever conducted on running injuries, a study of 4,358 male and 428 female joggers in Switzerland, researchers reported that 45.8% and 40%, respectively, had sustained a jogging injury during the preceding year.[10,11] Because of injuries, one in seven male joggers sought medical treatment, and one out of forty missed work. One in five male runners was forced to fully interrupt his

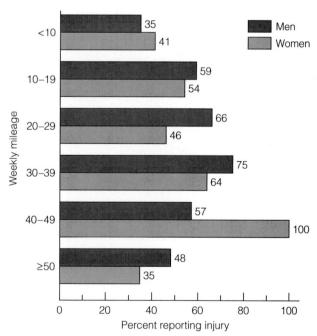

Figure 16.3 Percentage of runners injured by running distance among 326 men and 209 women during 10 years. Except for the highest-mileage runners, injury rates tend to rise with increases in weekly running mileage. *Source:* Koplan JP, Rothenberg RB, Jones EL. The natural history of exercise: A 10-yr follow-up of a cohort of runners. *Med Sci Sports Exerc* 27: 1180–1184, 1995.

exercise routine. Frequency of jogging injuries increased with increase in weekly distance jogged (see Figure 16.5).

Factors Associated with Injuries

Many potential factors have been suggested as influencing risk of injury for runners. These are usually divided into two general categories: personal characteristics of the runner (gender, age, running experience, previous injury, body composition, and psychological factors) and training habits (weekly mileage, frequency, speed, racing activity, warm-up, time of run, stretching, and running surface).[2,15] Of these, the most consistent predictors are excessive weekly running distance, previous injury, lack of running experience, and running to compete[2,4,5,15] (see Figure 16.6). Factors not apparently associated with running injuries are age, gender,

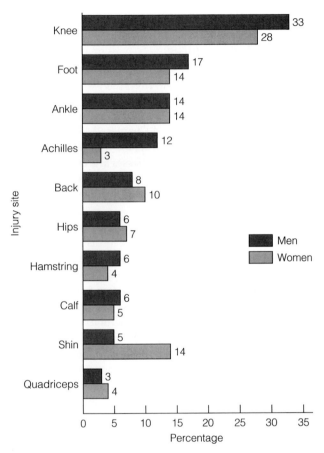

Figure 16.4 Injury sites in runners over a 10-year period among 326 men and 209 women. The knee is the most common site of injury in runners. *Source:* Koplan JP, Rothenberg RB, Jones EL. The natural history of exercise: A 10-yr follow-up of a cohort of runners. *Med Sci Sports Exerc* 27:1180–1184, 1995.

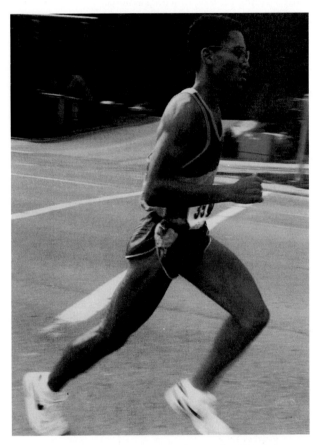

Figure 16.6 The most consistent predictors of running injuries are excessive weekly running distance, previous injury, lack of running experience, and running to compete.

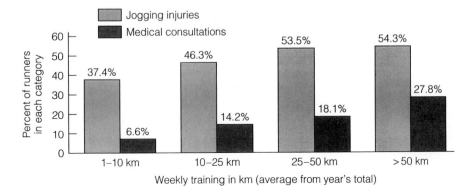

Figure 16.5 Percentage of Swiss male runners injured during previous 12 months. Frequency of jogging injuries and medical consultations as a result of jogging injuries increased according to weekly training distance of Swiss male runners. *Source:* Marti B, Vader JP, Minder CE, Abelin T. On the epidemiology of running injuries. *Am J Sports Med* 16:285–294, 1988.

stretching routines, type of running surface, type of terrain, and speed of training. Although some exercise physiologists have theorized that muscle tightness (lack of flexibility) may be related to injuries, support for this theory is lacking.[17]

Running is a traumatic form of exercise for the musculoskeletal system of the human body. Studies of triathletes have found that relatively few of their injuries involve their bicycling and swimming—most are from running. In one study, 70% of the injuries sustained by 168 triathletes occurred during running practice sessions.[18]

The sudden impact of the foot with the running surface causes a force equal to 2.5 times one's body weight.[15] The human body appears to be able to handle moderate amounts of running, but when running is excessive or when distances are suddenly increased, injuries become common.

The injuries most frequently associated with running are those classified as *overuse syndromes,* especially common among runners who run excessive distances in their training.[19]

Overtraining creates an imbalance between training and recovery.[1,19] It can cause staleness as the physical and emotional stress of the exercise program exceeds the individual's coping capacity (ability to respond to stress) (see Figure 16.7 and Box 16.1 for an overview of the terms and the signs and symptoms associated with overtraining).[1] One of the most effective ways of avoiding overtraining is to follow a well-balanced, progressive training schedule.

The running style (biomechanical factors) and anatomical structure of runners have been associated with running injuries, but the data are far from conclusive.[16,20–23] In one study, 48 trained runners with runner's knee were examined, treated, and followed for 8 months to identify the causes and response to treatment.[22] Most were found to have anatomic malalignment of the lower limb. Sixty-nine

percent were also predisposed to runner's knee because of suddenly increased running distance, hill running, interval training, or racing too often. Other researchers have found that the "Q angle" (the angle at which the femur comes down to the knee) is important in predicting who gets knee pain from running.[20] Other researchers, however, have been unable to establish that lower-extremity alignment is a risk factor for running injuries.[16]

Aerobic-Dance Injuries

Aerobic dance is probably the most popular organized fitness activity for women in the United States, ranking fourth overall in popularity in the United States, for young and old alike (see Figure 16.8 and Chapter 1). Aerobic dance traces its origins to Jacki Sorenson, the wife of a naval pilot, who began conducting exercise classes at a U.S. Navy base in Puerto Rico in 1969.[24] The growth of aerobic dance has been more recently stimulated by the production of videotaped dance exercise programs.

The original aerobic-dance programs consisted of an eclectic combination of various dance forms, including ballet, modern jazz, disco, and folk, as well as calisthenic-type exercises. More recent innovations include water aerobics in a swimming pool, nonimpact or low-impact aerobics (one foot on the ground at all times), specific dance aerobics, step aerobics, and "assisted" aerobics with weights worn on the wrists and/or ankles.

Exercise physiologists were concerned initially that the early aerobic-dance programs were conceived by people with little or no background in medicine, kinesiology, or exercise physiology. In addition, some of the activities and positions utilized in the aerobic-dance programs were potentially injurious. Today, most of the popular videotapes by Jane Fonda, Cindy Crawford, and other models and movie stars are designed using professional consultants who try to keep the various movements safe and within the range of most people.

The early major studies examining the injury potential of aerobic dance found that about 45% of students and 75% of instructors reported injuries.[24–28] Rates of injury for students were about 1 per 100 hours of dancing, and for instructors, about 1 per 400 hours. Most of these injuries, however, were mild, causing some pain and some disruption in participation, but generally not leading participants to stop dancing or to seek professional medical assistance. The lower extremities accounted for about 80% of all injuries.

What factors were associated with increased risk of aerobic-dance injuries? In one study of 1,123 female and 164 male aerobics students, those who exercised more than three times per week, wore improper shoes, and exercised on nonresilient surfaces suffered the most injuries.[28] Appar-

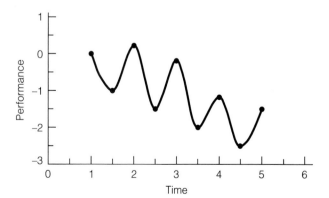

Figure 16.7 Overtraining syndrome. Schematic of training overload resulting in decreased performance. *Source:* Kreider RB, Fry AC, O'Toole ML. *Overtraining in Sport.* Champaign, IL: Human Kinetics, 1998. Reprinted by permission from Human Kinetics.

Box 16.1

Overreaching and Overtraining

Overreaching

Overreaching involves an accumulation of training or nontraining stress, resulting in a *short-term* decrement in performance capacity, with or without related physiological and psychological signs and symptoms of overtraining, in which restoration of performance capacity may take from several days to several weeks.

Overtraining

Overtraining involves an accumulation of training or nontraining stress, resulting in a *long-term* decrement in performance capacity, with or without related physiological and psychological signs and symptoms of overtraining, in which restoration of performance capacity may take several weeks or months.

Signs and Symptoms of Overtraining

Psychosocial

- Apathy
- Lethargy
- Sleep disturbance
- Lowered self-esteem
- Mood changes
- Feelings of depression
- Difficulty in concentrating
- Fear of competition

Performance

- Decreased performance
- Lack of desire to train
- Inability to meet previously attained performance
- Chronic fatigue
- Increased heart rate and RPE at set workload
- Decreased muscular strength
- Reduced toleration of pain during training
- Prolonged recovery following training

Physiological

- Immune suppression, with increased rates of infection
- Depressed muscle glycogen concentration
- Decreased body iron stores
- Elevated cortisol levels
- Decreased testosterone levels
- Loss of appetite and decreased body weight
- Amenorrhea or oligomenorrhea
- Gastrointestinal disturbances

Source: Kreider RB, Fry AC, O'Toole ML. *Overtraining in Sport.* Champaign, IL: Human Kinetics, 1998.

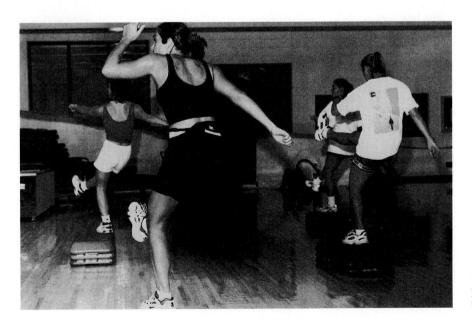

Figure 16.8 Aerobic dance is a popular activity, especially for millions of females.

ently, lower-leg injuries were the result of excessive physical trauma.

Since these studies were published during the mid-1980s, much has been done to reduce the injury risk of aerobic dancing. In particular, aerobic routines have been substituted for the high-impact (jumping and dancing on the balls of the feet) variety. In low-impact dance aerobics, the common denominator is that at least one foot is touching the floor throughout the aerobic portion of the workout. Movements are not ballistic, but focus on large-muscle upper-body and arm movements, combined with leg kicks, high-powered steps, side-to-side movements, and lunges, often with steps or small weights.

Although no large-scale studies have yet been published on the injury risk of low-impact aerobics, there is every reason to believe that it is much lower than during the early history of the aerobic-dance movement.

Bicycling Injuries

Bicyclers also suffer their share of injuries, but they are usually caused by accidents. Actual rates of injuries due to the cycling exercise itself appear to be quite low, although pain in the hands, seat, neck, and back are commonly reported.[29] Among the 96 million cyclists in the United States, there are about 1,000 deaths and 600,000 emergency room visits each year.[30,31] Head injuries account for approximately two thirds of bicycling deaths and bicycle-related hospital admissions. The large increase in off-road or mountain bicycling has increased the need for safety, with injuries reported by 50–90% of participants each year.[32]

Bicycle helmets have been shown to provide substantial protection against head injuries for cyclists of all ages involved in crashes[33] (see Figure 16.9). The Injury Prevention Program of the World Health Organization has been coordinating a worldwide initiative to increase the use of bicycle helmets, and in the United States, there is a push for legislation to mandate their use.[34,35] Also, because helmets are costly ($25 to $65), the requirement of a helmet with new bicycle purchases may prove helpful, especially when combined with legislation and education.

Swimming Injuries

Competitive swimmers may swim 8,000–20,000 yards per day, 5–7 days each week. Shoulder pain is the most common musculoskeletal complaint, usually resulting from supraspinatus or biceps tendonitis and impingement of subacromial tissues.[36,37] Symptoms include point tenderness on the anterior part of the tip of the shoulder. (It is painful to raise the bent arm overhead.) In severe cases, total rest may be necessary to alleviate the pain. Physical therapy may be helpful.

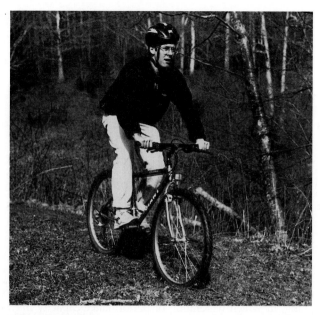

Figure 16.9 Bicycle helmets provide substantial protection against head injuries for cyclists of all ages.

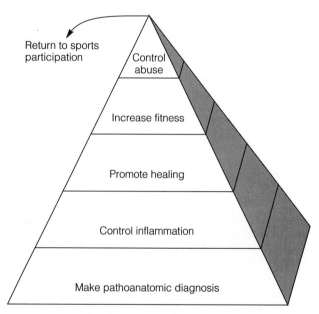

Figure 16.10 Management pyramid for overuse injuries. Management of overuse injuries is organized into five separate phases. *Source:* O'Connor FG, Howard TM, Fieseler CM, Nirschl RP. Managing overuse injuries: A systematic approach. *Physician Sportsmed* 25(5):88–113, 1997.

Knee pain can occur among breaststroke swimmers (involving pain and tenderness in the medial aspect of the knee joint, apparently related to the breaststroke "whip kick").[38] Leg strengthening and flexibility exercises may be helpful, and coaching on proper technique should be emphasized.

However, among competitive swimmers, about three in four breaststroke specialists report a history of "breaststroker's knee," indicating that regardless of technique, the breaststroke kick itself may be too stressful for the average human knee.[38]

Management of Overuse Injuries

Figure 16.10 and Box 16.2 summarize the various steps that can be used in the diagnosis and management of overuse injuries by a multidisciplinary, sports-medicine team.[39] The pyramid plan provides a functional approach to injuries and pain that offers patients the best chance for recovering from injury. Treatment of musculoskeletal pain and injury during the first 72 hours centers around rest, ice, compression, and elevation (RICE).[39-42] Additional therapy includes the use of ultrasound and orally administered analgesics and anti-inflammatory agents such as ibuprofen (Advil, Motrin IB, Nuprin) and aspirin (Bayer, Empirin, Norwich).[41] (Acetaminophen, e.g., Tylenol, does not reduce inflammation.) Controlling the *edema* (accumulation of fluid) and swelling that accompany the injury is of the utmost importance. Control of edema brings about more rapid and complete healing, allowing more normal joint function and reducing pain and necrotic tissue buildup.

Compression of the area appears to be the most effective deterrent to swelling. Applying external compression

---

Box 16.2

Management of Overuse Injuries

The diagnosis and management of overuse injuries require a multidisciplinary approach involving the sports-medicine physician, physical therapists, orthotists, athletic trainers, and coaches. Follow the five-step approach shown in the management pyramid (see Figure 16.10). Diagnosis should focus on the quality of the athlete's pain, based on a complete physical examination.

Nirschl Pain Phase Scale of Athletic Overuse Injuries

Phase 1. Stiffness or mild soreness after activity. Pain is usually gone within 24 hours.

Phase 2. Stiffness or mild soreness before activity that is relieved by warm-up. Symptoms are not present during activity but return afterward, lasting up to 48 hours.

Phase 3. Stiffness or mild soreness before specific sport or occupational activity. Pain is partially relieved by warm-up. It is minimally present during activity but does not cause the athlete to alter activity.

Phase 4. Similar to phase 3 pain but more intense, causing the athlete to alter performance of the activity. Mild pain occurs with activities of daily living but does not cause a major change in them.

Phase 5. Significant (moderate or greater) pain before, during, and after activity, causing alteration of activity. Pain occurs with activities of daily living but does not cause a major change in them.

Phase 6. Phase 5 pain that persists even with complete rest. Pain disrupts simple activities of daily living and prohibits doing household chores.

Phase 7. Phase 6 pain that also disrupts sleep consistently. Pain is aching in nature and intensifies with activity.

Recommendations Based on Pain Phase

Phases 1, 2, and 3. Avoid intensive exercise that could make the injury worse. Moderate exercise with appropriate warm-up and cool-down is recommended.

Phases 3 & 4. Mild-to-moderate exercise only, with duration and frequency cut in half to allow appropriate rest for healing. Control inflammation with RICE (rest, ice, compression, and elevation) and medications. Consider duplicating land workouts in a swimming pool.

Phases 5, 6, & 7. Control inflammation with RICE and medications. Promote healing with site-specific rehabilitation exercise under the care of a physical therapist or certified athletic trainer, (early exercise enhances tissue oxygenation and nutrition, minimizes unnecessary atrophy, and aligns collagen fibers to meet eventual sports-induced stresses). Also incorporate exercises for general body conditioning. During the healing process, control force loads to the rehabilitated tissue area by bracing or taping the injured part, controlling the intensity and duration of the activity, appropriately modifying equipment, and improving the athlete's sports technique.

Source: O'Connor FG, Howard TM, Fieseler CM, Nirschl RP. Managing overuse injuries: A systematic approach. *Physician Sportsmed* 25(5):88–113, 1997. Reprinted with permission of McGraw-Hill, Inc.

inhibits the seepage of fluid into underlying tissue spaces and disperses excess fluid.

Initial rest for the injured area is also important. Movement that causes severe pain should be avoided (athletes who want to continue exercising should engage in some form of substitute activity that does not cause pain).

POTENTIAL PROBLEMS OF EXCESS EXERCISE FOR WOMEN

While exercise is widely viewed as beneficial for women of all ages, for some the pressure to succeed in competitive sports leads them to train excessively and restrict eating in order to achieve unrealistically low body weights.[43–45] Certain susceptible women may develop *amenorrhea* (absence of menstruation for 3 to 6 consecutive cycles), leading to osteoporosis. This syndrome of disordered eating (and excessive exercising), amenorrhea, and osteoporosis is called the "female athlete triad" (see Figure 16.11).[45]

The Female Athlete Triad

For reasons that are not yet understood, large volumes of exercise have been associated with increased rates of *oligomenorrhea* (scanty or infrequent menstrual flow) and *amenorrhea* (absence of menstruation). Whereas only 2–5% of the sedentary population has this problem, approximately 5–20% of women who exercise regularly and vigorously and up to 50% of competitive athletes may develop it.[43–47] Another common problem among highly active young females in endurance or "appearance" sports (gymnastics, for example) is delayed menarche (>16 years).[48]

The rates vary widely, depending on the type of athlete and the amount of training. Runners and ballet dancers, for example, have much higher rates than swimmers and cyclists. Nearly half of female runners who train 80 or more miles per week are amenorrheic, compared to only about 5–10% of runners who run more moderate distances. Moderate amounts of exercise have little effect on menstrual function[49,50] (see Figure 16.12).

Although all physically active girls and women could be at risk for developing one or more components of the female athlete triad (see Box 16.3), participation in the following sports is a major risk factor:[43]

- Sports in which performance is subjectively scored (dance, figure skating, diving, gymnastics, aerobics)
- Endurance sports emphasizing a low body weight (distance running, cycling, cross-country skiing)
- Sports requiring body-contour-revealing clothing for competition (volleyball, swimming, diving, cross-country running, cross-country skiing, track, cheerleading)
- Sports using weight categories for participation (horse racing, some martial arts, wrestling, rowing)
- Sports emphasizing a prepubertal body habitus for performance success (figure skating, gymnastics, diving)

The female athlete triad syndrome is associated with increased risk of musculoskeletal problems and decreased bone mass. Researchers have reported that spinal bone mass is 20–30% lower for women with amenorrhea, with a high prevalence of stress fractures and musculoskeletal injuries[51–55] (see Figure 16.13).

The causes of menstrual dysfunction and the associated loss in bone mineral mass are still hotly debated but may

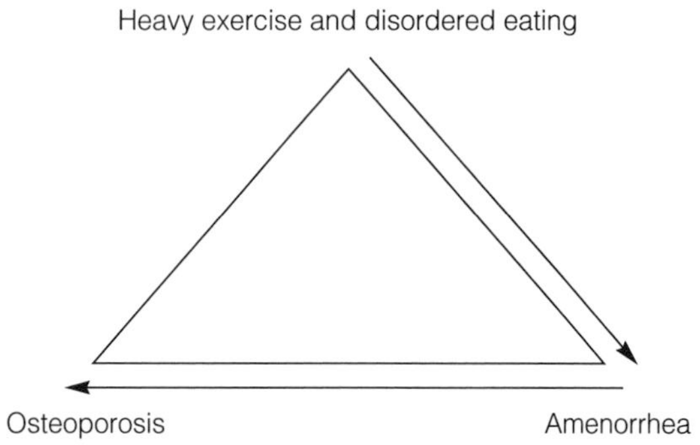

Heavy exercise and disordered eating

Osteoporosis   Amenorrhea

Figure 16.11 The female athlete triad. Female athletes with disordered eating habits and heavy exercise habits may be susceptible to amenorrhea, potentially leading to osteoporosis. *Source:* Yeager KK, Agostini R, Nattiv A, Drinkwater B. The female athlete triad: Disordered eating, amenorrhea, osteoporosis. *Med Sci Sports Exerc* 25:775–777, 1993.

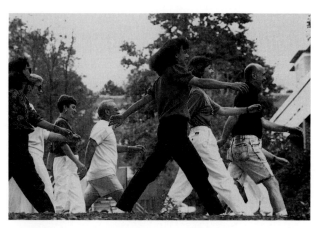

Figure 16.12 Moderate amounts and intensity of exercise, such as with brisk walking, have not been found to impair normal menstrual cycle function.

include the direct effect of exercise itself on the sex hormones or some indirect effect of exercise, such as psychological stress, or malnutrition.[43–47,55–62] The two most widely accepted hypotheses are that (1) heavy exercise causes the hypothalamus to release less gonadotropin-releasing hormone and (2) heavily exercising female athletes do not eat enough to match caloric expenditure (called "energy drain").

There are many parallels between the amenorrhea induced by anorexia nervosa and by strenuous athletic training, with both causing an increased secretion of antireproductive hormones, which inhibit the normal pulsatile secretion pattern of gonadotropins.[47,60]

Although the percentage of athletic women with disordered eating habits is not known for certain, estimates

---

Box 16.3

The Female Athlete Triad: ACSM Position Stand

Based on a comprehensive literature survey, research studies, case reports, and the consensus of experts, it is the position of the American College of Sports Medicine that . . .

1. The Female Athlete Triad is a serious syndrome consisting of disordered eating, amenorrhea, and osteoporosis. The components of the Triad are interrelated in etiology, pathogenesis, and consequences. Because of the recent definition of the Triad, prevalence studies have not yet been completed. However, it occurs not only in elite athletes but also in physically active girls and women participating in a wide range of physical activities. The Triad can result in declining physical performance, as well as medical and psychological morbidity and mortality.

2. Internal and external pressures placed on girls and women to achieve or maintain unrealistically low body weight underlies the development of these disorders.

3. The Triad is often denied, not recognized, and under reported. Sports-medicine professionals need to be aware of the interrelated pathogenesis and the varied presentation of components of the Triad. They should be able to recognize, diagnose, and treat or refer women with any one component of the Triad.

4. Women with one component of the Triad should be screened for the other components. Screening for the Triad can be done at the time of the pre-participation examination and during clinical evaluation of the following: menstrual change, disordered eating patterns, weight change, cardiac arrhythmias including bradycardia, depression, or stress fracture.

5. All sports-medicine professionals, including coaches and trainers, should learn about preventing and recognizing the symptoms and risks of the Triad. All individuals working with active girls and women should participate in athletic training that is medically and psychologically sound. They should avoid pressuring girls and women about losing weight. They should know basic nutrition information and have referral sources for nutritional counseling and medical and mental health evaluation.

6. Parents should avoid pressuring their daughters to diet and lose weight. Parents should be educated about the warning signs of the Triad and initiate medical care for their daughters if signs are present.

7. Sports-medicine professionals, athletic administrators, and officials of sport governing bodies share a responsibility to prevent, recognize, and treat the Triad. The sport governing bodies should work toward offering opportunities for educational programs for coaches to educate them and to lead them toward professional certification. They should work toward developing programs to monitor coaches and others to ensure safe training practices.

8. Physically active girls and women should be educated about proper nutrition, safe training practices, and the warning signs and risks of the Triad. They should be referred for medical evaluation at the first sign of any of the components of the Triad.

9. Further research is needed into the prevalence, causes, prevention, treatment, and sequelae of the Triad.

Source: ACSM Position Stand on the Female Athlete Triad. *Med Sci Sports Exerc* 29:i–ix, 1997. With permission from Williams and Wilkins.

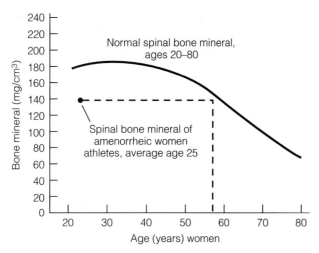

Figure 16.13 Several researchers have found that the spinal bone mineral mass of amenorrheic women athletes at age 25 is equal to that of women twice their age. *Source:* Drinkwater BL, Nilson K, Chestnut CH, et al. Bone mineral content of amenorrheic and eumenorrheic athletes. *N Eng J Med* 311:277–281, 1984.

range from 30% to 65%.[45,61,62] Whatever the percentages, the net result of athletic amenorrhea is that estrogen levels drop to postmenopausal levels, leading to a rapid loss of bone in the spine.[43,45]

All women who stop menstruating or menstruate irregularly because of their exercise program should be examined by a physician. Amenorrheic athletes should be encouraged to optimize their diets, increase calcium intake to 1,500 mg/day, modify their exercise to avoid energy drain, and perhaps receive estrogen/progesterone replacement therapy.[43,45] Amenorrhea appears to be rapidly reversible upon cessation of hard training.[63–66] Even the loss of bone mineral mass has been found to be reversible (though not always completely so) when runners reduce their running distances, gain weight, and resume regular menses.[63–65]

Exercise and Pregnancy

Earlier in this century, pregnant women were urged to reduce physical activity and stop working, especially during the later stages of pregnancy.[67] Exercise was thought to increase the risk of early labor by stimulating uterine activity. Today, concerns have been raised regarding female athletes who continue intensive training throughout their pregnancies. Nonetheless, Ingride Kristiansen, the famous runner from Norway, for example, ran to the day of labor and delivered a healthy baby boy. Five months later, she ran a 2:27 marathon, and then a few months later, a 2:24, and within 2 years held the world records for the 5K, 10K, and marathon. *Runner's World* magazine reported the story of a woman who ran up to 40 miles a week throughout her pregnancy. Nine days before giving birth, she completed a marathon race. The day before giving birth to a healthy baby boy, she competed in a 24-hour race, running 62.5 miles.

Many athletes have the attitude expressed by Joan Ullyot, a physician and marathon runner who has observed, "Gazelles run when they're pregnant. Why should it be any different for women?" These types of stories have concerned many experts and doctors who provide health care for women.[67–71]

Pregnancy stresses the body more than any other physiological event in a healthy woman's life.[67] A variety of cardiovascular, metabolic, hormonal, respiratory, and musculoskeletal adaptations take place during the 9 months of pregnancy. Can regular, moderate physical activity provide benefits to the mother and fetus? On the other hand, could high volumes of intensive exercise pose potential risks for pregnancy outcome?

Moderate amounts of exercise during pregnancy are recommended for the health and fitness of the mother and baby.[67–74] One large-scale study of some 2,000 women in Missouri showed that those who largely avoided exercise during pregnancy were more likely to give birth to very low birth weight infants (who are more prone to sickness and death).[73] In another study of some 400 pregnant women, aerobic exercise throughout pregnancy led to fewer discomforts later on.[74] A few studies even suggest that fit mothers gain less unnecessary body fat during pregnancy, experience shorter labor, and have fewer cesarean births.[67,70–72] There is limited evidence that moderate exercise during pregnancy may be a useful treatment for gestational diabetes.[75] In general, 30–45 minutes of moderate aerobic activity on a near-daily basis does not appear to expose the mother to serious metabolic consequences that might adversely affect her or the fetus.

Debate still centers on whether intense and prolonged exercise by the pregnant mother can cause harm to the growing fetus.[67,69,76,77] Concern has been expressed that during heavy exertion, body temperature may rise to high levels, while blood flow, glucose supply, and oxygen delivery to the fetus may be decreased, affecting normal development. In other words, the dual stresses of pregnancy and intense exercise may create conflicting physiological demands that could adversely affect pregnancy outcome.[67]

In 1985, the American College of Obstetricians and Gynecologists (ACOG) released guidelines for exercise during pregnancy.[78] They took a cautious approach, urging that pregnant women exercise moderately for only 15 minutes at a time, keeping the heart rate below 140 beats per minute. These guidelines caused an outcry among some experts, who claimed they were too conservative. In one review of the medical literature, researchers concluded that exercise performed for up to 40–45 minutes, three times a week at a heart rate of up to 140–145 beats per minute did not appear to adversely affect the mother or the fetus.[71]

In 1994, ACOG released their new guidelines, which removed the heart rate guideline.[79] According to ACOG, "There are no data in humans to indicate that pregnant women should limit exercise intensity and lower target heart rates because of potential adverse effects." However, ACOG did urge that regular, moderate exercise is sufficient to derive health benefits, and that pregnant women should listen to their bodies, stop exercising when fatigued, and not exercise to exhaustion (see Box 16.4).

In general, it appears that trained women, who were exercising regularly prior to conception, may continue their exercise program, although often specific symptoms and overall comfort level lead to changes in mode of exercise and decreases in duration, frequency, or intensity.[67–70] For women who were not exercising regularly before pregnancy, it is safe to begin a moderate exercise program, particularly in the second trimester.[67] Maintenance of regular physical activity during pregnancy helps keep the mother fit and healthy, causes no harm to the growing fetus, and may improve the birthing experience.

Although it appears that there are compensatory mechanisms that serve to protect the fetus for all of the potential physiological problems imposed by intensive exercise during pregnancy, atypical and high volumes of intensive exercise should be avoided until more is known about the health effects to both the pregnant mother and the fetus.

HEAT INJURIES

The American College of Sports Medicine has advised athletes that heat exhaustion and heat strokes are their number one enemies.[80] Risk factors for heat illness are listed in Box 16.5.[80–86] The four major forms of heat illness—

Box 16.4

Recommendations for Exercise in Pregnancy and Postpartum

There are no data in humans to indicate that pregnant women should limit exercise intensity and lower target heart rates because of potential adverse effects. For women who do not have any additional risk factors for adverse maternal or perinatal outcomes, the following recommendations may be made:

1. During pregnancy, women can continue to exercise and derive health benefits even from mild-to-moderate exercise routines. Regular exercise (at least three times per week) is preferable to intermittent activity.

2. Women should avoid exercise in the supine position after the first trimester. Such a position is associated with decreased cardiac output in most pregnant women; because the remaining cardiac output will be preferentially distributed away from splanchnic beds (including the uterus) during vigorous exercise, such regimens are best avoided during pregnancy. Prolonged periods of motionless standing should also be avoided.

3. Women should be aware of the decreased oxygen available for aerobic exercise during pregnancy. They should be encouraged to modify the intensity of their exercise according to maternal symptoms. Pregnant women should stop exercising when fatigued and not exercise to exhaustion. Weight-bearing exercises may under some circumstances be continued at intensities similar to those prior to pregnancy throughout pregnancy.

Non-weight-bearing exercises, such as cycling or swimming, will minimize the risk of injury and facilitate the continuation of exercise during pregnancy.

4. Morphological changes in pregnancy should serve as a relative contraindication to types of exercise in which loss of balance could be detrimental to maternal or fetal well-being, especially in the third trimester. Further, any type of exercise involving the potential for even mild abdominal trauma should be avoided.

5. Pregnancy requires an additional 300 Calories/day in order to maintain metabolic homeostasis. Thus, women who exercise during pregnancy should be particularly careful to ensure an adequate diet.

6. Pregnant women who exercise in the first trimester should augment heat dissipation by ensuring adequate hydration, appropriate clothing, and optimal environmental surroundings during exercise.

7. Many of the physiological and morphological changes of pregnancy persist 4–6 weeks postpartum. Thus, prepregnancy exercise routines should be resumed gradually, based on a woman's capability.

Source: American College of Obstetricians and Gynecologists. Exercise during pregnancy and the postpartum period. *Technical Bulletin* #189, Washington, DC, 1994.

Risk Factors and Symptoms for Heat Illness

Because of the potentially grave consequences of heat illness, all athletes and fitness professionals should be alert to these risk factors and symptoms.

Risk Factors

1. Obesity (or high body mass index)
2. Low degree of physical fitness
3. Dehydration
4. Lack of heat acclimatization
5. Previous history of heat stroke
6. Sleep deprivation
7. Certain medications, including diuretics and antidepressants
8. Sweat-gland dysfunction or sunburn
9. Sickness with fever, respiratory tract infection, diarrhea

Symptoms

1. Clumsiness
2. Stumbling
3. Headache
4. Nausea
5. Dizziness
6. Apathy
7. Confusion
8. Impairment of consciousness

Source: American College of Sports Medicine. Position stand on heat and cold illnesses during distance running. *Med Sci Sports Exerc* 27: i–x, 1996. With permission from Williams and Wilkins.

heat cramps, heat exhaustion, heat stroke, and exertional rhabdomyolysis—are reviewed in this section (see Chapter 9 for a review of exercise in the heat). Box 16.6 summarizes ACSM guidelines for conducting race events.[80]

Heat Cramps

Heat cramps involve muscular pains and spasms. First aid includes moving the victim to a cool place, having her or him lie down if she or he feels faint, and administering one or two glasses of liquid with ¼ teaspoon of salt added to each glass. The cause is most likely a salt deficit from heavy sweating during prolonged strenuous exercise.[82]

Heat Exhaustion

Heat exhaustion, primarily body fluid depletion due to lack of salt or water deprivation, is characterized by fatigue, weakness, and collapse. Heat exhaustion is the most common form of heat injury among athletes and soldiers.[82] There is profuse sweating, and the skin is often pale and clammy, while body temperature is usually close to normal. First aid includes moving the victim to the coolest possible place, removing clothing, and cooling (with cold water applications, fans to create a draft, or ice packs). Care should be taken to avoid chilling the victim. Oral electrolyte solutions will suffice for most cases, but some athletes may need 3–4 liters after prolonged exercise. IV solutions most commonly used are 5% dextrose in 0.45% NaCl.[84] Salt tablets are not recommended.

Heat Stroke

Heat stroke is distinguished by extremely high body temperature (>105°F) and disturbance of the sweating mechanism. The skin is hot, red, and dry (although sweating may persist), the pulse is rapid and strong, and the victim may be unconscious (or disoriented). First aid includes moving the victim to a cool place, removing clothing, and cooling as fast as possible with all available means, including cold water, ice, fans, or rubbing alcohol (ice water baths are best).[85] Speed is of the essence. Heat stroke is a life-threatening situation.

Exertional Rhabdomyolysis

Exertional rhabdomyolysis is the degeneration of skeletal muscle caused by excessive unaccustomed exercise on hot days. Symptoms include muscle pain, weakness, and swelling; dark urine (from a muscle pigment called myoglobin); and increased levels of muscle enzymes and chemicals in the blood. In rare cases, the myoglobin can precipitate in the kidneys, causing renal failure and death. Severe incidents of rhabdomyolysis tend to occur at the start of a training program when exercise is excessive and accompanied by heat stress and dehydration.

Measuring Temperature for Exercise Risk

The simplest measurement of environmental heat stress is the *wet bulb temperature* (WBT). It is obtained by putting a

Box 16.6

ACSM Recommendations for Race Managers and Medical Directors of Community Race Events

The American College of Sports Medicine advises that the following recommendations be employed by race managers and medical directors of community events that involve prolonged or intense exercise in mild and stressful environments.

1. *Race organization.* Distance races should be scheduled to avoid extremely hot and humid and very cold months. Summer events should be scheduled in the early morning or the evening. The heat stress index should be measured at the race site, using the wet bulb globe temperature (WBGT). If the WBGT is above 82°F, consideration should be given to canceling or postponing the race. An adequate supply of fluid must be available before the start of the race, along the race course, and at the end of the event. Encourage athletes to drink 150–300 ml every 15 minutes. Cool or cold (ice) water immersion is the most effective means of cooling a collapsed hyperthermic athlete. Race officials should be aware of the warning signs of heat illness and should warn athletes to slow down or stop if they appear to be in difficulty. Radio communication or cellular phones should be available throughout the race course for emergency responses.

2. *Medical director.* A sports-medicine physician should work closely with the race director to enhance overall safety and provide adequate medical care for all participants.

3. *Medical support.* The medical director should alert local hospitals and ambulance services. Medical support staff and facilities must be available at the race site.

4. *Competitor education.* Race organizers should conduct clinics and publish articles in the local media to educate runners about heat illness and measures to take to reduce risk. Signs at the race event should caution athletes about the environmental heat stress.

Source: American College of Sports Medicine. Position stand on heat and cold illnesses during distance running. *Med Sci Sports Exerc* 27: i–x, 1996. With permission from Williams and Wilkins.

wick around the bulb of a thermometer, wetting it, and then blowing air by it with a fan, to determine the effects of evaporation on the temperature reading. Because evaporation is affected by humidity, the WBT will help provide a guide to the degree of environmental stress. A WBT of 78°F or higher requires that exercise be postponed.

The *wet bulb globe temperature* (WGBT) consists of a dry bulb temperature reading, a wet bulb temperature reading, and a black globe temperature reading. The black globe, which is simply a thermometer placed with its bulb inside a copper toilet float painted black, measures the effect of radiant heat from the sun. All readings are taken in the open, allowing 30 minutes of exposure before readings are taken. To compute WBGT, use the following formula:

$$\text{WBGT (°F)} = (0.7 \times wb) + (0.2 \times g) + (0.1 \times db)$$

where wb = wet bulb temperature; g = globe temperature; and db = dry bulb temperature (°F).

The following standards have been developed, designed primarily for mass-participation runs:[80]

<WBGT	Low risk
65–73 WBGT	Moderate risk (warn the runners that conditions may worsen)
73–82 WBGT	High risk (warn runners; those at high risk should not run)
>82 WBGT	Very high risk (postpone race)

ENVIRONMENTAL POLLUTION

Air pollution has long been suspected of causing ill health and increased risk of lung cancer and other pulmonary diseases.[87–90] In 1952, 4,000 excess deaths occurred in London due to a thick accumulation of air pollutants emitted from burning fossil fuels and blocked by a severe temperature inversion layer.[87] Similar episodes have occurred in Belgium and Pennsylvania. In a 15-year study of more than 8,000 adults in six U.S. cities, Harvard researchers showed that death from lung cancer and cardiopulmonary disease was 26% higher in those living in the most polluted areas.[88] Mortality was most strongly associated with fine particulates including soot, acid condensates, and sulfate and nitrate particles that can be breathed deep into the lungs, posing a risk to health. According to the Centers for Disease Control (CDC) and Prevention, 66% of the U.S. population is at risk for excessive exposure to "inhalable particles" from air pollution.[89]

The CDC has listed people who exercise as "an important group at risk" for the effects of ozone and other air pollutants.[89] The long-term effect of exercising in air with fine particulates is unknown, but common sense would urge caution, especially on days with high levels.

During rest, the average human ventilates only 6 liters of air per minute. During heavy exercise, women can ventilate 60–90 liters of air per minute, and males 100–130 liters of air per minute. Obviously, the dosage of air pollutants entering the body is increased, and exercise can exaggerate the normal pulmonary effects of air pollution.[91]

There are two kinds of air pollutants: primary and secondary. *Primary air pollutants* include carbon monoxide (CO), carbon dioxide (CO_2), sulfur dioxide (SO_2), nitrogen oxide (NO), and particulate material such as lead, graphite carbon, and fly ash. *Secondary air pollutants* are formed by the chemical action of the primary pollutants and the natural chemicals in the atmosphere. Examples include ozone (O_3), sulfuric acid (H_2SO_4), nitric acid (HNO_3), peroxyacetyl nitrate, and a host of other inorganic and organic compounds.

Ozone is produced by the photochemical reaction of sunlight and hydrocarbons and nitrogen dioxide from car exhaust. *Stage 1* alerts are called when ozone reaches 0.2 ppm, *Stage 2* at 0.35 ppm. In the Los Angeles area, ozone levels reach 0.2 ppm levels for 1 hour or more on about 180 days per year.[91]

Ozone's toxicity is due to its action as an oxidant.[91–96] It is extremely reactive, affecting the pulmonary membranes.

Ozone has been shown to cause tissue injury and lung inflammation and reacts rapidly.[96] Symptoms include chest tightness, coughing, headache, dyspnea, nausea, throat irritation, and burning of the eyes (see Figure 16.14).

Heavy exercise in air polluted with ozone impairs the ability to exercise and reduces lung function, at least temporarily.[91–97] Statistically significant impairment of exercise performance can occur at 0.2 ppm. Individuals vary widely, however, in their response to ozone. Reported subjective symptoms have included shortness of breath, coughing, excess sputum, raspy throat, and wheezing.

Interestingly, sensitivity to ozone has been found to diminish with repeated exposure.[95] Results show that by the end of 4-day periods of repeated exercise in polluted air, significant improvements are experienced in $\dot{V}O_{2max}$ and performance time, with decreased subjective symptoms. Although habituation may benefit competitive performance, the long-term consequences of repeated exposures may be undesirable. There are data that high exposure to ozone over 10–20 years does impair pulmonary function.[97]

SUDDEN DEATH FROM HEART ATTACK

Of all the potential problem areas associated with exercise, the one that has caused the most controversy is the effect on the heart.

The Saga of Jim Fixx

In northern Vermont, late on the afternoon of Friday, July 20, 1984, a passing motorcyclist discovered a man lying dead beside the road. He was clad only in shorts and Nike running shoes. The man was Jim Fixx, author of *The Complete Book of Running*. This amazingly successful book had stayed on the best-seller list for nearly 2 years, helping to accelerate the running boom of the late 1970s. Jim Fixx had become one of the leading spokespersons on the health benefits of running. Now he lay dead—with his running shoes on—and this is why so many Americans were disturbed. Jim Fixx died of cardiac arrest pounding the pavement to gain the fitness and health he advocated for all.[98]

On autopsy, it was discovered that all of Jim Fixx's blood vessels were partially or nearly completely blocked from atherosclerotic plaque buildup. The left circumflex coronary artery was 99% occluded, and scar tissue indicated that three other heart attacks had occurred within 2 months of his death. How could a man in seemingly peak condition, having run 60–70 miles per week for more than 12 years, be stricken by a disease most strongly associated with a sedentary life?

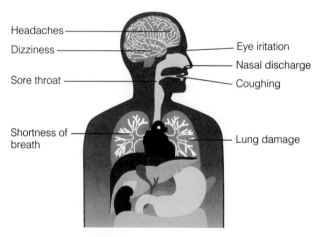

Figure 16.14 Ozone symptoms. Ozone reacts rapidly, causing multiple symptoms. *Ground-level ozone.* It is the main ingredient in urban smog. Naturally occurring ozone in the upper atmosphere protects life by filtering the ultraviolet radiation from the sun. Ground-level ozone is produced by vehicle or industrial emissions combining with sunlight and high heat during times of little or no wind. *Health hazard.* High concentrations of ozone can cause inflammation and irritation of the respiratory tract. Ozone can increase asthma and allergy problems and susceptibility to lung infections. Ozone damage to lungs can continue days after exposure has ended. *Most vulnerable people.* Those most likely to suffer ozone pollution effects: people with lung diseases, the elderly, children and healthy adults who exercise outdoors. Children are especially vulnerable because they often play outside and, in muggy heat, breathe more rapidly and inhale more air pollution.

As a matter of fact, Jim Fixx, despite his running, was at extremely high risk for heart disease—yet he chose to ignore the warning signals. Jim's father had died of a heart attack at age 43. (Family history of heart disease, especially before age 55 for men, is an extremely potent risk factor; see Chapter 10.)

Up to his mid-30s, Jim Fixx was smoking two packs of cigarettes per day, was a "steak-and-potatoes" man, weighed 220 pounds, and had a high-stress, executive job. At age 35, he suddenly tried to turn his life around by running a lot of miles. He lost weight and soon began racing marathons. He decided there was no need to see a doctor, however, even when experiencing heart disease warning signals such as throat and chest tightness. (Six months before Fixx's death, Ken Cooper had invited Fixx to undergo a stress test, but he declined.) In addition, Fixx was not handling well the strain, stress, and pressure of notoriety.

Seventeen years later, at age 52, Jim Fixx lay dead by the side of that Vermont back road, dead of a heart attack. Running may have lengthened his life a bit, but it probably ended up killing him as well.

Exercise and Heart Attack: A Double-Edged Sword

There's probably not a single fitness enthusiast in America who has not read the reports of famous athletes dying on basketball courts, runners found dead with their running shoes on, executives discovered slumped over their treadmills, or middle-aged fathers unearthed alongside their snow shovels. Examples besides Jim Fixx include basketball stars Reggie Lewis, "Pistol Pete" Maravich, and Hank Gathers, and MCI chair Bill McGowan. During the "blizzard of the century" in 1993, scores of people along the eastern seaboard died of sudden heart attack while shoveling their driveways.

Yet, as reviewed in Chapter 10, people who exercise regularly are less likely on average to die of heart disease than those who refrain (relative risk for inactivity is about 1.9). According to the Centers for Disease Control and Prevention, when all the evidence is considered, lack of exercise is just as responsible for the epidemic of heart disease in America as is high blood pressure, high blood cholesterol, and smoking.[99]

Whether exercise is beneficial or hazardous to the heart appears to depend on who the person is. In one study of 158 athletes who died young (average age 17) and in their prime, 134 of them had heart or blood vessel defects that were present at birth.[100] Most common was hypertrophic cardiomyopathy, a thickening of the heart's main pumping muscle (see Figure 16.15). In other words, when a young athlete dies during or shortly after exercise, it is most often due to a birth defect of the cardiovascular system. There are renewed calls by many experts that, despite the relative rarity of these types of deaths and the cost of testing,

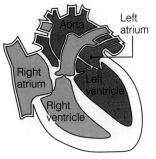

Normal heart   Heart with hypertrophic cardiomyopathy

- Often affects the left ventricle, which pumps blood to the aorta. The blood then goes through the aorta to the rest of the body.
- Often is hereditary.
- Condition usually develops before age 20.
- Considered cause of death in 36% of all cases of sudden deaths in athletes.

Abnormal thickening of the heart wall

Figure 16.15 Hypertrophic cardiomyopathy is an abnormal thickening of the left ventricle muscle wall that typically goes undetected during routine physical exams and can cause sudden death in young athletes. Medical experts consider hypertrophic cardiomyopathy the most common fatal heart defect among young athletes. An athlete with this condition can compete for years without showing any symptoms and suddenly suffer a heart attack. It is characterized as follows:

- Often affects the left ventricle, which pumps blood to the aorta. (The blood then goes through the aorta to the rest of the body.)
- Often is hereditary
- Condition usually develops before age 20
- Considered cause of death in 36% of all cases of sudden deaths in athletes

young athletes should be examined prior to sport participation.[101,102] (see Chapter 3).

For most individuals over age 30, however, who die during or shortly after exercise, the cause is entirely different—a narrowing of the coronary blood vessels of the heart because of cholesterol and fat deposits called *atherosclerosis* (as in Jim Fixx).[102] It appears that when people with these narrowed coronary blood vessels exert themselves heavily during exercise, the increase in heart rate and blood pressure may disrupt the deposits, setting in motion a chain of events that cause a complete blockage and heart attack.[102–105] In other words, middle-aged and older adults who die during exercise tend to be people who already have heart disease. They are at high risk to begin with, and then the vigorous exercise triggers a heart attack.

Researchers from Harvard University studied the heart attack episodes of 1,228 men and women and found that the risk was 5.9 times higher after heavy versus lighter or no exertion.[103] As shown in Figure 16.16 heavy physical exertion was especially risky for people who were habitually inactive. In other words, people who usually exercised very little, and then went out and exercised vigorously (e.g., shoveling snow), were much more likely to suffer a heart attack than those who were accustomed to exercise (see Figure 16.17). These researchers concluded that every year in the United States, 75,000 Americans suffer a heart attack after vigorous exercise and that these victims tend to be sedentary and at high risk for heart attack to begin with. Another study, from Germany, has also concluded that "a period of strenuous physical activity is associated with a temporary increase in the risk of having a myocardial infarction, particularly among patients who exercise infrequently."[104]

In one study of 36 marathon runners who had died suddenly or suffered a heart attack, researchers found that in most of the cases, a strong family history of heart disease, high blood cholesterol, or early warning symptoms (e.g., chest pain) were present.[106] Most of the runners had symptoms of heart disease but denied they had them and continued training and racing until they finally had a heart attack or died, as did Jim Fixx.[107]

It is important to understand that the risk of a heart attack during exercise is a rare event despite the media reports. Most researchers have found that in a given year, fewer than 10 out of 100,000 men will have a heart attack during exercise.[102,107–109] These victims tend to be men who were sedentary, already had heart disease or were at high risk for it, and then exercised too hard for their fitness level. If an individual is at low risk for heart disease, has not experienced any symptoms, and exercises moderately, risk is extremely low, and overall, risk for heart disease should be lowered because of the regular exercise program.

People at high risk for heart disease should avoid heavy exertion until being cleared by their physicians after taking

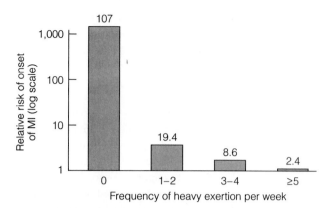

Figure 16.16 Risk of myocardial infarction after heavy exertion. During the hour after heavy exertion, the relative risk of myocardial infarction is much higher for sedentary people than for those who exercise frequently. *Source:* Mittleman MA, Maclure M, Tofler GH, Sherwood JB, Goldberg RJ, Muller JE. Triggering of acute myocardial infarction by heavy physical exertion: Protection against triggering by regular exertion. *N Engl J Med* 329:1677–1683, 1993.

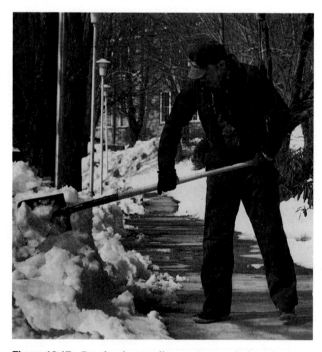

Figure 16.17 People who usually exercise very little and are at high risk for heart disease are much more likely to suffer a heart attack during exercise than are low-risk individuals accustomed to regular exercise.

a maximal treadmill ECG test (see Chapter 3). Even after clearance, they should avoid intense exercise until fitness has been gradually improved and heart disease risk factors have been brought under control. Figure 16.18 outlines recommendations for intensity of exercise using the rating of perceived exertion scale.

6	
7	Very, very light
8	
9	Very light
10	
11	Fairly light
12	
13	Somewhat hard
14	
15	Hard
16	
17	Very hard
18	
19	Very, very hard
20	Maximal

Light exercise
Some health benefits, but minimal fitness improvement

Moderate exercise
Both health and fitness benefits with minimal risk

Intense exercise
For those who desire high fitness. Can precipitate heart attack in high-risk individuals.

Figure 16.18 Exercise risk versus benefit using the rating of perceived exertion. The rating of perceived exertion scale can be used to guide exercisers according to their personal goals and fitness levels. Risk for heart attack is greatest when the perceived exertion is "hard" to "maximal." Risks and benefits are as follows: Light exercise (6–11)—some health benefits, but minimal fitness improvements; moderate exercise (12–14)—both health and fitness benefits with minimal risk; intense exercise (15–20)—for those who desire high fitness, can precipitate heart attack in those at high risk.

RISK FOR UPPER RESPIRATORY TRACT INFECTION

People who exercise report fewer colds than their sedentary peers.[110,111] For example, a 1989 *Runner's World* survey revealed that 61% of 700 recreational runners reported fewer colds since beginning to run, while only 4% felt they had experienced more. In another survey of 170 runners who had been training for 12 years, 90% reported that they definitely or mostly agreed with the statement that they "rarely get sick." A survey of 750 master athletes (ranging in age from 40 to 81 years) showed that 76% perceived themselves as less vulnerable to viral illnesses than their sedentary peers.

Very few studies have been carried out in the area of moderate exercise and colds, and more research is certainly needed to investigate this interesting question. Two randomized, controlled studies with young adult and elderly women have been conducted.[112,113] In both studies, women in the exercise groups walked briskly 35–45 minutes, 5 days a week, for 12–15 weeks during the winter/spring or fall, while the control groups remained physically inactive. The results were in the same direction reported by fitness enthusiasts—walkers experienced about half the days with cold symptoms as the sedentary controls did.

Other research has shown that during moderate exercise, several positive changes occur in the immune system.[111,114,115] Stress hormones, which can suppress immunity, are not elevated during moderate exercise. Although the immune system returns to pre-exercise levels very quickly after the exercise session is over, each session represents a boost that appears to reduce the risk of infection over the long term. Although public health recommendations must be considered tentative, the data on the relationship between moderate exercise and lowered risk of sickness are consistent with guidelines urging the general public to engage in near-daily brisk walking.[111]

In contrast, among elite athletes and their coaches, a common perception is that heavy exertion lowers resistance to colds.[111,116] For example, Liz McColgan, one of the best female runners in Scotland, blamed overtraining "which led to a cold and two subsequent illnesses" as the major reason for her poor performance in the 1992 World Cross Country Championships. Uta Pippig, winner of the 1994 Boston Marathon, caught a cold the week before the race, after training 140 miles a week for 10 weeks at high altitude. Claimed Pippig, "when you are on such a high level you can so quickly fall off." Alberto Salazar, once one of the best marathon runners in the world, reported that while training for the 1984 Olympic marathon, he caught 12 colds in 12 months. "My immune system was totally shot," he recalls. "I caught everything. I felt like I should have been living in a bubble." During the winter and summer Olympic Games, it has been regularly reported by clinicians that "upper respiratory infections abound" and that "the most irksome troubles with the athletes were infections."[111]

To determine whether these anecdotal reports were true, researchers studied a group of 2,311 marathon runners who ran the 1987 Los Angeles marathon.[117] During the week following the race, one out of seven runners came down sick, which was nearly six times the rate of runners who trained for but did not run the marathon (see Figure 16.19). During the 2-month period before the race, runners training more than 60 miles a week doubled their odds for sickness, compared to those training less than 20 miles a week. Researchers in South Africa have also confirmed that after marathon-type exertion, runners are at high risk for sickness.[118,119]

The immune systems of marathon runners have been studied under laboratory conditions before and after running 2–3 hours.[116] A steep drop in immune function occurs, which lasts at least 6–9 hours. Much of this immune suppression appears to be related to the elevation of stress hormones, which are secreted in high quantity during and following heavy exertion. Several exercise immunologists believe this allows viruses to spread and gain a foothold.[111,114,116] Heavy training day in and day out has also been related to a chronic suppression of neutrophil function.[120] This is a critical finding because neutrophils are an

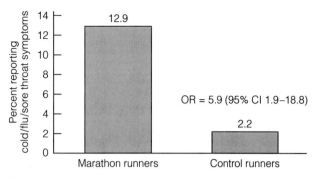

Figure 16.19 Risk of upper respiratory tract infection increases during the week after a marathon race. During the week after the Los Angeles marathon (March 1987), the odds for reporting an upper respiratory tract infection among runners who ran the race were 5.9 times greater than for those who applied but did not run. *Source:* Nieman DC, Johansen LM, Lee JW, Cermak J, Arabatzis K. Infectious episodes in runners before and after the Los Angeles marathon. *J Sports Med Phys Fit* 30:316–328, 1990.

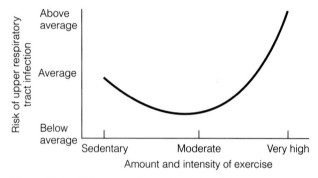

Figure 16.20 Whereas moderate physical activity may decrease the risk for upper respiratory tract infection, heavy exertion may increase this risk. *Source:* Nieman DC. Exercise, upper respiratory tract infection, and the immune system. *Med Sci Sports Exerc* 26:128–139, 1994.

important component of the immune system's "first-line defense."

Together, these studies on the relationship between exercise and infection have potential implications for public health, and for the athlete, they may mean the difference between being able to compete or performing at a subpar level or missing the event altogether because of illness. The relationship between exercise and infection may be modeled in the form of a "J" curve.[111] This model suggests that although the risk of infection may decrease below that of a sedentary individual when one engages in moderate exercise training, risk may rise above average during periods of excessive amounts of high-intensity exercise (see Figure 16.20).

Athletes must train hard to prepare for competition. Although this increases the risk for infection if the training becomes too intensive, there are several practical recom-

mendations the athlete can follow to minimize the impact of other stressors on the immune system:[111]

- Keep other life stresses to a minimum. Mental stress in and of itself has been linked to an increased risk of upper respiratory tract infection.

- Eat a well-balanced diet to keep vitamin and mineral pools in the body at optimal levels. Although there is insufficient evidence to recommend nutrient supplements, ultramarathon runners may benefit by taking vitamin C supplements before ultramarathon races.

- Avoid overtraining and chronic fatigue.

- Obtain adequate sleep on a regular schedule. Sleep disruption has been linked to suppressed immunity.

- Avoid rapid weight loss (which has also been linked to negative immune changes).

- Avoid putting hands to the eyes and nose (primary routes of introducing viruses into the body). Before important race events, avoid sick people and large crowds when possible.

- For athletes competing during the winter months, flu shots are recommended.

- Use carbohydrate beverages before, during, and after marathon-type race events or unusually heavy training bouts. This may lower the impact of stress hormones on the immune system.

Athletes and fitness enthusiasts are often uncertain of whether they should exercise or rest during sickness. Human studies are lacking to provide definitive answers.[111] Animal studies, however, generally support the finding that one or two periods of exhaustive exercise following injection of the animal with certain types of viruses or bacteria lead to more frequent appearance of infection and more severe symptoms.

With athletes, it is well established that the ability to compete is reduced during sickness. Also, several case histories have shown that sudden and unexplained downturns in athletic performance can sometimes be traced to a recent bout of sickness.[111] In some athletes, exercising when sick can lead to a severely debilitating state known as "postviral fatigue syndrome." The symptoms can persist for several months and include weakness, inability to train hard, easy fatigability, frequent infections, and depression.

Concerning exercising when sick, most clinical authorities in the area of exercise immunology recommend[111,114,116]

- If one has common cold symptoms (e.g., runny nose and sore throat without fever or general body aches and pains), intensive exercise training may be safely resumed a few days after the resolution of symptoms.

- Mild-to-moderate exercise (e.g., walking) when sick with the common cold does not appear to be harmful. In two studies using nasal sprays of a rhinovirus leading to common cold symptoms, subjects were able to engage in exercise during the course of the illness without any negative effects on severity of symptoms or performance capability.

- With symptoms of fever, extreme tiredness, muscle aches, and swollen lymph glands, 2–4 weeks should probably be allowed before resumption of intensive training.

EXERCISE-INDUCED ASTHMA

Of the various triggers for asthma, physical activity is one of the most common.[121–128] More than 80% of children and 60% of adult asthmatics get exercise-induced asthma (EIA) during or after exercise. In the 1972 Olympic Games, EIA gained considerable attention when an American swimmer lost a gold medal due to the use of a banned drug to treat asthma.[121] Recognition that EIA could be controlled with proper medication and education grew, following reports of the success of U.S. Olympians. Of 597 U.S. athletes in the 1984 Olympic summer games in Los Angeles, 11% reported a history of EIA. These athletes still won 41 medals. In the 1988 Olympic Games in Seoul, about 8% of U.S. athletes were confirmed asthmatics and won, proportionately, as many medals as did athletes without asthma.

Prevalence of Asthma

Asthma (Greek, "to pant") is an inflammation of the lungs, which causes airways to narrow, making it difficult to breathe. Inflammation makes the airways sensitive to allergens, chemical irritants, tobacco smoke, cold air, or exercise.[129–135] When exposed to these stimuli, an asthma attack can occur, causing the muscles around the windpipes to tighten, making the opening smaller. The lining of the windpipe swells (becomes inflamed) and produces mucus. This leads to coughing, wheezing, chest tightness, and difficulty in breathing, particularly at night or in the early morning (see Figure 16.21). Asthma symptoms come and go; they can last for a few moments or for days. Asthma attacks can be mild or severe and sometimes fatal.

Each year in America, more than 5,000 people die from asthma, with rates twice as high among blacks compared to whites.[134] Asthma is a major public health problem, affecting more than 100 million people worldwide and 5% of Americans (about 14–15 million).[129,130,134] In the United States, about 1 child in every 15 has asthma. During the 1980s, for unknown reasons, asthma rates rose 49%, a problem also recognized in many other nations. According to experts of the Global Initiative for Asthma, "this may be linked to

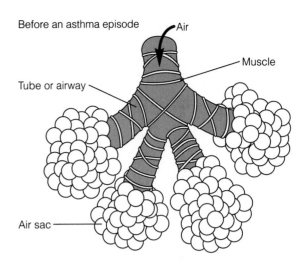

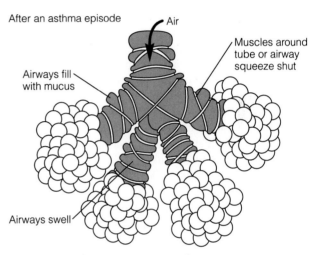

Figure 16.21 During an asthma episode, the muscles around the airways tighten, and the lining swells and produces mucus. *Source:* Flieger K. Controlling asthma. *FDA Consumer,* November 1996, 19–23.

factors including housing with reduced ventilation, exposure to indoor allergens (such as domestic dust mites in bedding, carpets, and stuffed furnishings, and animals with fur, especially cats), tobacco smoke, viral infections, air pollution, and chemical irritants."[133]

Prevention Guidelines

Asthma episodes can be prevented, but more studies are needed to determine whether development of the underlying inflammatory disease can be averted.[133,134] Controlling exposure to environmental allergens, irritants, and pollution may help prevent asthma. Asthma is no longer considered a condition with isolated and periodic attacks. Rather, asthma is now understood to be a chronic inflammatory affliction of the airways.[133–134] Inflammation makes the airways hypersensitive to a wide variety of irritants. Causes of the initial tendency toward inflammation in the airways are not yet known for certain, but one of the strongest risk factors is an inherited tendency to have allergic reactions.

Common allergens that are risk factors for developing asthma include dust mites, animals with fur, cockroaches, pollens, and molds.[133] Exposure to tobacco smoke, especially in infants, is a strong risk factor. Chemicals or air pollutants in the workplace can also lead to the development of asthma. Viral respiratory infections, small size at birth, and diet (e.g., certain foods such as shellfish, peanuts, eggs, and chocolate) may also contribute.

Many of these risk factors for developing asthma also aggravate it and are known as triggers because they provoke asthma attacks. Other triggers include wood smoke from open fires or stoves, physical activity, extreme emotional expressions (e.g., laughing or crying hard), cold air or weather changes, certain food additives (e.g., metabisulphite, monosodium glutamate), and aspirin. By avoiding triggers, a person with asthma lowers the risk of irritating the sensitive airways. The risk can be further reduced by taking medications that decrease airway inflammation.[133,134]

Although asthma cannot be cured, it can be controlled by establishing a lifelong management plan with a physician.[133,134] Patients can be educated to avoid triggers and to use appropriate medications. Various quick-relief and long-term preventive medications should be considered. The quick-relief medications include short-acting bronchodilators (e.g., inhaled beta$_2$-agonists) that act quickly to relieve airway tightness and acute symptoms such as coughing, chest tightness, and wheezing. Long-term preventive medications (e.g., inhaled corticosteroids) help control the inflammation that causes attacks. Many asthma medications are delivered by metered dose inhalers, which are highly effective.

The best way to stop asthma attacks is prevention. Identifying and controlling triggers is essential for successful control of asthma. The common triggers include[131,133,134]

- *Dust mites.* These are often a major component of house dust and feed on human skin sheddings. They are found in mattresses, blankets, rugs, soft toys, and stuffed furniture. Exposure to mite allergens in early childhood contributes strongly to the development of asthma. Hot laundering, airtight covers, removal of carpets, and avoiding fabric-covered furniture are recommended.

- *Allergens from animals with fur.* These furry animals include small rodents, cats, and dogs and can trigger asthma. Animals should be removed from the home.

- *Tobacco smoke.* This is a trigger whether the patient smokes or breathes in the smoke from others.

- *Cockroach allergen.* A common trigger in some locations, infested homes should be cleaned thoroughly and regularly.

- *Mold and other fungal spores and pollens.* These are particles from plants. Windows and doors should be closed, and those with asthma are advised to stay indoors when pollen and mold counts are highest. Air conditioning can be helpful.

- *Smoke from wood-burning stoves and other indoor air pollutants.* These produce irritating particles. Vent all furnaces and stoves to the outdoors, and keep rooms well ventilated.

- *Colds or viral respiratory infections.* These can trigger asthma, especially in children. Give an influenza vaccination every year to patients with moderate-to-severe asthma. At the first sign of a cold, use asthma medications to control symptoms.

- *Physical activity.* Intense activity is a common trigger for most people with asthma.

Exercise-Induced Asthma Symptoms and Phases

Although not entirely understood, most clinicians feel that EIA is triggered as the lining cells of the airway are cooled and dried during exercise.[134] As air is taken into the lungs, it is warmed and humidified, resulting in a cooling and drying of the airway lining. Certain chemicals are then released by the lining cells, causing the airways to tighten. This cooling and drying are worsened by several factors, including exercising in cool and dry air, a switch from nasal to mouth breathing, and fast and deep breathing from intense exercise. If pollutants and pollen are in the air, the risk of EIA is increased.[121–128]

EIA symptoms do not generally occur during the exercise bout itself or the first few minutes after exercise (see Figure 16.22). Following exercise, EIA goes through at least three phases.[121,124,125]

- *Early phase response.* Within several minutes after stopping exercise, the airways begin to tighten, leading to difficulty in breathing, wheezing, coughing, and chest tightness. The symptoms are most severe within 5–10 minutes after exercise. The EIA attack generally lasts 5–15 minutes.

  In the laboratory, clinicians diagnose EIA if the ability to exhale a certain amount of air from the lungs quickly (within 1 second) falls by 15% or more following 6–8 minutes of high-intensity exercise (90% of the maximal heart rate)[134] (see Box 16.7). Many asthmatics now use peak-flow meters, which are small devices that measure how well air moves out of the

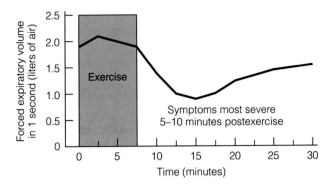

Figure 16.22 Pattern of exercise-induced asthma. EIA is diagnosed if FEV_1 falls by 15% or more following 6–8 minutes of high-intensity exercise. *Source:* Hendrickson CD, Lynch JM, Gleeson K. Exercise induced asthma: A clinical perspective. *Lung* 172:1–14, 1993.

Box 16.7

National Institutes of Health Guidelines for Exercise-Induced Asthma

Exercise-induced asthma, which untreated can limit and disrupt otherwise normal lives, should be anticipated in all asthma patients. EIA is a bronchospastic event that is caused by a loss of heat, water, or both from the lung during exercise because of hyperventilation of air that is cooler and dryer than that of the respiratory tree. EIA usually occurs during or minutes after vigorous activity, reaches its peak 5–10 minutes after stopping the activity, and usually resolves in another 20–30 minutes

Exercise may be the only precipitant of asthma symptoms for some patients. These patients should be monitored regularly to ensure that they have no symptoms of asthma or reductions in peak expiratory flow (PEF) in the absence of exercise because EIA is often a marker of inadequate asthma management and responds well to regular anti-inflammatory therapy.

Diagnosis

A history of cough, shortness of breath, chest pain or tightness, wheezing, or endurance problems during exercise suggests EIA. An exercise challenge can be used to establish the diagnosis. This can be performed in a formal laboratory setting or as a free-run challenge sufficiently strenuous to increase the baseline heart rate to 80% of maximum for 4–6 minutes. Alternatively, the patient may simply undertake the task that previously caused the symptoms. A 15% decrease in PEF or FEV_1 (forced expiratory volume in one second) (measurements taken before and after exercise at 5-minute intervals for 20–30 minutes) is compatible with EIA.

Management Strategies

One goal of management is to enable patients to participate in any activity they choose without experiencing asthma symptoms. EIA should not limit either partici-

pation or success in vigorous activities. Recommended treatments include the following:

Beta₂-agonists will prevent EIA in more than 80% of patients.

- Short-acting inhaled beta₂-agonists used shortly before exercise (or as close to exercise as possible) may be helpful for 2–3 hours.

- Salmeterol has been shown to prevent EIA for 10–12 hours.

Cromolyn and nedocromil, taken shortly before exercise, are also acceptable for preventing EIA.

A lengthy warm-up period before exercise may benefit patients who can tolerate continuous exercise with minimal symptoms. The warm-up may preclude a need for repeated medications.

Long-term-control therapy, if appropriate, may affect EIA. There is evidence that appropriate long-term control of asthma with anti-inflammatory medication will reduce airway responsiveness, and this is associated with a reduction in the frequency and severity of EIA.

Teachers and coaches need to be notified that a child has EIA, should be able to participate in activities, and may need inhaled medication before activity. Individuals involved in competitive athletics need to be aware that their medication use should be disclosed and should adhere to standards set by the U.S. Olympic Committee. The U.S. Olympic Committee's Drug Control Hotline is 800-233-0393.

Source: U.S. Department of Health and Human Services, PHS, NIH, NHLBI. *Guidelines for the Diagnosis and Management of Asthma*, NIH Publication No. 97-4051. Bethesda, MD: National Heart, Lung, and Blood Institute, 1997.

airways. Asthmatics should avoid exercising vigorously until the peak-flow reading returns to or exceeds 80% of the personal-best peak-flow reading.

- *Spontaneous recovery.* EIA symptoms gradually diminish, usually within 45–60 minutes.
- *Refractory period.* If the individual exercises again within 30–90 minutes of the first bout, the airway tightening is markedly less, and fewer EIA symptoms are experienced.

Some individuals with EIA appear to experience a late asthmatic attack about 3–6 hours after the first one. This late response is still debated, and many factors other than exercise may be responsible.[133,134]

Despite the fact that exercise may trigger asthma, the benefits that come from regular physical training are so important that most asthma experts urge that it be included as an important part of the management strategy of the asthmatic.[134] Regular exercise improves the overall physical fitness level of the individual with asthma, improves psychological mood state, decreases the risk for other chronic diseases, and improves heart and lung function. Also, several researchers have shown that as the individual with asthma becomes physically fit, EIA attacks are less frequent.

Many famous athletes have coped with asthma, including Jackie Joyner-Kersee, Bill Koch, Greg Louganis, Dominique Wilkins, Jim Ryun, Tom Dolan, and Nancy Hogshead.[127] Each learned how to follow her or his own personal asthma management plan, which included a mix of proper medications and control of asthma triggers. Individuals who follow their asthma management plans and keep their asthma under control can usually participate vigorously in the full range of sports and physical activities. Proper management of EIA includes[133,134] (see Box 16.7)

- Monitoring airflow with a peak-flow meter
- Avoiding allergic triggers
- Using medication before exercise
- Modifying exercise habits and practices

Asthma symptoms can change a lot. They are often worse at night than during the day. They may be more intense in the winter or during "allergy seasons" when pollen counts are high. To help monitor airflow, the new National Heart, Lung, and Blood Institute guidelines recommend that people with moderate-to-severe asthma use a peak-flow meter twice a day.[134] Often, decreases in airflow can provide an early warning of an asthma attack.

Drugs that relax the muscle spasm in the wall of the airways and help to open them (e.g., bronchodilators) are often the first line of treatment in preventing EIA.[134] Doctors recommend using the medication (typically beta$_2$-agonist) from 5 minutes to 1 hour before exercise. Beta$_2$-agonist medications will control EIA in more than 80% of asthmat-

ics and are helpful for several hours. However, because effectiveness does decrease with time, it is preferable to take the medication just before exercise. If breathing problems develop during exercise, a second dose may be needed.

Cromolyn sodium is often prescribed to treat athletes who have EIA.[132–134] This drug, which is also an inhalant, prevents the lining of the airways from swelling in response to cold air or allergic triggers. Cromolyn sodium can be used up to 15 minutes before engaging in physical activity. Corticosteroids should be used as preventive medicine, usually on an ongoing basis, to help control the underlying inflammation.[135]

In addition to proper medications, control of triggers, and use of peak-flow meters, several modifications to the exercise program have proven valuable:[121–128]

- *Adequate warm-up and cool-down periods.* These help prevent or lessen episodes of EIA. The warm-up helps asthmatics take advantage of the refractory period when episodes of EIA are reduced.
- *Type of exercise.* This plays a critical role in determining the degree of EIA. Outdoor running is regarded as most conducive to EIA, followed by treadmill running, cycling, walking, and swimming. Swimming rarely leads to EIA because warm and humid air near the surface of the water prevents cooling and drying of the airways.
- *Length of exercise.* Long, intense, continuous exercise (e.g., running and cycling) causes more EIA than repeated short bursts of exercise (generally less than 5 minutes each). Stop-and-go sports such as tennis, volleyball, or football may lead to less EIA for some asthmatics.
- *Intensity of exercise.* High-intensity exercise (above 80–90% of the maximal heart rate) causes more EIA than does exercise at more moderate levels (e.g., walking).
- *Nasal breathing.* Breathe slowly through the nose whenever possible. Nasal breathing warms and humidifies the air better than breathing through the mouth. Interestingly, research has shown that while breathing through the nose only, most people can reach an exercise intensity great enough to improve aerobic fitness.
- *Wear a mask or scarf in cold weather.* This can increase the temperature and humidity of the inhaled air, reducing cooling and drying of the airway lining.
- *Monitor the environment for potential allergens and irritants.* Examples include a recently mowed field, refinished gym floor, smoke in the air, or high pollen counts during a spring morning. If an allergen or irritant is present, a temporary change in time of day or location should be considered because the presence of irritants can trigger more severe EIA attacks.

SPORTS MEDICINE INSIGHT

Risks versus Benefits—A Summary

Broad claims have been made regarding the health benefits of physical activity—but claiming too much can ruin the message.[136–140] Many of the benefit claims are not supported by all researchers. In addition, benefits must be balanced against the risks, which rise exponentially with excessive exercise.

Table 16.1 is a summary of the major benefits of exercise described in Chapters 10 through 15, balanced against the potential risks outlined in this chapter. The summary represents the author's evaluation of present evidence and published data. The "surety rating" is an estimate of the strength of the data.

Notice from Table 16.1 that the highest "surety ratings" indicate that regular physical activity improves health in the following ways:

- Reduces the risk of dying prematurely (i.e., improves life expectancy)
- Reduces the risk of dying from coronary heart disease
- Reduces the risk of developing type 2 diabetes
- Helps prevent and treat high blood pressure
- Reduces the risk of developing colon cancer
- Reduces feelings of depression and anxiety, while improving mood state and self-esteem
- Helps control body weight
- Helps build and maintain healthy bones and muscles, and improves heart and lung fitness
- Improves the life quality of older adults, patients with disease, and people of all ages

Also notice that in some health and disease areas, very little evidence exists to support a prevention or treatment role for regular physical activity. As summarized in Table 16.1, there are few or no physical activity research data supporting the treatment or prevention of type 1 diabetes, arthritis, asthma, and most types of cancer. Regular exercise has also not been shown to slow the progression of HIV infection to AIDS. When change in dietary habits and weight loss is controlled, physical exercise has not been consistently linked to a decrease in LDL cholesterol. Also, more research is needed to confirm whether physical activity can promote regression of atherosclerosis, prevent stroke or hormone-dependent cancers such as breast and prostate cancer, treat osteoporosis, prevent and treat low-back pain, improve diet quality, enhance success in quitting cigarette smoking, improve immunity, and protect against the common cold.

Figure 16.23 depicts the relationship between exercise and risks versus benefits. The greatest gain in the risk–benefit relationship occurs at the lower end of the activity spectrum. In other words, the greatest benefits of exercise are gained by previously sedentary people just beginning moderate exercise programs. Risks are low at the lower levels of activity, but become increasingly frequent and severe at higher levels. Thus, such activities as brisk walking are highly recommended, producing many benefits with few risks.

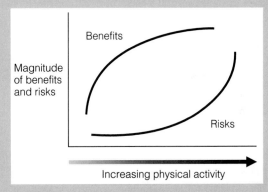

Figure 16.23 The increase in benefits from regular exercise are greatest at low levels and diminish with increasing activity. Risks, on the other hand, are low at lower levels and become increasingly frequent and severe at higher levels.

TABLE 16.1 The Health Benefits and Risks of Regular Physical Activity[a]

Physical Activity Benefit/Risk	Surety Rating	Physical Activity Benefit/Risk	Surety Rating
Fitness of Body		**Cardiovascular disease**	
Improved heart & lung fitness	****	Coronary heart disease prevention	****
Improved muscular strength/size	****	Regression of atherosclerosis	**
Risk: Musculoskeletal injury	****	Treatment of heart disease	***
Risk: Heat injury	****	Prevention of stroke	**

(continued)

TABLE 16.1 The Health Benefits and Risks of Regular Physical Activity[a] *(continued)*

Physical Activity Benefit/Risk	Surety Rating	Physical Activity Benefit/Risk	Surety Rating
Risk: Heart attack for those at high risk	****	**Diabetes**	
Cancer		Prevention of type 2	****
Prevention of colon cancer	****	Treatment of type 2	***
Prevention of breast cancer	**	Treatment of Type 1	*
Prevention of uterine cancer	**	Improvement of diabetic life quality	***
Prevention of prostate cancer	**	*Risk:* Hypoglycemia, type 1	****
Prevention of other cancers	*	**Infection and Immunity**	
Treatment of cancer	*	Prevention of the common cold	**
Osteoporosis		Improve overall immunity	**
Helps build up bone density	****	Slow progression of HIV to AIDS	*
Prevention of osteoporosis	***	Improve life quality of HIV-infected	***
Treatment of osteoporosis	**	*Risk:* Immune suppression, infection from overtraining	***
Blood Cholesterol/Lipoproteins		**Arthritis**	
Lowers total blood cholesterol	*	Prevention of arthritis	*
Lowers LDL cholesterol	*	Treatment/cure of arthritis	*
Lowers triglycerides	***	Improvement life quality/fitness	****
Raises HDL cholesterol	***	**High Blood Pressure**	
Low-Back Pain		Prevention of high blood pressure	****
Prevention of low-back pain	**	Treatment of high blood pressure	****
Treatment of low-back pain	**	**Asthma**	
Nutrition and Diet Quality		Prevention/treatment of asthma	*
Improvement in diet quality	**	Improvement in asthmatic's life quality	***
Increase in total energy intake	***	*Risk:* Exercise-induced asthma	****
Risk: Iron deficiency	***		
Cigarette Smoking			
Improves success in quitting	**		

SUMMARY

1. This chapter surveyed some of the risks involved with exercise, especially when performed excessively. These include musculoskeletal injuries, disruption of normal reproductive function of women, possible problems for women who are pregnant, heat injury, effects of air pollution on performance, sudden death from heart attack, increased risk of infectious episodes and exercise-induced asthma.

2. The potential for musculoskeletal injury was reviewed for running, aerobic dance, bicycling, and swimming. Most of the injuries are related to overtraining and accidents. The muscles, joints, and supporting ligaments and tendons of the legs and feet respond very poorly to excessive exercise, especially activities that require running and jumping.

3. Running is associated with a high rate of musculoskeletal injuries, with 24–77% of runners reporting injuries within a given year. Although most of the runners usually do not seek medical help, the pain is frequently serious enough to disrupt the running routine.

4. Researchers have tried to measure the factors responsible for the high prevalence of injuries among runners and have looked at both personal factors and training habits. Overtraining is a common cause of injury.

5. The major studies examining the injury potential of aerobic dance have found that about 45% of students and 75% of instructors report injuries. Most of these injuries, however, are mild, causing some

TABLE 16.1 The Health Benefits and Risks of Regular Physical Activity[a] *(continued)*

Physical Activity Benefit/Risk	Surety Rating	Physical Activity Benefit/Risk	Surety Rating
Sleep		**Psychological Well-Being**	
Improvement in sleep quality	***	Elevation in mood	****
Risk: Sleep disturbance from overtraining, overexertion	***	Buffers effects of mental stress	***
		Alleviate/prevent depression	****
Weight Management		Anxiety reduction	****
Prevention of weight gain	****	Improvement in self-esteem	****
Treatment of obesity	**	*Risk:* Exercise addiction	***
Helps maintain weight loss	****	*Risk:* Mood disturbance, overtraining	***
Risk: Musculoskeletal injury	****	**Special Issues for Women**	
Children and Youths		Improves total body fitness	****
Prevention of obesity	***	Improves fitness while pregnant	****
Control of disease risk factors	***	Improves birthing experience	**
Reduction of unhealthy habits	**	Improves health of fetus	**
Improves odds of adult activity	**	*Risk:* Female athlete triad	****
Elderly and the Aging Process		*Risk:* Harm to fetus	**
Improvement in physical fitness	****		
Counter loss in heart/lung fitness	**		
Counter loss of muscle	***		
Counter gain in fat	***		
Improvement in life expectancy	****		
Improvement in life quality	****		

[a]Table is based on a total physical fitness program that includes physical activity designed to improve both aerobic and musculoskeletal fitness.

****Strong consensus, with little or no conflicting data

*** Most data are supportive, but more research is needed for clarification

** Some data are supportive, but much more research is needed

* Few or no data support

pain and some disruption in participation, but generally falling short of leading participants to cease aerobic-dance activities or to seek professional medical assistance.

6. Studies have shown that exercise increases the rates of oligomenorrhea and amenorrhea; they vary widely, however, depending on the type of athlete and the amount of training. The causes are still hotly debated. Loss of bone mineral mass is a problem for oligomenorrheic athletes. The *female athlete triad* is the syndrome of disordered eating habits and heavy exercise leading to amenorrhea and osteoporosis.

7. Moderate exercise during pregnancy serves to maintain the fitness of the mother and has been associated with several favorable pregnancy outcomes.

8. The American College of Sports Medicine has advised athletes that the risk of heat exhaustion and heat stroke during high temperature and humidity is greatly increased. Heat injury is a major cause of death among exercising athletes, and appropriate measures should be taken, including postponing the exercise.

9. The air pollutant regarded as the most detrimental to athletic performance is ozone. Heavy exercise in air polluted with ozone has been shown to impair the ability to exercise and decrease lung function at least temporarily.

10. The principal cause of death among adults over 30 years of age during exercise is coronary heart attack. It happens rarely, however, and more often to those with underlying heart disease and those unaccustomed to exercise. Congenital forms of cardiovascular disease are the leading cause of athletic death in younger athletes.

11. Excessive exercise has been associated with increased risk of infectious health problems. Moderate exercise may be protective, but little research has been conducted so far to verify this.

12. During and following strenuous exercise, the majority of asthmatics experience exercise-induced asthma (EIA). EIA can be controlled with appropriate medications and exercise techniques.

13. The risks of exercise must be balanced with all of its documented benefits. The greatest gain in the risk–benefit relationship occurs at the lower end of the activity spectrum.

REFERENCES

1. Kreider RB, Fry AC, O'Toole ML. *Overtraining in Sport.* Champaign, IL: Human Kinetics, 1998.

2. Pate RR, Macera CA. Risk of exercising: Musculo-skeletal injuries. In Bouchard C, Shephard RJ (eds), *Exercise, Fitness, and Health: A Consensus of Current Knowledge.* Champaign, IL: Human Kinetics Books, 1994.

3. O'Toole ML. Prevention and treatment of injuries to runners. *Med Sci Sports Exerc* 24(9)(suppl):S360–S363, 1992.

4. Van Mechelen W. Running injuries: A review of the epidemiological literature. *Sports Med* 14:320–335, 1992.

5. Hoeberigs JH. Factors related to the incidence of running injuries: A review. *Sports Med* 13:408–422, 1992.

6. Koplan JP, Powell KE, Sikes RK, Shirley RW, Campbell GC. An epidemiologic study of the benefits and risks of running. *JAMA* 248:3118–3121, 1982.

7. Koplan JP, Siscovick DS, Goldbaum GM. The risks of exercise: A public health view of injuries and hazards. *Pub Health Rep* 100:189–195, 1985.

8. Powell KE, Kohl HW, Caspersen CJ, Blair SN. An epidemiological perspective on the causes of running injuries. *Physician Sportsmed* 14(6):100–114, 1986.

9. Koplan JP, Rothenberg RB, Jones EL. The natural history of exercise: A 10-yr follow-up of a cohort of runners. *Med Sci Sports Exerc* 27:1180–1184, 1995.

10. Marti B, Vader JP, Minder CE, Abelin T. On the epidemiology of running injuries. *Am J Sports Med* 16:285–294, 1988.

11. Marti B. Benefits and risks of running among women: An epidemiologic study. *Int J Sports Med* 9:92–98, 1988.

12. Blair SN, Kohl HW, Goodyear NN. Rates and risks for running and exercise injuries: Studies in three populations. *Res Quart Exerc Sport* 58:221–228, 1987.

13. Macera CA, Pate RR, Power KE, et al. Predicting lower-extremity injuries among habitual runners. *Arch Intern Med* 149:2565–2568, 1989.

14. Walter SD, Hart LE, McIntosh JM, Sutton JR. The Ontario cohort study of running-related injuries. *Arch Intern Med* 149:2561–2564, 1989.

15. Van Mechelen W. Can running injuries be effectively prevented? *Sports Med* 19:161–165, 1995.

16. Wen DY, Puffer JC, Schmalzried TP. Lower extremity alignment and risk of overuse injuries in runners. *Med Sci Sports Exerc* 29:1291–1298, 1997.

17. Jones BH, Cowan DN, Tomlinson JP, et al. Epidemiology of injuries associated with physical training among young men in the army. *Med Sci Sports Exerc* 25:197–203, 1993.

18. Ireland ML, Micheli LJ. Triathletes: Biographic data, training, and injury patterns. *Ann Sports Med* 3:117–120, 1987.

19. Kuipers H. How much is too much? Performance aspects of overtraining. *Res Quart Exerc Sport* 67(suppl):65–69, 1996.

20. Messier SP, Davis SE, Curl WW, Lowery RB, Pack RJ. Etiologic factors associated with patellofemoral pain in runners. *Med Sci Sports Exerc* 23:1008–1015, 1991.

21. Messier SP, Pittala KA. Etiologic factors associated with selected running injuries. *Med Sci Sports Exerc* 20:501–505, 1988.

22. Pretorius DM, Noakes TD, Irving G, Allerton K. Runner's knee: What is it and how effective is conservative management? *Phys Sportsmed* 14(12):71–81, 1986.

23. Messier SP, Edwards DG, Martin DF, et al. Etiology of iliotibial band friction syndrome in distance runners. *Med Sci Sports Exerc* 27:951–960, 1995.

24. Garrick JG, Requa RK. Aerobic dance: A review. *Sports Med* 6:169–179, 1988.

25. Garrick JG, Gillien DM, Whiteside P. The epidemic of aerobic dance injuries. *Am J Sports Med* 14:67–72, 1986.

26. Rothenberger LA, Chang JI, Cable TA. Prevalence and types of injuries in aerobic dancers. *Am J Sports Med* 16:403–407, 1988.

27. Mutoh Y, Sawai S, Takanashi Y, Skurko L. Aerobic dance injuries among instructors and students. *Physician Sportsmed* 16:81–88, 1988.

28. Richie DH, Kelso SF, Bellucci PA. Aerobic dance injuries: A retrospective study of instructors and participants. *Physician Sportsmed* 13:130–140, 1985.

29. Mellion MB. Common cycling injuries: Management and prevention. *Sports Med* 11:52–70, 1991.

30. Sacks JJ, Holmgreen P, Smith SM, Sosin DM. Bicycle-associated head injuries and deaths in the United States from 1984 through 1988: How many are preventable? *JAMA* 266:3016–3018, 1991.

31. Wasserman RC, Waller JA, Monty MJ, Emergy AB, Robinson DR. Bicyclists, helmets and head injuries: A rider-based study of helmet use and effectiveness. *Am J Public Health* 78:1220–1221, 1988.

32. Kronisch RL, Pfeiffer RP, Chow TK. Acute injuries in cross-country and downhill off-road bicycle racing. *Med Sci Sports Exerc* 28:1351–1355, 1996.

33. Thompson DC, Rivara FP, Thompson RS. Effectiveness of bicycle safety helmets in preventing head injuries. *JAMA* 276:1968–1973, 1996.

34. Dannenberg AL, Vernick JS. A proposal for the mandatory inclusion of helmets with new children's bicycles. *Am J Public Health* 83:644–646, 1993.

35. Dannenberg AL, Gielen AC, Beilenson PL, Wilson MH, Joffe A. Bicycle helmet laws and educational campaigns: An evaluation of strategies to increase children's helmet use. *Am J Public Health* 83:667–674, 1993.

36. Johnson JE, Sim FH, Scott SG. Musculoskeletal injuries in competitive swimmers. *Mayo Clin Proc* 62:289–304, 1987.

37. Koehler SM, Thorson DC. Swimmer's shoulder. *Physician Sportsmed* 24(11):39–50, 1996.

38. Vizsolyi P, Taunton J, Robertson G, et al. Breaststroker's knee: An analysis of epidemiological and biochemical factors. *Am J Sports Med* 15:63–71, 1987.

39. O'Connor FG, Howard TM, Fieseler CM, Nirschl RP. Managing overuse injuries: A systematic approach. *Physician Sportsmed* 25(5):88–113, 1997.

40. Rizzo TD. Using RICE for injury relief. *Physician Sportsmed* 24(10):33–34, 1996.

41. Hasson SM, Daniels JC, Divine JG, et al. Effect of ibuprofen use on muscle soreness, damage, and performance: A preliminary investigation. *Med Sci Sports Exerc* 25:9–17, 1993.

42. Wilkerson GB. External compression for controlling traumatic edema. *Physician Sportsmed* 13:97–106, 1985.

43. ACSM position stand on the female athlete triad. *Med Sci Sports Exerc* 29:i–ix, 1997.

44. Joy E, Clark N, Ireland ML, Martire J, Nattiv A, Varechok S. Team management of the female athlete triad: Part 1. What to look for, what to ask. *Physician Sportsmed* 25(3):12–16, 1997; Part 2. What to look for, what to ask. *Physician Sportsmed* 25(4):13–17, 1997.

45. Yeager KK, Agostini R, Nattiv A, Drinkwater B. The female athlete triad: Disordered eating, amenorrhea, osteoporosis. *Med Sci Sports Exerc* 25:775–777, 1993.

46. Loucks AB, Vaitukaitis J, Cameron JL, et al. The reproductive system and exercise in women. *Med Sci Sports Exerc* 24(suppl): S288–S292, 1992.

47. De Souza MJ, Metzger DA. Reproductive dysfunction in amenorrheic athletes and anorexic patients: A review. *Med Sci Sports Exerc* 23:995–1007, 1991.

48. Merzenich H, Boeing H, Wahrendorf J. Dietary fat and sports activity as determinants for age at menarche. *Am J Epidemiol* 138:217–224, 1993.

49. Bonen A. Recreational exercise does not impair menstrual cycles: A prospective study. *Int J Sports Med* 13:110–120, 1992.

50. Rogol AD, Weltman A, Weltman JY, et al. Durability of the reproductive axis in eumenorrheic women during 1 yr of endurance training. *J Appl Physiol* 74:1571–1580, 1992.

51. Rencken ML, Chestnut CH, Drinkwater BL. Bone density at multiple skeletal sites in amenorrheic athletes. *JAMA* 276:238–240, 1996.

52. Lloyd T, Triantafyllou SJ, Baker ER, et al. Women athletes with menstrual irregularity have increased musculoskeletal injuries. *Med Sci Sports Exerc* 18:374–379, 1986.

53. Barrow GW, Saha S. Menstrual irregularity and stress fractures in collegiate female distance runners. *Am J Sports Med* 16:209–216, 1988.

54. Drinkwater BL, Nilson K, Chestnut CH, et al. Bone mineral content of amenorrheic and eumenorrheic athletes. *N Engl J Med* 311:277–281, 1984.

55. Snead DB, Stubbs CC, Weltman JY, et al. Dietary patterns, eating behaviors, and bone mineral density in women runners. *Am J Clin Nutr* 56:705–711, 1992.

56. Perry AC, Crane LS, Applegate B, Marquez-Sterling S, Signorile JF, Miller PC. Nutrient intake and psychological and physiological assessment in eumenorrheic and amenorrheic female athletes: A preliminary study. *Int J Sport Nutr* 6:3–13, 1996.

57. Arena B, Maffulli N, Maffulli F, Morleo MA. Reproductive hormones and menstrual changes with exercise in female athletes. *Sports Med* 19:278–287, 1995.

58. Williams NI, Young JC, McArthur JW, Bullen B, Skrinar GS, Turnbull B. Strenuous exercise with caloric restriction: Effect on luteinizing hormone secretion. *Med Sci Sports Exerc* 27:1390–1398, 1995.

59. Dueck CA, Manore MM, Matt KS. Role of energy balance in athletic menstrual dysfunction. *Int J Sport Nutr* 6:165–190, 1996.

60. Keizer HA, Rogol AD. Physical exercise and menstrual cycle alterations: What are the mechanisms? *Sports Med* 10:218–235, 1990.

61. Myerson M, Gutin B, Warren MP, et al. Resting metabolic rate and energy balance in amenorrheic and eumenorrheic runners. *Med Sci Sports Exerc* 23:15–22, 1991.

62. Weight LM, Noakes TD. Is running an analog of anorexia? A survey of the incidence of eating disorders in female distance runners. *Med Sci Sports Exerc* 19:213–217, 1987.

63. Lindberg JS, Powell MR, Hunt MM, et al. Increased vertebral bone mineral in response to reduced exercise in amenorrheic runners. *West J Med* 146:39–42, 1987.

64. Drinkwater BL, Nilson K, Ott S, Chesnut CH. Bone mineral density after resumption of menses in amenorrheic athletes. *JAMA* 256:380–382, 1986.

65. Dueck CA, Matt KS, Manore MM, Skinner JS. Treatment of athletic amenorrhea with a diet and training intervention program. *Int J Sport Nutr* 6:24–40, 1996.

66. Cumming DC. Exercise-associated amenorrhea, low bone density, and estrogen replacement therapy. *Arch Intern Med* 156:2193–2195, 1996.

67. Sternfeld B. Physical activity and pregnancy outcome: Review and recommendations. *Sports Med* 23:33–47, 1997.

68. Araujo D. Expecting questions about exercise and pregnancy? *Physician Sportsmed* 25(4):20–24, 1997.

69. McMurray RG, Mottola MF, Wolfe LA, Artal RM, Millar L, Pivarnik JM. Recent advances in understanding maternal and fetal responses to exercise. *Med Sci Sports Exerc* 25:1305–1321, 1993.

70. Clapp JF, Rokey R, Treadway JL, Carpenter MW, Artal RM, Warrnes C. Exercise in pregnancy. *Med Sci Sports Exerc* 24 (suppl):S294–S300, 1992.

71. Lokey EA, Tran ZT, Wells CL, Myers BC, Tran AC. Effects of physical exercise on pregnancy outcomes: A meta-analytic review. *Med Sci Sports Exerc* 23:1234–1239, 1991.

72. Clapp JF, Little KD. Effect of recreational exercise on pregnancy weight gain and subcutaneous fat deposition. *Med Sci Sports Exerc* 27:170–177, 1995.

73. Schramm WF, Stockbauer JW, Hoffman HJ. Exercise, employment, other daily activities, and adverse pregnancy outcomes. *Am J Epidemiol* 143:211–218, 1996.

74. Sternfeld B, Quesenberry CP, Eskenazi B, Newman LA. Exercise during pregnancy and pregnancy outcome. *Med Sci Sports Exerc* 27:634–640, 1995.

75. Artal R. Exercise: An alternative therapy for gestational diabetes. *Physician Sportsmed* 24(3):54–66, 1996.

76. Wolfe LA, Ohtake PJ, Mottola MF, McGrath MJ. Physiological interactions between pregnancy and aerobic exercise. *Exerc Sport Sci Rev* 17:295–351, 1989.

77. Clapp JF, Dickstein S. Endurance exercise and pregnancy outcome. *Med Sci Sports Exerc* 16:556–562, 1984.

78. American College of Obstetricians and Gynecologists. *Exercise during Pregnancy and the Postnatal Period (ACOG Home Exercise Programs)*. Washington, DC: Author, 1985.

79. American College of Obstetricians and Gynecologists. *Exercise during Pregnancy and the Postpartum Period,* Technical Bulletin #189. Washington, DC: Author, 1994.

80. American College of Sports Medicine. Position stand on heat and cold illnesses during distance running. *Med Sci Sports Exerc* 27:i–x, 1996.

81. CDC. Heat-related deaths—United States, 1993. *MMWR* 42: 558–560, 1993.

82. Armstrong LE, Maresh CM. The exertional heat illnesses: A risk of athletic participation. *Med Exerc Nutr Health* 2:125–134, 1993.

83. Verdaguer-Codina J, Martin DE, Pujol-Amat P, Ruiz A, Inef L, Prat JA. Climatic heat stress studies at the Barcelona Olympic games, 1992. *Sports Med Train Rehab* 6:167–192, 1995.

84. Galloway SDR, Maughan RJ. Effects of ambient temperature on the capacity to perform prolonged cycle exercise in man. *Med Sci Sports Exerc* 29:1240–1249, 1997.

85. Sandon RP. Heat illness. *Physician Sportsmed* 25(6):35–40, 1997.

86. Gardner JW, Kark JA, Karni K, Sanborn JS, Gastaldo E, Burr P, Wenger CB. Risk factors predicting exertional heat illness in male Marine Corps recruits. *Med Sci Sports Exerc* 28:939–944, 1996.

87. Schenker M. Air pollution and mortality. *N Engl J Med* 329: 1807–1808, 1993.

88. Dockery DW, Pope A, Xu X, et al. An association between air pollution and mortality in six U.S. cities. *N Engl J Med* 329: 1753–1759, 1993.

89. CDC. Populations at risk from air pollution—United States, 1991. *MMWR* 42:301–304, 1993.

90. Borja-Aburto VH, Loomis DP, Bangdiwala SI, Shy CM, Rascon-Pacheco RA. Ozone, suspended particulates, and daily mortality in Mexico City. *Am J Epidemiol* 145:258–268, 1997.

91. Adams WC. Effects of ozone exposure at ambient air pollution episode levels on exercise performance. *Sports Med* 4: 395–424, 1987.

92. Hazucha MJ, Bates DV, Dromberg PA. Mechanisms of action of ozone on the human lung. *J Appl Physiol* 67:1535–1541, 1989.

93. Folinsbee LJ, et al. Pulmonary function changes after 1 h continuous heavy exercise in 0.21 ppm ozone. *J Appl Physiol* 57: 984–988, 1984.

94. Schelegle ES, Adams WC. Reduced exercise time in competitive simulations consequent to low level ozone exposure. *Med Sci Sports Exerc* 18:408–414, 1986.

95. Foxcroft WJ, Adams WC. Effects of ozone exposure on four consecutive days on work performance and $\dot{V}O_2$ max. *J Appl Physiol* 61:960–966, 1986.

96. Wiester MJ, Watkinson WP, Costa DL, et al. Ozone toxicity in the rat: III. Effect of changes in ambient temperature on pulmonary parameters. *J Appl Physiol* 81:1691–1700, 1996.

97. Kunzli N, Lurmann F, Segal M, Ngo L, Balmes J, Tager IB. Association between lifetime ambient ozone exposure and pulmonary function in college freshmen—results of a pilot study. *Environ Res* 72:8–23, 1997.

98. Cooper KH. *Running without Fear.* New York: Bantam Books, 1985.

99. Powell KE, Thompson PD, Caspersen CJ, Kendric JS. Physical activity and the incidence of coronary heart disease. *Ann Rev Public Health* 8:253–287, 1987.

100. Maron BJ, Shirani J, Poliac LC, Mathenge R, Roberts WC, Mueller FO. Sudden death in young competitive athletes. *JAMA* 276:199–204, 1996.

101. American Heart Association. Cardiovascular preparticipation screening of competitive athletes. *Circulation* 94:850–856, 1996.

102. Thompson PD. The cardiovascular complications of vigorous physical activity. *Arch Intern Med* 156:2297–2302, 1996.

103. Mittleman MA, Maclure M, Tofler GH, Sherwood JB, Goldberg RJ, Muller JE. Triggering of acute myocardial infarction by heavy physical exertion: Protection against triggering by regular exertion. *N Engl J Med* 329:1677–1683, 1993.

104. Willich SN, Lewis M, Löwel H, Arntz H-R, Schubert F, Schröder R. Physical exertion as a trigger of acute myocardial infarction. *N Engl J Med* 329:1684–1690, 1993.

105. Curfman GD. Is exercise beneficial—or hazardous—to your heart? *N Engl J Med* 329:1730–1731, 1993.

106. Noakes TD. Heart disease in marathon runners: A review. *Med Sci Sports Exerc* 19:187–194, 1987.

107. Maron BJ, Poliac LC, Roberts WO. Risk for sudden cardiac death associated with marathon running. *J Am Coll Cardiol* 28: 428–431, 1996.

108. Van Camp SP. Exercise-related sudden death: Risks and causes. *Physician Sportsmed* 16(5):97–112, 1988.

109. Siscovick DS, Weiss NS, Fletcher RH, Lasky T. The incidence of primary cardiac arrest during vigorous exercise. *N Engl J Med* 311:874–877, 1984.

110. Nieman DC. Exercise, upper respiratory tract infection, and the immune system. *Med Sci Sports Exerc* 26:128–139, 1994.

111. Nieman DC. Exercise immunology: Practical applications. *Int J Sports Med* 18(suppl 1):S91–S100, 1997.

112. Nieman DC, Nehlsen-Cannarella SL, Markoff PA, et al. The effects of moderate exercise training on natural killer cells and acute upper respiratory tract infections. *Int J Sports Med* 11: 467–473, 1990.

113. Nieman DC, Henson DA, Gusewitch G, Warren BJ, Dotson RC, Butterworth DE, Nehlsen-Cannarella SL. Physical activity and immune function in elderly women. *Med Sci Sports Exerc* 25:823–831, 1993.

114. Pedersen BK. *Exercise Immunology.* New York: Springer, 1997.

115. Pedersen BK, Ullum H. NK cell response to physical activity: Possible mechanisms of action. *Med Sci Sports Exerc* 26:140–146, 1994.

116. Nieman DC. Immune response to heavy exertion. *J Appl Physiol* 82:1385–1394, 1997.

117. Nieman DC, Johansen LM, Lee JW, Cermak J, Arabatzis K. Infectious episodes in runners before and after the Los Angeles marathon. *J Sports Med Phys Fit* 30:316–328, 1990.

118. Peters EM, Bateman ED. Respiratory tract infections: An epidemiological survey. *S Afr Med J* 64:582–584, 1983.

119. Peters EM, Goetzsche JM, Grobbelaar B, et al. Vitamin C supplementation reduces the incidence of postrace symptoms of upper-respiratory-tract infection in ultramarathon runners. *Am J Clin Nutr* 57:170–174, 1993.

120. Pyne DB. Regulation of neutrophil function during exercise. *Sports Med* 17:245–258, 1994.

121. Mahler DA. Exercise-induced asthma. *Med Sci Sports Exerc* 25: 554–561, 1993.

122. Virant FS. Exercise-induced bronchospasm: Epidemiology, pathophysiology, and therapy. *Med Sci Sports Exerc* 24:851–855, 1992.

123. Kyle JM, Walker RB, Hanshaw SL, Leaman JR, Frobase JK. Exercise-induced bronchospasms in the young athlete: Guidelines for routine screening and initial management. *Med Sci Sports Exerc* 24:856–859, 1992.

124. Giesbrecht GG, Younes M. Exercise- and cold-induced asthma. *Can J Appl Physiol* 20:300–314, 1995.

125. Hendrickson CD, Lynch JM, Gleeson K. Exercise induced asthma: A clinical perspective. *Lung* 172:1–14, 1993.

126. McKenzie DC. The asthmatic athlete: A brief review. *Clin J Sport Med* 1:110–114, 1991.

127. Papazian R. Being a sport with exercise-induced asthma. *FDA Consumer,* January–February 1994, 30–33.

128. Rupp NT. Diagnosis and management of exercise-induced asthma. *Physician Sportsmed* 24(1):77–87, 1996.

129. Asthma—United States, 1980–1990. *MMWR* 41:733–735, 1992.

130. Weiss KB, Wagener DK. Changing patterns of asthma mortality: Identifying target populations at high risk. *JAMA* 264:1683–1687, 1990.

131. Flieger K. Controlling asthma. *FDA Consumer,* November 1996, 19–23.

132. U.S. Department of Health and Human Services, PHS, NIH, NHLBI. *Asthma and Physical Activity in the School,* NIH Publication No. 95-3651. Bethesda, MD: National Heart, Lung, and Blood Institute Information Center, 1995.

133. U.S. Department of Health and Human Services, PHS, NIH, NHLBI. *Asthma Management and Prevention, Global Initiative for Asthma: A Practical Guide for Public Health Officials and Health Care Professionals,* NIH Publication No. 96-3659A. Bethesda, MD: National Heart, Lung, and Blood Institute, 1995.

134. U.S. Department of Health and Human Services, PHS, NIH, NHLBI. *Guidelines for the Diagnosis and Management of Asthma,* NIH Publication No. 97-4051. Bethesda, MD: National Heart, Lung, and Blood Institute, 1997.

135. Donahue JG, Weiss ST, Livingston JM, Goetsch MA, Greineder DK, Platt R. Inhaled steroids and the risk of hospitalization for asthma. *JAMA* 277:887–891, 1997.

136. Powell KE, Paffenbarger RS. Workshop on epidemiologic and public health aspects of physical activity: A summary. *Public Health Rep* 100:118–126, 1985.

137. Phelps JR. Physical activity and health maintenance—exactly what is known? *West J Med* 146:200–206, 1987.

138. Elrick H. Exercise is medicine. *Physician Sportsmed* 24(2):72–78, 1996.

139. Ready AE, Naimark B, Ducas J, et al. Influence of walking volume on health benefits in women post-menopause. *Med Sci Sports Exerc* 28:1097–1105, 1996.

140. Nieman DC. *The Exercise–Health Connection.* Champaign, IL: Human Kinetics, 1998.

PHYSICAL FITNESS ACTIVITY 16.1

Benefits versus Risks of Exercise

As noted at the end of this chapter, while heavy amounts of exercise are associated with various risks, moderate exercise can bring many health benefits. Not exercising at all is worse than too much exercise, and moderate exercise is a virtue. The well-documented benefits of moderate exercise are too valuable to be ignored.

Major benefits of regular, moderate exercise include the following:

1. Improved heart and lung fitness
2. Lower resting heart rate
3. Firmer, toned muscles
4. Reduced body fat (especially when dietary fat is low)
5. Reduced risk of high blood pressure
6. Increased high-density lipoprotein cholesterol, reduced triglycerides
7. Reduced risk of cancer
8. Reduced risk of heart disease
9. Reduced risk of diabetes
10. Elevation of psychological mood state, and reduced anxiety and depression
11. Increased self-esteem
12. Increased density of bones, and lowered risk of osteoporosis
13. Improved quality of life even into old age
14. Increased life expectancy
15. Less fatigue, increased energy for work, leisure, and emergencies

Review this list carefully, and then, drawing on your own experience, list five benefits that *you* personally feel are most valuable to you. List the benefit, and then explain why you chose it. List the benefits in order of importance, beginning with the most important.

1. _____
_____

2. _____
_____

3. _____
_____

4. _____
_____

5. _____
_____

Review the chapter again carefully. List three risks that *you* personally feel have been most bothersome for you. In other words, drawing on your own experience, what risks have caused you the most pain and grief? List the risk, then explain why you chose it. Again, list in order of importance.

1. _____
_____

2. _____
_____

3. _____
_____

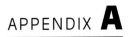

Physical Fitness Test Norms

Section 1. Physical Fitness Test Norms for Children, Adolescents, and College Students

NATIONAL CHILDREN AND YOUTH FITNESS STUDY I (NCYFS I)

In 1984, the Public Health Service (Office of Disease Prevention and Health Promotion, U.S. Department of Health and Human Services), in response to the landmark government report *Promoting Health/Preventing Disease: Objectives for the Nation*, launched the National Children and Youth Fitness Study to determine how fit and how active first- through twelfth-grade students actually are. Data on 10- to 18-year-olds were collected from a random sample of 10,275 students from 140 public and private schools in 19 states between February and May 1984. The NCYFS I was the first nationwide assessment of the physical fitness of American young people in nearly a decade and the most rigorous study of fitness among our youths ever conducted in the United States.

Test items of the NCYFS I include

- Triceps and subscapular skinfolds for body composition
- Walk/run (1 mile) for cardiorespiratory endurance
- Sit-and-reach test for lower back–hamstring flexibility
- Pull-up for upper-body muscular strength and endurance
- Bent-knee sit-ups (1 minute) for abdominal strength/endurance

---

Note: See description of methods in Chapters 4 to 6.

Source: Public Health Service. Summary of findings from National Children and Youth Fitness Study. *JOPHER*/January 1985, 44–90.

Interpretations of Norms

<25%	Unacceptable or Poor
25–50%	Minimal or Fair
50–75%	Acceptable or Good
>75%	Optimal or Excellent

TABLE 1 Sum of Triceps and Subscapular Skinfolds—Boys (total mm)

Age	10	11	12	13	14	15	16	17	18
99%	9	9	9	9	9	10	10	10	11
90	12	12	12	11	12	12	12	13	13
80	13	13	13	13	13	13	13	14	14
75	14	14	14	13	13	14	14	14	15
70	15	15	15	14	14	14	14	15	15
60	16	16	16	15	15	15	15	16	17
50	17	18	17	17	17	17	17	17	18
40	20	20	20	19	18	18	18	19	19
30	22	23	22	21	21	20	20	21	22
25	24	25	24	23	22	22	22	22	24
20	25	26	28	25	25	24	23	24	25
10	35	36	38	34	33	32	30	30	30

TABLE 2 Sum of Triceps and Subscapular Skinfolds—Girls (total mm)

Age	10	11	12	13	14	15	16	17	18
99%	10	11	11	12	12	13	13	16	14
90	13	14	15	15	17	19	19	20	19
80	15	16	17	18	19	21	21	22	21
75	16	17	18	19	20	23	22	23	22
70	17	18	18	20	21	24	23	24	23
60	18	19	21	22	24	26	24	26	25
50	20	21	22	24	26	28	26	28	27
40	22	24	24	26	28	30	28	31	28
30	25	28	27	29	31	33	32	34	32
25	27	30	29	31	33	34	33	36	34
20	29	33	31	34	35	37	35	37	36
10	36	40	40	43	40	43	12	42	42

TABLE 3 Chin-Ups—Boys (hands in underhand position, palms toward subject)

Age	10	11	12	13	14	15	16	17	18
99%	13	12	13	17	18	18	20	20	21
90	8	8	8	10	12	14	14	15	16
80	5	5	6	8	9	11	12	13	14
75	4	5	5	7	8	10	12	12	13
70	4	4	5	7	8	10	11	12	12
60	2	3	4	5	6	8	10	10	11
50	1	2	3	4	5	7	9	9	0
40	1	1	2	3	4	6	8	8	9
30	0	0	1	1	3	5	6	6	7
25	0	0	0	1	2	4	6	5	6
20	0	0	0	0	1	3	5	4	5
10	0	0	0	0	0	1	2	2	3

TABLE 4 Chin-Ups—Girls (hands in underhand position, palms toward subject)

Age	10	11	12	13	14	15	16	17	18
99%	8	8	8	5	8	6	8	7	6
90	3	3	2	2	2	2	2	2	2
80	2	1	1	1	1	1	1	1	1
75	1	1	1	1	1	1	1	1	1
70	1	1	1	0	1	1	1	1	1
60	0	0	0	0	0	0	0	0	0
50	0	0	0	0	0	0	0	0	0
40	0	0	0	0	0	0	0	0	0
30	0	0	0	0	0	0	0	0	0
20	0	0	0	0	0	0	0	0	0
10	0	0	0	0	0	0	0	0	0

TABLE 5 Bent-Knee Sit-Ups—Boys (number in 1 minute; arms crossed on chest)

Age	10	11	12	13	14	15	16	17	18
99%	60	60	61	62	64	65	65	68	67
90	47	48	50	52	52	53	55	56	54
80	43	43	46	48	49	50	51	51	50
75	40	41	44	46	47	48	49	50	50
70	38	40	43	45	45	46	48	49	48
60	36	38	40	41	43	44	45	46	44
50	34	36	38	40	41	42	43	43	43
40	32	34	35	37	39	40	41	41	40
30	30	31	33	34	37	37	39	39	38
25	28	30	32	32	35	36	38	37	36
20	26	28	30	31	34	35	36	35	35
10	22	22	25	28	30	31	32	31	31

TABLE 6 Bent-Knee Sit-Ups—Girls (number in 1 minute; arms crossed on chest)

Age	10	11	12	13	14	15	16	17	18
99%	50	53	66	58	57	56	59	60	65
90	43	42	46	46	47	45	49	47	47
80	39	39	41	41	42	42	42	41	42
75	37	37	40	40	41	40	40	40	40
70	36	36	39	39	40	39	39	39	40
60	33	34	36	35	37	36	37	37	38
50	31	32	33	33	35	35	35	36	35
40	30	30	31	31	32	32	33	33	33
30	27	28	30	28	30	30	30	31	30
25	25	26	28	27	29	30	30	30	30
20	24	24	27	25	27	28	28	29	28
10	20	20	21	21	23	24	23	24	24

TABLE 7   Sit-and-Reach, Flexibility Test—Boys (footline set at 0; measurement in inches, plus or minus)

Age	10	11	12	13	14	15	16	17	18
99%	6	6.5	6.5	7.5	8	9.5	10	9.5	10
90	4	4.5	4	4.5	5.5	6	7	7.5	7.5
80	3	3.5	3	3	4	5	6	6	6
75	2.5	3	3	3	3.5	4.5	5	5.5	5.5
70	2.5	2.5	2.5	2.5	3	4	5	5	5
60	2	2	1.5	1.5	2	3	4	4	4
50	1.5	1	1	1	1.5	2	3	3.5	3
40	0.5	1.5	0	0.5	1	1.5	2	2.5	2.5
30	0	0	−0.5	0	0	0.5	1.5	1.5	1.5
25	−0.5	−0.5	−1	−1	−1	0	1	1	1
20	−1	−1	−1.5	−1.5	−1	−0.5	0	−0.5	−0.5
10	−2	−2.5	−3.5	−3	−3	−2.5	−2	−1.5	−2

TABLE 8   Sit-and-Reach, Flexibility Test—Girls (footline set at 0; measurement in inches, plus or minus)

Age	10	11	12	13	14	15	16	17	18
99%	8.5	8.5	9	10	10	11	11	11	10.5
90	5.5	6	7	8	7.5	8	8.5	8.5	8.5
80	4.5	5	6	7	7	7	7.5	7.5	7.5
75	4.5	4.5	5	6	6.5	7	7	7	7
70	4	4.5	5	5.5	6	6.5	7	7	6.5
60	3	3.5	4	5	5.5	6	6	6	6
50	2.5	3	3.5	4	5	5	5.5	6	5.5
40	2	2	3	3.5	4	5	5	5	5
30	1	1.5	2.5	2.5	3	4	4.5	4	4
25	1	1	2	2	3	3.5	4	3.5	3.5
20	0	1	1.5	1.5	2	3	3.5	3	3
10	−1.5	−0.5	0	0	0.5	1.5	2	1.5	1

TABLE 9   1-Mile Run—Boys (min:sec)

Age	10	11	12	13	14	15	16	17	18
99%	6:55	6:21	6:21	5:59	5:43	5:40	5:31	5:14	5:33
90	8:13	7:25	7:13	6:48	6:27	6:23	6:13	6:08	6:10
80	8:35	7:52	7:41	7:07	6:58	6:43	6:31	6:31	6:33
75	8:48	8:02	7:53	7:14	7:08	6:52	6:39	6:40	6:42
70	9:02	8:12	8:03	7:24	7:18	7:00	6:50	6:46	6:57
60	9:26	8:38	8:23	6:46	7:34	7:13	7:07	7:10	7:15
50	9:52	9:03	8:48	8:04	7:51	7:30	7:27	7:31	7:35
40	10:15	9:25	9:17	8:26	8:14	7:50	7:48	7:59	7:53
30	10:44	10:17	9:57	8:54	8:46	8:18	8:04	8:24	8:12
20	11:25	10:55	10:38	9:20	9:28	8:50	8:34	8:55	9:10
10	12:27	12:07	11:48	10:38	10:34	10:13	9:36	10:43	10:50

TABLE 10 1-Mile Run—Girls (min:sec)

Age	10	11	12	13	14	15	16	17	18
99%	7:55	7:14	7:20	7:08	7:01	6:59	7:03	6:52	6:58
90	9:09	8:45	8:34	8:27	8:11	8:23	8:28	8:20	8:22
80	9:56	9:52	9:30	9:13	8:49	9:04	9:06	9:10	9:27
75	10:09	9:56	9:52	9:30	9:16	9:28	9:25	9:26	9:31
70	10:27	10:10	10:05	9:48	9:31	9:49	9:41	9:41	9:36
60	10:51	10:35	10:32	10:22	10:04	10:20	10:15	10:16	10:08
50	11:14	11:15	10:58	10:52	10:32	10:46	10:34	10:34	10:51
40	11:54	11:46	11:26	11:22	10:58	11:20	11:08	10:59	11:27
30	12:27	12:33	12:03	11:55	11:35	11:53	11:49	11:43	11:58
25	12:52	12:54	12:33	12:17	11:49	12:18	12:10	12:03	12:14
20	13:12	13:17	12:53	12:43	12:10	12:48	12:32	12:30	12:37
10	14:20	14:35	14:07	13:45	13:13	14:07	13:42	13:46	15:18

NATIONAL CHILDREN AND YOUTH FITNESS STUDY II (NCYFS II)

As described in Chapter 1, the second National Children and Youth Fitness Study (NCYFS II) was launched to study the physical fitness and physical activity habits of 4,678 children ages 6–9. The study was the first to assess the fitness and activity patterns of 6- to 9-year-olds.

Test items of the NCYFS II include

- Triceps, subscapular, and medial calf skinfolds for body composition.
- Walk/run for cardiorespiratory endurance (1 mile, age 8 or 9; or ½ mile, age 6 or 7)
- Sit-and-reach test for lower back–hamstring flexibility
- Modified pull-up for upper-body muscular strength and endurance
- Bent-knee sit-ups (1 minute) for abdominal strength/endurance

---

Interpretations of Norms: <25% = Unacceptable or Poor; 25–50% = Minimal or Fair; 50–75% = Acceptable or Good; >75% = Optimal or Excellent

Note: See description of methods in Chapters 4 to 6.

Source: Ross JG, Pate RR, Delpy LA, Gold RS, Svilar M. New health-related fitness norms. *JOPERD,* November/December 1987, 66–70.

TABLE 11 Triceps Skinfold (in millimeters)

	Age								
	Boys					**Girls**			
Percentile	6	7	8	9		6	7	8	9
99	5	5	5	5		5	6	6	6
95	6	5	6	6		7	7	7	7
90	6	6	6	6		8	7	8	8
85	7	7	7	7		8	8	8	9
80	7	7	7	7		9	8	9	10
75	7	7	7	8		9	9	9	10
70	7	7	8	8		9	9	10	11
65	8	8	8	9		10	10	10	11
60	8	8	8	10		10	10	11	12
55	8	8	9	10		11	11	12	12
50	8	9	9	10		11	11	12	13
45	9	9	10	11		12	12	13	14
40	9	10	10	12		12	12	14	14
35	10	10	11	13		13	13	15	15
30	10	11	12	14		13	13	16	16
25	10	11	13	15		14	14	17	18
20	11	12	14	16		14	15	18	19
15	12	14	15	18		15	17	19	21
10	13	16	19	21		17	19	21	22
5	16	20	23	23		20	22	25	25

TABLE 12 Subscapular Skinfold (in millimeters)

	Age								
	Boys					**Girls**			
Percentile	6	7	8	9		6	7	8	9
99	4	4	4	4		4	4	4	4
95	4	4	4	4		4	4	5	5
90	4	4	4	5		5	5	5	5
85	4	5	5	5		5	5	5	5
80	5	5	5	5		5	5	5	6
75	5	5	5	5		5	5	6	6
70	5	5	5	5		5	5	6	6
65	5	5	5	6		6	6	6	6
60	5	5	5	6		6	6	6	7
55	5	5	6	6		6	6	7	7
50	5	5	6	6		6	6	7	8
45	5	6	6	7		6	7	7	8
40	6	6	6	7		7	7	8	9
35	6	6	6	7		7	7	8	9
30	6	6	7	8		7	8	9	10
25	6	7	7	9		8	9	10	12
20	7	7	8	10		8	10	12	15
15	7	8	10	12		10	11	15	17
10	8	10	14	15		12	13	17	21
5	12	16	19	20		16	19	21	25

TABLE 13   Sum of Triceps and Medial Calf Skinfolds (in millimeters)

Percentile	Boys 6	Boys 7	Boys 8	Boys 9	Girls 6	Girls 7	Girls 8	Girls 9
99	9	9	9	9	11	11	11	12
95	11	11	11	11	13	13	14	14
90	12	12	12	12	15	15	15	16
85	12	13	13	13	16	16	16	18
80	13	13	13	14	17	17	18	19
75	14	14	14	15	18	18	19	20
70	14	14	15	16	18	18	20	21
65	15	16	17	18	20	20	22	23
60	15	16	17	18	20	20	22	23
55	16	16	17	19	21	21	23	25
50	16	17	18	21	21	22	24	26
45	17	18	19	22	22	23	26	27
40	17	19	20	23	23	24	27	29
35	18	20	21	25	24	25	29	30
30	20	21	23	27	25	26	31	32
25	20	22	24	29	27	28	33	35
20	22	24	27	31	28	31	35	37
15	23	27	31	35	30	33	38	41
10	27	32	37	40	33	37	43	45
5	33	39	44	47	38	43	49	52

TABLE 14 **Modified Pull-Ups (number completed)**

	Age								
	Boys					Girls			
Percentile	6	7	8	9		6	7	8	9
99	25	27	38	35		24	27	25	30
95	18	20	21	25		17	20	20	20
90	15	19	20	20		13	16	17	17
85	12	15	17	20		11	14	14	15
80	11	13	15	17		10	12	12	13
75	10	13	14	15		9	11	11	12
70	9	12	13	14		9	10	11	11
65	8	11	12	13		7	9	10	10
60	7	10	11	12		7	8	9	10
55	7	9	10	11		6	8	9	9
50	6	8	10	10		6	7	8	9
45	6	8	9	10		5	7	7	8
40	5	7	8	9		5	6	6	7
30	4	5	7	7		4	4	5	5
35	5	6	8	7		4	4	5	5
25	3	4	6	6		3	4	4	4
20	3	4	5	5		2	3	4	4
15	2	3	4	4		1	2	3	2
10	1	1	3	3		0	1	1	1
5	0	0	1	2		0	0	0	0

The child is positioned on his or her back with the shoulders directly below a bar that is set at a height 1 or 2 inches beyond the child's reach. An elastic band is suspended across the uprights parallel to and about 7–8 inches below the bar. In the start position, the child's buttocks are off the floor, the arms and legs are straight, and only the heels are in contact with the floor. An overhand grip (palm away from the body) is used, and the thumbs are placed around the bar. A pull-up is completed when the chin is hooked over the elastic band. The movement should be accomplished using only the arms, and the body must be kept rigid and straight. (See Chapter 6.)

TABLE 15   Timed Bent-Knee Sit-Ups (number in 1 minute)

	Age								
	Boys					**Girls**			
Percentile	**6**	**7**	**8**	**9**		**6**	**7**	**8**	**9**
99	36	42	43	48		36	40	44	43
95	31	35	38	42		31	35	37	39
90	28	32	35	39		28	33	34	36
85	26	30	33	36		26	30	32	34
80	25	29	32	35		24	28	30	32
75	24	28	30	33		23	27	29	31
70	22	27	29	32		22	26	28	30
65	21	26	28	31		21	24	27	29
60	20	25	27	30		20	23	26	28
55	19	24	26	29		19	22	25	26
50	19	23	26	28		18	21	25	26
45	17	21	24	26		17	20	23	24
40	17	21	24	26		17	20	23	24
35	16	20	23	24		15	17	20	22
30	15	19	21	24		15	17	20	22
25	14	18	20	23		14	16	19	21
20	12	16	19	22		12	15	17	19
15	11	14	17	19		10	13	16	17
10	9	12	15	16		6	11	13	15
5	4	7	11	13		1	7	9	10

Note: See Chapter 6 for details on methods.

TABLE 16 Sit-and-Reach, Flexibility Test (in inches; footline set at zero)

| | Age | | | | | | | |
| | Boys | | | | Girls | | | |
Percentile	6	7	8	9	6	7	8	9
99	5.5	6.0	6.0	5.5	6.5	6.0	7.0	7.0
95	4.5	4.5	4.5	4.0	5.5	5.5	5.5	6.0
90	4.0	4.0	4.0	3.5	4.5	5.0	5.0	5.0
85	3.5	4.0	3.5	3.0	4.0	4.5	4.5	4.5
80	3.0	3.5	3.0	2.5	4.0	4.0	4.0	4.0
75	3.0	3.0	2.5	2.5	3.5	4.0	4.0	4.0
70	2.5	2.5	2.5	2.0	3.0	3.0	3.0	3.0
65	2.0	2.0	2.0	2.0	3.0	3.0	3.0	3.0
60	2.0	2.0	2.0	1.5	3.0	3.0	3.0	3.0
55	1.5	1.5	1.5	1.0	2.5	3.0	2.5	2.5
50	1.5	1.5	1.5	1.0	2.0	2.5	2.0	2.0
45	1.0	1.0	1.0	0.5	2.0	2.5	2.0	2.0
40	0.5	0.5	0.5	0	2.0	2.0	1.5	2.0
35	0.5	0.5	0.5	0	1.5	2.0	1.5	1.5
30	0	0	0	−0.5	1.0	1.5	1.0	1.0
25	0	−0.5	−0.5	−1.0	0.5	1.0	0.5	0.5
20	−0.5	−0.5	−1.0	−1.5	0	0.5	0	0
15	−1.0	−1.0	−1.5	−2.0	0	0	−0.5	−0.5
10	−1.5	−2.0	−2.5	−2.5	−0.5	−0.5	−1.0	−1.0
5	−2.0	−3.0	−3.5	−4.0	−1.5	−1.5	−2.0	−3.0

TABLE 17   Distance Walk/Run (1 mile for children age 8 or 9; ½ mile for children age 6 or 7; min:sec)

	Age							
	Boys				**Girls**			
	Half Mile		**Mile**		**Half Mile**		**Mile**	
Percentile	**6**	**7**	**8**	**9**	**6**	**7**	**8**	**9**
99	3:53	3:34	7:42	7:31	4:05	4:03	8:18	8:06
95	4:15	3:56	8:18	7:54	4:29	4:18	9:14	8:41
90	4:27	4:11	8:46	8:10	4:46	4:32	9:39	9:08
85	4:35	4:22	9:02	8:33	4:57	4:38	9:55	9:26
80	4:45	4:28	9:19	8:48	5:07	4:46	10:08	9:40
75	4:52	4:33	9:29	9:00	5:13	4:54	10:23	9:50
70	4:59	4:40	9:40	9:13	5:20	5:00	10:35	10:15
65	5:04	4:46	9:52	9:29	5:25	5:06	10:46	10:31
60	5:10	4:50	10:04	9:44	5:31	5:11	10:59	10:41
55	5:17	4:54	10:16	9:58	5:39	5:18	11:14	10:56
50	5:23	5:00	10:39	10:10	5:44	5:25	11:32	11:13
45	5:28	5:05	11:00	10:27	5:49	5:32	11:46	11:30
40	5:33	5:11	11:14	10:41	5:55	5:39	12:03	11:46
35	5:41	5:17	11:30	10:59	6:00	5:46	12:14	12:09
30	5:50	5:28	11:51	11:16	6:07	5:55	12:37	12:26
25	5:58	5:35	12:14	11:44	6:14	6:01	12:59	12:45
20	6:09	5:46	12:39	12:02	6:27	6:10	13:26	13:13
15	6:21	6:06	13:16	12:46	6:39	6:20	14:18	13:44
10	6:40	6:20	14:05	13:37	6:51	6:38	14:48	14:31
5	7:15	6:50	15:24	15:15	7:16	7:09	16:35	15:40

THE 1985 SCHOOL POPULATION FITNESS SURVEY, PRESIDENT'S COUNCIL ON PHYSICAL FITNESS AND SPORTS

As described in Chapter 1, in 1985, the President's Council on Physical Fitness and Sports School Population Fitness Survey was conducted. Data were collected to assess the physical fitness status of American public school children ages 6–17. A four-stage probability sample was designed to select approximately 19,200 boys and girls from 57 school districts and 187 schools.

The test was not designed to measure all of the health-related fitness components (body composition was not assessed). In addition, several skill-related tests were included. Nine test items were selected for both boys and girls. Norms are given for boys and girls ages 6–17.

- Pull-ups
- Flexed-arm hang
- Curl-ups
- 1-mile run/walk
- V-sit reach
- Shuttle run
- 2-mile walk
- 50-yard dash
- Standing long jump

Source: Youth Physical Fitness in 1985. *The President's Council on Physical Fitness and Sports School Population Fitness Survey.* President's Council on Physical Fitness and Sports. 450 Fifth St., NW, Suite 7103, Washington, DC 20001.

Suggested Interpretation of Norms

90–100%	Excellent	30–40%	Fair
75–85%	Very good	15–25%	Poor
60–70%	Good	0–10%	Very poor
45–55%	Average		

The results from this survey form the basis for the norms used in the "President's Challenge" (see norms next page and discussion in Chapters 3 and 4). Those youngsters reaching the 85th percentile or above on all five items of the test become eligible to receive the Presidential Physical Fitness Award. The National Physical Fitness Award was added in 1987 and recognizes those who score at or above the 50th percentile for all five test items. The Participant Award, introduced in 1991, recognizes those who attempt all test items but whose scores fall below the 50th percentile on one or more of them.

Source: President's Council on Physical Fitness and Sports. *Get Fit, A Handbook for Youth Ages 6–17.* President's Challenge, Poplars Research Center, 400 E. 7th St., Bloomington, IN 47405.

TABLE 18   The President's Challenge, Qualifying Standards

			The Presidential Physical Fitness Award			
Age	Curl-Ups (timed 1 minute)	Shuttle Run (seconds)	V-Sit Reach (inches)	or Sit and Reach (centimeters)	1-Mile Run (minutes:seconds)	Pull-Ups
Boys						
6	33	12.1	+3.5	31	10:15	2
7	36	11.5	+3.5	30	9:22	4
8	40	11.1	+3.0	31	8:48	5
9	41	10.9	+3.0	31	8:31	5
10	45	10.3	+4.0	30	7:57	6
11	47	10.0	+4.0	31	7:32	6
12	50	9.8	+4.0	31	7:11	7
13	53	9.5	+3.5	33	6:50	7
14	56	9.1	+4.5	36	6:26	10
15	57	9.0	+5.0	37	6:20	11
16	56	8.7	+6.0	38	6:08	11
17	55	8.7	+7.0	41	6:06	13
Girls						
6	32	12.4	+5.5	32	11:20	2
7	34	12.1	+5.0	32	10:36	2
8	38	11.8	+4.5	33	10:02	2
9	39	11.1	+5.5	33	9:30	2
10	40	10.8	+6.0	33	9:19	3
11	42	10.5	+6.5	34	9:02	3
12	45	10.4	+7.0	36	8:23	2
13	46	10.2	+7.0	38	8:13	2
14	47	10.1	+8.0	40	7:59	2
15	48	10.0	+8.0	43	8:08	2
16	45	10.1	+9.0	42	8:23	1
17	44	10.0	+8.0	42	8:15	1

The National Physical Fitness Award

Age	Curl-Ups (timed 1 minute)	Shuttle Run (seconds)	V-Sit Reach or Sit and Reach (inches)	(centimeters)	1-Mile Run (minutes:seconds)	Pull-Ups or Flexed-Arm Hang (seconds)	
Boys							
6	22	13.3	+1.0	26	12:36	1	6
7	28	12.8	+1.0	25	11:40	1	8
8	31	12.2	+0.5	25	11:05	1	10
9	32	11.9	+1.0	25	10:30	2	10
10	35	11.5	+1.0	25	9:48	2	12
11	37	11.1	+1.0	25	9:20	2	11
12	40	10.6	+1.0	26	8:40	2	12
13	42	10.2	+0.5	26	8:06	3	14
14	45	9.9	+1.0	28	7:44	5	20
15	45	9.7	+2.0	30	7:30	6	30
16	45	9.4	+3.0	30	7:10	7	28
17	44	9.4	+3.0	34	7:04	8	30
Girls							
6	23	13.8	+2.5	27	13:12	1	5
7	25	13.2	+2.0	27	12:56	1	6
8	29	12.9	+2.0	28	12:30	1	8
9	30	12.5	+2.0	28	11:52	1	8
10	30	12.1	+3.0	28	11:22	1	8
11	32	11.5	+3.0	29	11:17	1	7
12	35	11.3	+3.5	30	11:05	1	7
13	37	11.1	+3.5	31	10:23	1	8
14	37	11.2	+4.5	33	10:06	1	9
15	36	11.0	+5.0	36	9:58	1	7
16	35	10.9	+5.5	34	10:31	1	7
17	34	11.0	+4.5	35	10:22	1	7

The Participant Physical Fitness Award

Boys and girls who attempt all five test items but whose scores fall below the fiftieth percentile on one or more of them are eligible to receive the Participant Award.

TABLE 19   The FITNESSGRAM® Standards for Healthy Fitness Zone (HFZ)[a]

		**Boys**										
Age	1 Mile min:sec		Pacer # laps		$\dot{V}O_{2max}$ ml/kg/min		Percent Fat		Body Mass Index		Curl-Up # completed	
5	*Completion of*		*Participate in*				25	10	20	14.7	2	10
6	*distance. Time*		*run. Lap count*				25	10	20	14.7	2	10
7	*standards not*		*standards not*				25	10	20	14.9	4	14
8	*recommended*		*recommended*				25	10	20	15.0	6	20
9							25	10	20	15.2	9	24
10	11:30	9:00	17	55	42	52	25	10	21	15.3	12	24
11	11:00	8:30	23	61	42	52	25	10	21	15.8	15	28
12	10:30	8:00	29	68	42	52	25	10	22	16.0	18	36
13	10:00	7:30	35	74	42	52	25	10	23	16.6	21	40
14	9:30	7:00	41	80	42	52	25	10	24.5	17.5	24	45
15	9:00	7:00	46	85	42	52	25	10	25	18.1	24	47
16	8:30	7:00	52	90	42	52	25	10	26.5	18.5	24	47
17	8:30	7:00	57	94	42	52	25	10	27	18.8	24	47
17+	8:30	7:00	57	94	42	52	25	10	27.8	19.0	24	47

Age	Trunk Lift inches		Push-Up # completed		Modified Pull-Up # completed		Pull-Up # completed		Flexed-Arm Hang seconds		Back Saver Sit & Reach[b] inches	Shoulder Stretch
5	6	12	3	8	2	7	1	2	2	8	8	
6	6	12	3	8	2	7	1	2	2	8	8	
7	6	12	4	10	3	9	1	2	3	8	8	
8	6	12	5	13	4	11	1	2	3	10	8	
9	6	12	6	15	5	11	1	2	4	10	8	*Passing = Touching the fingertips together behind the back*
10	9	12	7	20	5	15	1	2	4	10	8	
11	9	12	8	20	6	17	1	3	6	13	8	
12	9	12	10	20	7	20	1	3	10	15	8	
13	9	12	12	25	8	22	1	4	12	17	8	
14	9	12	14	30	9	25	2	5	15	20	8	
15	9	12	16	35	10	27	3	7	15	20	8	
16	9	12	18	35	12	30	5	8	15	20	8	
17	9	12	18	35	14	30	5	8	15	20	8	
17+	9	12	18	35	14	30	5	8	15	20	8	

[a]For each standard, the number on the left is lower end of HFZ; number on the right is upper end of HFZ.
[b]Test scored Pass / Fail; must reach this distance to pass.

TABLE 19   The FITNESSGRAM® Standards for Healthy Fitness Zone (HFZ)[a] *(continued)*

Girls

Age	1 Mile min:sec		Pacer # laps		$\dot{V}O_{2max}$ ml/kg/min		Percent Fat		Body Mass Index		Curl-Up # completed	
5	*Completion of*		*Participate in*				32	17	21	16.2	2	10
6	*distance. Time*		*run. Lap count*				32	17	21	16.2	2	10
7	*standards not*		*standards not*				32	17	21	16.2	4	14
8	*recommended*		*recommended*				32	17	22	16.2	6	20
9							32	17	23	16.2	9	22
10	12:30	9:30	7	35	39	47	32	17	23.5	16.6	12	26
11	12:00	9:00	9	37	38	46	32	17	24	16.9	15	29
12	12:00	9:00	13	40	37	45	32	17	24.5	16.9	18	32
13	11:30	9:00	15	42	36	44	32	17	24.5	17.5	18	32
14	11:00	8:30	18	44	35	43	32	17	25	17.5	18	32
15	10:30	8:00	23	50	35	43	32	17	25	17.5	18	35
16	10:00	8:00	28	56	35	43	32	17	25	17.5	18	35
17	10:00	8:00	34	61	35	43	32	17	26	17.5	18	35
17+	10:00	8:00	34	61	35	43	32	17	27.3	18.0	18	35

Age	Trunk Lift inches		Push-Up # completed		Modified Pull-Up # completed		Pull-Up # completed		Flexed-Arm Hang seconds		Back Saver Sit & Reach[b] inches	Shoulder Stretch
5	6	12	3	8	2	7	1	2	2	8	9	
6	6	12	3	8	2	7	1	2	2	8	9	
7	6	12	4	10	3	9	1	2	3	8	9	
8	6	12	5	13	4	11	1	2	3	10	9	*Passing = Touching the fingertips together behind the back*
9	6	12	6	15	4	11	1	2	4	10	9	
10	9	12	7	15	4	13	1	2	4	10	9	
11	9	12	7	15	4	13	1	2	6	12	10	
12	9	12	7	15	4	13	1	2	7	12	10	
13	9	12	7	15	4	13	1	2	8	12	10	
14	9	12	7	15	4	13	1	2	8	12	10	
15	9	12	7	15	4	13	1	2	8	12	12	
16	9	12	7	15	4	13	1	2	8	12	12	
17	9	12	7	15	4	13	1	2	8	12	12	
17+	9	12	7	15	4	13	1	2	8	12	12	

[a]For each standard, the number on the left is lower end of HFZ; number on the right is upper end of HFZ.
[b]Test scored Pass / Fail; must reach this distance to pass.

Source: Reprinted with permission from the Cooper Institute for Aerobics Research, Dallas, TX.

AAHPERD NORMS FOR COLLEGE STUDENTS

The American Association of Health, Physical Education, Recreation, and Dance (AAHPERD) released the results of their new testing program for college students in 1985. The study population consisted of 5,158 young adults in colleges from all geographic regions of the United States. The data for the study were collected under the supervision of 24 coinvestigators. The test items, in order, are as follows:

- Two-site skinfold test (triceps and subscapular)
- Mile run or 9-minute run for cardiorespiratory endurance
- Sit-and-reach test for flexibility
- Timed (1 minute) sit-ups for abdominal muscular endurance

AAHPERD allows authors to publish only a limited part of the norms. The reader is urged to purchase the book from AAHPERD, listed in the source note.

TABLE 20a   Health-Related Physical Fitness Test Items—Males

%	Mile Run	Sit-Ups	Sit and Reach	Sum of Skinfold	% Body Fat
99	5:06	68	26	10	2.9
75	6:12	50	16	16	6.6
50	6:49	44	11	21	9.4
25	7:32	38	6	26	13.1
5	9:47	30	−4	40	20.4

TABLE 20b   Health-Related Physical Fitness Test Items—Females

%	Mile Run	Sit-Ups	Sit and Reach	Sum of Skinfold	% Body Fat
99	6:04	61	28	11	7.9
75	8:15	42	18	24	19.0
50	9:22	35	14	30	22.8
25	10:41	0	9	37	27.1
5	12:43	21	1	51	33.7

Mile run: Run 1 mile in the fastest possible time.
Sit-ups: As many correctly executed sit-ups as possible in 60 seconds.
Sit and reach: Footline is set at 0 cm. Score is cm beyond feet when legs are straight.
Sum of skinfolds: Triceps plus subscapular skinfolds.
See Chapters 4 through 6 for details on how to administer tests.

Source (Tables 20a and b): AAHPERD. *Norms for College Students: Health Related Physical Fitness Test.* 1985. Reprinted by permission of the American Alliance for Health, Physical Education, Recreation, and Dance, 1900 Association Dr., Reston, VA 22091.

Section 2. *Cardiorespiratory Test Norms for Adults*

(See Chapter 4 for instructions.)

TABLE 21 YMCA Norms for Resting Heart Rate (beats/min)

Age (yr)	18–25		26–35		36–45		46–55		56–65		>65	
Gender	M	F	M	F	M	F	M	F	M	F	M	F
Excellent	40–54	42–57	36–53	39–57	37–55	40–58	35–56	43–58	42–56	42–59	40–55	49–59
Good	57–59	59–63	55–59	60–62	58–60	61–63	58–61	61–64	59–61	61–64	57–61	60–64
Above average	61–65	64–67	61–63	64–66	62–64	65–67	63–65	65–69	63–65	65–68	62–65	66–68
Average	66–69	68–71	65–67	68–70	66–69	69–71	66–70	70–72	68–71	69–72	66–69	70–72
Below average	70–72	72–76	69–71	72–74	70–72	72–75	72–74	73–76	72–75	73–77	70–73	73–76
Poor	74–78	77–81	74–78	77–81	75–80	77–81	77–81	77–82	76–80	79–81	74–79	78–83
Very poor	82–103	84–104	81–102	84–102	83–101	83–102	84–103	85–104	84–103	84–103	83–103	86–97

Source: YMCA. *Y'S Way to Fitness,* 4th ed., 1998. Reprinted with permission from the YMCA of the USA.

TABLE 22 YMCA 3-Minute Step Test Postexercise 1-Minute Heart Rate (beats/min)

Age (yr)	18–25		26–35		36–45		46–55		56–65		>65	
Gender	M	F	M	F	M	F	M	F	M	F	M	F
Excellent	50–76	52–81	51–76	58–80	49–76	51–84	56–82	63–91	60–77	60–92	59–81	70–92
Good	79–84	85–93	79–85	85–92	80–88	89–96	87–93	95–101	86–94	97–103	87–92	96–101
Above average	88–93	96–102	88–94	95–101	92–98	100–104	95–101	104–110	97–100	106–111	94–102	104–111
Average	95–100	104–110	96–102	104–110	100–105	107–112	103–111	113–118	103–109	113–118	104–110	116–121
Below average	102–107	113–120	104–110	113–119	108–113	115–120	113–119	120–124	111–117	119–127	114–118	123–126
Poor	111–119	122–131	114–121	122–129	116–124	124–132	121–126	126–132	119–128	129–135	121–126	128–133
Very poor	124–157	135–169	126–161	134–171	130–163	137–169	131–159	137–171	131–154	141–174	130–151	135–155

Note: Pulse is to be counted for 1 full minute following 3 minutes of stepping at 24 steps/minute on a 12-inch bench. See Chapter 4 for further instructions.

Source: YMCA. *Y'S Way to Fitness,* 4th ed., 1998. Reprinted with permission from the YMCA of the USA.

TABLE 23a Aerobic Power Tests—Men

%	Ages 20–29				Ages 30–39				
	Balke Treadmill (time)	$\dot{V}O_{2max}$ (ml/kg/min)	12-Minute Run (miles)	1.5-Mile Run (time)	Balke Treadmill (time)	$\dot{V}O_{2max}$ (ml/kg/min)	12-Minute Run (miles)	1.5-Mile Run (time)	
99	30:20	58.79	1.94	7:29	29:00	58.86	1.89	7:11	S
95	27:00	53.97	1.81	8:13	26:00	52.53	1.77	8:44	
90	25:11	51.35	1.74	9:09	24:30	50.36	1.71	9:30	
85	24:00	49.64	1.69	9:45	23:00	48.20	1.65	10:16	
80	23:00	48.20	1.65	10:16	22:00	46.75	1.61	10:47	E
75	22:10	46.99	1.62	10:42	21:00	45.31	1.57	11:18	
70	22:00	46.75	1.61	10:47	20:30	44.59	1.55	11:34	
65	21:00	45.31	1.57	11:18	20:00	43.87	1.53	11:49	
60	20:15	44.23	1.54	11:41	19:00	42.42	1.49	12:20	G
55	20:00	43.87	1.53	11:49	18:25	41.58	1.47	12:38	
50	19:03	42.49	1.50	12:18	18:00	40.98	1.45	12:51	
45	19:00	42.42	1.49	12:20	17:00	39.53	1.41	13:22	
40	18:00	40.98	1.45	12:51	16:32	38.86	1.39	13:36	F
35	17:30	40.26	1.43	13:06	16:00	38.09	1.37	13:53	
30	17:00	39.53	1.41	13:22	15:30	37.37	1.35	14:08	
25	16:00	38.09	1.37	13:53	15:00	36.65	1.33	14:24	
20	15:20	37.13	1.34	14:13	14:06	35.35	1.29	14:52	P
15	15:00	36.65	1.33	14:24	13:10	34.00	1.25	15:20	
10	13:30	34.48	1.27	15:10	12:09	32.53	1.21	15:52	
5	11:30	31.57	1.19	16:12	11:00	30.87	1.17	16:27	VP
1	8:23	27.09	1.06	17:48	8:00	26.54	1.13	18:00	

$n = 1675$ $n = 7094$

TABLE 23a   Aerobic Power Tests—Men *(continued)*

%	Ages 40–49 Balke Treadmill (time)	$\dot{V}O_{2max}$ (ml/kg/min)	12-Minute Run (miles)	1.5-Mile Run (time)	Ages 50–59 Balke Treadmill (time)	$\dot{V}O_{2max}$ (ml/kg/min)	12-Minute Run (miles)	1.5-Mile Run (time)	
99	28:00	55.42	1.85	7:42	26:00	52.53	1.77	8:44	S
95	24:30	50.36	1.71	9:30	22:15	47.11	1.62	10:40	
90	23:00	48.20	1.65	10:16	21:00	45.31	1.57	11:18	
85	21:00	45.31	1.57	11:18	19:00	42.42	1.49	12:20	
80	20:10	44.11	1.54	11:44	18:00	40.98	1.45	12:51	E
75	20:00	43.89	1.53	11:49	17:00	39.53	1.41	13:22	
70	18:32	41.75	1.47	12:34	16:15	38.45	1.38	13:45	
65	18:00	40.98	1.45	12:51	15:40	37.61	1.35	14:03	
60	17:15	39.89	1.42	13:14	15:00	36.65	1.33	14:24	G
55	17:00	39.53	1.41	13:22	14:30	36.10	1.31	14:40	
50	16:00	38.09	1.37	13:53	14:00	35.20	1.29	14:55	
45	15:30	37.37	1.35	14:08	13:15	34.12	1.26	15:08	
40	15:00	36.69	1.33	14:29	13:00	33.76	1.25	15:26	F
35	14:15	35.56	1.30	14:47	12:07	32.48	1.22	15:53	
30	13:57	35.13	1.29	14:56	12:00	32.31	1.21	15:57	
25	13:00	33.76	1.25	15:26	11:08	31.06	1.17	16:23	
20	12:30	33.04	1.23	15:41	10:30	30.15	1.15	16:43	P
15	12:00	32.31	1.21	15:57	10:00	29.43	1.13	16:58	
10	10:59	30.85	1.17	16:28	9:00	27.98	1.09	17:29	
5	6:21	28.29	1.10	17:23	7:00	25.09	1.01	18:31	VP
1	6:21	24.15	.98	18:51	4:54	22.06	.92	19:36	

n = 6837   *n* = 7094

TABLE 23a Aerobic Power Tests—Men *(continued)*

%	Age 60 +				
	Balke Treadmill (time)	**$\dot{V}O_{2max}$ (ml/kg/min)**	**12-Minute Run (miles)**	**1.5-Mile Run (time)**	
99	24:29	50.39	1.71	9:30	S
95	20:56	45.21	1.57	11:20	
90	19:00	42.46	1.49	12:20	
85	17:00	39.53	1.41	13:22	
80	16:00	38.09	1.37	13:53	E
75	15:00	36.65	1.30	14:24	
70	14:04	35.30	1.29	14:53	
65	13:22	39.29	1.26	15:19	
60	12:53	33.59	1.24	15:29	G
55	12:03	32.39	1.21	15:55	
50	11:40	31.83	1.19	16:07	
45	11:00	30.87	1.17	16:27	
40	10:30	30.15	1.15	16:43	F
35	10:00	29.43	1.13	16:58	
30	9:30	28.70	1.11	17:14	
25	8:54	27.89	1.08	17:32	
20	8:00	26.54	1.05	18:00	P
15	7:00	25.09	1.01	18:31	
10	5:35	23.05	.95	19:15	
5	4:00	20.76	.89	20:04	VP
1	2:17	18.28	.82	20:57	

Note: n = 1005; S, superior; E, excellent; G, good; F, fair; P, poor; VP, very poor.

TABLE 23b   Aerobic Power Tests—Women

%	Ages 20–29				Ages 30–39				
	Balke Treadmill (time)	**$\dot{V}O_{2max}$ (ml/kg/min)**	**12-Minute Run (miles)**	**1.5-Mile Run (time)**	**Balke Treadmill (time)**	**$\dot{V}O_{2max}$ (ml/kg/min)**	**12-Minute Run (miles)**	**1.5-Mile Run (time)**	
99	26:21	53.03	1.78	8:33	23:22	48.73	1.66	10:05	S
95	22:00	46.75	1.61	10:47	20:00	43.87	1.53	11:49	
90	20:12	44.15	1.54	11:43	18:00	40.98	1.45	12:51	
85	19:00	42.42	1.49	12:20	17:30	40.26	1.43	13:06	
80	18:00	40.98	1.45	12:51	16:20	38.57	1.38	13:43	E
75	17:00	39.53	1.41	13:22	15:30	37.37	1.35	14:08	
70	16:00	38.09	1.37	13:53	15:00	36.65	1.33	14:24	
65	15:30	37.37	1.35	14:08	14:10	35.44	1.29	14:50	
60	15:00	36.65	1.33	14:24	13:35	34.60	1.27	15:08	G
55	14:39	36.14	1.31	14:35	13:10	33.85	1.26	15:20	
50	14:00	35.20	1.29	14:55	13:00	33.76	1.25	15:26	
45	13:30	34.48	1.27	15:10	12:10	32.41	1.22	15:47	
40	13:00	33.76	1.25	15:26	12:00	32.31	1.21	15:57	F
35	12:17	32.72	1.22	15:48	11:09	31.09	1.17	16:23	
30	12:00	32.31	1.21	15:57	10:45	30.51	1.16	16:35	
25	11:03	30.94	1.17	16:26	10:00	29.93	1.13	16:58	
20	10:50	30.63	1.16	16:33	9:30	28.70	1.11	17:14	P
15	10:00	29.43	1.13	16:58	9:00	27.98	1.09	17:29	
10	9:17	28.39	1.10	17:21	8:00	26.54	1.05	18:00	
5	7:33	25.89	1.03	18:14	7:00	25.09	1.01	18:31	VP
1	5:15	22.57	.94	19:25	5:12	22.49	.93	19:27	

n = 764   *n* = 2049

TABLE 23b   Aerobic Power Tests—Women *(continued)*

%	Ages 40–49 Balke Treadmill (time)	$\dot{V}O_{2max}$ (ml/kg/ min)	12-Minute Run (miles)	1.5-Mile Run (time)	Ages 50–59 Balke Treadmill (time)	$\dot{V}O_{2max}$ (ml/kg/ min)	12-Minute Run (miles)	1.5-Mile Run (time)	
99	22:00	46.75	1.61	10:47	18:44	42.04	1.48	12:28	S
95	18:00	40.98	1.45	12:51	15:07	36.81	1.33	14:20	
90	17:00	39.53	1.41	13:22	14:00	35.20	1.29	14:55	
85	15:35	37.49	1.35	14:06	12:53	33.59	1.24	15:29	
80	14:45	36.28	1.32	14:31	12:00	32.31	1.21	15:57	E
75	13:56	35.11	1.29	14:57	11:43	39.90	1.20	16:05	
70	13:00	33.76	1.25	15:16	11:00	30.87	1.17	16:27	
65	12:30	33.04	1.23	15:41	10:14	29.76	1.14	16:51	
60	12:00	32.31	1.21	15:57	10:00	29.43	1.13	16:58	G
55	11:30	31.59	1.19	16:12	9:30	28.70	1.11	17:14	
50	11:00	30.87	1.17	16:27	9:10	28.22	1.10	17:24	
45	10:48	30.58	1.16	16:34	9:00	27.98	1.09	17:29	
40	10:01	29.45	1.13	16:58	8:13	26.85	1.06	17:55	F
35	10:00	29.43	1.12	16:59	7:43	26.13	1.04	18:09	
30	9:11	28.25	1.10	17:24	7:16	25.48	1.02	18:23	
25	9:00	27.98	1.09	17:29	7:00	25.09	1.01	18:31	
20	8:00	26.54	1.05	18:00	6:25	24.25	.98	18:49	P
15	7:20	25.57	1.02	18:21	6:00	23.65	.97	19:02	
10	7:00	25.09	1.01	18:31	5:05	22.33	.93	19:30	
5	5:55	23.53	.96	19:05	4:14	21.10	.90	19:57	VP
1	4:00	20.76	.89	20:04	2:36	18.74	.83	20:47	

n = 1630   *n* = 7094

		Age 60+			
%	**Balke Treadmill (time)**	**$\dot{V}O_{2max}$ (ml/kg/min)**	**12-Minute Run (miles)**	**1.5-Mile Run (time)**	
99	20:25	44.47	1.55	11:36	S
95	15:34	37.46	1.35	14:06	
90	14:00	35.20	1.29	14:55	
85	12:00	32.31	1.21	15:57	
80	11:15	31.23	1.18	16:20	E
75	11:00	30.87	1.17	16:27	
70	10:00	29.43	1.13	16:58	
65	9:00	27.98	1.09	17:29	
60	8:28	27.21	1.07	17:46	G
55	8:00	26.54	1.05	18:00	
50	7:30	25.82	1.03	18:16	
45	7:00	25.09	1.01	18:31	
40	6:35	24.49	.99	18:44	F
35	6:16	24.03	.98	18:54	
30	6:08	23.80	.97	18:59	
25	6:00	23.65	.97	19:02	
20	5:24	22.78	.94	19:21	P
15	5:00	22.21	.93	19:33	
10	4:00	20.76	.89	20:04	
5	3:15	19.68	.86	20:23	VP
1	2:00	17.87	.81	21:06	

Note: n = 202; S, superior; E, excellent; G, good; F, fair; P, poor; VP, very poor.

Source (Tables 23a–d): Data provided by the Institute for Aerobics Research, Dallas, TX, 1994. Reprinted by permission of the Cooper Institute for Aerobics Research, Dallas, TX.

TABLE 24 $\dot{V}O_{2max}$ Norms

	Low	**Fair**	**Avg**	**Good**	**High**	**Athletic**	**Olympic**
Women							
20–29	<28	29–34	35–43	44–48	49–53	54–59	60+
30–39	<27	28–33	34–41	42–47	48–52	53–58	59+
40–49	<25	26–31	32–40	41–45	46–50	51–56	57+
50–65	<21	22–28	29–36	37–41	42–45	46–49	50+
Men							
20–29	<38	39–43	44–51	52–56	57–62	63–69	70+
30–39	<34	35–39	40–47	48–51	52–57	58–64	65+
40–49	<30	31–35	36–43	44–47	48–53	54–60	61+
50–59	<25	26–31	32–39	40–43	44–48	49–44	56+
60–69	<21	22–26	27–35	36–39	40–44	45–49	50+

Note: $\dot{V}O_{2max}$ is expressed in tables as milliliters of oxygen per kilogram of body weight per minute.

Source: Adapted from Astrand, *ACTA Physiol Scand* 49(suppl):169,1960. Reprinted with permission from Blackwell Scientific Publications LTD.

TABLE 25 $\dot{V}O_{2max}$ Norms

Athletic Group	Sex	Age (yr)	Height (cm)	Weight (kg)	$\dot{V}O_{2max}$ (ml/kg/min)
Maximal Oxygen Uptake of Male and Female Athletes					
Baseball/softball				
	Male	21	182.7	83.3	52.3
	Male	28	183.6	88.1	52.0
	Female	19–23	—	—	55.3
Basketball				
	Female	19	167.0	63.9	42.3
	Female	19	169.1	62.6	42.9
	Female	19	173.0	68.3	49.6
Centers	Male	28	214.0	109.2	41.9
Forwards	Male	25	200.6	96.9	45.9
Guards	Male	25	188.0	83.6	50.0
Bicycling (competitive)				
	Male	24	182.0	74.5	68.2
	Male	24	180.4	79.2	70.3
	Male	25	180.0	72.8	67.1
	Male	—	180.3	67.1	74.0
	Male	—	—	—	74.0
	Male	—	—	—	69.1
	Female	20	165.0	55.0	50.2
	Female	—	167.7	61.3	57.4
Canoeing/paddling				
	Male	19	173.0	64.0	60.0
	Male	22	190.5	80.7	67.7
	Male	24	182.0	79.6	66.1
	Male	26	181.0	74.0	56.8
	Female	18	166.0	57.3	49.2
Dancing				
Ballet	Male	24	177.5	68.0	48.2
	Female	24	165.6	49.5	43.7
General	Female	21	162.7	51.2	41.5
Football				
	Male	19	186.8	93.1	56.5
	Male	20	184.9	96.4	51.3
Defensive backs	Male	25	182.5	84.8	53.1
Offensive backs	Male	25	183.8	90.7	52.2
Linebackers	Male	24	188.6	102.2	52.1
Offensive linemen	Male	25	193.0	112.6	49.9
Defensive linemen	Male	26	192.4	117.1	44.9
Quarterbacks/kickers	Male	24	185.0	90.1	49.0
Gymnastics				
	Male	20	178.5	69.2	55.5
	Female	15	159.7	48.8	49.8
	Female	19	163.0	57.9	36.3
Ice hockey				
	Male	11	140.5	35.5	56.6
	Male	22	179.0	77.3	61.5
	Male	24	179.3	81.8	54.6
	Male	26	180.1	86.4	53.6

Athletic Group	Sex	Age (yr)	Height (cm)	Weight (kg)	$\dot{V}O_{2max}$ (ml/kg/min)
Jockeys					
	Male	31	158.2	50.3	53.8
Orienteering					
	Male	25	179.7	70.3	71.1
	Male	31	—	72.2	61.6
	Male	52	176.0	72.7	50.7
	Female	23	165.8	60.0	60.7
	Female	29	—	58.1	46.1
Pentathlon					
	Female	21	175.4	65.4	45.9
Racquetball/handball					
	Male	24	183.7	81.3	60.0
	Male	25	181.7	80.3	58.3
Rowing					
	Male	—	—	—	65.7
	Male	23	192.7	89.9	62.6
	Male	25	189.9	86.9	66.9
Heavyweight	Male	23	192.0	88.0	68.9
Lightweight	Male	21	186.0	71.0	71.1
	Female	23	173.0	68.0	60.3
Skating					
Speed	Male	20	175.5	73.9	56.1
	Male	21	181.0	76.5	72.9
	Male	25	183.1	82.4	64.6
	Female	20	168.1	65.4	52.0
	Female	21	164.5	60.8	46.1
Figure	Male	21	166.9	59.6	58.5
	Female	17	158.8	48.6	48.9
Skiing					
Alpine	Male	16	173.1	65.5	65.6
	Male	21	176.0	70.1	63.8
	Male	22	177.8	75.5	66.6
	Male	26	176.6	74.8	62.3
	Female	19	165.1	58.8	52.7
Cross-country	Male	21	176.0	66.6	63.9
	Male	25	180.4	73.2	73.9
	Male	26	174.0	69.3	78.3
	Male	23	176.2	73.2	73.0
	Male	—	—	—	72.8
	Female	20	163.4	55.9	61.5
	Female	24	163.0	59.1	68.2
	Female	25	165.7	60.5	56.9
	Female	—	—	—	58.1
Nordic	Male	23	176.0	70.4	72.8
	Male	22	181.7	70.4	67.4
Ski jumping					
	Male	22	174.0	69.9	61.3

(continued)

TABLE 25 $\dot{V}O_{2max}$ **Norms** *(continued)*

	Maximal Oxygen Uptake of Male and Female Athletes				
Athletic Group	**Sex**	**Age (yr)**	**Height (cm)**	**Weight (kg)**	**$\dot{V}O_{2max}$ (ml/kg/min)**
Soccer					
	Male	26	176.0	75.5	58.4
Swimming					
	Male	12	150.4	41.2	52.5
	Male	13	164.8	52.1	52.9
	Male	15	169.6	59.8	56.6
	Male	15	166.8	59.1	56.8
	Male	20	181.4	76.7	55.7
	Male	20	181.0	73.0	50.4
	Male	21	182.9	78.9	62.1
	Male	21	181.0	78.3	69.9
	Male	22	182.3	79.1	56.9
	Male	22	182.3	79.7	55.9
	Female	12	154.8	43.3	46.2
	Female	13	160.0	52.1	43.4
	Female	15	164.8	53.7	40.5
Sprint	Male	19	181.1	75.0	58.3
Middle distance	Male	22	178.0	74.6	55.4
Long distance	Male	21	179.0	74.9	65.4
	Female	19	168.0	63.8	37.6
Tennis					
	Male	42	179.6	77.1	50.2
	Female	39	163.3	55.7	44.2
Track and field					
Run	Male	21	180.6	71.6	66.1
	Male	22	177.4	64.5	64.0
	Male	23	177.0	69.5	72.4
Sprint	Male	17–22	—	—	51.0
	Male	46	177.0	74.1	47.2
Middle distance	Male	25	180.1	67.8	70.1
	Male	25	179.0	72.3	69.8
Long distance	Male	10	144.3	31.9	56.6
	Male	17–22	—	—	65.5
	Male	26	176.1	64.5	72.2
	Male	26	178.9	63.9	77.4
	Male	26	177.0	66.2	78.1
	Male	27	178.7	64.9	73.2
	Male	32	177.3	64.3	70.3
	Male	35	174.0	63.1	66.6
	Male	36	177.3	69.6	65.1
	Male	40–49	180.7	71.6	57.5
	Male	55	174.5	63.4	54.4
	Male	50–59	174.7	67.2	54.4
	Male	60–69	175.7	67.1	51.4
	Male	70–75	175.6	66.8	40.0
	Male	—	—	—	72.5
	Female	16	162.6	48.6	63.2

Athletic Group	Sex	Age (yr)	Height (cm)	Weight (kg)	$\dot{V}O_{2max}$ (ml/kg/min)
	Female	16	163.3	50.9	50.8
	Female	21	170.2	58.6	57.5
	Female	32	169.4	57.2	59.1
	Female	44	161.5	53.8	43.4
	Female	—	—	—	58.2
Race walking	Male	27	178.7	68.5	62.9
Jumping	Male	17–22	—	—	55.0
Shot / discus	Male	17–22	—	—	49.5
	Male	26	190.8	110.5	42.8
	Male	27	188.2	112.5	42.6
	Male	28	186.1	104.7	47.5
Volleyball					
	Male	25	187.0	84.5	56.4
	Male	26	192.7	85.5	56.1
	Female	19	166.0	59.8	43.5
	Female	20	172.2	64.1	56.0
	Female	22	183.7	73.4	41.7
	Female	22	178.3	70.5	50.6
Weight lifting					
	Male	25	171.0	81.3	40.1
	Male	25	166.4	77.2	42.6
Power	Male	26	176.1	92.0	49.5
Olympic	Male	25	177.1	88.2	50.7
Bodybuilding	Male	27	178.8	88.1	46.3
	Male	29	172.4	83.1	41.5
Wrestling					
	Male	21	174.8	67.3	58.3
	Male	23	—	79.2	50.4
	Male	24	175.6	77.7	60.9
	Male	26	177.0	81.8	64.0
	Male	27	176.0	75.7	54.3

Source: Wilmore JH. Design issues and alternatives in assessing physical fitness among apparently healthy adults in a health examination survey of the general population. In Drury TF (ed), National Center for Health Statistics. *Assessing Physical Fitness and Physical Activity in Population-Based Surveys.* DHHS Pub. No. (PHS) 89-1253. Public Health Service. Washington, DC: U.S. Government Printing Office, 1989.

Section 3. Body Composition

TABLE 26 Disease Risk Associated with Body Mass Index and Waist Circumference

Classification	Obesity Class	BMI (kg/m²)	Disease Risk Relative to Normal Weight and Waist Circumference*	
			Men ≤40 in Women ≤35 in	>40 in >35 in
Underweight		<18.5	—	—
Normal		18.5–24.9	—	—
Overweight		25.0–29.9	Increased	High
Obesity	I	30.0–34.9	High	Very high
	II	35.0–39.9	Very high	Very high
Extreme obesity	III	≥40	Extremely high	Extremely high

*Disease risk for type 2 diabetes, hypertension, and cardiovascular disease.

Source: NHLBI Obesity Education Initiative Expert Panel. *Clinical Guidelines on the Identification, Evaluation, and Treatment of Overweight and Obesity in Adults.* National Heart, Lung, and Blood Institute: www.nhlbi.nih.gov/nhlbi/1998.

TABLE 27a Means, Standard Deviations, and Percentiles of Triceps Skinfold Thickness (mm) by Age for American Males of 1–74 Years

Age (yr)	n	Mean	SD	Percentiles								
				5	10	15	25	50	75	85	90	95
1.0–1.9	681	10.4	2.9	6.5	7.0	7.5	8.0	10.0	12.0	13.0	14.0	15.5
2.0–2.9	677	10.0	2.9	6.0	6.5	7.0	8.0	10.0	12.0	13.0	14.0	15.0
3.0–3.9	717	9.9	2.7	6.0	7.0	7.0	8.0	9.5	11.5	12.5	13.5	15.0
4.0–4.9	708	9.2	2.7	5.5	6.5	7.0	7.5	9.0	11.0	12.0	12.5	14.0
5.0–5.9	677	8.9	3.1	5.0	6.0	6.0	7.0	8.0	10.0	11.5	13.0	14.5
6.0–6.9	298	8.9	3.8	5.0	5.5	6.0	6.5	8.0	10.0	12.0	13.0	16.0
7.0–7.9	312	9.0	4.0	4.5	5.0	6.0	6.0	8.0	10.5	12.5	14.0	16.0
8.0–8.9	296	9.6	4.4	5.0	5.5	6.0	7.0	8.5	11.0	13.0	16.0	19.0
9.0–9.9	322	10.2	5.1	5.0	5.5	6.0	6.5	9.0	12.5	15.5	17.0	20.0
10.0–10.9	334	11.5	5.7	5.0	6.0	6.0	7.5	10.0	14.0	17.0	20.0	24.0
11.0–11.9	324	12.5	7.0	5.0	6.0	6.5	7.5	10.0	16.0	19.5	23.0	27.0
12.0–12.9	348	12.2	6.8	4.5	6.0	6.0	7.5	10.5	14.5	18.0	22.5	27.5
13.0–13.9	350	11.0	6.7	4.5	5.0	5.5	7.0	9.0	13.0	17.0	20.5	25.0
14.0–14.9	358	10.4	6.5	4.0	5.0	5.0	6.0	8.5	12.5	15.0	18.0	23.5
15.0–15.9	356	9.8	6.5	5.0	5.0	5.0	6.0	7.5	11.0	15.0	18.0	23.5
16.0–16.9	350	10.0	5.9	4.0	5.0	5.1	6.0	8.0	12.0	14.0	17.0	23.0
17.0–17.9	337	9.1	5.3	4.0	5.0	5.0	6.0	7.0	11.0	13.5	16.0	19.5
18.0–24.9	1752	11.3	6.4	4.0	5.0	5.5	6.5	10.0	14.5	17.5	20.0	23.5
25.0–29.9	1251	12.2	6.7	4.0	5.0	6.0	7.0	11.0	15.5	19.0	21.5	25.0
30.0–34.9	941	13.1	6.7	4.5	6.0	6.5	8.0	12.0	16.5	20.0	22.0	25.0
35.0–39.9	832	12.9	6.2	4.5	6.0	7.0	8.5	12.0	16.0	18.5	20.5	24.5
40.0–44.9	828	13.0	6.6	5.0	6.0	6.9	8.0	12.0	16.0	19.0	21.5	26.0
45.0–49.9	867	12.9	6.4	5.0	6.0	7.0	8.0	12.0	16.0	19.0	21.0	25.0
50.0–54.9	879	12.6	6.1	5.0	6.0	7.0	8.0	11.5	15.0	18.5	20.8	25.0
55.0–59.9	807	12.4	6.0	5.0	6.0	6.5	8.0	11.5	15.0	18.0	20.5	25.0
60.0–64.9	1259	12.5	6.0	5.0	6.0	7.0	8.0	11.5	15.5	18.5	20.5	24.0
65.0–69.9	1774	12.1	5.9	4.5	5.0	6.5	8.0	11.0	15.0	18.0	20.0	23.5
70.0–74.9	1251	12.0	5.8	4.5	6.0	6.5	8.0	11.0	15.0	17.0	19.0	23.0

TABLE 27b   Means, Standard Deviations, and Percentiles of Triceps Skinfold Thickness (mm) by Age for American Females of 1–74 Years

Age (yr)	n	Mean	SD	5	10	15	25	50	75	85	90	95
1.0–1.9	622	10.4	3.1	6.0	7.0	7.0	8.0	10.0	12.0	13.0	14.0	16.0
2.0–2.9	614	10.5	2.9	6.0	7.0	7.5	8.5	10.0	12.0	13.5	14.5	16.0
3.0–3.9	652	10.4	2.9	6.0	7.0	7.5	8.5	10.0	12.0	13.0	14.0	16.0
4.0–4.9	681	10.3	3.0	6.0	7.0	7.5	8.0	10.0	12.0	13.0	14.0	15.5
5.0–5.9	673	10.4	3.5	5.5	7.0	7.0	8.0	10.0	12.0	13.5	15.0	17.0
6.0–6.9	296	10.4	3.7	6.0	6.5	7.0	8.0	10.0	12.0	13.0	15.0	17.0
7.0–7.9	330	11.1	4.2	6.0	7.0	7.0	8.0	10.5	12.5	15.0	16.0	19.0
8.0–8.9	276	12.1	5.4	6.0	7.0	7.5	8.5	11.0	14.5	17.0	18.0	22.5
9.0–9.9	322	13.4	5.9	6.5	7.0	8.0	9.0	12.0	16.0	19.0	21.0	25.0
10.0–10.9	329	13.9	6.1	7.0	8.0	8.0	9.0	12.5	17.5	20.0	22.5	27.0
11.0–11.9	302	15.0	6.8	7.0	8.0	8.5	10.0	13.0	18.0	21.5	24.0	29.0
12.0–12.9	323	15.1	6.3	7.0	8.0	9.0	11.0	14.0	18.5	21.5	24.0	27.5
13.0–13.9	360	16.4	7.4	7.0	8.0	9.0	11.0	15.0	20.0	24.0	25.0	30.0
14.0–14.9	370	17.1	7.3	8.0	9.0	10.0	11.5	16.0	21.0	23.5	26.5	32.0
15.0–15.9	309	17.3	7.4	8.0	9.5	10.5	12.0	16.5	20.5	23.0	26.0	32.5
16.0–16.9	343	19.2	7.0	10.5	11.5	12.0	14.0	18.0	23.0	26.0	29.0	32.5
17.0–17.9	291	19.1	8.0	9.0	10.0	12.0	13.0	18.0	24.0	26.5	29.0	34.5
18.0–24.9	2588	20.0	8.2	9.0	11.0	12.0	14.0	18.5	24.5	28.5	31.0	36.0
25.0–29.9	1921	21.7	8.8	10.0	12.0	13.0	15.0	20.0	26.5	31.0	34.0	38.0
30.0–34.9	1619	23.7	9.2	10.5	13.0	15.0	17.0	22.5	29.5	33.0	35.0	41.5
35.0–39.9	1453	24.7	9.3	11.0	13.0	15.5	18.0	23.5	30.0	35.0	37.0	41.0
40.0–44.9	1391	25.1	9.0	12.0	14.0	16.0	19.0	24.5	30.5	35.0	37.0	41.0
45.0–49.9	962	26.1	9.3	12.0	14.5	16.5	19.5	25.5	32.0	35.5	38.0	42.5
50.0–54.9	1006	26.5	9.0	12.0	15.0	17.5	20.5	25.5	32.0	36.0	38.5	42.0
55.0–59.9	880	26.6	9.4	12.0	15.0	17.0	20.5	26.0	32.0	36.0	39.0	42.5
60.0–64.9	1389	26.6	8.8	12.5	16.0	17.5	20.5	26.0	32.0	35.5	38.0	42.5
65.0–69.9	1946	25.1	8.5	12.0	14.5	16.0	19.0	25.0	30.0	33.5	36.0	40.0
70.0–74.9	1463	24.0	8.5	11.0	13.5	15.5	18.0	24.0	29.5	32.0	35.5	38.5

Source (Tables a and b): Frisancho AR. *Anthropometric Standards for the Assessment of Growth and Nutritional Status.* Ann Arbor: University of Michigan Press, 1990. Used with permission.

TABLE 28 Relative Body Fat in Male and Female Athletes

Athletic Group	Sex	Age (yr)	Height (cm)	Weight (kg)	Relative Fat
Baseball					
	Male	20.8	182.7	83.3	14.2
	Male	—	—	—	11.8
	Male	27.4	183.1	88.0	12.6
Basketball					
	Female	19.1	169.1	62.6	20.8
	Female	19.4	167.0	63.9	26.9
Centers	Male	27.7	214.0	109.2	7.1
Forwards	Male	25.3	200.6	96.9	9.0
Guards	Male	25.2	188.0	83.6	10.6
Canoeing					
	Male	23.7	182.0	79.6	12.4
Football					
	Male	20.3	184.9	96.4	13.8
	Male	—	—	—	13.9
Defensive backs	Male	17–23	178.3	77.3	11.5
	Male	24.5	182.5	84.8	9.6
Offensive backs	Male	17–23	179.7	79.8	12.4
	Male	24.7	183.8	90.7	9.4
Linebackers	Male	17–23	180.1	87.2	13.4
	Male	24.2	188.6	102.2	14.0
Offensive linemen	Male	17–23	186.0	99.2	19.1
	Male	24.7	193.0	112.6	15.6
Defensive linemen	Male	17–23	186.6	97.8	18.5
	Male	25.7	192.4	117.1	18.2
Quarterbacks, kickers	Male	24.1	185.0	90.1	14.4
Gymnastics					
	Male	20.3	178.5	69.2	4.6
	Female	20.0	158.5	51.5	15.5
	Female	14.0	—	—	17.0
	Female	23.0	—	—	11.0
	Female	23.0	—	—	9.6
Ice hockey					
	Male	26.3	180.3	86.7	15.1
	Male	22.5	179.0	77.3	13.0
Jockeys					
	Male	30.9	158.2	50.3	14.1
Orienteering					
	Male	31.2	—	72.2	16.3
	Female	29.0	—	58.1	18.7
Pentathlon					
	Female	21.5	175.4	65.4	11.0
Racquetball					
	Male	25.0	181.7	80.3	8.1
Rowing					
Heavyweight	Male	23.0	192.0	88.0	11.0
Lightweight	Male	21.0	186.0	71.0	8.5
	Female	23.0	173.0	68.0	14.0

Athletic Group	Sex	Age (yr)	Height (cm)	Weight (kg)	Relative Fat
Skiing					
Alpine	Male	21.2	176.0	70.1	14.1
	Male	21.8	177.8	75.5	10.2
	Female	19.5	165.1	58.8	20.6
Cross-country	Male	21.2	176.0	66.6	12.5
	Male	25.6	174.0	69.3	10.2
	Male	22.7	176.2	73.2	7.9
	Female	24.3	163.0	59.1	21.8
	Female	20.2	163.4	55.9	15.7
Nordic combination	Male	22.9	176.0	70.4	11.2
	Male	21.7	181.7	70.4	8.9
Ski jumping					
	Male	22.2	174.0	69.9	14.3
Soccer					
	Male	26.0	176.0	75.5	9.6
Speed skating					
	Male	21.0	181.0	76.5	11.4
Swimming					
	Male	21.8	182.3	79.1	8.5
	Male	20.6	182.9	78.9	5.0
	Female	19.4	168.0	63.8	26.3
Sprint	Female	—	165.1	57.1	14.6
Middle distance	Female	—	166.6	66.8	24.1
Long distance	Female	—	166.3	60.9	17.1
Tennis					
	Male	—	—	—	15.2
	Male	42.0	179.6	77.1	16.3
	Female	39.0	163.3	55.7	20.3
Track and field					
	Male	21.3	180.6	71.6	3.7
	Male	—	—	—	8.8
Run	Male	22.5	177.4	64.5	6.3
Long distance	Male	26.1	175.7	64.2	7.5
	Male	26.2	177.0	66.2	8.4
	Male	40–49	180.7	71.6	11.2
	Male	55.3	174.5	63.4	18.0
	Male	50–59	174.7	67.2	10.9
	Male	60–69	175.7	67.1	11.3
	Male	70–75	175.6	66.8	13.6
	Male	47.2	176.5	70.7	13.2
	Female	19.9	161.3	52.9	19.2
	Female	32.4	169.4	57.2	15.2
Middle distance	Male	24.6	179.0	72.3	12.4
Sprint	Female	20.1	164.9	56.7	19.3
	Male	46.5	177.0	74.1	16.5
Discus	Male	28.3	186.1	104.7	16.4
	Male	26.4	190.8	110.5	16.3
	Female	21.1	168.1	71.0	25.0
Jumping and hurdling	Female	20.3	165.9	59.0	20.7

(continued)

TABLE 28 Relative Body Fat in Male and Female Athletes *(continued)*

Athletic Group	Sex	Age (yr)	Height (cm)	Weight (kg)	Relative Fat
Shot-put	Male	27.0	188.2	112.5	16.5
	Male	22.0	191.6	126.2	19.6
	Female	21.5	167.6	78.1	28.0
Volleyball					
	Female	19.4	166.0	59.8	25.3
	Female	19.9	172.2	64.1	21.3
Weight lifting					
	Male	24.9	166.4	77.2	9.8
Power	Male	26.3	176.1	92.0	15.6
Olympic	Male	25.3	177.1	88.2	12.2
Bodybuilding	Male	29.0	172.4	83.1	8.4
	Male	27.6	178.7	88.1	8.3
Wrestling					
	Male	26.0	177.8	81.8	9.8
	Male	27.0	176.0	75.7	10.7
	Male	22.0	—	—	5.0
	Male	23.0	—	79.3	14.3
	Male	19.6	174.6	74.8	8.8
	Male	15–18	172.3	66.3	6.9
	Male	20.6	174.8	67.3	4.0

Source: Wilmore JH. Design issues and alternatives in assessing physical fitness among apparently healthy adults in a health examination survey of the general population. In Drury TF (ed), National Center for Health Statistics. *Assessing Physical Fitness and Physical Activity in Population-Based Surveys.* DHHS Pub. No. (PHS) 89-1253. Public Health Service. Washington, DC: U.S. Government Printing Office, 1989.

Section 4. Musculoskeletal Test Norms for Adults

See descriptions given with each test. Also review Chapter 6.

TABLE 29 Timed (1 minute) Bent-Knee Sit-Up Norms by Age Groups and Gender

Age (yrs)	15–19		20–29		30–39		40–49		50–59		60–69	
Gender	M	F	M	F	M	F	M	F	M	F	M	F
Excellent	≥48	≥42	≥43	≥36	≥36	≥29	≥31	≥25	≥26	≥19	≥23	≥16
Above average	42–47	36–41	37–42	31–35	31–35	24–28	26–30	20–24	22–25	12–18	17–22	12–15
Average	38–41	32–35	33–36	25–30	27–30	20–23	22–25	15–19	18–21	5–11	12–16	4–11
Below average	33–37	27–31	29–32	21–24	22–26	15–19	17–21	7–14	13–17	3–4	7–11	2–3
Poor	≤32	≤26	≤28	≤20	≤21	≤14	≤16	≤6	≤12	≤2	≤6	≤1

Procedures: Subject lies in a supine position, knees bent at a right angle, and feet shoulder-width apart. The hands are placed at the side of the head with the fingers over the ears. The elbows are pointed toward the knees. The hands and elbows must be maintained in these positions for the entire duration of the test. Also, the ankles of the participant must be held throughout the test by the appraiser to ensure that the heels are in constant contact with the mat. The participant is required to sit up, touch the knees with the elbows and return to the starting position (shoulders touch the floor). The participant performs as many sit-ups as possible within 1 minute. A rocking or bouncing movement is not permitted. The buttocks must remain in contact with the mat at all times.

Source: The Canadian Physical Activity, Fitness & Lifestyle Appraisal: CSEP's Plan for Healthy Active Living, 1996. Reprinted by permission from the Canadian Society for Exercise Physiology.

TABLE 30 Push-up Norms by Age Groups and Gender

Age (yrs)	15–19		20–29		30–39		40–49		50–59		60–69	
Gender	M	F	M	F	M	F	M	F	M	F	M	F
Excellent	≥39	≥33	≥36	≥30	≥30	≥27	≥22	≥24	≥21	≥21	≥18	≥17
Above average	29–38	25–32	29–35	21–29	22–29	20–26	17–21	15–23	13–20	11–20	11–17	12–16
Average	23–28	18–24	22–28	15–20	17–21	13–19	13–16	11–14	10–12	7–10	8–10	5–11
Below average	18–22	12–17	17–21	10–14	12–16	8–12	10–12	5–10	7–9	2–6	5–7	1–4
Poor	≤17	≤11	≤16	≤9	≤11	≤7	≤9	≤4	≤6	≤1	≤4	≤1

Procedures: Males—The participant lies on his stomach, legs together. His hands, pointing forward, are positioned under the shoulders. The participant pushes up from the mat by fully straightening the elbows and using the toes as the pivotal point. The upper body must be kept in a straight line. The participant returns to the starting position, chin to the mat. Neither the stomach nor the thighs should touch the mat. *Females*—Same as for males, except the knees are the pivotal point. The lower legs remain in contact with the mat, ankles plantar-flexed.

Source: The Canadian Physical Activity, Fitness & Lifestyle Appraisal: CSEP's Plan for Healthy Active Living, 1996. Reprinted by permission from the Canadian Society for Exercise Physiology.

TABLE 31 Grip-Strength (kg) Norms by Age Groups and Gender for Combined Right and Left Hand

Age (yrs)	15–19		20–29		30–39		40–49		50–59		60–69	
Gender	M	F	M	F	M	F	M	F	M	F	M	F
Above average	103–112	64–70	113–123	65–70	113–122	66–72	110–118	65–72	102–109	59–64	98–101	54–59
Average	95–102	59–63	106–112	61–64	105–112	61–65	102–109	59–64	96–101	55–58	86–92	51–53
Below average	84–94	54–58	97–105	55–60	97–104	56–60	94–101	55–58	87–95	51–54	79–85	48–50
Poor	≤83	≤53	≤96	≤54	≤96	≤55	≤93	≤54	≤86	≤50	≤78	≤47

Procedures: Have the participant grasp the dynamometer in the right hand first. Adjust the grip of the dynamometer so the second joint of the fingers fits snugly under the handle. The participant holds the dynamometer in line with the forearm at the level of the thigh. The dynamometer is then squeezed vigorously so as to exert maximum force. During the test, neither the hand nor the dynamometer should touch the body or any other object. Measure both hands alternately, allowing two trials per hand. Record the scores for each hand to the nearest kilogram. Combine the maximum score for each hand.

Source: The Canadian Physical Activity, Fitness & Lifestyle Appraisal: CSEP's Plan for Healthy Active Living, 1996. Reprinted by permission from the Canadian Society for Exercise Physiology.

TABLE 32 Age Group and Gender Classifications for Partial Curl-Ups

Age	Excellent	Very Good	Good	Fair	Needs Improvement
15–19					
Male	25	23–24	21–22	16–20	≤15
Female	25	23–24	21–22	16–20	≤15
20–29					
Male	25	23–24	21–22	13–20	≤12
Female	25	23–24	19–22	13–18	≤12
30–39					
Male	25	23–24	21–22	13–20	≤12
Female	25	22–24	16–21	11–15	≤10
40–49					
Male	25	22–24	16–21	11–15	≤10
Female	25	21–24	13–20	6–12	≤5
50–59					
Male	25	19–24	14–19	9–13	≤8
Female	25	16–24	9–15	4–8	≤3
60–69					
Male	25	16–24	10–15	4–9	≤3
Female	≥18	11–17	6–10	2–5	≤1

Instructions:

1. Apply masking tape and string across a gym mat in two parallel lines 10 cm apart.

2. The individual to be tested should lie in a supine position with the head resting on the mat, arms straight and fully extended at the sides and parallel to the trunk, palms of the hands in contact with the mat, and the middle fingertip of both hands at the 0 mark line. The knees should be bent at a 90° angle. The heels must stay in contact with the mat, and the test is performed with the shoes on.

3. Set a metronome to a cadence of 50 beats per minute. The subject performs as many consecutive curl-ups as possible, without pausing, at a rate of 25 per minute. The test is terminated after 1 minute. During each curl-up, the upper spine should be curled up so that the middle fingertips of both hands reach the 10 cm mark. During the curl-up the palms and heels must remain in contact with the mat. Anchoring of the feet is not permitted. On the return, the shoulder blades and head must contact the mat, and the fingertips of both hands must touch the 0 mark. The movement is performed in a slow, controlled manner at a rate of 25 per minute.

4. The test is terminated before 1 minute if subjects experience undue discomfort, are unable to maintain the required cadence, or are unable to maintain the proper curl-up technique (e.g., heels come off the floor) over two consecutive repetitions despite cautions by the test supervisor.

Source: Canadian Society for Exercise Physiology. *The Canadian Physical Activity, Fitness & Lifestyle Appraisal: CSEP's Plan for Healthy Active Living.* Ottawa, Ontario: Author, 1996. Used with permission from the Canadian Society for Exercise Physiology.

TABLE 33a   Sit-and-Reach Test for Lower Back–Hamstring Flexibility Norms by Age Groups and Gender for Trunk Forward Flexion (cm)

Age (yrs)	15–19		20–29		30–39		40–49		50–59		60–69	
Gender	M	F	M	F	M	F	M	F	M	F	M	F
Excellent	≥39	≥43	≥40	≥41	≥38	≥41	≥35	≥38	≥35	≥39	≥33	≥35
Above average	34–38	38–42	34–39	37–40	33–37	36–40	29–34	34–37	28–34	33–38	25–32	31–34
Average	29–33	34–37	30–33	33–36	28–32	32–35	24–28	30–33	24–27	30–32	20–24	27–30
Below average	24–28	29–33	25–29	28–32	23–27	27–31	18–23	25–29	16–23	25–29	15–19	23–26
Poor	≤23	≤28	≤24	≤27	≤22	≤26	≤17	≤24	≤15	≤24	≤14	≤23

Procedures: Have the participant warm up for this test by performing slow aerobic activities and then stretching movements. The participant, barefoot, sits with legs fully extended with the soles of the feet placed flat against the flexibility box (see Chapter 6). Keeping knees fully extended, arms evenly stretched, palms down, the participant bends and reaches forward without jerking, pushing the sliding marker along the scale with the fingertips as far as possible. The position of maximum flexion must be held for approximately 2 seconds. The test is repeated twice. The footline is set at 26 cm.

Source: The Canadian Physical Activity, Fitness & Lifestyle Appraisal: CSEP's Plan for Healthy Active Living, 1996. Reprinted by permission from the Canadian Society for Exercise Physiology.

TABLE 33b

Classification	Sit and Reach (inches; footline at 0)
Excellent	≥ +7
Good	+4–6.75
Average	+0–3.75
Fair	−3–0.25
Poor	< −3

Note: There is some feeling that flexibility should not decrease with age if regular range-of-motion exercise is engaged in. The preceding norms are proposed.

TABLE 34a Push-Up Norms—Men

%	\n Age \n 20–29	30–39	40–49	50–59	60+	
99	100	86	64	51	39	S
95	62	52	40	39	28	
90	57	46	36	30	26	
85	51	41	34	28	24	
80	47	39	30	25	23	E
75	44	36	29	24	22	
70	41	34	26	21	21	
65	39	31	25	20	20	
60	37	30	24	19	18	G
55	35	29	22	17	16	
50	33	27	21	15	15	
45	31	25	19	14	12	
40	29	24	18	13	10	F
35	27	21	16	11	9	
30	26	20	15	10	8	
25	24	19	13	9.5	7	
20	22	17	11	9	6	P
15	19	15	10	7	5	
10	18	13	9	6	4	
5	13	9	5	3	2	VP
n =	1045	790	364	172	26	

Total *n* = 2397; S, superior; E, excellent; G, good; F, fair; P, poor; VP, very poor.

TABLE 34b Modified Push-Up Norms—Women

%	\n Age \n 20–29	30–39	40–49	50–59	60+	
99	70	56	60	31	20	S
95	45	39	33	28	20	
90	42	36	28	25	17	
85	39	33	26	23	15	
80	36	31	24	21	15	E
75	34	29	21	20	15	
70	32	28	20	19	14	
65	31	26	19	18	13	
60	30	24	18	17	12	G
55	29	23	17	15	12	
50	26	21	15	13	8	
45	25	20	14	13	6	
40	23	19	13	12	5	F
35	22	17	11	10	4	
30	20	15	10	9	3	
25	19	14	9	8	2	
20	17	11	6	6	2	P
15	15	9	4	4	1	
10	12	8	2	1	0	
5	9	4	1	0	0	VP
n =	579	411	246	105	12	

Total *n* = 1353; S, superior; E, excellent; G, good; F, fair; P, poor; VP, very poor.

Push-Up Test Procedures for Measurement of Muscular Endurance

1. The push-up test is administered with male subjects in the standard "up" position (hands shoulder-width apart, back straight, head up) and female subjects in the modified "knee push-up" position (ankles crossed, knees bent at 90° angle, back straight, hands shoulder-width apart, head up).

2. When testing male subjects, the tester places a fist on the floor beneath the subject's chest, and the subject must lower the body to the floor until the chest touches the tester's fist. The fist method is not used for female subjects, and no criteria are established for determining how much the torso must be lowered to count as a proper push-up.

3. For both men and women, the subject's back must be straight at all times and the subject must push up to a straight-arm position.

4. The maximal number of push-ups performed consecutively without rest is counted as the score.

Source (Tables 34a & b): Data provided by the Institute for Aerobics Research, Dallas, TX, 1994. Reprinted by permission of the Cooper Institute for Aerobics Research, Dallas, TX.

TABLE 35a Muscular Endurance—Men

1-Minute Sit-Up (number)[a]

%	<20	20–29	30–39	40–49	50–59	60+	
			Age				
99	>62	>55	>51	>47	>43	>39	S
95	62	55	51	47	43	39	
90	55	52	48	43	39	35	
85	53	49	45	40	36	31	
80	51	47	43	39	35	30	E
75	50	46	42	37	33	28	
70	48	45	41	36	31	26	
65	48	44	40	35	30	24	
60	47	42	39	34	28	22	G
55	46	41	37	32	27	21	
50	45	40	36	31	26	20	
45	42	39	36	30	25	19	
40	41	38	35	29	24	19	F
35	39	37	33	28	22	18	
30	38	35	32	27	21	17	
25	37	35	31	26	20	16	
20	36	33	30	24	19	15	P
15	34	32	28	22	17	13	
10	33	30	26	20	15	10	
5	27	27	23	17	12	7	VP
1	<27	<27	<23	<17	<12	<7	
n =	46	312	1431	1558	919	205	

Total n = 4471; S, superior; E, excellent; G, good; F, fair; P, poor; VP, very poor.

[a]Knees bent, with arms crossed over chest and feet held by a partner; sit up and touch elbows to knees.

TABLE 35b Muscular Endurance—Women

1-Minute Sit-Up (number)[a]

%	<20	20–29	30–39	40–49	50–59	60+	
			Age				
99	>55	>51	>42	>38	>30	>28	S
95	55	51	42	38	30	28	
90	54	49	40	34	29	26	
85	49	45	38	32	25	20	
80	46	44	35	29	24	17	E
75	40	42	33	28	22	15	
70	38	41	32	27	22	12	
65	37	39	30	25	21	12	
60	36	38	29	24	20	11	G
55	35	37	28	23	19	10	
50	34	35	27	22	17	8	
45	34	34	26	21	16	8	
40	32	32	25	20	14	6	F
35	30	31	24	19	12	5	
30	29	30	22	17	12	4	
25	29	28	21	16	11	4	
20	28	27	20	14	10	3	P
15	27	24	18	13	7	2	
10	25	23	15	10	6	1	
5	25	18	11	7	5	0	VP
1	<25	<18	<11	<7	<5	<0	
n =	15	144	289	249	137	26	

Total n = 860; S, superior; E, excellent; G, good; F, fair; P, poor; VP, very poor.

Source (Tables 35a and b): Data provided by the Institute for Aerobics Research, Dallas, TX, 1994. Reprinted by permission of the Cooper Institute for Aerobics Research, Dallas, TX.

TABLE 36a Upper-Body Strength—Men

1-Repetition Maximum Bench Press

$$\text{Bench Press Weight Ratio} = \frac{\text{Weight Pushed}}{\text{Body Weight}}$$

%	<20	20–29	30–39	40–49	50–59	60+	
99	>1.76	>1.63	>1.35	>1.20	>1.05	>.94	S
95	1.76	1.63	1.35	1.20	1.05	.94	
90	1.46	1.48	1.24	1.10	.97	.89	
85	1.38	1.37	1.17	1.04	.93	.84	
80	1.34	1.32	1.12	1.00	.90	.82	E
75	1.29	1.26	1.08	.96	.87	.79	
70	1.24	1.22	1.04	.93	.84	.77	
65	1.23	1.18	1.01	.90	.81	.74	
60	1.19	1.14	.98	.88	.79	.72	G
55	1.16	1.10	.96	.86	.77	.70	
50	1.13	1.06	.93	.84	.75	.68	
45	1.10	1.03	.90	.82	.73	.67	
40	1.06	.99	.88	.80	.71	.66	F
35	1.01	.96	.86	.78	.70	.65	
30	.96	.93	.83	.76	.68	.63	
25	.93	.90	.81	.74	.66	.60	
20	.89	.88	.78	.72	.63	.57	P
15	.86	.84	.75	.69	.60	.56	
10	.81	.80	.71	.65	.57	.53	
5	.76	.72	.65	.59	.53	.49	VP
1	<.76	<.72	<.65	<.59	<.53	<.49	
n =	60	425	1909	2090	1279	343	

Total *n* = 6106; S, superior; E, excellent; G, good; F, fair; P, poor; VP, very poor.

TABLE 36b Upper-Body Strength—Women

1-Repetition Maximum Bench Press

$$\text{Bench Press Weight Ratio} = \frac{\text{Weight Pushed}}{\text{Body Weight}}$$

%	<20	20–29	30–39	40–49	50–59	60+	
99	>.88	>1.01	>.82	>.77	>.68	>.72	S
95	.88	1.01	.82	.77	.68	.72	
90	.83	.90	.76	.71	.61	.64	
85	.81	.83	.72	.66	.57	.59	
80	.77	.80	.70	.62	.55	.54	E
75	.76	.77	.65	.60	.53	.53	
70	.74	.74	.63	.57	.52	.51	
65	.70	.72	.62	.55	.50	.48	
60	.65	.70	.60	.54	.48	.47	G
55	.64	.68	.58	.53	.47	.46	
50	.63	.65	.57	.52	.46	.45	
45	.60	.63	.55	.51	.45	.44	
40	.58	.59	.53	.50	.44	.43	F
35	.57	.58	.52	.48	.43	.41	
30	.56	.56	.51	.47	.42	.40	
25	.55	.53	.49	.45	.41	.39	
20	.53	.51	.47	.43	.39	.38	P
15	.52	.50	.45	.42	.38	.36	
10	.50	.480	.42	.38	.37	.33	
5	.41	.436	.39	.35	.305	.26	VP
1	<.41	<.436	<.39	<.35	<.305	<.26	
n =	20	191	379	333	189	42	

Total *n* = 1154; S, superior; E, excellent; G, good; F, fair; P, poor; VP, very poor.

Instructions:

1. Have your client warm up by completing 5–10 repetitions of the exercise at 40–60% of the estimated 1-RM.

2. During a 1-minute rest, have the client stretch the muscle group. This is followed by 3–5 repetitions of the exercise at 60–80% of the estimated 1-RM.

3. Then increase the weight conservatively and have the client attempt the 1-RM lift. If the lift is successful, the client should rest 3–5 minutes before attempting the next weight increment. Follow this procedure until the client fails to complete the lift. The 1-RM typically is achieved within three to five trials.

4. Record the 1-RM value as the maximum weight lifted for the last successful trial.

Source (Tables 36a and b): Data provided by the Institute for Aerobics Research, Dallas, TX, 1994. Reprinted with permission from the Cooper Institute for Aerobics Research, Dallas, TX.

TABLE 37a Leg Strength—Men

1-Repetition Maximum Leg Press

Leg Press Weight Ratio $= \dfrac{\text{Weight Pushed}}{\text{Body Weight}}$

%	<20	20–29	30–39	40–49	50–59	60+	
99	>2.82	>2.40	>2.20	>2.02	>1.90	>1.80	S
95	2.82	2.40	2.20	2.02	1.90	1.80	
90	2.53	2.27	2.07	1.92	1.80	1.73	
85	2.40	2.18	1.99	1.86	1.75	1.68	
80	2.28	2.13	1.93	1.82	1.71	1.62	E
75	2.18	2.09	1.89	1.78	1.68	1.58	
70	2.15	2.05	1.85	1.74	1.64	1.56	
65	2.10	2.01	1.81	1.71	1.61	1.52	
60	2.04	1.97	1.77	1.68	1.58	1.49	G
55	2.01	1.94	1.74	1.65	1.55	1.46	
50	1.95	1.91	1.71	1.62	1.52	1.43	
45	1.93	1.87	1.68	1.59	1.50	1.40	
40	1.90	1.83	1.65	1.57	1.46	1.38	F
35	1.89	1.78	1.62	1.54	1.42	1.34	
30	1.82	1.74	1.59	1.51	1.39	1.30	
25	1.80	1.68	1.56	1.48	1.36	1.27	
20	1.70	1.63	1.52	1.44	1.32	1.25	P
15	1.61	1.58	1.48	1.40	1.28	1.21	
10	1.57	1.51	1.43	1.35	1.22	1.16	
5	1.46	1.42	1.34	1.27	1.15	1.08	VP
1	<1.46	<1.42	<1.34	<1.27	<1.15	<1.08	
n =	60	424	1909	2089	1286	347	

Total n = 6115; S, superior; E, excellent; G, good; F, fair; P, poor; VP, very poor.

TABLE 37b Leg Strength—Women

1-Repetition Maximum Leg Press

Leg Press Weight Ratio $= \dfrac{\text{Weight Pushed}}{\text{Body Weight}}$

%	<20	20–29	30–39	40–49	50–59	60+	
99	>1.88	>1.98	>1.68	>1.57	>1.43	>1.43	S
95	1.88	1.98	1.68	1.57	1.43	1.43	
90	1.85	1.82	1.61	1.48	1.37	1.32	
85	1.81	1.76	1.52	1.40	1.31	1.32	
80	1.71	1.68	1.47	1.37	1.25	1.18	E
75	1.69	1.65	1.42	1.33	1.20	1.16	
70	1.65	1.58	1.39	1.29	1.17	1.13	
65	1.62	1.53	1.36	1.27	1.12	1.08	
60	1.59	1.50	1.33	1.23	1.10	1.04	G
55	1.51	1.47	1.31	1.20	1.08	1.01	
50	1.45	1.44	1.27	1.18	1.05	.99	
45	1.42	1.40	1.24	1.15	1.02	.97	
40	1.38	1.37	1.21	1.13	.99	.93	F
35	1.33	1.32	1.18	1.11	.97	.90	
30	1.29	1.27	1.15	1.08	.95	.88	
25	1.25	1.26	1.12	1.06	.92	.86	
20	1.22	1.22	1.09	1.02	.88	.85	P
15	1.19	1.18	1.05	.97	.84	.80	
10	1.09	1.14	1.00	.94	.78	.72	
5	1.06	.99	.96	.85	.72	.63	VP
1	<1.06	<.99	<.96	<.85	<.72	<.63	
n =	20	192	281	337	192	44	

Total n = 1166; S, superior; E, excellent; G, good; F, fair; P, poor; VP, very poor.

Instructions:

1. Have your client warm up by completing 5–10 repetitions of the exercise at 40–60% of the estimated 1-RM.

2. During a 1-minute rest, have the client stretch the muscle group. This is followed by 3–5 repetitions of the exercise at 60–80% of the estimated 1-RM.

3. Then increase the weight conservatively and have the client attempt the 1-RM lift. If the lift is successful, the client should rest 3–5 minutes before attempting the next weight increment. Follow this procedure until the client fails to complete the lift. The 1-RM typically is achieved within three to five trials.

4. Record the 1-RM value as the maximum weight lifted for the last successful trial.

Source (Tables 37a and b): Data provided by the Institute for Aerobics Research, Dallas, TX, 1994. Reprinted with permission from the Cooper Institute for Aerobics Research, Dallas, TX.

TABLE 38 YMCA Endurance Bench-Press Test—Total Lifts

Age (yr)	18–25		26–35		36–45		46–55		56–65		>65	
Gender	M	F	M	F	M	F	M	F	M	F	M	F
Excellent	44–64	42–66	41–61	40–62	36–55	33–57	28–47	29–50	24–41	24–42	20–36	18–30
Good	34–41	30–38	30–37	29–34	26–32	26–30	21–25	20–24	17–21	17–21	12–16	12–16
Above average	29–33	25–28	26–29	24–28	22–25	21–24	16–20	14–18	12–14	12–14	10	8–10
Average	24–28	20–22	21–24	18–22	18–21	16–20	12–14	10–13	9–11	8–10	7–8	5–7
Below average	20–22	16–18	17–20	14–17	14–17	12–14	9–11	7–9	5–8	5–6	4–6	3–4
Poor	13–17	9–13	12–16	9–13	9–12	6–10	5–8	2–6	2–4	2–4	2–3	0–2
Very poor	0–10	0–6	0–9	0–6	0–6	0–4	0–2	0–1	0–1	0–1	0–1	0

Note: See Chapter 6 for instructions. Women use a 35-pound bar; men, 80 pounds. Maximum repetitions in time to metronome at 30 lifts per minute.

Source: Adapted from YMCA. *Y'S Way to Fitness*, 4th ed., 1998. Reprinted with permission from the YMCA of the USA.

TABLE 39 Pull-Ups

Classification	Number of Pull-Ups
Excellent	15+
Good	12–14
Average	8–11
Fair	5–7
Poor	0–4

Note: See Chapter 6 for instructions. Norms are for college men.

Source: Johnson BL, Nelson JK. *Practical Measurement for Evaluation in Physical Education.* Minneapolis: Burgess Publishing Co., 1979. Reprinted with permission.

TABLE 40 Parallel Bar Dips

Classification	Number of Bar Dips
Excellent	25+
Good	18–24
Average	9–17
Fair	4–8
Poor	0–3

Note: See Chapter 6 for instructions.

Source: Adapted from Johnson BL, Nelson JK. *Practical Measurement for Evaluation in Physical Education.* Minneapolis; Burgess Publishing Co., 1979. Reprinted with permission from Burgess Publishing, 7110 Ohms Lane, Edina, MN 55435.

Addresses of Professional Organizations and Equipment Suppliers

ADDRESSES OF PROFESSIONAL ORGANIZATIONS

Major organizations with an emphasis in sports medicine include:

Aerobics and Fitness Association of America (AFAA)
15250 Ventura Blvd., Suite 310
Sherman Oaks, CA 91403
818-905-0040

Amateur Athletic Union of the United States (AAU)
AAU House
Box 68207
Indianapolis, IN 46268
317-872-2900

American Alliance for Health, Physical Education, Recreation and Dance (AAHPERD)
1900 Association Dr.
Reston, VA 22091
703-476-3400

American Athletic Trainers Association (AATA)
660 W. Duarte Rd.
Arcadia, CA 91006
818-445-1978

American College of Sports Medicine (ACSM)
Box 1440
Indianapolis, IN 46206-1440
317-637-9200

American Council on Exercise (ACE)
5820 Oberlin Dr., Suite 102
San Diego, CA 92121
619-535-8227

American Dietetic Association (ADA)
Practice Group of Sports and Cardiovascular Nutritionists (SCAN)
216 W. Jackson Blvd.
Chicago, IL 60606-6995
312-899-0040

American Medical Athletic Association (AMAA)
4405 East West Hwy., Suite 405
Bethesda, MD 20814
301-913-9517

American Orthopedic Society for Sports Medicine (AOSSM)
6300 N. River Rd., Suite 200
Rosemont, IL 60018
708-292-4900

Canadian Society for Exercise Physiology
1600 James Naismith Dr.
Gloucester, Ontario, Canada K1B 5N4
613-748-5763

Cooper Institute for Aerobics Research (CIAR)
12330 Preston Rd.
Dallas, TX 75230
214-701-8001

International Association of Fitness Professionals (IDEA)
6190 Cornerstone Court East, Suite 204
San Diego, CA 92121
619-535-8979

IRSA, The Association of Quality Clubs
253 Summer St.
Boston, MA 02110
800-228-IRSA

National Strength and Conditioning Association
530 Communications Circle, Suite 204
Colorado Springs, CO 80905

President's Council on Physical Fitness and Sports
(PCPFS)
701 Pennsylvania Ave., NW, Suite 250
Washington, DC 20004
202-272-3421

YMCA of the USA
101 N. Wacker Dr.
Chicago, IL 60606
312-977-0031

Note: Each year, the *Physician and Sportsmedicine* journal publishes
a "Sports Medicine Directory." Contact the Physician and Sports-
medicine, Centers Project, 4530 W. 77th St., Minneapolis, 55435,
for information.

ADDRESSES OF EQUIPMENT SUPPLIERS

Aerobics, Inc.
385 Main St.
Little Falls, NJ 07424
201-256-9700
treadmills

Cambridge Scientific Industries
Moose Lodge Rd., PO Box 265
Cambridge, MA 21613
800-638-9566
skinfold calipers, testing equipment

Concept II
RR1 Box 1100-A70
Morrisville, VT 05661
800-245-5676
rowing machines

County Technology, Inc.
PO Box 87
Gays Mills, WI 54631
608-735-4718
all types of testing equipment

Creative Health Products
5148 Saddle Ridge Rd.
Plymouth, MI 48170
800-742-4478
all types of testing equipment

Cybex
2100 Smithtown
Ronkonkoma, NY 11779-0903
516-585-9000
all types of testing equipment

Detecto Scale Company
333 N. Broadway, Suite 2006
Jericho, NY 11753
800-641-2008
weight scales

Futrex, Inc.
6 Montgomery Village Ave., Suite 620
Gaithersburg, MD 20879-3546
800-255-4206
fat-testing equipment

Heart Rate, Inc.
3188 Airway Ave.
Costa Mesa, CA 92626
714-850-9716
stair climber

Lafayette Instrument Co.
PO Box 5729
Lafayette, IN 47903
317-423-1505
skinfold calipers, fitness measuring equipment

Monark
948 Green Bay Rd.
Winnetka, IL 60093-1720
800-359-4609
cycles, rowers, ergometers

NordicTrack
104 Peavey Rd.
Chaska, MN 55318
800-468-4429
NordicTrack ski simulator, treadmills, weight-lifting
systems

Paramount Fitness Equipment Corp.
6450 E. Bandini Blvd.
Los Angeles, CA 90040
800-721-2121
weight training equipment, exercise bicycles and
treadmills

Polar Electro, Inc.
99 Seaview Blvd.
Port Washington, NY 11050
800-227-1314
heart rate meters

Precor Co.
20001 N. Creek Pkwy.
PO Box 3004
Bothell, WA 98041
206-486-9292
treadmills, bikes, rowers, ski simulator

Quinton Instrument Co.
3303 Monte Villa Pkwy.
Bothell, WA 98021-8972
800-426-0337
treadmills, bicycles, testing equipment, metabolic cart

Southwood Corp.
PO Box 410888
Charlotte, NC 28241-0888
800-627-6884
exercise and fitness outdoor trails

StairMaster Sports/Medical Products
12421 Willows Rd., NE, Suite 100
Kirkland, WA 98034
800-635-2936
stair climbing machines, cycles

TANITA Corp.
5200 Church St.
Skokie, IL 60077-1125
800-826-4828
bioelectrical impedance scales

Tectrix Fitness Equipment
68 Fairbanks
Irvine, CA 92718
800-767-8082
climbing machines

Trackmaster Treadmills
4300 Bayou Blvd., #36
Pensacola, FL 32503-2671
800-965-6455
treadmills

Trotter
10 Trotter Dr.
Medway, MA 02053-2275
800-677-6544
treadmills

Universal Gym Equipment, Inc.
515 N. Flagler Dr.
4th Floor Pavilion
West Palm Beach, FL 33401
800-843-3906
treadmills, cycles, weight-lifting equipment, rowers

Vacumed
4483 McGrath St., #102
Ventura, CA 93003
800-235-3333
metabolic cart, hydrostatic weighing equipment,
respiratory testing supplies

Valhalla Scientific, Inc.
7576 Trade St.
San Diego, CA 92121
800-395-4565
bioelectric impedance instrument

Wellsource, Inc.
15431 S.E. 82nd Dr., Suite D
PO Box 569
Clackamas, OR 97015
800-533-9355
computer software

Source: Fitness Management. A complete sourcebook for products and services can be obtained by writing to

Fitness Management
3923 W. 6th Street
Los Angeles, CA 90020
213-385-3926
http://www.fitnessworld.com

Calisthenics for Development of Flexibility and Muscular Strength and Endurance

FLEXIBILITY EXERCISES

The key to developing good flexibility is to hold each of the following positions just short of pain for 15–30 seconds. *Relax* totally, letting your muscles slowly go limp as the tension of the stretched muscle area slowly subsides. After the tension has subsided, it is a good idea to stretch just a bit farther to better develop your flexibility (hold this "developmental stretch" also for 15–30 seconds). Be sure that you do not stretch to the point of pain, for flexibility cannot be developed while the stretched muscle is in pain.

Flexibility exercises should be conducted *following* the aerobic phase. Research has shown that stretching is safer and more effective when done with warm muscles and joints. You can stretch farther without injury more often following stimulating aerobics than before.

Do not be worried if you seem "tighter" than other people in many of the following stretches. Flexibility is an individual matter, and each person should "make the most" of what she or he has, realizing there are genetic differences.

Flexibility 1

Lower Back–Hamstring Rope Stretch

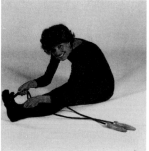

Start by sitting on the floor, one leg straight, the other relaxed off to the side (some people like the other leg bent at a 90° angle, foot against the other leg, some like it straight off to the side a bit, others slightly bent and loose). The rope should be doubled over the heel. (This exercise can also be done with both legs at one time.)

Stretch by reaching down the rope toward your foot with both hands until you feel a good tension in the back of your leg (some feel tension in the lower back also). Relax, breathe easily, letting the tension slowly subside, then reach a bit farther, holding this for 15–30 seconds also. Repeat with the other leg.

Benefits: This is perhaps the best stretch for the lower back and hamstrings (muscles on the back of your thigh). Your goal is to slowly work toward your foot as the weeks pass until you can at least hold onto your foot with one hand.

Flexibility 2

Calf Rope Stretch

Start just the same as for the lower back–hamstring rope stretch, but put the rope on the ball of your foot.

Stretch by pulling your upper foot (easy does it) toward your body until you feel a good tension in the top of your calf muscle. Relax and hold this position for 15–30 seconds, then reach a bit farther down the rope for a second 15- to 30-second stretch. Repeat with the other leg.

Benefits: Stretches the calf muscle.

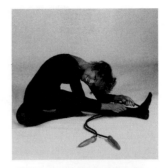

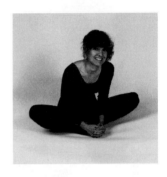

Flexibility 3

Groin Stretch

Start by sitting on the floor with the soles of your feet together, legs bent, knees up and out.

Stretch by pulling your feet with your hands to within a few inches of your crotch. Hold this position as you lean forward from the waist, keeping your chin up, and knees down as far as possible. Feel a good tension in the groin area, and hold. Be careful that you do not overstretch.

Benefits: Stretches the muscles in the groin area.

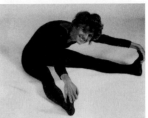

Flexibility 4

Quad Stretch

Start by lying on your right side, right hand supporting your head.

Stretch by bending your left leg, pulling the heel to your seat with the left hand grasping the ankle. Slowly move the entire left leg somewhat behind you until there is a good tension in front of the thigh, and hold. Repeat with the other leg.

Benefits: The muscles of the front of the thigh (quadriceps) are stretched in this exercise.

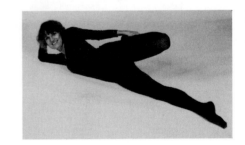

Flexibility 5

Spinal Twist

Start by sitting with your left leg straight out in front of you, your right leg bent, right foot crossed over the left knee.

Stretch by placing your left elbow on the outside of your right knee, pushing the right knee inward. At the same time, place your right hand on the ground behind you, and twist looking over your right shoulder. Keep pushing with your left elbow

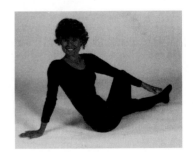

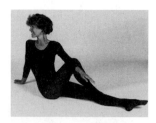

and twisting with your head over your right shoulder until you feel a good tension along your spine and hip, and hold for 15–30 seconds. Repeat on the other side.

Benefits: Stretches the muscles along the spine and side of the hips. Some people find this a hard stretch to coordinate. You may have to practice carefully with the pictures until you get used to all the important details.

Flexibility 6

Downward Dog

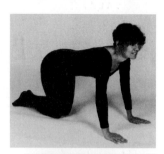

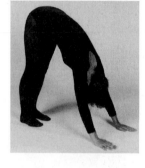

Start by getting on hands and knees.

Stretch by humping your seat straight up, with legs straight. Walk in with your hands toward your feet until your hands and feet are about 3 feet apart. Then try to keep your heels on the ground as you lean somewhat backward, keeping your legs straight, hands on the floor, and head down. You should feel a good tension all along your posterior leg. Hold for 15–30 seconds until the tension slowly subsides. The key is to keep the heels on the ground, but be careful not to hold a painful position, as this could injure your legs.

Benefits: This is an excellent stretch for the hamstrings and calves of your legs, as well as the lower back. Running tends to tighten the posterior leg muscles, and this exercise helps to counter this.

Flexibility 7

Upper-Body Stretch

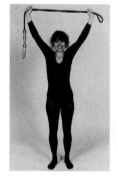

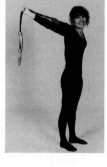

Start by grasping a rope or towel with your hands 2–4 feet apart.

Stretch by keeping your arms perfectly straight and slowly circling them up and behind you. Move slowly, feeling the tension in the front of your chest and shoulders. If you cannot keep your arms straight, or if the pain is too intense, put your hands farther apart. Repeat several times.

Benefits: Running tends to tighten the muscles in the front of the chest. This exercise helps to stretch those muscles, improving your posture.

Flexibility 8

Standing Side Stretch

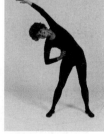

Start by standing with your feet 3 feet apart, hands on your hips.

Stretch by raising your right hand up and over your head as you lean way over to the left side. Keep your legs straight and lean straight to the side. Hold the position, feeling the stretch along your right side and inner left thigh. Repeat with the other side. If you do not feel a stretch in your thighs, put your feet farther apart.

Benefits: This exercise stretches the muscles along both sides and inner thighs.

MUSCLE ENDURANCE AND STRENGTH EXERCISES

The following exercises localize movement to specific muscle groups, developing the strength and muscle endurance in each of these areas. Do 5–15 reps of each (remembering that a rep = one–one, two, three; two–one, two, three; etc.).

Abdomen 1

Bent-Knee Sit-Ups

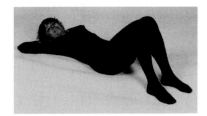

Start by lying on the ground, knees bent at a 90° angle. Most people need to tuck their feet under either another person or an object. If you are in good shape, you can put your hands behind your head. If your abdominal muscles are not in good shape, you can put your arms straight out in front of you (and even pull on your knees if you need to).

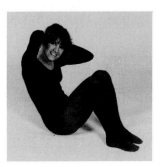

1. Sit up by flexing your abdominal muscles, and touch your elbows to your knees. If you need to, keep your arms out in front of you.
2. Lie back down, keeping your knees bent.

   Repeat.

Continue for 10–20 total sit-ups.

Benefits: The bent-knee sit-up is an excellent exercise for toning up the abdominal muscles. The knees are bent so that the strong hip flexors will have minimal action, allowing the abdominal muscles to act.

Abdomen 2

Ab-Curl Twisters

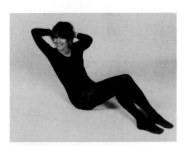

Start in the same basic position as the sit-up, except that you should have your torso two thirds the way up toward your knees.

1. Keeping your body in a two-thirds sit-up position, twist to your left.
2. Next twist to your right.

   Keep twisting back and forth, right and left, while leaning back, feeling a good tension in your abdominal area. If the movement becomes too hard, move closer to your knees.

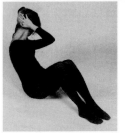

Continue for 5–10 full repetitions.

Benefits: The sides of the abdomen are given a great workout, as well as the middle abdominal muscles.

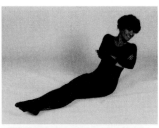

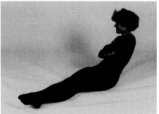

Abdomen 3

Straight-Leg Ab-Twisters

Start by sitting with your legs together, straight out in front of you, arms crossed over your chest.

1. Lean back at least one third of the way to the floor, hold this position throughout, and twist to the left, looking to the ground on the left side.
2. Next do the same to the right side.

Repeat, twisting left and right while leaning back, legs straight.

Continue for 5–10 repetitions.
   Benefits: This exercise also gives the sides of the abdomen a good workout while developing the muscle endurance of the middle abdominals as well.

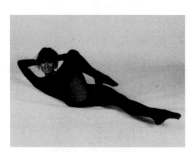

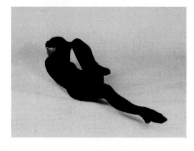

Abdomen 4

Steam Engine

Start by lying on your back, hands behind the head. Then lift the head off the ground and touch your left elbow to your right knee. The right leg is bent, foot off the ground, while the left leg is straight, off the ground as well.

1. While maintaining the basic starting position, twist your torso to the left while bending the left leg and straightening the right leg. Touch in one smooth movement your right elbow to your left knee.
2. Return to the starting position, twisting your torso to the right.

Repeat, twisting right and left, touching the elbow on each side to the knee of the opposite bent leg. The alternating leg should be straight and off the ground.

Continue for 5–20 repetitions.
   Benefits: This is probably the best abdominal exercise because the entire abdominal area is given a great workout. The abdominal muscles are best developed when the trunk is curled and twisted, as here.

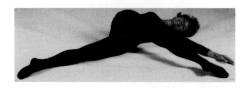

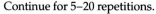

Abdomen 5

Wringer

Start by lying on the ground, legs straight and together, but arms straight and out to the sides.

1. Lift your leg up and over to your outstretched right hand. Try to keep your leg straight, plus keep your left shoulder as close to the ground as possible.
2. Return your left leg to the starting position.

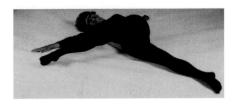

3. Repeat with your right leg, once again lifting it up and over to your left hand, which is straight out perpendicular from your body.

4. Return your right leg to the starting position.

Continue for 10–15 full repetitions.

Benefits: This exercise will not only develop the muscular endurance of the hip flexors and abdominal muscles, but also stretch the muscles along the sides of the body.

Abdomen 6

Gut Tucks

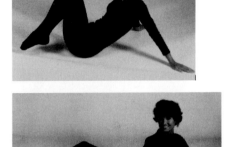

Start by sitting in a tuck position, with your legs drawn up close to your body and hands on the floor slightly behind you for balance and support.

1. Lift your feet several inches off the ground as you straighten your legs half-way. It is important not to straighten the legs all the way because this places too great a strain on the lower back.

2. Return your legs to the tuck position, with your legs drawn up close to your body, and hands on the floor slightly behind you for balance and support.

Repeat, half straightening your legs and then tucking them back in, keeping the feet off the ground as you support yourself with your hands, leaning back slightly.

Continue for 5–10 repetitions.

Benefits: This is an excellent abdominal exercise, firming up the muscles in the lower abdominal area especially.

Abdomen 7

Half-Pike Sit-Ups

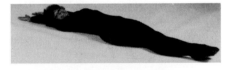

Start by lying on the ground on your back, body fully stretched out, legs together, and arms together over your head.

1. Lift your right leg up straight off the floor while lifting your arms, head, and shoulders up until you can touch your hands to your ankle or foot.

2. Return to the starting position.

3 & 4. Repeat with your left leg.

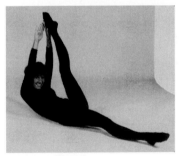

Continue for 10 repetitions.

Benefits: The hip flexors are given a good workout, while the abdominals are developed to a lesser extent because there is little abdominal curling going on.

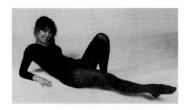

Abdomen 8

Single Leg Lifts

Start by supporting yourself on your elbows and seat, with your left leg bent, right leg straight.

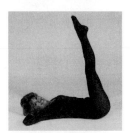

1. Lift your right leg, keeping it straight, up off the ground as high as you can.
2. Return your right leg to the starting position, but keep it several inches off the ground.

Repeat for 5–10 repetitions, then do the same with your left leg.

Continue lifting the straight leg up and down while keeping the other leg bent, supporting yourself with your elbows. It is important to stay in this position to prevent lower-back strain from lifting the straight leg.

Benefits: This exercise is especially good for the hip flexors, and secondarily for lower abdominal muscles.

Abdomen 9

Extended Leg Sit-Ups

Start by lying on your back, legs straight up in a "pike" position, with your hands joined together behind your head, elbows out.

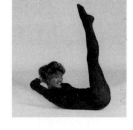

1. Lift your head, arms, and shoulders up as high as you can off the ground, making sure to keep the elbows out.
2. Return to the starting position.

Repeat, curling your upper body up and then down while keeping the legs straight up off the ground.

Continue for 5–10 repetitions.

Benefits: This is one of the best abdominal exercises you can do to develop a "flat tummy." The hip flexors are not involved because of the straight-leg-pike position which forces the abdominal muscles to curl your head and shoulders up.

Abdomen 10

Rowing

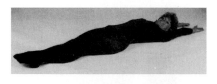

Start by lying on your back, arms and legs fully stretched and together.

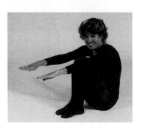

1. Draw your legs up to your body in a tuck position as you lift your upper body forward, reaching past your bent knees with your straight arms.
2. Return to the starting position.

Repeat, tucking your body into a tight ball, then returning to the starting position.

Continue for 5–10 repetitions.

Benefits: This is another excellent exercise for the abdominals and hip flexors. The tighter the ball you draw yourself into, the better.

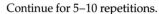

Arms–Shoulders 1

Push-Ups

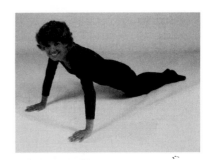

Start by supporting yourself on your knees and hands. It is important that your back be straight, seat not humped up. Your shoulders should be over your hands, arms straight. You should feel that you are supporting a good part of your weight on your hands. *Note:* If you are strong enough, support yourself between your feet and hands, keeping the trunk of your body perfectly straight and rigid. This can strain the lower back, so be certain that you possess sufficient strength.

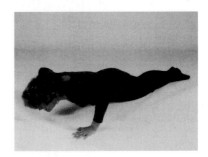

1. Lower yourself down to within a few inches off the ground, keeping your back rigid and straight, weight equally distributed between knees and hands.
2. Straighten your arms up, once again keeping the back rigid and straight. Avoid sagging or humping.

Repeat, lowering your body down and then pushing up, while the trunk is straight, and weight well felt on your arms and hands.

Continue for 5–15 repetitions (10–30 single push-ups).
Benefits: This exercise develops muscular strength and endurance of the muscles of the front of the chest (pectorals) and back of the upper arm (triceps). The muscles of the trunk are also developed as the body is kept in a straight and rigid position throughout the exercise.

Arms–Shoulders 2

Sitting Hand Pull Raises

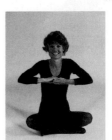

Start by sitting with your legs crossed, hands clasped together in the "Indian grip" (fingers hooked, hands opposite). Elbows should be out.

1. Pull hands apart, keeping them together with hooked fingers as you lift your hands and arms above your head. Keep pulling the hands hard the entire time.
2. Return the hands and arms to the starting position, still pulling hard.

Repeat, lifting the hands up and down as you try to pull them apart.

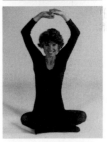

Continue for 5–10 repetitions.
Benefits: This calisthenic especially develops the muscles between the shoulder blades, the rhomboids. The muscles of the upper back and neck, the trapezius in particular, are also developed. The overall benefit is to improve back posture.

Arms–Shoulders 3

Isometric Rope Curls

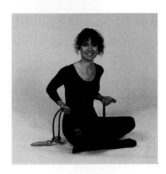

Start by sitting with legs crossed. Sit on top of your jumping rope and grasp the rope with both hands, palms up, arms at a 90° angle.

Forcefully lift up, contracting your arm muscles as tightly as possible. Hold for 5 seconds and then relax. *Isometric* means that there is muscle contraction without movement.

Repeat 3–5 times, contracting as forcefully as you can each time.

Benefits: This develops the biceps, the muscles on the front of your upper arms, plus other muscles of the forearm. This simple exercise will increase the strength of your arms.

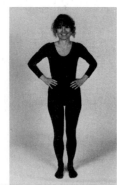

Hips–Thighs–Lower Back 1

Bear Hugs

Start by standing in a normal position, feet together.

1. Keeping your left foot in the same spot, step out straight to your right side, pointing your right foot in that direction. Reach out far enough so that your left leg remains straight, but your right leg is well bent. Wrap your arms around your right thigh as you finish stepping out to the right.

2. Return to the starting position.

3. & 4. Repeat with the left side.

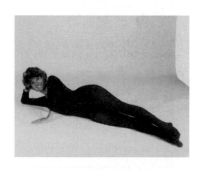

Continue stepping out to each side, hugging your thigh, and then returning back to the starting position. Be careful not to overdo the first several times, for this movement can cause quite a bit of soreness.

Continue for 5–10 repetitions.

Benefits: The hamstrings and gluteus maximus (back of upper thigh and buttock muscles) are well developed in this exercise. This exercise also develops the quadricep muscles in the front of your thigh.

Hips–Thighs–Lower Back 2

Lateral Leg Raises

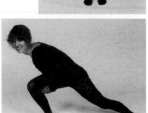

Start by lying on your right side, your head held propped up with your right hand, your left leg lying on top of your right leg.

1. Lift your left leg up as high as you can. Keep the leg straight.

2. Return the leg to the down position.

Repeat. Keep lifting the leg up, then down, concentrating on a full range of motion.

Repeat with the other leg.

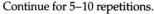

Continue for 5–10 repetitions.

Benefits: Develops the muscles on the side of your hip, the abductors. As the muscles here are developed, you will lose inches from your hip measurement.

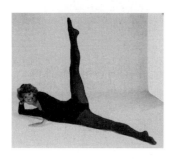

Hips–Thighs–Lower Back 3

Ballet Squats

Start by standing with your feet 3 feet apart, toes pointing out at a 45° angle. The arms should be straight, parallel to the ground, and out to the sides or angled forward.

1. Squat down until the thighs are parallel to the ground.
2. Straighten your legs only halfway. Do not stand all the way up, but keep the knees well bent.

Repeat, moving up and down between a half-squat and three-quarters squat position. The arms should be straight the entire time. The movement should be quick and almost bouncy.

Continue for 5–10 repetitions.
Benefits: The quadriceps, the muscles on the front of the thigh, are highly developed in this exercise. The buttock muscles also get a good workout.

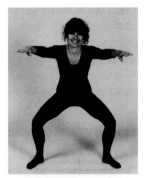
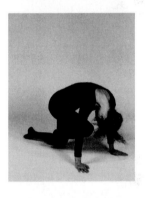

Hips–Thighs–Lower Back 4

Kneeling Leg Raises

Start by getting on hands and knees.

1. Lift your right leg slightly up and move it forward as you curl your head down, curling up the right side of your body. Your right knee should be close to your head.
2. Next lift your head up high as you also straighten and lift your right leg up high, arching your back.

Repeat, alternating curling and arching on one side of your body and then the other. Be careful not to strain your lower back by lifting your leg too high.

Continue for 5–10 repetitions.
Benefits: The major benefit is to the muscles of your back, especially near the neck and hip areas.

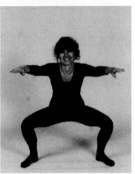
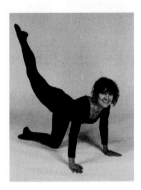

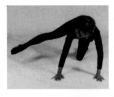
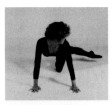

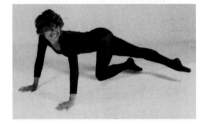

Hips–Thighs–Lower Back 5

Kneeling Leg Swings

Start by getting on hands and knees.

1. Straighten your right leg and swing it out to the side. Keep your leg straight, about 6–12 inches off the ground. Move your head and look right.

2. Next swing your right leg behind you and cross over to the left side as far as you can while looking left. Your leg should still be straight and off the ground 6–12 inches.

Repeat, swinging the leg back and forth, far to the right, and then crossing behind, while moving your head right, then left.

Repeat with the left leg.

Continue for 5–10 repetitions.

Benefits: This is an excellent exercise for developing the muscles along the sides of the abdomen and in the lower back. In addition, the muscles along the sides of the trunk are given a good stretch each time the head and leg curl to the opposite side.

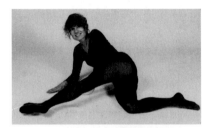

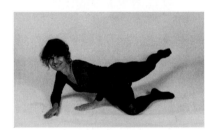

Hips–Thighs–Lower Back 6

Leg Pumps

Start by supporting yourself on your right side: right elbow, right hand, and bent right leg. Also put your left hand on the ground in front of you for support and balance. Your left leg should be straight, on top of the right.

1. Forcefully swing your straight left leg forward, keeping it several inches off the ground.

2. Next swing your leg way back behind you (keep it straight, off the ground several inches).

Repeat, swinging your leg forward and back over your bent right leg. Keep the top leg straight.

Repeat with the other leg.

Continue for 5–10 repetitions.

Benefits: This calisthenic develops the muscles on the side of the hip, the abductors, which will help to reduce the measurement of the hips. The muscles of the abdomen and lower back are also developed.

Hips–Thighs–Lower Back 7

Kneeling Bent-Leg Raises

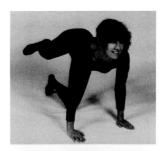

Start by supporting yourself on your hands and knees.

1. Lift your right leg, keeping it bent at a 90° angle, straight up to your side until it is parallel to the ground. Look at your leg with your head turned to the right side.

2. Return to the starting position.

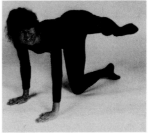

Repeat, raising the bent leg up while looking right, and then returning to the starting position.

Do the same on the left side.

Continue for 5 repetitions on each leg.
   Benefits: The muscles on the sides of the hips, the abductors, are developed in this exercise.

Hips–Thighs–Lower Back 8

Knee Leans

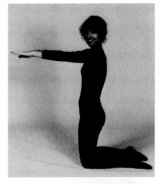

Start by kneeling, keeping your upper body straight, arms straight and reaching forward.

1. Keeping your body rigid and straight, lean back over your heels.

2. Return to the starting position.

Repeat, leaning back and then going forward, keeping the trunk rigid. To get the full effect, it is important that you do not bend at the waist. Be careful that you do not overdo the first several times, for these muscles can easily get sore with this movement.

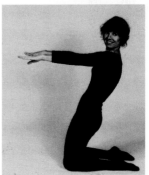

Continue for 5–10 repetitions.
   Benefits: This is an excellent exercise for developing the *quadricep muscles*, the big muscles on the front of your thighs.

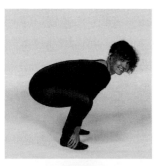

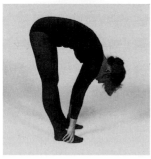

Hips–Thighs–Lower Back 9

Bent-over Squats

Start by squatting down, hands holding your feet (or if you are a stiff person, your ankles).

1. While holding your feet or ankles, straighten your legs so that your seat humps up above you. You should feel a good stretch as you straighten your legs.

2. Return to the starting position.

Repeat, straightening and bending the legs as you keep gripping your feet or ankles. Be careful that you do not overstretch. The movement should be slow and methodical.

Continue for 5–10 repetitions.

Benefits: This exercise does two things well—it develops the muscle endurance and strength of the quadricep muscles (front of the thigh), plus helps to stretch the muscles in the lower back and posterior leg.

Major Bones, Muscles, and Arteries of the Human Body

MAJOR BONES OF THE SKELETON

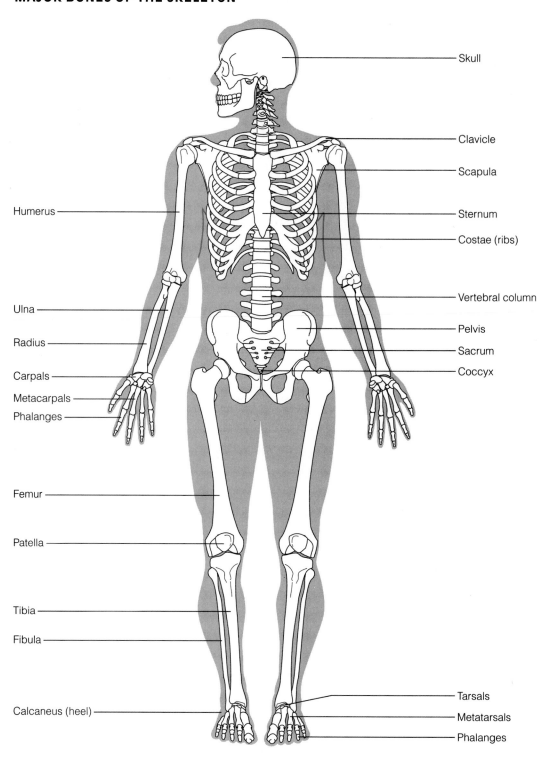

Skull

Clavicle

Scapula

Sternum

Costae (ribs)

Vertebral column

Pelvis

Sacrum

Coccyx

Humerus

Ulna

Radius

Carpals

Metacarpals

Phalanges

Femur

Patella

Tibia

Fibula

Calcaneus (heel)

Tarsals

Metatarsals

Phalanges

MAJOR MUSCLES OF THE BODY

(Anterior)

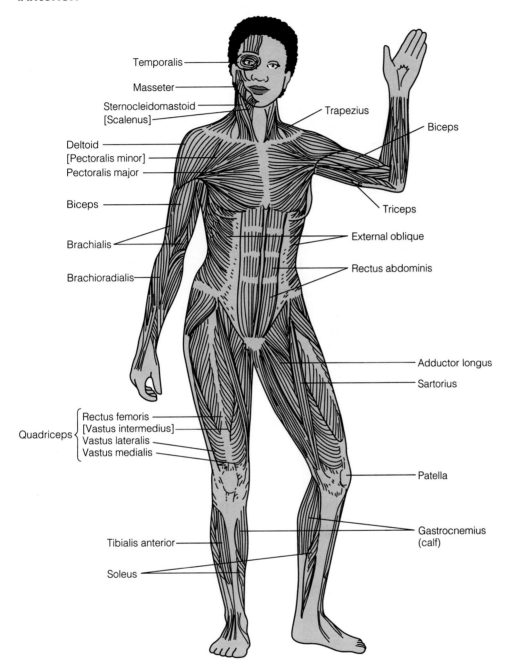

Temporalis

Masseter

Sternocleidomastoid
[Scalenus]

Trapezius

Biceps

Deltoid

[Pectoralis minor]

Pectoralis major

Triceps

Biceps

External oblique

Brachialis

Rectus abdominis

Brachioradialis

Adductor longus

Sartorius

Quadriceps
Rectus femoris
[Vastus intermedius]
Vastus lateralis
Vastus medialis

Patella

Gastrocnemius
(calf)

Tibialis anterior

Soleus

MAJOR MUSCLES OF THE BODY

(Posterior)

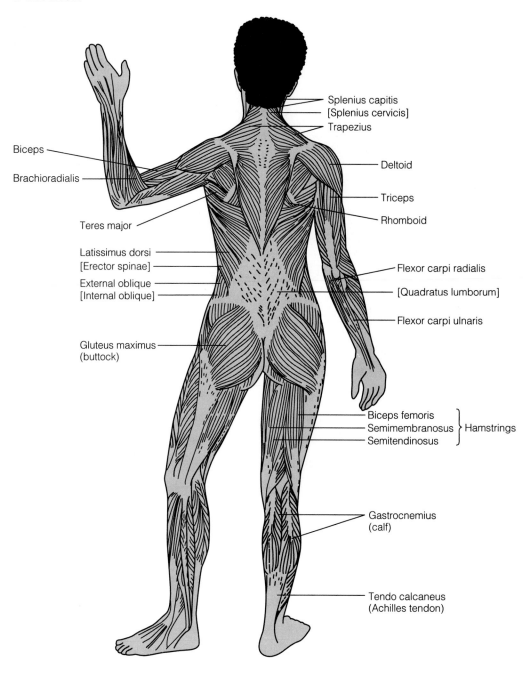

Splenius capitis
[Splenius cervicis]
Trapezius

Biceps

Brachioradialis

Deltoid

Triceps

Rhomboid

Teres major

Latissimus dorsi
[Erector spinae]
External oblique
[Internal oblique]

Flexor carpi radialis

[Quadratus lumborum]

Flexor carpi ulnaris

Gluteus maximus
(buttock)

Biceps femoris
Semimembranosus
Semitendinosus
} Hamstrings

Gastrocnemius
(calf)

Tendo calcaneus
(Achilles tendon)

MAJOR ARTERIES OF THE CIRCULATORY SYSTEM

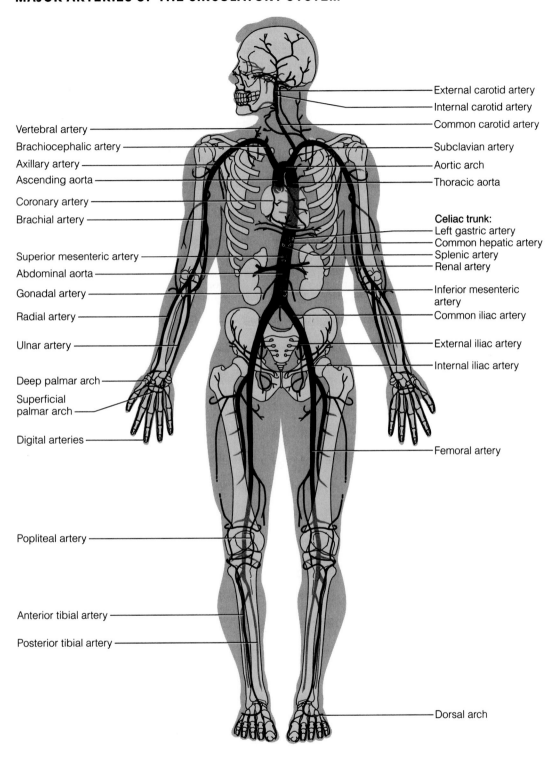

External carotid artery
Internal carotid artery
Common carotid artery
Subclavian artery
Aortic arch
Thoracic aorta

Celiac trunk:
Left gastric artery
Common hepatic artery
Splenic artery
Renal artery

Inferior mesenteric artery
Common iliac artery
External iliac artery
Internal iliac artery

Femoral artery

Dorsal arch

Vertebral artery
Brachiocephalic artery
Axillary artery
Ascending aorta
Coronary artery
Brachial artery

Superior mesenteric artery
Abdominal aorta
Gonadal artery
Radial artery
Ulnar artery

Deep palmar arch
Superficial palmar arch

Digital arteries

Popliteal artery

Anterior tibial artery
Posterior tibial artery

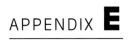
Compendium of Physical Activities

This "compendium of physical activities" was developed to provide researchers and practitioners with a comprehensive coding scheme and energy cost classification for a wide variety of human physical activities. MET values are listed beside the code number for each activity description. To determine energy cost in Calories per hour, multiply the MET value times the kilogram body weight of the individual. For example, bicycling at 14–15.9 mph (activity code #01040) demands 10 METs for a 70-kg individual, 700 Calories per hour.

Section 1. Codes and MET Values of Physical Activities

Code	MET		Physical Activities
01009	8.5	Bicycling,	Bicycling, BMX or mountain
01010	4.0	Bicycling,	Bicycling, <10 mph, general, leisure, to work or for pleasure (T 115)
01020	6.0	Bicycling,	Bicycling, 10–11.9 mph, leisure, slow, light effort
01030	8.0	Bicycling,	Bicycling, 12–13.9 mph, leisure, moderate effort
01040	10.0	Bicycling,	Bicycling, 14–15.9 mph, racing or leisure, fast, vigorous effort
01050	12.0	Bicycling,	Bicycling, 16–19 mph, racing/not drafting or >19 mph drafting, very fast, racing general
01060	16.0	Bicycling,	Bicycling, >20 mph, racing, not drafting
01070	5.0	Bicycling,	Unicycling
02010	5.0	Conditioning exercise,	Bicycling, stationary, general
02011	3.0	Conditioning exercise,	Bicycling, stationary, 50 W, very light effort
02012	5.5	Conditioning exercise,	Bicycling, stationary, 100 W, light effort

Code	MET		Physical Activities
02013	7.0	Conditioning exercise,	Bicycling, stationary, 150 W, moderate effort
02014	10.5	Conditioning exercise,	Bicycling, stationary, 200 W, vigorous effort
02015	12.5	Conditioning exercise,	Bicycling, stationary, 250 W, very vigorous effort
02020	8.0	Conditioning exercise,	Calisthenics (e.g., push-ups, pull-ups, sit-ups), heavy, vigorous effort
02030	4.5	Conditioning exercise,	Calisthenics, home exercise, light or moderate effort, general (T 150) (example: back exercises), going up & down from floor
02040	8.0	Conditioning exercise,	Circuit training, general
02050	6.0	Conditioning exercise,	Weight lifting (free weight, Nautilus or Universal-type), power lifting or bodybuilding, vigorous effort (T 210)
02060	5.5	Conditioning exercise,	Health club exercise, general (T 160)
02065	6.0	Conditioning exercise,	Stair-treadmill ergometer, general
02070	9.5	Conditioning exercise,	Rowing, stationary ergometer, general

Code	MET	Physical Activities	
02071	3.5	Conditioning exercise,	Rowing, stationary, 50 W, light effort
02072	7.0	Conditioning exercise,	Rowing, stationary, 100 W, moderate effort
02073	8.5	Conditioning exercise,	Rowing, stationary, 150 W, vigorous effort
02074	12.0	Conditioning exercise,	Rowing, stationary, 200 W, very vigorous effort
02080	9.5	Conditioning exercise,	Ski machine, general
02090	6.0	Conditioning exercise,	Slimnastics
02100	4.0	Conditioning exercise,	Stretching, hatha yoga
02110	6.0	Conditioning exercise,	Teaching aerobic exercise class
02120	4.0	Conditioning exercise,	Water aerobics, water calisthenics
02130	3.0	Conditioning exercise,	Weight lifting (free, Nautilus, or Universal-type), light or moderate effort, light workout, general
02135	1.0	Conditioning exercise,	Whirlpool, sitting
03010	6.0	Dancing,	Aerobic, ballet or modern, twist
03015	6.0	Dancing,	Aerobic, general
03020	5.0	Dancing,	Aerobic, low impact
03021	7.0	Dancing,	Aerobic, high impact
03025	4.5	Dancing,	General
03030	5.5	Dancing,	Ballroom, fast, (disco, folk, square) (T 125)
03040	3.0	Dancing,	Ballroom, slow (e.g., waltz, foxtrot, slow dancing)
04001	4.0	Fishing and hunting,	Fishing, general
04010	4.0	Fishing and hunting,	Digging worms, with shovel
04020	5.0	Fishing and hunting,	Fishing from river bank and walking
04030	2.5	Fishing and hunting,	Fishing from boat, sitting
04040	3.5	Fishing and hunting,	Fishing from river bank, standing (T 660)
04050	6.0	Fishing and hunting,	Fishing in stream, in waders (T 670)
04060	2.0	Fishing and hunting,	Fishing, ice, sitting
04070	2.5	Fishing and hunting,	Hunting, bow and arrow or crossbow
04080	6.0	Fishing and hunting,	Hunting, deer, elk, large game (T 710)
04090	2.5	Fishing and hunting,	Hunting, duck, wading
04100	5.0	Fishing and hunting,	Hunting, general
04110	6.0	Fishing and hunting,	Hunting, pheasants or grouse (T 680)
04120	5.0	Fishing and hunting,	Hunting, rabbit, squirrel, prairie chick, raccoon, small game (T 690)
04130	2.5	Fishing and hunting,	Pistol shooting or trap shooting, standing
05010	2.5	Home activities,	Carpet sweeping, sweeping floors
05020	4.5	Home activities,	Cleaning, heavy or major (e.g., wash car, wash windows, mop, clean garage), vigorous effort
05030	3.5	Home activities,	Cleaning, house or cabin, general
05040	2.5	Home activities,	Cleaning, light (dusting, straightening up, vacuuming, changing linen, carrying out trash), moderate effort
05041	2.3	Home activities,	Wash dishes—standing or in general (not broken into stand/walk components)
	2.3	Home activities,	Wash dishes; clearing dishes from table—walking
05050	2.5	Home activities,	Cooking or food preparation—standing or sitting or in general (not broken into stand/walk components)
05051	2.5	Home activities,	Serving food, setting table —implied walking or standing
05052	2.5	Home activities,	Cooking or food preparation—walking
05055	2.5	Home activities,	Putting away groceries (e.g., carrying groceries, shopping without a grocery cart)
05056	8.0	Home activities,	Carrying groceries upstairs
05060	3.5	Home activities,	Food shopping, with grocery cart
05065	2.0	Home activities,	Standing—shopping (non-grocery shopping)
05066	2.3	Home activities,	Walking—shopping (non-grocery shopping)
05070	2.3	Home activities,	Ironing
05080	1.5	Home activities,	Sitting, knitting, sewing, light wrapping (presents)
05090	2.0	Home activities,	Implied standing—laundry, fold or hang clothes, put clothes in washer or dryer, packing suitcase
05095	2.3	Home activities,	Implied walking—putting away clothes, gathering clothes to pack, putting away laundry
05100	2.0	Home activities,	Making bed
05110	5.0	Home activities,	Maple syruping/sugar bushing (including carrying buckets, carrying wood)
05120	6.0	Home activities,	Moving furniture, household
05130	5.5	Home activities,	Scrubbing floors, on hands and knees
05140	4.0	Home activities,	Sweeping garage, sidewalk, or outside of house
05145	7.0	Home activities,	Moving household items, carrying boxes

Code	MET		Physical Activities
05146	3.5	Home activities,	Standing—packing / unpacking boxes, occasional lifting of household items— light-moderate effort
05147	3.0	Home activities,	Implied walking—putting away household items— moderate effort
05150	9.0	Home activities,	Move household items upstairs, carrying boxes or furniture
05160	2.5	Home activities,	Standing—light (pump gas, change lightbulb, etc.)
05165	3.0	Home activities,	Walking—light, noncleaning (ready to leave, shut / lock doors, close windows, etc.)
05170	2.5	Home activities,	Sitting—playing with child(ren)—light
05171	2.8	Home activities,	Standing—playing with child(ren)—light
05175	4.0	Home activities,	Walk / run—playing with child(ren)—moderate
05180	5.0	Home activities,	Walk / run—playing with child(ren)—vigorous
05185	3.0	Home activities,	Childcaresitting / kneeling— dressing, bathing, grooming, feeding, occasional lifting of child—light effort
05186	3.5	Home activities,	Child care: standing— dressing, bathing, grooming, feeding, occasional lifting of child—light effort
06010	3.0	Home repair,	Airplane repair
06020	4.5	Home repair,	Automobile body work
06030	3.0	Home repair,	Automobile repair
06040	3.0	Home repair,	Carpentry, general, workshop (T 620)
06050	6.0	Home repair,	Carpentry, outside house (T 640), installing rain gutters
06060	4.5	Home repair,	Carpentry, finishing or refinishing cabinets or furniture
06070	7.5	Home repair,	Carpentry, sawing hardwood
06080	5.0	Home repair,	Caulking, chinking log cabin
06090	4.5	Home repair,	Caulking, except log cabin
06100	5.0	Home repair,	Cleaning gutters
06110	5.0	Home repair,	Excavating garage
06120	5.0	Home repair,	Hanging storm windows
06130	4.5	Home repair,	Laying or removing carpet
06140	4.5	Home repair,	Laying tile or linoleum
06150	5.0	Home repair,	Painting, outside house (T 650)
06160	4.5	Home repair,	Painting, papering, plastering, scraping, inside house, hanging sheet rock, remodeling (T 630)
06170	3.0	Home repair,	Put on and removal of tarp, sailboat
06180	6.0	Home repair,	Roofing
06190	4.5	Home repair,	Sanding floors with a power sander
06200	4.5	Home repair,	Scrape and paint sailboat or powerboat
06210	5.0	Home repair,	Spreading dirt with a shovel
06220	4.5	Home repair,	Wash and wax hull of sailboat, car, powerboat, airplane
06230	4.5	Home repair,	Washing fence
06240	3.0	Home repair,	Wiring, plumbing
07010	0.9	Inactivity, quiet	Lying quietly, reclining (watch television), lying quietly in bed—awake
07020	1.0	Inactivity, quiet	Sitting quietly (riding in a car, listening to a lecture or music, watch television or a movie)
07030	0.9	Inactivity, quiet	Sleeping
07040	1.2	Inactivity, quiet	Standing quietly (standing in a line)
07050	1.0	Inactivity, light	Recline—writing
07060	1.0	Inactivity, light	Reclining—talking or talking on phone
07070	1.0	Inactivity, light	Recline—reading
08010	5.0	Lawn and garden,	Carrying, loading or stacking wood, loading / unloading or carrying lumber
08020	6.0	Lawn and garden,	Chopping wood, splitting logs
08030	5.0	Lawn and garden,	Clearing land, hauling branches
08040	5.0	Lawn and garden,	Digging sandbox
08050	5.0	Lawn and garden,	Digging, spading, filling garden (T 590)
08060	6.0	Lawn and garden,	Gardening with heavy power tools, tilling a garden (see Occupation, shoveling)
08080	5.0	Lawn and garden,	Laying crushed rock
08090	5.0	Lawn and garden,	Laying sod
08095	5.5	Lawn and garden,	Mowing lawn, general
08100	2.5	Lawn and garden,	Mowing lawn, riding mower (T 550)
08110	6.0	Lawn and garden,	Mowing lawn, walk, hand mower (T 570)
08120	4.5	Lawn and garden,	Mowing lawn, walk, power mower (T 590)
08130	4.5	Lawn and garden,	Operating snow blower, walking
08140	4.0	Lawn and garden,	Planting seedlings, shrubs
08150	4.5	Lawn and garden,	Planting trees
08160	4.0	Lawn and garden,	Raking lawn (T 600)
08170	4.0	Lawn and garden,	Raking roof with snow rake
08180	3.0	Lawn and garden,	Riding snow blower

Code	MET	Physical Activities	
08190	4.0	Lawn and garden,	Sacking grass, leaves
08200	6.0	Lawn and garden,	Shoveling, snow, by hand (T 610)
08210	4.5	Lawn and garden,	Trimming shrubs or trees, manual cutter
08215	3.5	Lawn and garden,	Trimming shrubs or trees, power cutter
08220	2.5	Lawn and garden,	Walking, applying fertilizer or seeding a lawn
08230	1.5	Lawn and garden,	Watering lawn or garden, standing or walking
08240	4.5	Lawn and garden,	Weeding, cultivating garden (T 580)
08245	5.0	Lawn and garden,	Gardening, general
08250	3.0	Lawn and garden,	Implied walking/standing—picking up yard, light
09010	1.5	Miscellaneous,	Sitting, card playing, playing board games
09020	2.0	Miscellaneous,	Standing—drawing (writing), casino gambling
09030	1.3	Miscellaneous,	Sitting—reading, book, newspaper, etc.
09040	1.8	Miscellaneous,	Sitting—writing, desk work
09050	1.8	Miscellaneous,	Standing—talking or talking on the phone
09055	1.5	Miscellaneous,	Sitting—talking or talking on the phone
09060	1.8	Miscellaneous,	Sitting—studying, general, including reading, and/or writing
09065	1.8	Miscellaneous,	Sitting—in class, general, including note-taking or class discussion
09070	1.8	Miscellaneous,	Standing—reading
10010	1.8	Music playing,	Accordion
10020	2.0	Music playing,	Cello
10030	2.5	Music playing,	Conducting
10040	4.0	Music playing,	Drums
10050	2.0	Music playing,	Flute (sitting)
10060	2.0	Music playing,	Horn
10070	2.5	Music playing,	Piano or organ
10080	3.5	Music playing,	Trombone
10090	2.5	Music playing,	Trumpet
10100	2.5	Music playing,	Violin
10110	2.0	Music playing,	Woodwind
10120	2.0	Music playing,	Guitar, classical, folk (sitting)
10125	3.0	Music playing,	Guitar, rock and roll band (standing)
10130	4.0	Music playing,	Marching band, playing an instrument, baton twirling (walking)
10135	3.5	Music playing,	Marching band, drum major (walking)
11010	4.0	Occupation,	Bakery, general
11020	2.3	Occupation,	Bookbinding
11030	6.0	Occupation,	Building road (including hauling debris, driving heavy machinery)
11035	2.0	Occupation,	Building road, directing traffic (standing)
11040	3.5	Occupation,	Carpentry, general
11050	8.0	Occupation,	Carrying heavy loads, such as bricks
11060	8.0	Occupation,	Carrying moderate loads up stairs, moving boxes (16–40 pounds)
11070	2.5	Occupation,	Chambermaid
11080	6.5	Occupation,	Coal mining, drilling coal, rock
11090	6.5	Occcupation,	Coal mining, erecting supports
11100	6.0	Occupation,	Coal mining, general
11110	7.0	Occupation,	Coal mining, shoveling coal
11120	5.5	Occupation,	Construction, outside, remodeling
11130	3.5	Occupation,	Electrical work, plumbing
11140	8.0	Occupation,	Farming, baling hay, cleaning barn, poultry work
11150	3.5	Occupation,	Farming, chasing cattle, nonstrenuous
11160	2.5	Occupation,	Farming, driving harvester
11170	2.5	Occupation,	Farming, driving tractor
11180	4.0	Occupation,	Farming, feeding small animals
11190	4.5	Occupation,	Farming, feeding cattle
11200	8.0	Occupation,	Farming, forking straw bales
11210	3.0	Occupation,	Farming, milking by hand
11220	1.5	Occupation,	Farming, milking by machine
11230	5.5	Occupation,	Farming, shoveling grain
11240	12.0	Occupation,	Firefighter, general
11245	11.0	Occupation,	Firefighter, climbing ladder with full gear
11246	8.0	Occupation,	Firefighter, hauling hoses on ground
11250	17.0	Occupation,	Forestry, ax chopping, fast
11260	5.0	Occupation,	Forestry, ax chopping, slow
11270	7.0	Occupation,	Forestry, barking trees
11280	11.0	Occupation,	Forestry, carrying logs
11290	8.0	Occupation,	Forestry, felling trees
11300	8.0	Occupation,	Forestry, general
11310	5.0	Occupation,	Forestry, hoeing
11320	6.0	Occupation,	Forestry, planting by hand
11330	7.0	Occupation,	Forestry, sawing by hand
11340	4.5	Occupation,	Forestry, sawing, power
11350	9.0	Occupation,	Forestry, trimming trees
11360	4.0	Occupation,	Forestry, weeding
11370	4.5	Occupation,	Furriery
11380	6.0	Occupation,	Horse grooming

Code	MET		Physical Activities
11390	8.0	Occupation,	Horse racing, galloping
11400	6.5	Occupation,	Horse racing, trotting
11410	2.6	Occupation,	Horse racing, walking
11420	3.5	Occupation,	Locksmith
11430	2.5	Occupation,	Machine tooling, machining, working sheet metal
11440	3.0	Occupation,	Machine tooling, operating lathe
11450	5.0	Occupation,	Machine tooling, operating punch press
11460	4.0	Occupation,	Machine tooling, tapping and drilling
11470	3.0	Occupation,	Machine tooling, welding
11480	7.0	Occupation,	Masonry, concrete
11485	4.0	Occupation,	Masseur, masseuse (standing)
11490	7.0	Occupation,	Moving, pushing heavy objects, 75 lbs or more (desks, moving van work)
11500	2.5	Occupation,	Operating heavy duty equipment/automated, not driving
11510	4.5	Occupation,	Orange grove work
11520	2.3	Occupation,	Printing (standing)
11525	2.5	Occupation,	Police, directing traffic (standing)
11526	2.0	Occupation,	Police, driving a squad car (sitting)
11527	1.3	Occupation,	Police, riding in a squad car (sitting)
11528	8.0	Occupation,	Police, making an arrest (standing)
11530	2.5	Occupation,	Shoe repair, general
11540	8.5	Occupation,	Shoveling, digging ditches
11550	9.0	Occupation,	Shoveling, heavy (more than 16 lbs · min⁻¹)
11560	6.0	Occupation,	Shoveling, light (less than 10 lbs · min⁻¹)
11570	7.0	Occupation,	Shoveling, moderate (10–15 lbs · min⁻¹)
11580	1.5	Occupation	Sitting—light office work, in general (chemistry lab work, light use of hand-tools, watch repair or micro-assembly, light assembly/repair)
11585	1.5	Occupation,	Sitting—meetings, general, and/or with talking involved
11590	2.5	Occupation,	Sitting; moderate (heavy levers, riding mower/fork-lift, crane operation)
11600	2.5	Occupation,	Standing; light (bartending, store clerk, assembling, filing, xeroxing, put up Christmas tree)
11610	3.0	Occupation,	Standing; light/moderate (assemble/repair heavy parts, welding, stocking, auto repair, pack boxes for moving, etc.), patient care (as in nursing)
11620	3.5	Occupation,	Standing; moderate (assembling at fast rate, lifting 50 lbs, hitch/twisting ropes)
11630	4.0	Occupation,	Standing; moderate/heavy (lifting more than 50 lb, masonry, painting, paper hanging)
11640	5.0	Occupation,	Steel mill, fettling
11650	5.5	Occupation,	Steel mill, forging
11660	8.0	Occupation,	Steel mill, hand rolling
11670	8.0	Occupation,	Steel mill, merchant mill rolling
11680	11.0	Occupation,	Steel mill, removing slag
11690	7.5	Occupation,	Steel mill, tending furnace
11700	5.5	Occupation,	Steel mill, tipping molds
11710	8.0	Occupation,	Steel mill, working in general
11720	2.5	Occupation,	Tailoring, cutting
11730	2.5	Occupation,	Tailoring, general
11740	2.0	Occupation,	Tailoring, hand sewing
11750	2.5	Occupation,	Tailoring, machine sewing
11760	4.0	Occupation,	Tailoring, pressing
11766	6.5	Occupation,	Truck driving, loading and unloading truck (standing)
11770	1.5	Occupation,	Typing, electric, manual or computer
11780	6.0	Occupation,	Using heavy power tools such as pneumatic tools (jackhammers, drills, etc.)
11790	8.0	Occupation,	Using heavy tools (not power) such as shovel, pick, tunnel bar, spade
11791	2.0	Occupation,	Walking on job, less than 2.0 mph (in office or lab area), very slow
11792	3.5	Occupation,	Walking on job, 3.0 mph, in office, moderate speed, not carrying anything
11793	4.0	Occupation,	Walking on job, 3.5 mph, in office, brisk speed, not carrying anything
11795	3.0	Occupation,	Walking, 2.5 mph, slowly and carrying light objects less than 25 lbs
11800	4.0	Occupation,	Walking, 3.0 mph, moderately and carrying light objects less than 25 lbs
11810	4.5	Occupation,	Walking, 3.5 mph, briskly and carrying objects less than 25 lbs

Code	MET	Physical Activities	
11820	5.0	Occupation,	Walking or walk downstairs or standing, carrying objects about 25–49 lbs
11830	6.5	Occupation,	Walking or walk downstairs or standing, carrying objects about 50–74 lbs
11840	7.5	Occupation,	Walking or walk downstairs or standing, carrying objects about 75–99 lbs
11850	8.5	Occupation,	Walking or walk downstairs or standing, carrying objects about 100 lbs and over
11870	3.0	Occupation,	Working in scene shop, theater actor, backstage, employee
12010	6.0	Running,	Job/walk combination (jobbing component of less than 10 min) (T 180)
12020	7.0	Running,	Jogging, general
12030	8.0	Running,	Running, 5 mph (12 mile · mile⁻¹)
12040	9.0	Running,	Running, 5.2 mph (11.5 min · mile⁻¹)
12050	10.0	Running,	Running, 6 mph (10 min · mile⁻¹)
12060	11.0	Running,	Running, 6.7 mph (9 min · mile⁻¹)
12070	11.5	Running,	Running, 7 mph (8.5 min · mile⁻¹)
12080	12.5	Running,	Running, 7.5 mph (8 min · mile⁻¹)
12090	13.5	Running,	Running, 8 mph (7.5 min · mile⁻¹)
12100	14.0	Running,	Running, 8.6 mph (7 min · mile⁻¹)
12110	15.0	Running;	Running, 9 mph (6.5 min · mile⁻¹)
12120	16.0	Running,	Running, 10 mph (6 min · mile⁻¹)
12130	18.0	Running,	Running, 10.9 mph (5.5 min · mile⁻¹)
12140	9.0	Running,	Running, cross-country
12150	8.0	Running,	Running, general (T 200)
12160	8.0	Running,	Running, in place
12170	15.0	Running,	Running, stairs, up
12180	10.0	Running,	Running, on a track, team practice
12190	8.0	Running,	Running, training, pushing wheelchair, marathon wheeling
12195	3.0	Running,	Running, wheeling, general
13000	2.5	Self-care,	Standing—getting ready for bed, in general
13009	1.0	Self-care	Sitting on toilet
13010	2.0	Self-care,	Bathing (sitting)

Code	MET	Physical Activities	
13020	2.5	Self-care,	Dressing, undressing (standing or sitting)
13030	1.5	Self-care,	Eating (sitting)
13035	2.0	Self-care,	Talking and eating or eating only (standing)
13040	2.5	Self-care,	Sitting or standing—grooming (washing, shaving, brushing teeth, urinating, washing hands, put on make-up)
13050	4.0	Self-care,	Showering, toweling off (standing)
14010	1.5	Sexual activity,	Active, vigorous effort
14020	1.3	Sexual activity,	General, moderate effort
14030	1.0	Sexual activity,	Passive, light effort, kissing, hugging
15010	3.5	Sports,	Archery (nonhunting)
15020	7.0	Sports,	Badminton, competitive (T 450)
15030	4.5	Sports,	Badminton, social singles and doubles, general
15040	8.0	Sports,	Basketball, game (T 490)
15050	6.0	Sports,	Basketball, nongame, general (T 480)
15060	7.0	Sports,	Basketball, officiating (T 500)
15070	4.5	Sports,	Basketball, shooting baskets
15075	6.5	Sports,	Basketball, wheelchair
15080	2.5	Sports,	Billiards
15090	3.0	Sports,	Bowling (T 390)
15100	12.0	Sports,	Boxing, in ring, general
15110	6.0	sports,	Boxing, bunching bag
15120	9.0	Sports,	Boxing, sparring
15130	7.0	Sports,	Broomball
15135	5.0	Sports,	Children's games (hopscotch, 4-square, dodgeball, playground apparatus, t-ball, tetherball, marbles, jacks, arcade games)
15140	4.0	Sports,	Coaching: football, soccer, basketball, baseball, swimming, etc.
15150	5.0	Sports,	Cricket (batting, bowling)
15160	2.5	Sports,	Croquet
15170	4.0	Sports,	Curling
15180	2.5	Sports,	Darts, wall or lawn
15190	6.0	Sports,	Drag racing, pushing or driving a car
15200	6.0	Sports,	Fencing
15210	9.0	Sports,	Football, competitive
15230	8.0	Sports,	Football, touch, flag, general (T 510)
15235	2.5	Sports,	Football or baseball, playing catch
15240	3.0	Sports,	Frisbee playing, general

Code	MET		Physical Activities	Code	MET		Physical Activities
15250	3.5	Sports,	Frisbee, ultimate	15640	6.0	Sports,	Softball, pitching
15255	4.5	Sports,	Golf, general	15650	12.0	Sports,	Squash (T 530)
15260	5.5	Sports,	Golf, carrying clubs (T 090)	15660	4.0	Sports,	Table tennis, ping pong (T 410)
15270	3.0	Sports,	Golf, miniature, driving range	15670	4.0	Sports,	Tai chi
15280	5.0	Sports,	Golf, pulling clubs (T 080)	15675	7.0	Sports,	Tennis, general
15290	3.5	Sports,	Golf, using power cart (T 070)	15680	6.0	Sports,	Tennis, doubles (T 430)
				15690	8.0	Sports,	Tennis, singles (T 420)
15300	4.0	Sports,	Gymnastics, general	15700	3.5	Sports,	Trampoline
15310	4.0	Sports,	Hacky sack	15710	4.0	Sports,	Volleyball, competitive, in gymnasium (T 400)
15320	12.0	Sports,	Handball, general (T 520)				
15330	8.0	Sports,	Handball, team	15720	3.0	Sports,	Volleyball, noncompetitive; 6–9 member team, general
15340	3.5	Sports,	Hang gliding				
15350	8.0	Sports,	Hockey, field	15725	8.0	Sports,	Volleyball, beach
15360	8.0	Sports,	Hockey, ice	15730	6.0	Sports,	Wrestling (one match = 5 min)
15370	4.0	Sports,	Horseback riding, general				
15380	3.5	Sports,	Horseback riding, saddling horse	15731	7.0	Sports,	Wallyball, general
				16010	2.0	Transportation,	Automobile or light truck (not a semi) driving
15390	6.5	Sports,	Horseback riding, trotting				
15400	2.5	Sports,	Horseback riding, walking	16020	2.0	Transportation,	Flying airplane
15410	3.0	Sports,	Horseshoe pitching, quoits	16030	2.5	Transportation,	Motor scooter, motorcycle
15420	12.0	Sports,	Jai alai	16040	6.0	Transportation,	Pushing plane in and out of hangar
15430	10.0	Sports,	Judo, jujitsu, karate, kick boxing, tae kwan do				
				16050	3.0	Transportation,	Driving heavy truck, tractor, bus
15440	4.0	Sports,	Juggling				
15450	7.0	Sports,	Kickball	17010	7.0	Walking,	Backpacking, general (T 050)
15460	8.0	Sports,	Lacrosse				
15470	4.0	Sports,	Moto-cross	17020	3.5	Walking,	Carrying infant or 15-lb load (e.g., suitcase), level ground or downstairs
15480	9.0	Sports,	Orienteering				
15490	10.0	Sports,	Paddleball, competitive				
15500	6.0	Sports,	Paddleball, casual, general (T 460)	17025	9.0	Walking,	Carrying load upstairs, general
				17026	5.0	Walking,	Carrying 1- to 15-lb load, upstairs
15510	8.0	Sports,	Polo				
15520	10.0	Sports,	Racketball, competitive	17027	6.0	Walking,	Carrying 16- to 24-lb load, upstairs
15530	7.0	Sports,	Racketball, casual, general (T 470)				
				17028	8.0	Walking,	Carrying 25- to 49-lb load, upstairs
15535	11.0	Sports,	Rock climbing, ascending rock				
				17029	10.0	Walking,	Carrying 50- to 74-lb load, upstairs
15540	8.0	Sports,	Rock climbing, rapelling				
15550	12.0	Sports,	Rope jumping, fast	17030	12.0	Walking,	Carrying 74+-lb load, upstairs
15551	10.0	Sports,	Rope jumping, moderate, general				
				17035	7.0	Walking,	Climbing hills with 0- to 9-lb load
15552	8.0	Sports,	Rope jumping, slow				
15560	10.0	Sports,	Rugby	17040	7.5	Walking,	Climbing hills with 10- to 20-lb load
15570	3.0	Sports,	Shuffleboard, lawn bowling				
15580	5.0	Sports,	Skateboarding	17050	8.0	Walking,	Climbing hills with 21- to 42-lb load
15590	7.0	Sports,	Skating, roller (T 360)				
15600	3.5	Sports,	Sky diving	17060	9.0	Walking,	Climbing hills with 42+-lb load
15605	10.0	Sports,	Soccer, competitive				
15610	7.0	Sports,	Soccer, casual, general (T 540)	17070	3.0	Walking,	Downstairs
				17080	6.0	Walking,	Hiking, cross country (T 040)
15620	5.0	Sports,	Softball or baseball, fast or slow pitch, general (T 440)				
				17090	6.5	Walking,	Marching, rapidly, military
15630	4.0	Sports,	Softball, officiating	17100	2.5	Walking,	Pushing or pulling stroller with child

Code	MET		Physical Activities
17110	6.5	Walking,	Race walking
17120	8.0	Walking,	Rock or mountain climbing (T 060)
17130	8.0	Walking,	Up stairs, using or climbing up ladder (T 030)
17140	4.0	Walking,	Using crutches
17150	2.0	Walking,	Walking, less than 2.0 mph, level ground, strolling, household walking, very slow
17160	2.5	Walking,	Walking, 2.0 mph, level, slow pace, firm surface
17170	3.0	Walking,	Walking, 2.5 mph, firm surface
17180	3.0	Walking,	Walking, 2.5 mph, downhill
17190	3.5	Walking,	Walking, 3.0 mph, level, moderate pace, firm surface
17200	4.0	Walking,	Walking, 3.5 mph, level, brisk, firm surface
17210	6.0	Walking,	Walking, 3.5 mph, uphill
17220	4.0	Walking,	Walking, 4.0 mph, level, firm surface, very brisk pace
17230	4.5	Walking,	Walking, 4.5 mph, level, firm surface, very, very brisk
17250	3.5	Walking,	Walking, for pleasure, work break, walking the dog
17260	5.0	Walking,	Walking, grass track
17270	4.0	Walking,	Walking, to work or class (T 015)
18010	2.5	Water activities,	Boating, power
18020	4.0	Water activities,	Canoeing, on camping trip (T 270)
18030	7.0	Water activities,	Canoeing, portaging
18040	3.0	Water activities,	Canoeing, rowing, 2.0–3.9 mph, light effort
18050	7.0	Water activities,	Canoeing, rowing, 4.0–5.9 mph, moderate effort
18060	12.0	Water activities,	Canoeing, rowing, >6 mph, vigorous effort
18070	3.5	Water activities,	Canoeing, rowing, or pleasure, general (T 250)
18080	12.0	Water activities,	Canoeing, rowing, in competition, or crew or sculling (T 260)
18090	3.0	Water activities,	Diving, springboard or platform
18100	5.0	Water activities,	Kayaking
18110	4.0	Water activities,	Paddleboat
18120	3.0	Water activities,	Sailing, boat and board sailing, windsurfing, ice sailing, general (T 235)
18130	5.0	Water activities,	Sailing, in competition
18140	3.0	Water activities,	Sailing, Sunfish / Laser / Hoby Cat, keel boats, ocean sailing, yachting
18150	6.0	Water activities,	Skiing, water (T 220)
18160	7.0	Water activities,	Skimobiling
18170	12.0	Water activities,	Skindiving or scuba diving as frogman
18180	16.0	Water activities,	Skindiving, fast
18190	12.5	Water activities,	Skindiving, moderate
18200	7.0	Water activities,	Skindiving, scuba diving, general (T 310)
18210	5.0	Water activities,	Snorkeling (T 320)
18220	3.0	Water activities,	Surfing, body or board
18230	10.0	Water activities,	Swimming laps, freestyle, fast, vigorous effort
18240	8.0	Water activities,	Swimming laps, freestyle, slow, moderate or light effort
18250	8.0	Water activities,	Swimming, backstroke, general
18260	10.0	Water activities,	Swimming, breastroke, general
18270	11.0	Water activities,	Swimming, butterfly, general
18280	11.0	Water activities,	Swimming, crawl, fast (75 yards · min⁻¹), vigorous effort
18290	8.0	Water activities,	Swimming, crawl, slow (50 yards · min⁻¹), moderate or light effort
18300	6.0	Water activities,	Swimming, lake, ocean, river (T 280, T 295)
18310	6.0	Water activities,	Swimming, leisurely, not lap swimming, general
18320	8.0	Water activities,	Swimming, sidestroke, general
18330	8.0	Water activities,	Swimming, synchronized
18340	10.0	Water activities,	Swimming, treading water, fast vigorous effort
18350	4.0	Water activities,	Swimming, treading water, moderate effort, general
18360	10.0	Water activities,	Water polo
18365	3.0	Water activities,	Water volleyball
18370	5.0	Water activities,	Whitewater rafting, kayaking, or canoeing
19010	6.0	Winter activities,	Moving ice house (set up / drill holes, etc.
19020	5.5	Winter activities,	Skating, ice, 9 mph or less
19030	7.0	Winter activities,	Skating, ice, general (T 360)
19040	9.0	Winter activities,	Skating, ice, rapidly, more than 9 mph
19050	15.0	Winter activities,	Skating, speed, competitive
19060	7.0	Winter activities,	Ski jumping (climb up carrying skis)
19075	7.0	Winter activities,	Skiing, general
19080	7.0	Winter activities,	Skiing, cross-country, 2.5 mph, slow or light effort, ski walking
19090	8.0	Winter activities,	Skiing, cross-country, 4.0–4.9 mph, moderate speed and effort, general

Code	MET	Physical Activities	
19100	9.0	Winter activities,	Skiing, cross-country, 5.0–7.0 mph, brisk speed, vigorous effort
19110	14.0	Winter activities,	Skiing, cross-country, >8.0 mph, racing
19130	16.5	Winter activities,	Skiing, cross-country, hard snow, uphill, maximum
19150	5.0	Winter activities,	Skiing, downhill, light effort

Code	MET	Physical Activities	
19160	6.0	Winter activities,	Skiing, downhill, moderate effort, general
19170	8.0	Winter activities,	Skiing, downhill, vigorous effort, racing
19180	7.0	Winter activities,	Sledding, tobogganing, bobsledding, luge (T 370)
19190	8.0	Winter activities,	Snowshoeing
19200	3.5	Winter activities,	Snowmobiling

Section 2. Guidelines for Assigning Activities by Major Purpose or Intent

1. *Conditioning exercises* include activities with the intent of improving physical condition. This includes stationary ergometers (bicycling, rowing machines, treadmills, etc.), health-club exercise, calisthenics, and aerobics.

2. *Home repair* includes all activity associated with the repair of a house and does not include housework. This is not an occupational task.

3. Sleeping, lying, sitting, and standing are classified as *inactivity*.

4. *Home activities* include all activities associated with maintaining the inside of a house and include house cleaning, laundry, grocery shopping, and cooking.

5. *Lawn and garden* includes all activity associated with maintaining the yard and includes yardwork, gardening, and snow removal.

6. *Occupation* includes all job-related physical activity where one is paid (gainful employment). Specific activities may be cross-referenced in other categories (such as reading, writing, driving a car, walking) and should be coded in this major heading if related to employment. Housework is occupational only if the person is earning money for the task.

7. *Self-care* includes all activity related to grooming, eating, bathing, etc.

8. *Transportation* includes energy expended for the primary purpose of going somewhere in a motorized vehicle.

Section 3. Guidelines for Coding Specific Activities

A. General guidelines: All activities should be coded as "general" if no other information about the activity is given. This applies primarily to intensity ratings. If any additional information is given, activities should be coded accordingly.

B. Specific guidelines

   1. Bicycling

      a. Stationary cycling using cycle ergometers (all types), wind trainers, or other conditioning devices should be classified under the major heading of Conditioning Exercise, stationary cycling specific activities (codes 02010 to 02015).

      b. The list does not account for differences in wind conditions.

      c. If bicycling is performed in a race, classify it as general racing if no descriptions are given about drafting (code 01050). If information is given about the speed or drafting, code as 01050 (bicycling, 16–19 mph, racing/not drafting or >19 mph drafting, very fast) or 01060 (bicycling, ≥ 20 mph, racing, not drafting).

      d. Using a mountain bike in the city should be classified as bicycling, general (code 01010). Cycling on mountain trails or on a BMX course is coded 01009.

   2. Conditioning Exercises

      a. If a calisthenics program is described as a light or moderate type of activity (e.g., performing back exercises) but indicates a vigorous effort on the part of the participant, code the activity as calisthenics, general (code 02030).

      b. Exercise performed at a health club that is not described should be classified as health club, general (code 02060). Other activities performed at a health club (e.g., weight lifting, aerobic dance, circuit training, treadmill running, etc.) should be classified under separate major headings.

   c. Regardless of whether aerobic dance, conditioning, circuit training, or water calisthenics programs are described by their component parts (i.e., 10 min jogging in place, 10 min sit-ups, 10 min stretching, etc.), code the activity as one activity (e.g., water aerobics, code 02120).

   d. Effort, speed, or intensity breakdowns for the specific activities of stair–treadmill ergometer (code 02065), ski machine (code 02080), water aerobics or water calisthenics (code 02120), circuit training (code 02040), and slimnastics (code 02090) are not given. Code these as general, even though effort or intensities may vary in the descriptions of the activity.

3. Dancing

   a. If the type of dancing performed is not described, code it as dancing, general (code 03025).

4. Home Activities

   a. House cleaning should be coded as light (code 05040) or heavy (code 05020). Examples for each are given in the description of the specific activities.

   b. Making the bed on a daily basis is coded 05100. Changing the bed sheets is coded as cleaning, light (code 05040).

5. Home Repair

   a. Any painting outside of the house (i.e., fence, the house, barn) is coded, painting, outside house (code 60150).

6. Inactivity

   a. Sitting and reading a book or newspaper is listed under the major heading of Miscellaneous, reading, book, newspaper, etc. (code 09030).

   b. Sitting and writing is listed under the major heading of Miscellaneous, writing (code 09040).

7. Lawn and Garden

   a. Working in the garden with a specific type of tool (e.g., hoe, spade) is coded as digging, spading, filling garden (code 08050).

   b. Removing snow may be done by one of three methods: shoveling snow by hand (code 08200), walking and operating a snow blower (code 08130), or riding a snow blower (code 08180).

8. Music Playing

   a. Most variation in music playing will be according to the setting (i.e., rock and roll band, orchestra, marching band, concert band, standing on the stage, performance, practice, in a church, etc.). The compendium does not consider differences in the setting (except for marching band and guitar playing).

9. Occupation

   a. Types of occupational activities not listed separately under specific activities (e.g., chemistry laboratory experiments), should be placed into the types of energy expenditure classifications best describing the activity. See sitting: light (code 11580), sitting: moderate (code 11590), standing: light (code 11600), standing: light to moderate (code 11610), standing: moderate (code 11620), standing: moderate to heavy (code 11630).

   b. Driving an automobile or a light truck for employment (taxi cab, salesperson, contractor, ambulance driver, bus driver), should be listed under the major heading of Transportation, automobile or light truck (not a semi) driving (code 06010).

   c. Performing skin or SCUBA diving as an occupation is listed under the major heading of Water Activities, and the specific activity of skindiving or SCUBA diving as a frogman (code 18170).

10. Running

   a. Running is not classified as treadmill or outdoor running. Running on a treadmill or outdoors should be coded by the speed of the run (codes 12030 to 12130). If speed is not given, code it as running, general (code 12150).

11. Self-care

   a. The compendium does not account for effort ratings. All items are considered to be general.

12. Transportation

   a. Being a passenger in an automobile is coded under the major heading of Inactivity, sitting quietly (code 07020).

13. Walking

   a. Household walking is coded 17150, regardless of whether the subject identified a walking speed.

   b. If the walking speed is unidentified, use 3.0 mph, level, moderate, firm surface as the standard speed (code 17190). This should not be used for household walking.

   c. Walking during a household move, shopping, or for household work is coded under the major heading of Home Activities. Walking for job-related activities is coded under Occupational Activities.

   d. If a subject is backpacking, regardless of descriptors attached, the code is backpacking, general (code 17010).

   e. The compendium does not account for variations in speed or effort while carrying luggage or a child.

   f. Mountain climbing should be classified as general (rock or mountain climbing, code 17120) if no descriptors are given. If the weight of the load is described, code the activity as climbing hills with the appropriate load (codes 17030 to 17060).

   g. Walking on a grassy area (golf course, in a park, etc.) should be coded as walking, grass track (code 17260). The compendium does not account for variations in walking speed on a grassy area, so ignore recordings of walking speed or effort. If the walking is not on a grassy area, code the activity according to the walking speed (codes 17150 to 17230).

   h. Walking to work or to class should be coded as 17270. The compendium does not account for walking speed or effort in this activity. Even though a speed or effort is given for the walking, do not code walking to work or to class in any other walking category.

   i. Hiking and cross-country walking (code 17080) should be used only if the walking activity lasted 3 hours or more. Do not use this category for backpacking, but for day hikes.

14. Water Activities

   a. Swimming should be coded as leisurely, not lap swimming, general (code 18310) if descriptors about stroke, speed, or swimming location are not given.

   b. Lap swimming should be coded as swimming laps, freestyle, slow (code 18240) if the activity is described as lap swimming, light or moderate effort, but stroke or speed are not indicated. Swimming laps should be coded as swimming, laps, freestyle, fast (code 18230) if the activity is described as lap swimming, vigorous effort, but stroke or speed are not indicated.

   c. Swimming crawl should be coded as swimming, crawl, slow (50 yards . min^{-1}) if speed is not given and the effort is rated light or moderate (code 18290). Swimming crawl should be coded as swimming, crawl, fast (75 yards . min^{-1}) if speed is not given, but the effort is rated as vigorous (code 18280).

   d. The swimming strokes of backstroke (code 18250), breaststroke (code 18260), butterfly (code 18270), and sidestroke (code 18230) are coded as general for speed and intensity.

   e. If a swimming activity is not identified as lake, ocean, or river swimming (code 18300), assume that the swimming was performed in a swimming pool.

   f. If canoeing is related to a canoe trip, code as canoeing, on a camping trip (code 18020). Otherwise, code it according to the speed and effort listed.

Source: Ainsworth BE, Haskell WL, Leon AS, Jacobs DR, Montoye HJ, Sallis JF, Paffenbarger RS. Compendium of physical activities: Classification of energy costs of human physical activities. *Med Sci Sports Exerc* 25(1):71–80, 1993. Reprinted with permission of Barbara E. Ainsworth and the publisher, Williams & Wilkins.

Glossary

acclimatization   The body's gradual adaptation to a changed environment, such as higher temperatures.

acromegaly   A chronic disease caused by excess production of growth hormone, leading to elongation and enlargement of bones of the extremities and certain head bones.

acute   Sudden, short-term.

acute muscle soreness   Occurs during and immediately following exercise; the muscular tension developed during exercise, which reduces blood flow to the active muscles, causing lactic acid and potassium to build up, stimulating pain receptors.

adenosine triphosphate (ATP)   Energy released from the separation of high-energy phosphate bonds; the immediate energy source for muscular contraction.

adherence   Sticking to something; used to describe a person's continuation in an exercise program.

adipose tissue   Fat tissue.

aerobic   Using oxygen.

aerobic activities   Activities using large-muscle groups at moderate intensities, which permit the body to use oxygen to supply energy and to maintain a steady state for more than a few minutes.

aerobic dance   The original aerobic-dance programs consisted of an eclectic combination of various dance forms, including ballet, modern jazz, disco, and folk, as well as calisthenic-type exercises; more recent innovations include water aerobics (done in a swimming pool), nonimpact or low-impact aerobics (one foot on the ground at all times), specific dance aerobics, and "assisted" aerobics, whereby weights are worn on the wrists and / or ankles.

aerobic power   See *maximal oxygen uptake.*

agility   Relates to the ability to rapidly change the position of the entire body in space, with speed and accuracy.

aging   Refers to the normal yet irreversible biological changes that occur during the total years that a person lives.

alcohol dependent   Dependency on alcohol, which leads to negative consequences such as arrest, accident, or impairment of health or job performance.

alcoholism   A chronic, progressive, and potentially fatal disease, characterized by *tolerance* (brain adaptation to the presence of alcohol) and *physical dependency* (withdrawal symptoms occur when consumption of alcohol is decreased); alcohol-related problems may include symptoms of alcohol dependence such as memory loss, inability to stop drinking until intoxicated, inability to cut down on drinking, binge drinking, and withdrawal symptoms.

alveoli   Air sacs of the lung.

Alzheimer's disease   Disease that progresses from short-term memory loss to a final stage requiring total care; a form of senile dementia, associated with atrophy of parts of the brain.

amenorrhea   Absence of menstruation.

amino acid   An organic compound that makes up protein; 20 amino acids are necessary for metabolism and growth, but only 11 are "essential" in that they must be provided from the food eaten.

anabolic   The building up of a body substance.

anabolic steroids   A group of synthetic, testosterone-like hormones that promote anabolism, including muscle hypertrophy; their use in athletics is considered unethical and carries numerous serious health risks.

anaerobic   Not using oxygen.

anaerobic activities   Activities using muscle groups at high intensities that exceed the body's capacity to use oxygen to supply energy, thereby creating an oxygen debt by using energy produced without oxygen; see *oxygen debt.*

anaerobic threshold   The point at which blood lactate concentrations start to rise above resting values; can be expressed as a percent of $\dot{V}O_{2max}$.

androgenic   Causing masculinization.

android   A type of obesity characterized by the predominance of body fat in the upper half of the body.

anemia   Low hemoglobin concentration in the blood.

aneurysm   Localized abnormal dilatation of a blood vessel due to weakness of the wall.

angina   A gripping, choking, or suffocating pain in the chest (angina pectoris) caused most often by insufficient flow of oxygen to the heart muscle during exercise or excitement.

anorexia (anorexia nervosa) Lack of appetite; a psychological and physiological condition characterized by inability or refusal to eat, leading to severe weight loss, malnutrition, hormone imbalances, and other potentially life-threatening biological changes.

anthropometry The science dealing with the measurement (size, weight, proportions) of the human body.

anticipatory response Prior to exercise, heart rates can rise due to anticipation of the exercise bout.

apoprotein The protein part of the lipoprotein; important in activating or inhibiting certain enzymes involved in the metabolism of fats.

aquacise Aerobic dance in the water.

arrhythmia Any abnormal rate or rhythm of the heart beat.

arteriosclerosis Commonly called hardening of the arteries; includes a variety of conditions that cause the artery walls to thicken and lose elasticity.

arteriovenous oxygen difference ($\bar{a} - \bar{v}O_2$ difference) The difference between the oxygen content of arterial blood and that of venous blood.

artery Vessel that carries blood away from the heart to the tissues of the body

asthma A disease characterized by wheezing caused by a spasm of the bronchial tubes or by swelling of their mucous membranes.

atherosclerosis A very common form of arteriosclerosis, in which the arteries are narrowed by deposits of cholesterol and other material in the inner walls of the artery.

atrioventricular (AV) node A small mass of specialized conducting tissue at the bottom of the right atrium, through which the electrical impulse stimulating the heart to contract must pass to reach the ventricles.

auscultation Process of listening for sounds within the body using a stethoscope.

balance Relates to the maintenance of equilibrium while stationary or moving.

ballistic movement A flexibility exercise movement in which a part of the body is sharply moved against the resistance of antagonist muscles or against the limits of a joint.

basal metabolic rate The minimum energy required to maintain the body's life functions at rest; usually expressed in Calories per day.

bee pollen A substance gleaned from honey, which is claimed by some to have unusual nutritional qualities enhancing performance; double-blind placebo studies do not support this claim.

behavior modification Considers in great detail the eating behavior to be changed, events that trigger the eating, and the behavior's consequences.

binge eating The consumption of large quantities of rich foods within short periods of time.

blood doping An ergogenic procedure wherein an athlete's own blood is infused, or type-matched donor blood is transfused, to enhance endurance performance.

blood pressure The pressure exerted by the blood on the wall of the arteries; measures are in millimeters of mercury (such as 120/80 mm Hg).

bodybuilding An activity in which competitors work to develop the mass, definition, and symmetry of their muscles, rather than the strength, skill, or endurance required for more common athletic events.

body composition The proportions of fat, muscle, and bone making up the body; usually expressed as percent of body fat and percent of lean body mass.

body density The specific gravity of the body, which can be tested by underwater weighing; compares the weight of the body to the weight of the same volume of water; result can be used to estimate the percentage of body fat.

body mass index (BMI) Calculation of body weight and height indices for determining degree of obesity.

bradycardia Slow heart beat of less than 60 beats per minute at rest.

branched-chain amino acids Valine, isoleucine, leucine.

BTPS The volume of air at the temperature and pressure of the body, and 100% saturated with water vapor.

bundle of His A bundle of fibers of the impulse-conducting system of the heart; from its origin in the A-V node, enters the interventricular septum, where it divides into two branches (bundle branches), the fibers of which pass to the right and left ventricles, becoming continuous with the Purkinje fibers of the ventricles.

caffeine A methylxanthine found in many plants; has unpredictable effects on endurance performance, but may increase muscle utilization of free fatty acids, sparing muscle glycogen stores.

calisthenics A system of exercise movements, without equipment, for the building of muscular strength and endurance, and flexibility; the Greeks formed the word from *kalos* (beautiful) and *sthenos* (strength).

caloric cost The number of Calories burned to produce the energy for a task; usually measured in Calories (kilocalories) per minute.

calorie The energy required to raise the temperature of 1 kilogram of water 1° Celsius; used as a unit of metabolism (as in diet and energy expenditure); equals 1,000 calories (spelled with a capital C to make that distinction); also called a kilocalorie (kcal).

cancer A large group of diseases characterized by uncontrolled growth and spread of abnormal cells.

carbohydrate Chemical compound of carbon, oxygen and hydrogen, usually with the hydrogen and oxygen in the right proportions to form water; common forms are starches, sugars, and dietary fibers.

carbohydrate loading A dietary scheme emphasizing high amounts of carbohydrate to increase muscle glycogen stores before long endurance events.

carbon dioxide A colorless, odorless gas formed in the tissues by the oxidation of carbon and eliminated by the lungs.

carbon monoxide Produced mainly during combustion of fossil fuels such as coal and gasoline; a tasteless, odorless, colorless gas.

cardiac output The volume of blood pumped out by the heart in a given unit of time; equals the stroke volume times the heart rate.

cardiac rehabilitation A program to prepare cardiac patients to return to productive lives with a reduced risk of recurring health problems.

cardiopulmonary resuscitation (CPR) A first-aid method to restore breathing and heart action through mouth-to-mouth breathing and rhythmic chest compressions; CPR instruction is offered by local American Heart Association and American Red Cross units and is a minimum requirement for most fitness-instruction certifications.

cardiorespiratory endurance The same as aerobic endurance; can be defined as the ability to continue or persist in strenuous tasks involving large-muscle groups for extended periods of time; the ability of the circulatory and respiratory systems to adjust to and recover from the effects of whole-body exercise or work.

cardiovascular Pertaining to the heart and blood vessels.

carotid artery The principal artery in both sides of the neck. A convenient place to detect a pulse.

catecholamine Epinephrine and norepinephrine hormones.

cellulite A commercially created name for lumpy fat deposits; actually behaves no differently from other fat; distinguished by straining against irregular bands of connective tissue.

cerebral thrombosis Clot that forms inside the cerebral artery.

cholesterol An alcohol steroid found in animal fats; a pearly, fatlike substance implicated in the narrowing of the arteries in atherosclerosis; all Americans are being urged to decrease their serum cholesterol levels to less than 200 mg/dl.

chronic Continuing over time.

chronic diseases Lifestyle-related diseases, such as heart disease, cancer, and stroke, and also accidents, which together account for 75% of all deaths in America.

circuit training A series of exercises, performed one after the other, with little rest between.

circuit weight training programs Involve 8–12 repetitions with various weight machines at 7–14 stations, moving quickly from one station to the next.

citric acid cycle See *Krebs cycle.*

collateral circulation Blood circulation through small side branches that can supplement (or substitute for) the main vessel's delivery of blood to certain tissues.

compliance Staying with a prescribed exercise program.

concentric action Muscle action in which the muscle is shortening under its own power; commonly called "positive" work or, redundantly, "concentric contraction."

continuous passive motion (CPM) Motorized machines that continuously move isolated muscle groups through their range of motion without requiring any effort by the user.

contraindication Any condition indicating that a particular course of action (or exercise) would be inadvisable.

cool-down A gradual reduction of the intensity of exercise to allow physiological processes to return to normal; also called warm-down.

coordination Relates to the ability to use the senses, such as sight and hearing, together with body parts in performing motor tasks smoothly and accurately.

coronary arteries The arteries circling the heart like a crown, which supply blood to the heart muscle; three major branches.

coronary heart disease (CHD) Atherosclerosis of the coronary arteries.

cortical bone Compact outer shaft bone.

creatine phosphokinase (CPK) A muscle enzyme that can rise dramatically in the blood after unaccustomed exercise, indicating considerable muscle cell damage.

cross-sectional study A study made at one point in time (cf. *longitudinal study*).

cryokinetics A treatment that alternates cold and exercise for rehabilitation of traumatic musculoskeletal injuries in athletes.

dehydration Condition resulting from the excessive loss of body water.

delayed-onset muscle soreness (DOMS) Occurs from 1 to 5 days following unaccustomed or severe exercise, involving actual damage to the muscle cells.

detraining The process of losing the benefits of training by returning to a sedentary life.

DHEA An unapproved drug (dehydroepiandrosterone or dehydroandrosterone) derived from human urine and other sources; manufacturers tout DHEA as a "natural" weight-loss product, but this claim has not been substantiated.

diabetes mellitus A group of disorders that share glucose intolerance (high serum levels of glucose) in common; there are two common types: type 1 and type 2. Type 1 can occur at any age, but especially in the young, and is characterized by an abrupt onset of symptoms, and a need for insulin to sustain life; type 2 is most common, usually occurring in people who are obese and over age 40.

diastolic blood pressure The blood pressure when the heart is resting between beats.

dietary fiber Complex plant cell-wall materials that cannot be digested by the enzymes in the human small intestine; examples include cellulose, hemicellulose, pectin, mucilages, and lignin.

diuretic Any agent that increases the flow of urine, ridding the body of water.

drug dependence Criteria are highly controlled or compulsive use, psychoactive effects, and drug-reinforced behavior.

dry-bulb thermometer An ordinary instrument for indicating temperature. Does not take into account humidity and other factors that combine to determine the heat stress experienced by the body.

duration The time spent in a single exercise session; frequency, intensity, and duration (time) are the F.I.T. factors, which affect improvement of cardiorespiratory endurance.

dynamometer A device for measuring force; common dynamometers include devices to test hand, leg, and back strength.

dyspnea Difficult or labored breathing.

eccentric action Muscle action in which the muscle resists while it is forced to lengthen; commonly called "negative" work, or "eccentric contraction," but because the muscle is lengthening, the word "contraction" is misapplied.

economy Refers to ease of administration, the use of inexpensive equipment, the need for little time, and the simplicity of the test so that the person taking it can easily understand the purpose and results.

ectomorphic A lean, thin, and linear body type.

efficiency The ratio of energy consumed to the work accomplished.

ECG lead A pair of electrodes placed on the body and connected to an electrocardiograph (ECG recorder).

elderly Individuals who reach or pass the age of 65; this group now represents the fastest-growing minority in the United States.

electrical muscle stimulators (EMS) EMS devices give a painless electrical stimulation to the muscle; manufacturers claim that muscles are toned without exercise; other claimed benefits include face lifts without surgery, slimming and trimming, weight loss, bust development, spot reducing, and removal of cellulite; the Food and Drug Administration considers claims for EMS devices promoted for such purposes to be misbranded and fraudulent.

electrocardiogram (ECG, EKG) A graph of the electrical activity caused by the stimulation of the heart muscle; the millivolts of electricity are detected by electrodes on the body surface and recorded by an electrocardiograph.

electrolyte Scientists call minerals like sodium, chloride, and potassium "electrolytes" because, in water, they can conduct electrical currents; sodium and potassium ions carry positive charges, while chloride ions are negatively charged.

electron transport system An additional metabolic pathway from which the products of the Krebs cycle enter and yield ATP; this cycle requires oxygen.

embolus A blood clot that breaks loose and travels to smaller arterial vessels, where it may lodge and block the blood flow.

endurance The capacity to continue a physical performance over a period of time.

enzyme Complex proteins that induce and accelerate the speed of chemical reactions without being changed themselves; present in digestive juices, enzymes act on food substances, breaking them down into simpler molecules.

epidemiological studies Statistical study of the relationships among various factors that determine the frequency and distribution of disease in human populations.

epinephrine A hormone primarily excreted from the adrenal medulla; also called a catecholamine; involved in many important body functions, including the elevation of blood glucose levels during exercise or stress.

ergogenic aids A physical, mechanical, nutritional, psychological, or pharmacological substance or treatment that either directly improves physiological variables associated with exercise performance or removes subjective restraints that may limit physiological capacity.

ergometer A device that can measure work consistently and reliably; stationary exercise cycles were the first widely available devices equipped with ergometers.

estrogen replacement One of the mainstays of prevention and management of osteoporosis, especially for women who are postmenopausal; also effective in preventing cardiovascular disease.

ethyl alcohol (ethanol) Grain alcohol; a social drug that is called a "sedative–hypnotic" because of its dramatic effects on the brain; ethanol (CH_3CH_2OH) is a small water-soluble molecule that is absorbed rapidly and completely from the stomach and small intestine.

exercise   Physical exertion of sufficient intensity, duration, and frequency to achieve or maintain fitness or other health or athletic objectives.

exercise-induced bronchospasm (EIB)   Defined as a diffuse bronchospastic response in both large and small airways following heavy exercise; postexercise symptoms include difficulty in breathing, coughing, shortness of breath, and wheezing.

exercise oxygen economy   The oxygen cost of exercise, usually expressed as $\dot{V}O_2$ at a certain running or exercise pace.

exercise prescription   A recommendation for a course of exercise to meet desirable individual objectives for fitness; includes activity types, as well as duration, intensity, and frequency of exercise.

exercise program director   Certification by the American College of Sports Medicine indicates the competency to design, implement, and administer preventive and rehabilitative exercise programs, to educate staff in conducting tests and leading physical activity, and to educate the community about such programs; must have all the competencies of fitness instructor, exercise technologist, and exercise specialist.

exercise specialist   Certified by the American College of Sports Medicine as having the competency and skill to supervise preventive and rehabilitative exercise programs and prescribe activities for patients; must also pass the ACSM standards for exercise technologist.

exercise technologist   Certified by the American College of Sports Medicine as competent to administer graded exercise tests, calculate the data, and implement any needed emergency procedures; must have current CPR certification.

expiratory reserve volume (ERV)   The amount of air that can be pushed out of the lung following an expired resting tidal volume.

extension   Moving the two ends of a jointed body part away from each other, as in straightening the arm.

extensor   A muscle that extends a jointed body part.

extracellular   Outside of the body cell.

Fartlek training   Similar to interval training; a free form of training done on trails or roads.

fast-twitch fibers   Muscle fiber type that contracts quickly and is used most in intensive, short-duration exercises, such as weightlifting or sprints; also called Type II fibers.

fats   Serve as a source of energy; in food, the fat molecule is formed from one molecule of glycerol and is combined with three of fatty acids; a high caloric value, yielding about 9 Calories per gram, as compared with 4 Calories for carbo-

hydrates and proteins; *saturated fats* have no double bonds, are generally hard at room temperature, and have been associated with increased risk of heart disease; *monounsaturated fats* and *polyunsaturated fats* have one and two double bonds, respectively, are generally liquid at room temperature, and have been associated with decreased risk of heart disease.

fat cell theory   A theory that may explain obesity; fat cell number can increase two to three times normal if an individual ingests excessive Calories; once formed, the extra fat cells cannot be removed by the body; this can happen any time during the life span of an individual but appears to be particularly important during infancy when fat cells are still dividing.

fat-free weight   Lean body mass or bone, muscle, and water.

fatigue   A loss of power to continue a given level of physical performance.

fitness   See *physical fitness.*

fitness instructor   Directs classes or individuals in the performance of exercise; certification by the American College of Sports Medicine indicates the competency to identify risk factors, conduct submaximal exercise tests, recommend exercise programs, lead classes, counsel exercisers, and work with persons without known disease; CPR certification is required.

flexibility   The range of motion around a joint.

flexion   Moving the two ends of a jointed body part closer to each other, as in bending the arm.

food supplements   Substances or pills that are added to the diet; most reputable nutritionists state that vitamin or mineral supplementation is unwarranted for people eating a balanced diet.

forced vital capacity (FVC)   The total amount of air that can be breathed into the lung on top of the residual volume.

frame size   Elbow breadth measurement for determination of small, medium, or large skeletal mass.

frequency   How often a person repeats a complete exercise session (e.g., three times per week); frequency, along with duration and intensity, affects the cardiorespiratory response to exercise.

functional capacity   See *maximal oxygen uptake.*

functional residual capacity (FRC)   The combined expiratory reserve volume and residual volume.

gastric stapling   Surgery to radically reduce the volume of the stomach to less than 50 ml.

genetic factors   One theory advanced to explain the high prevalence of obesity in Western countries; some studies have demonstrated that certain people are more prone to obesity than others due to genetic factors; such people have to be unusually careful in their dietary and exercise habits to counteract these inherited tendencies.

glucagon   A hormone that is secreted by the pancreas; helps to raise blood glucose levels by stimulating the breakdown of liver glycogen.

gluconeogenesis   The formation of glucose and glycogen from noncarbohydrate sources such as amino acids, glycerol, and lactate.

glucose   Blood sugar; the transportable form of carbohydrate, which reaches the cells.

glucose polymers   Four to six glucose units produced by partial breakdown of corn starch.

glycogen   The storage form of carbohydrate; used in the muscles for the production of energy.

glycolysis   A metabolic pathway that converts glucose to lactic acid to produce energy in the form of ATP.

glycosuria   Glucose in the urine.

Golgi tendon organ   Organs at the junction of muscle and tendon which send inhibitory impulses to the muscle when the muscle's contraction reaches certain levels; the purpose may be to protect against separating the tendon from bone when a contraction is too great.

graded exercise test (GXT)   A treadmill or cycle-ergometer test with the workload gradually increased until exhaustion or a predetermined endpoint.

grapefruit pills   For several decades, grapefruit has been promoted as having special fat-burning properties; this myth has spread far and wide; grapefruit pills contain grapefruit extract, diuretics, and bulk-forming agents, and some contain phenylpropanolamine (PPA), along with herbs or other ingredients.

growth hormone   A hormone released from the pituitary, which elevates blood glucose; as its name indicates, this hormone helps regulate growth.

growth hormone releasers   Various products sold with the claim that if they are taken before retiring, weight loss will occur overnight due to the increased release of growth hormone from the amino acids arginine and ornithine contained in the products—an erroneous concept.

gynoid   A form of obesity characterized by excess body fat in the lower half of the body, especially the hips, buttocks, and thighs.

haptoglobin   A mucoprotein to which hemoglobin released into plasma is bound; increased in certain inflammatory conditions, and decreased during hemolysis.

HDL-C:TC   The ratio of HDL-C to total cholesterol, which has been found to be highly predictive of heart disease.

health   The World Health Organization has defined *health* as a state of complete physical, mental, and social well-being, and not merely the absence of disease.

health fraud   Defined as the promotion, for financial gain, of fraudulent or unproven devices, treatments, services, plans, or products (including, but not limited to, diets and nutritional supplements) that alter or claim to alter the human condition.

health promotion   The science and art of helping people change their lifestyle to move toward optimal health.

health-related fitness   Elements of fitness such as cardiorespiratory fitness, muscular strength and endurance, flexibility, and body composition that are related to improvement of health.

heart attack   Also called myocardial infarction; often occurs when a clot blocks an atherosclerotic coronary blood vessel.

heart rate   Number of heart beats per minute.

heart rate reserve   The difference between the resting heart rate and the maximal heart rate.

heat cramps   Muscle twitching or painful cramping, usually following heavy exercise with profuse sweating; the legs, arms, and abdominal muscles are the most often affected.

heat exhaustion   Caused by dehydration; symptoms include a dry mouth, excessive thirst, loss of coordination, dizziness, headaches, paleness, shakiness, and cool and clammy skin.

heat stroke   A life-threatening illness when the body's temperature-regulating mechanisms fail; body temperature may rise to over 104°F, skin appears red, dry, and warm to the touch; the victim has chills, sometimes nausea and dizziness, and may be confused or irrational; seizures and coma may follow unless temperature is brought down to 102° within an hour.

Hegsted formula   Used to predict change in serum cholesterol from saturated fats (S) and polyunsaturated fats (P) and cholesterol in the diet: change in serum cholesterol = $(2.16 \times$ change in S$) - (1.65 \times$ change in P$) + (0.097 \times$ change in dietary cholesterol$)$.

hematocrit   Expressed as the percentage of total blood volume, consisting of red blood cells and other solids.

heme iron   Forty percent of the iron in animal products is called heme iron; the remaining 60% of the iron in animal products and all the iron in vegetable products are called nonheme iron; heme iron is more easily absorbed by the body.

hemoconcentration   Increase in the thickness of blood due to loss of plasma volume.

hemoglobin   The iron-containing pigment of the red blood cells; its function is to carry oxygen from the lungs to the tissues. Low levels of hemoglobin is called anemia.

hemolysis   Breakdown of red blood cells, with liberation of hemoglobin, and loss through the kidneys.

hemorrhage Abnormal internal or external discharge of blood.

hepatic lipase (HL) An enzyme of the liver, which removes HDL from circulation.

high blood pressure See *hypertension.*

high-density lipoprotein cholesterol (HDL-C) Cholesterol is carried by the high-density lipoprotein to the liver; the liver then uses the cholesterol to form bile acids, which are finally excreted in the stool; thus, high levels of HDL-C have been associated with low cardiovascular disease risk.

homeostasis State of equilibrium of the internal environment of the body.

hormone A substance secreted from an organ or gland, which is transported by the blood to another part of the body.

human growth hormone Hormone that is liberated by the anterior pituitary and is important for regulating growth.

hypercholesterolemia High blood cholesterol levels.

hyperglycemia Excessive levels of glucose in the blood.

hyperplastic obesity A high number of fat cells, two to three times normal.

hypertension A condition in which the blood pressure is chronically elevated above optimal levels; diagnosis in adults is confirmed when the average of two or more diastolic measurements on at least two separate visits is 90 mm Hg or higher; if the diastolic blood pressure is below 90 mm Hg, systolic hypertension is diagnosed when the average of multiple systolic blood pressure measurements on two or more separate visits is consistently greater than 140 mm Hg.

hyperthermia Body temperatures exceeding normal.

hypertonic Describes a solution concentrated enough to draw water out of body cells.

hypertriglyceridemia High blood triglyceride levels.

hypertrophy An enlargement of a muscle by the increase in size of the cells.

hypochromic Condition of the red blood cells in which they have a reduced hemoglobin content.

hypoglycemia Blood sugar levels below 50 mg/dl, accompanied by symptoms of dizziness, nausea, trembling, irritation, and so on.

hyponatremia Low sodium levels in the bloodstream, which can be caused by excessive sweating and inadequate electrolyte replacement during ultramarathons.

hypothalamus A portion of the brain lying below the thalamus; secretions from the hypothalamus are important in the control of important body functions, including the regulation of water balance, appetite, and body temperature.

hypothermia Body temperature below normal; usually due to exposure to cold temperatures, especially after exhausting ready energy supplies.

hypotonic Describes a solution dilute enough to allow its water to be absorbed by body cells.

hypoxia Insufficient oxygen flow to the tissues.

iliac crest The upper, wide portion of the hip bone.

impaired glucose tolerance Borderline hyperglycemia (between 115 and 140 mg/dl).

indirect calorimetry Measurement of energy expenditure by analysis of expired air.

infarction Death of a section of tissue, due to the obstruction of blood flow (ischemia) to the area.

informed consent A procedure for obtaining a client's signed consent to a fitness center's testing and exercise program; includes a description of the objectives and procedures, with associated benefits and risks, stated in plain language, with a consent statement and signature line in a single document.

inspiration Breathing air into the lungs.

inspiratory reserve volume (IRV) The amount of air that can be breathed into the lung on top of a resting inspired tidal volume.

insulin A hormone secreted by special cells (beta cells) in the pancreas; essential for the maintenance of blood glucose levels.

intensity The level of exertion during exercise; intensity, duration, and frequency are important for improving cardiorespiratory endurance.

interval training An exercise session in which the intensity and duration of exercise are consciously alternated between harder and easier work; often used to improve aerobic capacity and/or anaerobic endurance in exercisers who already have a base of endurance in training.

intima The inner layer of arteries.

intracellular Inside the cell.

iron deficiency The most common single nutritional deficiency in the world today; characterized by low iron stores in the body; severe iron deficiency or anemia is characterized by low blood hemoglobin.

iron-deficient erythropoiesis Stage 2 of iron deficiency, following the exhaustion of bone marrow iron stores, and characterized by a diminishing iron supply to developing red blood cells; iron-deficient erythropoiesis (formation of red blood cells) occurs and is measured by increased total iron-binding capacity and reduced serum iron and percent saturation (<16% is abnormal).

ischemia Inadequate blood flow to a body part, caused by constriction or obstruction of a blood vessel, leading to insufficient oxygen supply.

isokinetic contraction A muscle contraction against a resistance that moves at a constant velocity, so that the maximum force of which the muscle is capable throughout the range of motion may be applied.

isometric action Muscle action in which the muscle attempts to contract against an immovable object; sometimes called "isometric contraction," although there is not appreciable shortening of the muscle.

isotonic contraction A muscle contraction against a constant resistance, as in lifting a weight.

Karvonen formula A method to calculate the training heart rate using a percentage of the heart rate reserve, which is the difference between the maximal and resting heart rates.

ketosis An elevated level of ketone bodies in the tissues; seen in sufferers of starvation or diabetes, and a symptom brought about in dieters on very-low-carbohydrate diets.

kilocalorie (kcal) A measure of the heat required to raise the temperature of 1 kilogram of water 1° Celsius; a Calorie, used in diet and metabolism measures, equals 1 kilocalorie or 1,000 calories.

kilogram (kg) A unit of weight equal to 1,000 grams; (2.204623 pounds).

kilogram-meters (kgm) The amount of work required to lift 1 kilogram 1 meter.

kilopond-meters (kpm) Equivalent to kilogram-meters, in normal gravity.

Korotkoff sounds Blood pressure sounds.

Krebs cycle Final common metabolic pathway for fats, proteins, and carbohydrates, which yields additional ATP; carbon dioxide and water are produced.

lactate Lactic acid.

lactate dehydrogenase (LDH) A muscle enzyme that can leak out of ruptured muscle cells into the blood.

lactate system Exercise of 1–3 minutes duration; depends on the lactate system or anaerobic glycolysis for ATP.

lactic acid The end product of the metabolism of glucose (glycolysis) for the anaerobic production of energy.

late-onset (PEL) hypoglycemia Typically, PEL hypoglycemia happens during the night and occurs 6–15 hours after the completion of unusually strenuous exercise or play in diabetics.

law of diminishing returns Appears to be a certain amount of training that most humans will respond quickly and fruitfully to, but every step beyond that level brings less return for the time and effort invested.

L-carnitine An amine responsible for transporting fatty acids into the mitochondria for oxidation; L-carnitine supplements have been claimed to increase the amount of fatty acid oxidation during exercise, sparing the glycogen; however, L-carnitine supplements have never been shown in reputable, double-blind, controlled studies to improve the athletic performance of a healthy individual.

lean body weight The weight of the body, less the weight of its fat.

lecithin:cholesterol acyltransferase (LCAT) An enzyme from the liver that "matures" incomplete HDL by connecting fatty acids to the free cholesterol in the HDL particle. The incomplete HDL (HDL_3) swells into a mature sphere (HDL_3); the LCAT enzyme then grabs more cholesterol from the tissues and other circulating lipoproteins to form even bigger HDL particles (HDL_2).

life expectancy The average number of years of life expected in a population at a specific age, usually at birth.

life span The maximal obtainable age by a particular member of the species, which is primarily related to one's genetic makeup.

lipid A general term used for several different compounds, which include both solid fats and liquid oils; the three major classes of lipids are triglycerides, phospholipids, and sterols.

lipoprotein A soluble aggregate of cholesterol, phospholipids, triglycerides, and protein; this package allows for easy transport through the blood; the four types of lipoproteins are chylomicrons, low-density lipoprotein (LDL), very low-density lipoprotein (VLDL), and high-density lipoprotein (HDL).

lipoprotein lipase (LPL) An enzyme that breaks down VLDL, providing fatty acids for the muscle or adipose tissue.

longitudinal study A study that observes the same subjects over a period of time (cf. *cross-sectional study*).

lordosis Forward pelvis tilt, often caused from weak abdominals and inflexible posterior thigh muscles, allowing the pelvis to tilt forward, causing curvature in the lower back.

low-back pain (LBP) Pain in the lower back, often caused from weak abdominal muscles and tight lower back and hamstring muscles.

low-density lipoprotein (LDL) Transports cholesterol from the liver to other body cells; often referred to as "bad" cholesterol because it may be taken up by muscle cells in arteries and has been implicated in the development of atherosclerosis.

low-impact aerobics At least one foot is touching the floor throughout.

lumen Inside opening of an artery.

lung diffusion The rate at which gases diffuse from the lung air sacs to the blood in the pulmonary capillaries.

Mason-Likar The 12-lead exercise ECG system.

maximal anaerobic power The ability to exercise for a short time period at high power levels; important for various sports where sprinting and power movements are common.

maximal heart rate The highest heart rate of which an individual is capable; a broad rule of thumb for estimating maximal heart rate is 220 (beats per minute) minus the person's age (in years).

maximal oxygen uptake The highest rate of oxygen consumption of which a person is capable; usually expressed in milliliters of oxygen per kilogram of body weight per minute; also called maximal aerobic power, maximal oxygen consumption, maximal oxygen intake.

mean arterial pressure Equals ⅓ (systolic blood pressure − diastolic blood pressure) + diastolic blood pressure.

mean corpuscular volume Stage 3 iron-deficient anemia, characterized by a drop in hemoglobin; the bone marrow produces an increasing number of smaller and less brightly colored red blood cells; measured when the mean corpuscular volume (MCV) falls below 80 fl.

media Middle layer of muscle in artery wall.

medical history A list of a person's previous illnesses, present conditions, symptoms, medications, and health risk factors; used to help classify an individual as apparently healthy, at risk for disease, or with known disease.

mesomorphic An athletic, muscular body type.

MET A measure of energy output equal to the basal metabolic rate of a resting subject; assumed to be equal to an oxygen uptake of 3.5 milliliters per kilogram of body weight per minute, or approximately 1 kilocalorie per kilogram of body weight per hour.

microcyte A small red blood cell.

mild obesity Defined as being 20–40% overweight.

mineral Of the nearly 45 dietary nutrients known to be necessary for human life, 17 are minerals; although mineral elements represent only a small fraction of human body weight, they play important roles throughout the body; they help form hard tissues such as bones and teeth, aid in normal muscle and nerve activity, act as catalysts in many enzyme systems, help control body water levels, and are integral parts of organic compounds such as hemoglobin and the hormone thyroxine; evidence is growing that certain minerals are related to prevention of disease and proper immune system function.

minute ventilation The volume of air that is breathed into the body each minute.

mitochondria The slender filaments or rods inside of cells, containing enzymes important to producing energy from fat and carbohydrates.

mode Type of exercise.

moderate obesity Defined as being 40–100% overweight.

monosaccharides The simplest carbohydrate, containing only one molecule of sugar; glucose, fructose, and galactose are the primary monosaccharides.

monounsaturated fatty acids See *fats.*

motor neuron A nerve cell that conducts impulses from the central nervous system to a group of muscle fibers, producing movement.

motor unit A motor neuron and the muscle fibers activated by it.

muscle glycogen supercompensation The practice of exercise tapering, combined with a high-carbohydrate diet, that stores very high levels of glycogen in the muscles before long endurance events.

muscle spindle Organ in a muscle that senses changes in the muscle's length, especially stretches; rapid stretching of a muscle results in messages being sent to the nervous system to contract the muscle, thereby limiting the stretch.

muscular endurance Defined as the ability of the muscles to apply a submaximal force repeatedly or to sustain a muscular contraction for a certain period of time.

musculoskeletal fitness Comprises three components: flexibility, muscular strength, and muscular endurance.

myocardial infarction A common form of heart attack, in which the blockage of a coronary artery causes the death of a part of the heart muscle.

myofilaments Within the muscle cell; actin and myosin protein fibers are myofilaments.

myoglobin A muscle protein molecule that contains iron; carries oxygen from the blood to the muscle cell.

net energy expenditure Equals the Calories expended during the exercise session minus the Calories expended for the resting metabolic rate and other activities that would have occupied the individual had the person not been formally exercising.

nonpharmacological approaches Use of nondrug methods to treat hypertension, hypercholesterolemia, or other health problems.

non-weight-bearing activities Activities such as bicycling, swimming, and brisk walking, which do not overstress the musculoskeletal system.

norms Represent the average achievement level of a particular group to which the measured scores can be compared.

nutritional assessment Involves the use of a wide variety of clinical and biochemical methods to assess the state of health as characterized by body composition, tissue function, and metabolic activity.

obesity Excessive accumulation of body fat.

oligomenorrhea Scanty or infrequent menstrual flow.

omega-3 fatty acids A type of fat found in fish oils and associated with lower blood cholesterol levels, lower blood pressure, and reduced blood clotting.

one-repetition maximum, 1-RM The maximum resistance with which a person can execute one repetition of an exercise movement.

oral glucose tolerance test (OGTT) The OGTT is a 75-gram glucose solution given after an overnight fast of 10–16 hours.

osmolarity The concentration of a solution participating in osmosis.

osteoarthritis A noninflammatory joint disease of older persons; cartilage in the joint wears down, and bone grows at the edges of the joints; results in pain and stiffness, especially after prolonged exercise.

osteoblasts Bone cells that build bone.

osteoclasts The cells that break down bone.

osteoporosis Defined as an age-related disorder characterized by decreased bone mineral content and increased risk of fractures.

overload Subjecting a part of the body to efforts greater than it is accustomed to, in order to elicit a training response; increases may be in intensity or duration.

overuse Excessive repeated exertion or shock, which results in injuries such as stress fractures of bones or inflammation of muscles and tendons.

oxygen debt The oxygen required to restore the capacity for anaerobic work after an effort has used those reserves; measured by the extra oxygen that is consumed during the recovery from the work.

oxygen deficit The energy supplied anaerobically while oxygen uptake has not yet reached the steady state that matches energy output; becomes oxygen debt at end of exercise.

oxygen uptake The amount of oxygen used up at the cellular level during exercise; can be measured by determining the amount of oxygen exhaled (in carbon dioxide), as compared to the amount inhaled, or estimated by indirect means.

ozone In the lower atmosphere, produced by the photochemical reaction of sunlight on hydrocarbons and nitrogen dioxide from car and industrial exhaust.

pangamic acid So-called vitamin B_{15}, which is claimed to enhance performance; reputable nutritionists do not support this claim or even the fact that a vitamin B_{15} exists.

parasympathetic The craniosacral division of the autonomic nervous system.

parcourse An outdoor circuit system that combines calisthenics with running.

passive smoking Breathing of air that has cigarette smoke in it.

pellagra A disease of niacin deficiency.

percentage of total Calories Concept used by nutritionists to represent the percentage of protein, carbohydrate, and fat Calories present in the diet; calculated from the fact that 1 gram of carbohydrate, protein, and fat equals 4 Calories, 4 Calories, and 9 Calories, respectively.

percent saturation During iron-deficient erythropoiesis (stage 2 iron deficiency), percent saturation falls (<16 percent is abnormal).

phenylpropanolamine (PPA) The active ingredient in most nonprescription weight-control products; related to amphetamines and has similar side effects, such as nervousness, insomnia, headaches, nausea, tinnitus (ringing in the ears), and elevated blood pressure.

phospholipids Substances found in all body cells; similar to lipids, but containing only two fatty acids and one phosphorus-containing substance.

physical activity Any form of muscular movement.

physical fitness A dynamic state of energy and vitality that enables one to carry out daily tasks, to engage in active leisure-time pursuits, and to meet unforeseen emergencies without undue fatigue; in addition, physically fit individuals have a decreased risk of hypokinetic diseases and are more able to function at the peak of intellectual capacity while experiencing joie de vivre.

physical work capacity (PWC) An exercise test that measures the amount of work done at a given, submaximal heart rate; work is measured in oxygen uptake, kilogram-meters per minute, or other units, and can be used to estimate maximal heart rate and oxygen uptake.

placebo An inactive substance given to satisfy a patient's demand for medicine.

platelets The clotting material in the blood.

polarized Charged heart cells in the resting state (negative ions inside the cell, positive outside); when electrically stimulated, they depolarize (positive ions inside the heart cell, negative ions outside) and contract.

polydipsia Excessive thirst.

polyphagia Unsatisfied hunger.

polyunsaturated fat Dietary fat comprising molecules that have more than one double bond open to receive more hydrogen; found in safflower oil, corn oil, soybeans, sesame seeds, sunflower seeds.

polyuria Excessive urination.

power Work performed per unit of time; measured by the formula: work equals force times distance divided by time; a combination of strength and speed.

pre-event meal A meal 3–5 hours before an exercise event, emphasizing low-fiber, high-carbohydrate foods.

premature ventricular contraction (PVC) One of the most common ECG abnormalities during the exercise test, where a spot on the ventricle becomes the pacemaker, superseding the SA node.

primary air pollutants Include carbon monoxide (CO), carbon dioxide (CO_2), sulfur dioxide (SO_2), nitrogen oxide (NO), and particulate material such as lead, graphite carbon, and fly ash.

primary osteoporosis May occur in two types: Type I osteoporosis (postmenopausal), which is the accelerated decrease in bone mass that occurs when estrogen levels fall after menopause; and Type II osteoporosis (age-related) which is the inevitable loss of bone mass with age in both men and women.

progressive resistance exercise Exercise in which the amount of resistance is increased to further stress the muscle after it has become accustomed to handling a lesser resistance.

pronation Of the body, assuming a face-down position; of the hand, turning the palm backward or downward; of the foot, lowering the inner (medial) side of the foot so as to flatten the arch; the opposite of supination.

proprioceptive neuromuscular facilitation (PNF) stretch Muscle stretches that use the proprioceptors (muscle spindles) to send inhibiting (relaxing) messages to the muscle that is to be stretched; for example, the contraction of an agonist muscle sends inhibiting signals that relax the antagonist muscle, allowing it to stretch.

protein A complex nitrogen-carrying compound, which occurs naturally in plants and animals and yields amino acids when broken down; the component amino acids are essential for the growth and repair of living tissue; also a source of heat and energy for the body.

protoporphyrin A derivative of hemoglobin; formed from heme by deletion of an atom of iron.

prudent diet Defined in this book as the diet adhering to the 1988 *Surgeon General's Report on Nutrition and Health.*

puberty The period in life when one becomes functionally capable of reproduction.

P wave Transmission of electrical impulse through the atria.

QRS complex Impulse through the ventricles.

Quetelet index Body weight in kilograms, divided by height in meters, squared; the most widely accepted body mass index.

radial pulse The pulse at the wrist.

rating of perceived exertion (RPE) A means to quantify the subjective feeling of the intensity of an exercise; Borg scales, charts that describe a range of intensity from resting to maximal energy outputs, are used as a visual aid to exercisers in keeping their efforts in the effective training zone.

reaction time Relates to the time elapsed between stimulation and the beginning of the reaction to it.

recommended dietary allowance (RDA) Established by the National Research Council of the National Academy of Sciences; the premier nutrient standard worldwide; used for nutrition policies and decision making; also used for purposes ranging from development of new food products to setting standards for federal nutrition assistance programs.

relative risk An expression of disease risk that usually compares death rates from groups varying in a certain health-related practice.

relative weight The body weight divided by the midpoint value of the weight range.

relaxation therapy A treatment that involves teaching a patient to accomplish a state of both muscular and mental deactivation by the systematic use of relaxation or meditation exercises to reduce high blood pressure.

reliability Deals with how consistently a certain element is measured by the particular test.

residual volume The volume of air remaining in the lungs after a maximum expiration; must be calculated in the formula for determining body composition through underwater weighing.

respiratory exchange ratio (R) The ratio between the amount of carbon dioxide produced and the amount of oxygen consumed by the body during exercise.

resting metabolic rate (RMR) Represents the energy expended by the body to maintain life and normal body functions, such as respiration and circulation.

R.I.C.E. Recommended treatment of musculoskeletal pain and injury during the first 48–72 hours; stands for rest, ice, compression, and elevation.

risk factors Characteristics associated with higher risk of developing a specific health problem.

sarcolemma The membrane of the muscle cell.

sarcomere The smallest functional skeletal muscle subunit capable of contraction.

satiety The feeling of fullness and satisfaction.

saturated fat Dietary fat comprising molecules saturated with hydrogen; usually hard at room temperature and readily converted into cholesterol in the body; sources include animal products as well as hydrogenated vegetable oils.

scurvy A disease of vitamin C deficiency.

secondary air pollutants Formed by chemical action of the primary pollutants and the natural chemicals in the atmosphere; examples include ozone (O_3), sulfuric acid

(H$_2$SO$_4$), nitric acid (HNO$_3$), peroxyacetyl nitrate, and a host of other inorganic and organic compounds.

secondary osteoporosis   A loss of bone mineral mass that may develop at any age, as a consequence of hormonal, digestive, and metabolic disorders, as well as prolonged bed rest and weightlessness (space flight).

senile dementia   A form of organic brain syndrome, a mental disorder associated with impaired brain function in the elderly.

serum erythropoietin   A hormone that regulates red blood cell production.

serum iron   During iron-deficient erythropoiesis (stage 2 iron deficiency) serum iron levels fall.

set   A group of repetitions of an exercise movement done consecutively, without rest, until a given number, or momentary exhaustion, is reached.

severe obesity   Defined as more than 100% overweight.

skeletal muscle   Muscle connected to a bone.

skill-related fitness   Elements of fitness such as agility, balance, speed, and coordination; important for participation in various dual and team sports but has little significance for the day-to-day tasks of Americans or their general health.

skinfold measurements   The most widely used method for determining obesity: calipers are used to measure the thickness of a double fold of skin at various sites.

slow-twitch fibers   Muscle fiber type that contracts slowly and is used most in moderate-intensity, endurance exercises, such as distance running; also called Type I fibers.

smokeless tobacco   Use of smokeless tobacco takes two forms: (1) dipping—placing a pinch of moist or dry powdered tobacco (snuff) between the cheek or lip and the lower gum; (2) chewing—placing a golfball-size amount of loose-leaf tobacco between the cheek and lower gum, where it is sucked and chewed.

sodium   An electrolyte that is the major cation (positive ion) of fluids outside the body cells; sodium and chloride ions tend to concentrate outside of body cell walls (extracellular), while potassium tends to concentrate inside of body cell walls (intracellular); this arrangement is essential in maintaining the balance of tissue fluids inside and outside of cells; sodium, potassium, and chloride work with bicarbonate in regulating the acid–base balance of the body; has an important role in regulating normal muscle tone; the Food and Nutrition Board has established safe and adequate daily dietary intakes for sodium of 1100–3300 mg.

sodium bicarbonate   A substance used by some athletes to enhance performance in events lasting 1–3 minutes; sodium bicarbonate ingestion increases the pH of the body, allowing greater lactic acid to be produced and buffered.

sodium-to-potassium ratio (Na:K)   A ratio of the dietary sodium-to-potassium intake, which may be important as an indicator of hypertension risk.

specificity   The principle that the body adapts very specifically to the training stimuli it is required to deal with; the body will perform best at the specific speed, type of contraction, using the muscle group and energy source it has been accustomed to in training.

speed   Relates to the ability to perform a movement within a short period of time.

sphygmomanometer   Blood pressure measurement device; consists of an inflatable, compression bag enclosed in an unyielding covering called the cuff, plus an inflating bulb, a manometer from which the pressure is read, and a controlled exhaust to deflate the system during measurement of blood pressure.

spirulina   A dark green powder or pill derived from marine algae, which has been promoted as a weight-loss product.

spot reducing   An effort to reduce fat at one location on the body by concentrating exercise, manipulation, wraps, and so forth on that location; research indicates that any fat loss is generalized over the body, however.

stadiometer   A vertical ruler with a horizontal headboard that can be brought into contact with the most superior (highest) point on the head.

starch   A polysaccharide made up of glucose monosaccharides.

starch blockers   An enzyme inhibitor claimed to block the digestion and absorption of ingested carbohydrate; several studies have shown these not only to be ineffective, but also a possible risk to health.

step-care therapy   An approach with lifestyle techniques and various drugs to treat hypertension.

sterols   A type of lipid such as cholesterol, estrogen, testosterone, and vitamin D.

stethoscope   Device for amplifying physiological sounds (e.g., heart and lungs); made up of rubber tubing attached to a device that amplifies sounds, such as blood passing through the blood vessels during measurement of blood pressure. (See *auscultation*.)

strength   The amount of muscular force that can be exerted.

stress   The general physical and psychological response of an individual to any real or perceived adverse stimulus, internal or external, that tends to disturb the individual's homeostasis.

stretching   Lengthening a muscle to its maximum extension; moving a joint to the limits of its extension.

stroke   A form of cardiovascular disease that affects the blood vessels supplying oxygen and nutrients to the brain.

stroke volume   The volume of blood pumped out of the heart (by the ventricles) in one contraction.

ST segment depression   An indication of atherosclerotic blockage in the coronary arteries.

submaximal   Less than maximum; submaximal exercise requires less than one's maximum oxygen uptake, heart rate, or anaerobic power; usually refers to intensity of the exercise, but may be used to refer to duration.

sugars   Categorized as *monosaccharides* (glucose, fructose, galactose) and *disaccharides* (lactose, mannose, sucrose).

supination   Assuming a horizontal position facing upward; in the case of the hand, it also means turning the palm forward; the opposite of pronation.

supplementation   Use of vitamin or mineral pills to supplement the regular diet.

systolic blood pressure   The pressure of the blood upon the walls of the blood vessels when the heart is contracting; a normal systolic blood pressure ranges between 90 and 139 mm Hg; when the systolic blood pressure is measured on more than one occasion to be more than 140 mm Hg, high blood pressure is diagnosed.

tachycardia   Excessively rapid heart rate. Usually describes a pulse of more than 100 beats per minute at rest.

target heart rate (THR)   The heart rate at which one aims to exercise. For example, the American College of Sports Medicine recommends that healthy adults exercise at a THR of 60–90% of maximum heart rate reserve; also called training heart rate.

testosterone   An androgen hormone produced by the testicles and adrenal cortex; accelerates growth in tissues.

thermic effect of food (TEF)   The increase in energy expenditure above the resting metabolic rate that can be measured for several hours after a meal.

thrombosis   Formation or existence of a blood clot within the blood vessel system.

tidal volume   The amount of air per breath.

total iron-binding capacity (TIBC)   During iron-deficient erythropoiesis (inadequate formation of red blood cells), total iron-binding capacity is increased.

total lung capacity (TLC)   Represents the total amount of air in the lung.

total peripheral resistance   The sum of all the forces that oppose blood flow in the body's blood vessel system. During exercise, total peripheral resistance decreases because the blood vessels in the active muscles increase in size.

trabecular bone   Spongy, internal end bone.

triglyceride   A type of fat made of glycerol with three fatty acids; most animal and vegetable fats are triglycerides.

T wave   Electrical recovery or repolarization of the ventricles.

type 1 diabetes mellitus   The form of diabetes mellitus in which the pancreas does not make or secrete insulin; the patient must use an external source of insulin to sustain life; also called insulin-dependent diabetes mellitus (IDDM) or juvenile-onset diabetes.

type 2 diabetes mellitus   See *diabetes mellitus.*

underwater weighing   The most widely used laboratory procedure for measuring body density; in this procedure, whole-body density is calculated from body volume according to Archimedes' principle of displacement, which states that an object submerged in water is buoyed up by the weight of the water displaced.

US-RDA   A set of standards developed by the Food and Drug Administration (FDA) for use in regulating nutrition labeling; although these standards were taken from the RDA, they are based on very few categories, and only 19 vitamins and minerals were chosen.

validity   Refers to the degree to which a test measures what it was designed to measure.

Valsalva maneuver   A strong exhaling effort against a closed glottis, which builds pressure in the chest cavity, interfering with the return of blood to the heart; may deprive the brain of blood and cause fainting.

vasoconstriction   The narrowing of a blood vessel to decrease blood flow to a body part.

vasodilation   The enlarging of a blood vessel to increase blood flow to a body part.

very low-calorie diet (VLCD)   Also called the protein-sparing modified fast; provides 400–700 Calories per day for weight loss; protein is emphasized to help avoid loss of muscle tissue; patients can use either special formula beverages or natural foods such as fish, fowl, or lean meat (along with mineral and vitamin supplements).

very low-density lipoproteins (VLDL)   Transport triglycerides to body tissues.

vital capacity   The amount of air that can be expired after a maximum inspiration; the maximum total volume of the lungs, less the residual volume.

vitamin   Nutrients essential for life itself; the body uses these organic substances to accomplish much of its work; do not supply energy but do help release energy from carbohydrates, fats, and proteins; play a vital role in chemical reactions throughout the body; there are two types of vitamins—fat-soluble (A,D,E,K) and water-soluble (eight B vitamins and vitamin C); 13 vitamins have been discovered, the most recent in 1948.

$\dot{V}O_{2max}$ Maximum volume of oxygen consumed per unit of time; In scientific notation, a dot appears over the V to indicate "per unit of time."

waist-to-hip circumference (WHR) Ratio of waist and hip circumferences. A relatively high WHR predicts increased complications from obesity.

warm-up A gradual increase in the intensity of exercise to allow physiological processes to prepare for greater energy outputs; changes include rise in body temperature, cardio-respiratory changes, increase in muscle elasticity and contractility, and so on.

watt A measure of power equal to 6.12 kilogram-meters per minute.

weight-reducing clothing Special weight-reducing clothing, including heated belts, rubberized suits, and oilskins, rely chiefly on dehydration and localized pressure.

wet-bulb thermometer A thermometer, the bulb of which is enclosed in a wet wick, so that evaporation from the wick will lower the temperature reading more in dry air than in humid air; the comparison of wet- and dry-bulb readings can be used to calculate relative humidity.

wet-globe temperature A temperature reading that approximates the heat stress that the environment will impose on the human body; takes into account not only temperature and humidity, but also radiant heat from the sun and cooling breezes that would speed evaporation and convection of heat away from the body; reading is provided by an instrument that encloses a thermometer in a wetted, black copper sphere. Cf. *dry-bulb thermometer, wet-bulb thermometer.*

white blood cells Immune system cells that circulate in the blood, including monocytes, neutrophils, basophils, eosinophils, and lymphocytes.

Index

AAHPERD. *See* American Alliance for Health, Physical Education, Recreation, and Dance

abdominal muscles, testing, 162–164, 173–174

abdominal obesity (android obesity), 146, 467–469

abdominal skinfold measurement, 131–132

absenteeism, worksite exercise programs affecting, 17–18

acclimatization, to exercise in heat, 293

ACSM. *See* American College of Sports Medicine

actin microfilaments, 197

activity. *See* physical activity

adenosine triphosphate. *See* ATP

aerobic dance
  for cardiorespiratory conditioning, 231
  injuries associated with, 582–584

aerobic energy system, in ATP production, 281–284

aerobic training, 216–237
  aerobic dance for, 231
  brisk walking for, 230–231
  cardiorespiratory changes with, 192–195
    during maximal exercise, 194–195
    at rest, 192–193
    during submaximal exercise, 193
  by elderly, 549, 553
  frequency of sessions in, 219–220
  health risks vs. benefits of, 592–595
  indoor exercise equipment for, 233
  intensity of sessions in, 220–228
  low-impact exercises for, 231–232
  mode of exercise in, 229–234
  physiologic changes with, 192–195
  racquet sports for, 233
  rate of progression in, 233–234
  skeletal muscle changes with, 191–192
  supervision during, 237
  systems of, 234
  time (duration) of sessions in, 228–229
  types of exercise for, 229–233
    rating, 230–231
  warm-down period after, 237
  warm-up session before, 216–219
  weight loss and, 488–496
  work activities for, 233

See also cardiorespiratory fitness / endurance; exercise

age
  adaptation to exercise affected by, 200, 201
  health/ "risk," calculating, 575–577
  See also aging

agility, definition of, 36

aging, 545–578
  body composition changes associated with, 548, 554–555
  cardiorespiratory training and, 549, 553
  changes associated with, 547–549
  definition of, 547–548
  exercise and, 550–556
    life expectancy affected by, 549–550
  health habits and, 549–550
  muscular strength and resistance training and, 554
  osteoporosis and, 556–563
  physical training and, 552–555
  statistics and, 545–547
  theories of, 548
  trends in, 545–547
  $\dot{V}O_{2max}$ and, 549, 551–552
  See also elderly

air pollution, exercise and, 591–597

alcohol
  abuse of (alcoholism), definition of, 366
  blood levels of, 367
  cancer rates affected by, 368, 425, 427–428
  consumption by American adults, 366–368
  coronary heart disease and, 367–368
  hypertension and, 365–368
  organ systems affected by, 366–368
  in prudent diet, 275–276
  testing for, 410
  violence and injuries associated with use of, 366–367
  "wellness revolution" affecting use of, 22–23

Alzheimer's disease, 547

amenorrhea, excess exercise causing, 586–588

American Alliance for Health, Physical Education, Recreation, and Dance, fitness testing programs of, 40–41, 64–65

American College of Sports Medicine
  bench-stepping equation developed by, 95
  cycle equation developed by, 99, 101
  certification for health/fitness professionals and, 50–55, 66–69
  exercise prescription recommendations of, 211–216
  fitness classification categories of, 50–52
  health/fitness facility standards and guidelines established by, 9, 60–62
  program of for improving exercise habits, 22
  $\dot{V}O_{2max}$ estimation equations for walking and running of, 103

American Heart Association
  risk factors, 348–350
  risk stratification, 51–52

amino acids, exercise affecting metabolism of, 305–307

anabolic steroids, for muscle building, 316–318

anaerobic energy system, in ATP production, 281–283

anaerobic power, maximal, Wingate test for, 104–105

anaerobic threshold, response to exercise and, 191, 203

analgesics, for musculoskeletal pain and injury, 585

androgenic steroids, for muscle building, 316–318

android obesity, 146, 467–469

anemia, iron-deficiency, 298–302

aneurysm, stroke caused by, 341

angina pectoris, 350

angiography, coronary, 350

angioplasty, percutaneous transluminal coronary, 350–351

anorexia nervosa, 496–500, 587
  assessment checksheet for, 512–513
  diagnostic criteria for, 499

anticipatory response, and pre-exercise heart rate elevation, 184

anti-inflammatory agents
  for arthritis treatment, 565
  for musculoskeletal pain and injury, 585

antioxidants
  and effect of exercise on cancer, 304